THE WASHINGTON MANUAL®
OF MEDICAL T

Department of Medicine
Washington University
School of Medicine
St. Louis, Missouri

Editors

Pavat Bhat, MD

Alexandra Dretler, MD

Mark Gdowski, MD

Rajeev Ramgopal, MD

Dominique Williams, MD

Wolters Kluwer

Philadelphia • Baltimore • New York • London
Buenos Aires • Hong Kong • Sydney • Tokyo

Executive Editor: Rebecca S. Gaertner
Product Development Editor: Kristina Oberle
Editorial Coordinator: Katie Sharp
Marketing Manager: Stephanie Kindlick
Production Project Manager: David Saltzberg
Design Coordinator: Teresa Mallon
Manufacturing Coordinator: Beth Welsh
Prepress Vendor: Absolute Service, Inc.

35th edition

Adhesive binding:
ISBN: 978-1-4698-9024-1
ISBN: 1-4698-9024-0

Spiral binding:
ISBN: 978-1-4963-3851-8
ISBN: 1-4963-3851-0

RRS1512

We dedicate this manual to the outstanding medicine house staff at Washington University and Barnes-Jewish Hospital—their wisdom, dedication, and compassion continue to inspire us each and every day.

Contents

9 Obstructive Lung Disease 249
Jeffrey J. Atkinson, Junfang Jiao, and Mario Castro

10 Pulmonary Diseases 279
Murali Chakinala, Tonya D. Russell, Patrick Aguilar, Adrian Shifren, Andrea Loiselle, Alexander Chen, Ali Sadoughi, Allen Burks, Praveen Chenna, Brad Bemiss, and Daniel B. Rosenbluth

11 Allergy and Immunology 332
Sean Brady, Junfang Jiao, Jennifer M. Monroy, and Andrew L. Kau

12 Fluid and Electrolyte Management 354
Anubha Mutneja, Steven Cheng, and Judy L. Jang

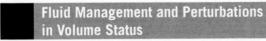

Fluid Management and Perturbations 354
in Volume Status

13 Renal Diseases 389

Rajesh Rajan, Seth Goldberg, and Daniel W. Coyne

14 Treatment of Infectious Diseases 416

Allison L. Nazinitsky, Stephen Y. Liang, and Nigar Kirmani

15 Antimicrobials 478

David J. Ritchie, Matthew P. Crotty, and Nigar Kirmani

17 Solid Organ Transplant Medicine 527

Rupinder Sodhi and Rowena Delos Santos

18 Gastrointestinal Diseases 538

C. Prakash Gyawali and Amit Patel

19 Liver Diseases 576
Maria Samuel, Kristen Singer, and Mauricio Lisker-Melman

20 Disorders of Hemostasis and Thrombosis 616
Kristen M. Sanfilippo, Brian F. Gage, Tzu-Fei Wang, and Roger D. Yusen

23 Diabetes Mellitus and Related Disorders   730
Cynthia J. Herrick and Janet B. McGill

26 Medical Emergencies 808
Rebecca Bavolek, Evan S. Schwarz, and Jason Wagner

27 **Neurologic Disorders 824**
Robert C. Bucelli and Beau M. Ances

 28 **Toxicology 869**
S. Eliza Halcomb, Evan S. Schwarz, and Michael E. Mullins

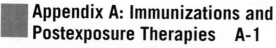

Appendix A: Immunizations and Postexposure Therapies   A-1

Abigail L. Carlson and Carlos A. Q. Santos

Appendix B: Infection Control and Isolation Recommendations A-15

Abigail L. Carlson and Carlos A. Q. Santos

Appendix C: Advanced Cardiac Life Support Algorithms A-22

Mark Gdowski

Contributors

Patrick Aguilar
Fellow
Division of Pulmonary and Critical Care Medicine

Zarmeena Ali, MD
Instructor in Medicine
Division of Rheumatology

Beau M. Ances, MD, PhD, MS
Associate Professor
Department of Neurology

Jeffrey J. Atkinson, MD
Assistant Professor of Medicine
Division of Pulmonary and Critical Care Medicine

Philip M. Barger, MD
Associate Professor of Medicine
Division of Cardiovascular Medicine

Rebecca Bavolek, MD
Instructor in Emergency Medicine
Division of Emergency Medicine

Brad Bemiss, MD
Postdoctorate Research Scholar
Division of Pulmonary and Critical Care Medicine

Morey Blinder, MD
Associate Professor of Medicine
Division of Hematology

Sean Brady, MD
Fellow
Division of Allergy and Immunology

Angela L. Brown, MD
Assistant Professor of Medicine
Division of Cardiology

Robert C. Bucelli, MD, PhD
Assistant Professor
Department of Neurology

Allen Burks, MD
Fellow
Division of Pulmonary and Critical Care Medicine

Abigail L. Carlson, MD
Fellow
Division of Infectious Diseases

Mario Castro, MD
Professor of Medicine
Division of Pulmonary and Critical Care Medicine

Murali Chakinala, MD
Associate Professor of Medicine
Division of Pulmonary and Critical Care Medicine

Alexander Chen, MD
Assistant Professor of Medicine
Division of Pulmonary and Critical Care Medicine

Catherine Chen, MD
Fellow
Division of Pulmonary and Critical Care Medicine

Steven Cheng, MD
Assistant Professor of Medicine
Division of Renal Diseases

Praveen Chenna, MD
Assistant Professor of Medicine
Division of Pulmonary and Critical Care Medicine

William E. Clutter, MD
Associate Professor of Medicine
Division of Medical Education

Daniel H. Cooper, MD
Assistant Professor of Medicine
Division of Cardiovascular Medicine

Daniel W. Coyne, MD
Professor of Medicine
Division of Renal Diseases

Matthew P. Crotty, PharmD
Infectious Diseases Pharmacy Resident
BJH Department of Pharmacy

Vladimir Despotovic, MD
Assistant Professor of Medicine
Division of Pulmonary and Critical Care Medicine

Siddhartha Devarakonda, MD
Fellow
Division of Hematology and Oncology

Mitchell N. Faddis, MD, PhD
Associate Professor of Medicine
Division of Cardiovascular Medicine

Brian F. Gage, MD
Professor of Medicine
Division of General Medical Sciences

Mark Gdowski, MD
Instructor in Medicine
Division of Medical Education

Anne C. Goldberg, MD
Associate Professor of Medicine
Division of Endocrinology and Metabolism

Seth Goldberg, MD
Assistant Professor of Medicine
Division of Nephrology

Jacob S. Goldstein
Fellow
Cardiovascular Division

María González-Mayda, MD
Assistant Professor of Medicine
Division of Rheumatology

Ramaswamy Govindan, MD
Professor of Medicine
Division of Medical Oncology

C. Prakash Gyawali, MD
Professor of Medicine
Division of Gastroenterology

S. Eliza Halcomb, MD
Assistant Professor
Division of Emergency Medicine

Cynthia J. Herrick, MD
Instructor in Medicine
Division of Endocrinology, Metabolism, and
   Lipid Research

Ronald Jackups, MD
Assistant Professor of Pathology and Immunology
Laboratory and Genomic Medicine

Judy L. Jang, MD
Assistant Professor of Medicine
Division of Renal Diseases

Junfang Jiao, MD
Fellow
Division of Allergy and Immunology

Eric Johnson, MD
Instructor in Medicine
Division of Hospital Medicine

Andrew L. Kau, MD
Instructor in Medicine
Division of Allergy and Immunology

Daniel S. Kim, MD
Instructor in Medicine
Division of Medical Education

Nigar Kirmani, MD
Professor of Medicine
Division of Infectious Diseases

Marin H. Kollef, MD
Professor of Medicine
Division of Pulmonary and Critical Care Medicine

Shane J. LaRue, MD
Instructor in Medicine
Cardiovascular Division

Stephen Y. Liang, MD
Instructor in Medicine
Division of Infectious Diseases

Brian R. Lindman, MD
Assistant Professor of Medicine
Division of Cardiovascular Medicine

Mauricio Lisker-Melman, MD
Professor of Medicine
Division of Gastroenterology

Andrea Loiselle, MD
Instructor in Medicine
Division of Pulmonary and Critical Care Medicine

Caline Mattar, MD
Fellow
Division of Infectious Diseases

Janet B. McGill, MD
Professor of Medicine
Division of Endocrinology

Adam Meyer, MD
Instructor in Medicine
Division of Hospital Medicine

Jennifer M. Monroy, MD
Assistant Professor of Medicine
Division of Allergy and Immunology

Daniel Morgensztern, MD
Associate Professor of Medicine
Division of Medical Oncology

Clare E. Moynihan, MD
Fellow
Division of Endocrinology and Metabolism

Michael E. Mullins, MD
Associate Professor of Emergency Medicine
Department of Medicine

Anubha Mutneja, MD
Fellow
Division of Renal Diseases

Allison L. Nazinitsky, MD
Fellow
Division of Infectious Diseases

Amit Patel, MD
Fellow
Division of Gastroenterology

Rachel Presti, MD
Assistant Professor of Medicine
Division of Infectious Diseases

Rajesh Rajan, MD
Fellow
Division of Renal Diseases

Dominic Reeds, MD
Associate Professor of Medicine
Division of Geriatrics and Nutritional Science

Tom Regenbogen, MD
Fellow
Division of Medical Oncology

Hilary E. L. Reno, MD
Assistant Professor of Medicine
Division of Infectious Diseases

David J. Ritchie, PharmD
Clinical Pharmacist
Division of Infectious Diseases

Daniel B. Rosenbluth, MD
Professor of Medicine and Pediatrics
Division of Pulmonary and Critical Care Medicine

Tonya D. Russell, MD
Associate Professor of Medicine
Division of Pulmonary and Critical Care Medicine

Ali Sadoughi, MD
Fellow
Division of Pulmonary and Critical Care Medicine

Maria Samuel, MD
Fellow
Division of Gastroenterology

Kristen M. Sanfilippo, MD
Instructor in Medicine
Division of Hematology

Carlos A. Q. Santos, MD
Assistant Professor of Medicine
Division of Infectious Diseases

Rowena Delos Santos, MD
Assistant Professor of Medicine
Division of Renal Diseases

Evan S. Schwarz, MD
Assistant Professor of Emergency Medicine
Division of Emergency Medicine

Adrian Shifren, MD
Assistant Professor of Medicine
Division of Pulmonary and Critical Care Medicine

Kristen Singer, MD
Resident
Department of Internal Medicine

Marc A. Sintek, MD
Fellow
Cardiovascular Division

Rupinder Sodhi, MD
Fellow
Division of Renal Diseases

Mark Thoelke, MD
Associate Professor
Division of Hospital Medicine

Justin M. Vader, MD
Assistant Professor of Medicine
Cardiovascular Division

Tiphanie Vogel, MD
Fellow
Division of Rheumatology

Jason Wagner, MD
Assistant Professor of Emergency Medicine
Division of Emergency Medicine

Tzu-Fei Wang, MD
Assistant Professor of Internal Medicine
Division of Hematology
The Ohio State University

Peter H. Yen, MD
Resident
Department of Medicine

Roger D. Yusen, MD, MPH
Associate Professor of Medicine
Division of Pulmonary and Critical Care Medicine

Amy Zhou
Fellow
Division of Medical Oncology

Chairman's Note

The tremendous advances in medical research place an enormous burden on physicians to keep up with new evidence guiding clinical practice, particularly in novel therapies that will improve patient outcomes. The *Washington Manual® of Medical Therapeutics* provides an easily accessible source of current information that focuses on practical clinical approaches to the diagnosis, investigation, and treatment of common medical conditions that internists encounter on a regular basis. The electronic online version and the pocket-book size of the *Washington Manual®* ensure that it will continue to be of enormous assistance to interns, residents, medical students, and other practitioners in need of readily accessible clinical information. The *Washington Manual®* continues to address an important need in an era of information overload.

I acknowledge the authors, who include the outstanding house officers, fellows, and attendings at Washington University/Barnes-Jewish Hospital. Their efforts and exceptional skills are evident in the quality of the final product. In particular, I am proud of our editors: Drs. Pavan Bhat, Alexandra Dretler, Mark Gdowski, Rajeev Ramgopal, and Dominique Williams, and series editor Dr. Tom De Fer, who have worked tirelessly to produce another outstanding edition of the *Washington Manual® of Medical Therapeutics*. I also recognize Dr. Melvin Blanchard, Chief of the Division of Medical Education in the Department of Medicine at Washington University, for his guidance and advice. I am confident that this edition will meet its desired goal of providing practical knowledge that can be directly applied to improving patient care.

Victoria J. Fraser, MD
Adolphus Busch Professor of Medicine
Chairman, Department of Medicine
Washington University School of Medicine
St. Louis, Missouri

Preface

It is our distinct pleasure to introduce the 35th edition of *The Washington Manual® of Medical Therapeutics.* "The *Manual,*" as it is known here at Washington University, has a proud tradition of being edited by the Internal Medicine Chief Residents. Since its inception as a simple handbook for local medical students and house staff, the *Manual* has grown to be one of the best-selling medical texts in the world. Concurrently, the *Manual* has grown in size and complexity, mirroring the practice of medicine.

From the first edition edited by Wayland MacFarlane in 1943, numerous revisions have occurred, transforming the *Manual* from a short textbook to a portable reference, and now a text with both written and electronic forms with availability on portable electronic devices. Throughout the many revisions, however, the editors have sought to retain the virtues that made the work a success from the start: a concise discussion of pathophysiology, an evidence-based presentation of current therapies, and a sensible format. Additionally, with each new edition, the content is carefully updated to reflect the ever-changing advances in medical technology and therapeutics.

The Washington Manual® of Medical Therapeutics has established a tradition of excellence that we aspire to preserve. No discussion of the *Manual* would be complete without mention of the fantastic Washington University medicine house staff, fellows, medical students, and attendings with whom we work daily. Their brilliance, compassion, and dedication are truly remarkable and inspiring. We are honored that they turn to the *Manual* for guidance. We are deeply indebted for the substantial support and direction that Dr. Tom De Fer, the series editor, provided in the creation of this edition of the *Manual.* We also sincerely thank Katie Sharp and the editorial staff at Wolters Kluwer for their assistance and patience with our busy schedules.

We have had the honor and pleasure of serving as chief residents of Shatz-Strauss, Karl-Flance, Kipnis-Daughaday, and North Campus firms, and the Primary Care Medicine Clinic in the Barnes-Jewish Center for Outpatient Health. Our firm chiefs, Drs. Megan Wren, Emily Fondahn, Geoffrey Cislo, and E.-P. Barrette, have been instrumental over the course of the year, serving as mentors and role models. Our program director, Dr. Melvin Blanchard, provided guidance and support in the production of the *Manual.* Our Chairman of Medicine, Dr. Vicky Fraser, served as an outstanding role model and provided support in the creation of this text. We thank our families for their support, patience, and inspiration. To Muffie, Rob, Charlotte, and Doug; the whole Gdowski family but especially Henry; Carolyn, John, and Stanley; Caroline, Priya, Kolari, and Shashi; and the entire Ramgopal and Martin families—our gratitude is beyond measure.

Pavan Bhat, MD
Alexandra Dretler, MD
Mark Gdowski, MD
Rajeev Ramgopal, MD
Dominique Williams, MD

1

Inpatient Care in Internal Medicine

Mark Thoelke, Eric Johnson, and Adam Meyer

General Care of the Hospitalized Patient

GENERAL PRINCIPLES

- Although a general approach to common problems can be outlined, **therapy must be individualized**. All diagnostic and therapeutic procedures should be explained carefully to the patient, including the potential risks, benefits, and alternatives.
- The period of hospitalization represents a complex interplay of multiple caregivers that subjects the patient to potential harm by **medical errors and iatrogenic complications**. Every effort must be made to minimize these risks. Basic measures include:
  - Use of standardized abbreviations and dose designations
  - Excellent communication between physicians and other caregivers
  - Institution of appropriate prophylactic precautions
  - Prevention of nosocomial infections, including attention to hygiene and discontinuation of unnecessary catheters
  - Medicine reconciliation at all transfers of care
- **Hospital orders**
  - Computer order entry offers admission order sets that should be entered promptly after evaluation of a patient. A contact number should be made available.
  - Daily rounds should include assessment for ongoing need of IV fluids, telemetry, catheters, and supplemental oxygen, all of which can limit mobility.
  - Routine daily labs, such as CBC and BMP, should be discouraged because significant iatrogenic anemia may develop.
- **Discharge**
  - **Discharge planning** begins at the time of admission. Assessment of the patient's social situation and potential discharge needs should be made at this time.
  - **Early coordination** with nursing, social work, and case coordinators/managers facilitates efficient discharge and a complete postdischarge plan.
  - **Patient education** should occur regarding changes in medications and other new therapies. Compliance with treatment is influenced by the patient's understanding of that treatment.
  - **Prescriptions** should be written for all new medication, and the patient should be provided with a complete medication list including instructions and indications.
  - **Communication** with physicians who will be resuming care of the patient is important for optimal follow-up care and should be a component of the discharge process.

PROPHYLACTIC MEASURES

Venous Thromboembolism Prophylaxis

GENERAL PRINCIPLES

Epidemiology

Venous thromboembolism (VTE) is a preventable cause of death in hospitalized patients. In the largest observational study to date attempting to risk-stratify medical patients, 1.2% of medical patients developed VTE within 90 days of admission. A total of 10–31% of patients were deemed to be at high risk for VTE, defined as having **2 or more points** by weighted risk factors below (*Chest 2011;140:706*).

Risk Factors
- 3 points: previous VTE, thrombophilia
- 1 point: cancer, age >60

Prevention
- **Ambulation** several times a day should be encouraged.
- **Pharmacologic prophylaxis** results in a 50% decrease in VTE risk, although this includes many asymptomatic calf vein thromboses that do not progress. No overall mortality benefit from prophylaxis has been demonstrated.
- Acutely ill patients at high risk of VTE, without bleeding or high risk of bleeding, should be treated with low-dose unfractionated heparin (UFH), 5000 units SC q12h or q8, or low-molecular-weight heparin (LMWH); enoxaparin, 40 mg SC daily, or dalteparin, 5000 units SC daily; or fondaparinux, 2.5 mg SC daily.
- Aspirin alone is not sufficient for prophylaxis in hospitalized patients (*Chest 2012;141:e195S*).
- At-risk patients with contraindications to anticoagulation prophylaxis may receive mechanical prophylaxis with intermittent pneumatic compression or graded compression stockings, although evidence of benefit is lacking (*Ann Intern Med 2011;155:625*).

Decubitus Ulcers

GENERAL PRINCIPLES

Epidemiology
Decubitus ulcers typically occur within the first 2 weeks of hospitalization and can develop within 2–6 hours. Once they develop, decubitus ulcers are difficult to heal and have been associated with increased mortality (*J Gerontol A Biol Sci Med Sci 1997;52:M106*). Risk factors for the development of decubitus ulcers include, advanced age, paralysis, and severe illness (*Clin Dermatol 2010;28(5):527*).

Prevention
Prevention is the key to management of decubitus ulcers. It is recognized that not all decubitus ulcers are avoidable (*J Wound Ostomy Continence Nurs 2014;41:313*). Preventative measures include:
- **Risk factor assessment**, including immobility, limited activity, incontinence, impaired nutritional status, impaired circulation, and altered level of consciousness.
- **Advanced static mattresses or** overlays should be used in at-risk patients (*Ann Intern Med 2015;162:359*).
- **Skin care**, including daily inspection with particular attention to bony prominences including heels, minimizing exposure to moisture, and applying moisturizers to dry sacral skin.
- **Nutritional supplements** may be provided to patients at risk.
- **Frequent repositioning** (minimum of every 2 hours, or every 1 hour for wheelchair-bound patients) is suggested.

DIAGNOSIS

Clinical Presentation
National Pressure Ulcer Advisory Panel Staging
- **Suspected deep tissue injury:** Purple or maroon localized area of discolored intact skin or blood-filled blister due to damage of underlying soft tissue from pressure and/or shear.

The area may be preceded by tissue that is painful, firm, mushy, boggy, warmer, or cooler as compared to adjacent tissue.

- **Stage I:** Intact skin with nonblanchable redness of a localized area usually over a bony prominence. Darkly pigmented skin may obscure findings.
- **Stage II:** Partial thickness loss of dermis presenting as a shallow open ulcer with a red pink wound bed without slough. May also present as a blister.
- **Stage III:** Full thickness tissue loss. Subcutaneous fat may be visible but bone, tendon, or muscle are not exposed. Slough may be present but does not obscure the depth of tissue loss. May include undermining and tunneling.
- **Stage IV:** Full thickness tissue loss with exposed bone, tendon, or muscle. Slough or eschar may be present on some parts of the wound bed. Often includes undermining and tunneling.
- **Unstageable:** Full thickness tissue loss in which the base of the ulcer is covered by slough (yellow, tan, gray, green, or brown) and/or eschar (tan, brown, or black) in the wound bed.

TREATMENT

Optimal treatment of pressure ulcers remains poorly defined. There is evidence to support the following (*Ann Intern Med 2015;162:370*).
- **Hydrocolloid or foam** dressings may reduce wound size.
- **Protein or amino acid supplementation** is recommended, although there are insufficient data to recommend a specific supplement regimen (*Cochrane Database Syst Rev 2014*).
- **Electrical stimulation** may accelerate healing.
- **Other adjunctive therapies** with less supporting evidence include radiant heat, negative pressure, and platelet-derived growth factor. Topical agents (silver sulfadiazine) may optimizing healing or lead to minor slough debridement (Santyl, Xenaderm).
- There is no role for antibiotics to aid healing of a noninfected ulcer.

Other Precautions

GENERAL PRINCIPLES

- **Fall precautions** should be written for patients who have a history of falls or are at high risk of a fall (e.g., dementia, weakness, orthostasis). Falls are the most common accident in hospitalized patients, frequently leading to injury. **Fall risk should not be equated with bedrest**, which may lead to debilitation and higher risk of future falls.
- **Seizure precautions**, which include padded bed rails and an oral airway at the bedside, should be considered for patients with a history of seizures or those at risk of seizing.
- **Restraint orders** are written for patients who are at risk of injuring themselves or interfering with their treatment due to disruptive or dangerous behaviors. Restraint orders must be renewed every 24 hours. Physical restraints may exacerbate agitation. Bed alarms, sitters, and sedatives are alternatives in appropriate settings.

ACUTE INPATIENT CARE

An approach to selected common complaints is presented in this section. An evaluation should generally include a directed history and physical examination, review of the medical problem list (including chronic conditions), review of medications with attention to recent medication changes, and consideration of recent procedures.

Chest Pain

GENERAL PRINCIPLES

Common causes of chest pain range from life-threatening causes such as myocardial infarction (MI) and pulmonary embolism to other causes including esophageal reflux, peptic ulcer disease, pneumonia, costochondritis, shingles, trauma, and anxiety.

DIAGNOSIS

History and Physical Examination

• History should include previous cardiac or vascular disease history, cardiac risk factors, and factors that would predispose the patient to a pulmonary embolus.
• Physical examination is ideally conducted during an episode of pain and includes vital signs (bilateral blood pressure [BP] measurements if considering aortic dissection), cardiopulmonary and abdominal examination, and inspection and palpation of the chest.

Diagnostic Testing

Assessment of oxygenation status, chest radiography, and ECG is appropriate in most patients. Serial cardiac biomarkers should be obtained if there is suspicion of ischemia. Spiral CT and ventilation/perfusion scans are employed to diagnose pulmonary embolus.

TREATMENT

• If cardiac ischemia is a concern, see Chapter 4, Ischemic Heart Disease, for details.
• If a gastrointestinal (GI) source is suspected, Maalox and diphenhydramine (1:1 mix) can be administered.
• Musculoskeletal pain typically responds to acetaminophen or NSAID therapy.
• Prompt empiric anticoagulation if there is high suspicion for MI or pulmonary embolism.

Dyspnea

GENERAL PRINCIPLES

Dyspnea is most commonly caused by a cardiopulmonary abnormality, such as congestive heart failure (CHF), cardiac ischemia, bronchospasm, pulmonary embolus, infection, mucus plugging, and aspiration. Dyspnea must be promptly and carefully evaluated.

DIAGNOSIS

History and Physical Examination

• Initial evaluation should include a review of the medical history for underlying pulmonary or cardiovascular disease and a directed history.
• A detailed cardiopulmonary examination should take place, including vital signs.

Diagnostic Testing

• Oxygen assessment by pulse oximetry or arterial blood gas and chest radiography are useful in most patients.
• Other diagnostic measures should be directed by the findings in the initial evaluation.

TREATMENT

Oxygen should be administered promptly if needed. Other therapeutic measures should be directed by the findings in the initial evaluation.

Acute Hypertensive Episodes

GENERAL PRINCIPLES

- Acute hypertensive episodes in the hospital are most often caused by inadequately treated essential hypertension. If there is evidence of end-organ damage, IV medications are indicated. Oral agents are more appropriate for hypertensive urgency without end-organ damage.
- Volume overload and pain may exacerbate hypertension and should be recognized appropriately and treated.
- Hypertension associated with withdrawal syndromes (e.g., alcohol, cocaine) and rebound hypertension associated with sudden withdrawal of antihypertensive medications (i.e., clonidine, α-adrenergic antagonists) should be considered. These entities should be treated as discussed in Chapter 3, Preventive Cardiology.

Fever

GENERAL PRINCIPLES

Fever accompanies many illnesses and is a valuable marker of disease activity. Infection is a primary concern. Drug reaction, malignancy, VTE, vasculitis, central fever, and tissue infarction are other possibilities but are diagnoses of exclusion.

DIAGNOSIS

History and Physical Examination

- History should include chronology of the fever and associated symptoms, medications, potential exposures, and a complete social and travel history.
- Physical examination should include oral or rectal temperature. In the hospitalized patient, special attention should be paid to any IV lines, abnormal fluid accumulation, and indwelling devices such as urinary catheters.
- For management of neutropenic fever, see Chapter 22, Cancer.

Diagnostic Testing

- Testing includes blood and urine cultures, complete blood count (CBC) with differential, serum chemistries with liver function tests, urinalysis, and stool cultures if appropriate.
- Diagnostic evaluation generally includes chest radiography.
- Cultures of abnormal fluid collections, sputum, cerebrospinal fluid, and stool should be sent if clinically indicated. Cultures are ideally obtained prior to initiation of antibiotics; however, antibiotics should not be delayed if serious infection is suspected.

TREATMENT

- Antipyretic drugs may be given to decrease associated discomfort. Aspirin, 325 mg, and acetaminophen, 325–650 mg PO or PR q4h, are the drugs of choice.
- Empiric antibiotics should be considered in hemodynamically unstable patients in whom infection is a primary concern, as well as in neutropenic and asplenic patients.

• Heat stroke and malignant hyperthermia are medical emergencies that require prompt recognition and treatment (see Chapter 26, Medical Emergencies).

Pain

GENERAL PRINCIPLES

Pain is subjective, and therapy must be individualized. Chronic pain may not be associated with any objective physical findings. Pain scales should be employed for quantitation.

TREATMENT

• Acute pain usually requires temporary therapy.
• For chronic pain, use a combination of long-acting medication with bolus as needed.
• If pain is refractory to conventional therapy, then nonpharmacologic modalities, such as nerve blocks, sympathectomy, and cognitive behavioral therapy, may be appropriate.

Medications

• Acetaminophen
  ○ Effects: Antipyretic and analgesic actions; no anti-inflammatory or antiplatelet properties.
  ○ Dosage: 325–1000 mg q4–6h (maximum dose, 4 g/d), available in oral, IV, and rectal suppository. Dosage in patients with liver disease should not exceed 2 g/d.
  ○ Adverse effects: The principal *advantage* of acetaminophen is its lack of gastric toxicity. Hepatic toxicity may be serious, and acute overdose with 10–15 g can cause fatal hepatic necrosis (see Chapter 19, Liver Diseases, and Chapter 26, Medical Emergencies).
• Aspirin
  ○ Effects: Aspirin has analgesic, antipyretic, anti-inflammatory, and antiplatelet effects. Aspirin should be used with caution in patients with hepatic or renal disease or bleeding disorders, those who are pregnant, and those who are receiving anticoagulation therapy. Antiplatelet effects may last for up to 1 week after a single dose.
  ○ Dosage: 325–650 mg q4h PRN (maximum dose, 4 g/d), available in oral and rectal suppository. Enteric coated formulation may minimize GI side effects.
  ○ Adverse effects: Dose-related side effects include tinnitus, dizziness, and hearing loss. Dyspepsia and GI bleeding can develop and may be severe. Hypersensitivity reactions, including bronchospasm, laryngeal edema, and urticaria, are uncommon, but patients with asthma and nasal polyps are more susceptible. Chronic use can result in interstitial nephritis and papillary necrosis.
• NSAIDs
  Effects: NSAIDs have analgesic, antipyretic, and anti-inflammatory properties mediated by inhibition of cyclooxygenase. All NSAIDs have similar efficacy and toxicities, with a side effect profile similar to that of aspirin. Patients with allergic or bronchospastic reactions to aspirin should not be given NSAIDs. See Chapter 25, Arthritis and Rheumatologic Diseases, for further information on NSAIDs.
• Opioid analgesics
  ○ Effects: Opioid analgesics are pharmacologically similar to opium or morphine and are the drugs of choice when analgesia without antipyretic action is desired.
  ○ Dosage: Table 1-1 lists equianalgesic dosages.
    ▪ Constant pain requires continuous (basal) analgesia with supplementary, PRN doses for breakthrough pain at doses of roughly 5–15% of the daily basal dose. If frequent PRN doses are required, the maintenance dose should be increased or the dosing interval should be decreased.

TABLE 1-1	Equipotent Doses of Opioid Analgesics			
Drug	Onset (min)	Duration (hr)	IM/IV/SC (mg)	PO (mg)
Fentanyl	7–8	1–2	0.1	NA
Levorphanol	30–90	4–6	2	4
Hydromorphone	15–30	2–4	1.5–2.0	7.5
Methadone	30–60	4–12	10	20
Morphine	15–30	2–4	10	30[a]
Oxycodone	15–30	3–4	NA	20
Codeine	15–30	4–6	120	200

NA, not applicable.
Note: Equivalences are based on single-dose studies.
[a]An IM:PO ratio of 1:2 to 1:3 used for repetitive dosing.

- When changing to a new narcotic due to poor response or patient intolerance, the new medication should be started at 50% the equianalgesic dose to account for incomplete cross-tolerance.
- Parenteral and transdermal administration are useful in the setting of dysphagia, emesis, or decreased GI absorption.
- Agents with short half-lives, such as morphine, should be used. Narcotic-naïve patients should be started on the lowest possible doses, whereas patients with demonstrated tolerance will require higher doses.
- Patient-controlled analgesia often is used to control pain in a postoperative or terminally ill patient. Opioid-naïve patients should not have basal rates prescribed due to risk of overdose.
- Selected opiates
  - Codeine is usually given in combination with aspirin or acetaminophen.
  - Oxycodone and hydrocodone are both available orally in combination with acetaminophen; oxycodone is available without acetaminophen in immediate-release and sustained-release formulations. Care should be taken to avoid acetaminophen overdose with these formulations.
  - Morphine sulfate preparations include both immediate release and sustained release. The liquid form can be useful in patients who have difficulty in swallowing pills. Morphine should be used with caution in renal insufficiency.
  - Methadone is very effective when administered orally and suppresses the symptoms of withdrawal from other opioids because of its extended half-life. Despite its long elimination half-life, its analgesic duration of action is much shorter.
  - Hydromorphone is a potent morphine derivative, five to seven times the strength of morphine, and caution should be used when ordering this medication.
  - Fentanyl is available in a transdermal patch with sustained release over 72 hours. Initial onset of action is delayed. Respiratory depression may occur more frequently with fentanyl.
- Precautions
  - Opioids are relatively contraindicated in acute disease states in which the pattern and degree of pain are important diagnostic signs (e.g., head injuries, abdominal pain). They also may increase intracranial pressure.

○ Opioids should be used with caution in patients with hypothyroidism, Addison disease, hypopituitarism, anemia, respiratory disease (e.g., chronic obstructive pulmonary disease [COPD], asthma, kyphoscoliosis, severe obesity), severe malnutrition, debilitation, or chronic cor pulmonale.

○ Opioid dosage should be adjusted for patients with impaired hepatic or renal function.

○ Drugs that potentiate the adverse effects of opioids include phenothiazines, antidepressants, benzodiazepines, and alcohol.

○ Tolerance develops with chronic use and coincides with the development of physical dependence, which is characterized by a withdrawal syndrome (anxiety, irritability, diaphoresis, tachycardia, GI distress, and temperature instability) when the drug is stopped abruptly. It may occur after only 2 weeks of therapy.

○ Administration of an opioid antagonist may precipitate withdrawal after only 3 days of therapy. Tapering the medication slowly over several days can minimize withdrawal.

• Adverse and toxic effects
  ○ Central nervous system (CNS) effects include sedation, euphoria, and pupillary constriction.
  ○ Respiratory depression is dose related and pronounced after IV administration.
  ○ Cardiovascular effects include peripheral vasodilation and hypotension.
  ○ GI effects include constipation, nausea, and vomiting. Stool softeners and laxatives should be prescribed to prevent constipation. Opioids may precipitate toxic megacolon in patients with inflammatory bowel disease.
  ○ Genitourinary effects include urinary retention.
  ○ Pruritus occurs most commonly with spinal administration.

• Opioid overdose
  Naloxone, an opioid antagonist, should be readily available for administration in the case of accidental or intentional overdose. For details of administration, see Chapter 26, Medical Emergencies.

• Alternative medications
  ○ Tramadol is an opioid agonist and a centrally acting non-opioid analgesic that acts on pain processing pathways.
    ▪ Dosage: 50–100 mg PO q4–6h can be used for acute pain. For elderly patients and those with renal or liver dysfunction, dosage reduction is recommended.
    ▪ Adverse effects: Concomitant use of alcohol, sedatives, or narcotics should be avoided. Nausea, dizziness, constipation, and headache may also occur. Respiratory depression has not been described at prescribed dosages but may occur with overdose. Tramadol should not be used in patients who are taking a monoamine oxidase inhibitor, as it can contribute to serotonin syndrome.
  ○ Anticonvulsants (e.g., gabapentin, pregabalin, carbamazepine, oxcarbazepine), tricyclic antidepressants (e.g., amitriptyline), and duloxetine are PO agents that can be used to treat neuropathic pain.
  ○ Topical anesthetics (e.g., lidocaine) may provide analgesia to a localized region (e.g., postherpetic neuralgia).

Altered Mental Status

GENERAL PRINCIPLES

Mental status changes have a broad differential diagnosis that includes neurologic (e.g., stroke, seizure, delirium), metabolic (e.g., hypoxemia, hypoglycemia), toxic (e.g., drug effects, alcohol withdrawal), and other etiologies. Infection (e.g., urinary tract infections, pneumonia) is a common cause of mental status changes in the elderly and in patients with underlying neurologic disease. Sundown syndrome refers to the appearance of worsening confusion in the evening and is associated with dementia, delirium, and unfamiliar environments.

DIAGNOSIS

History and Physical Examination

- Focus particularly on medications, underlying dementia, cognitive impairment, neurologic or psychiatric disorders, and a history of alcohol and/or drug use.
- Family and nursing personnel may be able to provide additional details.
- Physical examination generally includes vital signs, a search for sites of infection, a complete cardiopulmonary examination, and a detailed neurologic examination including mental status evaluation.

Diagnostic Testing

- Testing includes blood glucose, serum electrolytes, creatinine, CBC, urinalysis, and oxygen assessment.
- Other evaluation, including lumbar puncture, toxicology screen, cultures, thyroid function tests, noncontrast head CT, electroencephalogram, chest radiograph, or ECG should be directed by initial findings.

TREATMENT

Management of specific disorders is discussed in Chapter 27, Neurologic Disorders, available in the online version.

Medications

Agitation and psychosis may be features of a change in mental status. The antipsychotic haloperidol and the benzodiazepine lorazepam are commonly used in the acute management of these symptoms. Second-generation antipsychotics (risperidone, olanzapine, quetiapine, clozapine, ziprasidone, aripiprazole, paliperidone) are alternative agents that may lead to decreased incidence of extrapyramidal symptoms. All of these agents pose risks to elderly patients and those with dementia if given long term.

- Haloperidol is the initial drug of choice for acute management of agitation and psychosis. The initial dose of 0.5–5 mg (0.25 mg in elderly patients) PO and 2–10 mg IM/IV can be repeated every 30–60 minutes. Haloperidol has fewer active metabolites and fewer anticholinergic, sedative, and hypotensive effects than other antipsychotics but may have more extrapyramidal side effects. In low dosages, haloperidol rarely causes hypotension, cardiovascular compromise, or excessive sedation.
- Prolongation of the QT interval. Use should be discontinued with prolongation of QTc >450 msec or 25% above baseline.
- Postural hypotension may occasionally be acute and severe after administration. IV fluids should be given initially for treatment. If vasopressors are required, dopamine should be avoided because it may exacerbate the psychotic state.
- Neuroleptic malignant syndrome (see Chapter 27, Neurologic Disorders).
- Lorazepam is a benzodiazepine that is useful for agitation and psychosis in the setting of hepatic dysfunction and sedative or alcohol withdrawal. The initial dose is 0.5–1 mg IV. Lorazepam has a short duration of action and few active metabolites. Excessive sedation and respiratory depression can occur.

Nonpharmacologic Therapies

Patients with delirium of any etiology often respond to frequent reorientation, observance of the day–night light cycle, and maintenance of a familiar environment.

Insomnia and Anxiety

GENERAL PRINCIPLES

- Insomnia and anxiety may be attributed to a variety of underlying medical or psychiatric disorders, and symptoms may be exacerbated by hospitalization.
- Causes of insomnia include environmental disruptions, mood and anxiety disorders, substance abuse disorders, common medications (i.e., β-blockers, steroids, bronchodilators), sleep apnea, hyperthyroidism, and nocturnal myoclonus.
- Anxiety may be seen in anxiety disorder, depression, substance abuse disorders, hyperthyroidism, and complex partial seizures.

DIAGNOSIS

The diagnosis of insomnia and anxiety is a clinical one. No laboratory or imaging tests help in establishing the diagnosis; however, they can help to rule out other etiologies.

TREATMENT

- Benzodiazepines are frequently used in management of anxiety and insomnia. Table 1-2 provides a list of selected benzodiazepines and their common uses and dosages.
  - Pharmacology: Most benzodiazepines undergo oxidation to active metabolites in the liver. Lorazepam, oxazepam, and temazepam undergo glucuronidation to inactive metabolites; therefore, these agents may be particularly useful in the elderly and in those with liver disease. Benzodiazepines with long half-lives may accumulate substantially in the elderly, in whom the half-life may be increased manyfold.
  - Dosages: Relief of anxiety and insomnia is achieved at the doses outlined in Table 1-2. Therapy should be started at the lowest recommended dosage with intermittent dosing schedules.
  - Side effects include drowsiness, dizziness, fatigue, psychomotor impairment, and anterograde amnesia. Benzodiazepine toxicity is heightened by malnutrition, advanced age, hepatic disease and concomitant use of alcohol, other CNS depressants, and CYP3A4 inhibitors. The elderly may experience falls, paradoxical agitation, and delirium.
    - IV administration of diazepam and midazolam can be associated with hypotension, bradycardia, and respiratory or cardiac arrest.
    - Respiratory depression can occur even with oral administration in patients with respiratory compromise.
    - Tolerance to benzodiazepines can develop and dependence may develop after only 2–4 weeks of therapy.
    - Seizures and delirium may also occur with sudden discontinuation of benzodiazepines. A *withdrawal syndrome* consisting of agitation, irritability, insomnia, tremor, palpitations, headache, GI distress, and perceptual disturbance begins 1–10 days after a rapid decrease in dosage or abrupt cessation of therapy. Short-acting and intermediate-acting drugs should be decreased by 10–20% every 5 days, with a slower taper in the final few weeks. Long-acting preparations can be tapered more quickly.
  - Overdose
  Flumazenil, a benzodiazepine antagonist, should be readily available in case of accidental or intentional overdose. For details of administration, see Chapter 26, Medical Emergencies.
- Trazodone
  - Trazodone is a serotonin receptor antagonist antidepressant that may be useful for the treatment of severe anxiety or insomnia. Common dosing is 50–100 mg at bedtime.

TABLE 1-2	Characteristics of Selected Benzodiazepines			
Drug	**Route**	**Common Uses**	**Usual Dosage**	**Half-life (hr)**[a]
Alprazolam	PO	Anxiety disorders	0.75–4.0 mg/ 24 h (in three doses)	12–15
Chlordiazepoxide	PO	Anxiety disorders, alcohol withdrawal	15–100 mg/24 h (in divided doses)	5–30
Clonazepam	PO	Anxiety disorders, seizure disorders	0.5–4.0 mg/24 h (in two doses)	18–28
Diazepam	PO	Anxiety disorders, seizure disorders, preanesthesia	6–40 mg/24 h (in one to four doses)	20–50
	IV		2.5–20.0 mg (slow IV push)	20–50
Flurazepam	PO	Insomnia	15–30 mg at bedtime	50–100
Lorazepam[b]	PO	Anxiety disorders	1–10 mg/24 h (in two to three doses)	10–20
	IV or IM	Preanesthetic medication	0.05 mg/kg (4 mg max)	10–20
Midazolam	IV	Preanesthetic and intraoperative medication	0.01–0.05 mg/kg	1–12
	IM		0.08 mg/kg	1–12
Oxazepam[b]	PO	Anxiety disorders	10–30 mg/24 h (in three to four doses)	5–10
Temazepam[b]	PO	Insomnia	15–30 mg at bedtime	8–12
Triazolam	PO	Insomnia	0.125–0.250 mg at bedtime	2–5

[a]Half-life of active metabolites may differ.
[b]Metabolites are inactive.

- ○ It is highly sedating and can cause postural hypotension. It is rarely associated with priapism.
- ○ Levels may be substantially increased when used with CYP3A4 inhibitors.
- Nonbenzodiazepine hypnotics
These agents appear to act on the benzodiazepine receptor and have been shown to be safe and effective for initiating sleep. All should be used with caution in patients with impaired respiratory function.
- ○ Zolpidem is an imidazopyridine hypnotic agent that is useful for the treatment of insomnia. It has no withdrawal syndrome, rebound insomnia, or tolerance. Side effects

include headache, daytime somnolence, and GI upset. The starting dose is 5 mg PO every night at bedtime.

○ Zaleplon has a half-life of approximately 1 hour and no active metabolites. Side effects include dizziness and impaired coordination. The starting dose is 10 mg PO at bedtime (5 mg for the elderly or patients with hepatic dysfunction).

○ Eszopiclone offers a longer half-life compared to the previous agents. Side effects include headache and dizziness. Starting dose is 1 mg PO at bedtime.

○ Ramelteon is a melatonin analog. The usual dose is 8 mg PO at bedtime.

• Antihistamines
Over-the-counter antihistamines can be used for insomnia and anxiety, particularly in patients with a history of drug dependence. Anticholinergic side effects limit the utility, especially in the elderly.

PERIOPERATIVE MEDICINE

The role of the medical consultant is to estimate the level of risk associated with a given procedure, determine the need for further evaluation based upon this risk estimate, and prescribe interventions to mitigate risk. Although preoperative consultations often focus on cardiac risk, it is essential to remember that poor outcomes can result from significant disease in other organ systems. Evaluation of the entire patient is necessary to provide optimal perioperative care.

Preoperative Cardiac Evaluation

GENERAL PRINCIPLES

Perioperative cardiac complications are generally defined as cardiac death, MIs (both ST and non-ST elevation), CHF, and clinically significant rhythm disturbances.

Epidemiology

• Overall, an estimated 50,000 perioperative infarctions and 1 million other cardiovascular complications occur annually (*N Engl J Med 2001;345:1677*). Of those who have a perioperative MI, the risk of in-hospital mortality is estimated at 10–15% (*Chest 2006;130:584*).

• Perioperative MI (PMI) is believed to occur via two distinct mechanisms. Type I PMI results from erosion or rupture of unstable atherosclerotic plaque, leading to coronary thrombosis and subsequent myocardial injury. Type II PMI occurs when myocardial oxygen demand exceeds supply in the absence of overt thrombosis.

• Although angiographic data suggest that existing stenoses may underpin some perioperative events, a significant number of PMIs are "stress" related (Type II) and not due to plaque rupture (*Am J Cardiol 1996;77:1126*; *J Cardiothorac Vasc Anesth 2003;17:90*).

• Autopsy data indicate that fatal PMIs occur predominantly in patients with multivessel and especially left main coronary artery disease, via the same mechanism as non-PMIs (*Int J Cardiol 1996;57:37*).

DIAGNOSIS

Clinical Presentation

History
The aim is to identify patient factors and comorbid conditions that will affect perioperative risk. Current guidelines focus on identification of active cardiac disease and known risk factors for perioperative events, which include:

• Unstable coronary syndromes including severe angina

• Recent MI (defined as >7 but <30 days)

- Decompensated CHF (New York Heart Association class IV, worsening or new-onset heart failure [HF])
- Significant arrhythmia including non-sinus rhythm (rate controlled and stable)
- Severe valvular disease
- Clinical risk factors for coronary artery disease (CAD)
- Preexisting, stable CAD
- Compensated or prior CHF
- Diabetes mellitus
- Prior cerebrovascular accident (CVA) or transient ischemic attack (TIA)
- Chronic kidney disease
- Poorly controlled hypertension
- Abnormal ECG (e.g., left ventricular hypertrophy, left bundle branch block, ST-T wave abnormalities)
- Age >70 years identified in several studies as a significant risk factor (*JAMA 2001; 285:1865; Eur Heart J 2008;29:394*) but not uniformly accepted as independent

Physical Examination

Specific attention should be paid to the following:
- Vital signs, with particular evidence of hypertension. Systolic blood pressure (SBP) <180 and diastolic blood pressure (DBP) <110 are generally considered acceptable. The management of stage III hypertension (SBP >180 or DBP >110) is controversial. However, postponing elective surgery to allow adequate BP control in this setting seems reasonable; how long to wait after treatment is implemented remains unclear.
- Evidence of decompensated CHF (elevated jugular venous pressure, rales, S3, edema).
- Murmurs suggestive of significant valvular lesions. According to the 2014 American Heart Association (AHA)/American College of Cardiology (ACC) Guideline for the Management of Patients with Valvular Heart Disease, the risk of noncardiac surgery is increased in all patients with significant valvular heart disease, although symptomatic aortic stenosis (AS) is thought to carry the greatest risk. The estimated rate of cardiac complications in patients with undiagnosed severe AS undergoing noncardiac surgery is 10–30%. However, aortic valve replacement is also associated with considerable risk. Risk–benefit analysis appears to favor proceeding to intermediate-risk elective noncardiac surgery (see below) with appropriate intra- and postoperative hemodynamic monitoring (including intraoperative right heart catheter or transesophageal echocardiogram) as opposed to prophylactic aortic valve replacement in the context of asymptomatic severe disease. The same recommendations (albeit with less supporting evidence) apply to asymptomatic severe mitral regurgitation, asymptomatic severe AR with normal ejection fraction, and asymptomatic severe mitral stenosis (assuming valve morphology is not amenable to percutaneous balloon mitral commissurotomy, which should otherwise be considered to optimize cardiac status prior to proceeding to surgery). Symptomatic severe valvular disease of any type should prompt preoperative cardiology consultation. See the section on Valvular Heart Disease in Chapter 6.

Diagnostic Criteria

The 2014 ACC/AHA Guideline on Perioperative Cardiovascular Evaluation and Management of Patients Undergoing Noncardiac Surgery offers a stepwise approach to preoperative evaluation and risk stratification (Figure 1-1).
- Step 1: Establish the urgency of surgery. Many surgeries are unlikely to allow for a time-consuming evaluation.
- Step 2: Assess for active cardiac conditions (see History, above).
- Step 3: Determine the surgery-specific risk as follows:
  - Low-risk surgeries (<1% expected risk of adverse cardiac events) include superficial procedures, cataract/breast surgery, endoscopic procedures, and most procedures that can be performed in an ambulatory setting.

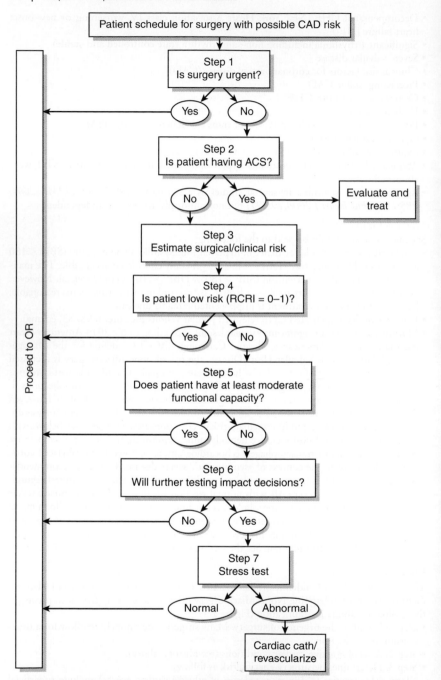

Figure 1-1. Cardiac evaluation algorithm for noncardiac surgery. (Modified from *Circulation 2014;130:e278–e333.*)

- ○ Intermediate risk surgeries (1–5% risk of adverse cardiac events) include carotid endarterectomy, intraperitoneal/intrathoracic surgery, orthopedic surgery, head and neck surgery, and prostate surgery.
  - ○ Vascular surgery involving extremity revascularization or aortic repair generally carries the highest risk (>5% risk of adverse cardiac events).
- Step 4: Assess the patient's functional capacity.
  Poor functional capacity (<4 metabolic equivalents [METs]) is associated with an increased risk of perioperative cardiac events (*Arch Intern Med 1999;159:2185*; *Chest 1999;116:355*). Although exercise testing is the gold standard, functional capacity can be reliably estimated by patient self-report (*Am J Cardiol 1989;64:651*). Examples of activities that suggest at least moderate functional capacity (>4 METs) include climbing one to two flights of stairs or walking a block at a brisk pace. Patients with a functional capacity of >4 METs without symptoms can proceed to surgery with relatively low risk.
- Step 5: Assess the patient's clinical risk factors.
  - ○ The number of risk factors combined with the surgery-specific risk (intermediate vs. vascular) determines further management. The following risk factors are adapted from the Revised Cardiac Risk Index (RCRI) (*Circulation 1999;100:1043*):
    - Ischemic heart disease
    - History of TIA or CVA
    - History of CHF
    - Preoperative serum creatinine ≥2 mg/dL
    - Diabetes mellitus requiring insulin
  - ○ Patients with no clinical risk factors are at inherently low risk (<1% risk of cardiac events) and may proceed to surgery without further testing. Patients with one or two clinical risk factors are generally at intermediate risk and may proceed to surgery, although stress testing might help refine risk assessment in selected cases. Patients with three or more clinical risk factors are at high risk of adverse cardiac events, particularly when undergoing vascular surgery. In this population especially, stress testing may provide a better estimate of cardiovascular risk and may be considered if knowledge of this increased risk would change management (*J Am Coll Cardiol 2006;48:964*). A positive stress test in a high-risk patient portends a substantially increased risk of a perioperative cardiac event, whereas a negative study suggests a lower risk than that predicted by clinical factors alone (*JAMA 2001;285:1865*).

Revascularization

- The best available data on preoperative revascularization come from the Coronary Artery Revascularization Prophylaxis (CARP) trial, a prospective study of patients scheduled to undergo vascular surgery (*N Engl J Med 2004;351:2795*). Patients with angiographically proven significant CAD were randomized to revascularization versus no revascularization. There was no difference between the groups in the occurrence of MI or death at 30 days or in mortality with long-term follow-up. Patients with three or more clinical risk factors and extensive ischemia on stress testing were evaluated in a separate small study (*J Am Coll Cardiol 2007;49:1763*). High event rates were seen in both study arms, and no benefit was seen with revascularization. Taken together, these studies suggest that the risk of adverse cardiac events is not altered by attempts at preoperative revascularization, even in high-risk populations. A notable possible exception are patients with left main disease, who appeared to have benefited from preoperative revascularization in a subset analysis of the CARP trial data (*Am J Cardiol 2008;102:809*).
- Based on these cumulative results, a strategy of routinely pursuing coronary revascularization as a method of decreasing perioperative cardiac risk cannot be recommended. However, careful screening of patients is still essential to identify those high-risk subsets who may obtain a survival benefit from revascularization independent of their need for noncardiac surgery.

Special Considerations

- Patients with drug-eluting coronary stents: see Perioperative Anticoagulation and Antithrombotic Management.
- Multiple studies have reported a correlation between delayed repair of hip fracture and increased morbidity and mortality (*Br Med J (Clin Res Ed) 1986;293(6556):1203; Clin Orthop 1984;(186):45*). For urgent surgical procedures (i.e., those that should be done within 48 hours of diagnosis), the value of additional testing is typically outweighed by the risk of worsened short- and long-term outcomes incurred with surgical delay. Unnecessary preoperative cardiac testing may be an independent risk factor for postoperative complications in hip fracture patients (*Am J Orthop 2008;37(1):32*). In such cases, it is advisable to optimize the patient's medical status and modifiable risk factors and then proceed to the operating room.

Diagnostic Testing

- **12-Lead ECG.** The value of a routine ECG is controversial. Per the 2014 ACC/AHA guidelines (level of evidence: B):
  - ECG is "reasonable" in patients with known CAD, significant arrhythmia, peripheral arterial disease, cerebrovascular disease, or other significant structural heart disease prior to intermediate-risk surgery and above (Class IIa);
  - "May be considered" for asymptomatic patients without known coronary heart disease prior to intermediate- and high-risk surgery (Class IIb);
  - Is "not useful" for asymptomatic patients undergoing low-risk surgical procedures (Class III).
- **Resting echocardiogram.** In general, the indications for preoperative echocardiographic evaluation are no different from those in the nonoperative setting. Murmurs found on physical exam suggestive of significant underlying valvular disease (see above) should be evaluated by echocardiogram. Assessment of left ventricular function should be considered when there is clinical concern for underlying undiagnosed CHF or if there is concern for deterioration since the last exam.
- **Noninvasive stress testing.** The decision to pursue a stress evaluation should be guided by an assessment of preoperative risk as detailed above. For further details on stress testing see Chapter 4, Ischemic Heart Disease.

TREATMENT

Medications

- β-Blockers
  - Multiple studies have provided support for perioperative β-blockade in patients with or at risk for CAD undergoing noncardiac surgeries. The most pronounced benefit has been observed in high-risk patients undergoing vascular surgery where β-blocker dose was titrated to heart rate control (*J Am Coll Cardiol 2006;48:964; Circulation 2006;114(suppl):I344*). However, a subsequent analysis has called into question the role of dose titration (*J Am Coll Cardiol 2014 Aug 1, E-pub ahead of print*). Although reduction in perioperative cardiac events has been observed consistently, it warrants mentioning that few data support the effectiveness of perioperative β-blockade in reducing mortality.
  - According to the 2014 ACC/AHA guidelines:
    - In patients with three or more RCRI risk factors (see above) or evidence of myocardial ischemia on preoperative stress testing, starting preoperative β-blockade is reasonable (level of evidence: B).
    - β-blockade should not be started on the day of surgery, as it is at minimum ineffective and may actually be harmful (level of evidence: B).
    - Patients already taking β-blockers should be continued on their medication (level of evidence: B).

- Statins
  - Statins are believed to improve cardiovascular outcomes by enhancing endothelial function, reducing vascular inflammation, and stabilizing atherosclerotic plaque in addition to their lipid-lowering effects. Multiple trials have shown a decrease in perioperative cardiac events and/or mortality with statin use in patients undergoing vascular surgery. Moreover, a recent cohort study of statin therapy in patients undergoing intermediate-risk noncardiac, nonvascular surgery revealed a fivefold reduced risk of 30-day all-cause mortality along with a statistically significant reduction in the composite end point of 30-day all-cause mortality, atrial fibrillation (AF), and nonfatal MI (*Clin Cardiol 2013;36(8):456*).
  - Per the 2014 ACC/AHA guidelines:
    - Patients currently taking statins should be maintained on therapy (level of evidence: B).
    - Patients undergoing vascular surgery, and those with risk factors undergoing intermediate risk surgery, may benefit from initiation of statin therapy perioperatively (level of evidence: B and C, respectively). Optimal dose, duration of therapy, and target low-density lipoprotein (LDL) levels for perioperative risk reduction are unclear.
- Aspirin
  For discussion, see Perioperative Anticoagulation and Antithrombotic Management.

MONITORING/FOLLOW-UP

Postoperative Infarction and Surveillance

- Most events will occur within 48–72 hours of surgery, with the majority in the first 24 hours (*CMAJ 2005;173:779*).
- Most are not heralded by chest pain and may be **clinically asymptomatic** (*Anesthesiology 1990;72:153*). Although overall 30-day mortality has been linked to postoperative troponin elevation (*JAMA 2012;307:2295*), the cause of death is not predictable, and no specific course of therapy may be offered.
- The 2014 ACC/AHA (*Circulation 2014;130;e278*) guidelines offer the following:
  - Routine postoperative ECGs and troponins are not recommended.
  - The benefit of troponin measurements and ECGs in high cardiac risk patients is uncertain.
  - Symptomatic infarctions should be addressed according to standard therapy of acute coronary syndromes (see Chapter 4, Ischemic Heart Disease). The major caveat is that bleeding risk with anticoagulants must be carefully considered.

Perioperative Anticoagulation and Antithrombotic Management

GENERAL PRINCIPLES

- Patients on chronic anticoagulation for AF, VTE, or mechanical heart valves often need to undergo procedures that pose risk of bleeding.
- The indication for anticoagulation and risk of interruption must be weighed against the risk of bleeding of the procedure (including possible neuraxial anesthesia).
- Until better research is available, decisions regarding perioperative anticoagulation will have to be made with the help of guidelines with relatively weak strength of evidence (*Chest 2012;141:326S*).

TREATMENT

- Recommended management varies according to the indication for anticoagulation, medication used, and surgical bleeding risk.

- **For patients being treated with oral anticoagulants/vitamin K antagonists (VKA):**
  - **Low bleeding risk** procedures permit continuation of **oral anticoagulation** through the perioperative period (e.g., minor dental and dermatologic procedures, cataract extraction, endoscopy without biopsy, arthrocentesis). Pacemaker and implantable cardioverter defibrillator (ICD) placement lead to less hematoma if anticoagulation is not interrupted (*N Engl J Med 2013;368:2084*).
  - **Significant bleeding risk procedures** require the anticoagulation to be discontinued.
    - Although the international normalized ratio (INR) at which surgery can be safely performed is subjective, an INR of <1.5 is typically a reasonable goal.
    - The VKA (e.g., warfarin) will typically need to be stopped 5 days preoperatively.
    - The INR should be checked the day before surgery. If a level <1.5 is not obtained, 1–2.5 mg oral vitamin K effectively achieves an INR <1.5 on the day of surgery.
    - The VKA can generally be resumed 12–24 hours postoperatively if postoperative bleeding has been controlled (*Chest 2012;141:326S*).
  - **High bleeding risk procedures** (e.g., intracranial or spinal) with potential catastrophic outcomes due to bleeding will preclude any anticoagulation in the perioperative period. Other procedures with high bleeding risk (e.g., sessile polypectomy; bowel resection; kidney, liver, or spleen biopsy; extensive orthopedic or plastic surgery) should lead to a delay of at least 48 hours prior to resumption of anticoagulation.
- **Bridging therapy** refers to the administration of an alternative anticoagulation during the time the INR is anticipated to be below the therapeutic range. The potential decrease in thrombosis must be weighed against the increased risk of bleeding (*Circulation 2012;126:1630*).
- **High thrombotic risk patients** below should typically be treated with bridging therapy.
  - Mechanical mitral valve
  - Older-generation mechanical valve (e.g., Starr-Edwards ball-in-cage valve)
  - Any mechanical valve with a history of cardioembolism within the preceding 6 months
  - Nonvalvular AF with either a history of embolism in the last 3 months or CHADS$_2$ score ≥5 (see Chapter 7, Cardiac Arrhythmias)
  - Valvular AF
  - Recent VTE (<3 months)
  - Known thrombophilic state (e.g., protein C deficiency)
- For **moderate thrombotic risk patients** as below, bridging may be considered in patients with low bleeding risk. Deep venous thrombosis (DVT) prophylaxis dosing is acceptable.
  - Mechanical aortic valve (bileaflet) with one or more associated risk factors: AF, CHF, hypertension, age ≥75, DM, and prior CVA or TIA
  - AF with a CHADS$_2$ score of 3 or 4, or history of prior embolism
  - History of VTE within preceding 3–12 months
  - Non–high-risk thrombophilia (e.g., heterozygous factor V Leiden mutation)
  - History of recurrent VTE
  - Active malignancy
- **Low thrombotic risk** patients are **not** believed to require bridging therapy. Treatment with DVT prophylaxis doses of LMWH or UFH is an alternative. This group includes patients with:
  - Mechanical aortic valve (bileaflet) without associated risk factors, as above
  - Nonvalvular AF with a CHADS$_2$ score ≤2 and no history of embolism
  - Prior VTE >12 months prior (without history of recurrent VTE or known hypercoagulable state)
- **Choices for bridging therapy** are generally the LMWHs and UFH, including patients with mechanical heart valves (*Chest 2012;141:326S*). There is less experience in this setting with other agents (e.g., fondaparinux), and their use cannot be considered routine.
  - **LMWHs** have the advantages of relatively predictable pharmacokinetics and ability to be administered SC. Monitoring of anticoagulant effect is typically not required.

Renal dosing is available for patients not on dialysis. Subcutaneous administration allows for outpatient therapy in appropriate patients. This decreases the length and cost of hospitalization. The last dose should be given 24 hours prior to surgery.

- ○ **UFH** is the agent of choice for patients with end-stage renal disease (ESRD). It is typically administered IV and requires frequent monitoring of the activated partial thromboplastin time. UFH should be stopped at least 4 hours prior to the planned surgical procedure to allow the anticoagulant effect to wane. Fixed-dose subcutaneous UFH has been proven efficacious for treatment of VTE and may be considered as an option (*JAMA 2006;295:1152*).
- ○ **Novel oral anticoagulants** have relatively short half-lives (dabigatran = 14 hours, rivaroxaban = 9 hours, apixaban = 12 hours), obviating the need for bridging anticoagulation. Agents should be held for two or three half-lives for low bleed risk procedures and three or four half-lives for high bleed risk procedures, keeping in mind the effects of renal function on clearance. Reversal agents are currently being developed.
- **Patients being treated with antiplatelet agents**
  - ○ Continuing antiplatelet agents perioperatively also carries a risk of bleeding, whereas discontinuation may increase cardiovascular events. Irreversible agents must be withheld for 5–7 days before effects fully abate. Clinicians are again left with little evidence and sometimes conflicting guidelines.
  - ○ **Low bleeding risk procedures** (e.g., minor dermatologic or dental procedures) allow continuation of aspirin (acetylsalicylic acid [ASA]) being given for secondary prevention of cardiovascular disease.
  - ○ **Noncardiac surgery patients** should generally have clopidogrel (or other thienopyridines) held 5 days preoperatively. Prompt reinitiation with a loading dose of 300 mg should take place postoperatively. Further stratification drives decisions regarding ASA:
    - ▪ **Moderate to high cardiac risk**, in which case ASA should be continued perioperatively
    - ▪ **Low cardiac risk**, in which case ASA should be held 7 days preoperatively
  - ○ **Coronary artery bypass graft** candidates should generally continue ASA perioperatively and have clopidogrel held 5 days preoperatively.
  - ○ **Coronary stents** pose a particular risk of in-stent thrombosis and infarction if dual antiplatelet therapy is prematurely withheld. Whenever possible, surgery should be deferred until the minimum period of dual antiplatelet therapy is completed (balloon angioplasty without stent, 14 days; drug-eluting stents, 12 months; bare metal stents, 6 weeks).
  - ○ **Urgent surgeries** within the previous time frames should proceed with continued dual antiplatelet treatment, if possible. If the bleeding risk is felt to be high, ASA alone should be continued. Heparin bridging has not been shown to be of benefit. Bridging with IV glycoprotein IIb/IIIa antagonists or reversible oral agents (e.g., ticagrelor) is not routinely recommended (*Chest 2012;141:326S*).

PERIOPERATIVE MANAGEMENT OF SPECIFIC CONDITIONS

Hypertension

GENERAL PRINCIPLES

- **Severe hypertension** (BP >180/110) preoperatively often results in wider fluctuations in intraoperative BP and has been associated with an increased rate of perioperative cardiac events (see the previous section, Preoperative Cardiac Evaluation).

- Antihypertensive agents that the patient has taken prior to admission for surgery may have an impact on the perioperative period.
  - When the patient is receiving β-blockers or clonidine chronically, withdrawal of these medications may result in tachycardia and rebound hypertension, respectively.
  - Evidence suggests that holding angiotensin-converting enzyme inhibitors and angiotensin II receptor blockers on the day of surgery may reduce perioperative hypotension. This is believed to be due to the effect of this class of medication in blunting the compensatory activation of the renin–angiotensin system perioperatively.

DIAGNOSIS

BP monitoring should be done as part of a patient's routine vital signs. A portable or wall blood pressure cuff should be used. In the setting of severe hypertension, BP should be checked in both arms and with two different types of BP cuffs in order to ensure accuracy.

TREATMENT

- Hypertension in the postoperative period is a common problem with multiple possible causes.
  - All **remediable causes of hypertension**, such as pain, agitation, hypercarbia, hypoxia, hypervolemia, and bladder distention, should be excluded or treated.
  - Poor control of essential hypertension secondary to discontinuation of medications the patient was previously taking in the immediate postoperative period is not uncommon; thus, reviewing the patient's home medication list is recommended.
  - A rare cause of perioperative hypertension is **pheochromocytoma**, particularly if its presence was unrecognized. Patients can develop an acute hypertensive crisis perioperatively which should be treated, with **phentolamine** or **nitroprusside** recommended in this situation. When the diagnosis of pheochromocytoma is suspected, preoperative treatment to minimize risk is recommended and can be classically accomplished by titration of **phenoxybenzamine** preoperatively.
- Many parenteral antihypertensive medications are available for patients who are unable to take medications orally. Transdermal clonidine also is an option, but the onset of action is delayed.

Pacemakers and ICDs

GENERAL PRINCIPLES

- The use of electrocautery intraoperatively can have adverse effects on the function of implanted cardiac devices.
- A variety of errors can occur, from resetting the device to inadvertent discharge of an ICD.
- Complications are rare but are more likely with abdominal and thoracic surgeries.
- The type of device (i.e., pacemaker or ICD) and manufacturer should be determined.
- The initial indication for placement and the patient's underlying rhythm should be determined. Ideally, this can be determined from the history and an ECG.
- The device should be interrogated within 3–6 months of a significant surgical procedure.

TREATMENT

If the patient is pacemaker dependent, the device should be reprogrammed to an asynchronous mode (e.g., VOO, DOO) for the surgery.
- The application of a magnet will cause most pacemakers to revert to an asynchronous pacing mode; however, if this is the planned management, it should be tested preoperatively, especially in the pacemaker-dependent patient.

- It should be noted that the effect of a magnet on ICDs is typically different from the effect on pacemakers in that it affects the anti-tachycardia function but does not alter the pacing function of most models. If the pacing function of an ICD needs to be altered perioperatively, the device will need to be reprogrammed.
- The anti-tachycardia function of an ICD will typically need to be programmed off for surgical procedures in which electrocautery may cause interference with device function, leading to the potential for unintentional discharge. The effect of a magnet on this function is variable, so programming is the preferred management. Continuous monitoring for arrhythmia is essential during the period when this function is suspended.
- Continuous ECG and pulse monitoring is recommended during surgery. Pulse monitoring should not be affected by electrocautery interference.
- Postoperative interrogation may be necessary, particularly if the device settings were changed perioperatively or if the patient is pacemaker dependent.
- **Consultation with an electrophysiologist** is strongly recommended if there is any uncertainty regarding the perioperative management of a device.

Pulmonary Disease and Preoperative Pulmonary Evaluation

GENERAL PRINCIPLES

Postoperative pulmonary complications are probably more common than cardiac complications, and the occurrence of one may predispose to the other (*Am J Med 2003;115:515*; *Am J Respir Crit Care Med 2005;171:514*). Clinically significant pulmonary complications include pneumonia, bronchospasm, atelectasis, exacerbation of underlying chronic lung disease, and respiratory failure. Postoperative respiratory failure can be a life-threatening complication, with a 30-day mortality rate as high as 26.5% (*J Am Coll Surg 2007;204:1188*).

Risk Factors

- Both patient-dependent and surgery-specific risk factors determine overall risk (*Ann Intern Med 2006;144:575*).
- Procedure-related risk factors
  - Surgical site is generally considered the greatest determinant of risk of pulmonary complications, with upper abdominal and thoracic surgeries associated with highest risk (*N Engl J Med 1999;340:937*). Neurosurgery and surgeries involving the mouth and palate also impart increased risk (*Ann Surg 2000;232:242*; *J Am Coll Surg 2007;204:1188*).
  - Duration of surgery correlates positively with risk in multiple studies (*Chest 1997;111:564*; *Acta Anaesthesiol Scand 2001;45:345*; *Am J Respir Crit Care Med 2003;167:741*).
  - Type of anesthesia may influence pulmonary risk as well. Although somewhat controversial due to conflicting data and study heterogeneity, it seems that neuraxial anesthesia affords reduced risk of pneumonia, respiratory failure, and possibly short-term mortality in comparison to general anesthesia (*Br Med J 2000;321:1493*; *Lancet 2008;372(9638):562*).
- Patient-dependent risk factors
  - COPD has reliably been found to be a risk factor for postoperative pulmonary complications. Disease severity correlates with risk of serious complications (*Chest 1993;104:1445*). However, even patients with advanced lung disease can safely undergo surgery if deemed medically necessary (*Br Med J 1975;3:670*; *Arch Intern Med 1992;152:967*). In contradistinction to hepatic disease, there is no identified threshold that precludes surgery.
  - Interstitial lung disease likely places patients at elevated risk but is not well studied in patients undergoing general surgery (*Chest 2007;132:1637*). Well-controlled asthma

and restrictive physiology associated with obesity do not appear to be significant risk factors (*Ann Intern Med 2006;144:575; Br J Anaesth 2009;103(1):i57*).

○ Pulmonary hypertension is associated with significant morbidity in patients undergoing surgery (*J Am Coll Cardiol 2005;45:1691; Br J Anaesth 2007;99:184*).

○ Data from the systematic review that formed the basis for the American College of Physicians guideline regarding pulmonary risk stratification for noncardiothoracic surgery suggest that heart failure may increase the risk of pulmonary complications to a greater degree than that seen with COPD (pooled adjusted odds ratios 2.93 and 2.36, respectively) (*Ann Intern Med 2006;144:581*).

○ Poor general health status is associated with increased perioperative pulmonary risk. Multiple indices of general health status including degree of functional dependence and American Society of Anesthesiologists class have been linked to poor pulmonary outcomes (*Ann Intern Med 2006;144:581*). Odds ratios for postoperative respiratory failure of 2.53 and 2.29 were observed for hypoalbuminemia (<3 g/dL) and azotemia (BUN >30 mg/dL), respectively, in a large cohort (*Ann Surg 2000;232:242*).

○ The above-mentioned systematic review for the American College of Physicians identified age >50 years as an independent predictor of postoperative pulmonary complications after adjustment for age-related comorbidities; risk was noted to increase linearly with increasing age. Large observational studies informing risk prediction models currently in use (see below) have further validated this observation, in contrast to postsurgical cardiac risk.

○ Smoking is a well-established risk factor for both postoperative pulmonary and nonpulmonary complications (*Ann Surg 2014;259:52*). As with malignancy, risk appears to be dose-dependent and associated with active use (*Chest 1998;113(4):883; Am J Respir Crit Care Med 2003;167:741*).

○ Obstructive sleep apnea (OSA) is increasingly being recognized as a risk factor for perioperative complications, both pulmonary and cardiac (*Chest 2008;133:1128*). A meta-analysis showed that OSA increased the odds of various postoperative complications by a factor of 2–4 (*Br J Anaesth 2012;109:897*); the most frequent pulmonary complication appears to be hypoxemia (*Anesthesiology 2008;108:822*). Unrecognized sleep apnea may pose an even greater risk (*Mayo Clin Proc 2001;76:897*). It is estimated that over half of patients with OSA presenting for surgery are undiagnosed (*Br J Anaesth 2013;110:629; Sleep Med 2013;14:407*).

DIAGNOSIS

Clinical Presentation

History

Preoperative pulmonary evaluation should focus on the above-mentioned patient-dependent risk factors.

• Any history of lung disease should be elucidated. If chronic lung disease is present, an effort should be made to determine the patient's baseline and whether there has been any recent deterioration, such as increased cough, wheezing, or sputum production.

• Symptoms of current upper respiratory tract infection should be ascertained. Although not an absolute contraindication to surgery, it seems prudent to postpone purely elective procedures until such infections have resolved.

• A full smoking history should be obtained.

• Patients should be questioned regarding symptoms potentially consistent with OSA (snoring, daytime somnolence, observed apneas). See the section on Obstructive Sleep Apnea–Hypopnea Syndrome in Chapter 10.

• As myriad nonpulmonary comorbidities impact the likelihood of pulmonary complications (as delineated previously), a complete medical history is vital.

Physical Examination
- Body mass index (BMI) should be calculated. Although obesity itself is not associated with postoperative pulmonary complications, prevalence of OSA increases with increasing BMI. Uncontrolled hypertension may also suggest undiagnosed sleep apnea. Measurement of oxygen saturation by pulse oximetry assists in risk stratification (*Anesthesiology 2010;113:1338*).
- A Mallampati score should be determined. A study of 137 adults being evaluated for OSA found that every 1-point increase in the Mallampati score increased the odds of OSA by 2.5 (95% confidence interval 1.2–5.0) (*Sleep 2006;29:903*).
- Attention should be paid to evidence of chronic lung disease such as increased anteroposterior dimension of the chest, digital clubbing, and the presence of adventitious lung sounds (see Chapter 9, Obstructive Lung Disease, and Chapter 10, Pulmonary Diseases). Persistent coughing after a voluntary cough is also a marker of increased risk (*Am J Respir Crit Care Med 2003;167:741*).
- Again, signs of decompensated heart failure (see the section on Preoperative Cardiac Evaluation in this chapter, and Chapter 5, Heart Failure and Cardiomyopathy) should be actively sought.

Risk Stratification

Several risk indices have been developed for quantitating risk of postoperative respiratory failure (defined here as failure to wean from mechanical ventilation within 48 hours of surgery) or pneumonia (*Ann Surg 2000;232:242; Chest 2011;140:1207; Mayo Clin Proc 2013;88:1241*). The Arozullah respiratory failure index was based on multivariate analysis of a cohort of 81,719 patients and validated on another 99,390 patients. It offers the advantage of manual calculation at the bedside. The Gupta calculators for postoperative pneumonia and respiratory failure are derived from a data set of 211,410 patients and validated on another 257,385. Although considerably more complicated than the Arozullah index, these calculators are accessible online and may be downloaded for free.

Diagnostic Testing

- **Pulmonary function tests (PFTs)**
  The value of preoperative PFTs is debatable outside of lung resection surgery, where its role is relatively well defined (see the section on Chronic Obstructive Pulmonary Disease in Chapter 9, and the section on Lung Cancer in Chapter 22). In other surgical contexts, measurements gleaned from PFTs either fail to predict pulmonary complications or add little beyond what can be gathered clinically (*Chest 1997;111:1536*). Although routine PFTs do not appear warranted per the current guidelines (*Ann Intern Med 2006;144:575*), they should be considered for patients with unexplained dyspnea or exercise intolerance or for patients with known lung disease and an unclear baseline.
- **Arterial blood gas (ABG) analysis**
  No data exist that suggest that ABG results contribute to preoperative pulmonary risk estimation beyond other clinically derived variables as discussed earlier. Nevertheless, an ABG should be obtained when otherwise indicated; for example, to determine if a patient's lung disease is compensated (see the section on Respiratory Failure in Chapter 8).
- **Chest radiography**
  In general, a chest radiograph is recommended only if otherwise indicated (e.g., for evaluation of unexplained dyspnea). Many findings deemed abnormal are chronic and do not alter management (*Can J Anesth 2005;52:568*).

TREATMENT

Treatment should be focused on modifiable patient-related and procedure-related risk factors.
- The effect of preoperative smoking cessation on pulmonary complications has been largely described in cardiothoracic surgeries, where a benefit to quitting smoking at least

2 months prior to surgery has been shown (*Mayo Clin Proc 1989;64:609*). The effect on a general surgical population is less clear, because most of the observed benefit in this latter group relates to improvements in nonpulmonary outcomes, such as fewer wound complications (*Ann Surg 2008;248:739*). Nevertheless, given the long-term benefits of smoking cessation, all patients should be counseled to stop smoking even if <8 weeks from surgery. Previous concerns about a paradoxical increase in complications appear unfounded (*Arch Intern Med 2011;171(11):983*).

• COPD and asthma therapy should be optimized (see Chapter 9, Obstructive Lung Disease). Nonemergent surgery may need to be postponed to allow recovery of pulmonary function to baseline.

• OSA should be treated prior to elective high-risk surgery when possible. Data in the preoperative setting are limited, but in a recent open-label trial, patients with moderate OSA who were randomized to auto-titrated continuous positive airway pressure treatment had improved postoperative oxygen saturation and markedly decreased apnea-hypopnea indices compared with control patients, even despite observed low compliance (*Anesthesiology 2013;119:837*).

• Alternative procedures with reduced pulmonary risk should be considered for high-risk patients if feasible. Laparoscopic procedures may yield fewer pulmonary complications (*Br J Anaesth 1996;77:448*; *Ann Intern Med 2006;144:581*); regional nerve block also appears to be associated with decreased risk (*Am Rev Respir Dis 1979;119:293*). If general anesthesia is absolutely necessary, duration should be minimized to the degree possible.

Anemia and Transfusion Issues in Surgery

GENERAL PRINCIPLES

• Transfusion-associated risks include transmission of blood-borne infections, transfusion-related acute lung injury, transfusion reactions, and immunosuppressive effects.

• Preoperative anemia is present in 5–35% of patients depending on the definition of anemia and type of surgery studied (*Lancet 2011 Oct 15;378(9800):1396–407*).

DIAGNOSIS

• A history of anemia, hematologic disease, or bleeding diathesis should be noted on history or review of medical records.

• Any clinical signs of anemia (e.g., pallor) or coagulopathy (e.g., petechiae) should prompt further evaluation.

• There is no standardized preoperative evaluation for anemia.
  ○ For low-risk procedures, there is no evidence that routine testing of asymptomatic individuals before low-risk procedures increases safety (*Ann Surg 2012;256(3):518–28*).
  ○ For higher risk procedures, particularly those with higher bleeding risk, a baseline CBC and coagulation profile are typically obtained. Further testing should be performed as indicated.

TREATMENT

Volume resuscitation and control of active bleeding are the initial therapy of anemia, particularly in the perioperative period when acute blood loss is a common occurrence.

• Guidelines for perioperative blood transfusions are variable.

• Preoperative anemia, hematocrit <39% in men and <36% in women, is independently associated with an increase in 30-day morbidity/mortality risk. (*Lancet 2011 Oct 15;378(9800)*).

- Postoperatively, in a cohort of patients who refused transfusion, no mortality was observed for hemoglobin >7 g/dL. A marked increase in risk was seen at hemoglobin <5 g/dL threshold (*Transfusion 2002;42:812*).
- The benefit of transfusion at physiologically tolerable levels of anemia is unclear.
  - The TRICC trial, a study of intensive care unit patients, showed no mortality difference between transfusion thresholds of hemoglobin <7 g/dL or <10 g/dL. Subgroup analysis showed improved mortality in younger, less critically ill patients when using transfusion threshold of hemoglobin <7 g/dL. (*N Engl J Med 1999;336:933*). The applicability of this study to the perioperative setting is uncertain.
  - The FOCUS trial showed no mortality difference between a restrictive (hemoglobin <8 g/dL) and liberal (hemoglobin <10 g/dL) transfusion threshold in high-risk (known or have risk factors for cardiovascular disease) patients after hip surgery (*N Engl J Med 2011;365(26):2453–2462*).
  - In general, no transfusion is indicated for hemoglobin >10 g/dL in a stable patient.
  - In stable patients, transfusion may be considered at hemoglobin of 7–8 g/dL.
  - In stable patients with cardiovascular disease, a transfusion threshold of 8 g/dL should be utilized.
  - In patients with concern for active cardiac ischemia, transfusions may be indicated to achieve a hemoglobin of 8–10 g/dL, but there is no consistent recommendation.

Other Nonpharmacologic Therapies

Measures to reduce the need for allergenic blood should be utilized where feasible.
- Preoperative autologous blood donation should be considered for elective procedures where the anticipated need for transfusion is high.
- Preoperative erythropoietin is generally not indicated, but can be considered in patients who may refuse blood products due to personal or religious reasons (*Transfusion 1994; 34(1):66*).
- Avoidance of perioperative hypothermia may also limit blood loss, and thereby decrease transfusion requirements (*Anesthesiology 2008;108:71*).

SPECIAL CONSIDERATIONS

Patients with sickle cell anemia should generally be transfused to a hemoglobin of 10 g/dL preoperatively to decrease the incidence of complications (*Lancet 2013;381:930*).

Liver Disease

GENERAL PRINCIPLES

- Patients with hepatic dysfunction face an increased risk of morbid outcomes when undergoing surgery and may develop acute hepatic decompensation postoperatively.
- The myriad systemic effects of hepatic dysfunction result in an increased frequency of other complications as well, such as bleeding and infection.

Classification

- Both Child-Turcotte-Pugh (CTP) and Model for End-stage Liver Disease (MELD) scores (see Chapter 19, Liver Diseases) are well-validated statistical models for predicting surgical risk.
- A large review of patients undergoing a variety of surgical procedures clearly identified a demarcation between CTP class A (score <7) and those with class B and C disease (*Anesthesiology 1999;90:42*). The 30-day mortality was 9.4% in the CTP class A group versus 16.7% in classes B and C group combined. Other complications were also significantly more common.

- Patients with CTP class C disease have particularly elevated operative risk; perioperative mortality exceeds 80% with abdominal surgery in this group (*Surgery 1997;122:730*).
- The 30-day mortality correlated linearly with the MELD score in a study of 772 cirrhotic patients who underwent major digestive, orthopedic, or cardiovascular surgery (*Gastroenterology 2007;132:1261*). MELD score >20 predicted >50% mortality.
- The superiority of either model as a nontransplant surgical risk predictor is a subject of continuing debate. It has been suggested that patients with CTP class A or MELD <10 cirrhosis can safely undergo elective surgery, those with class B or MELD of 10–15 may undergo elective surgery with caution, and those with class C or MELD >15 should not undergo elective surgery (*Natl Clin Pract Gastroenterol Hepatol 2007;4:266*).

DIAGNOSIS

Clinical Presentation

History

Historical details suggesting risk for hepatic disease (e.g., alcohol/drug use, prior blood transfusion, family history of cirrhosis) should be elicited.

Physical Examination

Findings potentially consistent with liver dysfunction should be noted. Some should be obvious, such as icterus and abdominal distention with ascites, but other abnormalities such as spider nevi, palmar erythema, and testicular atrophy may be more subtle.

Diagnostic Testing

- Because significant disease is usually clinically manifest, routine laboratory screening for hepatic dysfunction in patients presenting for surgery is not recommended (*Med Clin North Am 2003;87:211*).
- Patients with known or suspected liver disease should undergo a thorough evaluation of liver function including hepatic enzyme levels, albumin and bilirubin measurements, and evaluation for coagulopathy.
- Renal function, including electrolytes, blood urea nitrogen (BUN), and creatinine measurements, should also be evaluated.

TREATMENT

- Patients with acute viral or alcoholic hepatitis tolerate surgery poorly, and delaying surgery until recovery is recommended if possible.
- Patients with chronic hepatitis without evidence of hepatic decompensation generally tolerate surgery well.
- Based on the aforementioned high perioperative mortality rates in patients with advanced cirrhosis, nonoperative alternatives should be strongly considered.
- For patients who do require surgery, steps should be taken to optimize preoperative status:
  ○ Coagulopathy should be corrected to the degree possible.
    ▪ Vitamin K should be administered if the INR is elevated. However, as the coagulopathy may prove refractory to this measure in the setting of impaired hepatic synthetic function, fresh frozen plasma and/or cryoprecipitate may ultimately be required.
    ▪ Thrombocytopenia also is a common finding and should be corrected if severe. The general recommendation for most surgical procedures is a minimum platelet count of 50,000. However, coexisting platelet dysfunction due to liver disease should be considered, particularly if there is clinical evidence of bleeding.

○ Renal and electrolyte abnormalities should be addressed and careful attention should be paid to volume status.
  ▪ Nephrotoxic agents, such as NSAIDs and aminoglycosides, should be avoided.
  ▪ Patients with cirrhosis often have hypokalemia and alkalosis. These conditions should be corrected preoperatively to minimize the risk of cardiac arrhythmias and to limit encephalopathy.
  ▪ If hyponatremia develops, free water restriction may be required.
  ▪ Ascites should be treated. Ascites has been found to be an independent risk factor for postoperative pulmonary complications (*J Am Coll Surg 2007;204:1188*). If time permits, diuretic therapy should be instituted. Paracentesis should be considered preoperatively if diuretics are ineffective or if circumstances prevent their use.
○ Encephalopathy should be treated aggressively.
  ▪ Lactulose titrated to two to three soft bowel movements per day should be started in patients with encephalopathy.
  ▪ Protein restriction has been recommended for individuals who respond poorly to lactulose, but this should be done cautiously because excessive restriction may actually contribute to malnutrition.
  ▪ Sedatives and opioids can precipitate or worsen encephalopathy. They should be used sparingly, and dose reductions should be considered.
○ Adequate nutrition should be provided. Malnutrition often accompanies advanced cirrhosis, and deficiencies of fat-soluble vitamins and electrolytes are not uncommon in the context of chronic cholestasis and alcohol abuse, respectively.

Diabetes Mellitus

GENERAL PRINCIPLES

• Medical and surgical patients with hyperglycemia are at increased risk for poor outcomes (*J Clin Endocrinol Metab 2002;87:978*).
• Poor preoperative glucose control, as indicated by elevated hemoglobin A1C levels, is associated with an increased risk of surgical infections (*Arch Surg 2006;141:375*). Hyperglycemia postoperatively also appears to be associated with an increased risk of postoperative infection (*JPEN J Parenter Enteral Nutr 1998;22:77*).
• There is some suggestion, particularly in patients undergoing cardiothoracic surgery, that more aggressive medical management of hyperglycemia mitigates the risk of infection and possibly mortality (*Ann Thorac Surg 1997;63:356; J Thorac Cardiovasc Surg 2003;125:1007*).
• The fact that hyperglycemia is a marker for poor outcomes appears to be relatively clear. However, whether aggressive management truly improves outcomes is uncertain. Trial results have been mixed.
  ○ In a population of mostly surgical patients requiring critical care, impressive reductions in mortality were demonstrated in a single institution study (*N Engl J Med 2001;345:1359*). The results of this trial prompted widespread adoption of aggressive insulin protocols in surgical intensive care units.
  ○ However, a recent larger multicenter trial of both surgical and medical critical care patients was unable to show improvements in outcome and actually found a slight increase in risk with aggressive treatment of hyperglycemia (*N Engl J Med 2009;360:1283*).
  ○ Diabetics are at **increased risk for cardiovascular disease**. Appropriate risk stratification for cardiac complications of surgery is vital to the perioperative evaluation of these patients.

Classification

- Establishing the etiology of hyperglycemia has important implications for subsequent patient care.
  - **Stress hyperglycemia** can occur in the perioperative setting because of the body's response to surgery with the release of counterregulatory hormones and cytokines that impede glucose metabolism. These patients need adequate glucose control during the perioperative period but are unlikely to require such treatment later.
  - Type 2 diabetes is notoriously underdiagnosed, and the notation of perioperative hyperglycemia may be the first indication of its presence.
- It is essential to distinguish between type 1 and type 2 diabetes mellitus.
  - **Type 1 diabetics** will require a continuous supply of insulin regardless of glucose level and oral intake.
  - The insulin requirement, if any, of **type 2 diabetics** during the perioperative period will vary.

DIAGNOSIS

- A **hemoglobin A1C** level should be obtained.
  - This can assist in differentiating perioperative stress hyperglycemia from undiagnosed diabetes.
  - Knowledge of recent glycemic control in known diabetics also is helpful in determining what therapy is required.
- Evaluating **renal function** also is recommended given the increased prevalence of renal disease in diabetics.
- Cardiovascular risk stratification may require other evaluations (see the previous section, Preoperative Cardiac Evaluation).

TREATMENT

- Elective surgery in patients with uncontrolled diabetes mellitus should preferably be scheduled after acceptable glycemic control has been achieved.
- If possible, the operation should be scheduled for early morning to minimize prolonged fasting.
- Frequent monitoring of blood glucose levels is required in all situations.
- **Type 1 diabetes**
  - Some form of basal insulin is required at all times.
  - On the evening prior to surgery, the regularly scheduled basal insulin should be continued. If taken in the morning, it is still recommended to give the regularly scheduled basal insulin without dose adjustment (*Diabetes Care 2004;27:553*). However, patients who are very tightly controlled may be at increased risk for hypoglycemia and will need to be monitored closely. A decrease in the last preoperative basal insulin dose may be considered in this circumstance.
  - Glucose infusions (e.g., D5-containing fluids) can be administered to avoid hypoglycemia while the patient is NPO and until tolerance of oral intake postoperatively is established.
  - For complex procedures and procedures requiring a prolonged NPO status, a continuous insulin infusion will likely be necessary.
  - **Caution should be exercised with the use of subcutaneous insulin** in the intraoperative and critical care settings, as alterations in tissue perfusion may result in variable absorption.
- **Type 2 diabetes**
  - Treatment of type 2 diabetics varies according to their preoperative requirements and the complexity of the planned procedure (*Med Clin North Am 2003;87:175*).

○ Consideration should be given to the efficacy of the patient's current regimen. If the patient is not well controlled at baseline, then an escalation in therapy may be required.

- **Diet-controlled type 2 diabetes** can generally be managed without insulin therapy. Glucose values should be checked regularly and elevated levels (>180 mg/dL) can be treated with intermittent doses of short-acting insulin.
- **Type 2 diabetes managed with oral therapy**
  □ **Short-acting sulfonylureas** and **other oral agents** should be withheld on the operative day.
  □ **Metformin** and **long-acting sulfonylureas** (e.g., chlorpropamide) should be withheld 1 day before planned surgical procedures. Metformin is generally held for 48 hours postoperatively provided there is no acute renal injury. Other oral agents can be resumed when patients are tolerating their pre-procedure diet.
  □ Most patients can be managed without an insulin infusion.
  □ Glucose values should be checked regularly and elevated levels (>180 mg/dL) can be treated with intermittent doses of short-acting insulin.
- **Type 2 diabetes managed with insulin**
  □ If it is anticipated that the patient will be able to eat postoperatively, basal insulin is still given on the morning of surgery.
  □ If given as long-acting insulin (e.g., glargine insulin) and the patient usually takes the dose in the morning, 50–100% of the usual dose can be given.
  □ If the patient utilizes intermediate-acting insulin (e.g., NPH), one-half to two-thirds of the usual morning dose is given to avoid periprocedural hyperglycemia.
  □ Dextrose-containing IV fluids may be required to avoid hypoglycemia.
  □ Patients undergoing major procedures will typically require an insulin drip perioperatively.
  □ The usual insulin treatment can be reintroduced once oral intake is established postoperatively.

- **Target glucose levels**
  ○ There are no generally agreed-upon target glucose levels applicable to the entire post-surgical population.
    - Earlier literature recommends aggressive glucose control in the critical care setting (*Diabetes Care 2008;31S:S12; N Engl J Med 2009;360:1283–1297*).
    - In a general medical–surgical population, recurring glucose values >200 mg/dL were associated with a poor outcome (*J Clin Endocrinol Metab 2002;87:978*).
  ○ Pending further research, a goal of maintaining glucose levels <180 mg/dL in the post-operative setting seems reasonable. It should be noted that this may still require intensive treatments such as insulin infusion.
  ○ In patients treated with sliding scale insulin, it is essential to monitor the response to therapy. Patients who are hyperglycemic consistently are unlikely to have adequate glucose control with intermittent treatment alone, and a basal/bolus regimen should be introduced if hyperglycemia is persistent (*Diabetes Care 2007;30:2181*).

Adrenal Insufficiency and Corticosteroid Management

GENERAL PRINCIPLES

- Surgery is a potent activator of the hypothalamic–pituitary axis, and patients with adrenal insufficiency may lack the ability to respond appropriately to surgical stress.
- Patients receiving corticosteroids as anti-inflammatory therapy may rarely develop post-operative adrenal insufficiency. Case reports of presumed adrenal insufficiency from the 1950s led to the widespread use of perioperative "stress-dose" steroids in this population (*JAMA 1952;149:1542; Ann Intern Med 1953;39:116*).

- The dose and duration of exogenous corticosteroids required to produce clinically significant tertiary adrenal insufficiency is highly variable, but general principles can be outlined (*Med Clin North Am 2003;87:175*).
  ○ Daily therapy with 5 mg or less of prednisone (or its equivalent), alternate-day corticosteroid therapy, and any dose given for <3 weeks should not result in clinically significant adrenal suppression.
  ○ Patients receiving >20 mg/d prednisone (or equivalent) for >3 weeks and patients who are clinically "cushingoid" in appearance can be expected to have significant suppression of adrenal responsiveness.
  ○ The function of the hypothalamic–pituitary axis cannot be readily predicted in patients receiving doses of prednisone 5–20 mg for >3 weeks.

DIAGNOSTIC TESTING

Cosyntropin stimulation test may also be performed to determine adrenal responsiveness, measuring cortisol levels at 30 minutes after 250 μg of cosyntropin. This can be done any time of day and there is no need for baseline cortisol. Levels >18 μg/dL at 30 minutes generally suggest an intact hypothalamic–pituitary axis.

TREATMENT

- If there is concern for secondary adrenal insufficiency, it is reasonable **to simply continue to provide baseline steroid supplementation** perioperatively (*Arch Surg 2008; 143:1222*). It may be prudent to switch to an IV formulation to ensure it is not withheld while the patient is NPO.
- For patients with primary adrenal insufficiency, a stress stratification scheme has been developed, based on expert opinion. Please refer to Chapter 24, Endocrine Diseases, for details of treatment.

Chronic Renal Insufficiency and ESRD

GENERAL PRINCIPLES

- **Chronic renal insufficiency (CRI)** is an independent risk factor for **perioperative cardiac complications**, so all patients with renal disease need appropriate cardiac risk stratification (*JAMA 2001;285:1865*).
- **Patients with ESRD** have a substantial mortality risk when undergoing surgery (*Arch Intern Med 1994;154:1674*).
- Most general anesthetic agents have no appreciable nephrotoxicity or effect on renal function other than that mediated through hemodynamic changes (*Anesthesiol Clin 2006;24:523*).

TREATMENT

- **Volume status**
  ○ Every effort should be made to **achieve euvolemia** preoperatively to reduce the incidence of volume-related complications intraoperatively and postoperatively (*Med Clin North Am 2003;87:193*).
  ○ Although this typically entails removing volume, some patients may be hypovolemic and require hydration.

- ○ Patients with CRI not receiving hemodialysis may require treatment with loop diuretics.
- ○ Patients being treated with **hemodialysis** should undergo dialysis preoperatively, which is commonly performed on the day prior to surgery. Hemodialysis can be performed on the day of surgery as well, but the possibility should be considered that transient electrolyte abnormalities and hemodynamic changes post dialysis can occur.
- **Electrolyte abnormalities**
  - ○ **Hyperkalemia** in the preoperative setting should be treated, particularly because tissue breakdown associated with surgery may elevate the potassium level further postoperatively.
    - ▪ For patients on dialysis, preoperative dialysis should be utilized.
    - ▪ For patients with CRI not undergoing dialysis, alternative methods of potassium excretion will be necessary.
      - □ **Loop diuretics** can be utilized, particularly if the patient is also hypervolemic.
      - □ **Sodium polystyrene sulfonate (SPS) resins** can also be utilized. The possibility that **intestinal necrosis** with SPS resins occurs more frequently in the perioperative setting has been suggested (*Am J Kidney Dis 1992;20:159*).
  - ○ Although chronic **metabolic acidosis** has not been associated with elevated perioperative risk, some local anesthetics have reduced efficacy in acidotic patients. Preoperative metabolic acidosis should be corrected with sodium bicarbonate infusions or dialysis.
- **Bleeding diathesis**
  - ○ **Platelet dysfunction** has long been associated with uremia.
    - ▪ The value of a preoperative bleeding time in predicting postoperative bleeding has been questioned (*Blood 1991;77:2547*). A preoperative bleeding time is, therefore, not recommended.
    - ▪ Patients with evidence of perioperative bleeding should, however, be treated.
      - □ **Dialysis** for patients with ESRD will improve platelet function.
      - □ **Desmopressin** (0.3 μg/kg IV or intranasally) can be utilized.
      - □ **Cryoprecipitate,** 10 units over 30 minutes IV, is an additional option.
      - □ In patients with coexisting anemia, **red blood cell transfusions** can improve uremic bleeding.
      - □ For patients **with a history of prior uremic bleeding**, preoperative desmopressin or **conjugated estrogens** (0.5 mg/kg/d IV for 5 days) should be considered.
  - ○ **Heparin** given with dialysis can increase bleeding risk. Heparin-free dialysis should be discussed with the patient's nephrologist when surgery is planned.

Acute Renal Failure

GENERAL PRINCIPLES

Surgery has been associated with an increased risk of **acute renal failure (ARF)** (*Med Clin North Am 2003;87:193*).
- Patients with **CRI** are at increased risk of ARF.
- ARF among patients with normal preoperative renal function is a relatively rare event but is associated with increased mortality when it occurs (*Anesthesiology 2007; 107:892*).

DIAGNOSIS

- The approach to ARF in the perioperative setting is not substantially different from that in the nonoperative setting (see Chapter 13, Renal Diseases).

- However, certain additional factors have to be considered when evaluating the cause in the perioperative setting:
  - **Intraoperative hemodynamic changes**, particularly hypotension, should be considered.
    - Intraoperative factors associated with ARF postoperatively include vasopressor use and diuretic use (*Anesthesiology 2007;107:892*).
    - A careful review of the operative record is advised.
  - Certain procedures can have an adverse effect on the renal function (e.g., aortic clamping procedures). Therefore, careful attention to the details of the procedure is necessary.
  - The possibility that bleeding is responsible for a prerenal state deserves special attention.

TREATMENT

For a detailed discussion regarding the management of acute renal failure, please refer to Chapter 13, Renal Diseases.

2

Nutrition Support

Dominic Reeds and Peter H. Yen

Nutrient Requirements

GENERAL PRINCIPLES

- **Energy**
  - **Total daily energy expenditure** (TEE) is composed of resting energy expenditure (normally ~70% of TEE), the thermic effect of food (normally ~10% of TEE), and energy expenditure of physical activity (normally ~20% of TEE).
  - It is impossible to determine **daily energy requirements** precisely with predictive equations because of the complexity of factors that affect metabolic rate. Judicious use of predictive equations can provide a reasonable estimate that should be modified as needed based on the patient's clinical course.
  - **Malnutrition** and **hypocaloric feeding** may decrease resting energy expenditure to values 15–20% below those expected for actual body size, whereas metabolic stressors, such as inflammatory diseases or trauma, often increase energy requirements (usually by ~50% of pre-illness values).
  - The **Harris–Benedict equation** provides a reasonable estimate of resting energy expenditure (in kilocalories [kcal] per day) in healthy adults. The equation takes into account the effect of body size and lean tissue mass (which is influenced by gender and age) on energy requirements and can be used to estimate total daily energy needs in hospitalized patients:
    - Men = $66 + (13.7 \times W) + (5 \times H) - (6.8 \times A)$
    - Women = $665 + (9.6 \times W) + (1.8 \times H) - (4.7 \times A)$

    where W is the weight in kilograms, H the height in centimeters, and A is the age in years (*Publication No. 279. Carnegie Institute of Washington. Philadelphia: JB Lippincott, 1919:223*).
  - Energy requirements per kilogram of body weight are inversely related to body mass index (BMI) (Table 2-1). The lower range within each category should be considered in insulin-resistant, critically ill patients unless they are depleted in body fat.
  - **Ideal body weight** can be estimated based on height:
    - For men: 106 lb + 6 lb for each inch over 5 ft
    - For women, 100 lb + 5 lb for each inch over 5 ft
- **Protein**
  - Protein intake of 0.8 g/kg/d meets the requirements of 97% of the adult population.
  - Protein requirements are affected by several factors, such as the amount of nonprotein calories provided, overall energy requirements, protein quality, the patient's baseline nutritional status, and the presence of metabolic stressors (Table 2-2).
  - Inadequate amounts of any of the essential amino acids result in inefficient utilization.
  - Illness increases the efflux of amino acids from skeletal muscle; however, increasing protein intake to >1.2 g/kg/d of prehospitalization body weight in critically ill patients may not reduce the loss of lean body mass (*Crit Care Med 1998;26(9):1529*).
- **Essential fatty acids**
  - The liver can synthesize most fatty acids, but humans lack the desaturase enzyme needed to produce the ω-3 and ω-6 fatty acid series. Therefore, linoleic acid should constitute at least 2% and linolenic acid at least 0.5% of the daily caloric intake to prevent essential fatty acid deficiency.

TABLE 2-1	Estimated Energy Requirements for Hospitalized Patients Based on Body Mass Index
Body Mass Index (kg/m²)	**Energy Requirements (kcal/kg/d)**
15	35–40
15–19	30–35
20–24	20–25
25–29	15–20
≥30	<15

Note: These values are recommended for critically ill patients and all obese patients; add 20% of total calories in estimating energy requirements in non–critically ill patients.

- ○ The plasma pattern of increased triene-to-tetraene ratio (>0.4) can be used to detect essential fatty acid deficiency.
  - ○ Patients who are unable to receive IV or oral lipid solutions may receive a daily topical application of 1 tbsp of safflower oil to provide essential fatty acids.
- **Carbohydrates**
  Certain tissues, such as bone marrow, erythrocytes, leukocytes, renal medulla, eye tissues, and peripheral nerves, cannot metabolize fatty acids and require glucose (~40 g/d) as a fuel. Endogenous protein and glycerol from lipid stores can undergo gluconeogenesis to supply glucose-requiring organs.
- **Major minerals**
  Major minerals are important for ionic equilibrium, water balance, and normal cell function.
- **Micronutrients (trace elements and vitamins)**
  Trace elements and vitamins are essential constituents of enzyme complexes. The recommended dietary intake for trace elements, fat-soluble vitamins, and water-soluble vitamins is set at 2 standard deviations above the estimated mean so that it will cover the needs of 97% of the healthy population. See Table 2-3 for specifics regarding the assessment of micronutrient nutritional states as well as signs and symptoms of micronutrient deficiency and toxicity.

TABLE 2-2	Recommended Daily Protein Intake
Clinical Condition	**Protein Requirements (g/kg IBW/d)[a]**
Normal	0.8
Metabolic stress (illness/injury)	1.0–1.5
Acute renal failure (undialyzed)	0.8–1.0
Hemodialysis	1.2–1.4
Peritoneal dialysis	1.3–1.5

IBW, ideal body weight.
[a]Additional protein intake may be needed to compensate for excess protein loss in specific patient populations such as those with burn injury, open wounds, and protein-losing enteropathy or nephropathy. Lower protein intake may be necessary in patients with chronic renal insufficiency who are not treated by dialysis and certain patients with hepatic encephalopathy.

TABLE 2-3	Trace Minerals, Fat-Soluble Vitamins, and Water-Soluble Vitamins: Recommended Daily Intake, Deficiency, At-Risk Populations, Toxicity, and Status Evaluation				
Nutrient	Recommended Daily Enteral Intake[1]/ *Parenteral Intake*[2]	Signs and Symptoms of Deficiency[4]	Populations At Risk for Deficiency[1,4]	Signs and Symptoms of Toxicity[4]	Status Evaluation[4,5]
Chromium (Cr^{3+})	30–35 µg/ *10–15 µg*	Glucose intolerance, peripheral neuropathy[a]	None[a,4]	PO: gastritis IV: skin irritation Cr^{6+}: (steel, welding) lung carcinogen if inhaled	Chromium$_s$
Copper (Cu^{2+})	900 µg/ *300–500 µg*	Hypochromic normo-cytic or macrocytic anemia (rarely microcytic), neutro-penia, thrombocy-topenia, diarrhea, osteoporosis/ pathologic fractures[a] Intrinsic: Menkes disease[18]	Chronic diarrhea, high-zinc/low-protein diets[7,8]	PO: gastritis, nausea, vomiting, coma, movement/ neurologic abnor-malities, hepatic necrosis Intrinsic: Wilson disease	Copper$_{s,u}$ Ceruloplasmin$_p$
Iodine (I^-)	150 µg/ ***70–140 µg (not routinely added)***	Thyroid hyperplasia (goiter) + functional hypothyroidism Intrinsic in utero: cretinism, poor CNS development, hypothyroidism	Those without access to fortified salt, grain, milk, or cooking oil[11]	Deficiency: causes hypothyroidism Excess: acutely causes hypo-thyroidism; chronic excess: hyperthyroidism	TSH$_s$, iodine$_u$ (24-hour intake and iodine: Cr ratio are more representative than a single sample) Thyroglobulin$_s$[13]

(continued)

TABLE 2-3 Trace Minerals, Fat-Soluble Vitamins, and Water-Soluble Vitamins: Recommended Daily Intake, Deficiency, At-Risk Populations, Toxicity, and Status Evaluation (*Continued*)

Nutrient	Recommended Daily Enteral Intake[1]/ *Parenteral Intake*[2]	Signs and Symptoms of Deficiency[4]	Populations At Risk for Deficiency[1,4]	Signs and Symptoms of Toxicity[4]	Status Evaluation[4,5]
Iron ($Fe^{2+,3+}$)	8 mg/*1.0–1.5 mg (not routinely added)*	Fatigue, hypochromic microcytic anemia, glossitis, koilonychia	Reproductive age females, pregnant females, chronic anemias, hemoglobinopathies, post–gastric bypass/duodenectomy, alcoholics	PO or IV: hemosiderosis, followed by deposition in liver, heart, pancreas, and glands Intrinsic: Hereditary hemochromatosis	Ferritin$_s$, TIBC$_s$, % transferrin saturation$_c$, iron$_s$
Manganese (Mn^{2+})	2.3 mg/*60–100 µg*	Hypercholesterolemia, dermatitis, dementia, weight loss[b]	Chronic liver disease, iron-deficient populations	PO: None[b] Inhalation: hallucination, Parkinsonian-type symptoms[9]	No reliable markers Manganese$_s$ does not reflect bodily stores, especially in the CNS
Selenium (SeO_4^{2-})	55 µg/*20–60 µg*	Myalgias, cardiomyopathy[a] Intrinsic: Keshan disease (Chinese children), Kashin-Beck disease, myxedematous endemic cretinism	Endemic areas of low soil content include certain parts of China and New Zealand[13]	PO: Nausea, diarrhea, AMS, irritability, fatigue, peripheral neuropathy, hair loss, white splotchy nails, halitosis (garlic-like odor)	Selenium$_s$, glutathione peroxidase activity$_b$

Nutrient	Dose	Deficiency	Conditions	Toxicity	Monitoring
Zinc (Zn^{2+})	11 mg/**2.5–5.0 mg**	Poor wound healing, diarrhea (high fistula risk), dysgeusia, teratogenicity, hypogonadism, infertility, acro-oroficial skin lesions (glossitis, alopecia), behavioral changes Intrinsic: Acrodermatitis enteropathica	Chronic diarrhea, cereal-based diets, alcoholics, chronic liver disease, sickle cell, HIV, pancreatic insufficiency/any intestinal malabsorptive states, fistulas/ostomies, nephrotic syndrome, diabetes, post-gastric bypass/duodenectomy, anorexia, pregnancy[12] Intrinsic: Acrodermatitis enteropathica	PO: Nausea, vomiting, gastritis, diarrhea, low HDL, gastric erosions Competition with GI absorption can precipitate Cu^{2+} *deficiency* Inhaled: Hyperpnea, weakness, diaphoresis	$Zinc_{s,p}$ alkaline phosphatase$_s$ (good for those on TPN, but in general $Zinc_{s,p}$ hair, RBC, WBC levels can be misleading) Zinc radioisotope studies (most accurate tests at present; limited by cost and availability)[12]
Molybdenum$_b$	45 µg/**45 µg**	CNS toxicity, hyperoxypurinemia, hypouricemia, low urinary sulfate excretion[a,10] (also reported with parenteral sulfite infusion) Intrinsic: Molybdenum cofactor deficiency, isolated sulfite oxidase deficiency	None[a]	PO or any exposure: Hyperuricemia + gout Inhaled: Pneumoconiosis (industrial exposure)	Molybdenum$_b$

(continued)

TABLE 2-3	Trace Minerals, Fat-Soluble Vitamins, and Water-Soluble Vitamins: Recommended Daily Intake, Deficiency, At-Risk Populations, Toxicity, and Status Evaluation *(Continued)*				
Nutrient	Recommended Daily Enteral Intake[1]/ *Parenteral Intake*[2]	Signs and Symptoms of Deficiency[4]	Populations At Risk for Deficiency[1,4]	Signs and Symptoms of Toxicity[4]	Status Evaluation[4,5]
Vitamin A *Retinol*	900 µg/*3300 IU*	Conjunctival xerosis, keratomalacia, follicular hyperkeratosis, night blindness, *Bitot's spots*, corneal + retinal dysfunction	Any malabsorptive state involving proximal small bowel, vegetarians, chronic liver disease	Acute: Teratogenic, skin exfoliation, intracranial hypertension, hepatocellular necrosis Chronic: Alopecia, ataxia, cheilitis, dermatitis, conjunctivitis, pseudotumor cerebri, hyperlipidemia, hyperostosis	$Retinol_s$, retinol $esters_p$, electroretinogram, liver biopsy (diagnostic for toxicity), retinol binding protein (useful in ESRD; accurately assesses blood levels)[14]
Vitamin D *Ergocalciferol*	5–15 µg/*200 IU*	Rickets/osteomalacia	Any malabsorptive state involving proximal small bowel, chronic liver disease Of note: Those with higher skin melanin content (i.e., darker skin) have low baseline 25-OH vitamin D levels; it is unclear whether this merits their inclusion as an "at-risk" population[15]	Hypercalcemia, hyperphosphatemia, which can lead to $CaPO_4$ precipitation, systemic calcification +/− AMS +/− AKI	25-OH vitamin D_s Of note: lively debate between IOM and Endocrine Society regarding definitions of deficiency, goal serum 25-OH levels, and at-risk populations[15,16]

Nutrient	Dose	Deficiency	At-risk	Toxicity	Lab
Vitamin E (α,γ)- *Tocopherol*	15 mg/*10 IU*	Hemolytic anemia, posterior column degeneration, ophthalmoplegia, peripheral neuropathy Seen in severe malabsorption, abetalipoproteinemia	Any malabsorptive state involving proximal small bowel, chronic liver disease	Possible increased risk in hemorrhagic CVA, functional inhibition of vitamin K-mediated procoagulants	Tocopherol Must account for cholesterol/triglyceride ratio: otherwise, higher cholesterol/triglyceride ratio overestimates vitamin E, lower cholesterol/triglyceride ratio underestimates vitamin E[2,c]
Vitamin K *Phylloquinone*	120 μg/*150 IU*	Hemorrhagic disease of newborn, coagulopathy	Any malabsorptive state involving proximal small bowel, chronic liver disease	In utero: Hemolytic anemia, hyperbilirubinemia, kernicterus IV: flushing, dyspnea, hypotension (possibly related to dispersal agent)	Prothrombin time[p]
Vitamin B$_1$ *Thiamine*	1.2 mg/*6 mg*	Irritability, fatigue, headache *Wernicke encephalopathy, Korsakoff psychosis, "wet" beriberi, "dry" beriberi*	Alcoholics, severely malnourished	IV: Lethargy and ataxia	RBC transketolase activity[b], thiamine[b&u]

(continued)

TABLE 2-3	Trace Minerals, Fat-Soluble Vitamins, and Water-Soluble Vitamins: Recommended Daily Intake, Deficiency, At-Risk Populations, Toxicity, and Status Evaluation *(Continued)*				
Nutrient	**Recommended Daily Enteral Intake[1]/ *Parenteral Intake*[2]**	**Signs and Symptoms of Deficiency[4]**	**Populations At Risk for Deficiency[1,4]**	**Signs and Symptoms of Toxicity[4]**	**Status Evaluation[4,5]**
Vitamin B_2 *Riboflavin*	1.3 mg/*3.6 mg*	Cheilosis, angular stomatitis, glossitis, seborrheic dermatitis, normocytic normochromic anemia	Alcoholics, severely malnourished	None[b]	RBC glutathione reductase activity[p]
Vitamin B_3 *Niacin*	16 mg/*40 mg*	*Pellagra* dysesthesias, glossitis, stomatitis, vaginitis, vertigo Intrinsic: Hartnup disease	Alcoholics, malignant carcinoid syndrome, severely malnourished	Flushing, hyperglycemia, hyperuricemia, hepatocellular injury[b]	N-methyl-nicotinamide[u]
Vitamin B_5 *Pantothenic acid*	5 mg/*15 mg*	Fatigue, abdominal pain, vomiting, insomnia, paresthesias[b]	Alcoholics[6]	PO: Diarrhea	Pantothenic acid[u]
Vitamin B_6 *Pyridoxine*	1.3–1.7 mg/*6 mg*	Cheilosis, stomatitis, glossitis, irritability, depression, confusion, normochromic normocytic anemia	Alcoholics, diabetics, celiac sprue, chronic isoniazid or penicillamine use[6]	Peripheral neuropathy, photosensitivity	Pyridoxal phosphate[p]

Vitamin B[7] *Biotin*	30 µg/**60 µg**	Mental status changes, myalgias, hyperesthesias, anorexia[c,5] (excessive egg white consumption results in avidin-mediated biotin inactivation)	Alcoholics[6]	None[b,5]	Biotin[p], methyl-citrate[u], 3-methyl-crotonyglycine[u], 3-hydroxyisovalerate[u]
Vitamin B[9] *Folic acid*	400 µg/**600 µg**	Bone marrow suppression, macrocytic megaloblastic anemia, glossitis, diarrhea Can be precipitated by sulfasalazine + phenytoin	Alcoholics, celiac or tropical sprue, chronic sulfasalazine use[6]	PO: May lower seizure threshold in those taking anticonvulsants	Folic acid[s], RBC folic acid[p]
Vitamin B[12] *Cobalamin*	2.4 µg/**5 µg**	Bone marrow suppression, macrocytic megaloblastic anemia, glossitis, diarrhea, posterolateral column demyelination, AMS, depression, psychosis	Vegetarians, atrophic gastritis, pernicious anemia, celiac sprue, Crohn disease, patients post gastrectomy or ileal resection	None[b]	Cobalamin (B[12])[s], methylmalonic acid[s&p]

(continued)

TABLE 2-3	Trace Minerals, Fat-Soluble Vitamins, and Water-Soluble Vitamins: Recommended Daily Intake, Deficiency, At-Risk Populations, Toxicity, and Status Evaluation (*Continued*)				
Nutrient	**Recommended Daily Enteral Intake[1]/** *Parenteral Intake[2]*	**Signs and Symptoms of Deficiency[4]**	**Populations At Risk for Deficiency[1,4]**	**Signs and Symptoms of Toxicity[4]**	**Status Evaluation[4,5]**
Vitamin C *Ascorbic acid*	90 mg/***200 mg***	*Scurvy*, ossification abnormalities Tobacco lowers plasma and WBC vitamin C[2] Sudden cessation of high-dose vitamin C can precipitate scurvy	Fruit-deficient diet, smokers,[1] ESRD[3]	Nausea, diarrhea, increased oxalate synthesis (theoretical nephrolithiasis risk)	Ascorbic acid$_p$, leukocyte ascorbic acid

AKI, acute kidney injury; AMS, altered mental status; CNS, central nervous system; CVA, cerebrovascular accident; ESRD, end-stage renal disease; IOM, Institute of Medicine; GI, gastrointestinal; HDL, high-density lipoprotein (cholesterol); RBC, red blood cell; TIBC, total iron bonding capacity; TPN, total parenteral nutrition; TSH, thyroid-stimulating hormone; WBC, white blood cell.

Subscript: b, blood; c, calculated; p, plasma; s, serum; u, urine.

[a]Only reported in patients on long-term TPN.

[b]Never demonstrated in humans.

[c]Only able to induce under experimental conditions and/or only been able to induce in animals.

[1]Trumbo P, Yates AA, Schlicker S, et al. Institute of Medicine, Food and Nutrition Board. Dietary reference intakes for vitamin A, vitamin K, arsenic, boron, chromium, copper, iodine, iron, manganese, molybdenum, nickel, silicon, vanadium, and zinc. *J Am Diet Assoc.* 2001;101(3):294–301.

[2]Mirtallo J, Canada T, Johnson D, et al. Safe practices for parenteral nutrition. *JPEN J Parenter Enteral Nutr.* 2004;28:S39–S74.

[3]Deicher R, Hörl WH. Vitamin C in chronic kidney disease and hemodialysis patients. *Kidney Blood Press Res.* 2003;26:100–6.

[4]Office of Dietary Supplements: National Institutes of Health. Dietary supplement fact sheet: chromium. Office of Dietary Supplements: National Institutes of Health. http://ods.od.nih.gov/pdf/factsheets/Chromium-HealthProfessional.pdf. August 5, 2005. Accessed 1/6/15–1/11/15.

Ibid. Dietary supplement fact sheet: iodine. Office of Dietary Supplements: National Institutes of Health. http://ods.od.nih.gov/pdf/factsheets/Iodine -HealthProfessional.pdf. June 24, 2011. Accessed 1/6/15–1/11/15.

Ibid. Dietary supplement fact sheet: iron. Office of Dietary Supplements: National Institutes of Health. http://ods.od.nih.gov/factsheets/Iron-HealthProfessional/. August 22, 2014. Accessed 1/6/15–1/11/15.

Ibid. Dietary supplement fact sheet: selenium. Office of Dietary Supplement: National Institutes of Health. http://ods.od.nih.gov/factsheets/Selenium -HealthProfessional/. November 22, 2013. Accessed 1/6/15–1/11/15.

Ibid. Dietary supplement fact sheet: vitamin A. Office of Dietary Supplements: National Institutes of Health. http://ods.od.nih.gov/factsheets/VitaminA-HealthProfessional/. April 23, 2006. Accessed 1/6/15–1/11/15.

Ibid. Dietary supplement fact sheet: vitamin B12. Office of Dietary Supplements: National Institutes of Health. http://ods.od.nih.gov/factsheets/VitaminB12-HealthProfessional/. June 24, 2011. Accessed 1/6/15–1/11/15.

Ibid. Dietary supplement fact sheet: vitamin C. Office of Dietary Supplements: National Institutes of Health. http://ods.od.nih.gov/factsheets/VitaminC-HealthProfessional/. June 24, 2011. Accessed 1/6/15–1/11/15.

Ibid. Dietary supplement fact sheet: vitamin D. Office of Dietary Supplements: National Institutes of Health. http://ods.od.nih.gov/factsheets/VitaminD-HealthProfessional/. June 24, 2011. Accessed 1/6/15–1/11/15.

Ibid. Dietary supplement fact sheet: vitamin B6. Office of Dietary Supplements: National Institutes of Health. http://ods.od.nih.gov/factsheets/VitaminB6-HealthProfessional/. September 15, 2011. Accessed 1/6/15–1/11/15.

Ibid. Dietary Supplement fact sheet: vitamin E. Office of Dietary Supplements: National Institutes of Health. http://ods.od.nih.gov/factsheets/VitaminE-HealthProfessional/. October 11, 2011. Accessed 1/6/15–1/11/15.

Ibid. Dietary Supplement fact sheet: zinc. Office of Dietary Supplements: National Institutes of Health. http://ods.od.nih.gov/factsheets/Zinc-HealthProfessional/. September 20, 2011. Accessed 1/6/15–1/11/15.

[5]Feldman M, Friedman LS, Brandt LJ. *Sleisenger and Fordtran's Gastrointestinal and Liver Disease*, 9th ed. Philadelphia: Saunders Elsevier, 2010.

[6]Said HM. Intestinal absorption of water-soluble vitamins in health and disease. *Biochem J.* 2011;437:357–72.

[7]Stern BR. Essentiality and toxicity in copper health risk assessment: overview, update and regulatory considerations. *J Toxicol Environ Health A.* 2010;73:114–27.

[8]Abumrad NN, Schneider AJ, Steel D, et al. Amino acid intolerance during prolonged total parenteral nutrition reversed by molybdate therapy. *Am J Clin Nutr.* 1981;34(11):2551–9.

[9]Santamaria AB, Sulsky, SI. Risk assessment of an essential element: manganese. *J Toxicol Environ Health A.* 2010;73:128–55.

[10]Linus Pauling Institute. http://lpi.oregonstate.edu/.
Higdon J, Drake VL, Turnlund JR. Micronutrient information center: molybdenum. Linus Pauling Institute, Micronutrient Research and Optimum Health. http://lpi.oregonstate.edu/infocenter/minerals/molybdenum/. Accessed 1/6/15–1/11/15.
Higdon J, Drake VL, Mock D. Micronutrient information center: biotin. Linus Pauling Institute, Micronutrient Research and Optimum Health. http://lpi.oregonstate.edu/infocenter/vitamins/biotin/. Accessed 1/6/15–1/11/15.

[11]Zimmermann MB. Iodine deficiency. *Endocr Rev.* 2009 Jun;30(4):376–408.

[12]Semrad C. Zinc and intestinal function. *Curr Gastroenterol Rep.* 1999;1:398–403.

[13]Fairweather-Tait SJ, Collings R, Hurst R. Selenium bioavailability: current knowledge and future research requirements. *Am J Clin Nutr.* 2010;91(suppl):1484S–91S.

[14]Mahmood K, Samo AH, Lairamani KL, et al. Serum retinol binding protein as an indicator of vitamin A status in cirrhotic patients with night blindness. *Saudi J Gastroenterol.* 2008;14(1):7–11.

[15]Rosen CJ, Abrams SA, Aloia JF, et al. IOM committee members respond to Endocrine Society vitamin D guideline. *J Clin Endocrinol Metab.* 2012;97:1146–52.

[16]Holick MF, Binkley NC, Bischoff-Ferrari HA, et al. Evaluation, treatment, and prevention of vitamin D deficiency: an Endocrine Society clinical practice guideline. *J Clin Endocrinol Metab.* 2001;96:1911–30.

[17]Ford L, Farr J, Morris P, et al. The value of measuring serum cholesterol-adjusted vitamin E in routine practice. *Ann Clin Biochem.* 2006;43:130–4.

[18]Uauy R, Olivares O, Gonzales M. Essentiality of copper in humans. *Am J Clin Nutr.* 1998;67(suppl):952S–59S.

SPECIAL CONSIDERATIONS

- Both the amount and location of prior gut resection influence nutrient needs. Patients with a reduced length of functional small bowel may require additional vitamins and minerals if they are not receiving parenteral nutrition. Table 2-4 provides guidelines for supplementation in these patients.
- Distal ileum inflammation, resection, inflammatory bowel disease (IBD), and bypass (ileojejunal bypass) can cause B_{12} deficiency and bile salt loss. Diarrhea in this setting may be improved with oral cholestyramine given with the first meal of the day.
- Proximal gut resection (stomach or duodenum) via partial gastrectomy, Billroth I and II, duodenal switch/biliopancreatic diversion, Roux-en-Y gastric bypass, pancreaticoduodenectomy (Whipple), and sleeve gastrectomy may impair absorption of divalent cations such as iron, calcium, and copper. Copper deficiency is extremely common in post–gastric bypass patients who do not receive routine supplementation (*Int J Obes (Lond) 2012;36(3):328*).
- Patients with excessive gastrointestinal (GI) tract losses require additional fluids and electrolytes. An assessment of fluid losses due to diarrhea, ostomy output, and fistula volume should be made to help determine fluid requirements. Intestinal mineral losses may be calculated by multiplying the volume of fluid loss by the fluid electrolyte concentration (Table 2-5).

TABLE 2-4	Guidelines for Vitamin and Mineral Supplementation in Patients with Severe Malabsorption	
Supplement	**Dose**	**Route**
Prenatal multivitamin with minerals[a]	1 tablet daily	PO
Vitamin D[a]	50,000 units 2–3 times per wk	PO
Calcium[a]	500 mg elemental calcium tid–qid	PO
Vitamin B_{12}[b]	1 mg daily	PO
	100–500 μg q1–2 mo	SC
Vitamin A[b]	10,000–50,000 units daily	PO
Vitamin K[b]	5 mg/d	PO
	5–10 mg/wk	SC
Vitamin E[b]	30 units/d	PO
Magnesium gluconate[b]	108–169 mg elemental magnesium qid	PO
Magnesium sulfate[b]	290 mg elemental magnesium 1–3 times per week	IM/IV
Zinc gluconate or zinc sulfate[b]	25 mg elemental zinc daily plus 100 mg elemental zinc per liter intestinal output	PO
Ferrous sulfate[b]	60 mg elemental iron tid	PO
Iron dextran[b]	Daily dose based on formula or table	IV

[a]Recommended routinely for all patients.
[b]Recommended for patients with documented nutrient deficiency or malabsorption.

TABLE 2-5	Electrolyte Concentrations in Gastrointestinal Fluids			
Location	Na (mEq/L)	K (mEq/L)	Cl (mEq/L)	HCO_3 (mEq/L)
Stomach	65	10	100	–
Bile	150	4	100	35
Pancreas	150	7	80	75
Duodenum	90	15	90	15
Mid–small bowel	140	6	100	20
Terminal ileum	140	8	60	70
Rectum	40	90	15	30

Assessment of Nutritional Status

GENERAL PRINCIPLES

- Patients should be assessed for protein-energy malnutrition as well as specific nutrient deficiencies.
- A thorough history and physical exam combined with appropriate laboratory studies is the best approach to evaluate nutritional status.

DIAGNOSIS

Clinical Presentation

History
- Assess for changes in diet pattern (size, number, and content of meals). If present, the reason for altered food intake should be investigated.
- Unintentional weight loss of >10% body weight in the last 6 months is associated with a poor clinical outcome (*Am J Med 1980;69:491*).
- Look for evidence of **malabsorption** (diarrhea, weight loss).
- For symptoms of specific **nutrient deficiencies**, see Table 2-3.
- Consider factors that may increase metabolic stress (e.g., infection, inflammatory disease, malignancy).
- Assess patient's functional status (e.g., bedridden, suboptimally active, very active).

Physical Examination
- By World Health Organization (WHO) criteria, patients can be classified by BMI as underweight (<18.5 kg/m²), normal weight ($18.5–24.9$ kg/m²), overweight ($25.0–29.9$ kg/m²), class I obesity ($30.0–34.9$ kg/m²), class II obesity ($35.0–39.9$ kg/m²), or class III obesity (≥ 40.0 kg/m²) (*Obes Res 1998;6(suppl 2):S53*).
- Patients who are **extremely underweight** (BMI <14 kg/m²) or those **with rapid, severe weight loss** (even with supranormal BMI) have a high risk of death and should be considered for admission to the hospital for nutritional support.
- Look for **tissue depletion** (loss of body fat and skeletal muscle wasting).
- Assess **muscle function** (strength testing of individual muscle groups).
- **Fluid status:** Evaluate patients for dehydration (e.g., hypotension, tachycardia, mucosal xerosis) or excess body fluid (edema or ascites).

• Evaluate patients for sources of protein or nutrient losses: large wounds, burns, nephrotic syndrome, surgical drains, etc. Quantify the volume of drainage and the concentration of fat and protein content.

Diagnostic Testing

• Perform laboratory studies to determine specific nutrient deficiencies only when clinically indicated because the plasma concentration of many nutrients may not reflect true body stores (Table 2-3).
• Plasma albumin and prealbumin concentrations should not be used to assess patients for protein-calorie malnutrition or to monitor the adequacy of nutrition support. Although levels of these plasma proteins correlate with clinical outcome, inflammation and injury can alter their synthesis and degradation, limiting their usefulness for nutritional assessment (*Crit Care Med 1982;10:305*; *Gastroenterology 1990;99:1845*).
• Most hospitalized patients are vitamin D deficient, and caregivers should have a low threshold for checking plasma 25-OH vitamin D levels (*N Engl J Med 1998;338:777*).

Enteral Nutrition

GENERAL PRINCIPLES

Whenever possible, **oral/enteral** feeding is preferred to **parenteral** feeding because it limits mucosal atrophy, maintains IgA secretion, and prevents cholelithiasis. Additionally, oral/enteral feeds are less expensive than parenteral nutrition.

• **Types of feedings**
  Hospital diets include a regular diet and those modified in either nutrient content (amount of fiber, fat, protein, or sodium) or consistency (liquid, puréed, soft). There are ways that food intake can often be increased:
  ○ Encourage patients to eat.
  ○ Provide assistance at mealtime.
  ○ Allow some food to be supplied by relatives and friends.
  ○ Limit missed meals for medical tests and procedures.
  ○ Avoid unpalatable diets. Milk-based formulas (e.g., Carnation Instant Breakfast) contain milk as a source of protein and fat and tend to be more palatable than other defined formula diets.
  ○ Use calorically dense supplements (e.g., Ensure, Boost).
• **Defined liquid formulas**
  ○ **Polymeric formulas** (e.g., Osmolite, Jevity) are appropriate for most patients. They contain nitrogen in the form of whole proteins and include blenderized food, milk-based, and lactose-free formulas. Other formulas are available with modified nutritional content including high-nitrogen, high-calorie, fiber-enriched, and low-potassium/phosphorus/magnesium formulas.
  ○ **Semielemental *oligomeric* formulas** (e.g., Peptamen) contain hydrolyzed protein in the form of small peptides and free amino acids. Although these formulas may have benefit in those with exocrine pancreatic insufficiency or short gut, pancreatic enzyme replacement is a less expensive, equally effective intervention in most of these patients.
  ○ **Elemental monomeric formulas** (e.g., Vivonex, Glutasorb) contain nitrogen in the form of free amino acids and small amounts of fat (<5% of total calories) and are hyperosmolar (550–650 mOsm/kg). These formulas are not palatable and therefore require either tube feeding or mixing with other foods or flavorings for oral ingestion. Free amino acids are poorly absorbed, and these formulas have not been shown to be clinically superior to oligomeric or polymeric formulas in patients with adequate

pancreatic digestive function. These formulas may exacerbate osmotic diarrhea in patients with short gut.

- ○ **Oral rehydration solutions** stimulate sodium and water absorption by taking advantage of the sodium–glucose cotransporter present in the brush border of intestinal epithelium. Oral rehydration therapy (using 90–120 mEq/L solutions to avoid intestinal sodium secretion and negative sodium and water balance) can be especially useful in patients with short bowel syndrome (*Clin Ther 1990;12(suppl A):129*). The characteristics of several oral rehydration solutions are listed in Table 2-6.
- • **Tube feeding**
  - ○ Tube feeding is useful in patients who have a **functional GI tract** but who cannot or will not ingest adequate nutrients.
  - ○ The type of tube feeding approach selected (nasogastric, nasoduodenal, nasojejunal, gastrostomy, jejunostomy, pharyngostomy, and esophagostomy tubes) depends on physician experience, clinical prognosis, gut patency and motility, risk of aspirating gastric contents, patient preference, and anticipated duration of feeding.
  - ○ Short-term (<6 weeks) tube feeding can be achieved by placement of a soft, small-bore nasogastric or nasoenteric feeding tube. Although nasogastric feeding is usually the most appropriate route, orogastric feeding may be needed in those who are intubated or in patients with nasal injury or deformity. Nasoduodenal and nasojejunal feeding tubes can be placed at the bedside with a success rate approaching 90% when inserted by experienced personnel (*Nutr Clin Pract 2001;16:258*).
  - ○ Long-term (>6 weeks) tube feeding usually requires a gastrostomy or jejunostomy tube that can be placed percutaneously by endoscopic or radiographic assistance. Alternatively, they can be placed surgically, depending on the clinical situation and local expertise.
- • **Feeding schedules:** Patients who have feeding tubes in the stomach can often tolerate intermittent bolus or gravity feedings, in which the total amount of daily formula is divided into four to six equal portions.
  - ○ **Bolus feedings** are given by syringe as rapidly as tolerated.
  - ○ **Gravity feedings** are infused over 30–60 minutes.
  - ○ The patient's upper body should be elevated by 30–45 degrees during feeding and for at least 2 hours afterward. Tubes should be flushed with water after each feeding. Intermittent feedings are useful for patients who cannot be positioned with continuous head-of-the-bed elevation or who require greater freedom from feeding. Patients who experience nausea and early satiety with bolus gravity feedings may require continuous infusion at a slower rate.
  - ○ **Continuous feeding** can often be started at 20–30 mL/h and advanced by 10 mL/h every 6 hours until the feeding goal is reached. Patients who have gastroparesis often tolerate gastric tube feedings when they are started at a slow rate (e.g., 10 mL/h) and advanced by small increments (e.g., 10 mL/h every 8–12 hours). Patients with severe gastroparesis may require passage of the feeding tube tip past the ligament of Treitz. **Continuous feeding should always be used when feeding directly into the duodenum or jejunum to avoid distention, abdominal pain, and dumping syndrome.**
  - ○ **Jejunal feeding** may be possible in closely monitored patients with mild to moderate **acute pancreatitis** (*J Am Coll Nutr 1995;14(6):662*).
- • **Contraindications:** The intestinal tract cannot be used effectively in some patients due to:
  - ○ Persistent nausea or vomiting
  - ○ Intolerable postprandial abdominal pain or diarrhea
  - ○ Mechanical obstruction or severe hypomotility
  - ○ Severe malabsorption
  - ○ Presence of high-output fistula

TABLE 2-6   Enteral Feeding Formulas: Comparing Composition

Formula	kcal/mL	% Protein	% Lipid	% Carbohydrate	K⁺ (mEq/L)	PO₄³⁻ (mg/L)	Purpose/Niche
Osmolite	1.0	16.7	29	54.3	40.2	760	Standard polymeric
Jevity	1.5	17	29	53.6	40.2	1200	Standard polymeric
TwoCal HN	2	16.7	40.1	43.2	62.6	1050	Volume restricted
Nepro with Carb Steady	1.8	18	48	34	27.2	700	ESRD
Glucerna	1.2	20	45	35	51.8	800	Glucose intolerance/diabetes
Promote	1.0	25	23	52	50.8	1200	High protein
Peptamen AF	1.2	25	39	36	41	800	Short gut, exocrine pancreatic insufficiency
Vivonex RTF	1.0	20	10	70	31	670	Fat malabsorption
Oxepa	1.5	16.7	55.2	28.1	50.1	1060	SIRS, ARDS, sepsis

ARDS, acute respiratory distress syndrome; ESRD, end-stage renal disease; SIRS, systemic inflammatory response syndrome.
Table adapted from Barnes-Jewish Hospital Enteral Nutrition Formulary (8/2009).

COMPLICATIONS

- **Mechanical complications**
  - ○ **Nasogastric feeding tube misplacement** occurs more commonly in unconscious patients. Intubation of the tracheobronchial tree has been reported in up to 15% of patients. Intracranial placement can occur in patients with skull fractures.
  - ○ **Erosive tissue damage** can lead to nasopharyngeal erosions, pharyngitis, sinusitis, otitis media, pneumothorax, and GI tract perforation.
  - ○ **Tube occlusion** is often caused by inspissated feedings or pulverized medications given through small-diameter (<#10 French) tubes. Frequent flushing of the tube with 30–60 mL of water and avoiding administration of pill fragments or "thick" medications help to prevent occlusion. Techniques used to unclog tubes include the use of a small-volume syringe (10 mL) to flush warm water or pancreatic enzymes (Viokase dissolved in water) through the tube.
- **Hyperglycemia**
  - ○ The precise level at which glucose should be maintained in hospitalized patients remains controversial.
  - ○ Subcutaneously administered insulin can usually maintain good glycemic control. IV insulin drip protocols should be used to control blood glucose in critically ill patients with anasarca and hemodynamic instability to ensure adequate insulin absorption.
  - ○ Intermediate-duration insulin (e.g., NPH) can often be used safely once tube feedings reach 1000 kcal/d. Long-duration insulin (e.g., detemir, glargine) should be used with caution in critically ill patients because changes in clinical status may affect pharmacokinetics and increase the risk of sustained hypoglycemia.
  - ○ Patients who are receiving bolus feeds should receive short-acting insulin at the time of the feed.
  - ○ Patients who are being given continuous (24 hours per day) feeding should receive intermediate-duration insulin every 8 hours when clinically stable. If tube feeds are interrupted and insulin has been given, an infusion of dextrose-containing fluid should be given at a rate to match the infusion rate of the scheduled tube feeds until the insulin has worn off.
- **Pulmonary aspiration**
  - ○ The etiology of **pulmonary aspiration** can be difficult to determine in tube-fed patients because aspiration can occur from refluxed tube feedings or oropharyngeal secretions that are unrelated to feedings. Recent evidence suggests that oral secretions play a far greater role in the development of ventilator-associated pneumonia than aspiration of tube feedings (*JAMA 2013;309(3):249–56*).
  - ○ Addition of food coloring to tube feeds **should not be used** for the diagnosis of aspiration. This method is insensitive for diagnosis, and several case reports suggest that food coloring can be absorbed by the GI tract in critically ill patients and can lead to serious complications and death (*N Engl J Med 2000;343:1047*).
  - ○ Gastric residuals are poorly predictive of aspiration risk.
  - ○ Prevention of reflux: Decrease gastric acid secretion with pharmacologic therapy (H2 blocker, proton pump inhibitor), elevate head of bed during feeds, and avoid gastric feeding in high-risk patients (e.g., those with gastroparesis, frequent vomiting, gastric outlet obstruction).
- **GI complications**
  - ○ Nausea, vomiting, and abdominal pain are common.
  - ○ **Diarrhea** is often associated with antibiotic therapy (*JPEN J Parenter Enteral Nutr 1991;15:27*) and the use of liquid medications that contain nonabsorbable carbohydrates, such as sorbitol (*Am J Med 1990;88:91*). If diarrhea from tube feeding persists after proper evaluation of possible causes, a trial of antidiarrheal agents or fiber is

justified. Diarrhea is common in patients who receive tube feeding and occurs in up to 50% of critically ill patients.

○ Diarrhea in patients with short gut, who do not have other causes such as *Clostridium difficile* infection, may be minimized by use of small, frequent meals that do not contain concentrated sweets (e.g., soda). Intestinal transit time should be maximized to allow nutrient absorption using tincture of opium, loperamide, or diphenoxylate. Low-dose clonidine (0.025–0.05 mg orally bid) may be used to reduce diarrhea in hemodynamically stable patients with short bowel syndrome (*JPEN J Parenter Enteral Nutr 2004;28(4):265*).

○ **Intestinal ischemia/necrosis** has been reported in patients receiving tube feeding. These cases have occurred predominantly in critically ill patients receiving vasopressors for blood pressure support in conjunction with enteral feeding. There are no reliable clinical signs for diagnosis, and the mortality rate is high. **Caution should be used when enterally feeding critically ill patients requiring vasopressors.**

Parenteral Nutrition

GENERAL PRINCIPLES

• Parenteral nutrition should be considered if energy intake cannot, or it is anticipated that it cannot, be met by enteral nutrition (<50% of daily requirements) for more than 7–10 days. This guideline originates from two intensive care unit (ICU)-focused meta-analyses citing increased complications (*Am J Clin Nutr 2001;74:534*) and increased overall mortality (*JAMA 1998;280:2013*) in ICU patients receiving early parenteral nutrition (i.e., within 7 days of admission), compared to those receiving no nutrition support (*JPEN J Parenter Enteral Nutr 2009;33(3):285*). Recent studies have found that critically ill patients who are unable to meet caloric goals by enteral nutrition alone for the first 8 days of hospitalization have longer durations of stay and greater mortality rates than those in whom total parenteral nutrition (TPN) is withheld for the first 8 days after admission (*N Engl J Med 2011;365:506*).

• **Recommendations**
  ○ **Central parenteral nutrition (CPN)**
    ▪ The infusion of hyperosmolar (usually >1500 mOsm/L) nutrient solutions requires a large-bore, high-flow vessel to minimize vessel irritation and damage.
    ▪ Percutaneous subclavian vein **catheterization** and peripherally inserted central venous catheterization (PICC) are the most commonly used techniques for CPN access. The internal jugular, saphenous, and femoral veins are also used, although they are less desirable due to decreased patient comfort and difficulty in maintaining sterility. Tunneled catheters are preferred in patients who are likely to receive >8 weeks of TPN to reduce the risk of mechanical failure.
    ▪ PICCs (which reduce the risk of pneumothorax) are increasingly used to provide CPN in patients with adequate antecubital vein access. These catheters are not suitable for patients in whom CPN is anticipated to be necessary for an extended duration (>6 months).
  ○ **CPN macronutrient solutions**
    ▪ Crystalline **amino acid solutions** containing 40–50% essential and 50–60% nonessential amino acids (usually with little or no glutamine, glutamate, aspartate, asparagine, tyrosine, and cysteine) are used to provide protein needs (Table 2-2). Infused amino acids are oxidized and should be included in the estimate of energy provided as part of the parenteral formulation.
    ▪ Some amino acid solutions have been modified for specific disease states such as those enriched in branched-chain amino acids for use in patients who have hepatic

encephalopathy and solutions that contain mostly essential amino acids for use in patients with renal insufficiency.

- **Glucose** (dextrose) in IV solutions is hydrated; each gram of dextrose monohydrate provides 3.4 kcal. Although there is no absolute requirement for glucose in most patients, providing >150 g of glucose per day maximizes protein balance.
- **Lipid emulsions** are available as a 10% (1.1 kcal/mL) or 20% (2.0 kcal/mL) solution and provide energy as well as a source of essential fatty acids. Emulsion particles are similar in size and structure to chylomicrons and are metabolized like nascent chylomicrons after acquiring apoproteins from contact with circulating endogenous high-density lipoprotein cholesterol particles. Lipid emulsions are as effective as glucose in conserving body nitrogen economy once absolute tissue requirements for glucose are met. The optimal percentage of calories that should be infused as fat is not known, but 20–30% of total calories is reasonable for most patients. The rate of infusion should not exceed 1.0 kcal/kg/h (0.11 g/kg/h) because most complications associated with lipid infusions have been reported when providing more than this amount (*Curr Opin Gastroenterol 1991;7:306*). A rate of 0.03–0.05 g/kg/h is adequate for most patients who are receiving continuous CPN. Lipid emulsions should not be given to patients who have triglyceride concentrations of >400 mg/dL. Moreover, patients at risk for hypertriglyceridemia should have serum triglyceride concentrations checked at least once during lipid emulsion infusion to ensure adequate clearance. Underfeeding obese patients by the amount of lipid calories that would normally be given (e.g., 20–30% of calories) facilitates mobilization of endogenous fat stores for fuel and may improve insulin sensitivity. IV lipids should still be administered twice per week to these patients to provide essential fatty acids.

- **Peripheral parenteral nutrition**
  - Peripheral parenteral nutrition is often considered to have limited usefulness because of the high risk of thrombophlebitis.
  - Appropriate adjustments in the management of peripheral parenteral nutrition can increase the life of a single infusion site to >10 days. The following guidelines are recommended:
    - Provide at least 50% of total energy as a lipid emulsion piggybacked with the dextrose–amino acid solution.
    - Add 500–1000 units of heparin and 5 mg of hydrocortisone per liter (to decrease phlebitis).
    - Place a fine-bore 22- or 23-gauge polyvinylpyrrolidone-coated polyurethane catheter in as large a vein as possible in the proximal forearm using sterile technique.
    - Place a 5-mg glycerol trinitrate ointment patch (or 0.25 inch of 2% nitroglycerin ointment) over the infusion site.
    - Infuse the solution with a volumetric pump.
    - Keep the total infused volume <3500 mL/d.
    - Filter the solution with an inline 1.2-m filter (*Nutrition 1994;10:49*).

- **Long-term home parenteral nutrition**
  - Long-term home parenteral nutrition is usually given through a **tunneled catheter** or an implantable subcutaneous port inserted in the subclavian vein.
  - **Nutrient formulations** can be infused overnight to permit daytime activities in patients who are able to tolerate the fluid load. IV lipids may not be necessary in patients who are able to ingest and absorb adequate amounts of fat.
  - Patient selection for appropriate patients for home TPN is crucial due to the high rates of complications (~50% at 6 months). Risk factors for complications include use of a nontunneled or multilumen catheter, blood draws from the catheter, infusion of nonparenteral medications, use of lipid infusions, anticoagulation, older age, and open wounds (*JPEN J Parenter Enteral Nutr 2014;38:6; JPEN J Parenter Enteral Nutr;in press*).

COMPLICATIONS

- **Mechanical complications**
  - Complications at time of line placement include pneumothorax, air embolism, arterial puncture, hemothorax, and brachial plexus injury.
  - Thrombosis and pulmonary embolus: Radiologically evident subclavian vein thrombosis occurs commonly; however, clinical manifestations (upper extremity edema, superior vena cava syndrome) are rare. Fatal microvascular pulmonary emboli can be caused by nonvisible precipitate in parenteral nutrition solutions. Inline filters should be used with all solutions to minimize the risk of these emboli.
- **Metabolic complications:** Usually caused by overzealous or inadequate nutrient administration.
  - Fluid overload.
  - Hypertriglyceridemia.
  - Hypercalcemia.
  - Specific nutrient deficiencies. Consider providing supplemental **thiamine** (100 mg for 3–5 days) during initiation of CPN in patients at risk for thiamine deficiency (e.g., alcoholism).
  - Hypoglycemia.
  - **Hyperglycemia.** Tight blood glucose control (between 90–120 mg/dL) historically was the standard dogma in ICU populations (*N Engl J Med 2001;345:1359*); however, this practice has been called into question in light of a 2009 randomized controlled trial illustrating significantly higher overall mortality and incidence of critical hypoglycemia in patients whose blood glucose was being tightly controlled (*N Engl J Med 2009;360(13):1283*). Management of patients with hyperglycemia or type 2 diabetes (*Mayo Clin Proc 1996;71:587*) can be performed in the following way:
    - If blood glucose is >200 mg/dL, consider obtaining better control of blood glucose before starting CPN.
    - If CPN is started, (a) limit dextrose to <200 g/d, (b) add 0.1 unit of regular insulin for each gram of dextrose in CPN solution (e.g., 15 units for 150 g), (c) discontinue other sources of IV dextrose, and (d) order routine, regular insulin with blood glucose monitoring by fingerstick every 4–6 hours or IV regular insulin infusion with blood glucose monitoring by fingerstick every 1–2 hours.
    - In outpatients who use insulin, an estimate of the reduction in blood sugar that will be caused by the administration of 1 unit of insulin may be calculated by dividing 1500 by the total daily insulin dose (e.g., for a patient receiving 50 units of insulin as an outpatient, 1 unit of insulin may be predicted to reduce plasma glucose concentration by 1500/50 = 30 mg/dL).
    - If blood glucose remains >200 mg/dL and the patient has been requiring SC insulin, add 50% of the supplemental short-acting insulin given in the last 24 hours to the next day's CPN solution and double the amount of SC insulin sliding-scale dose for blood glucose values >200 mg/dL.
    - The insulin-to-dextrose ratio in the CPN formulation should be maintained while the CPN dextrose content is changed.
- **Infectious complications**
  - Catheter-related sepsis is the most common life-threatening complication in patients who receive CPN and is most commonly caused by skin flora: *Staphylococcus epidermidis* and *Staphylococcus aureus.*
  - In **immunocompromised patients** and those with long-term (>2 weeks) CPN, *Enterococcus, Candida* species, *Escherichia coli, Pseudomonas, Klebsiella, Enterobacter, Acinetobacter, Proteus,* and *Xanthomonas* should be considered.
  - The principles of **evaluation and management** of suspected catheter-related infection are outlined in Chapter 14, Treatment of Infectious Diseases.

○ Although antibiotics are often infused through the central line, the **antibiotic lock technique** has been used successfully to treat and prevent central catheter–related infections (*Nutrition 1998;14:466; Antimicrob Agents Chemother 1999;43:2200*). This technique involves local delivery of antibiotics in the catheter without systemic administration.

- **Hepatobiliary complications.** Although these abnormalities are usually benign and transient, more serious and progressive disease may develop in a small subset of patients, usually after 16 weeks of CPN therapy or in those with short bowel (*Diseases of the Liver. 7th ed. Philadelphia: JB Lippincott; 1993:1505*).
  ○ Biochemical: Elevated aminotransferases and alkaline phosphatase are commonly seen.
  ○ Histologic alterations: Steatosis, steatohepatitis, lipidosis, phospholipidosis, cholestasis, fibrosis, and cirrhosis have all been seen.
  ○ Biliary complications usually occur in patients who receive CPN for >3 weeks.
    - Acalculous cholecystitis
    - Gallbladder sludge
    - Cholelithiasis
  ○ Routine efforts to prevent hepatobiliary complications in all patients receiving long-term CPN include providing a portion (20–40%) of calories as fat, cycling CPN so that the glucose infusion is stopped for at least 8–10 hours per day, encouraging enteral intake to stimulate gallbladder contraction and maintain mucosal integrity, avoiding excessive calories, and preventing hyperglycemia.
  ○ If abnormal liver biochemistries or other evidence of liver damage occurs, evaluation for other possible causes of liver disease should be performed.
  ○ If mild hepatobiliary complications are noted, parenteral nutrition does not need to be discontinued, but the same principles used in preventing hepatic complications can be applied therapeutically.
  ○ When cholestasis is present, copper and manganese should be deleted from the CPN formula to prevent accumulation in the liver and basal ganglia. A 4-week trial of metronidazole or ursodeoxycholic acid has been reported to be helpful in some patients.

- **Metabolic bone disease**
  ○ Metabolic bone disease has been observed in patients receiving long-term (>3 months) CPN.
  ○ Patients may be asymptomatic. Clinical manifestations include bone fractures and pain (*Annu Rev Nutr 1991;11:93*). Demineralization may be seen in radiologic studies. Osteopenia, osteomalacia, or both may be present.
  ○ The precise causes of metabolic bone disease are not known, but several mechanisms have been proposed, including aluminum toxicity, vitamin D toxicity, and negative calcium balance.
  ○ Several therapeutic options should be considered in patients who have evidence of bone abnormalities.
  ○ Remove vitamin D from the CPN formulation if the parathyroid hormone and 1,25-hydroxy vitamin D levels are low.
  ○ Reduce protein to <1.5 g/kg/d because amino acids cause hypercalciuria.
  ○ Maintain normal magnesium status because magnesium is necessary for normal parathormone action and renal conservation of calcium.
  ○ Provide oral calcium supplements of 1–2 g/d.
  ○ Consider bisphosphonate therapy to decrease bone resorption.

SPECIAL CONSIDERATIONS

Monitoring nutrition support
- Adjustment of the nutrient formulation is often needed as medical therapy or clinical status changes.

- When nutrition support is initiated, other sources of **glucose** (e.g., peripheral IV dextrose infusions) should be stopped and the volume of other IV fluids adjusted to account for CPN.
- Vital signs should be checked every 8 hours.
- In certain patients, body weight, fluid intake, and fluid output should be followed daily.
- Serum electrolytes (including phosphorus) should be measured every 1–2 days after CPN is started until values are stable and then rechecked weekly.
- Serum glucose should be checked up to every 4–6 hours by fingerstick until blood glucose concentrations are stable and then rechecked weekly.
- If lipid emulsions are being given, **serum triglycerides** should be measured during lipid infusion in patients at risk for hypertriglyceridemia to demonstrate adequate clearance (triglyceride concentrations should be <400 mg/dL).
- Careful attention to the catheter and catheter site can help to prevent **catheter-related infections**.
  - Gauze dressings should be changed every 48–72 hours or when contaminated or wet, but transparent dressings can be changed weekly.
  - Tubing that connects the parenteral solutions with the catheter should be changed every 24 hours.
  - A 0.22-μm filter should be inserted between the IV tubing and the catheter when **lipid-free CPN** is infused and should be changed with the tubing.
  - A 1.2-μm filter should be used when a total nutrient admixture containing a **lipid emulsion** is infused.
  - When a **single-lumen** catheter is used to deliver CPN, the catheter should not be used to infuse other solutions or medications (with the exception of compatible antibiotics) and should not be used to monitor central venous pressure.
  - When a **triple-lumen** catheter is used, the distal port should be reserved solely for the administration of CPN.

Refeeding the Severely Malnourished Patient

COMPLICATIONS

Initiating nutritional therapy in patients who are severely malnourished and have had minimal nutrient intake can have adverse clinical consequences and precipitate the refeeding syndrome.

- **Hypophosphatemia, hypokalemia, and hypomagnesemia:** Rapid and marked decreases in these electrolytes occur during initial refeeding because of insulin-stimulated increases in cellular mineral uptake from extracellular fluid. For example, plasma phosphorus concentration can fall below 1 mg/dL and cause death within hours of initiating nutritional therapy if adequate phosphate is not given (*Am J Clin Nutr 1981;34:393*).
- **Fluid overload** and **congestive heart failure** are associated with decreased cardiac function and insulin-induced increased sodium and water reabsorption in conjunction with nutritional therapy containing water, glucose, and sodium. Renal mass may be reduced, limiting the ability to excrete salt or water loads.
- **Cardiac arrhythmias:** Patients who are severely malnourished often have bradycardia. Sudden death from ventricular tachyarrhythmias can occur during the first week of refeeding in severely malnourished patients and may be associated with a prolonged QT interval (*Ann Intern Med 1985;102:49*) or plasma electrolyte abnormalities. Patients with ECG changes should be monitored on telemetry, possibly in an ICU.
- **Glucose intolerance:** Starvation causes insulin resistance such that refeeding with high-carbohydrate meals or large amounts of parenteral glucose can cause marked elevations in blood glucose concentration, glycosuria, dehydration, and hyperosmolar coma.

TABLE 2-7	Major Mineral Daily Requirements, Deficiency, Toxicity, and Diagnostic Evaluation			
Mineral	Recommended Daily Enteral[1] Intake/Parenteral[2] Intake	Signs and Symptoms of Deficiency	Signs and Symptoms of Toxicity	Diagnostic Evaluation
Sodium	1.2–1.5 g[3,5]/1–2 mEq/kg	Encephalopathy, seizure, weakness, dehydration, cerebral edema	Encephalopathy, seizure	$Sodium_p$ (correct for hyperglycemia) $Sodium_u$ (will often only provide a rough estimate [i.e., too low, too high])
Potassium	4700 mg[4,5]/1–2 mEq/kg	Abdominal cramping, diarrhea, paresthesias, QT prolongation, weakness	QRS widening, QT shortening (sine wave morphology in extreme cases), peaked T waves	$Potassium_{w,b}$
Calcium	1000–1200 mg/10–15 mEq	QRS widening, paresthesias (Trousseau sign), tetany (Chvostek sign), osteomalacia	Encephalopathy, head-ache, abdominal pain, nephrolithiasis, metastatic calcification	$Calcium_{w,b}$, 24-hour $calcium_u$ (correct for $albumin_s$)

(continued)

TABLE 2-7 Major Mineral Daily Requirements, Deficiency, Toxicity, and Diagnostic Evaluation (*Continued*)

Mineral	Recommended Daily Enteral[1] Intake/Parenteral[2] Intake	Signs and Symptoms of Deficiency	Signs and Symptoms of Toxicity	Diagnostic Evaluation
Magnesium	420 mg/8–20 mEq	Tachyarrhythmia, weakness, muscle cramping, peripheral and central nervous system overstimulation (seizure, tetany)	Hyporeflexia, nausea, vomiting, weakness, encephalopathy, decreased respiratory drive, hypocalcemia, hyperkalemia, heart block	Magnesium$_s$, magnesium$_u$
Phosphorus	700 mg/20–40 mmol	Weakness, fatigue, increased cell membrane fragility (hemolytic anemias, leukocyte + platelet dysfunction), encephalopathy	Metastatic calcification, theoretic higher risk of nephrolithiasis, secondary hyperparathyroidism	Phosphorus$_p$

Subscript: b, blood; p, plasma; s, serum; u, urine; w, whole blood.
[1]Trumbo P, Yates AA, Schlicker S, et al. Institute of Medicine, Food and Nutrition Board. Dietary reference intakes for vitamin A, vitamin K, arsenic, boron, chromium, copper, iodine, iron, manganese, molybdenum, nickel, silicon, vanadium, and zinc. *J Am Diet Assoc.* 2001;101(3):294–301.
[2]Mirtallo J, Canada T, Johnson D, et al. Safe practices for parenteral nutrition. *JPEN J Parenter Enteral Nutr.* 2004;28:S39–S74.
[3]Higdon J, Drake V, Obarzanek E. Micronutrient Information Center: sodium (chloride). Linus Pauling Institute: Micronutrient Research for Optimum Health. http://lpi.oregonstate.edu/infocenter/minerals/sodium/. Accessed 1/6/15–1/11/15.
[4]Higdon J, Drake V, Pao-Hwa L. Micronutrient Information Center: potassium. Linus Pauling Institute: Micronutrient Research for Optimum Health. http://lpi.oregonstate.edu/infocenter/minerals/potassium/. Accessed 1/6/15–1/11/15.
[5]*Note:* Adequate daily intake.

In addition, carbohydrate refeeding in patients who are depleted in thiamine can precipitate Wernicke encephalopathy.

- **Recommendations**
  - ○ Careful **evaluation** of cardiovascular function and plasma electrolytes (history, physical examination, ECG, and blood tests) and correction of abnormal plasma electrolytes are **important before initiation of feeding**.
  - ○ Refeeding by the oral or enteral route involves the frequent or continuous administration of small amounts of food or an isotonic liquid formula.
  - ○ Parenteral supplementation or complete parenteral nutrition may be necessary if the intestine cannot tolerate feeding.
  - ○ During initial refeeding, fluid intake should be limited to approximately 800 mL/d plus insensible losses. Adjustments in fluid and sodium intake are needed in patients who have evidence of fluid overload or dehydration.
  - ○ Changes in body weight provide a useful guide for evaluating the efficacy of fluid administration. Weight gain >0.25 kg/d or 1.5 kg/wk probably represents fluid accumulation in excess of tissue repletion. Initially, approximately 15 kcal/kg, containing approximately 100 g carbohydrate and 1.5 g protein per kilogram of actual body weight, should be given daily.
  - ○ The rate at which the caloric intake can be increased depends on the severity of the malnutrition and the tolerance to feeding. In general, increases of 2–4 kcal/kg every 24–48 hours are appropriate.
  - ○ Sodium should be restricted to approximately 60 mEq or 1.5 g/d, but liberal amounts of phosphorus, potassium, and magnesium should be given to patients who have normal renal function.
  - ○ All other nutrients should be given in amounts needed to meet the recommended dietary intake (Table 2-7).
  - ○ Body weight, fluid intake, urine output, plasma glucose, and electrolyte values should be **monitored daily** during early refeeding (first 3–7 days) so that nutritional therapy can be appropriately modified when necessary.

Preventive Cardiology

3

Angela L. Brown, Daniel S. Kim, Clare E. Moynihan, and Anne C. Goldberg

Hypertension

GENERAL PRINCIPLES

Definition

Hypertension is defined as the presence of a blood pressure (BP) elevation to a level that places patients at increased risk for target organ damage in several vascular beds including the retina, brain, heart, kidneys, and large conduit arteries (Table 3-1, Table 3-2).

Classification

- **Normal BP** is defined as systolic blood pressure (SBP) <120 mm Hg and diastolic blood pressure (DBP) <80 mm Hg; pharmacologic intervention is not indicated.
- **Prehypertension** is defined as SBP of 120–139 mm Hg or DBP of 80–89 mm Hg. These patients should engage in comprehensive lifestyle modifications to delay progression or prevent the development of hypertension. Pharmacologic therapy should be initiated in prehypertensive patients with evidence of target organ damage or diabetes.
- **In stage 1** (SBP 140–159 mm Hg or DBP 90–99 mm Hg) **and stage 2** (SBP >160 mm Hg or DBP >100 mm Hg) **hypertension**, pharmacologic therapy should be initiated in addition to lifestyle modification to lower BP to <140/90 mm Hg in patients without diabetes or chronic kidney disease and age <60 years. For those age ≥60 years without diabetes or chronic kidney disease, pharmacologic therapy should be initiated in addition to lifestyle modification to lower BP to <150/90 mm Hg. In patients with diabetes or chronic kidney disease and age ≥18 years, BP should be lowered to <140/90 mm Hg.
- Patients with BP levels >20/10 mm Hg above their treatment target will often require more than one medication to achieve adequate control, and a two-drug regimen may be initiated as initial therapy. Patients with an average BP of 200/120 mm Hg or greater require immediate therapy and, if symptomatic end-organ damage is present, hospitalization.
- **Hypertensive crisis** includes hypertensive emergencies and urgencies. It usually develops in patients with a previous history of elevated BP but may arise in those who were previously normotensive. The severity of a hypertensive crisis correlates not only with the absolute level of BP elevation but also with the rapidity of development because autoregulatory mechanisms have not had sufficient time to adapt.
  - **Hypertensive urgencies** are defined as a substantial increase in BP, usually with a DBP >120 mm Hg, and occur in approximately 1% of hypertensive patients. Hypertensive urgencies (i.e., upper levels of stage 2 hypertension, hypertension with optic disk edema, progressive end-organ complications rather than damage, and severe perioperative hypertension) warrant BP reduction within several hours (*JAMA 2003;289:2560*).
  - **Hypertensive emergencies** include **accelerated hypertension**, typically defined as an SBP >210 mm Hg and DBP >130 mm Hg presenting with headaches, blurred vision, or focal neurologic symptoms and **malignant hypertension** (which requires the presence of papilledema). Hypertensive emergencies require immediate BP reduction by 20–25% to prevent or minimize end-organ damage (i.e., hypertensive encephalopathy, intracranial hemorrhage, unstable angina [UA] pectoris, acute myocardial infarction [MI], acute left ventricular failure with pulmonary edema, dissecting aortic aneurysm, progressive renal failure, or eclampsia).
- **Isolated systolic hypertension**, defined as an SBP >140 mm Hg and normal DBP, occurs frequently in the elderly (beginning after the fifth decade and increasing with age).

TABLE 3-1	Manifestations of Target Organ Disease
Organ System	**Manifestation**
Large vessel	Aneurysmal dilation Accelerated atherosclerosis Aortic dissection
Cardiac	*Acute:* Pulmonary edema, myocardial infarction *Chronic:* Clinical or ECG evidence of CAD; LVH by ECG or echocardiogram
Cerebrovascular	*Acute:* Intracerebral bleeding, coma, seizures, mental status changes, TIA, stroke *Chronic:* TIA, stroke
Renal	*Acute:* Hematuria, azotemia *Chronic:* Serum creatinine >1.5 mg/dL, proteinuria >1+ on dipstick
Retinopathy	*Acute:* Papilledema, hemorrhages *Chronic:* Hemorrhages, exudates, arterial nicking

CAD, coronary artery disease; LVH, left ventricular hypertrophy; TIA, transient ischemic attack.

Nonpharmacologic therapy should be initiated with medications added as needed to lower SBP to the appropriate level based on age and comorbidities.

Epidemiology

- The **public health burden** of hypertension is enormous, affecting an estimated 67 million American adults (*Circulation 2014;130:1692*). Indeed, for nonhypertensive individuals aged 55–65 years, the lifetime risk of developing hypertension is 90% (*JAMA 2002;287:1003*).
- Data derived from the Framingham Study have shown that hypertensive patients have a *fourfold* increase in cerebrovascular accidents as well as a *sixfold* increase in congestive heart failure (CHF) when compared to normotensive control subjects.

TABLE 3-2	Classification of Blood Pressure for Adults Age 18 Years and Older[a]	
Category	**Systolic Pressure (mm Hg)**	**Diastolic Pressure (mm Hg)**
Normal	<120 and	<80
Prehypertension	120–139 or	<80–89
Hypertension, stage 1	140–159 or	90–99
Hypertension, stage 2	>160 or	>100

[a]Not taking antihypertensive drugs and not acutely ill. When systolic and diastolic pressures fall into different categories, the higher category should be selected to classify the individual's blood pressure status.
From National High Blood Pressure Education Program. *The Seventh Report of the Joint National Committee on Prevention, Detection, Evaluation, and Treatment of High Blood Pressure.* Bethesda, MD: National Heart, Lung, and Blood Institute (US); 2004.

- Disease-associated morbidity and mortality, including atherosclerotic cardiovascular disease, stroke, heart failure (HF), and renal insufficiency, increase with higher levels of SBP and DBP.
- Over the last three decades, aggressive treatment of hypertension has resulted in a substantial decrease in death rates from stroke and coronary heart disease (CHD). Unfortunately, rates of end-stage renal disease (ESRD) and hospitalization for CHF have continued to increase. BP control rates have improved but remain poor, with only 50.1% of treated hypertensive patients below their goal BP level (*JAMA 2010;303:2043*).

Etiology

- BP rises with age. Other contributing factors include overweight/obesity, increased dietary sodium intake, decreased physical activity, increased alcohol consumption, and lower dietary intake of fruits, vegetables, and potassium.
- Of all hypertensive patients, more than 90% have primary or essential hypertension; the remainder have secondary hypertension due to causes such as renal parenchymal disease, renovascular disease, pheochromocytoma, Cushing syndrome, primary hyperaldosteronism, coarctation of the aorta, obstructive sleep apnea, and uncommon autosomal dominant or autosomal recessive diseases of the adrenal–renal axis that result in salt retention.

DIAGNOSIS

Clinical Presentation

- BP elevation is usually discovered in asymptomatic individuals during routine health visits.
- Optimal detection and evaluation of hypertension require accurate noninvasive BP measurement, which should be obtained in a seated patient with the arm resting level with the heart. A calibrated, appropriately fitting BP cuff (inflatable bladder encircling at least 80% of the arm) should be used because falsely high readings can be obtained if the cuff is too small.
- Two readings should be taken, separated by 2 minutes. SBP should be noted with the appearance of Korotkoff sounds (phase I) and DBP with the disappearance of sounds (phase V).
- In certain patients, the Korotkoff sounds do not disappear but are present at 0 mm Hg. In this case, the initial muffling of Korotkoff sounds (phase IV) should be taken as the DBP. One should be careful to avoid reporting spuriously low BP readings due to an auscultatory gap, which is caused by the disappearance and reappearance of Korotkoff sounds in hypertensive patients and may account for up to a 25-mm Hg gap between true and measured SBP. Hypertension should be confirmed in both arms, and the higher reading should be used.

History

- History should seek to discover secondary causes of hypertension and note the presence of medications and supplements that can affect BP (e.g., decongestants, oral contraceptives, appetite suppressants, sympathomimetics, venlafaxine, tricyclic antidepressants, monoamine oxidase inhibitors [MAOIs], chlorpromazine, some herbal supplements [ma huang], steroids, NSAIDs, cyclosporine, caffeine, thyroid hormones, cocaine, alcohol use, erythropoietin).
- A diagnosis of secondary hypertension should be considered in the following situations:
  - Age at onset younger than 30 or older than 60 years
  - Hypertension that is difficult to control after therapy has been initiated
  - Stable hypertension that becomes difficult to control
  - Clinical occurrence of a hypertensive crisis
  - The presence of signs or symptoms of a secondary cause such as hypokalemia or metabolic alkalosis that is not explained by diuretic therapy

- In patients who present with significant hypertension at a young age, a careful family history may give clues to forms of hypertension that follow simple Mendelian inheritance.

Physical Examination

Physical examination should include investigation for target organ damage or a secondary cause of hypertension by noting the presence of carotid bruits, an S_3 or S_4, cardiac murmurs, neurologic deficits, elevated jugular venous pressure, rales, retinopathy, unequal pulses, enlarged or small kidneys, cushingoid features, and abdominal bruits. Overweight/obesity should be assessed by measurement of height and weight and/or abdominal waist circumference.

Differential Diagnosis

- Hypertension may be part of several important syndromes of withdrawal from drugs, including alcohol, cocaine, and opioid analgesics. Rebound increases in BP also may be seen in patients who abruptly discontinue antihypertensive therapy, particularly β-adrenergic antagonists and central α_2-agonists (see Complications).
- Cocaine and other sympathomimetic drugs (e.g., amphetamines, phencyclidine hydrochloride) can produce hypertension in the setting of acute intoxication and when the agents are discontinued abruptly after chronic use. Hypertension is often complicated by other end-organ insults, such as ischemic heart disease, stroke, and seizures. Phentolamine is effective in acute management, and sodium nitroprusside or nitroglycerin can be used as an alternative. β-Adrenergic antagonists should be avoided due to the risk of unopposed α-adrenergic activity, which can exacerbate hypertension.

Diagnostic Testing

- Tests are needed to help identify patients with possible target organ damage, to help assess cardiovascular risk, and to provide a baseline for monitoring the adverse effects of therapy.
- Basic laboratory data should include urinalysis, hematocrit, plasma glucose, serum potassium, serum creatinine, calcium, and uric acid and fasting lipid levels.
- Other testing includes ECG and chest radiography. Echocardiography may be of value for certain patients to assess cardiac function or detection of left ventricular hypertrophy (LVH).

TREATMENT

- The goal of treatment is to prevent long-term sequelae (i.e., target organ damage) while controlling other modifiable cardiovascular risk factors.
  - In isolated systolic hypertension, the therapeutic goal should be to lower SBP to <140 mm Hg. SBP >140 mm Hg is associated with increased cerebrovascular and cardiac events.
  - In patients with chronic kidney disease or diabetes, BP should be reduced to a goal of <140/90 mm Hg.
  - In patients age ≥60 without chronic kidney disease or diabetes, BP should be reduced to a goal of <150/90 mm Hg. Discretion is warranted in prescribing medication to lower BP that may affect cardiovascular risk adversely in other ways (e.g., glucose control, lipid metabolism, uric acid levels).
- In the absence of hypertensive crisis, BP should be reduced gradually to avoid end-organ (e.g., cerebral) ischemia.
- Lifestyle modifications should be encouraged in all hypertensive patients regardless of whether they require medication (Table 3-3). These changes may have beneficial effects on other cardiovascular risk factors. Some of these lifestyle modifications include cessation of smoking, reduction in body weight if the patient is overweight, judicious consumption of alcohol, adequate nutritional intake of minerals and vitamins, reduction in sodium intake, and increased physical activity.

TABLE 3-3	Lifestyle Modifications and Effects
Modification	**Approximate SBP Reduction**
Weight reduction (for every 10-kg weight loss)	5–20 mm Hg
Adoption of DASH eating plan	8–14 mm Hg
Dietary sodium reduction (intake <2 g/d)	2–8 mm Hg
Physical activity (150 min/wk)	4–9 mm Hg
Moderation of alcohol consumption (intake <2 drinks/d)	2–4 mm Hg

DASH, Dietary Approaches to Stop Hypertension; SBP, systolic blood pressure.

• Barring an overt need for immediate pharmacologic therapy, most patients should be given the opportunity to achieve a reduction in BP over an interval of 3–6 months by applying nonpharmacologic modifications and pharmacologic therapies if needed.

Medications
• **Initial drug therapy**
  ○ Initial drug choice may be affected by coexistent factors such as age, race, angina, HF, renal insufficiency, LVH, obesity, hyperlipidemia, gout, and bronchospasm. Cost and drug interactions should also be considered. The BP response is usually consistent within a given class of agents; therefore, if a drug fails to control BP, another agent from the same class is unlikely to be effective. At times, however, a change within drug class may be useful in reducing adverse effects. The lowest possible effective dosage should be used to control BP, adjusted every 1–2 months as needed (Table 3-4).
    ▪ Diuretics, calcium channel blockers (CCBs), angiotensin-converting enzyme (ACE) inhibitors, and angiotensin receptor blockers (ARBs) should be considered first-line therapy for the general nonblack population, including those with diabetes (those with chronic kidney disease are discussed below). Multiple large randomized controlled trials have shown comparable effects on decreasing overall cardiovascular and cerebrovascular mortality for all four drug classes (*JAMA 2014;311(5):507*).
    ▪ In the general black population, including those with diabetes, a diuretic or CCB can be considered for first-line therapy. Data from the ALLHAT trial have shown decreased cardiovascular and cerebrovascular morbidity and mortality with the use of thiazide diuretics or CCB over an ACE inhibitor (*JAMA 2002;288:2981*).
  ○ In patients with chronic kidney disease, initial or combination therapy with an ACE inhibitor or ARB should be considered.
• **Additional therapy.** When a second drug is needed, it should generally be chosen from among the other first-line agents.
• **Adjustments of a therapeutic regimen.** Before considering a modification of therapy because of inadequate response to the current regimen, other possible contributing factors should be investigated. Poor patient compliance, use of antagonistic drugs (i.e., sympathomimetics, venlafaxine, tricyclic antidepressants, MAOIs, chlorpromazine, some herbal supplements [ma huang], steroids, NSAIDs, cyclosporine, caffeine, thyroid hormones, cocaine, erythropoietin), inappropriately high sodium intake, or increased alcohol consumption should be considered and may be the cause of inadequate BP response. Secondary causes of hypertension should be considered when a previously effective regimen becomes inadequate and other confounding factors are absent.

TABLE 3-4 Commonly Used Antihypertensive Agents by Functional Class

Drugs by Class	Properties	Initial Dose	Dosage Range (mg)
β-Adrenergic Antagonists			
Atenolol[a]	Selective	50 mg PO daily	25–100
Betaxolol[a]	Selective	10 mg PO daily	5–40
Bisoprolol[a]	Selective	5 mg PO daily	2.5–20
Metoprolol	Selective	50 mg PO bid	50–450
Metoprolol XL	Selective	50–100 mg PO daily	50–400
Nebivolol[a,b]	Selective with vaso-dilatory properties	5 mg PO daily	5–40
Nadolola	Nonselective	40 mg PO daily	20–240
Propranolol	Nonselective	40 mg PO bid	40–240
Propranolol LA	Nonselective	80 mg PO daily	60–240
Timolol	Nonselective	10 mg PO bid	20–40
Pindolol	ISA	5 mg PO daily	10–60
Labetalol	α- and β-antagonist properties	100 mg PO bid	200–1200
Carvedilol	α- and β-antagonist properties	6.25 mg PO bid	12.5–50
Carvedilol CR[b]	α- and β-antagonist properties	10 mg PO daily	10–80
Acebutolol[a]	ISA, selective	200 mg PO bid, 400 mg PO daily	200–1200
Calcium Channel Antagonists			
Amlodipine	DHP	5 mg PO daily	2.5–10
Diltiazem		30 mg PO qid	90–360
Diltiazem LA		180 mg PO daily	120–540
Diltiazem CD		180 mg PO daily	120–480
Diltiazem XR		180 mg PO daily	120–540
Diltiazem XT		180 mg PO daily	120–480
Isradipine	DHP	2.5 mg PO bid	2.5–10
Nicardipine[b]	DHP	20 mg PO tid	60–120
Nifedipine	DHP	10 mg PO tid	30–120
Nifedipine XL (or CC)	DHP	30 mg PO daily	30–90
Nisoldipine	DHP	20 mg PO daily	20–40

(continued)

TABLE 3-4	Commonly Used Antihypertensive Agents by Functional Class *(Continued)*

Drugs by Class	Properties	Initial Dose	Dosage Range (mg)
Verapamil		80 mg PO tid	80–480
Verapamil SR		120 mg PO daily	120–480
Angiotensin-Converting Enzyme Inhibitors[c]			
Benazepril		10 mg PO bid	10–40
Captopril		25 mg PO bid–tid	50–450
Enalapril		5 mg PO daily	2.5–40
Fosinopril		10 mg PO daily	10–40
Lisinopril		10 mg PO daily	5–40
Moexipril		7.5 mg PO daily	7.5–30
Quinapril		10 mg PO daily	5–80
Ramipril		2.5 mg PO daily	1.25–20
Trandolapril		1–2 mg PO daily	1–4
Perindopril		4 mg PO daily	2–16
Angiotensin II Receptor Blockers[c]			
Azilsartan[b]		40 mg PO daily	40–80
Candesartan		8 mg PO daily	8–32
Eprosartan		600 mg PO daily	600–800
Irbesartan		150 mg PO daily	150–300
Olmesartanb		20 mg PO daily	20–40
Losartan		50 mg PO daily	25–100
Telmisartan		40 mg PO daily	20–80
Valsartan		80 mg PO daily	80–320
Direct Renin Inhibitors[c]			
Aliskiren[b]		150 mg PO daily	150–300
Diuretics[c]			
Chlorthalidone	Thiazide diuretic	25 mg PO daily	12.5–50
Hydrochlorothiazide	Thiazide diuretic	12.5 mg PO daily	12.5–50
Hydroflumethiazide[b]	Thiazide diuretic	50 mg PO daily	50–100
Indapamide	Thiazide diuretic	1.25 mg PO daily	2.5–5
Methyclothiazide	Thiazide diuretic	2.5 mg PO daily	2.5–5
Metolazone	Thiazide diuretic	2.5 mg PO daily	1.25–5

(continued)

TABLE 3-4	Commonly Used Antihypertensive Agents by Functional Class (Continued)		

Drugs by Class	Properties	Initial Dose	Dosage Range (mg)
Bumetanide	Loop diuretic	0.5 mg PO daily (or IV)	0.5–5
Ethacrynic acid[b]	Loop diuretic	50 mg PO daily (or IV)	25–100
Furosemide	Loop diuretic	20 mg PO daily (or IV)	20–320
Torsemide	Loop diuretic	5 mg PO daily (or IV)	5–10
Amiloride	Potassium-sparing diuretic	5 mg PO daily	5–10
Triamterene[b]	Potassium-sparing diuretic	50 mg PO bid	50–200
Eplerenone	Aldosterone antagonist	25 mg PO daily	25–100
Spironolactone	Aldosterone antagonist	25 mg PO daily	25–100
α-Adrenergic Antagonists			
Doxazosin		1 mg PO daily	1–16
Prazosin		1 mg PO bid–tid	1–20
Terazosin		1 mg PO at bedtime	1–20
Centrally Acting Adrenergic Agents			
Clonidine		0.1 mg PO bid	0.1–1.2
Clonidine patch		TTS 1/wk (equivalent to 0.1 mg/d release)	0.1–0.3
Guanfacine		1 mg PO daily	1–3
Guanabenz		4 mg PO bid	4–64
Methyldopa[a]		250 mg PO bid–tid	250–2000
Direct-Acting Vasodilators			
Hydralazine[a]		10 mg PO qid	50–300
Minoxidil		5 mg PO daily	2.5–100
Miscellaneous			
Reserpine		0.5 mg PO daily	0.01–0.25

DHP, dihydropyridine; ISA, intrinsic sympathomimetic activity; TTS, transdermal therapeutic system.
[a]Adjusted in renal failure.
[b]Available only in brand name. Assume all drugs are available in generic form unless otherwise denoted by superscript "b."
[c]Renal function should be considered for all angiotensin-converting enzyme inhibitors before initiation.

- **Diuretics** (see Table 3-4) are effective agents in the therapy of hypertension and have been shown to reduce the incidence of stroke and cardiovascular events. Several classes of diuretics are available, generally categorized by their site of action in the kidney.
- **Thiazide** and thiazide-like diuretics (e.g., hydrochlorothiazide, chlorthalidone) block sodium reabsorption predominantly in the distal convoluted tubule by inhibition of the thiazide-sensitive Na/Cl cotransporter. Thiazide diuretics can produce weakness, muscle cramps, and impotence. Metabolic side effects include hypokalemia, hypomagnesemia, hyperlipidemia (with increases in low-density lipoproteins [LDLs] and triglyceride levels), hypercalcemia, hyperglycemia, hyperuricemia, hyponatremia, and rarely, azotemia. Thiazide-induced pancreatitis has also been reported. Metabolic side effects may be limited when thiazides are used in low doses (e.g., hydrochlorothiazide, 12.5–25.0 mg/d).
- **Loop diuretics** (e.g., furosemide, bumetanide, ethacrynic acid, torsemide) block sodium reabsorption in the thick ascending loop of Henle through inhibition of the Na/K/2Cl cotransporter and are the most effective agents in patients with renal insufficiency (estimated glomerular filtration rate <35 mL/min/1.73 m^2). Loop diuretics can cause electrolyte abnormalities such as hypomagnesemia, hypocalcemia, and hypokalemia, and can also produce irreversible ototoxicity (usually dose related and more common with parenteral therapy).
- **Spironolactone and eplerenone, potassium-sparing agents**, act by competitively inhibiting the actions of aldosterone on the kidney. Triamterene and amiloride are potassium-sparing drugs that inhibit the epithelial Na$^+$ channel in the distal nephron to inhibit reabsorption of Na$^+$ and secretion of potassium ions. Potassium-sparing diuretics are weak agents when used alone; thus, they are often combined with a thiazide for added potency. Aldosterone antagonists may have an additional benefit in improving myocardial function in HF; this effect may be independent of its effect on renal transport mechanisms. Spironolactone and eplerenone can produce hyperkalemia; however, the gynecomastia that may occur in men and breast tenderness in women are not seen with eplerenone. Triamterene (usually in combination with hydrochlorothiazide) can cause renal tubular damage and renal calculi. Unlike thiazides, potassium-sparing and loop diuretics do not cause adverse lipid effects.
- **Calcium channel antagonists** (see Table 3-4) generally have no significant central nervous system (CNS) side effects and can be used to treat diseases, such as angina pectoris, that can coexist with hypertension. **Due to the concern that the use of short-acting dihydropyridine calcium channel antagonists may increase the number of ischemic cardiac events, they are not indicated for hypertension management** (*JAMA 1995;274:620*); long-acting agents are considered safe in the management of hypertension (*Am J Cardiol 1996;77:81*).
  - ○ **Classes of calcium channel antagonists** include diphenylalkylamines (e.g., verapamil), benzothiazepines (e.g., diltiazem), and dihydropyridines (e.g., nifedipine). The dihydropyridines include many newer second-generation drugs (e.g., amlodipine, felodipine, isradipine, and nicardipine), which are more vasoselective and have longer plasma half-lives than nifedipine. Verapamil and diltiazem have negative cardiac inotropic and chronotropic effects. Nifedipine also has a negative inotropic effect, but in clinical use, this effect is much less pronounced than that of verapamil or diltiazem because of peripheral vasodilation and reflex tachycardia. Less negative inotropic effects have been observed with the second-generation dihydropyridines. All calcium channel antagonists are metabolized in the liver; thus in patients with cirrhosis, the dosing interval should be adjusted accordingly. Some of these drugs also inhibit the metabolism of other hepatically cleared medications (e.g., cyclosporine). Verapamil and diltiazem should be used with caution in patients with cardiac conduction abnormalities, and they can worsen HF in patients with decreased left ventricular function.

- ○ **Side effects** of verapamil include constipation, nausea, headache, and orthostatic hypotension. Diltiazem can cause nausea, headache, and rash. Dihydropyridines can cause lower extremity edema, flushing, headache, and rash. Calcium channel antagonists have no significant effects on glucose tolerance, electrolytes, or lipid profiles.
- **Inhibitors of the renin–angiotensin system** (see Table 3-4) include ACE inhibitors, ARBs, and a direct renin inhibitor.
  - ○ **ACE inhibitors** may have beneficial effects in patients with concomitant HF or kidney disease. One study has also suggested that ACE inhibitors (ramipril) may significantly reduce the rate of death, MI, and stroke in patients without HF or low ejection fraction (*N Engl J Med 2000;342:145*). Additionally, they can reduce hypokalemia, hypercholesterolemia, hyperglycemia, and hyperuricemia caused by diuretic therapy and are particularly effective in states of hypertension associated with a high renin state (e.g., scleroderma renal crisis). **Side effects** associated with the use of ACE inhibitors are infrequent. They can cause a dry cough (up to 20% of patients), angioneurotic edema, and hypotension, but they do not cause levels of lipids, glucose, or uric acid to increase. ACE inhibitors that contain a sulfhydryl group (e.g., captopril) may cause taste disturbance, leukopenia, and a glomerulopathy with proteinuria. Because ACE inhibitors cause preferential vasodilation of the efferent arteriole in the kidney, worsening of renal function may occur in patients who have decreased renal perfusion or who have preexisting severe renal insufficiency. ACE inhibitors can cause hyperkalemia and should be used with caution in patients with a decreased glomerular filtration rate (GFR) who are taking potassium supplements or who are receiving potassium-sparing diuretics.
  - ○ **ARBs** are a class of antihypertensive drugs that are effective in diverse patient populations (*N Engl J Med 1996;334:1649*). ARBs are useful alternatives in patients with HF who are unable to tolerate ACE inhibitors (*N Engl J Med 2001;345:1667*). **Side effects** of ARBs occur rarely but include angioedema, allergic reaction, and rash.
  - ○ The **direct renin inhibitor** class consists of one agent, aliskiren, that is indicated solely for the treatment of hypertension (see Table 3-4). It may be used in combination with other antihypertensive agents; however, combined use with ACE inhibitors or ARBs is contraindicated in patients with diabetes (*Food and Drug Administration [FDA] Drug Safety Communication, April 2012*).
- **β-Adrenergic antagonists** (see Table 3-4) are part of medical regimens that have been proven to decrease the incidence of stroke, MI, and HF. β-Adrenergic antagonists work via competitive inhibition of the effects of catecholamines at β-adrenergic receptors, which decreases heart rate and cardiac output. These agents also decrease plasma renin and cause a resetting of baroreceptors to accept a lower level of BP. β-Adrenergic antagonists cause release of vasodilatory prostaglandins, decrease plasma volume, and may also have a CNS-mediated antihypertensive effect.
  - ○ **Classes of β-adrenergic antagonists** can be subdivided into those that are cardioselective, with primarily β_1-blocking effects, and those that are nonselective, with β_1- and β_2-blocking effects. At low doses, the cardioselective agents can be given with caution to patients with mild chronic obstructive pulmonary disease, diabetes mellitus (DM), or peripheral vascular disease. At higher doses, these agents lose their β_1 selectivity and may cause unwanted effects in these patients. β-Adrenergic antagonists can also be categorized according to the presence or absence of partial agonist or intrinsic sympathomimetic activity (ISA). β-Adrenergic antagonists with ISA cause less bradycardia than do those without it. In addition, there are agents with mixed properties having both α- and β-adrenergic antagonist actions (labetalol and carvedilol). Nebivolol is a highly selective β-adrenergic antagonist that is vasodilatory through an unclear mechanism.
  - ○ **Side effects** include high-degree atrioventricular (AV) block, HF, Raynaud phenomenon, and impotence. Lipophilic β-adrenergic antagonists, such as propranolol, have a

higher incidence of CNS side effects including insomnia and depression. Propranolol can also cause nasal congestion. β-Adrenergic antagonists can cause adverse effects on the lipid profile; increased triglyceride and decreased high-density lipoprotein (HDL) levels occur mainly with nonselective β-adrenergic antagonists but generally do not occur when β-adrenergic antagonists with ISA are used. Pindolol, a selective β-adrenergic antagonist with ISA, may actually increase HDL and nominally increase triglycerides. Side effects of labetalol include hepatocellular damage, postural hypotension, a positive antinuclear antibody (ANA) test, a lupus-like syndrome, tremors, and potential hypotension in the setting of halothane anesthesia. Carvedilol appears to have a similar side effect profile to other β-adrenergic antagonists. Both labetalol and carvedilol have negligible effects on lipids. Rarely, reflex tachycardia may occur because of the initial vasodilatory effect of labetalol and carvedilol. Because β-receptor density is increased with chronic antagonism, abrupt withdrawal of these agents can precipitate angina pectoris, increases in BP, and other effects attributable to an increase in adrenergic tone.

- **Selective α-adrenergic antagonists** such as prazosin, terazosin, and doxazosin have replaced nonselective α-adrenergic antagonists such as phenoxybenzamine (see Table 3-4) in the treatment of essential hypertension. Based on the ALLHAT trial, these drugs appear to be less efficacious than diuretics, CCBs, and ACE inhibitors in reducing primary end points of cardiovascular disease when used as monotherapy (*JAMA 2002;283:1967; JAMA 2002;288:2981*).

  Side effects of these agents include a "first-dose effect," which results from a greater decrease in BP with the first dose than with subsequent doses. Selective α_1-adrenergic antagonists can cause syncope, orthostatic hypotension, dizziness, headache, and drowsiness. In most cases, side effects are self-limited and do not recur with continued therapy. Selective α_1-adrenergic antagonists may improve lipid profiles by decreasing total cholesterol and triglyceride levels and increasing HDL levels. Additionally, these agents can improve the negative effects on lipids induced by thiazide diuretics and β-adrenergic antagonists. Doxazosin specifically may be less effective at lowering SBP than thiazide diuretics and may be associated with a higher risk of HF and stroke in patients with hypertension and at least one additional risk factor for coronary artery disease (CAD) (*JAMA 2002;283:1967*).

- **Centrally acting adrenergic agents** (see Table 3-4) are potent antihypertensive agents. In addition to its oral dosage forms, clonidine is available as a transdermal patch that is applied weekly.

  Side effects may include bradycardia, drowsiness, dry mouth, orthostatic hypotension, galactorrhea, and sexual dysfunction. Transdermal clonidine causes a rash in up to 20% of patients. These agents can precipitate HF in patients with decreased left ventricular function, and abrupt cessation can precipitate an acute withdrawal syndrome (AWS) of elevated BP, tachycardia, and diaphoresis. Methyldopa produces a positive direct antibody (Coombs) test in up to 25% of patients, but significant hemolytic anemia is much less common. If hemolytic anemia develops secondary to methyldopa, the drug should be withdrawn. Severe cases of hemolytic anemia may require treatment with glucocorticoids. Methyldopa also causes positive ANA test results in approximately 10% of patients and can cause an inflammatory reaction in the liver that is indistinguishable from viral hepatitis; fatal hepatitis has been reported. Guanabenz and guanfacine decrease total cholesterol levels, and guanfacine can also decrease serum triglyceride levels.

- **Direct-acting vasodilators** are potent antihypertensive agents (see Table 3-4) now reserved for refractory hypertension or specific circumstances such as the use of hydralazine in pregnancy.

  ○ Hydralazine in combination with nitrates is useful in treating patients with hypertension and HF with reduced ejection fraction (see Chapter 5, Heart Failure and Cardiomyopathy). **Side effects** of hydralazine therapy may include headache, nausea, emesis, tachycardia, and postural hypotension. Asymptomatic patients may have a positive ANA test result, and a hydralazine-induced systemic lupus-like syndrome may develop in approximately 10% of patients. Patients at greater risk for the latter complication include those treated with excessive doses (e.g., >400 mg/d), those with impaired renal or cardiac function, and those with the slow acetylation phenotype. Hydralazine should be discontinued if clinical evidence of a lupus-like syndrome develops and a positive ANA test result is present. The syndrome usually resolves with discontinuation of the drug, leaving no adverse long-term effects.

○ **Side effects** of minoxidil include weight gain, hypertrichosis, hirsutism, ECG abnormalities, and pericardial effusions.

• **Reserpine, guanethidine, and guanadrel** (see Table 3-4) were among the first effective antihypertensive agents available. Currently, these drugs are not regarded as first- or second-line therapy because of their significant side effects.

  Side effects of reserpine include severe depression in approximately 2% of patients. Sedation and nasal stuffiness also are potential side effects. Guanethidine can cause severe postural hypotension through a decrease in cardiac output, a decrease in peripheral resistance, and venous pooling in the extremities. Patients who are receiving guanethidine with orthostatic hypotension should be cautioned to arise slowly and to wear support hose. Guanethidine can also cause ejaculatory failure and diarrhea.

• **Parenteral antihypertensive agents** are indicated for the immediate reduction of BP in patients with hypertensive emergencies. Judicious administration of these agents (Table 3-5) may also be appropriate in patients with hypertension complicated by HF or MI. These drugs are also indicated for individuals who have perioperative hypertensive urgency or are in need of emergency surgery. If possible, an accurate baseline BP should be determined before the initiation of therapy. In the setting of hypertensive emergency, the patient should be admitted to an intensive care unit (ICU) for close monitoring, and an intra-arterial monitor should be used when available. Although parenteral agents are indicated as a first-line treatment in hypertensive emergencies, oral agents may also be effective in this group; the choice of drug and route of administration must be individualized. If parenteral agents are used initially, oral medications should be administered shortly thereafter to facilitate rapid weaning from parenteral therapy.

○ **Sodium nitroprusside**, a direct-acting arterial and venous vasodilator, is the drug of choice for most hypertensive emergencies (see Table 3-5). It reduces BP rapidly and is easily titratable, and its action is short lived when discontinued. Patients should be monitored very closely to avoid an exaggerated hypotensive response. Therapy for more than 48–72 hours with a high cumulative dose or renal insufficiency may cause accumulation of thiocyanate, a toxic metabolite. Thiocyanate toxicity may cause paresthesias, tinnitus, blurred vision, delirium, or seizures. Serum thiocyanate levels should be kept at <10 mg/dL. Patients on high doses (>2–3 mg/kg/min) or those with renal dysfunction should have serum levels of thiocyanate drawn after 48–72 hours of therapy. In patients with normal renal function or those receiving lower doses, levels can be drawn after 5–7 days. Hepatic dysfunction may result in accumulation of cyanide, which can cause metabolic acidosis, dyspnea, vomiting, dizziness, ataxia, and syncope. Hemodialysis should be considered for thiocyanate poisoning. Nitrites and thiosulfate can be administered intravenously for cyanide poisoning.

○ **Nitroglycerin** given as a continuous IV infusion (see Table 3-5) may be appropriate in situations in which sodium nitroprusside is relatively contraindicated, such as in patients with severe coronary insufficiency or advanced renal or hepatic disease. It is the preferred agent for patients with moderate hypertension in the setting of acute coronary ischemia or after coronary artery bypass surgery because of its more favorable effects on pulmonary gas exchange and collateral coronary blood flow. In patients with severely elevated BP, sodium nitroprusside remains the agent of choice. Nitroglycerin reduces

TABLE 3-5	Parenteral Antihypertensive Drug Preparations				
Drug	**Administration**	**Onset**	**Duration of Action**	**Dosage**	**Adverse Effects and Comments**
Fenoldopam	IV infusion	<5 min	30 min	0.1–0.3 µg/kg/min	Tachycardia, nausea, vomiting
Sodium nitroprusside	IV infusion	Immediate	2–3 min	0.5–10 µg/kg/min (initial dose, 0.25 µg/kg/min for eclampsia and renal insufficiency)	Hypotension, nausea, vomiting, apprehension; risk of thiocyanate and cyanide toxicity is increased in renal and hepatic insufficiency, respectively; levels should be monitored; must shield from light
Diazoxide	IV bolus	15 min	6–12 h	50–100 mg q5–10min, up to 600 mg	Hypotension, tachycardia, nausea, vomiting, fluid retention, hyperglycemia; may exacerbate myocardial ischemia, heart failure, or aortic dissection
Labetalol	IV bolus	5–10 min	3–6 h	20–80 mg q5–10min, up to 300 mg	Hypotension, heart block, heart failure, bronchospasm, nausea, vomiting, scalp tingling, paradoxical pressor response; may not be effective in patients receiving α- or β-antagonists
	IV infusion			0.5–2 mg/min	

Drug	Route	Onset	Duration	Dose	Adverse effects
Nitroglycerin	IV infusion	1–2 min	3–5 min	5–250 µg/min	Headache, nausea, vomiting. Tolerance may develop with prolonged use.
Esmolol	IV bolus IV infusion	1–5 min	10 min	500 µg/kg/min for first 1 min 50–300 µg/kg/min	Hypotension, heart block, heart failure, bronchospasm
Phentolamine	IV bolus	1–2 min	3–10 min	5–10 mg q5–15min	Hypotension, tachycardia, headache, angina, paradoxical pressor response
Hydralazine (for treatment of eclampsia)	IV bolus	10–20 min	3–6 h	10–20 mg q20min (if no effect after 20 mg, try another agent)	Hypotension, fetal distress, tachycardia, headache, nausea, vomiting, local thrombophlebitis. Infusion site should be changed after 12 h.
Methyldopate (for treatment of eclampsia)	IV bolus	30–60 min	10–16 h	250–500 mg	Hypotension
Nicardipine	IV infusion	1–5 min	3–6 h	5 mg/h, increased by 1.0–2.5 mg/h q15min, up to 15 mg/h	Hypotension, headache, tachycardia, nausea, vomiting
Enalaprilat	IV bolus	5–15 min	1–6 h	0.6255 mg q6h	Hypotension

preload more than afterload and should be used with caution or avoided in patients who have inferior MI with right ventricular infarction and are dependent on preload to maintain cardiac output.

○ **Labetalol** can be administered parenterally (see Table 3-5) in hypertensive crisis, even in patients in the early phase of an acute MI, and is the drug of choice in hypertensive emergencies that occur during pregnancy. When given intravenously, the β-adrenergic antagonist effect is greater than the α-adrenergic antagonist effect. Nevertheless, symptomatic postural hypotension may occur with IV use; thus, patients should be treated in a supine position. Labetalol may be particularly beneficial during adrenergic excess (e.g., clonidine withdrawal, pheochromocytoma, post–coronary bypass grafting). Because the half-life of labetalol is 5–8 hours, intermittent IV bolus dosing may be preferable to IV infusion. IV infusion can be discontinued before oral labetalol is begun. When the supine DBP begins to rise, oral dosing can be initiated at 200 mg PO, followed in 6–12 hours by 200–400 mg PO, depending on the BP response.

○ **Esmolol** is a parenteral, short-acting, cardioselective β-adrenergic antagonist (see Table 3-5) that can be used in the treatment of hypertensive emergencies in patients in whom β-blocker intolerance is a concern. Esmolol is also useful for the treatment of aortic dissection. β-Adrenergic antagonists may be ineffective when used as monotherapy in the treatment of severe hypertension and are frequently combined with other agents (e.g., with sodium nitroprusside in the treatment of aortic dissection).

○ **Nicardipine** is an effective IV calcium antagonist preparation (see Table 3-5) approved for use in postoperative hypertension. Side effects include headache, flushing, reflex tachycardia, and venous irritation. Nicardipine should be administered via a central venous line. If it is given peripherally, the IV site should be changed q12h. Fifty percent of the peak effect is seen within the first 30 minutes, but the full peak effect is not achieved until after 48 hours of administration.

○ **Enalaprilat** is the active de-esterified form of enalapril (see Table 3-5) that results from hepatic conversion after an oral dose. Enalaprilat (as well as other ACE inhibitors) has been used effectively in cases of severe and malignant hypertension. However, variable and unpredictable results have also been reported. ACE inhibition can cause rapid BP reduction in hypertensive patients with high renin states such as renovascular hypertension, concomitant use of vasodilators, and scleroderma renal crisis; thus, enalaprilat should be used cautiously to avoid precipitating hypotension. Therapy can be changed to an oral preparation when IV therapy is no longer necessary.

○ **Diazoxide and hydralazine** are only rarely used in hypertensive crises and offer little or no advantage to the agents discussed previously. It should be noted, however, that hydralazine is a useful agent in pregnancy-related hypertensive emergencies because of its established safety profile.

○ **Fenoldopam** is a selective agonist to peripheral dopamine-1 receptors, and it produces vasodilation, increases renal perfusion, and enhances natriuresis. Fenoldopam has a short duration of action; the elimination half-life is <10 minutes. The drug has important application as parenteral therapy for high-risk hypertensive surgical patients and the perioperative management of patients undergoing organ transplantation.

• **Oral loading of antihypertensive agents** has been used successfully in patients with hypertensive crisis when urgent but not immediate reduction of BP is indicated.

○ **Oral clonidine loading** is achieved by using an initial dose of 0.2 mg PO followed by 0.1 mg PO q1h to a total dose of 0.7 mg or a reduction in diastolic pressure of 20 mm Hg or more. BP should be checked at 15-minute intervals over the first hour, 30-minute intervals over the second hour, and then hourly. After 6 hours, a diuretic can be added, and an 8-hour clonidine dosing interval can be begun. Sedative side effects are significant.

○ Sublingual nifedipine has an onset of action within 30 minutes but can produce wide fluctuations and excessive reductions in BP. Because of the potential for adverse cardiovascular events (stroke/MI), sublingual nifedipine should be avoided in the acute management of elevated BP. Side effects include facial flushing and postural hypotension.

SPECIAL CONSIDERATIONS

* **Hypertensive crisis.** In hypertensive emergency, control of acute or ongoing end-organ damage is more important than the absolute level of BP. BP control with a rapidly acting parenteral agent should be accomplished as soon as possible (within 1 hour) to reduce the chance of permanent organ dysfunction and death. A reasonable goal is a 20–25% reduction of mean arterial pressure or a reduction of the diastolic pressure to 100–110 mm Hg over a period of minutes to hours. A precipitous fall in BP may occur in patients who are elderly, volume depleted, or receiving other antihypertensive agents. BP control in hypertensive urgencies can be accomplished more slowly. The initial goal of therapy in urgency should be to achieve a DBP of 100–110 mm Hg. Excessive or rapid decreases in BP should be avoided to minimize the risk of cerebral hypoperfusion or coronary insufficiency. Normal BP can be attained gradually over several days as tolerated by the individual patient.

* **Aortic dissection**
Acute proximal aortic dissection (type A) is a surgical emergency, whereas uncomplicated distal dissection (type B) can be treated successfully with medical therapy alone. All patients, including those treated surgically, require acute and chronic antihypertensive therapy to provide initial stabilization and to prevent complications (e.g., aortic rupture, continued dissection). Medical therapy of chronic stable aortic dissection should seek to maintain SBP at or below 130–140 mm Hg if tolerated. Antihypertensive agents with negative inotropic properties, including calcium channel antagonists, β-adrenergic antagonists, methyldopa, clonidine, and reserpine, are preferred for management in the postacute phase.
  ○ **Sodium nitroprusside** is considered the initial drug of choice because of the predictability of response and absence of tachyphylaxis. The dose should be titrated to achieve an SBP of 100–120 mm Hg or the lowest possible BP that permits adequate organ perfusion. Nitroprusside alone causes an increase in left ventricular contractility and subsequent arterial shearing forces, which contribute to ongoing intimal dissection. Thus, when using sodium nitroprusside, adequate simultaneous **β-adrenergic antagonist therapy** is essential, regardless of whether systolic hypertension is present. Traditionally, propranolol has been recommended. **Esmolol**, a cardioselective class intravenous β-adrenergic antagonist with a very short duration of action, may be preferable, especially in patients with relative contraindications to β-antagonists. If esmolol is tolerated, a longer acting β-adrenergic antagonist should be used.
  ○ **IV labetalol** has been used successfully as a single agent in the treatment of acute aortic dissection. Labetalol produces a dose-related decrease in BP and lowers contractility. It has the advantage of allowing for oral administration after the acute stage of dissection has been managed successfully.

* **The elderly hypertensive patient** (age >60 years) is generally characterized by increased vascular resistance, decreased plasma renin activity, and greater LVH than in younger patients. Often, elderly hypertensive patients have coexisting medical problems that must be considered when initiating antihypertensive therapy. Drug doses should be increased slowly to avoid adverse effects and hypotension. Diuretics as initial therapy have been shown to decrease the incidence of stroke, fatal MI, and overall mortality in this age group (*JAMA 1991;265:3255*). Calcium channel antagonists decrease vascular resistance, have no adverse effects on lipid levels, and are also good choices for elderly patients. ACE inhibitors and ARBs may be effective agents in this population.

○ **African American hypertensive patients** generally have a lower plasma renin level, higher plasma volume, and higher vascular resistance than do Caucasian patients. Thus, African American patients respond well to diuretics, alone or in combination with calcium channel antagonists. ACE inhibitors, ARBs, and β-adrenergic antagonists are also effective agents in this population, particularly when combined with a diuretic.

○ **The obese hypertensive patient** is characterized by more modest elevations in vascular resistance, higher cardiac output, expanded intravascular volume, and lower plasma renin activity at any given level of arterial pressure. Weight reduction is the primary goal of therapy and is effective in reducing BP and causing regression of LVH.

○ **The diabetic patient** with nephropathy may have significant proteinuria and renal insufficiency, which can complicate management (see Chapter 13, Renal Diseases). Control of BP is the most important intervention shown to slow loss of renal function. ACE inhibitors should be used as first-line therapy, because they have been shown to decrease proteinuria and to slow progressive loss of renal function independent of their antihypertensive effects. ACE inhibitors may also be beneficial in reducing the rates of death, MI, and stroke in diabetics who have cardiovascular risk factors but lack left ventricular dysfunction. Hyperkalemia is a common side effect in diabetic patients treated with ACE inhibitors, especially in those with moderate to severe impairment of their GFR. ARBs are also effective antihypertensive agents and have been shown to slow the rate of progression to ESRD, thus supporting a renal protective effect (*N Engl J Med 2001;345(12):861*).

○ **The patient with chronic renal insufficiency** has hypertension that usually is partially volume dependent. Retention of sodium and water exacerbates the existing hypertensive state, and diuretics are important in the management of this problem. When estimated GFR is <30–35 mL/min/1.73 m^2, loop diuretics are the most effective class. In the presence of proteinuria, ACE inhibitors/ARBs should be considered because higher urinary excretion of protein is associated with a more rapid decline in GFR, regardless of the cause of renal insufficiency.

○ **The hypertensive patient with LVH** is at increased risk for sudden death, MI, and all-cause mortality. Although there is no direct evidence, regression of LVH could be expected to reduce the risk for subsequent complications. ACE inhibitors appear to have the greatest effect on regression (*Am J Hypertens 1998;11(6 Pt 1):631*).

○ **The hypertensive patient with CAD** is at increased risk for UA and MI. β-Adrenergic antagonists can be used as first-line agents in these patients because they can decrease cardiac mortality and subsequent reinfarction in the setting of acute MI and can decrease progression to MI in those who present with UA. β-Adrenergic antagonists also have a role in secondary prevention of cardiac events and in increasing long-term survival after MI. Care should be exercised in those with cardiac conduction system disease. ACE inhibitors are beneficial in patients with CAD and decrease mortality in individuals who present with acute MI, especially those with left ventricular dysfunction (*Eur Heart J 1999;20(2):136; N Engl J Med 1991;325(5):293; Lancet 1995;345(8951):669; Lancet 1994;343(8906):1115*).

• **The hypertensive patient with HF** is at risk for progressive left ventricular dilatation and sudden death. In this population, ACE inhibitors decrease mortality (*N Engl J Med 1992;327:685*), and in the setting of acute MI, they decrease the risk of recurrent MI, hospitalization for HF, and mortality (*N Engl J Med 1992;327:669*). ARBs have similar beneficial effects, and they appear to be an effective alternative in patients who are unable to tolerate an ACE inhibitor (*N Engl J Med 2001;345:1667*). Nitrates and hydralazine also decrease mortality in patients with HF irrespective of hypertension, but hydralazine can cause reflex tachycardia and worsening ischemia in patients with unstable coronary syndromes and should be used with caution. Nondihydropyridine calcium channel antagonists should generally be avoided in patients in whom negative inotropic effects would affect their status adversely.

- **In the pregnant patient with hypertension**, there is concern for potential maternal and fetal morbidity and mortality associated with elevated BP and the clinical syndromes of preeclampsia and eclampsia. The possibility of teratogenic or other adverse effects of antihypertensive medications on fetal development also should be considered.
- **Classification of hypertension** during pregnancy has been proposed by the American College of Obstetrics and Gynecology (*Obstet Gynecol 2013;122(5):1122*).
  - **Preeclampsia-eclampsia.** Diagnosis is established if there is *new-onset* hypertension after 20 weeks of gestation and the presence of proteinuria. Elevated SBP ≥140 mm Hg or DBP ≥90 mm Hg on two occasions at least 4 hours apart or a one-time measurement of SBP ≥160 mm Hg or DBP ≥110 mm Hg qualifies as hypertension. If no proteinuria is present, then hypertension along with one of the following qualifies: platelets <100,000/μL, creatinine >1.1 mg/dL (or doubling from baseline), liver transaminases greater than twice the normal, pulmonary edema, or cerebral/visual symptoms. Eclampsia encompasses these parameters in addition to generalized seizures.
  - **Chronic (preexisting) hypertension.** This disorder is defined by a BP ≥140/90 mm Hg before the 20th week of pregnancy.
  - **Chronic hypertension with superimposed preeclampsia.** This classification is used when a woman with chronic hypertension develops worsening hypertension and new proteinuria and/or other features of preeclampsia as outlined previously.
  - **Gestational hypertension.** This disorder is defined by a BP ≥140/90 mm Hg after the 20th week of pregnancy without proteinuria or other features of preeclampsia.
- **Therapy.** Treatment of hypertension in pregnancy should begin if SBP is ≥160 mm Hg or DBP is ≥100 mm Hg.
  - Nonpharmacologic therapy, such as weight reduction and vigorous exercise, is not recommended during pregnancy.
  - Alcohol and tobacco use should be strongly discouraged.
  - Pharmacologic intervention with labetalol, nifedipine, or methyldopa is recommended as first-line therapy because of its proven safety. Other antihypertensives have theoretical disadvantages, but none except the ACE inhibitors have been proven to increase fetal morbidity or mortality.
  - If a patient is suspected of having preeclampsia or eclampsia, urgent referral to an obstetrician who specializes in high-risk pregnancy is recommended.
- **MAOIs.** MAOIs used in association with certain drugs or foods can produce a catecholamine excess state and accelerated hypertension. Interactions are common with tricyclic antidepressants, meperidine, methyldopa, levodopa, sympathomimetic agents, and antihistamines. Tyramine-containing foods that can lead to this syndrome include certain cheeses, red wine, beer, chocolate, chicken liver, processed meat, herring, broad beans, canned figs, and yeast. Nitroprusside, labetalol, and phentolamine have been used effectively in the treatment of accelerated hypertension associated with MAOI use (see Table 3-5).

COMPLICATIONS

Withdrawal syndrome associated with discontinuation of antihypertensive therapy. In substituting therapy in patients with moderate-to-severe hypertension, it is reasonable to increase doses of the new medication in small increments while tapering the previous medication to avoid excessive BP fluctuations. On occasion, an AWS develops, usually within the first 24–72 hours. Occasionally, BP rises to levels that are much higher than those of baseline values. The most severe complications of AWS include encephalopathy, stroke, MI, and sudden death. AWS is associated most commonly with centrally acting adrenergic agents (particularly clonidine) and β-adrenergic antagonists but has been reported with other agents as well, including diuretics. Discontinuation of antihypertensive medications should be done with caution in patients with preexisting cerebrovascular or cardiac disease. Management of AWS by reinstitution of the previously administered drug is generally effective.

MONITORING/FOLLOW-UP

- BP measurements should be performed on multiple occasions under nonstressful circumstances (e.g., rest, sitting, empty bladder, comfortable temperature) to obtain an accurate assessment of BP in a given patient.
- Hypertension should not be diagnosed on the basis of one measurement alone, unless it is >210/120 mm Hg or accompanied by target organ damage. Two or more abnormal readings should be obtained, preferably over a period of several weeks, before therapy is considered.
- Care should also be used to exclude pseudohypertension, which usually occurs in elderly individuals with stiff, noncompressible vessels. A palpable artery that persists after cuff inflation (Osler sign) should alert the physician to this possibility.
- Home and ambulatory BP monitoring can be used to assess a patient's true average BP, which correlates better with target organ damage. Circumstances in which ambulatory BP monitoring might be of value include:
  - Suspected "white-coat hypertension" (increases in BP associated with the stress of physician office visits), which should be evaluated carefully.
  - Evaluation of possible drug resistance, where suspected.

Dyslipidemia

GENERAL PRINCIPLES

- Lipids are sparingly soluble molecules that include cholesterol, fatty acids, and their derivatives.
- Plasma lipids are transported by lipoprotein particles composed of **apolipoproteins**, **phospholipids, free cholesterol, cholesterol esters**, and **triglycerides**.
- Human plasma lipoproteins are separated into **five major classes** based on density:
  - Chylomicrons (least dense)
  - Very-low-density lipoproteins (VLDLs)
  - Intermediate-density lipoproteins (IDLs)
  - Low-density lipoproteins (LDLs)
  - High-density lipoproteins (HDLs)
- A sixth class, lipoprotein(a) [Lp(a)], resembles LDL in lipid composition and has a density that overlaps LDL and HDL.
- Physical properties of plasma lipoproteins are summarized in Table 3-6.
- Nearly 90% of patients with CHD have some form of dyslipidemia. Increased levels of LDL cholesterol, remnant lipoproteins, and Lp(a) and decreased levels of HDL cholesterol have all been associated with an increased risk of premature vascular disease (*Circulation 1992;85:2025; Circulation 1998;97:2519*).
- **Clinical dyslipoproteinemias**
  - Most dyslipidemias are multifactorial in etiology and reflect the effects of genetic influences coupled with diet, inactivity, smoking, alcohol use, and comorbid conditions such as obesity and DM.
  - Differential diagnosis of the major lipid abnormalities is summarized in Table 3-7.
  - The major genetic dyslipoproteinemias are reviewed in Table 3-8 (*Circulation 1974;49:476; J Lipid Res 1990;31:1337; Clin Invest 1993;71:362*).
    - Familial hypercholesterolemia and familial combined hyperlipidemia are disorders that contribute significantly to premature cardiovascular disease.

TABLE 3-6	Physical Properties of Plasma Lipoproteins[a]		
Lipoprotein	**Lipid Composition**	**Origin**	**Apolipoproteins**
Chylomicrons	TG, 85%; chol, 3%	Intestine	A-I, A-IV; B-48; C-I, C-II, C-III; E
VLDL	TG, 55%; chol, 20%	Liver	B-100; C-I, C-II, C-III; E
IDL	TG, 25%; chol, 35%	Metabolic product of VLDL	B-100; C-I, C-II, C-III; E
LDL	TG, 5%; chol, 60%	Metabolic product of IDL	B-100
HDL	TG, 5%; chol, 20%	Liver, intestine	A-I, A-II; C-I, C-II, C-III; E
Lp(a)	TG, 5%; chol, 60%	Liver	B-100; Apo(a)

Chol, cholesterol; HDL, high-density lipoprotein; IDL, intermediate-density lipoprotein; LDL, low-density lipoprotein; Lp(a), lipoprotein(a); TG, triglyceride; VLDL, very-low-density lipoprotein.
[a]Remainder of particle is composed of phospholipid and protein.

TABLE 3-7	Differential Diagnosis of Major Lipid Abnormalities	
Lipid Abnormality	**Primary Disorders**	**Secondary Disorders**
Hypercholesterolemia	Polygenic, familial hypercholesterolemia, familial defective apo B-100	Hypothyroidism, nephrotic syndrome, anorexia nervosa
Hypertriglyceridemia	Lipoprotein lipase deficiency, apo C-II deficiency, apo A-V deficiency, familial hypertriglyceridemia, dysbetalipoproteinemia	Diabetes mellitus, obesity, metabolic syndrome, alcohol use, oral estrogen, renal failure, hypothyroidism, retinoic acid, lipodystrophies
Combined hyperlipidemia	Familial combined hyperlipidemia, dysbetalipoproteinemia	Diabetes mellitus, obesity, metabolic syndrome, nephrotic syndrome, hypothyroidism, lipodystrophies
Low HDL	Familial hypoalphalipoproteinemia, Tangier disease (ABCA1 deficiency), apoA1 mutations, lecithin:cholesterol acyltransferase (LCAT) deficiency	Diabetes mellitus, obesity, metabolic syndrome, hypertriglyceridemia, smoking, anabolic steroids

apo, apolipoprotein; HDL, high-density lipoprotein.

TABLE 3-8	Review of Major Genetic Dyslipoproteinemias			
Type of Genetic Dyslipidemia	**Typical Lipid Profile**	**Type of Inheritance Pattern**	**Phenotypic Features**	**Other Information**
Familial hypercholesterolemia (FH)	• Increased LDL cholesterol (>190 mg/dL) cholesterol • Homozygous form or compound heterozygous form (rare) can have LDL cholesterol >500 mg/dL	Autosomal dominant (prevalence of 1 in 200–500 for heterozygote form and 1 in 250,000 for homozygous form)	• Premature CAD • Tendon xanthomas • Premature arcus corneae (full arc before age 40) • Homozygous form: planar and tendon xanthomas and CAD in childhood and adolescence	Mutations of the LDL receptor, apolipoprotein B-100, and gain-of-function mutations of proprotein convertase/kexin subtype 9 (PCSK9) lead to impaired uptake and degradation of LDL
Familial combined hyperlipidemia (FCH)	• High levels of VLDL, LDL, or both • LDL apo B-100 level >130 mg/dL	Autosomal dominant (prevalence of 1–2%)	• Premature CAD • Patients do *not* develop tendon xanthomas	Genetic and metabolic defects are not established
Familial dysbetalipoproteinemia	• Symmetric elevations of cholesterol and triglycerides (300–500 mg/dL) • Elevated VLDL-to-triglyceride ratio (>0.3)	Autosomal recessive	• Premature CAD • Tuberous or tubero-eruptive xanthomas • Planar xanthomas of the palmar creases are essentially pathognomonic	Mutation of ApoE gene Many homozygotes are normolipidemic, and emergence of hyperlipidemia often requires a secondary metabolic factor such as diabetes mellitus, hypothyroidism, or obesity

Familial hypertriglyceridemia (can result in chylomicronemia syndrome)	• Most patients have triglyceride levels in the range of 150–500 mg/dL • Clinical manifestations may occur when triglyceride levels exceed 1500 mg/dL	• Familial hypertriglyceridemia is an autosomal dominant disorder caused by overproduction of VLDL triglycerides and manifests in adults	• Eruptive xanthomas • Lipemia retinalis • Pancreatitis • Hepatosplenomegaly	Patients may develop the chylomicronemia syndrome in the presence of secondary factors such as obesity, alcohol use, or diabetes
Familial hyperchylomicronemia	• Similar to familial hypertriglyceridemia	• Onset before puberty indicates deficiency of lipoprotein lipase or apo C-II, both autosomal recessive	• Similar to familial hypertriglyceridemia	Homozygosity for mutations in apoAV and GHIHBP1 also found (rare)

CAD, coronary artery disease; GHIHBP1, glycosylphosphatidylinositol–anchored high-density lipoprotein–binding protein 1; LDL, low-density lipoprotein; VLDL, very low-density lipoprotein.

- Familial hypercholesterolemia is an underdiagnosed, autosomal co-dominant condition with a prevalence of 1 in 200 to 1 in 500 people that causes elevated LDL cholesterol levels from birth (*Curr Opin Lipidol 2012;23:282; Eur Heart J 2013;34:3478*). It is associated with significantly increased risk of early cardiovascular disease when untreated (*J Clin Lipidol 2011;5:133*).
- Familial combined hyperlipidemia has a prevalence of 1–2% and typically presents in adulthood, although obesity and high dietary fat and sugar intake have led to increased presentation in childhood and adolescence (*J Clin Endocrinol Metab 2012;97:2969*).
- **Standards of care for hyperlipidemia**
  - LDL cholesterol–lowering therapy, particularly with hydroxymethylglutaryl-coenzyme A (HMG-CoA) reductase inhibitors (commonly referred to as statins), lowers the risk of CHD-related death, morbidity, and revascularization procedures in patients **with** (secondary prevention) (*Lancet 1994;344:1383; N Engl J Med 1996;335:1001; N Engl J Med 1998;339:1349; Lancet 2002;360:7*) **or without** (primary prevention) (*Lancet 2002;360:7; N Engl J Med 1995;333:1301; JAMA 1998;279:1615; Lancet 2003;361:1149; Lancet 2004;364:685*) known CHD.
  - Prevention of atherosclerotic cardiovascular disease (ASCVD) is the primary goal of the 2013 American College of Cardiology (ACC)/American Heart Association (AHA) Guidelines. These guidelines address risk assessment (*Circulation 2014;129:S49*), lifestyle modifications (*Circulation 2014;129:S76*), evaluation and treatment of obesity (*Circulation 2014;129:S102*), and evaluation and management of blood cholesterol (*Circulation 2014;129:S1*).

DIAGNOSIS

Screening

- Screening for hypercholesterolemia should be done **in all adults age 20 years or older** (*Circulation 2014;129:S49*).
- Screening is best performed with a lipid profile (total cholesterol, LDL cholesterol, HDL cholesterol, and triglycerides) obtained after a 12-hour fast.
- If a fasting lipid panel cannot be obtained, total and HDL cholesterol should be measured. Non-HDL cholesterol ≥220 mg/dL may indicate a genetic or secondary cause. A fasting lipid panel is required if non-HDL cholesterol is ≥220 mg/dL or triglycerides are ≥500 mg/dL.
- If the patient does not have an indication for LDL-lowering therapy, screening can be performed every 4–6 years between ages 40–75 (*Circulation 2014;129:S49*).
- Patients hospitalized for an acute coronary syndrome or coronary revascularization should have a lipid panel obtained within 24 hours of admission if lipid levels are unknown.
- Individuals with hyperlipidemia should be evaluated for potential **secondary causes**, including hypothyroidism, DM, obstructive liver disease, chronic renal disease such as nephrotic syndrome, and medications such as estrogens, progestins, anabolic steroids/androgens, corticosteroids, cyclosporine, retinoids, atypical antipsychotics, and antiretrovirals (particularly protease inhibitors).

RISK ASSESSMENT

- The 2013 guidelines identify four groups in whom the benefits of LDL cholesterol–lowering therapy with HMG-CoA reductase inhibitors (statins) clearly outweigh the risks (*Circulation 2014;129:S1*):
  1. Patients with clinical ASCVD
  2. Patients with LDL cholesterol ≥190 mg/dL
  3. Patients with DM age 40–75 years with LDL cholesterol between 70–189 mg/dL
  4. Patients with a calculated ASCVD risk ≥7.5%

- For patients **without** clinical ASCVD or an LDL cholesterol ≥190 mg/dL, the guidelines advise calculating a patient's risk for ASCVD based on age, sex, ethnicity, total and HDL cholesterol, SBP (treated or untreated), presence of DM, and current smoking status (*Circulation 2014;129:S49*).
- The ACC/AHA risk calculator is available at http://my.americanheart.org/cvriskcalculator.
  - For patients of ethnicities other than African American or non-Hispanic white, risk cannot be as well assessed. Use of the non-Hispanic white risk calculation is suggested, with the understanding that risk may be lower than calculated in East Asian Americans and Hispanic Americans and higher in American Indians and South Asians.
  - Ten-year risk should be calculated beginning at age 40 in patients without ASCVD or LDL cholesterol ≥190 mg/dL.
  - Lifetime risk may be calculated in patients age 20–39 and patients age 40–59 with a 10-year risk <7.5% to inform decisions regarding lifestyle modification.

TREATMENT

- The 2013 guidelines recognize lifestyle factors, including diet (*Circulation 2014;129:S76*) and weight management (*Circulation 2014;129:S102*) as an important component of risk reduction for all patients.
- Patients should be advised to adopt a diet that is high in fruits and vegetables, whole grains, fish, lean meat, low-fat dairy, legumes, and nuts, with lower intake of red meat, saturated and trans fats, sweets, and sugary beverages (Table 3-9).
Saturated fat should comprise no more than 5–6% of total calories (*Circulation 2014;129:S76*).
- Physical activity, including aerobic and resistance exercise, is recommended in all patients (*Circulation 2014;129:S76*).
- For all obese patients (body mass index ≥30) and for overweight patients (body mass index ≥25) who have additional risk factors, sustained weight loss of 3–5% or greater reduces ASCVD risk (*Circulation 2014;129:S102*).
- Consultation with a registered dietitian may be helpful to plan, start, and maintain a saturated fat–restricted and weight loss–promoting diet.
- Prior to the start of treatment, there should be a risk discussion between the patient and the clinician. Topics for discussion include:
  - Potential for ASCVD risk reduction benefits
  - Potential for adverse effects and drug–drug interactions
  - Heart-healthy lifestyle and management of other risk factors
  - Patient preferences
- **Clinical ASCVD**
  - Clinical ASCVD includes acute coronary syndromes, history of MI, stable angina, arterial revascularization (coronary or otherwise), stroke, transient ischemic attack, or atherosclerotic peripheral arterial disease.
  - Secondary prevention is an indication for high-intensity statin therapy, which has been shown to reduce events more than moderate-intensity statin therapy. Statin regimens are listed in Table 3-10.
  - If high-dose statin therapy is contraindicated or poorly tolerated or there are significant risks to high-intensity therapy (including age >75 years), moderate-intensity therapy is an option.
- **LDL cholesterol ≥190 mg/dL**
  - These individuals have elevated lifetime risk because of long-term exposure to very high LDL cholesterol levels, and the risk calculator does not account for this.
  - LDL cholesterol should be reduced by at least 50%, primarily with high-intensity statin therapy. If high-intensity therapy is not tolerated, maximum tolerated intensity should be used.

TABLE 3-9	Nutrient Composition of the Therapeutic Lifestyle Change Diet
Nutrient	**Recommended Intake**
Saturated fat[a]	<5–6% of total calories
Polyunsaturated fat	Up to 10% of total calories
Monounsaturated fat	Up to 20% of total calories
Total fat	25–35% of total calories
Carbohydrate[b]	50–60% of total calories
Fiber	20–30 g/d
Protein	Approximately 15% of total calories
Cholesterol	<200 mg/d
Total calories (energy)[c]	Balance energy intake and expenditure to maintain desirable body weight/prevent weight gain

[a]Trans fatty acids are another low-density lipoprotein–raising fat that should be kept at a low intake.
[b]Carbohydrates should be derived predominantly from foods rich in complex carbohydrates, including grains (especially whole grains), fruits, and vegetables.
[c]Daily energy expenditure should include at least moderate physical activity (contributing approximately 200 kcal/d).
From *Circulation* 2014;129:S76.

- Even high-intensity statin therapy may not be sufficient to reduce LDL cholesterol by 50%, and nonstatin therapies are often required to achieve this goal (*J Clin Lipidol 2011;5:S18*).
- LDL apheresis is an optional therapy in patients with homozygous familial hypercholesterolemia and those with severe heterozygous familial hypercholesterolemia with insufficient response to medication. Lomitapide, a microsomal triglyceride transfer protein

TABLE 3-10	Statin Therapy Regimens by Intensity	
High Intensity (↓ LDL ≥50%)	**Medium Intensity (↓ LDL 30–50%)**	**Low Intensity (↓ LDL <30%)**
Atorvastatin 40–80 mg	Atorvastatin 10–*20* mg	*Fluvastatin 20–40 mg*
Rosuvastatin 20–*40* mg	Fluvastatin 40 mg bid, *80 mg XL*	Lovastatin 20 mg
	Lovastatin 40 mg	*Pitavastatin 1 mg*
	Pitavastatin 2–4 mg	Pravastatin 10–20 mg
	Pravastatin 40–*80* mg	*Simvastatin 10 mg*
	Rosuvastatin *5*–10 mg	
	Simvastatin 20–40 mg	

LDL, low-density lipoprotein; ↓, decreased. Italicized doses have not been studied in randomized controlled trials but achieve this level of LDL reduction in clinical use.
From *Circulation* 2014;129:S1.

inhibitor, and mipomersen, an apolipoprotein B antisense oligonucleotide, are new medications indicated for the treatment of patients with homozygous familial hypercholesterolemia (*Eur Heart J 2013;34:3478*).

- ○ Because hyperlipidemia of this degree is often genetically determined, discuss screening of other family members (including children) to identify candidates for treatment. In addition, screen for and treat secondary causes of hyperlipidemia (*Curr Opin Lipidol 2012;23:282*).
- **Patients with diabetes, aged 40–75, LDL cholesterol between 70–189 mg/dL**
  - ○ Using the AHA/ACC risk calculator, calculate 10-year risk of an ASCVD event in these patients (categories: ≥7.5% or <7.5%).
  - ○ If the risk is ≥7.5%, consider high-intensity statin therapy. Otherwise, these patients have an indication for moderate-intensity statin therapy.
- **Patients without diabetes, aged 40–75, LDL cholesterol between 70–189 mg/dL**
  - ○ Using the AHA/ACC risk calculator, calculate 10-year risk of an ASCVD event in these patients (categories: ≥7.5%, between 5.0–7.5%, and <5.0%).
  - ○ A 10-year risk ≥7.5% is an indication for moderate- or high-intensity statin therapy. The decision between moderate- and high-intensity therapy should be made with the patient based on anticipated individualized risks and benefits.
  - ○ A 10-year risk between 5.0–7.5% is reasonable for moderate-intensity statin therapy.
- **Other patient populations**
  - ○ Some patients not described above may still benefit from statin therapy: if the decision on treatment is unclear, the guidelines offer assessment of family history, high-sensitivity C-reactive protein (hs-CRP), coronary artery calcium (CAC) score, or arterial-brachial index (ABI) as options to further define risk (*Circulation 2014;129:S49*; *Circulation 2014;129:S1*).
    - ■ A family history of premature ASCVD is defined as an event in a first-degree male relative before age 55 or in a first-degree female relative before age 65.
    - ■ Higher risk is also indicated by an hs-CRP ≥2 mg/L; CAC ≥300 Agatston units or ≥75th percentile for age, sex, and ethnicity; or ABI ≤0.9.
    - ■ The role of other biomarkers in risk assessment remains uncertain.
    - ■ Depending on patient preference and assessment of risks and benefits, lower LDL cholesterol levels can be considered for treatment (particularly LDL cholesterol ≥160 mg/dL).
    - ■ Patients with diabetes younger than 40 or older than 75 are reasonable candidates for statin therapy based on individual evaluation.
  - ○ Use of statin therapy should be individualized for patients older than 75. In randomized controlled trials, patients older than 75 continued to have benefit from statin therapy, particularly for secondary prevention (*Lancet 2002;360:7*; *Lancet 2002;360:1623*). In addition, many ASCVD events occur in this age group, and patients without other comorbidities may benefit substantially from cardiovascular risk reduction.
  - ○ No official recommendation was made in the guidelines regarding initiation or continuation of statin therapy in patients on maintenance hemodialysis or with New York Heart Association class II–IV ischemic systolic HF. Evidence from randomized controlled trials has not shown a benefit from statin therapy in these subpopulations (*Circulation 2014;129:S1*).
- **Hypertriglyceridemia**
  - ○ Hypertriglyceridemia may be an **independent cardiovascular risk factor** (*Circulation 2007;115:450*; *Ann Intern Med 2007;147:377*; *Circulation 2011;123:2292*).
  - ○ Hypertriglyceridemia is often observed in the metabolic syndrome (*Circulation 2011;123:2292*), and there are many potential etiologies for hypertriglyceridemia, including obesity, DM, renal insufficiency, genetic dyslipidemias, and therapy with oral estrogen, glucocorticoids, β-blockers, tamoxifen, cyclosporine, antiretrovirals, and retinoids.

○ The classification of serum triglyceride levels is as follows (*Circulation 2011;123:2292*): normal: <150 mg/dL; borderline high: 150–199 mg/dL; high: 200–499 mg/dL; and very high: ≥500 mg/dL. The Endocrine Society has added two further categories: severe: 1000–1999 mg/dL (greatly increases the risk of pancreatitis); and very severe: ≥2000 mg/dL (*J Clin Endocrinol Metab 2012;97:2969*).

○ Treatment of hypertriglyceridemia depends on the degree of severity.

▪ For patients with very high triglyceride levels, triglyceride reduction through a very low–fat diet (≤15% of calories), exercise, weight loss, and drugs (fibrates, niacin, ω-3 fatty acids) is the primary goal of therapy to prevent acute pancreatitis.

▪ When patients have a lesser degree of hypertriglyceridemia, controlling the LDL cholesterol level is the primary aim of initial therapy. Lifestyle changes are indicated to lower triglyceride levels (*J Clin Endocrinol Metab 2012;97:2969*).

• **Low HDL cholesterol**

○ Low HDL cholesterol is an **independent ASCVD risk factor** that is identified as a non-LDL cholesterol risk and is included as a component of the ACC/AHA scoring algorithm (*Circulation 2014;129:S49*).

○ Etiologies for low HDL cholesterol include genetic conditions, physical inactivity, obesity, insulin resistance, DM, hypertriglyceridemia, cigarette smoking, high-carbohydrate (>60% of calories) diets, and certain medications (β-blockers, anabolic steroids/androgens, progestins).

○ Because therapeutic interventions for low HDL cholesterol are of limited efficacy, the guidelines recommend considering low HDL cholesterol as a component of overall risk, rather than a specific therapeutic target.

○ There are no clinical trial data showing a benefit of pharmacologic methods of elevating HDL cholesterol.

• **Starting and monitoring therapy**

○ Before starting therapy, guidelines recommend checking alanine aminotransferase (ALT), hemoglobin A1C (if diabetes status is unknown), labs for secondary causes (if indicated), and creatine kinase (if indicated).

○ Evaluate for patient characteristics that increase the risk of adverse events from statins, including impaired hepatic and renal function, history of statin intolerance, history of muscle disorders, unexplained elevations of ALT >3× the upper limit of normal, drugs affecting statin metabolism, Asian ethnicity, and age >75 years (*Circulation 2014;129:S1*).

○ **A repeat fasting lipid panel** is indicated 4–12 weeks after starting therapy to assess adherence, with reassessment every 3–12 months as indicated.

○ In contrast to previous guidelines, therapeutic targets are not recommended because specific targets and a "treat to target" strategy have not been evaluated in randomized controlled trials.

○ In patients without the anticipated level of LDL cholesterol reduction based on intensity of statin therapy (≥50% for high intensity, 30–50% for moderate intensity), assess adherence to therapy and lifestyle modifications, evaluate for intolerance, and consider secondary causes. After evaluation, if the therapeutic response is still insufficient on maximally tolerated statin therapy, it is reasonable to consider adding a nonstatin agent.

○ Creatine kinase should not be routinely checked in patients on statin therapy but is reasonable to measure in patients with muscle symptoms.

○ In 2012, the FDA stated that liver enzyme tests should be performed before starting statin therapy and only as clinically indicated thereafter. The FDA concluded that serious liver injury with statins is rare and unpredictable and that routine monitoring of liver enzymes does not appear to be effective in detecting or preventing serious liver injury. Elevations of liver transaminases 2–3× the upper limit of normal are dose dependent, may decrease on repeat testing even with continuation of statin therapy, and are reversible with discontinuation of the drug.

Treatment of Elevated LDL Cholesterol

- **HMG-CoA reductase inhibitors (statins)**
  - ○ Statins (see Table 3-10) are the treatment of choice for elevated LDL cholesterol and usually lower levels by 30–50% with moderate-intensity and ≥50% with high-intensity statin therapy (*J Clin Lipidol 2011;5:S18*; *N Engl J Med 1999;341:498*; *Circulation 2014;129:S1*).
  - ○ The lipid-lowering effect of statins appears within the first week of use and becomes stable after approximately 4 weeks of use.
  - ○ Common side effects (5–10% of patients) include gastrointestinal upset (e.g., abdominal pain, diarrhea, bloating, constipation) and muscle pain or weakness, which can occur without creatine kinase elevations. Other potential side effects include malaise, fatigue, headache, and rash (*N Engl J Med 1999;341:498*; *Ann Pharmacother 2002;36:1907*; *Circulation 2002;106:1024*).
  - ○ Myalgias are the most common cause of statin discontinuation and are often dose-dependent. They occur more often with increasing age and number of medications and decreasing renal function and body size (*Circulation 2002;106:1024*; *Endocrinol Metab Clin North Am 2009;38:121*).
    - ▪ The AHA/ACC guidelines recommend discontinuing statins in patients who develop muscle symptoms until they can be evaluated. For severe symptoms, evaluate for rhabdomyolysis (*Circulation 2014;129:S1*).
    - ▪ For mild to moderate symptoms, evaluate for conditions increasing the risk of muscle symptoms, including renal or hepatic impairment, hypothyroidism, vitamin D deficiency, rheumatologic disorders, and primary muscle disorders. Statin-induced myalgias are likely to resolve within 2 months of discontinuing the drug.
    - ▪ If symptoms resolve, the same or lower dose of the statin can be reintroduced.
    - ▪ If symptoms recur, use a low dose of a different statin and increase as tolerated.
    - ▪ If the cause of symptoms is determined to be unrelated, restart the original statin.
  - ○ Statins have been associated with an increased incidence of DM. However, the total benefit of statin use usually outweighs the potential adverse effects from an increase in blood sugar (*Lancet 2010;375:735*).
  - ○ Statins have very rarely been associated with reversible cognitive impairment and have not been associated with irreversible or progressive dementia.
  - ○ Because some of the statins undergo metabolism by the cytochrome P450 enzyme system, taking these statins in combination with other drugs metabolized by this enzyme system increases the risk of **rhabdomyolysis** (*N Engl J Med 1999;341:498*; *Ann Pharmacother 2002;36:1907*; *Circulation 2002;106:1024*). Among these drugs are fibrates (greater risk with gemfibrozil), itraconazole, ketoconazole, erythromycin, clarithromycin, cyclosporine, nefazodone, and protease inhibitors (*Circulation 2002;106:1024*).
  - ○ Statins may also interact with large quantities of grapefruit juice to increase the risk of myopathy.
  - ○ Simvastatin can increase the levels of warfarin and digoxin and has significant dose-limiting interactions with amlodipine, amiodarone, dronedarone, verapamil, diltiazem, and ranolazine. Rosuvastatin may also increase warfarin levels.
  - ○ Because a number of drug interactions are possible depending on the statin and other medications being used, drug interaction programs and package inserts should be consulted (*J Clin Lipidol 2014;8:S30*).
  - ○ The use of statins is contraindicated during pregnancy and lactation.
- **Bile acid sequestrant resins**
  - ○ Currently available bile acid sequestrant resins include the following:
    - ▪ **Cholestyramine:** 4–24 g/d PO in divided doses before meals.
    - ▪ **Colestipol:** tablets, 2–16 g/d PO; granules, 5–30 g/d PO in divided doses before meals.
    - ▪ **Colesevelam:** 625-mg tablets, three tablets PO bid or six tablets PO daily (maximum of seven tablets daily) with food; or one packet of oral suspension daily.

- ○ Bile acid sequestrants typically lower LDL cholesterol levels by 15–30% and thereby lower the incidence of CHD (*N Engl J Med 1999;341:498; JAMA 1984;251:351*).
- ○ These agents should not be used as monotherapy in patients with triglyceride levels >250 mg/dL because they can raise triglyceride levels. They may be combined with nicotinic acid or statins.
- ○ Common side effects of resins include constipation, abdominal pain, bloating, nausea, and flatulence.
- ○ Bile acid sequestrants may decrease oral absorption of many other drugs, including warfarin, digoxin, thyroid hormone, thiazide diuretics, amiodarone, glipizide, and statins.
  - ▪ Colesevelam interacts with fewer drugs than do the older resins but can affect the absorption of thyroxine.
  - ▪ Other medications should be given at least 1 hour before or 4 hours after resins.
- **Nicotinic acid (niacin)**
  - ○ Niacin can lower LDL cholesterol levels by ≥15%, lower triglyceride levels by 20–50%, and raise HDL cholesterol levels by up to 35% (*Circulation 2007;115:450; Arch Intern Med 1994;154:1586*).
  - ○ Crystalline niacin is given 1–3 g/d PO in two to three divided doses with meals. Extended-release niacin is dosed at night, with a starting dose of 500 mg PO, and the dose may be titrated monthly in 500-mg increments to a maximum of 2000 mg PO (administer dose with milk, applesauce, or crackers).
  - ○ Common side effects of niacin include flushing, pruritus, headache, nausea, and bloating. Other potential side effects include elevation of liver transaminases, hyperuricemia, and hyperglycemia.
    - ▪ Flushing may be decreased with the use of aspirin 325 mg 30 minutes before the first few doses.
    - ▪ Hepatotoxicity associated with niacin is partially dose dependent and appears to be more prevalent with some over-the-counter time-release preparations.
  - ○ Avoid use of niacin in patients with gout, liver disease, active peptic ulcer disease, and uncontrolled DM.
    - ▪ Niacin can be used with care in patients with well-controlled DM (hemoglobin A1C level ≤7%).
    - ▪ Serum transaminases, glucose, and uric acid levels should be monitored every 6–8 weeks during dose titration and then every 4 months.
  - ○ The use of niacin in patients with well-controlled LDL cholesterol levels (with statins) has not been shown to be of benefit in clinical trials (*N Engl J Med 2011;365:2255; Eur Heart J 2013;34:1279*). Niacin can be useful as an additional agent in patients with severely elevated LDL cholesterol levels.
- **Ezetimibe**
  - ○ Ezetimibe is currently the only available cholesterol-absorption inhibitor. It appears to act at the brush border of the small intestine and inhibits cholesterol absorption.
  - ○ Ezetimibe may provide an additional 25% mean reduction in LDL cholesterol when combined with a statin and provides an approximately 18% decrease in LDL cholesterol when used as monotherapy (*Am J Cardiol 2002;90:1092; Eur Heart J 2003;24:729; Am J Cardiol 2002;90:1084; Mayo Clin Proc 2004;79:620*).
  - ○ The recommended dosing is 10 mg PO once daily. No dosage adjustment is required for renal insufficiency and mild hepatic impairment or in elderly patients. It is not recommended for use in patients with moderate to severe hepatic impairment.
  - ○ Side effects are infrequent and include gastrointestinal symptoms (e.g., diarrhea, abdominal pain) and myalgias.
  - ○ In clinical trials, there was no excess of rhabdomyolysis or myopathy when compared with statin or placebo alone.

○ Liver enzymes should be monitored when used in conjunction with fenofibrate but are not required in monotherapy or with a statin.
○ A clinical outcome trial showed decreased reduction of cardiovascular events with the combination of simvastatin and ezetimibe compared to placebo in patients with chronic renal failure (*Lancet 2011;377:2181*). The recently completed IMPROVE-IT trial showed a reduction in cardiovascular end points when ezetimibe was added to simvastatin in high-risk patients with already low LDL levels (*American Heart Association Scientific Sessions 2014*).
○ Ezetimibe is useful in patients with familial hypercholesterolemia who do not achieve adequate LDL cholesterol reductions with statin therapy alone (*J Clin Lipidol 2011;5:S38*).

Treatment of Hypertriglyceridemia

• **Nonpharmacologic treatment**
Nonpharmacologic treatments are important in the therapy of hypertriglyceridemia. Approaches include the following:
○ Changing oral estrogen replacement to transdermal estrogen
○ Decreasing alcohol intake
○ Encouraging weight loss and exercise
○ Controlling hyperglycemia in patients with DM
○ Avoiding simple sugars and very high–carbohydrate diets (*Circulation 2011;123:2292; J Clin Endocrinol Metab 2012;97:2969*)
• **Pharmacologic treatment**
○ Pharmacologic treatment of severe hypertriglyceridemia consists of a fibric acid derivative (fibrates), niacin, or ω-3 fatty acids.
○ Patients with severe hypertriglyceridemia (>1000 mg/dL) should be treated with pharmacotherapy in addition to reduction of dietary fat, alcohol, and simple carbohydrates to decrease the risk of pancreatitis.
○ Statins may be effective for patients with mild to moderate hypertriglyceridemia and concomitant LDL cholesterol elevation (*Circulation 2011;123:2292; J Clin Endocrinol Metab 2012;97:2969; N Engl J Med 2007;357:1009*).
○ **Fibric acid derivatives**
  ▪ Currently available fibric acid derivatives include the following:
    □ **Gemfibrozil:** 600 mg PO bid before meals
    □ **Fenofibrate:** available in several forms, dosage typically 48–145 mg/d PO
  ▪ Fibrates generally lower triglyceride levels by 30–50% and increase HDL cholesterol levels by 10–35%. They can lower LDL cholesterol levels by 5–25% in patients with normal triglyceride levels but may actually increase LDL cholesterol levels in patients with elevated triglyceride levels (*N Engl J Med 2007;357:1009; Lancet 2005;366:1849*).
  ▪ Common side effects include dyspepsia, abdominal pain, cholelithiasis, rash, and pruritus.
  ▪ Fibrates may potentiate the effects of warfarin (*N Engl J Med 1999;341:498*). Gemfibrozil given in conjunction with statins may increase the risk of rhabdomyolysis (*Circulation 2002;106:1024; Am J Med 2004;116:408; Am J Cardiol 2004;94:935; Am J Cardiol 2005;95:120*).
○ **ω-3 Fatty acids**
  ▪ High doses of ω-3 fatty acids from fish oil can lower triglyceride levels (*J Clin Invest 1984;74:82; J Lipid Res 1990;31:1549*).
  ▪ The active ingredients are eicosapentaenoic acid (EPA) and docosahexaenoic acid (DHA).
  ▪ To lower triglyceride levels, 1–6 g of ω-3 fatty acids, either EPA alone or with DHA, are needed daily.
  ▪ Main side effects are burping, bloating, and diarrhea.

- Prescription forms of ω-3 fatty acids are available and are indicated for triglyceride levels >500 mg/dL. One preparation contains EPA and DHA; four tablets contain about 3.6 g of ω-3 acid ethyl esters and can lower triglyceride levels by 30–40%. Other preparations contain only EPA or contain unesterified EPA and DHA.
- In practice, ω-3 fatty acids are being used as an adjunct to statins or other drugs in patients with moderately elevated triglyceride levels.
- The combination of ω-3 fatty acids plus a statin has the advantage of avoiding the risk of myopathy seen with statin–fibrate combinations (*Am J Cardiol 2008;102:429*; *Am J Cardiol 2008;102:1040*).

Treatment of Low HDL Cholesterol

- Low HDL cholesterol often occurs in the setting of hypertriglyceridemia and metabolic syndrome. Management of accompanying high LDL cholesterol, hypertriglyceridemia, and the metabolic syndrome may result in improvement of HDL cholesterol (*Circulation 2001;104:3046*).
- Nonpharmacologic therapies are the mainstay of treatment, including the following:
  ○ Smoking cessation
  ○ Exercise
  ○ Weight loss
- In addition, medications known to lower HDL levels, such as β-blockers (except carvedilol), progestins, and androgenic compounds, should be avoided.
- No clinical outcomes trials have shown a clear benefit to pharmacologic treatment for raising HDL cholesterol.

4 Ischemic Heart Disease

Marc A. Sintek and Philip M. Barger

Coronary Heart Disease and Stable Angina

GENERAL PRINCIPLES

Definition

- Coronary artery disease (CAD) refers to the luminal narrowing of a coronary artery, usually due to atherosclerosis. CAD is the leading contributor to ischemic heart disease (IHD). IHD includes angina pectoris, myocardial infarction (MI), and silent myocardial ischemia.
- Cardiovascular disease (CVD) includes IHD, cardiomyopathy, heart failure, arrhythmia, hypertension, cerebrovascular accident (CVA), diseases of the aorta, peripheral vascular disease (PVD), valvular heart disease, and congenital heart disease.
- Stable angina is defined as angina symptoms or angina equivalent symptoms that are reproduced by consistent levels of activity and relieved by rest.
- American Heart Association/American College of Cardiology (AHA/ACC) guidelines provide a more through overview of stable IHD (*J Am Coll Cardiol 2012;60:e44*; update *J Am Coll Cardiol 2014;64:1929*).

Epidemiology

- In the United States, IHD is the cause of one of every six deaths (*Circulation 2013;127:e6*).
- The lifetime risk of IHD at age 40 is one in two for men and one in three for women.
- There are more than 15 million Americans with IHD, 50% of whom have chronic angina.
- CVD has become an important cause of death worldwide, accounting for nearly 30% of all deaths, and has become increasingly significant in developing nations.
- Death due to CVD continues to decline in large part due to adherence to current guidelines.

Etiology

- CAD most commonly results from luminal accumulation of atheromatous plaque.
- Other causes of obstructive CAD include congenital coronary anomalies, myocardial bridging, vasculitis, and prior radiation therapy.
- Apart from obstructive CAD, other causes of angina include cocaine use, valvular and nonvalvular aortic stenosis, hypertrophic cardiomyopathy, left ventricular hypertrophy (LVH), malignant hypertension, dilated cardiomyopathy, spontaneous coronary dissection, and coronary vasospasm/Prinzmetal angina.
- Any factor that reduces myocardial oxygen supply or increases demand can cause or exacerbate angina (Table 4-1).

Pathophysiology

- Stable angina results from progressive luminal obstruction of angiographically visible epicardial coronary arteries or, less commonly, obstruction of the microvasculature, which results in a mismatch between myocardial oxygen supply and demand.
- Atherosclerosis is an inflammatory process, initiated by lipid deposition in the arterial intima layer followed by recruitment of inflammatory cells and proliferation of arterial smooth muscle cells to form an atheroma.
  - The coronary lesions responsible for stable angina differ from the vulnerable plaques associated with acute MI. The stable angina lesion is fixed and is less prone to fissuring, hence producing symptoms that are more predictable (*Circulation 2012;125:1147*).

TABLE 4-1	Conditions That May Provoke or Exacerbate Ischemia/Angina Independent of Worsening Atherosclerosis

Increased Oxygen Demand	Decreased Oxygen Supply
Noncardiac	
Hyperthermia	Anemia
Hyperthyroidism	Sickle cell disease
Sympathomimetic toxicity	Hypoxemia
(i.e., cocaine use)	*Pneumonia*
Hypertension	*Asthma exacerbation*
Anxiety	*Chronic obstructive pulmonary disease*
	Pulmonary hypertension
	Pulmonary fibrosis
	Obstructive sleep apnea
	Pulmonary embolus
	Sympathomimetic toxicity (i.e., cocaine use, pheochromocytoma)
	Hyperviscosity
	Polycythemia
	Leukemia
	Thrombocytosis
	Hypergammaglobulinemia
Cardiac	
Hypertrophic cardiomyopathy	Aortic stenosis
Aortic stenosis	Elevated left ventricular end-diastolic
Dilated cardiomyopathy	pressure
Tachycardia	Hypertrophic cardiomyopathy
Ventricular	Microvascular disease
Supraventricular	

Adapted from AHA/ACC Guidelines on Stable Ischemic Heart Disease. *J Am Coll Cardiol* 2012;60:e44.

- All coronary lesions are eccentric and do not uniformly alter the inner circumference of the artery.
- Epicardial coronary lesions causing less than 40% luminal narrowing generally do not significantly impair coronary flow.
- Moderate angiographic lesions (40–70% obstruction) may interfere with flow and are routinely underestimated on coronary angiograms given the eccentricity of CAD.

Risk Factors

- Of IHD events, >90% can be attributed to elevations in at least one major risk factor (*JAMA 2003;290:891*).
- Assessment of traditional CVD risk factors includes:
  - Age
  - Blood pressure (BP)
  - Blood sugar (Note: Diabetes is considered an IHD risk equivalent.)
  - Lipid profile (low-density lipoprotein [LDL], high-density lipoprotein [HDL], triglycerides); direct LDL for nonfasting samples or very high triglycerides

- ○ Tobacco use (Note: Smoking cessation restores the risk of IHD to that of a nonsmoker within approximately 15 years.) (*Arch Intern Med 1994;154(2):169*)
- ○ Family history of premature CAD: Defined as first-degree male relative with IHD before age 55 years or female relative before age 65 years
- ○ Measures for obesity, particularly central obesity; body mass index goal is between 18.5–24.9 kg/m^2; waist circumference goal is <40 inches for men and <35 inches for women
- As of 2013, AHA/ACC guidelines recommend assessing 10-year atherosclerotic cardiovascular disease (ASCVD) risk for patients age 40–79 years using new race and age-specific pooled cohort equations (*J Am Coll Cardiol 2014;63:2935*).
  - ○ The ASCVD risk calculator is available online (*http://tools.cardiosource.org/ASCVD-Risk-Estimator/*).
  - ○ If there remains uncertainty about lower risk estimates, high-sensitivity C-reactive protein (≥2 mg/dL), coronary artery calcium score (≥300 Agatston units or ≥75th percentile), or ankle-brachial index (<0.9) may be obtained to revise risk estimates upward.
  - ○ Traditional risk factors noted above should be assessed in patients younger than age 40 and every 4–6 years after 40; 10-year ASCVD risk should be calculated every 4–6 years in patients 40–79 years of age.
  - ○ Lifetime risk can be assessed using the ASCVD risk calculator and may be helpful in the setting of counseling patients about lifestyle modifications.

Prevention

Primary prevention: See Chapter 3, Preventive Cardiology

Clinical Presentation

History
- Angina: **Typical angina has three features**: (1) substernal chest discomfort with a characteristic quality and duration that is (2) provoked by stress or exertion and (3) relieved by rest or nitroglycerin.
  - ○ **Atypical angina** has two of these three characteristics.
  - ○ **Noncardiac chest pain** meets one or none of these characteristics.
- Chronic stable angina is reproducibly precipitated in a predictable manner by exertion or emotional stress and relieved within 5–10 minutes by sublingual nitroglycerin or rest.
- The severity of angina may be quantified using the Canadian Cardiovascular Society (CCS) classification system (Table 4-2).

TABLE 4-2	Canadian Cardiovascular Society (CCS) Classification System
Class	**Definition**
CCS 1	Angina with strenuous or prolonged activity
CCS 2	Angina with moderate activity (walking greater than two level blocks or one flight of stairs)
CCS 3	Angina with mild activity (walking less than two level blocks or one flight of stairs)
CCS 4	Angina that occurs with any activity or at rest

Anginal symptoms may include typical chest discomfort or anginal equivalents.
From Sangareddi V, Anand C, Gnanavelu G, et al. Canadian Cardiovascular Society classification of effort angina: an angiographic correlation. *Coron Artery Dis* 2004;15:111–4.

TABLE 4-3	Pretest Probability of Coronary Artery Disease by Age, Gender, and Symptoms							
Age (y)	**Asymptomatic**		**Nonanginal Chest Pain**		**Atypical/Probable Angina Pectoris**		**Typical/Definite Angina Pectoris**	
Gender	**Women**	**Men**	**Women**	**Men**	**Women**	**Men**	**Women**	**Men**
30–39	<5	<5	2	4	12	34	26	76
40–49	<5	<10	3	13	22	51	55	87
50–59	<5	<10	7	20	31	65	73	93
60–69	<5	<5	14	27	51	72	86	94
	Very Low <5%		**Low <10%**		**Intermediate 10–80%**		**High >80%**	

Data from Gibbons RJ, Balady GJ, Bricker JT, et al. ACC/AHA 2002 guideline update for exercise testing: summary article. A report of the ACC/AHA Task Force on Practice Guidelines (Committee to Update the 1997 Exercise Testing Guidelines). *Circulation* 2002;106:1883.

- Associated symptoms may include dyspnea, diaphoresis, nausea, vomiting, dizziness, jaw pain, and left arm pain.
- Female patients and those with diabetes or chronic kidney disease may have minimal or atypical symptoms that serve as anginal equivalents. Such symptoms include dyspnea (most common), epigastric pain, and nausea.
- The clinician's assessment of the pretest probability of IHD is the important driver for further diagnostic testing in patients without known CAD and is largely ascertained from the clinical history (Table 4-3). Patients with a low pretest probability (<5%) of CAD are unlikely to benefit from further diagnostic testing aimed at detecting CAD.

Physical Examination
- Clinical exam should include measurement of BP, heart rate, and arterial pulses.
- Exam findings of a mitral regurgitation (MR) murmur or aortic stenosis murmur can alert the clinician to additional CVD that may be contributing to symptoms of angina.
- Stigmata of hyperlipidemia such as corneal arcus and xanthelasmas should be noted.
- Signs of heart failure, such as an S_3 gallop, inspiratory crackles on lung exam, elevated jugular venous pulsation, and peripheral edema, are also high-risk exam findings.
- Vascular exam should include palpitation of radial, femoral, popliteal, posterior tibial, and dorsalis pedis pulses bilaterally to compare differences. Auscultation with the bell of the stethoscope should be performed to evaluate for femoral or carotid bruits.
- Pain that is reproducible on physical exam suggests a musculoskeletal cause of chest pain but does not exclude the presence of CAD.

Differential Diagnosis
- A wide range of disorders may manifest with chest discomfort and may include both cardiovascular and noncardiovascular etiologies (Table 4-4).
- A careful history focused on cardiac risk factors, physical exam, and initial laboratory evaluation usually narrows the differential diagnosis.
- In patients with established IHD, always look for exacerbating factors that contribute to ischemia (see Table 4-1).

TABLE 4-4	Differential Diagnosis of Chest Pain Excluding Epicardial Atherosclerosis
Diagnosis	**Comments**
Cardiovascular	
Aortic stenosis	Anginal episodes can occur with severe aortic stenosis.
HCM	Subendocardial ischemia may occur with exercise and/or exertion.
Prinzmetal angina	Coronary vasospasm that may be elicited by exertion or emotional stress.
Pericarditis	Pleuritic chest pain associated with pericardial inflammation from infectious or autoimmune disease.
Aortic dissection	May mimic anginal pain and/or involve the coronary arteries.
Cocaine use	Results in coronary vasospasm and/or thrombus formation.
Other	
Anemia	Marked anemia can result in a myocardial O_2 supply–demand mismatch.
Thyrotoxicosis	Increase in myocardial demand may result in an O_2 supply–demand mismatch.
Esophageal disease	GERD and esophageal spasm can mimic angina (responsive to NTG).
Biliary colic	Gallstones can usually be visualized on abdominal sonography.
Respiratory diseases	Pneumonia with pleuritic pain, pulmonary embolism, pulmonary hypertension
Musculoskeletal	Costochondritis, cervical radiculopathy

GERD, gastroesophageal reflux disease; HCM, hypertrophic cardiomyopathy; NTG, nitroglycerin.

Diagnostic Testing

- **General diagnostic testing**
  - A resting ECG can be helpful in determining the presence of prior infarcts or conduction system disease and may alert the clinician to the possibility of CAD in patients with chest pain.
  - Chest radiography can be used to evaluate for cardiomegaly, heart failure, or vascular disease (pulmonary and aortic) that can be important in the management of patients with chest pain or IHD.
  - A transthoracic echocardiogram (TTE) can be useful in determining presence of left ventricular (LV) dysfunction or valvular heart disease that may affect the management and diagnosis of IHD. TTE can also be used to assess for resting wall motion abnormalities that may be the result of prior MI.
  - Evidence of vascular disease or prior MI on the diagnostic testing modalities noted above should raise the pretest probability of IHD in patients presenting with chest pain.

- **Stress testing overview**
  - All stress testing requires a cardiovascular stress and way of imaging cardiac changes consistent with ischemia; stress and imaging methods are chosen by the clinician to meet the diagnostic needs of the patient.
  - Many stress testing modalities provide not only detection of ischemia/CAD but also prognostic information based on the burden of ischemia.
  - Table 4-5 provides an overview of the sensitivity and specificity for each stress and imaging modality along with advantages and disadvantages for the clinician to consider.
- **Stress testing indications**
  - Patients without known CAD:
    - Not indicated in asymptomatic patients as a screening test
    - Patients with anginal symptoms who are intermediate risk
    - Asymptomatic intermediate-risk patients who plan on beginning a vigorous exercise program or those with high-risk occupations (e.g., airline pilot)
    - Atypical symptoms in patients with a high risk of IHD (i.e., diabetes or vascular disease patients)
  - Patients with known CAD:
    - Post-MI risk stratification (see section on ST-segment elevation MI)
    - Preoperative risk assessment if it will change management prior to surgery
    - Recurrent anginal symptoms despite medical therapy or revascularization
    - Routine screening in asymptomatic patients after revascularization is controversial
- **Contraindications to stress testing**
  - Acute MI within 2 days
  - Unstable angina not previously stabilized by medical therapy
  - Cardiac arrhythmias causing symptoms or hemodynamic compromise
  - Symptomatic severe aortic stenosis
  - Symptomatic heart failure
  - Acute pulmonary embolus, myocarditis, pericarditis, or aortic dissection
- **Exercise stress testing**
  - The test of choice for evaluating most patients of intermediate risk for CAD (see Table 4-3).
  - Bruce protocol: Consists of 3-minute stages of increasing treadmill speed and incline. BP, heart rate, and ECG are monitored throughout the study and the recovery period.
  - The study is considered positive if:
    - New ST-segment depressions of >1 mm in multiple contiguous leads
    - Hypotensive response to exercise
    - Sustained ventricular arrhythmias are precipitated by exercise
  - The Duke Treadmill Score provides prognostic information for patients presenting with chronic angina (Table 4-6).
  - When exercise testing is combined with imaging (stress echocardiography or perfusion imaging) and the test is normal at the target heart rate for age, the risk of infarction or death from CVD is <1% annually in patients with no prior history of IHD. In patients who cannot exercise and require pharmacologic testing, the annual risk of infarction or death in a normal study doubles (2% per year), further underscoring the importance of the inability to perform physical activity as a contribution to increased cardiovascular risk.
- **Stress testing with imaging**
  - Recommended for patients with the following baseline ECG abnormalities:
    - Preexcitation (Wolf-Parkinson-White syndrome)
    - LVH
    - Left bundle branch block (LBBB) or paced rhythm

TABLE 4-5	Diagnostic Accuracy of Common Stress Testing Modalities in Patients Without Known Ischemic Heart Disease				
Test Type	Sensitivity	Specificity	Advantages	Disadvantages
ECG				
Exercise	61%	70–77%	• Easy to perform • Inexpensive	• Less diagnostic accuracy; especially in women • No viability assessment
Pharmacologic	—	—		
Echocardiography				
Exercise	70–85%	77–89%	• Gather other important information on diastolic function, valvular disorders, and pulmonary pressures • Can assess viability with pharmacologic stress	• Limited by image quality • Diagnostic accuracy reduced with resting wall motion abnormalities
Pharmacologic (dobutamine)	85–90%	79–90%		
Nuclear Perfusion Imaging				
Exercise	82–88%	70–88%	• More sensitive for small areas of ischemia/infarct • Very accurate ejection fraction assessment • Easy to compare to prior studies	• Significant radiation • May underestimate severe balanced ischemia • No other valve or other structural information • Viability may require separate testing
Pharmacologic (adencsine, regadenoson, or dobutamine)	82–91%	75–90%		
Cardiac MRI				
Exercise	—	—	• Excellent assessment of viability • Anatomic detail of heart and great vessels superb	• Expensive • Requires closed MRI • Exercise option not typically available
Pharmacologic[a]	91%	81%		

All diagnostic accuracies unadjusted for referral bias; data from *J Am Coll Cardiol* 2012;60:e44.
[a]Vasodilator stress only; dobutamine has sensitivity of 83% and specificity of 86%.

TABLE 4-6	Exercise Stress Testing: Duke Treadmill Score	

Duke Treadmill Score (DTS) = Minutes exercised − [5 × maximum ST-segment deviation] − [4 × angina score]. Angina score: 0 = none, 1 = not test limiting, 2 = test limiting

DTS

5	Annual mortality 0.25%	Low-risk study
−10 to 4	Annual mortality 1.25%	Intermediate-risk study
<−10	Annual mortality >5%	High-risk study

In general, β-blockers, other nodal blocking agents, and nitrates should be discontinued prior to stress testing.
Data from *N Engl J Med* 1991;325:849.

- Intraventricular conduction delay (IVCD)
- Resting ST-segment or T-wave changes
- Patients unable to exercise or who do not have an interpretable ECG at rest or with exercise
- May be considered in patients with high pretest probability of IHD who have not met the threshold of invasive angiography
  ○ **Myocardial perfusion imaging:** Commonly uses tracers that emit radiation detected by a camera in conjunction with exercise or pharmacologic stress. Perfusion imaging compares rest perfusion to stress perfusion images to discern areas of ischemia or infarct. It can be limited by body habitus, breast attenuation, and quality of the acquisition and processing of images. Severe CAD may cause balanced reduction in perfusion and an underestimation of ischemic burden.
  ○ **Echocardiographic imaging:** Exercise or dobutamine stress testing can be performed with echocardiography to aid in the diagnosis of CAD. Echocardiography adds to the sensitivity and specificity of the test by revealing areas with wall motion abnormalities. The technical quality of this study can be limited by imaging quality (i.e., obesity).
  ○ **Magnetic resonance perfusion imaging:** MRI sequences obtained with contrast and vasodilator stress testing. Exercise testing requires an MRI-compatible ergometer and has been done in select cases with success. Advantage of having viability assessment without additional testing and provides evaluation for other causes of myocardial dysfunction that may mimic IHD (i.e., sarcoidosis or infiltrative cardiomyopathies). Cannot be performed in patients with implanted cardiac devices (i.e., defibrillators and pacemakers).
- **Pharmacologic stress testing**
  ○ In patients who are unable to exercise, pharmacologic stress testing may be preferable.
  ○ Dipyridamole, adenosine, and regadenoson are vasodilators that are commonly used in conjunction with myocardial perfusion scintigraphy. These are the agents of choice in patients with LBBB or paced rhythm on ECG due to the increased incidence of false-positive stress tests with either exercise or dobutamine infusion. Technically, these agents do not impose a physiologic stress. Relative ischemia across a coronary vascular bed is elucidated as healthy vessels dilate more than diseased vessels with fixed obstruction. This in turn leads to relative changes in perfusion that are reflected in the postvasodilator images.
  ○ Dobutamine is a positive inotrope commonly used with echocardiographic stress tests and may be augmented with atropine to achieve target heart rate for age.

Diagnostic Procedures
- **Coronary angiography**
  - The gold standard for evaluating epicardial coronary anatomy because it quantifies the presence and severity of atherosclerotic lesions and provides prognostic information based on the extent and severity of CAD.
  - Coronary angiography is invasive and is associated with a small risk of death, MI, CVA, bleeding, arrhythmia, and vascular complications. Therefore, it is reserved for patients whose risk–benefit ratio favors an invasive approach such as:
    - ST-segment elevation MI (STEMI) patients
    - Most unstable angina (UA)/non–ST-segment elevation MI (NSTEMI) patients
    - Symptomatic patients with high-risk stress tests who are expected to benefit from revascularization
    - Class III and IV angina despite medical therapy (see Table 4-2)
    - Survivors of sudden cardiac death or those with serious ventricular arrhythmias
    - Signs or symptoms of heart failure or decreased LV function
    - Angina that is inadequately controlled with medical therapy for the patient's lifestyle
    - Previous coronary artery bypass grafting (CABG) or percutaneous coronary intervention (PCI)
    - Suspected/known left main ($\geq$50% stenosis) or severe three-vessel CAD
    - To diagnose CAD in patients with angina who have not undergone stress testing due to a high pretest probability of having CAD (see Table 4-3)
  - Can be both diagnostic and therapeutic if PCI is needed.
  - Can be used to evaluate patients who are suspected of having a nonatherosclerotic cause of ischemia (e.g., coronary anomaly, coronary dissection, radiation vasculopathy).
  - Intravascular ultrasound (IVUS) can be used to directly visualize plaque burden and plaque anatomy.
  - Functional significance of intermediate stenotic lesions (50–70% narrowing) can further be assessed by fractional flow reserve (FFR).
    - FFR is calculated by determining the ratio of pressure distal to the coronary obstruction to that of the aortic pressure at maximal hyperemia (flow).
    - An FFR $\leq$0.8 is considered flow limiting, and PCI improves urgent revascularization for UA or MI and potentially improves cardiovascular mortality compared to medical therapy (*N Engl J Med 2014;371:1208*).
  - Measurement of LV filling pressures (diastolic function) and aortic and mitral valve gradients, assessment of regional wall motion and LV function, and assessment for certain aortopathies can be accomplished by placing a catheter in the LV cavity or aorta directly and making the appropriate pressure measurements and/or injection of contrast.
- **Contrast-induced nephropathy (CIN)** occurs in up to 5% of patients undergoing coronary angiography and is more common in patients with baseline renal insufficiency and diabetics. In most patients, creatinine returns to baseline within 7 days. The following are considerations in the prevention of CIN:
  - The volume of contrast media used should be minimized, and patients with a creatinine clearance <60 mL/min should be considered for a staged procedure.
  - Adequate hydration with isotonic crystalloid should be given prior to angiography. We recommend 3 mL/kg bolus of normal saline at least 6 hours prior to the procedure with a 1-mL/kg continuous infusion rate until procedure start.
  - IV diuretics should be held if possible.
  - High-potency statins should be continued or initiated on the evening prior to and morning of the procedure (*J Am Coll Cardiol 2014;63:12S*). We recommend atorvastatin 40–80 mg or continuation of comparable home statin therapy.
  - All patients should receive some CIN prophylactic therapy: oral hydration, IV hydration, held diuretics, or statin therapy.

○ Nonionic low-osmolar contrast agents should be used.
○ *N*-Acetyl-L-cysteine may not be useful in the prevention of CIN.
○ National Cardiovascular Data Registry Acute Kidney Injury Risk Model is a robust risk stratification tool for acute kidney injury and the need for hemodialysis after cardiac catheterization (*J Am Heart Assoc 2014;3:e001380*) (Table 4-7).

• **Cardiac CT**
○ A noninvasive technique used to establish a diagnosis of CAD. Like cardiac angiography, it exposes the patient to both radiation and contrast material. CT has a high negative predictive value and hence is better suited for symptomatic patients with low to intermediate pretest probability for CAD to rule out disease, such as a patient with repeated emergency room admissions for chest pain or patients with equivocal stress test results.
○ Recent results from the PROMISE trial suggest no advantage of CT imaging over stress testing for patients with intermediate risk of IHD presenting with chest pain in reducing major adverse clinical events. Patients imaged with CT were less likely to have normal coronary angiography, and CT appears to be a safe diagnostic test when evaluating chest pain in this population (*N Engl J Med 2015;372:1291*).
○ May aid in identification of congenital anomalies of the coronary arteries.
○ Due to diminished study quality, it is not useful in patients with extensive coronary calcification, coronary stents, or small-caliber vessels.

TREATMENT

• The major goal of treatment is to reduce symptoms.
• An absolute reduction in incidence of MI or cardiac death in patients with stable IHD is accomplished mainly through medical therapy and not revascularization.
• A combination of lifestyle modification, medical therapy, and coronary revascularization can be used. A recommended strategy for the evaluation and management of the patient with stable angina can be found in Figure 4-1.
• **Medical treatment** is aimed at improving myocardial oxygen supply, reducing myocardial oxygen demand, controlling exacerbating factors (i.e., anemia), and limiting the development of further atherosclerotic disease.
• Medical treatment often is sufficient to control anginal symptoms in chronic stable angina.

Medications

• **Antiplatelet therapy**
○ **Acetylsalicylic acid (ASA)** (75–162 mg/d) reduces cardiovascular events, including repeat revascularization, MI, and cardiac death, by approximately 33% (*BMJ 1994;308:81*; *Lancet 1992;114:1421*).
○ ASA 81 mg appears to be sufficient for most patients (primary or secondary prevention for both IHD and CVA).
○ ASA desensitization may be performed in patients with ASA allergy.
○ **Clopidogrel** (75 mg/d) can be used in those allergic/intolerant of ASA.

• **Anti-ischemic therapy**
○ **β-Adrenergic antagonists** (Table 4-8) control anginal symptoms by decreasing heart rate and myocardial work, leading to reduced myocardial oxygen demand.
  ▪ β-Blockers with intrinsic sympathomimetic activity should be avoided.
  ▪ Dosage can be adjusted to result in a resting heart rate of 50–60 bpm.
  ▪ Use with caution or avoid in patients with active bronchospasm, atrioventricular (AV) block, resting bradycardia, or poorly compensated heart failure (HF).

TABLE 4-7	NCDR AKI Risk Model: Risk of AKI and AKI Resulting in HD in Patients Undergoing PCI (points are determined by the points column and total points are converted to risk in the risk conversion column)

Points			Risk Conversion			
	AKI	AKI+HD	Points Total	Risk AKI (%)	Points Total	Risk HD (%)
Variables			0	1.9	≤6	<1
			5	2.6	7	1.5
Age ≤50	0		10	3.6	8	2.6
50–59	2		15	4.9	9	4.4
60–69	4		20	6.7	10	7.6
70–79	6		25	9.2	11	12.6
80–89	8		30	12.4	12	20.3
>90	10		35	16.5	13	31.0
Heart failure within 2 wk	11	2	40	21.7		
GFR ≤30	18	5	45	27.9		
GFR 31–44	8	3	50	35.1		
GFR 45–59	3	1	55	43		
Diabetes mellitus	7	1	>60	51.4		
Any prior heart failure	4	—				
Any prior cerebrovascular disease/stoke	4	—				
Anemia (Hgb <10 g/dL)	10	—				
NSTEMI/UA presentation	6	1				
STEMI presentation	15	2				
Shock prior to procedure	16	–				
Cardiac arrest prior to procedure	8	3				
IABP use	11	–				

AKI, acute kidney injury; GFR, glomerular filtration rate; HD, hemodialysis; Hgb, hemoglobin; IABP, intra-aortic balloon counterpulsation; NCDR, National Cardiovascular Data Registry; NSTEMI, non–ST-segment elevation myocardial infarction; PCI, percutaneous coronary intervention; STEMI, ST-segment elevation myocardial infarction; UA, unstable angina. GFR calculated using the Modification of Diet in Renal Disease (MDRD) formula; AKI defined as at least a ≥0.3 mg/dL increase or ≥1.5-fold relative increase in creatinine after procedure or initiation of dialysis (HD) after procedure. Patients were excluded if on dialysis at the time of the procedure.

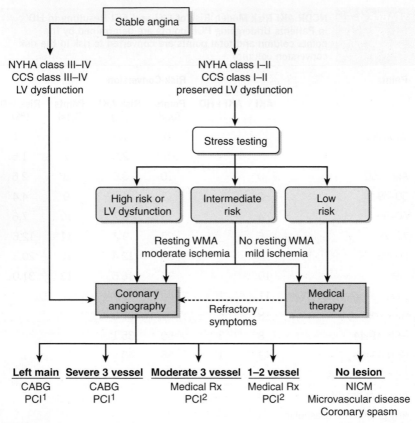

Figure 4-1. Approach to the evaluation and management of the patient with stable angina. Patients with clinical heart failure, severe limiting angina, and those with left ventricle (LV) dysfunction should undergo coronary angiography to define underlying coronary artery disease. Patients without these features may undergo further risk stratification with stress testing. Following stress testing, patients may undergo either coronary angiography or empiric medical therapy depending on their risk profile. Patients initially treated with medical therapy who have refractory symptoms should undergo angiography. [1]CABG generally preferred due to known survival advantage over medical therapy alone; however, if the coronary lesions are not complex, PCI may offer similar results to CABG but with a higher need for future revascularizations. [2]PCI should be reserved for patients who have high-grade lesions, have severe ischemia, and are refractory to medical therapy. CABG, coronary artery bypass grafting; CCS, Canadian Cardiovascular Society Classification (angina); NICM, nonischemic cardiomyopathy; NYHA, New York Heart Association; PCI, percutaneous coronary intervention; WMA, wall motion abnormality.

- **Calcium channel blockers** can be used either in conjunction with or in lieu of β-blockers in the presence of contraindications or adverse effects as a second-line agent (Table 4-9).
  - Calcium antagonists are often used in conjunction with β-blockers if the latter are not fully effective at relieving anginal symptoms. Both long-acting dihydropyridines and nondihydropyridine agents can be used.

TABLE 4-8	β-Blockers Commonly Used for Ischemic Heart Disease	
Drug	**β-Receptor Selectivity**	**Dose**
Propranolol	β_1 and β_2	20–80 mg bid
Metoprolol	β_1	50–200 mg bid
Atenolol	β_1	50–200 mg daily
Nebivolol	β_1	5–40 mg daily
Nadolol	β_1 and β_2	40–80 mg daily
Timolol	β_1 and β_2	10–30 mg tid
Acebutolol[a]	β_1	200–600 mg bid
Bisoprolol	β_1	10–20 mg daily
Esmolol (IV)	β_1	50–300 µg/kg/min
Labetalol	Combined α, β_1, β_2	200–600 mg bid
Pindolol[a]	β_1 and β_2	2.5–7.5 mg tid
Carvedilol	Combined α, β_1, β_2	3.125–25 mg bid

[a]β-blockers with intrinsic sympathomimetic activity.

TABLE 4-9	Calcium Channel Blockers Commonly Used for Ischemic Heart Disease	
Drug	**Duration of Action**	**Usual Dosage**
Dihydropyridines		
Nifedipine	Long	30–180 mg/d
Amlodipine	Long	5–10 mg/d
Felodipine (SR)	Long	5–10 mg/d
Isradipine	Medium	2.5–10 mg/d
Nicardipine	Short	20–40 mg tid
Nondihydropyridines		
Diltiazem		
Immediate release	Short	30–90 mg qid
Slow release	Long	120–360 mg/d
Verapamil		
Immediate release	Short	80–160 mg tid
Slow release	Long	120–480 mg/d

TABLE 4-10	Nitrate Preparations Commonly Used for Ischemic Heart Disease		
Preparation	**Dosage**	**Onset (min)**	**Duration**
Sublingual nitroglycerin	0.3–0.6 mg PRN	2–5	10–30 min
Aerosol nitroglycerin	0.4 mg PRN	2–5	10–30 min
Oral isosorbide dinitrate	5–40 mg tid	30–60	4–6 h
Oral isosorbide mononitrate	10–20 mg bid	30–60	6–8 h
Oral isosorbide mononitrate SR	30–120 mg daily	30–60	12–18 h
2% Nitroglycerin ointment	0.5–2.0 in. tid	20–60	3–8 h
Transdermal nitroglycerin patches	5–15 mg daily	>60	12 h
Intravenous nitroglycerin	10–200 μg/min	<2	During infusion

- Calcium channel blockers are effective agents for the treatment of coronary vasospasm.
- Nondihydropyridine agents (verapamil/diltiazem) should be avoided in patients with systolic dysfunction due to their negative inotropic effects.
- The use of short-acting dihydropyridines (nifedipine) should be avoided due to the potential to increase the risk of adverse cardiac events.
  - **Nitrates**, either long-acting formulations for chronic use or sublingual/topical preparations for acute anginal symptoms. More often used as adjunctive antianginal agents (Table 4-10).
    - Sublingual preparations should be used at the first indication of angina or prophylactically before engaging in activities that are known to precipitate angina. Patients should seek prompt medical attention if angina occurs at rest or fails to respond to the third sublingual dose.
    - Nitrate tolerance resulting in reduced therapeutic response may occur with all nitrate preparations. The institution of a nitrate-free period of 10–12 hours (usually at night) can enhance treatment efficacy.
    - For patients with CAD, nitrates have not shown a mortality benefit.
    - Nitrates are contraindicated (even in patients with acute coronary syndrome [ACS]) for use in patients who are on phoshodiesterase-5 inhibitors due to risk of severe hypotension. A washout period of 24 hours for sildenafil and vardenafil and 48 hours for tadalafil is required prior to nitrate use.
  - **Ranolazine** is indicated for angina refractory to standard medical therapy and has shown benefit in improving symptoms and quality of life. Ranolazine interacts with simvastatin metabolism and should not be used together.
- **Other secondary prevention medications**
  - **Angiotensin-converting enzyme inhibitors (ACE Inhibitors) and angiotensin receptor blockers (ARBs)** have cardiovascular protective effects that reduce the recurrence of ischemic events.
    - ACE inhibitor therapy, or ARBs in those intolerant to ACE inhibitors, should be used in all patients with an LV ejection fraction (EF) <40% and in those with hypertension, diabetes, or chronic kidney disease.
    - It is reasonable to use ACE inhibitor in all stable angina patients.
  - **Statins** have a marked effect in secondary prevention, and all patients with IHD who can tolerate therapy should be on a high-potency statin (see Chapter 3, Preventive Cardiology). Note, in secondary prevention of coronary heart disease, apart from statins, no other cholesterol agents have proven consistent mortality benefit.

Ezetimibe can be safely used if statins cannot be tolerated or further reductions in LDL cholesterol are warranted.
○ **Influenza vaccination** is recommended for all patients with IHD.

Revascularization

* **Coronary revascularization**
  ○ In general, medical therapy with at least two classes of antianginal agents should be attempted before medical therapy is considered a failure and coronary revascularization pursued.
  ○ Relief of angina symptoms is the most common objective of all revascularization procedures.
  ○ The indication for all revascularization procedures should consider the acuity of presentation, the extent of ischemia, and the ability to achieve full revascularization. The selection of revascularization should be tailored to the individual patient and, in complex cases, include the use of a multidisciplinary heart team. The heart team includes but is not limited to a cardiac surgeon, interventional cardiologist, noninvasive cardiologist, primary care physician, and other important members of the patient's care.
  ○ The choice between PCI and CABG surgery is dependent on the coronary anatomy, medical comorbidities, and patient preference.
    ▪ In general, patients with complex and diffuse disease do better with CABG, whereas PCI in select patients with the proper coronary anatomy can provide comparable results as CABG. Due to the more invasive nature of CABG, patient comorbidities often necessitate PCI for revascularization.
    ▪ The Syntax Score is a validated angiographic model that can aid the clinician in determining outcomes after PCI or CABG. In general, patients with a low or intermediate Syntax Score do as well or better with PCI compared to CABG (*Eur Heart J 2011;32:2125*) (available at *http://www.syntaxscore.com/*).
    ▪ The Society of Thoracic Surgeons (STS) score can help determine the risk of mortality and morbidity associated with CABG and should be determined for all patients when considering surgical revascularization (available at *http://riskcalc.sts.org/*).
  ○ Revascularization is shown to **improve survival** in the following circumstances as compared to medical therapy:
    ▪ CABG for >50% left main coronary artery disease that has not been grafted (unprotected). PCI is a reasonable alternative for patients with left main disease if the patient is a poor surgical candidate (STS score >5) and has a favorable morphology for PCI (low Syntax Score). PCI, in the right clinical context, can offer rates of MI, CVA, or death similar to CABG (*N Engl J Med 2009;360:961*).
    ▪ CABG for three-vessel disease or two-vessel disease that includes the proximal left anterior descending LAD (artery).
    ▪ CABG for patients with two-vessel disease not including the LAD artery if there is extensive ischemia (>20% myocardium at risk) or in patients with isolated proximal LAD artery disease when an internal mammary artery revascularization is performed.
    ▪ CABG, as compared to PCI or medical therapy, in patients with multivessel disease and diabetes, if a left internal mammary artery to the LAD artery can be placed (*N Engl J Med 1996;335:217*). PCI *may* offer similar survival outcomes in diabetics with multivessel disease and a low Syntax Score (<22) but does have a higher need for repeat revascularization (*J Am Coll Cardiol 2010;55:1067*).
    ▪ PCI or CABG in patients who have survived sudden cardiac death due to ischemic ventricular tachycardia.
    ▪ PCI or CABG in patients with ACS.
  ○ Due to the morbidity of a repeat CABG, PCI is often used to improve symptoms in patients with recurrent angina after CABG.

- ○ The use of internal mammary artery grafts is associated with 90% graft patency at 10 years, compared with 40–50% for saphenous vein grafts. The long-term patency of a radial artery graft is 80% at 5 years. After 10 years of follow-up, 50% of patients develop recurrent angina or other adverse cardiac events related to late vein graft failure or progression of native CAD.
- ○ The risks of elective PCI include <1% mortality, a 2–5% rate of nonfatal MI, and <1% need for emergent CABG for an unsuccessful procedure. Patients undergoing PCI have shorter hospitalizations but require more frequent repeat revascularization procedures compared to CABG.
- ○ Elderly patients represent a unique population when considering revascularization due to comorbidities, frailty, the physiology of aging as it relates to drug metabolism and cardiopulmonary function, and concern over polypharmacy. In general, this population has been underrepresented in most trials but still derives benefit from revascularization to relieve symptoms. Frailty should be heavily considered when considering a procedure or counseling about the benefits of revascularization.
- ○ It is reasonable to revascularize selected patients with severe LV dysfunction (EF <35%), but in general, there is no definitive clinical trial evidence that CABG or PCI will improve LV function or improve mortality compared to medical therapy (*N Engl J Med 2011;364:1407*).
- ○ Viability testing (nuclear perfusion imaging or MRI) may provide some assistance to the clinician when trying to determine the possible benefit of revascularization in patients with prior MI or severe LV dysfunction but is still largely unproven.

PATIENT EDUCATION

- Compliance with medications, diet, and exercise should be stressed to patients. All patients should be encouraged to participate in cardiac rehab as well as meet with a registered dietician.
- Patients with known CAD should present for evaluation if any change in chest pain pattern, frequency, or intensity develops.
- Patients should also be reevaluated if they report the presence of any HF symptoms.

Monitoring/Follow-Up

- Close patient follow-up is a critical component of the treatment of CAD because lifestyle modification and secondary risk factor reduction require serial reassessment and interventions.
- All patients should be aggressively treated for the traditional risk factors mentioned above.
- Relatively minor changes in anginal symptoms can be safely treated with titration and/or addition of antianginal medications.
- Significant changes in anginal complaints (frequency, severity, or time to onset with activity) should be evaluated by either stress testing (usually in conjunction with an imaging modality) or cardiac angiography as warranted.
- Cardiac rehabilitation or an exercise program should be offered or instituted.

Acute Coronary Syndromes, Unstable Angina, and Non–ST-Segment Elevation Myocardial Infarction

GENERAL PRINCIPLES

Definition

- NSTEMI and UA are closely related conditions whose pathogenesis and clinical presentations are similar but differ in severity.

- If coronary flow is not severe enough or the occlusion does not persist long enough to cause myocardial necrosis (as indicated by positive cardiac biomarkers), the syndrome is labeled UA.
- NSTEMI is defined by an elevation of cardiac biomarkers and the absence of ST-segment elevation on the ECG.
- NSTEMI, like STEMI, can lead to cardiogenic shock.
- AHA/ACC guidelines provide a more through overview of NSTEMI/UA (*J Am Coll Cardiol 2014;65:e139*).

Epidemiology

- The annual incidence of ACS is >780,000 events, with 70% being NSTEMI/UA.
- Among patients with ACS, approximately 60% have UA and 40% have MI (one-third of MIs present with an acute STEMI).
- At 1 year, patients with UA/NSTEMI are at considerable risk for death (~6%), recurrent MI (~11%), and need for revascularization (~50–60%). It is important to note that although the short-term mortality of STEMI is greater than that of NSTEMI, the long-term mortality is similar (*J Am Coll Cardiol 2007;50:e1*; *JAMA 1996;275:1104*).
- Patients with NSTEMI/UA tend to have more comorbidities, both cardiac and noncardiac, than STEMI patients.
- Women with NSTEMI/UA have worse short-term and long-term outcomes and more complications compared to men. Much of this has been attributed to delays in recognition of symptoms and underutilization of guideline-directed medical therapy and invasive management.

Etiology and Pathophysiology

- Myocardial ischemia results from decreased myocardial oxygen supply and/or increased demand. In the majority of cases, NSTEMI is due to a sudden decrease in blood supply via partial occlusion of the affected vessel. In some cases, markedly increased myocardial oxygen demand may lead to NSTEMI (demand ischemia), as seen in severe anemia, hypertensive crisis, acute decompensated HF, surgery, or any other significant physiologic stressor.
- UA/NSTEMI most often represents severe coronary artery narrowing or acute atherosclerotic plaque rupture/erosion and superimposed thrombus formation. Alternatively, it may also be due to progressive mechanical obstruction from advancing atherosclerotic disease, in-stent restenosis, or bypass graft disease.
- Plaque rupture may be triggered by local and/or systemic inflammation as well as shear stress. Rupture allows exposure of lipid-rich subendothelial components to circulating platelets and inflammatory cells, serving as a potent substrate for thrombus formation. A thin fibrous cap (thin-cap fibroatheroma) is felt to be more vulnerable to rupture and is most frequently represented as only moderate stenosis on angiography.
- Less common causes include dynamic obstruction of the coronary artery due to vasospasm (Prinzmetal angina, cocaine), coronary artery dissection (more common in women), coronary vasculitis, and embolus.

Clinical Presentation

History

- ACS symptoms include all the qualities of typical angina except the episodes are more severe, of longer duration, and may occur at rest.
- The three principal presentations for UA are **rest angina** (angina occurring at rest and prolonged, usually >20 minutes), **new-onset angina**, and **progressive angina** (previously diagnosed angina that has become more frequent, lasts longer, or occurs with less

TABLE 4-11	Killip Classification	
Class	**Definition**	**Mortality[a]**
I	No signs or symptoms of heart failure	6%
II	Heart failure: S_3 gallop, rales, or JVD	17%
III	Severe heart failure: pulmonary edema	38%
IV	Cardiogenic shock: SBP <90 mm Hg and signs of hypoperfusion and/or signs of severe heart failure	81%

JDV, jugular venous distention; SBP, systolic blood pressure.
[a]In-hospital mortality of patients in 1965–1967 with no reperfusion therapy (n = 250).
Adapted from *Am J Cardiol* 1967;20:457.

exertion). New-onset and progressive angina should occur with at least mild to moderate activity, CCS class III severity.
- ○ Female sex, diabetes, HF, end-stage kidney disease, and older age are traits that have been associated with a greater likelihood of atypical ACS symptoms. However, the most common presentation in these populations is still typical anginal chest pain.
- ○ Jaw, neck, arm, back, or epigastric pain and/or dyspnea can be anginal equivalents.
- ○ Pleuritic pain, pain that radiates down the legs or originates in the mid/lower abdomen, pain that can be reproduced by extremity movement or palpation, and pain that lasts seconds in duration are unlikely to be related to ACS.

Physical Examination
- Physical examination should be directed at identifying hemodynamic instability, pulmonary congestion, and other causes of acute chest discomfort.
- Objective evidence of HF, including peripheral hypoperfusion, heart murmur (particularly MR murmur), elevated jugular venous pulsation, pulmonary edema, hypotension, and peripheral edema worsen the prognosis.
- Killip classification can be useful to risk stratify and identify patients with features of cardiogenic shock (Table 4-11).
- Examination may also give clues to other causes of ischemia such as thyrotoxicosis or aortic dissection (see Table 4-4).

Diagnostic Testing
Electrocardiography
- Prior to or immediately on arrival to the emergency department, a baseline ECG should be obtained in all patients with suspected ACS. A normal tracing does not exclude the presence of disease.
- The presence of Q waves, ST-segment changes, or T-wave inversions is suggestive of CAD.
- Isolated Q waves in lead III only are a normal finding.
- Serial ECGs should be obtained to assess for dynamic ischemic changes.
- Comparison to prior ECGs is important when evaluating an ECG for dynamic changes.
- The posterior circulation (i.e., circumflex coronary artery distribution) is poorly assessed with standard ECG lead placement and should always be considered when evaluating patients with ACS. Posterior placed leads or urgent echocardiography may more accurately assess the presence of ischemia when the suspicion is high.

- Approximately 50% of patients with UA/NSTEMI have significant ECG abnormalities, including transient ST-segment elevations, ST depressions, and T-wave inversions (*J Am Coll Cardiol 2007;50:e1*).
  - ST-segment depression in two contiguous leads is a sensitive indicator of myocardial ischemia, especially if dynamic and associated with symptoms.
    - Threshold value for abnormal J-point depression should be 0.5 mm in leads V_2 and V_3 and 1 mm in all other leads.
    - ST-segment depression in multiple leads plus ST-segment elevation in aVR and/or V_1 suggests ischemia due to multivessel or left main disease.
  - Deeply inverted T waves (>5 mm) with QT prolongation in leads V_2 to V_4 (Wellens waves) are suggestive of a critical lesion in the LAD artery distribution.
  - Nonspecific ST-segment changes or T-wave inversions (those that do not meet voltage criteria) are nondiagnostic and unhelpful in management of acute ischemia but are associated with a higher risk for future cardiac events.

Laboratories
- A complete blood count, basic metabolic panel, fasting glucose, and lipid profile should be obtained in all patients with suspected CAD. Other conditions may be found to be contributing to ischemia (e.g., anemia) or mimicking ischemia (e.g., hyperkalemia-related ECG changes) or may alter management (e.g., severe thrombocytopenia).
- Cardiac biomarkers are essential in the diagnosis of UA/NSTEMI and should be obtained in all patients who present with chest discomfort suggestive of ACS. In patients with negative cardiac markers within 6 hours of the onset of pain, a second sample should be drawn 8–12 hours after symptom onset. Troponin is the recommended biomarker for assessment of myocardial necrosis.
  - Troponin T and I assays are highly specific and sensitive markers of myocardial necrosis. Serum troponin levels are usually undetectable in normal individuals, and any elevation is considered abnormal.
  - MI size and prognosis are directly proportional to magnitude of increase in troponin (*N Engl J Med 1996;335:1333*; *Circulation 1998;98:1853*).
- Creatine kinase (CK)-MB is also an acceptable marker of myocardial necrosis, but lacks specificity because it is present in both skeletal and cardiac muscle cells.
  - Specificity can be improved by using the CK-MB/total CK fraction. A CK-MB fraction >5% is suggestive of myocardial injury.
  - CK-MB is a useful assay for detecting postinfarct ischemia because a fall and subsequent rise in enzyme levels suggest reinfarction, especially if accompanied by recurrent ischemic symptoms or ECG changes.
  - CK-MB and troponin levels should not routinely be measured after PCI or cardiac surgery because their prognostic value is uncertain. Patients who have symptoms should be assessed with appropriate tests including biomarkers.
- Brain natriuretic peptide (BNP) can be a useful biomarker of myocardial stress in patients with ACS, and elevations are associated with worse outcomes (*Circulation 2002;105:1760*). Severe elevations of BNP in the setting of ACS in patients without known HF should raise concern for a large infarction and urgent angiography.

TREATMENT

- Acute treatment should be aimed at reducing the symptoms of chest pain.
- Risk stratification can be helpful in determining the appropriate testing, pharmacologic interventions, and timing or need for coronary angiography.

- Risk of death or MI progression is elevated with the following **high-risk ACS characteristics**:
  - Recurrent/accelerating angina despite adequate medical therapy
  - Signs or symptoms of new HF, pulmonary edema, or shock (high Killip Classification)
  - New or worsening MR
  - New LBBB
  - Ventricular tachycardia noted on monitoring
- These findings (on presentation **or anytime during the index hospitalization**) should prompt the performance of **urgent** coronary angiography with intention to offer revascularization.
- Several clinical tools can estimate a patient's risk of recurrent MI and cardiac mortality, such as the Thrombolysis in Myocardial Infarction (TIMI) and Global Registry of Acute Coronary Events (GRACE) risk scores. The TIMI risk score can be used to determine the risk of death or nonfatal MI up to 1 year after an ACS event and, given the ease of use, is our recommended risk stratification tool. Patients can be classified as low, intermediate, or high risk on the basis of their clinical profile (Figure 4-2).
  - Patients with a TIMI risk of 0 and negative troponins have a very low 30-day rate of major adverse cardiac events.
  - Patients with a TIMI risk score of ≥3 benefit from aggressive medical therapy and invasive evaluation.
- In the stabilized patient, two treatment strategies are available: the **ischemia-driven approach** (formerly termed *conservative*) versus the **routine invasive approach** (*early* defined as <24 hours of presentation or *delayed* >24 hours). The planned approach should always be individualized to the patient (Figure 4-3). All patients should receive aggressive antithrombotic, antiplatelet, and ischemic medical therapy no matter the final revascularization strategy. Table 4-12 summarizes the selection approach.
  - In the ischemia-driven approach, if the patient does not develop high-risk ACS features, has normal subsequent cardiac enzymes, has no dynamic ECG changes, and responds to medical therapy, a noninvasive stress test should be obtained for further risk stratification.
    - Patients should be angina free for at least 12 hours prior to stress testing.
    - If a patient with positive cardiac enzymes is selected for noninvasive testing, a submaximal or pharmacologic stress test 72 hours after the peak value may be performed.
    - Coronary angiography is reserved for patients who develop high-risk ACS features, have a high-risk stress test, develop angina at low levels of stress, or are noted to have an LVEF <40%.
  - In the **routine invasive strategy**, the patient is planned for a coronary angiography with intent to revascularize. An early (<24 hours from presentation) invasive approach is recommended for patients with high-risk scores or other high-risk features (see Table 4-12).
  - Note: Refractory chest pain, hemodynamic instability, or serious ventricular arrhythmias are indications for an urgent/emergent invasive strategy similar to STEMI; this is not to be confused with a routine invasive strategy.
  - An early invasive strategy is also warranted in low- or intermediate-risk patients with repeated ACS presentations despite appropriate therapy.
  - A routine invasive strategy is not recommended for the following:
    - Patients with severe comorbid illnesses such as chronic kidney disease, end-stage liver or lung disease, or metastatic/uncontrolled cancer whereby the benefits of the procedure are likely outweighed by the risk from the routine invasive procedure
    - Acute chest pain with a low likelihood of ACS and negative biomarkers, especially in women
  - As opposed to stable IHD, a routine invasive approach with possible PCI has been shown to **reduce the incidence of recurrent MI, hospitalizations, and death**. In general, patients with ACS should undergo a routine invasive strategy unless it is clear that the risk outweighs the possible benefit in a given patient.

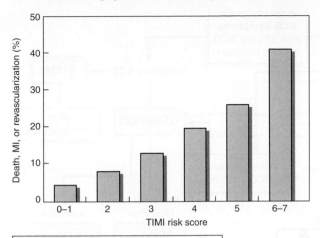

TIMI risk score (1 point for each)
1. Age >65 years
2. Known CAD (stenosis >50%)
3. 2+ episodes of chest pain in 24 hours
4. ST-segment or T-wave changes
5. Elevated cardiac biomarkers
6. ASA in the last 7 days
7. 3+ CAD risk factors

| Ischemia driven strategy | Routine invasive strategy |

β-Blocker, nitrates, oxygen ⟶
UFH, LMWH ⟶
ASA ⟶
Dual antiplatelet therapy ⟶
Triple antiplatelet therapy ⟶

TIMI risk score

Figure 4-2. Fourteen-day rates of death, MI, or urgent revascularization from the TIMI 11B and ESSENCE trials based on increasing TIMI risk score. Coronary artery disease (CAD) risk factors include family history of CAD, diabetes, hypertension, hyperlipidemia, and tobacco use. ASA, aspirin; LMWH, low–molecular-weight heparin; MI, myocardial infarction; TIMI, Thrombolysis in Myocardial Infarction; UFH, unfractionated heparin. (Data from *JAMA* 2000;284:835–42.)

Medications

Patients presenting with UA/NSTEMI should receive medications that reduce myocardial ischemia through reduction in myocardial oxygen demand, improvement in coronary perfusion, and prevention of further thrombus formation.
• This approach should include antiplatelet, anticoagulant, and antianginal medications.
• Supplemental oxygen should be provided if the patient is hypoxemic (<90%) or having difficulty breathing. Routine use of oxygen is not needed and possibly harmful (*Heart 2009;95:198*).

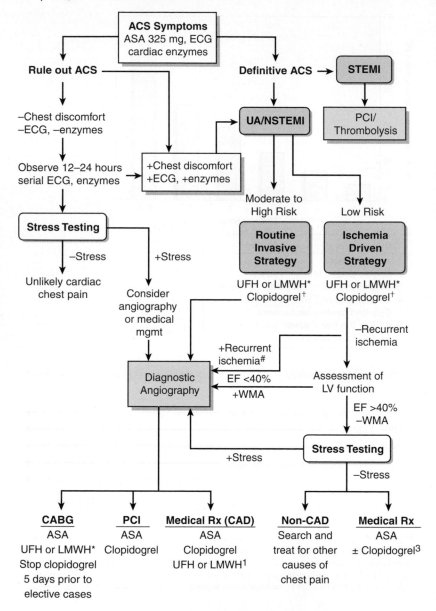

TABLE 4-12	Appropriate Selection of Routine Invasive Versus Ischemia-Driven Revascularization Strategy in Patients with NSTEMI/UA
Immediate/ urgent invasive (within 2 h)	Refractory angina Worsening signs or symptoms of heart failure or mitral regurgitation Hemodynamic instability or shock Sustained VT or VF
Ischemia-driven	Low-risk score (TIMI ≤1 or GRACE <109) Low-risk biomarker-negative female patients Patient or clinician preference in the absence of high-risk features
Early invasive (within 24 h)	None of the above but a high-risk score (TIMI ≥3 or GRACE >140) Rapid rate of rise in biomarkers New or presumably new ST depressions
Delayed invasive (24–72 h)	None of the above but presence of diabetes Renal insufficiency (GFR <60) LV ejection fraction <40% Early postinfarction angina Prior PCI within 6 months Prior CABG TIMI score ≥2 or GRACE score 109–140 and no indication for early invasive strategy

CABG, coronary artery bypass graft; GFR, glomerular filtration rate; GRACE, Global Registry of Acute Coronary Events; LV, left ventricular; NSTEMI, non–ST-segment elevation myocardial infarction; PCI, percutaneous coronary intervention; TIMI, Thrombolysis in Myocardial Infarction; UA, unstable angina; VF, ventricular fibrillation; VT, ventricular tachycardia.

- **Antiplatelet therapy**
  - Table 4-13 summarizes available agents and dosing recommendations for use in ACS.
  - Dual antiplatelet therapy is recommended for patients with NSTEMI/UA.
  - **Aspirin** blocks platelet aggregation within minutes.
    - A chewable 162–325-mg dose of ASA should be administered immediately at symptom onset or at first medical contact, unless a contraindication exists. This should be followed by ASA 81 mg daily indefinitely.

←————————————————————————————————————

Figure 4-3. Diagnostic and therapeutic approach to patients presenting with acute coronary syndrome (ACS) focusing on antiplatelet and antithrombotic therapy. *Bivalirudin is an appropriate alternative to UFH and LMWH, or at time of PCI, patients on UFH may be switched to bivalirudin. †Choose either clopidogrel, ticagrelor, or prasugrel as the second antiplatelet agent. #Indicators of recurrent ischemia include worsening chest pain, increasing cardiac enzymes, heart failure signs/symptoms, arrhythmia (VT/VF), and dynamic ECG changes. ¹UFH for 48 hours or LMWH until discharge or up to 8 days and clopidogrel or ticagrelor for 1 year. P2Y12 inhibitor includes antiplatelet agents clopidogrel, ticagrelor, or prasugrel. ASA, aspirin; CABG, coronary artery bypass grafting; CAD, coronary artery disease; EF, ejection fraction; glycoprotein IIb/IIIa inhibitor; LMWH, low–molecular-weight heparin; NSTEMI, non–ST-segment elevation myocardial infarction; PCI, percutaneous coronary intervention; Rx, treatment; STEMI, ST-segment elevation myocardial infarction; UA, unstable angina; UFH, unfractionated heparin; VT/VF, ventricular tachycardia/ventricular fibrillation; WMA, wall motion abnormality. (Data from the ACC/AHA 2007 Guidelines for the Management of Patients With Unstable Angina/Non-ST-Elevation Myocardial Infarction.)

TABLE 4-13	Antiplatelet Agents in UA/NSTEMI	
Medication	**Dosage**	**Comments**
Aspirin (ASA)	162–325 mg initial, then 75–100 mg	In patients taking ticagrelor, the maintenance dose of ASA *should not* exceed 100 mg.
Clopidogrel	300–600 mg loading dose, 75 mg daily	In combination with ASA, clopidogrel (300–600 mg loading dose, then 75 mg/d) decreased the composite end point of cardiovascular death, MI, or stroke by 18–30% in patients with UA/NSTEMI (*N Engl J Med 2001;345:494; Lancet 2001;358:527; JAMA 2002;288:2411*).
Ticagrelor	180 mg loading dose, then 90 mg bid	Ticagrelor reduced incidence of vascular death, MI, or CVA (9.8% vs. 11.0%) but with higher major bleeding not related to CABG (4.5% vs. 3.8%) as compared to clopidogrel (*N Engl J Med 2009;361:1045*).
Prasugrel	60 mg loading dose, 10 mg daily	Prasugrel has increased antiplatelet potency compared to clopidogrel. Prasugrel reduced the incidence of cardiovascular death, MI, and stroke (9.9% vs. 12.1%) at the expense of increased major (2.4% vs. 1.1%) and fatal bleeding (0.4% vs. 0.1%), compared to clopidogrel (*N Engl J Med 2007;357:2001*).
Eptifibatide	180 μg/kg IV bolus, 2 μg/kg/min[a]	Eptifibatide reduces the risk of death or MI in patients with ACS undergoing either invasive or noninvasive therapy in combination with ASA and heparin (*N Engl J Med 1998;339:436; Circulation 2000;101:751*). Compared to abciximab and tirofiban, eptifibatide has the most consistent effects on platelet inhibition with shortest on-time and drug half-life (*Circulation 2002;106:1470–6*).
Tirofiban	0.4 μg/kg IV bolus, 0.1 μg/kg/min[a]	Tirofiban reduces the risk of death or MI in patients with ACS undergoing either invasive or noninvasive therapy in combination with ASA and heparin (*Circulation 1997;96:1445; N Engl J Med 1998;338:1498; N Engl J Med 1998;338:1488*).

(continued)

TABLE 4-13	Antiplatelet Agents in UA/NSTEMI (*Continued*)

Medication	Dosage	Comments
Abciximab	0.25 mg/kg IV bolus, 10 μg/min[b]	Abciximab reduces the risk of death or MI in patients with ACS undergoing coronary intervention (*N Engl J Med 1994;330:956; Lancet 1997;349:1429; N Engl J Med 1997;336:1689*). It should not be used in patients in whom percutaneous intervention is not planned (*Lancet 2001;357:1915*). Platelet inhibition may be reversed by platelet transfusion.

ACS, acute coronary syndrome; CABG, coronary artery bypass grafting; CVA, cerebrovascular accident; ESRD, end-stage renal disease; GFR, glomerular filtration rate; HD, hemodialysis; MI, myocardial infarction; NSTEMI, non–ST-segment elevation myocardial infarction; UA, unstable angina.
[a]Infusion doses should be decreased by 50% in patients with a GFR <30 mL/min and avoided in patients on HD.
[b]Abciximab may be used in patients with ESRD because it is not cleared by the kidney.

- If an ASA allergy is present, clopidogrel may be substituted. An allergy consultation should be obtained for possible desensitization, preferably prior to the need for a coronary stent.
- After PCI, ASA 81 mg is the current recommended dose in the setting of dual antiplatelet therapy.
  ○ **Clopidogrel** is a prodrug whose metabolite blocks the P2Y12 receptor and inhibits platelet activation and aggregation by blocking the adenosine diphosphate receptor site on platelets.
    - The addition of clopidogrel to ASA reduced cardiovascular mortality and recurrent MI both acutely and at 11 months of follow-up (*N Engl J Med 2001;345:494*).
    - A loading dose should always be given in naïve patients.
    - In patients unable to take oral medications or unable to absorb oral medications due to ileus, rectal administration is unproven but has been reported. This may be particularly important after PCI when dual antiplatelet therapy is critical.
    - Can be used as part of the protocol in both the ischemia-driven and early invasive strategies.
  ○ **Prasugrel** is also a prodrug that blocks the P2Y12 adenosine receptor; its conversion to its active metabolite occurs faster and to a greater extent than clopidogrel.
    - Results in faster, greater, and more uniform platelet inhibition compared to clopidogrel at the expense of higher risk of bleeding (*Circulation 2007;116:2923*).
    - It decreases risk of CVD death, MI, CVA, and acute stent thrombosis as compared to clopidogrel in ACS patients, including STEMI patients.
    - It should be used with caution or avoided in patients older than 75 years and who weigh less than 60 kg. It is **contraindicated** in those with prior stroke or transient ischemic attack.
    - Used only in the **invasive approach of ACS** and **only after coronary anatomy is known and PCI is planned**. There is no benefit over clopidogrel when tested before initiation of PCI.
  ○ **Ticagrelor** is not a prodrug and blocks the P2Y12 adenosine receptor directly.
    - Reduces the risk of death, MI, CVA, and stent thrombosis as compared to clopidogrel in ACS patients, including STEMI patients (*N Engl J Med 2009;361:1045*).

- After the loading dose of ASA, the maintenance dose of ASA **must be <100 mg** (*Circulation 2011;124:544*).
- Can be used as part of the protocol in both the ischemia-driven and early invasive strategies.
  - Use of **proton pump inhibitors (PPIs)** with P2Y12 receptor antagonists.
    - PPIs should be used in patients who will require both ASA therapy and a P2Y12 antagonist with prior history of gastrointestinal bleeding and may be considered in those at increased risk of bleeding (such as older individuals, patients with known ulcers or *Helicobacter pylori* infection, and patients also on warfarin, steroids, or NSAIDs) (*Circulation 2010;122:2619*).
    - Pharmacologic studies have raised concerns about the potential of PPIs to blunt the efficiency of clopidogrel. However, in a prospective randomized trial, no apparent cardiovascular interaction was noted between PPIs and clopidogrel (*N Engl J Med 2010;363:1909*).
  - **Glycoprotein IIb/IIIa (GPIIb/IIIa) antagonists** (abciximab, eptifibatide, or tirofiban) block the interaction between platelets and fibrinogen, thus targeting the final common pathway for platelet aggregation.
    - GPIIb/IIIa inhibitors play a limited role in ACS management with the introduction of more potent oral antiplatelet agents.
    - Routine use of GPIIb/IIIa antagonists on initial presentation, before angiography, in patients undergoing the invasive approach *should be avoided* due to increased risk of major bleeding and a lack of improvement in outcomes.
    - GPIIb/IIIa agents may be considered in the following:
      - Patients who require add-on therapy for *worsening* ischemia any time prior to angiography or as part of conservative therapy even if the patient is already being treated with dual oral antiplatelet therapy and anticoagulation.
      - Discretional use during PCI due to the presence of complex coronary lesions or coronary thrombus.
    - Abciximab is reserved for use only during PCI and started no sooner than 4 hours prior to the planned procedure.
    - Eptifibatide has been used as a bridging, short-acting antiplatelet agent in patients who have had recent PCI and require surgery where dual antiplatelet therapy is prohibited. An infusion is started to bridge in absence of oral therapy, stopped before surgery, and promptly restarted after surgery when deemed safe. Although common practice, this strategy is of unproven benefit.
    - Thrombocytopenia, which can be severe, is an uncommon complication of these agents and should prompt discontinuation.
  - **Antiplatelet agents and timing of CABG**
    - Due to increased risk of bleeding, it is currently recommended that clopidogrel be withheld for at least 5 days prior to CABG, prasugrel 7 days prior, and ticagrelor 5 days prior.
    - GPIIb/IIIa antagonists can be an alternative to clopidogrel, ticagrelor, and prasugrel for upstream use (prior to angiography) in appropriate patients with UA/NSTEMI who are known to require surgical revascularization.
    - In general, dual antiplatelet therapy should not be withheld during the initial management of ACS for concern over need for surgical revascularization. There is a larger risk of withholding beneficial therapy to patients in this setting than causing harm by complicating surgical revascularization.
- **Anticoagulant therapy**
  - See Table 4-14 for recommended use and dosing in ACS.
  - Anticoagulation accompanied by dual antiplatelet therapy is required for all UA/NSTEMI patients, whether along the early invasive or conservative pathway.

TABLE 4-14	Anticoagulant Medications	
Medication	**Dosage**	**Comments**
Heparin (UFH)	60 units/kg IV bolus (maximum dose: 4000 units), 12–14 units/kg/h	Heparin therapy, when used in conjunction with ASA, has been shown to reduce the early rate of death or MI by up to 60% (*JAMA 1996;276:811*). The aPTT should be adjusted to maintain a value of 1.5–2.0 times control.
Enoxaparin (LMWH)	1 mg/kg SC bid[a]	LMWH is at least as efficacious as UFH and may further reduce the rate of death, MI, or recurrent angina (*N Engl J Med 1997;337:447*). LMWH may increase the rate of bleeding (*JAMA 2004;292:45*) and cannot be reversed in the setting of refractory bleeding. LMWH does not require monitoring for clinical effect.
Fondaparinux	2.5 mg SC daily	Fondaparinux has efficacy similar to that of LMWH with possibly reduced bleeding rates (*N Engl J Med 2006;354:1464*).
Bivalirudin[b]	0.75 mg/kg IV bolus, 1.75 mg/kg/h	When used in conjunction with ASA and clopidogrel, bivalirudin is at least as effective as the combination of ASA, UFH, clopidogrel, and GPIIb/IIIa antagonists with decreased bleeding rates (*N Engl J Med 2006;355:2203*). May increase risk for stent thrombosis. Monitoring is required with a goal aPTT of 1.5–2.5 times control.

aPTT, activated partial thromboplastin time; ASA, aspirin; GFR, glomerular filtration rate; GP, glycoprotein; LMWH, low–molecular-weight heparin; MI, myocardial infarction; UFH, unfractionated heparin.
[a]LMWH should be given at reduced dose (50%) in patients with a serum creatinine >2 mg/dL or GFR <30 mL/min.
[b]Bivalirudin requires dosage adjustment in patients with a GFR less than 30 mL/min or those on hemodialysis.

- **Unfractionated heparin (UFH)** works by binding antithrombin III, which catalyzes the inactivation of thrombin and other clotting factors.
  - Most commonly used and easily monitored but also most inconsistent in its anticoagulation and metabolism.
  - Heparin-induced thrombocytopenia (HIT) is a concern with prior use.
  - Easily reversed in the event of a severe hemorrhagic complication.
  - Always requires aggressive bolus dosing and anticoagulation monitoring in the setting of ACS.
  - Recommended anticoagulant to be used in the setting of ACS.
- **Low–molecular-weight heparin (LMWH)** inhibits mostly factor Xa but also affects thrombin activity and offers an ease of administration (weight-based, twice-daily subcutaneous dose). The risk of HIT is lower but not absent.

- As compared to UFH, LMWH has a more predictable anticoagulant effect.
- It has a similar efficacy as UFH but is associated with a higher risk of postprocedural bleeding (*JAMA 2004;292:45*).
- LMWH must be adjusted for renal dysfunction and should be avoided in patients with severe impairments.
- Enoxaparin 0.3 mg/kg IV should be administered at the time of PCI in patients who have received less than two therapeutic doses or if the last dose was received more than 8 hours before PCI.
  ○ **Fondaparinux** is a synthetic polysaccharide that selectively inhibits factor X and can be subcutaneously administered on a daily routine.
- Associated with less bleeding and similar major adverse cardiovascular outcomes when compared to enoxaparin.
- Associated with an increased risk of thrombosis during PCI and should not be used without additional antithrombin anticoagulation; as such, it is not recommended for the routine management of ACS.
- In patients not undergoing invasive management, fondaparinux may significantly reduce bleeding and improve outcomes compared to LMWH (*JAMA 2015;313:707*).
  ○ **Bivalirudin** is a direct thrombin inhibitor given as a continuous IV infusion and requires partial thromboplastin time (PTT) monitoring when used for >4 hours.
- It does not cause HIT and is used in the treatment of patients who develop HIT or patients with ACS who have history of HIT.
- Bivalirudin can be given in conjunction with ASA and clopidogrel in patients presenting with UA/NSTEMI who will undergo a routine invasive strategy.
- Bivalirudin alone compared to UFH/LMWH + GPIIb/IIIa inhibitor was associated with less bleeding (*N Engl J Med 2006;355:2203*). Recent evidence has shown that in ACS without significant GPIIb/IIIa inhibitor use, bivalirudin is associated with increased risk of stent thrombosis and target lesion revascularization (*Lancet 2014;384:1849*).
- Caution should be used with routine use of bivalirudin in ACS unless there is a high risk of bleeding.
- **Anti-ischemic therapy** (please also refer to Treatment section of stable angina)
  ○ **Nitroglycerin**
- Treatment can be initiated at the time of presentation with sublingual nitroglycerin. **NOTE:** 40% of patients with chest pain *not* due to CAD will get relief with nitroglycerin (*Ann Intern Med 2003;139:979*) (see Table 4-10).
- Patients with ongoing ischemic symptoms or those who require additional agents to control significant hypertension can be treated with IV nitroglycerin until pain relief, hypertension control, or both are achieved.
- Rule out right ventricular (RV) infarct prior to administration of nitrates because this can precipitate profound hypotension.
  ○ **β-Adrenergic blockers (BBs)** (please also refer to the Treatment section for stable angina)
- Oral therapy should be started early in the absence of contraindications.
- Treatment with an IV preparation should be reserved for treatment of arrhythmia, ongoing chest pain, or advanced hypertension rather than routine use.
- Routine use of IV BBs is associated with increased risk of cardiogenic shock and should be avoided.
- Contraindications to BB therapy include advanced AV block, active bronchospasm, decompensated HF, cardiogenic shock, hypotension, and bradycardia.
  ○ **Morphine** 2–4 mg IV may be used as an adjunct to BB, nitrates, and calcium channel blockers. Care must be used not to mask further clinical evaluation by heavy use of narcotic medications.

- **Adjunctive medical therapy**
  - **ACE inhibitors** (refer to Treatment section for stable angina) are effective antihypertensive agents and have been shown to reduce mortality in patients with CAD and LV systolic dysfunction. ACE inhibitors should be used in patients with LV dysfunction (EF <40%), hypertension, or diabetes presenting with ACS. **ARBs** are appropriate in patients who cannot tolerate ACEIs.
  - **Aldosterone antagonists** should be added, if there are no contraindications (potassium >5 mEq/L or creatinine clearance [CrCl] <30 mL/min), after initiation of ACE inhibitors to patients with diabetes or who have an LVEF <40%.
  - **3-Hydroxy-3-methylglutaryl–coenzyme A (HMG-CoA) reductase inhibitors (statins)** are potent lipid-lowering agents that reduce the incidence of ischemia, MI, and death in patients with CAD. High-dose statins should be routinely administered within 24 hours of presentation in patients presenting with ACS. A lipid profile should be obtained in all patients.
    - Statin therapy reduces adverse outcomes through lipid lowering and potentially through pleiotropic effects (anti-inflammatory/atherosclerotic plaque–stabilizing effects).
    - Aggressive statin therapy reduces the risk of recurrent ischemia, MI, and death in patients presenting with ACS (*JAMA 2001;285:1711*).
    - A reduction in adverse CVD outcomes following early initiation of a high-dose statin with achievement of an LDL <70 mg/dL can be seen as early as 30 days following initial presentation with ACS (*N Engl J Med 2004;350:1495*). Aggressive LDL lowering also reduces the incidence of periprocedural MI following PCI (*J Am Coll Cardiol 2007;49:1272*).
  - **NSAIDs** are associated with an increased risk of death, MI, myocardial rupture, hypertension, and HF in large meta-analyses (*Circulation 2006;113:2906*). Adverse outcomes have been observed for both nonselective and cyclooxygenase-2 (COX-2) selective agents.
    - NSAIDs should be discontinued in patients presenting with UA/NSTEMI.
    - Acetaminophen is an acceptable alternative for the treatment of osteoarthritis and other musculoskeletal pain.
  - **Blood glucose** should not be tightly controlled in diabetic patients who have suffered ACS because it may increase mortality. Goal is <180 mg/dL while avoiding hypoglycemia at all costs.

Revascularization

- **PCI**
  See "Revascularization" section on pp. 103–104 for invasive management strategies.
- **CABG**
  - The indications for PCI and CABG in patients with UA/NSTEMI are similar to those for individuals with chronic stable angina (please see section on revascularization on pp. 103–104).
  - The urgency of revascularization should weigh heavily in the decision for CABG; patients in cardiogenic shock may benefit from PCI and mechanical support compared to emergency cardiac surgery.
  - NSTEMI in the setting of critical left main coronary artery disease should prompt urgent surgical revascularization and consideration of intra-aortic balloon counterpulsation (IABP) for stabilization prior to the induction of anesthesia.

Monitoring/Follow-Up

The highest rate of progression to MI or development of recurrent MI is in the first 2 months after presentation with the index episode. Beyond that time, most patients have a clinical course similar to those with chronic stable angina.

- Patients should be discharged on dual antiplatelet, BB, and statin therapy.
- Most patients should be discharged on ACE inhibitors.

- Patients should be evaluated for the need of aldosterone antagonists.
- Screen for life stressors and depression. Refer for depression treatment as needed.
- Smoking cessation and risk factor modification should be stressed.
- Referral to cardiac rehabilitation should also be pursued.

ST-Segment Elevation Myocardial Infarction

GENERAL PRINCIPLES

Definition

- STEMI is defined as a clinical syndrome of myocardial ischemia in association with persistent ECG ST elevations (see ECG section) and subsequent release of biomarkers of necrosis.
- STEMI is a medical emergency.
- Compared to UA/NSTEMI, STEMI is associated with a higher in-hospital and 30-day morbidity and mortality. Left untreated, the mortality rate of STEMI can exceed 30%, and the presence of mechanical complications (papillary muscle rupture, ventricular septal defect [VSD], and free wall rupture) increases the mortality rate to 90%.
- Ventricular fibrillation accounts for approximately 50% of mortality and often occurs within the first hour from symptom onset.
- Keys to treatment of STEMI include rapid recognition and diagnosis, coordinated mobilization of health care resources, and prompt reperfusion therapy.
- Mortality is directly related to total ischemia time.
- AHA/ACC guidelines provide a more thorough overview of STEMI (*J Am Coll Cardiol 2013;61:e78*).

Epidemiology

- STEMI accounts for approximately 25–30% of ACS cases annually, and the incidence has been declining.
- Over the last several decades, there has been a dramatic improvement in short-term mortality to the current rate of 6–10%.
- Approximately 30% of STEMI presentations occur in women, but outcomes and complications continue to be worse compared with male counterparts.

Pathophysiology

- STEMI is caused by acute, total occlusion of an epicardial coronary artery, most often due to atherosclerotic plaque rupture/erosion and subsequent thrombus formation.
- As compared to NSTEMI/UA, thrombotic occlusion is complete such that there is total transmural ischemia/infarct in the distribution of the large occluded artery.

DIAGNOSIS

Clinical Presentation
History
- Chest pain from STEMI resembles angina but lasts longer, is more intense, and is not relieved by rest or sublingual nitroglycerin. Chest discomfort may be accompanied by dyspnea, diaphoresis, palpitations, nausea, vomiting, fatigue, and/or syncope.
- Severe tearing chest pain or focal neurologic deficits should raise concern for aortic dissection. Aortic dissection can mimic ACS; in addition, dissections of the ascending aorta may involve the right coronary artery and cause ST elevations on the ECG.
- It is imperative to determine the time of symptom onset because this is critical in determining the appropriate means of reperfusion.

- STEMI may have an atypical presentation particularly in female, elderly, and postoperative patients, as well as those with diabetes and chronic or end-stage kidney disease. Such patients may experience atypical or no chest pain and may instead present with confusion, dyspnea, unexplained hypotension, or HF.
- STEMI should always be considered as an etiology when any patient is hemodynamically compromised (i.e., postoperative, delirium, or shock).
- The initial history by the clinician should always include an inquiry about prior cardiac procedures or surgery. Prior PCI or CABG can have profound implications for acute revascularization management.
- The clinician should assess for absolute and relative contraindications to thrombolytic therapy (see the following text) and potential issues complicating primary PCI (IV contrast allergy, PVD/peripheral revascularization, renal dysfunction, central nervous system [CNS] disease, pregnancy, bleeding diathesis, or severe comorbidity).
- Inquire about recent cocaine use. In this setting, aggressive medical therapy with nitroglycerin, coronary vasodilators, and benzodiazepines should be administered before reperfusion therapy is considered.

Physical Examination

Physical examination should be directed at identifying hemodynamic instability, pulmonary congestion, mechanical complications of MI, and other causes of acute chest discomfort.
- The Killip classification (see Table 4-11) can be a useful guide when evaluating patients with ACS. The Forrester classification uses hemodynamic data to risk stratify patients and is less frequently used.
- The identification of a new systolic murmur may suggest the presence of ischemic MR or a VSD.
- A limited neurologic exam to detect baseline cognitive and motor deficits and a vascular examination (lower extremity pulses and bruits) will aid in determining candidacy and planning for reperfusion treatment.
- Cardiogenic shock due to right ventricular MI (RVMI) may be clinically suspected by the presence of hypotension, elevated jugular venous pressure, and absence of pulmonary congestion.
- Bilateral arm BPs should be obtained to assess for the presence of aortic dissection.

DIAGNOSTIC TESTING

Electrocardiography

The ECG is paramount to the diagnosis of STEMI and should be obtained within 10 minutes of presentation. If the diagnosis of STEMI is in doubt, serial ECGs may help elucidate the diagnosis. Classic findings include:
- Peaked upright T waves are the first ECG manifestation of myocardial injury.
- ST elevations correlate with the territory of injured myocardium (Table 4-15).
- **Diagnostic ECG criteria for STEMI** (*J Am Coll Cardiol 2009;53:1003*)
  ○ When ST elevations reach threshold values in two or more anatomically contiguous leads, a diagnosis of STEMI can be made.
  ○ In men >40 years of age, threshold value for abnormal ST-segment elevation at the J point is ≥2 mm in leads V_2 and V_3 and >1 mm in all other leads. In men <40 years of age, threshold value for abnormal ST-segment elevation at the J point in leads V_2 and V_3 is >2.5 mm.
  ○ In women, the threshold value of abnormal ST-segment elevation at the J point is >1.5 mm in leads V_2 and V_3 and >1 mm in all other leads.
  ○ In right-sided leads (V_3R and V_4R), the threshold for abnormal ST elevation at the J point is 0.5 mm, except in males <30 years in whom it is 1 mm. Right-sided leads

TABLE 4-15	Electrocardiogram-Based Anatomic Distribution	
ST Elevation	**Myocardial Territory**	**Coronary Artery**
$V_1–V_6$ or LBBB	Anterior and septal walls	Proximal LAD or left main
$V_1–V_2$	Septum	Proximal LAD or septal branch
$V_2–V_4$	Anterior wall	LAD
$V_5–V_6$	Lateral wall	LCX
II, III, aVF	Inferior wall	RCA or LCX
I, aVL	High lateral wall	Diagonal or proximal LCX

LAD, left anterior descending artery; LBBB, left bundle branch block; LCX, left circumflex artery; RCA, right coronary artery.

should be obtained in all patients with evidence of inferior wall ischemia to rule out RV ischemia. RV infarction can occur with proximal right coronary artery (RCA) lesions.
- In posterior leads (V_7, V_8, and V_9), the threshold for abnormal ST elevation at the J point is 0.5 mm.
  - All patients with ST-segment depression in leads V_1 to V_3, inferior wall ST elevation, or tall R waves in V_1 to V_3 should have posterior leads placed in order to diagnose a posterior wall MI. Posterior STEMIs are usually due to occlusion of the circumflex artery and are often misdiagnosed as UA/NSTEMI. R waves in V_1 or V_2 represent Q waves of the posterior territory.
  - Ischemia of the circumflex artery may also be electrocardiographically silent.
- The presence of reciprocal ST-segment depression opposite of the infarct territory increases the specificity for acute MI.
- New LBBB suggests a large anterior wall MI with a worse prognosis.
- ECG criteria for STEMI in patients with preexisting LBBB or RV pacing can be found in Table 4-16. Above criteria do not apply.
- **ECG changes that mimic MI.** ST-segment elevation and Q waves may result from numerous etiologies other than acute MI, including prior MI with aneurysm formation, aortic dissection, LV hypertrophy, pericarditis, myocarditis, or pulmonary embolism, or they may be a normal finding (Table 4-17). It is critical to obtain prior ECGs to clarify the diagnosis.

TABLE 4-16	Criteria for ST-segment Elevation for Prior LBBB or RV-Paced Rhythm

ECG Change

ST-segment elevation >1 mm in the presence of a positive QRS complex (concordant with the QRS)
ST-segment elevation >5 mm in the presence of a negative QRS complex (disconcordant with the QRS)
ST-segment depression >1 mm in $V_1–V_3$

LBBB, left bundle branch block; RV, right ventricular.
Sgarbossa's (GUSTO) criteria: *Am J Cardiol* 1996;77:423; *N Engl J Med* 1996;334:481; *Pacing Clin Electrophysiol* 2001;24:1289.

TABLE 4-17	Differential Diagnosis of ST-Segment Elevation on ECG Excluding STEMI

Cardiac Etiologies	Other Etiologies
Prior MI with aneurysm formation	Pulmonary embolism
Aortic dissection with coronary involvement	Hyperkalemia
Pericarditis	
Myocarditis	
LV hypertrophy or aortic stenosis (with strain)[a]	
Hypertrophic cardiomyopathy	
Coronary vasospasm (cocaine, Prinzmetal angina)	
Early repolarization (normal variant)	
Brugada syndrome	

LV, left ventricular; MI, myocardial infarction; ST-segment elevation myocardial infarction.
[a]Strain may occur in numerous settings including systemic hypertension, hypotension, tachycardia, exercise, and sepsis.

○ **Q waves.** Development of new pathologic Q waves is considered diagnostic for transmural MI but may occur in patients with prolonged ischemia or poor collateral supply. The presence of Q waves only is not an indication for acute reperfusion therapy; however, it is very helpful to have an old ECG to compare to in order to determine chronicity. Diagnostic criteria include:
  ▪ In leads V_2 and V_3, a pathologic Q wave is ≥ 0.02 second or a QS complex in V_2 or V_3. An isolated Q wave in lead V_1 or lead III is normal.
  ▪ In leads other than V_1 through V_3, presence of a Q wave ≥ 0.03 second and ≥ 0.1 mV deep or a QS complex in any two contiguous leads suggests prior MI.
  ▪ R wave ≥ 0.04 second in V_1 and V_2 and R/S ratio ≥ 1 with a positive T wave suggest prior posterior MI (in the absence of RV hypertrophy or right bundle branch block [RBBB]).

Laboratories and Imaging
• STEMI diagnosis and initiation of treatment are done in a patient who reports prolonged chest discomfort or anginal equivalent with qualifying ECG findings. Attempting to wait for results of cardiac biomarkers will add unnecessary delay.
• Blood samples should be sent for cardiac enzymes (troponin, CK-MB), complete blood cell count, coagulation studies (PTT, prothrombin time [PT], international normalized ratio [INR]), creatinine, electrolytes including magnesium, and type and screen. A fasting lipid profile should be obtained in all patients with STEMI for secondary prevention (note, however, that lipid levels may be falsely lowered during the acute phase of MI).
• Initial cardiac enzymes (including troponin assays) may be normal, depending on the time in relation to symptom onset. Myoglobin is the first enzyme to rise.
• CK-MB can be used to confirm that myocardial injury occurred within the previous 48 hours because troponin levels may remain elevated for up to 2 weeks after MI.
• The risk of subsequent cardiac death is directly proportional to the increase in cardiac-specific troponins, even when CK-MB levels are not elevated. Measuring enzymes until the peak level has been attained can be used to determine infarct size.
• Routine use of cardiac noninvasive imaging is not recommended for the initial diagnosis of STEMI. When the diagnosis is in question, a TTE can be performed to document regional wall motion abnormalities. If not adequately evaluated by TTE, a transesophageal echocardiogram (TEE) can be obtained to assess for acute complications of MI and presence of aortic dissection.

- A portable chest radiograph is useful to assess for pulmonary edema and evaluate for other causes of chest pain including aortic dissection. Importantly, a normal mediastinal width does not exclude aortic dissection, especially if clinically suspected.

TREATMENT

- **Before presentation to the hospital.** The general public should be informed of the signs and symptoms consistent with an acute MI that should lead them to seek urgent medical care. Availability of "911" access and emergency medical services facilitates delivery of patients to emergency medical care.
- **Acute management.** Prompt treatment should be initiated as soon as the diagnosis is suspected, as mortality and risk of subsequent HF are directly related to ischemia time (Figure 4-4).

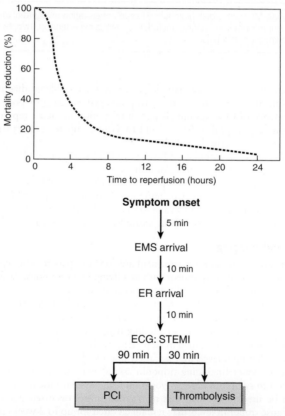

Figure 4-4. The benefit of coronary reperfusion is inversely related to ischemia time. **Top.** Graphic representation of mortality benefit of coronary reperfusion as a function of ischemia time. (Data from *JAMA 2005;293:979.*) **Bottom.** Recommended timeline of events following chest pain onset according to AHA/ACC guidelines (Data from *Circulation 2008;117:296*). AHA/ACC, American Heart Association/American College of Cardiology; ECG, electrocardiogram; EMS, emergency medical service; ER, emergency room; PCI, percutaneous coronary intervention; STEMI, ST-segment elevation myocardial infarction.

- All medical centers should have in place and use an AHA/ACC guideline–based STEMI protocol. Centers that are not primary PCI capable should have protocols in place to meet accepted time-to-therapy guidelines, with either rapid transfer to a PCI-capable facility or administration of thrombolytics with subsequent transfer to a PCI center.
- **In the emergency department**, an acute MI protocol should be activated that includes a targeted clinical examination and a 12-lead ECG completed within 10 minutes of arrival.
- **Immediate management.** The goal of immediate management in patients with STEMI is to identify candidates for reperfusion therapy and to immediately initiate that process. Other priorities include relief of ischemic pain, as well as recognition and treatment of hypotension, pulmonary edema, and arrhythmia.
- **General measures**
  - Supplemental oxygen should be administered if saturations are <90%. If necessary, institution of mechanical ventilation decreases the work of breathing and reduces myocardial oxygen demand.
  - Two peripheral IV catheters should be inserted upon arrival.
  - Serial ECGs should be obtained for patients who do not have ST-segment elevation on the initial ECG but experience ongoing chest discomfort as they may have an evolving STEMI. Telemetry should be placed to monitor for arrhythmias.

Medications

Upstream medical therapy should include administration of ASA and anticoagulants as well as agents that reduce myocardial ischemia (Table 4-18).
- Chewable **ASA** 162–325 mg should be given immediately to *all* patients with suspected acute MI; 325 mg is preferred for those who are ASA naïve. After PCI, the subsequent dose of ASA is 81 mg/d and is to be given indefinitely (*Eur Heart J 2009;30:900*).
- A loading dose of a **P2Y12 inhibitor** should be given to all STEMI patients, as part of dual antiplatelet therapy, as soon as possible after presentation. Cost and bleeding risk can be taken into consideration when choosing which agent. *Please also refer to the antiplatelet section on UA/NSTEMI for background information and dosing on agents listed in the following text.*
  - If the patient is to receive fibrinolytic therapy, along with ASA and an anticoagulant, patients should receive:
    - Clopidogrel 300-mg loading dose if given during the first 24 hours of therapy; if started 24 hours after administration of fibrinolytics, a 600-mg loading dose is preferred. Maintenance is 75 mg/d.
    - Patients older than 75 years should not be given the loading dose.
  - If the patient is going for PCI, **one** of the following should be added to ASA and anticoagulant:
    - **Clopidogrel** 600-mg loading, then 75 mg daily for 12 months.
    - **Prasugrel** 60-mg loading, then 10 mg daily for minimum of 12 months (contraindicated in patients with prior CVA and avoided in those >75 years and with weight <60 kg). Prasugrel generally should be given after diagnostic angiography (or within an hour of PCI) when it is certain the patient will not need CABG surgery given a higher incidence of bleeding related to surgery as compared to clopidogrel (*Lancet 2009;373:723*).
    - **Ticagrelor** 180-mg loading dose, then 90 mg bid (Note: maintenance ASA is 81 or 100 mg daily **only**) for a minimum of 12 months.
- **GPIIb/IIIa inhibitors** do not have a routine role in the initial presentation of STEMI patients or as part of adjunctive therapy with thrombolytics.
  - It may be reasonable to use GPIIb/IIIa inhibitors as an alternative to a P2Y12 antagonist in patients who present with acute complications of MI requiring surgery (ischemic MR, ruptured papillary muscle, or VSD).
  - In general, GPIIb/IIIa use should be left to the discretion of the invasive cardiologist.

TABLE 4-18	Upstream Medical Therapy	
Medication	**Dosage**	**Comments**
Aspirin (ASA)	162–325 mg	Non–enteric-coated formulations (chewed or crushed) given orally or rectally facilitate rapid drug absorption and platelet inhibition.
Clopidogrel	600 mg loading dose, 75–150 mg/d	600 mg loading dose followed by 150 mg maintenance dose for 7 d may reduce the incidence of stent thrombosis and MI compared to the standard 300 mg loading dose and 75 mg maintenance dose. Caution should be used in the elderly because clinical trials validating clopidogrel use in STEMI either did not include elderly patients or did not use a loading dose.
Prasugrel	60 mg loading dose, 10 mg/d	Compared to clopidogrel, prasugrel is a quicker acting and more potent antiplatelet agent with improved efficacy but did significantly increase CABG bleeding rates. Prasugrel should not be used in patients >75 y old, <60 kg, or with a history of stroke/TIA.
Ticagrelor	180 mg loading, then 90 mg bid	ASA dose should not exceed 100 mg. Ticagrelor has shown mortality benefit over clopidogrel at the expense of higher bleeding rates.
Unfractionated heparin (UFH)	60 units/kg IV bolus, 12 units/kg/h	UFH should be given to all patients undergoing PCI and those receiving thrombolytics with the exception of streptokinase. The maximum IV bolus is 4000 units.
Enoxaparin (LMWH)	30 mg IV bolus, 1 mg/kg SC bid	Patients >75 y old should not be given a loading dose and receive 0.75 mg/kg SC bid. An additional loading dose of 0.3 mg/kg should be given if the last dose of LMWH was >8 h prior to PCI. The use of LMWH is only validated in thrombolysis and rescue PCI.
Bivalirudin	0.75 mg/kg IV bolus, 1.75 mg/kg/h	Bivalirudin has been validated in patients undergoing PCI and has not been studied in conjunction with thrombolysis. Patients who received a heparin bolus prior to bivalirudin had a lower incidence of stent thrombosis than those who only received bivalirudin.
Fondaparinux	2.5 mg IV bolus, 2.5 mg SC daily	Shown to be superior to UFH when used during thrombolysis with decreased bleeding rates. Fondaparinux increases the risk of catheter thrombosis when used during PCI (*JAMA 2006;295:1519*).

(*continued*)

TABLE 4-18	Upstream Medical Therapy (*Continued*)	
Medication	**Dosage**	**Comments**
Nitroglycerin	0.4 mg SL or aerosol infusion; 10–200 μg/ min IV	Sublingual or aerosol nitroglycerin can be given every 5 min for a total of three doses in the absence of hypotension. IV nitroglycerin can be used for uncontrolled chest discomfort.
Metoprolol	25 mg PO qid, uptitrate as needed	β-Blockers should be avoided in patients with evidence of heart failure, hemodynamic instability, marked first-degree AV block, advanced heart block, and bronchospasm.

AV, atrioventricular; CABG, coronary artery bypass graft; LMWH, low–molecular-weight heparin; MI, myocardial infarction; PCI, percutaneous coronary intervention; SL, sublingual; STEMI, ST-segment elevation myocardial infarction; TIA, transient ischemic attack.

- **Anticoagulant therapy** should be initiated on presentation in all patients with STEMI regardless of the choice of PCI or thrombolytic therapy. *Please also refer to the medication section for UA/NSTEMI for background information on agents listed in the following text.*
  - **Patients who will receive fibrinolytic therapy should be started on either:**
    - **UFH** with monitoring to ensure the activated PTT is twice the upper limit of normal. UFH should be continued for at least 48 hours after fibrinolysis. If angiography with intent to perform PCI is anticipated to occur early after fibrinolysis, then UFH may be preferable.
      Dosing for UFH: bolus dose of 60 units/kg (maximum 4000 units), then 12 units/ kg/h (maximum 1000 units/h) to keep PTT at 50–70 seconds.
    - **Enoxaparin**, if the serum creatinine is <2.5 mg/dL in men or 2.0 mg/dL in women, an initial 30-mg IV bolus is given followed 15 minutes later with 1 mg/kg SC bid. Give for the entirety of the index hospitalization but not to exceed 8 days.
      - In patients 75 years or older, no bolus is given and subcutaneous dose is 0.75 mg/kg bid.
      - If CrCL <30 mL/min, the subcutaneous dose is 1 mg/kg daily.
    - **Fondaparinux** with an initial IV dose is 2.5 mg, followed by subcutaneous 2.5 mg daily. Agent should not be used if CrCl <30 mL/min. Give for the entirety of the index hospitalization but not to exceed 8 days.
    - **Bivalirudin** can be used for HIT-positive patients but has not been studied extensively in STEMI patients and patient with fibrinolysis.
  - **Anticoagulant choice for patients who will receive primary PCI:**
    - **UFH** is often preferred during PCI by many operators due to the availability and real-time therapeutic monitoring with activating clotting times (ACTs) in the catheterization laboratory. Additional bolus doses of UFH are given at PCI, with the dose and ACT goal dependent on whether a GPIIb/IIIa antagonist has been given.
    - **Enoxaparin** use in STEMI patients as an anticoagulant for PCI is unclear.
      - Additional IV dose may be needed at PCI depending on timing of the last dose and total number of doses given.
      - Patients on therapeutic enoxaparin should not be given UFH.
    - **Bivalirudin** can be given to patients already treated with ASA and clopidogrel on presentation.
      - Bivalirudin is an acceptable alternative to the use of combined heparin and GPIIb/ IIIa inhibitor during PCI with lower bleeding rates but higher rate of stent thrombosis (*N Engl J Med 2008;358:2218*; *JAMA 2003;19:853*).

   □ It is the agent of choice in patients with known HIT.
   □ It can be given with or without prior treatment with UFH. If patient is being treated
     with UFH, discontinue UFH for 30 minutes prior to starting bivalirudin.
   □ Dose is 0.75 mg/kg bolus, then 1.75 mg/kg/h infusion.
  ▪ **Fondaparinux** is not indicated for use in STEMI patients as a sole anticoagulant and
    has to be given along with UFH due to risk of catheter-related thrombosis.
• **Anti-ischemic therapy** (also refer to the Medications section for UA/NSTEMI for back-
  ground information on agents listed here)
  ○ **Nitroglycerin** should be administered to patients with ischemic chest pain, to aid in
    control of hypertension, or as part of the management of HF. Nitroglycerin should
    either be avoided or used with caution in patients with:
    ▪ Hypotension (systolic BP [SBP] <90 mm Hg)
    ▪ RV infarct
    ▪ Heart rate >100 bpm or <50 bpm
    ▪ Documented use of phosphodiesterase inhibitors in previous 48 hours
  ○ **Morphine** (2–4 mg IV) can be used for refractory chest pain that is not responsive
    to nitroglycerin. Adequate analgesia decreases levels of circulating catecholamines and
    reduces myocardial oxygen consumption.
  ○ **BBs** improve myocardial ischemia, limit infarct size, and reduce major adverse cardiac
    events including mortality, recurrent ischemia, and malignant arrhythmias.
    ▪ Oral BBs should be started in all patients with STEMI within the first 24 hours who
      do not have signs of new HF, evidence of cardiogenic shock (Killip class II or greater),
      age older than 70 years, SBP <120 mm Hg, pulse >110 or <60 bpm, or advanced
      heart block (*Lancet 2005;366:1622*).
    ▪ IV BBs can increase mortality in patients with STEMI and should be reserved for
      management of arrhythmias or acute treatment of accelerated hypertension in pa-
      tients without the earlier mentioned features. Sinus tachycardia in the setting of a
      STEMI may be a compensatory response to maintain cardiac output and should not
      prompt IV BB use.

Acute Coronary Reperfusion

• The majority of patients who suffer an acute STEMI have thrombotic occlusion of a
  coronary artery. Early restoration of coronary perfusion limits infarct size, preserves LV
  function, and reduces mortality.
• All other therapies are secondary and should not delay the timely goal of achieving coronary reperfusion.
• Unless spontaneous resolution of ischemia occurs (as determined by resolution of chest
  discomfort and normalization of ST elevation), the choice of reperfusion strategy includes thrombolysis, primary PCI, or emergent CABG (Figure 4-5).
  ○ Normalization of the ECG and symptoms should not preclude the patient being referred
    for urgent diagnostic angiography. Morphine may mask ongoing ischemic symptoms.
  ○ Note: Ongoing symptoms are not criteria for treatment of STEMI in the first 12 hours
    of symptom onset. Patients who arrive within 12 hours of their symptoms, despite
    symptom resolution, but with continued ECG changes of STEMI are still candidates
    for immediate reperfusion (either primary PCI or fibrinolytics). We recommend angi-
    ography with intent for PCI/CABG in such a circumstance.
• The choice of reperfusion therapy should be considered of secondary importance to the
  overall goal of achieving reperfusion in a timely manner.
  ○ **Primary PCI**
    ▪ Primary PCI is the preferred reperfusion strategy when available within 90 min-
      utes of first medical contact. Compared to fibrinolytic therapy, PCI offers supe-
      rior vessel patency and perfusion (TIMI 3 flow) with less reinfarction, less risk of

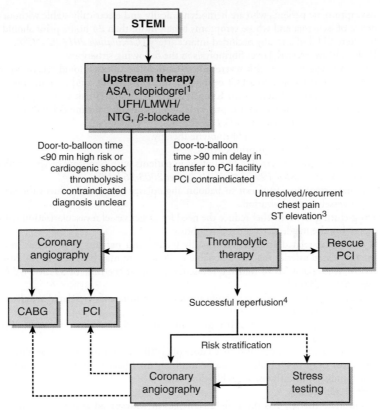

Figure 4-5. Strategies for coronary reperfusion and risk assessment. [1]If fibrinolytics are to be given, use clopidogrel only. If primary PCI is planned, give ticagrelor, prasugrel, or clopidogrel. [2]UFH may be used with either PCI or thrombolytic therapy, whereas bivalirudin has only been studied with PCI and LMWH has only been validated for fibrinolytic therapy and rescue PCI. In patients who are to receive fibrinolysis, LMWH and fondaparinux are preferred to UFH. [3]Patients who do not experience chest pain relief, have recurrent chest pain, have unstable arrhythmias, develop heart failure, or have ST-segment elevations that do not normalize 60–90 minutes following fibrinolysis should undergo rescue PCI. [4]Signs of successful reperfusion include chest pain relief, 50% reduction in ST-segment elevation, and idioventricular rhythm. P2Y12 inhibitors include antiplatelet agents: clopidogrel, prasugrel, and ticagrelor. ASA, aspirin; CABG, coronary artery bypass graft; LMWH, low–molecular-weight heparin; NTG, nitroglycerin; PCI, percutaneous coronary intervention; STEMI, ST-segment elevation myocardial infarction; UFH, unfractionated heparin.

intracranial hemorrhage, and improved survival regardless of lesion location or patient age. STEMI patients with symptom onset <12 hours prior have a better prognosis and outcome after PCI. PCI should still be routinely offered to patients with STEMI who have ongoing symptoms that began 12–24 hours prior to presentation.

▪ PCI may also be considered, although evidence of benefit is limited, in patients who are now asymptomatic but had symptoms in the previous 12- to 24-hour period.

- Asymptomatic patients who are hemodynamically and electrically stable without evidence of ischemia and whose symptoms began more than 24 hours prior should not be offered PCI of a totally occluded infarct artery (*Circulation 2011;22:2320*).
- **PCI** is always preferred over fibrinolysis in the following situations:
  □ Patients who present with severe HF or cardiogenic shock should receive primary PCI (even if transfer to a PCI center may cause delays beyond current time goals for reperfusion). Patients with Killip class III/IV or TIMI risk score ≥5 represent high-risk groups where PCI is preferred despite a potential time delay (*Eur Heart J 2010;31:676; Circulation 2005;112:2017*).
  □ Have a contraindication to fibrinolytic therapy.
  □ Have had recent PCI or prior CABG.
  □ PCI is generally preferred to fibrinolysis in patients with symptom onset >12 hours prior (*N Engl J Med 1997;336:1621; Lancet 2003;361:13*).
- Coronary stenting is superior to balloon angioplasty alone and reduces the rates of target vessel revascularization.
- Drug-eluting stents further reduce the need for target vessel revascularization without increasing the incidence of stent thrombosis.
- If the infarct-related artery is successfully treated and patients have lesions in non–infarct-related arteries that are amenable to PCI, there may be a benefit for death or recurrent nonfatal MI to undergo revascularization at the time of STEMI (*N Engl J Med 2013;369:1115*).
- Patients in shock should have significant lesions in non–infarct-related arteries intervened on if feasible.
- Transradial approach in STEMI reduces bleeding and may have a mortality benefit compared to transfemoral access.
- Facilitated PCI, a strategy of reduced dose of GPIIb/IIIa inhibitors and/or fibrinolytic agent just prior to PCI, should not be routinely used because it does not improve efficacy and significantly increases bleeding rates.
  ○ **Fibrinolytic therapy**
    - Fibrinolytic therapy has the main advantages of widespread availability and ease of delivery. The primary disadvantage of fibrinolytic therapy is the risk of intracranial hemorrhage, uncertainty of whether normal coronary flow has been restored, and risk of reocclusion of the infarct-related artery.
    - Fibrinolysis is indicated when primary PCI is not available in a timely fashion (i.e., delay >120 minutes).
    - Fibrinolytic therapy is indicated for use if given within 12 hours of the symptom onset with qualifying ECG changes of ST elevation, new LBBB, or true posterior MI. When given, it should be administered within 30 minutes of initial patient contact. Fibrinolytic therapy is most successful when given in the first 3 hours of symptom onset, after which the benefit tapers.
    - Patients presenting to a hospital without PCI capability should be transferred for primary PCI, rather than being given fibrinolytics, if time from first medical contact to PCI will not be >120 minutes. This seems particularly relevant to patients arriving 3–12 hours from symptom onset.
    - In patients transferred for PCI, primary PCI significantly lowered the incidence of death, MI, or stroke compared to on-site thrombolysis (*N Engl J Med 2003;249:733; J Am Coll Cardiol 2002;39:1713; Eur Heart J 2000;21:823*).
    - All patients should be transferred to a PCI-capable facility after fibrinolysis (early routine angiography); this should occur urgently if patients are in shock or have failed reperfusion.
    - Rescue PCI is PCI in the setting of failed fibrinolysis and has shown benefit over conservative management. Given the risk of bleeding, this decision must be tailored to the individual patient and clinical status (e.g., amount of myocardium in jeopardy, shock, other comorbid illness).

- Available thrombolytic agents include the fibrin-selective agents such as **alteplase (recombinant tissue plasminogen activator [rt-PA])**, **reteplase** (r-PA), and **tenecteplase** (TNK-tPA). **Streptokinase** is the only nonselective agent in use. Further details and dosing information can be found in Table 4-19.
  □ TNK-tPA is the current agent of choice due to similar efficacy, lower risk of bleeding, and convenient single bolus administration as compared to rt-PA. Streptokinase is the cheapest and still widely used worldwide.

TABLE 4-19	Fibrinolytic Agents	
Medication	**Dosage**	**Comments**
Streptokinase (SK)	1.5 million units IV over 60 min	Produces a generalized fibrinolytic state (not clot specific). SK reduces mortality following STEMI: 18% relative risk reduction and 2% absolute risk reduction (*Lancet 1987;2:871*). Allergic reactions including skin rashes, fever, and anaphylaxis may be seen in 1–2% of patients. Isolated hypotension occurs in 10% of patients and usually responds to volume expansion. Because of the development of antibodies, patients who were previously treated with SK should be given an alternate thrombolytic agent.
Recombinant tissue plasminogen activator (rt-PA)	15 mg IV bolus 0.75 mg/kg over 30 min (maximum 50 mg) 0.50 mg/kg over 60 min (maximum 35 mg)	Fibrin-selective agent with improved clot specificity compared to SK. Does not cause allergic reactions or hypotension. Mortality benefit compared to SK at the expense of an increased risk of intracranial hemorrhage (*N Engl J Med 1993;329:673*).
Reteplase (r-PA)	Two 10-unit IV boluses administered 30 min apart	Fibrin selective agent with a longer half-life but reduced clot specificity compared to rt-PA. Mortality benefit equivalent to that of rt-PA (*N Engl J Med 1997;337:1118*).
Tenecteplase (TNK-tPA)	0.50 mg/kg IV bolus (total dose 30–50 mg)	Genetically engineered variant of rt-PA with slower plasma clearance, improved fibrin specificity, and higher resistance to PAI-1. Mortality benefit equivalent to that of rt-PA with reduced bleeding rates (*Lancet 1999;354:716*). Monitoring is required with a goal aPTT of 1.5–2.5 times control.

aPTT, activated partial thromboplastin time; PAI-1, plasminogen activator inhibitor-1; STEMI, ST-segment elevation myocardial infarction.

□ Fibrin-selective agents should be used in combination with anticoagulant therapy, ASA, and clopidogrel (see earlier). GPIIb/IIIa inhibitors should not be used in conjunction. Prasugrel and ticagrelor have not been studied for use with fibrinolytics.

- Fibrinolytic therapy is contraindicated:
  □ In patients with ECG evidence of ST-segment depressions (unless posterior MI suspected).
  □ In those who are asymptomatic with initial symptoms occurring >24 hours prior (*this is in contrast to patients who are asymptomatic with symptom onset <12 hours prior; see earlier*).
  □ In patients with other contraindications to fibrinolysis (Table 4-20).
  □ In patients with presence of five or more risk factors for intracranial hemorrhage.
- The most common complication of fibrinolytic therapy is bleeding. Intracranial hemorrhage occurs in >4% of patients with five or more of the following risk factors for intracranial hemorrhage (*Stroke 2000;31:1802*).
  □ Age ≥75 years
  □ Weight ≤65 kg in women and ≤80 kg in men
  □ Female gender
  □ African American race
  □ Prior history of stroke
  □ SBP ≥160 mm Hg
  □ INR >4 or PT >24
  □ Use of alteplase
- Any patient who experiences a sudden change in neurologic status should undergo urgent head CT, and all anticoagulant and thrombolytic therapies should be discontinued. Fresh frozen plasma should be given to patients with intracerebral hemorrhage. Cryoprecipitate may also be used to replenish fibrinogen and factor VIII levels. Platelet transfusions and protamine can be useful in patients with markedly prolonged bleeding times. Neurologic and neurosurgical consultation should be obtained immediately.
- Major bleeding complications that require blood transfusion occur in approximately 10% of patients.

TABLE 4-20	Contraindications to Thrombolytic Therapy
Absolute Contraindications	**Relative Contraindications**
History of intracranial hemorrhage or hemorrhagic stroke	Prior ischemic stroke >3 mo ago
Ischemic stroke within 3 mo	Allergy or previous use of streptokinase (>5 d ago)[a]
Known structural cerebrovascular lesion (AVMs, aneurysms, tumor)	Recent internal bleeding (2–4 wk)
Closed head injury within 3 mo	Prolonged/traumatic CPR more than 10 min
Aortic dissection	Major surgery within 3 wk
Severe uncontrolled hypertension (SBP >180 mm Hg, DBP >110 mm Hg)	Active peptic ulcer disease
	Noncompressible vascular punctures
	History of intraocular bleeding
Active bleeding or bleeding diathesis	Pregnancy
Acute pericarditis	Uncontrolled hypertension
	Use of oral anticoagulants

AVM, arteriovenous malformation; CPR, cardiopulmonary resuscitation; DBP, diastolic blood pressure; SBP, systolic blood pressure.
[a]Thrombolytics other than streptokinase may be used.

- **Postfibrinolysis care**
  - All patients should receive appropriate dual antiplatelet therapy and at least 48 hours of anticoagulation after fibrinolysis.
  - Routine coronary angiography within 24 hours of thrombolysis has reduced adverse cardiac events compared to rescue PCI (*Lancet 2004;264:1045*). Immediate transfer for angiography (3–24 hours after fibrinolysis) at a PCI-capable facility is also proven to be beneficial (*Lancet 2008;371:559*).
  - Evidence for successful fibrinolysis includes:
    - Relief of chest pain or angina symptoms
    - >50% reduction in ST-segment elevations at 90 minutes
    - Reperfusion arrhythmia (i.e., accelerated idioventricular rhythm) up to 2 hours after completion of infusion
- **Rescue PCI after failed fibrinolysis**
  - Thrombolytic therapy does not achieve coronary artery patency in 30% of patients. In contrast, primary PCI results in restoration of normal coronary flow (TIMI 3) in >95% of cases.
  - Rescue PCI reduces the incidence of death, reinfarction, and HF by nearly 50% (*Circulation 1994;90:2280*; *N Engl J Med 2005;353:2758*).
  - Evidence of failed fibrinolysis includes:
    - Persistence or reoccurrence of ischemic symptoms
    - ST segments resolve <50% 90 minutes after fibrinolysis
    - Electrical or hemodynamic instability
    - Development of HF symptoms
  - **Emergency CABG** is a high-risk procedure that should be considered only if the patient has severe left main disease or refractory ischemia in the setting of failed PCI or coronary anatomy that is not amenable to PCI. Emergency surgery should also be considered for patients with acute mechanical complications of MI including papillary muscle rupture, severe ischemic MR, VSD, ventricular aneurysm formation in the setting of intractable ventricular arrhythmias, or ventricular free wall rupture.

Peri-Infarct Management

- **The coronary care unit (CCU)** was the first major advance in the modern era of treatment of acute MI. All patients with STEMI should be observed in a specialized CCU or intensive care unit setting for at least 24 hours after MI.
- Bed rest is appropriate intermediate care for the first 24 hours after presentation with an acute MI. After 24 hours, clinically stable patients can progressively advance their activity as tolerated.
- Patients should have continuous telemetry monitoring to detect for recurrent ischemia and arrhythmias.
- Daily evaluation should include assessment for recurrent chest discomfort, new HF symptoms, and routine ECGs. Physical exam should focus on new murmurs and any evidence of HF.
- A baseline echocardiogram should be obtained to document EF, wall motion abnormalities, valvular lesions, and presence of ventricular thrombus.
- **Cardiac pacing** may be required in the setting of an acute MI. Rhythm disturbance may be transient in nature, in which case temporary pacing is sufficient until a stable rhythm returns (see the following text). As compared to inferior wall MIs where AV block is transient and stable, AV block with anterior wall MIs can be unstable with wide QRS escape rhythms with 80% mortality and usually requires temporary and then permanent pacemakers.

Post-STEMI Medical Therapy

- See also Medications section for UA/NSTEMI.
- **ASA** should be continued indefinitely. Dose of 81 mg/d has been shown to be effective after PCI; however, the range of 75–162 mg/d has also been endorsed.

- **Clopidogrel** (75 mg/d), **prasugrel** (10 mg/d), or **ticagrelor** (90 mg bid) should be given for a minimum of 12 months regardless of whether a bare metal stent (BMS) or drug-eluting stent was used (*this is in contrast to non-ACS patients who receive a BMS and the minimum duration of therapy is 1 month*).
- **BBs** confer a mortality benefit following acute MI. Treatment should begin as soon as possible (preferably within the first 24 hours) and continued indefinitely unless contraindicated.
- **ACE inhibitors** provide a reduction in short-term mortality, incidence of HF, and recurrent MI when initiated within the first 24 hours of an acute MI (*Lancet 1994;343:1115*; *Lancet 1995;345:669*).
  - Patients with EF <40%, large anterior MI, and prior MI derive the most benefit from ACE inhibitor therapy.
  - Contraindications include hypotension, history of angioedema with use, pregnancy, acute renal failure, and hyperkalemia.
  - ARBs can be used in patients who are intolerant of ACE inhibitors.
- **HMG-CoA reductase inhibitors** should be started in all patients in the absence of contraindications. Several trials have shown the benefit of early and aggressive use of high-dose statins following acute MI. The goal is at least 50% reduction in LDL or LDL <70 mg/dL.
- **Aldosterone receptor antagonists (spironolactone and eplerenone)** have shown benefit in post-MI patients with LVEF <40% and in diabetics (*N Engl J Med 1999;341:709*; *N Engl J Med 2003;348:1309*). Caution should be used in patients with hyperkalemia and renal insufficiency.
- **Warfarin** should not be routinely prescribed to patients with apical hypokinesis in the setting of an anterior MI in the absence of LV thrombus or other indications for anticoagulation. Such therapy is associated with increased bleeding and death. The actual risk of developing LV thrombus is low because many patients will have recovery of hypokinesis (*J Am Coll Cardiol 2015;8:155*).

SPECIAL CONSIDERATIONS

Risk Assessment

- Asymptomatic patients who present >24 hours after symptom onset, patients who receive medical therapy alone, and patients who receive an incomplete revascularization should undergo further risk assessment. Patients may be evaluated using either noninvasive stress testing or an invasive (coronary angiography) strategy.
- **Stress testing** can be used to determine prognosis, residual ischemia, and functional capacity. Patients who are successfully revascularized do not need stress testing prior to discharge unless needed for referral to cardiac rehabilitation.
  - A submaximal exercise stress test can be performed as early as 2–3 days following MI in stable patients who have had no further ischemic signs/symptoms or signs of HF.
  - Alternatively, stress testing can be performed after hospital discharge (2–6 weeks) for low-risk patients and for patients starting cardiac rehabilitation.
  - Coronary angiography should be performed in patients with limiting angina, significant ischemic burden, and poor functional capacity.
- Patients treated medically or with fibrinolytics who experience complications of MI, including recurrent angina/ischemia, HF, significant ventricular arrhythmia, or a mechanical complication of the MI, should proceed directly to coronary angiography to define their anatomy and offer an appropriate revascularization strategy.
- **Special clinical situations**
  - **RVMI** is seen in patients with an acute inferior MI secondary to complete occlusion of the proximal RCA. RV function is very preload dependent, and frequently, hypotension responds to fluid resuscitation.
    - The clinical triad of hypotension, elevated jugular venous pressure, and clear lung fields in the setting of STEMI should prompt an evaluation for RV infarct.

- One-mm ST elevations in the V_1 or V_4R leads are the most sensitive marker of RV involvement.
- LV filling pressures are typically normal or decreased, the right atrial pressures are elevated (>10 mm Hg), and the cardiac index is depressed. In some patients, elevated right atrial pressures may not be evident until IV fluids are administered.
- Initial therapy is IV fluids. If hypotension persists, inotropic support with dobutamine and/or IABP may be necessary. Right-sided mechanical support devices are available when pharmacologic support fails.
- Invasive hemodynamic monitoring is critical in the persistently hypotensive patient because it guides volume status and the need for inotropic and mechanical support.
- In patients with heart block and AV dyssynchrony, sequential AV pacing has a marked beneficial effect.
  ○ **Restenosis and stent thrombosis** are disease entities unique to patients who have previously undergone PCI.
  - Restenosis is a result of neointimal hyperplasia and occurs more frequently in patients with BMS placement, diabetics, patients with long areas of prior stenting, and patients with stenting in small arteries. Restenosis presents most frequently as stable progressive angina and is not affected by the discontinuation of dual antiplatelet therapy.
  - Stent thrombosis is the thrombotic occlusion of a previously placed coronary stent and presents as ACS or sudden cardiac death. Stent thrombosis is associated with a high mortality rate and poor prognosis (*JAMA 2005;293:2126*; *J Am Coll Cardiol 2009;53:1399*).
    □ Acute stent thrombosis occurs within 24 hours and is due to mechanical procedural complications as well as inadequate anticoagulation and antiplatelet therapies.
    □ Subacute stent thrombosis (24 hours to 30 days) is a consequence of inadequate platelet inhibition and mechanical stent complications. Cessation of P2Y12 inhibitor (clopidogrel, prasugrel, ticagrelor) therapy during this time yields a 30- to 100-fold risk of stent thrombosis.
    □ Late (30 days to 1 year) stent thrombosis and very late stent thrombosis occur principally with drug-eluting stents.
    □ Neoatherosclerosis is atherosclerotic plaque unique to prior PCI, occurs in previously placed stents, and can predispose a patient to angina or plaque rupture with subsequent ACS.
  ○ **Ischemic MR** is a poor prognostic indicator following MI. Papillary muscle rupture is associated with inferior and posterior infarcts. The anterior papillary muscle has a dual blood supply and is less vulnerable to rupture. The mechanism of chronic MR after STEMI includes papillary muscle dysfunction or leaflet tethering due to posterior wall akinesis.
  - Acute MR from papillary muscle rupture is a severe complication of MI associated with high mortality (see below).
  - Progressive MR following MI may develop as a result of LV chamber dilation, apical remodeling, or posterior wall dyskinesis. These changes lead to leaflet tethering or mitral annular dilation.
  - Echocardiography is the diagnostic modality of choice.
  - Transient ischemic MR occurs secondary to papillary muscle ischemia and results in transient severe MR and pulmonary edema. It can be hard to detect on exam or imaging when ischemia is not induced.
  - Initial treatment of MR involves aggressive afterload reduction and revascularization. *Stable* patients should receive a trial of medical therapy and undergo surgery only if they fail to improve.
  ○ **STEMI** in the setting of recent **cocaine use** presents a unique and challenging management situation (*Circulation 2008;117:1897–907*). ST elevation can result from

myocardial ischemia due to coronary vasospasm, in situ thrombus formation, and/or increased myocardial oxygen demand. The common pathophysiology is excessive stimulation of α- and β-adrenergic receptors. Chest pain due to cocaine use usually occurs within 3 hours but may be seen several days following use.

- Oxygen, ASA, and heparin (UFH or LMWH) should be administered to all patients with cocaine-associated STEMI.
- Nitrates should be used preferentially to treat vasospasm. Additionally, benzodiazepines may confer additional relief by decreasing sympathetic tone.
- **BBs** are contraindicated; both selective and nonselective BBs should be avoided.
- Phentolamine (α-adrenergic antagonist) and calcium channel blockers may reverse coronary vasospasm and are recommended as second-line agents.
- The use of reperfusion therapy is controversial and should be reserved for those patients whose symptoms persist despite initial medical therapy.
  □ Primary PCI is the preferred approach for the patient with persistent symptoms and ECG changes despite aggressive medical therapy. It is important to note that coronary angiography and intervention carry a significant risk of worsening vasospasm.
  □ Fibrinolytic therapy should be reserved for patients who are clearly having a STEMI and who cannot undergo PCI.

COMPLICATIONS

Myocardial damage predisposes the patient to several potential adverse consequences and complications that should be considered if the patient experiences new clinical signs and/or symptoms. These include recurrent chest pain, cardiac arrhythmias, cardiogenic shock, and mechanical complications of MI.

- **Recurrent chest pain** may be due to ischemia in the territory of the original infarction, pericarditis, myocardial rupture, or pulmonary embolism.
  ○ Recurrent angina is experienced by 20–30% of patients after MI who receive fibrinolytic therapy and up to 10% of patients in the early time period following percutaneous revascularization. These symptoms may represent recurrence of ischemia or infarct extension.
    ■ Assessment of the patient may include evaluation for new murmurs or friction rubs, ECG to assess for new ischemic changes, cardiac enzymes (troponin and CK-MB), echocardiography, and repeat coronary angiography if indicated.
    ■ Patients with recurrent chest pain should continue to receive ASA, P2Y12 inhibition, heparin, nitroglycerin, and BB therapy.
    ■ If recurrent angina is refractory to medical treatment, urgent repeat coronary angiography and intervention should be considered.
  ○ **Acute pericarditis** occurs 24–96 hours after MI in approximately 10–15% of patients. The associated chest pain is often pleuritic and may be relieved in the upright position. A friction rub may be noted on clinical examination, and the ECG may show diffuse ST-segment elevation and PR-segment depression. Lead AVR may have PR elevation. Treatment is directed at pain management.
    ■ High-dose ASA (up to 650 mg qid maximum) is generally considered a first-line agent. NSAIDs such as ibuprofen may be used if ASA is not effective but should be avoided early after acute MI.
    ■ Colchicine along with ASA may also be beneficial for recurrent symptoms and may also be superior to each agent alone.
    ■ Glucocorticoids (prednisone 1 mg/kg daily) may be useful if symptoms are severe and refractory to initial therapy. Steroids should be used sparingly because they may lead to an increased risk of recurrence of pericarditis. Use should also be deferred until at least 4 weeks after acute MI due to their adverse impact on infarct healing and risk of ventricular aneurysm.

- Heparin should be avoided in the setting of pericarditis with or without pericardial effusion because it may lead to pericardial hemorrhage.
  - **Dressler syndrome** is thought to be an autoimmune process characterized by malaise, fever, pericardial pain, leukocytosis, elevated erythrocyte sedimentation rate, and often a pericardial effusion. In contrast to acute pericarditis, Dressler syndrome occurs 1–8 weeks after MI. Treatment is identical to acute pericarditis.
- **Arrhythmias.** Cardiac rhythm abnormalities are common following MI and may include conduction block, atrial arrhythmias, and ventricular arrhythmias. Arrhythmias that result in hemodynamic compromise require prompt, aggressive intervention. If the arrhythmia precipitates refractory angina or HF, urgent therapy is warranted. For all rhythm disturbances, exacerbating conditions should be addressed, including electrolyte imbalances, hypoxia, acidosis, and adverse drug effects. Details on specific arrhythmias can be found in Table 4-21.
  - **Atropine** should be attempted for all bradyarrhythmias in the setting of STEMI. Bradycardia is a common complication of intense vagal input to the AV node as a result of baroreceptor activation in the myocardium (also called Bezold-Jarisch reflex).
  - **Transcutaneous and transvenous pacing.** Conduction system disease that progresses to complete heart block or results in symptomatic bradycardia can be effectively treated with cardiac pacing. A transcutaneous pacing device can be used under emergent circumstances; however, a temporary transvenous system should be used for longer duration therapy.
    - Absolute indications for temporary transvenous pacing include asystole, symptomatic bradycardia, recurrent sinus pauses, complete heart block, and incessant polymorphic ventricular tachycardia (VT).
    - Temporary transvenous pacing may also be warranted for new trifascicular block, new Mobitz II block, and patients with LBBB who require a pulmonary artery catheter, given the risk of developing complete heart block.
  - **Implantable cardioverter-defibrillators (ICDs)** should not routinely be implanted in patients with reduced LV function following MI or those with VT/ventricular fibrillation (VF) in the setting of ischemia or immediately following reperfusion.
    - Routine insertion of ICDs into patients with reduced LV function immediately following MI does not improve outcomes (*N Engl J Med 2004;351:2481*).
    - In contrast, patients who continue to have depressed LV function (EF <35% and New York Heart Association [NYHA] class II or III or EF <30% regardless of NYHA class) >40 days following MI benefit from ICD therapy (*N Engl J Med 2005;352:225; N Engl J Med 2002;346:877*).
    - ICD therapy is also indicated for patients with recurrent episodes of sustained VT or VF despite coronary reperfusion.
- **Cardiogenic shock** is an infrequent, but serious, complication of MI and is defined as hypotension in the setting of inadequate ventricular function to meet the metabolic needs of the peripheral tissue. Risk factors include prior MI, older age, diabetes, and anterior infarction. Organ hypoperfusion may manifest as progressive renal failure, dyspnea, diaphoresis, or mental status changes. Hemodynamic monitoring reveals elevated filling pressures (wedge pressure >20 mm Hg), depressed cardiac index (<2.5 L/kg/min), and hypotension.
  - Patients with cardiogenic shock in the setting of MI have a mortality rate in excess of 50%. Such patients require invasive hemodynamic monitoring and advanced therapeutic modalities including inotropic and mechanical support.
  - **Dobutamine and milrinone** are the most frequently used medications for inotropic support. They both possess vasodilatory properties (i.e., afterload reducing) and are arrhythmogenic. Milrinone should be avoided in the setting of renal insufficiency.
  - **Dopamine** can be used as both a vasopressor and inotrope but increases the risk of atrial arrhythmias in patients with shock and is not a preferred first-line agent.

TABLE 4-21	Arrhythmias Complicating Myocardial Infarction	
Arrhythmia	**Treatment**	**Comments**
Intraventricular conduction delays	None	The left anterior fascicle is most commonly affected because of isolated coronary blood supply. Bifascicular and trifascicular block may progress to complete heart block and other rhythm disturbances.
Sinus bradycardia	None Atropine 0.5 mg Temporary pacing[a]	Sinus bradycardia is common in patients with RCA infarcts. In the absence of hypotension or significant ventricular ectopy, observation is indicated.
AV block	Temporary pacing[a]	First-degree AV block usually does not require specific treatment. Mobitz I second-degree block occurs more often with inferior MI. The block is usually within the His bundle and does not require treatment unless symptomatic bradycardia is present. Mobitz II second-degree AV block originates below the His bundle and is more commonly associated with anterior MI. Because of the significant risk of progression to complete heart block, patients should be observed in the CCU and treated with temporary pacing if symptomatic. Third-degree AV block complicates large anterior and RV infarcts. In patients with anterior MI, third-degree heart block often occurs 12–24 h after initial presentation and may appear suddenly. Temporary pacing is recommended because of the risk of progression to ventricular asystole.
Sinus tachycardia	None[b]	Sinus tachycardia is common in patients with acute MI and is often due to enhanced sympathetic activity resulting from pain, anxiety, hypovolemia, anxiety, heart failure, or fever. Persistent sinus tachycardia suggests poor underlying ventricular function and is associated with excess mortality.
Atrial fibrillation and flutter	β-Blockers Anticoagulation Cardioversion	Atrial fibrillation and flutter are observed in up to 20% of patients with acute MI. Because atrial fibrillation and atrial flutter are usually transient in the acute MI period, long-term anticoagulation is often not necessary after documentation of stable sinus rhythm.
Accelerated junctional rhythm	None	Accelerated junctional rhythm occurs in conjunction with inferior MI. The rhythm is usually benign and warrants treatment only if hypotension is present.

(continued)

TABLE 4-21	**Arrhythmias Complicating Myocardial Infarction (*Continued*)**

Arrhythmia	Treatment	Comments
Ventricular premature depolarizations (VPDs)	β-Blockers if symptomatic[c]	VPDs are common in the course of an acute MI. Prophylactic treatment with lidocaine or other antiarrhythmics has been associated with increased overall mortality and is not recommended (*N Engl J Med 1989;321:406*).
Accelerated idioventricular rhythm (AIVR)	None	Commonly seen within 48 h of successful reperfusion and is not associated with an increased incidence of adverse outcomes. If hemodynamically unstable, sinus activity may be restored with atropine or temporary atrial pacing.
Ventricular tachycardia (VT)	Cardioversion for sustained VT Lidocaine or amiodarone for 24–48 h[d]	Nonsustained ventricular tachycardia (NSVT, <30 s) is common in the first 24 h after MI and is only associated with increased mortality when occurring late in the post-MI course. Sustained VT (>30 s) during the first 48 h after acute MI is associated with increased in-hospital mortality.
Ventricular fibrillation (VF)	Unsynchronized cardioversion Lidocaine or amiodarone for 24–48 h[d]	VF occurs in up to 5% of patients in the early post-MI period and is life threatening.

AV, atrioventricular; CCU, coronary care unit; MI, myocardial infarction; RCA, right coronary artery; RV, right ventricular.
[a]Atropine and temporary pacing should only be used for symptomatic or hemodynamically unstable patients.
[b]The use of β-blockers in the setting of sinus tachycardia and poor left ventricular function may result in decompensated heart failure.
[c]β-Blockers should be used with caution in the setting of bradycardia and frequent VPDs as they may increase the risk of polymorphic VT.
[d]Lidocaine should be used as a 1 mg/kg bolus followed by a 1–2 mg/kg/h infusion. Amiodarone should be given as a 150–300 mg bolus followed by an infusion of 1 mg/kg/h for 6 h and then 0.5 mg/kg/h for 18 h.

- **Norepinephrine and phenylephrine** may be required to maintain systemic BP. The use of any vasoconstrictive agents in the setting of cardiogenic shock should prompt an evaluation for mechanical circulatory support
- **Epinephrine** is a potent vasopressor and inotrope and is frequently used as an adjunct to other medical therapies. There may be some preferential benefit to RV function, and thus, epinephrine may be used for shock secondary to RV infarct or severe RV dysfunction.
- **Mechanical circulatory support** includes both temporary and durable support devices. Temporary support devices include IABP, Impella catheter, TandemHeart System, or extracorporeal membrane oxygenation. Temporary support is offered as bridge to recovery or as bridge to decision about long-term durable mechanical support such as an LV assist device (see Chapter 5, Heart Failure and Cardiomyopathy). The choice of

temporary support device is not always clear and should be made by a team familiar with the management of cardiogenic shock.

- ○ All patients with cardiogenic shock should undergo echocardiography to evaluate for mechanical complications of MI (see the following text).
- ○ **LV thrombus** occurs most often in setting of anterior MI and should be treated with anticoagulation. Warfarin is the recommended long-term anticoagulation agent; novel oral anticoagulants such as dabigatran should be avoided because there have been no studies documenting safety in this setting. Patients should receive warfarin for 3–6 months unless other indications warrant its continued use.
- • **Mechanical complications**
  - ○ **Aneurysm.** After MI, the affected area of the myocardium may undergo infarct expansion and thinning, forming an aneurysm. The wall motion may become dyskinetic, making the endocardial surface susceptible to mural thrombus formation.
    - ▪ LV aneurysm is suggested by persistent ST elevation on the ECG and may be diagnosed by imaging studies including ventriculography, echocardiography, and MRI.
    - ▪ Anticoagulation is warranted to lower the risk of embolic events, especially if a mural thrombus is present.
    - ▪ Surgical intervention may be appropriate if the aneurysm results in HF or ventricular arrhythmias that are not satisfactorily managed with medical therapy.
  - ○ **Ventricular pseudoaneurysm.** Incomplete rupture of the myocardial free wall can result in formation of a ventricular pseudoaneurysm. In this case, blood escapes through the myocardial wall and is contained within the visceral pericardium. In the post-CABG patient, hemorrhage from frank ventricular rupture may be contained within the fibrotic pericardial space producing a pseudoaneurysm.
    - ▪ Echocardiography (TTE with contrast or TEE) is the preferred diagnostic test to assess for a pseudoaneurysm, often allowing differentiation from a true aneurysm.
    - ▪ Prompt surgical intervention for pseudoaneurysms is advised because of the high incidence of myocardial rupture.
  - ○ **Free wall rupture** represents a catastrophic complication of acute MI, accounting for 10% of early deaths. Rupture typically occurs within the first week after MI and presents with sudden hemodynamic collapse. This complication can occur after anterior or inferior MI and is more commonly seen in hypertensive women with their first large transmural MI, in patients receiving late therapy with fibrinolytics, and patients given NSAIDs or glucocorticoids.
    - ▪ Echocardiography may identify patients with particularly thinned ventricular walls at risk for rupture.
    - ▪ Emergent surgical correction is necessary.
    - ▪ Despite optimal intervention, mortality of free wall rupture remains >90%.
  - ○ **Papillary muscle rupture** (*please also refer to earlier MR section*) is a rare complication after MI and is associated with abrupt clinical deterioration. The posterior medial papillary muscle is most commonly affected due to its isolated vascular supply, but anterolateral papillary muscle rupture has been reported. Of note, papillary muscle rupture may be seen in the setting of a relatively small acute MI or even NSTEMI.
    - ▪ The diagnostic test of choice is echocardiography with Doppler imaging and/or TEE because physical exam reveals a murmur in only ~50% of cases.
    - ▪ Initial medical therapy should include aggressive afterload reduction. Patients with refractory HF and those with hemodynamic instability may require inotropic support with dobutamine and/or IABP. Surgical repair is indicated in the majority of patients.
  - ○ **Ventricular septal rupture** is most commonly associated with anterior MI occurring 3–5 days after MI. The perforation may follow a direct course between the ventricles or a serpiginous route through the septal wall.
    - ▪ Diagnosis can be made by echocardiography with Doppler imaging and often requires TEE.

- Diagnosis should be suspected in the postinfarct patient who develops HF symptoms and a new holosystolic murmur.
- Stabilization with afterload reduction, inotropic support, and/or IABP may be necessary for hemodynamically unstable patients until definitive therapy with surgical repair can be performed.
- In hemodynamically stable patients, surgery is best deferred for at least a week to improve patient outcome. Left untreated, mortality approaches 90%.
- Percutaneous device closure in the cardiac catheterization laboratory can be performed in select patients with an unacceptable surgical risk.

MONITORING/FOLLOW-UP

Routine office visits 1 month after discharge and every 3–12 months thereafter are suggested for the patient presenting with an acute MI.

- Patients should be instructed to seek more frequent or urgent follow-up evaluation if they experience any noticeable changes in their clinical status.
- Specific plans for long-term follow-up care should be individualized based on clinical status, anatomy, prior interventions, and change in symptoms.
- All patients should be referred for cardiac rehabilitation.

5 Heart Failure and Cardiomyopathy

Shane J. LaRue and Justin M. Vader

HEART FAILURE

General Principles

DEFINITION

Heart failure (HF) is a **clinical syndrome** in which either structural or functional abnormalities of the heart impair its ability to fill with or eject blood, resulting in dyspnea, fatigue, and fluid retention (*Circulation 2013;128:e240–e327*). HF is a progressive disorder and is associated with extremely high morbidity and mortality.

CLASSIFICATION

- HF may be due to abnormalities in myocardial contraction (systolic dysfunction), relaxation and filling (diastolic dysfunction), or both.
- Left ventricular (LV) ejection fraction (EF) is used to subdivide HF patients into groups for therapeutic and prognostic purposes. These groups are:
  - EF <40%: HF with reduced EF (HFrEF)
  - EF 40–50%: HF with borderline EF
  - EF >50%: HF with preserved EF (HFpEF)
- HF is classified in terms of natural history by American College of Cardiology/American Heart Association (ACC/AHA) HF stage and in terms of symptom status by New York Heart Association (NYHA) Functional Class (Tables 5-1 and 5-2).

EPIDEMIOLOGY

- In the United States, over 5.7 million people are living with HF (*Circulation 2014;131: e29–e322*).
- Approximately 870,000 new cases of HF are diagnosed each year.
- HF accounts for over 1 million hospitalizations per year.
- Estimated 1- and 5-year mortality are 30% and 50%, respectively (*Circulation 2010;123(4): 410–528*).

ETIOLOGY

- Coronary artery disease (CAD) is the most frequent cause of HF in the United States. Other risk factors with high population attributable risk include tobacco use, hypertension, diabetes, and obesity (*Circulation 2014;131:e29–e322*).
- Other causes include valvular heart disease, toxin induced (alcohol, cocaine, chemotherapy), myocarditis (infectious or autoimmune), familial cardiomyopathy, infiltrative disease (amyloidosis, sarcoidosis, hemochromatosis), peripartum cardiomyopathy (PPCM), hypertrophic cardiomyopathy (HCM), constrictive pericardial disease, high-output states

TABLE 5-1	American College of Cardiology/American Heart Association Guidelines of Evaluation and Management of Chronic Heart Failure in Adults	
Stage	**Description**	**Treatment**
A	No structural heart disease and no symptoms but risk factors: CAD, HTN, DM, cardio toxins, familial cardiomyopathy	Lifestyle modification—diet, exercise, smoking cessation; treat hyperlipidemia and use ACE inhibitor for HTN
B	Abnormal LV systolic function, MI, valvular heart disease, but no HF symptoms	Lifestyle modifications, ACE inhibitor, β-adrenergic blockers
C	Structural heart disease and HF symptoms	Lifestyle modifications, ACE inhibitor, β-adrenergic blockers, diuretics, digoxin
D	Refractory HF symptoms to maximal medical management	Therapy listed under A, B, and C, and mechanical assist device, heart transplantation, continuous IV inotropic infusion, hospice care in selected patients

ACE, angiotensin-converting enzyme; CAD, coronary artery disease; DM, diabetes mellitus; HF, heart failure; HTN, hypertension; LV, left ventricular; MI, myocardial infarction.
From Hunt SA, Abraham WT, Chin MH, et al. ACC/AHA guidelines for the evaluation and management of chronic heart failure in the adult: executive summary. *J Am Coll Cardiol* 2005;46:1116–43.

(i.e., arteriovenous malformation or fistula), generalized myopathy (Duchenne or Becker muscular dystrophy), tachycardia-induced cardiomyopathy, and idiopathic cardiomyopathy.
• HF exacerbations may be precipitated by dietary and medication noncompliance; however, myocardial ischemia, hypertension, arrhythmias (particularly atrial fibrillation), infection, volume overload, alcohol/toxins, thyroid disease, drugs (NSAIDs calcium channel blockers, doxorubicin), and pulmonary embolism are also potential triggers.

TABLE 5-2	New York Heart Association (NYHA) Functional Classification
NYHA Class	**Symptoms**
I (mild)	No symptoms or limitation while performing ordinary physical activity (walking, climbing stairs, etc.).
II (mild)	Mild symptoms (mild shortness of breath, palpitations, fatigue, and/or angina) and slight limitation during ordinary physical activity.
III (moderate)	Marked limitation in activity due to symptoms, even during less than ordinary activity (walking short distances [20–100 m]). Comfortable only at rest.
IV (severe)	Severe limitations with symptoms even while at rest. Mostly bedbound patients.

PATHOPHYSIOLOGY

- HF begins with an initial insult leading to myocardial injury.
- Regardless of etiology, the myocardial injury leads to a pathologic remodeling, which manifests as an increase in LV volume (dilatation) and/or mass (hypertrophy).
- Compensatory adaptations initially maintain cardiac output; specifically, there is activation of the renin–angiotensin–aldosterone system (RAAS) and vasopressin (antidiuretic hormone), which lead to increased sodium retention and peripheral vasoconstriction. The sympathetic nervous system is also activated, with increased levels of circulating catecholamines, resulting in increased myocardial contractility. Over time, these neurohormonal pathways result in direct cellular toxicity, fibrosis, arrhythmias, and pump failure.
- Cardiac dysfunction and pathologic remodeling alter the ventricular pressure–volume relationship, leading to an increase in chamber pressures, resulting in pulmonary and systemic venous congestion.

Diagnosis

CLINICAL PRESENTATION

History

- Affected patients most commonly present with symptoms of HF, including:
  - Dyspnea (on exertion and/or at rest)
  - Fatigue
  - Exercise intolerance
  - Orthopnea, paroxysmal nocturnal dyspnea
  - Systemic or pulmonary venous congestion (lower extremity swelling or cough/wheezing)
  - Presyncope, palpitations, and angina may also be present
- Other possible presentations include incidental detection of asymptomatic cardiomegaly or symptoms related to coexisting arrhythmia, conduction disturbance, thromboembolic complications, or sudden death.
- Clinical manifestations of HF vary depending on the severity and rapidity of cardiac decompensation, underlying etiology, age, and comorbidities of the patient.
- Extreme decompensation may present as cardiogenic shock (resulting from both low arterial and high venous pressures), characterized by hypoperfusion of vital organs, leading to renal failure (decreased urine output), mental status changes (confusion and lethargy), or "shock liver" (elevated liver function tests).

Physical Examination

- The goal of the physical exam in HF is to estimate intracardiac pressures, ventricular compliance, cardiac output, and end-organ perfusion.
- Elevated right-sided pressures result in lower extremity edema, jugular venous distension (JVD), abdominojugular reflux, pleural and pericardial effusions, hepatic congestion, and ascites.
  - JVD is the most specific and reliable physical exam indicator of right-sided volume overload and is representative of left-sided filling pressures except in cases of disproportionate right heart dysfunction (e.g., pulmonary hypertension, severe tricuspid regurgitation, and pericardial disease).
  - JVD is best visualized with oblique light and the patient at 45 degrees. Venous pulsations are differentiated from carotid pulsation by their biphasic nature, respiratory variability, and compressibility.
  - Abdominojugular reflux suggests an impaired ability of the right ventricle to handle augmented preload and may be due to constriction or pulmonary hypertension in addition to myocardial disease.

- Elevated left-sided pressures may result in pulmonary rales, but rales are absent in the majority of HF patients with elevated left-sided filling pressures.
- In the setting of systolic dysfunction, a third (S_3) or fourth (S_4) heart sound as well as the holosystolic murmurs of tricuspid or mitral regurgitation (MR) may be present; carotid upstrokes may also be diminished.
- Low cardiac output is suggested by a proportional pulse pressure (pulse pressure/diastolic blood pressure) $\leq 25\%$, diminished carotid upstroke, and cool extremities.

DIAGNOSTIC TESTING

Laboratories

- Initial laboratory studies should include complete blood count (CBC), urinalysis, serum electrolytes, blood urea nitrogen (BUN), creatinine, calcium, magnesium, fasting glucose, liver function tests, fasting lipid profile, and thyroid function tests.
- B-type natriuretic peptide (BNP) and the biologically inactive cleavage product N-terminal prohormone BNP (NT-proBNP) are released by myocytes in response to stretch, volume overload, and increased filling pressures. Elevated BNP/NT-proBNP is present in patients with asymptomatic LV dysfunction as well as symptomatic HF.
- BNP and NT-proBNP levels have been shown to correlate with HF severity and to predict survival (*N Engl J Med 2002;347:161*; *Eur Heart J 2006;27(3):330*). A serum BNP >400 pg/mL is consistent with HF; however, specificity is reduced in patients with renal dysfunction. A serum BNP level <100 pg/mL has a good negative predictive value to exclude HF in patients presenting with dyspnea (*Curr Opin Cardiol 2006;21:208*). Age-specific cut points have also been identified, for example, NT-proBNP levels of 450 pg/mL, 900 pg/mL, and 1800 pg/mL optimally identified acute HF for patients age <50, 50–75, and >75, respectively (*Eur Heart J 2006;27(3):330*).
- Additional laboratory testing in a patient with new-onset HF without CAD may include diagnostic tests for HIV, hepatitis, and hemochromatosis. When clinically suspected, serum tests for rheumatologic diseases (antinuclear antibody [ANA], antineutrophil cytoplasmic antibody [ANCA], etc.), amyloidosis (serum protein electrophoresis [SPEP], urine protein electrophoresis [UPEP]), or pheochromocytoma (catecholamines) should be considered (*Circulation 2013;62:e147*).

Electrocardiography

An ECG should be performed to look for evidence of ischemia (ST-T wave abnormalities), hypertrophy (increased voltage), infiltration (reduced voltage), previous myocardial infarction (MI) (Q waves), conduction block (PR interval), interventricular conduction delays (QRS), and arrhythmias (supraventricular and ventricular).

Imaging

- Chest radiography should be performed to evaluate the presence of pulmonary edema or cardiomegaly and rule out other etiologies of dyspnea (e.g., pneumonia, pneumothorax). Although chest radiograph findings of cephalization and interstitial edema are highly specific for identifying patients presenting with acute HF (specificity of 98% and 99%, respectively), they have limited sensitivity (41% and 27%, respectively) (*Am J Med 2004; 116(6):363*).
- An echocardiogram should be performed to assess right ventricular (RV) and LV systolic and diastolic function, valvular structure and function, and chamber size and to exclude cardiac tamponade.
- LV function may also be evaluated using radionuclide ventriculography (i.e., multigated acquisition [MUGA] scan) or cardiac catheterization with ventriculography and invasive hemodynamics.

• Cardiac MRI may also be useful in assessing ventricular function and evaluating the presence of intracardiac shunting, valvular heart disease, infiltrative cardiomyopathy, myocarditis, and previous MI.

Diagnostic Procedures

• Coronary angiography should be performed in patients with angina or evidence of ischemia by ECG or stress testing, unless the patient is not a candidate for revascularization (*J Am Coll Cardiol 2013;62:e147–e239*).
• Stress nuclear imaging or echocardiography may be an acceptable alternative for assessing ischemia in patients presenting with HF who have known CAD and no angina, unless they are ineligible for revascularization (*J Am Coll Cardiol 2013;62:e147–e239*).
• Right heart catheterization with placement of a pulmonary artery catheter may help guide therapy in patients with hypotension and evidence of shock.
• Cardiopulmonary exercise testing with measurement of peak oxygen consumption (VO_2) is useful in assessing functional capacity and in identifying candidates for heart transplantation (*J Heart Lung Transplant 2003;22:70*; *Circulation 2009;83:778*).
• Endomyocardial biopsy should be considered when seeking a specific diagnosis that would influence therapy, specifically in patients with rapidly progressive and unexplained cardiomyopathy, those in whom active myocarditis, especially giant cell myocarditis, is considered, and those with possible infiltrative processes such as cardiac amyloidosis and sarcoidosis (*Circulation 2007;116:2216–33*).

Treatment of Heart Failure

PHARMACOTHERAPY

• In general, pharmacologic therapy in chronic HF is aimed at blocking the neurohormonal pathways that contribute to cardiac remodeling and the progression of HF, while reducing symptoms, hospitalizations, and mortality.
• The cornerstone of medical therapy for HF includes RAAS blockade, β-adrenergic blockade, vasodilators, and diuretic therapy for volume overload.
• Pharmacotherapy is determined by the presence of a preserved or reduced LVEF. Several pharmacotherapies for HFrEF have been demonstrated to reduce death and hospitalization and improve quality of life in HF. No pharmacotherapy has been demonstrated to improve mortality in patients with HFpEF.

Chronic Medical Therapy with Reduced Ejection Fraction (HFrEF)

• **β-Adrenergic receptor antagonists (β-blockers)** (Table 5-3). β-Blockers are a critical component of HF therapy and work by blocking the toxic effects of chronic adrenergic stimulation on the heart.
  ○ Large randomized trials have documented the beneficial effects of β-blockers on functional status, disease progression, and survival in patients with NYHA class II–IV symptoms.
  ○ Improvement in EF, exercise tolerance, and functional class are common after the institution of a β-blocker (*Circulation 1995;92(6):1499*).
  ○ Typically, 2–3 months of therapy is required to observe significant effects on LV function, but reduction of cardiac arrhythmia and incidence of sudden cardiac death (SCD) may occur much earlier (*JAMA 2003;289:712*).
  ○ β-Blockers should be instituted at a low dose and titrated with careful attention to blood pressure and heart rate. Some patients experience volume retention and worsening HF symptoms that typically respond to transient increases in diuretic therapy.

TABLE 5-3	Drugs Commonly Used for Treatment of Heart Failure	
Drug	**Initial Dose**	**Target**
Angiotensin-Converting Enzyme Inhibitors		
Captopril	6.25–12.5 mg q6–8h	50 mg tid
Enalapril	2.5 mg bid	10 mg bid
Fosinopril	5–10 mg daily; can use bid	20 mg daily
Lisinopril	2.5–5.0 mg daily; can use bid	10–20 mg bid
Quinapril	2.5–5.0 mg bid	10 mg bid
Ramipril	1.25–2.5 mg bid	5 mg bid
Trandolapril	0.5–1.0 mg daily	4 mg daily
Angiotensin Receptor Blockers		
Valsartan[a]	40 mg bid	160 mg bid
Losartan	25 mg daily; can use bid	25–100 mg daily
Irbesartan	75–150 mg daily	75–300 mg daily
Candesartan[a]	2–16 mg daily	2–32 mg daily
Olmesartan	20 mg daily	20–40 mg daily
Thiazide Diuretics		
HCTZ	25–50 mg daily	25–50 mg daily
Metolazone	2.5–5.0 mg daily or bid	10–20 mg total daily
Loop Diuretics		
Bumetanide	0.5–1.0 mg daily or bid	10 mg total daily (maximum)
Furosemide	20–40 mg daily or bid	400 mg total daily (maximum)
Torsemide	10–20 mg daily or bid	200 mg total daily (maximum)
Aldosterone Antagonists		
Eplerenone	25 mg daily	50 mg daily
Spironolactone	12.5–25.0 mg daily	25 mg daily
β-Blockers		
Bisoprolol	1.25 mg daily	10 mg daily
Carvedilol	3.125 mg q12h	25–50 mg q12h
Metoprolol succinate	12.5–25.0 mg daily	200 mg daily
Digoxin	0.125–0.25 mg daily	0.125–0.25 mg daily

HCTZ, hydrochlorothiazide.
[a]Valsartan and candesartan are the only U.S. Food and Drug Administration–approved angiotensin II receptor blockers in the treatment of heart failure.

- ○ The survival benefit of β-blockers is proportional to the heart rate reduction achieved (*Ann Intern Med 2009;150(11):784–94*).
- ○ Individual β-blockers have unique properties, and the beneficial effect of β-blockers may not be a class effect. Therefore, one of three β-blockers with proven benefit on mortality in large clinical trials should be used (*Circulation 2013;128:e240–e327*):
  - **Carvedilol** (*N Engl J Med 2001;344:1651*; *Lancet 2003;362:7*)
  - **Metoprolol succinate** (*JAMA 2000;283:1295*)
  - **Bisoprolol** (*Lancet 1999;353:9*)
- **Angiotensin-converting enzyme (ACE) inhibitors** (see Table 5-3) attenuate vasoconstriction, vital organ hypoperfusion, hyponatremia, hypokalemia, and fluid retention attributable to compensatory activation of the renin–angiotensin system. They are the first choice for antagonism of the RAAS.
  - ○ Multiple large clinical trials have clearly demonstrated that ACE inhibitors improve symptoms and survival in patients with LV systolic dysfunction (*Circulation 2013;128:e240–e327*).
  - ○ ACE inhibitors may also prevent the development of HF in patients with asymptomatic LV dysfunction and in those at high risk of developing structural heart disease or HF symptoms (e.g., patients with CAD, diabetes mellitus, hypertension).
  - ○ Currently, no consensus has been reached regarding the optimal dosing of ACE inhibitors in HF, although higher doses have been shown to reduce morbidity without improving overall survival (*Circulation 1999;100:2312*).
  - ○ Absence of an initial beneficial response to treatment with an ACE inhibitor does not preclude long-term benefit.
  - ○ Most ACE inhibitors are excreted by the kidneys, necessitating careful dose titration in patients with renal insufficiency. ACE inhibitors should not be administered if creatinine >3 mg/dL, if potassium >5 mEq/L, or in patients with bilateral renal artery stenosis. Renal function and potassium levels should be monitored with dose adjustment and periodically with chronic use.
  - ○ A rise in serum creatinine up to 30% above baseline may be seen when initiating an ACE inhibitor and should not result in reflexive discontinuation of therapy (*N Engl J Med 2002;347:1256–61*).
  - ○ Additional adverse effects may include cough, rash, angioedema, dysgeusia, increase in serum creatinine, proteinuria, hyperkalemia, and leukopenia.
  - ○ Oral potassium supplements, potassium salt substitutes, and potassium-sparing diuretics should be used with caution during treatment with an ACE inhibitor.
  - ○ Agranulocytosis and angioedema are more common with captopril than with other ACE inhibitors, particularly in patients with associated collagen vascular disease or serum creatinine >1.5 mg/dL.
  - ○ **ACE inhibitors are contraindicated in pregnancy. Enalapril and captopril may be safely used by breastfeeding mothers.**
- **Angiotensin II receptor blockers (ARBs)** (see Table 5-3) inhibit the renin–angiotensin system via specific blockade of the angiotensin II receptor.
  - ○ ARBs reduce morbidity and mortality associated with HF in patients who are not receiving an ACE inhibitor (*Lancet 2000;355:1582*; *N Engl J Med 2001;345:1667*; *Lancet 2003;362:777*) and therefore should be instituted when ACE inhibitors are not tolerated (*Circulation 2013;128:e240–e327*).
  - ○ In contrast to ACE inhibitors, ARBs do not increase bradykinin levels and therefore are not associated with cough.
  - ○ Renal precautions and monitoring for ARB use are similar to ACE inhibitor use.
  - ○ Use of ARBs is contraindicated in patients taking ACE inhibitors and aldosterone antagonists due to a high risk for hyperkalemia.
  - ○ **ARBs are contraindicated in pregnancy and breastfeeding.**

- **Aldosterone receptor antagonists** attenuate aldosterone-mediated sodium retention, vascular reactivity, oxidant stress, inflammation, and fibrosis.
  - **Spironolactone** is a nonselective aldosterone receptor antagonist that has been shown to improve survival and decrease hospitalizations in NYHA class III–IV patients with low EF (*N Engl J Med 1999;341:709*) and is therefore indicated in such patients if the creatinine is <2.5 mg/dL and potassium is <5.0 mEq/L (see Table 5-3) (*Circulation 2013;128:e240–e327*).
  - **Eplerenone** is a selective aldosterone receptor antagonist without the estrogenic side effects of spironolactone. It has proven beneficial in patients with HF following MI (*N Engl J Med 2003;348:1309*) and in less symptomatic HF patients (NYHA Class II) with reduced EF (*N Engl J Med 2011;364:11*).
  - The potential for development of life-threatening hyperkalemia exists with the use of these agents. Serum potassium must be monitored closely after initiation; concomitant use of ACE inhibitors and NSAIDs and the presence of renal insufficiency increase the risk of hyperkalemia.
  - Gynecomastia may develop in 10–20% of men treated with spironolactone; eplerenone should be used in this case.
- **Vasodilator therapy** alters preload and afterload conditions to improve cardiac output.
  - **Hydralazine** acts directly on arterial smooth muscle to produce vasodilation and to reduce afterload.
  - **Nitrates** are predominantly venodilators and help relieve symptoms of venous and pulmonary congestion. They also reduce myocardial ischemia by decreasing ventricular filling pressures and by directly dilating coronary arteries.
  - A **combination of hydralazine and isosorbide dinitrate** (starting dose: 37.5/20 mg three times daily), when added to standard therapy with β-blockers and ACE inhibitors, has been shown to reduce mortality in African American patients (*N Engl J Med 2004;351:2049*).
  - In the absence of ACE inhibitors, ARBs, aldosterone receptor antagonists, and β-blockers, the combination of nitrates and hydralazine improves survival in patients with HFrEF (*N Engl J Med 1986;314:1547*) and should therefore be considered for use in all HFrEF patients unable to tolerate RAAS blockade.
  - Reflex tachycardia and increased myocardial oxygen consumption may occur in the setting of hydralazine use, requiring cautious use in patients with ischemic heart disease.
  - Nitrate therapy may precipitate hypotension in patients with reduced preload.
- **Digitalis glycosides** increase myocardial contractility and may attenuate the neurohormonal activation associated with HF.
  - Digoxin has been show to decrease rates of HF hospitalizations without improving overall mortality (*N Engl J Med 1997;336:525*).
  - Digoxin has a **narrow therapeutic index**, and serum levels should be followed closely, particularly in patients with unstable renal function.
  - The usual daily dose is 0.125–0.25 mg and should be decreased in patients with renal insufficiency.
  - Clinical benefits may not be related to the serum levels. Although serum digoxin levels of 0.8–2.0 ng/mL are considered therapeutic, toxicity can occur in this range.
  - Women and patients with higher serum digoxin levels (1.2–2.0 ng/mL) have an increased mortality risk (*N Engl J Med 2002;347:1403; JAMA 2003;289:871*).
  - Discontinuation of digoxin in patients who are stable on a regimen of digoxin, diuretics, and an ACE inhibitor may result in clinical deterioration (*N Engl J Med 1993;329:1*).
  - Drug interactions with digoxin are common and may lead to toxicity. Agents that may increase levels include erythromycin, tetracycline, quinidine, verapamil, flecainide, and

amiodarone. Electrolyte abnormalities (particularly hypokalemia), hypoxemia, hypothyroidism, renal insufficiency, and volume depletion may also exacerbate toxicity.
  ○ Digoxin is not dialyzable, and toxicity is only treatable by the administration of digoxin immune Fab.
• **α-Adrenergic receptor antagonists** have not been shown to improve survival in HF, and hypertensive patients treated with doxazosin as first-line therapy are at increased risk of developing HF (*JAMA 2000;283:1967*).
• **Calcium channel blockers** have no favorable effects on mortality in HFrEF.
  ○ Dihydropyridine calcium channel blockers such as amlodipine may be used in hypertensive HF patients already on maximal guideline-directed medical therapy (GDMT); however, these agents do not improve mortality (*N Engl J Med 1996;335:1107–14; JACC Heart Failure 2013;1(4):308–14*).
  ○ Nondihydropyridine calcium channel blockers should be avoided in HFrEF because their negative inotropic effects may potentiate worsening HF.
• **Diuretic therapy** (see Table 5-3), in conjunction with restriction of dietary sodium and fluids, often leads to clinical improvement in patients with symptomatic HF. Frequent assessment of the patient's weight and careful observation of fluid intake and output are essential during initiation and maintenance of therapy. Frequent complications of therapy include hypokalemia, hyponatremia, hypomagnesemia, volume contraction alkalosis, intravascular volume depletion, and hypotension. Serum electrolytes, BUN, and creatinine levels should be followed after institution of diuretic therapy. Hypokalemia may be life threatening in patients who are receiving digoxin or in those who have severe LV dysfunction that predisposes them to ventricular arrhythmias. Potassium supplementation or a potassium-sparing diuretic should be considered in addition to careful monitoring of serum potassium levels.
  ○ **Potassium-sparing diuretics (amiloride)** do not exert a potent diuretic effect when used alone.
  ○ **Thiazide diuretics (hydrochlorothiazide, chlorthalidone)** can be used as initial agents in patients with normal renal function in whom only a mild diuresis is desired. **Metolazone**, unlike other oral thiazides, exerts its action at the proximal and distal tubule and may be useful in combination with a loop diuretic in patients with a low glomerular filtration rate.
  ○ **Loop diuretics (furosemide, torsemide, bumetanide, ethacrynic acid)** should be used in patients who require significant diuresis and in those with markedly decreased renal function.
    ▪ Furosemide reduces preload acutely by causing direct venodilation when administered intravenously, making it useful for managing severe HF or acute pulmonary edema (*Circulation 1997;96(6):1847*).
    ▪ Use of loop diuretics may be complicated by hyperuricemia, hypocalcemia, ototoxicity, rash, and vasculitis. Furosemide, torsemide, and bumetanide are sulfa derivatives and may rarely cause drug reactions in sulfa-sensitive patients; ethacrynic acid can be used in such patients.
    ▪ Dose equivalence of oral loop diuretics is approximately 50 mg ethacrynic acid = 40 mg furosemide = 20 mg torsemide = 1 mg bumetanide.
• **New and emerging agents**
  ○ **LCZ-696 (Entresto™)** is a combination of the ARB valsartan and neprilysin inhibitor sacubitril recently approved for use in patients with HFrEF and NYHA Class II-IV symptoms. Neprilysin is a neutral endopeptidase involved in the degradation of vasoactive peptides including the natriuretic peptides, bradykinin, and adrenomedullin. Inhibition of neprilysin increased the availability of these peptides, which exert favorable effects in HF. In a large trial, this agent was shown to be superior to enalapril in reducing death and rehospitalization among NYHA class II-IV patients with HFrEF.

○ **Ivabradine** is an inhibitor of the I_{Kf} channel involved in generating "pacemaker" currents in cardiac tissue. Use of ivabradine in outpatients with HFrEF was shown to reduce HF hospitalization and HF death (*Lancet 2010;9744:875–85*), and it is indicated for the reduction of HF hospitalization in patients with EF <35%, stable HF symptoms, and sinus rhythm with a resting heart rate ≥70 bpm who are already taking β-blockers at the highest tolerated dose.

Chronic Medical Therapy with Preserved Ejection Fraction (HFpEF)

• No pharmacotherapy has been demonstrated to improve mortality in HFpEF.
• Control of blood pressure is recommended. The use of ACE inhibitors, ARBs, spironolactone, and β-blockers is reasonable. Use of these particular agents may be associated with a small reduction in HF hospitalization rates.
• Treatment of atrial fibrillation through rate or rhythm control in accordance with practice guidelines is recommended.
• Treatment of coronary disease and angina through pharmacotherapy and/or revascularization in accordance with practice guidelines is recommended.

Parenteral Agents

• **Parenteral vasodilators** should be reserved for patients with severe HF not responding to oral medications. Intravenous (IV) vasodilator therapy may be guided by central hemodynamic monitoring (pulmonary artery catheterization) to assess efficacy and avoid hemodynamic instability. Parenteral agents should be started at low doses, titrated to the desired hemodynamic effect, and discontinued slowly to avoid rebound vasoconstriction.
• **Nitroglycerin** is a potent vasodilator with effects on venous and, to a lesser extent, arterial vascular beds. It relieves pulmonary and systemic venous congestion and is an effective coronary vasodilator. Nitroglycerin is the preferred vasodilator for treatment of HF in the setting of acute MI or unstable angina.
• **Sodium nitroprusside** is a direct arterial vasodilator with less potent venodilatory properties. Its predominant effect is to reduce afterload, and it is particularly effective in patients with HF who are hypertensive or who have severe aortic or mitral valvular regurgitation. Nitroprusside should be used cautiously in patients with myocardial ischemia because of a potential reduction in regional myocardial blood flow (**coronary steal**).
  ○ The initial dose of **0.25 μg/kg/min** can be titrated (**maximum dose of 10 μg/kg/min**) to the desired hemodynamic effect or until hypotension develops.
  ○ The half-life of nitroprusside is 1–3 minutes, and its metabolism results in the release of cyanide, which is metabolized by the liver to thiocyanate and is then excreted via the kidney.
  ○ Toxic levels of thiocyanate (>10 mg/dL) may develop in patients with renal insufficiency. Thiocyanate toxicity may manifest as nausea, paresthesias, mental status changes, abdominal pain, and seizures.
  ○ **Methemoglobinemia** is a rare complication of treatment with nitroprusside.
• **Recombinant BNP (nesiritide)** is an arterial and venous vasodilator.
  ○ IV infusion of nesiritide reduces right atrial and LV end-diastolic pressures and systemic vascular resistance and results in an increase in cardiac output.
  ○ It is administered as a 2-μg/kg IV bolus, followed by a continuous IV infusion starting at 0.01 μg/kg/min.
  ○ Nesiritide is approved for use in acute HF exacerbations and relieves HF symptoms early after its administration (*JAMA 2002;287:1531*). It does not have an effect on survival or rehospitalization in patients with HF (*N Engl J Med 2011;365:32*).
  ○ *Hypotension* is the most common side effect of nesiritide, and its use should be avoided in patients with systemic hypotension (systolic blood pressure <90 mm Hg) or evidence of cardiogenic shock. Episodes of hypotension should be managed with discontinuation of nesiritide and cautious volume expansion or vasopressor support if necessary.

- **Inotropic agents**
  - **Sympathomimetic agents** are potent drugs reserved for the treatment of severe HF. Beneficial and adverse effects are mediated by stimulation of myocardial β-adrenergic receptors. The most important adverse effects are related to the arrhythmogenic nature of these agents and the potential for exacerbation of myocardial ischemia. Treatment should be guided by careful hemodynamic and ECG monitoring. Patients with refractory chronic HF may benefit symptomatically from continuous ambulatory administration of IV inotropes as palliative therapy or as a bridge to mechanical ventricular support or cardiac transplantation. However, this strategy may increase the risk of life-threatening arrhythmias or indwelling catheter–related infections (*Circulation 2013;128:e240–e327*).
  - **Norepinephrine**, rather than **dopamine** (Table 5-4), should be used for stabilization of the hypotensive HF patient. Although a large randomized trial found no mortality difference between dopamine and norepinephrine in a cohort of undifferentiated shock patients, there were more adverse events (primarily arrhythmic) in the dopamine group, and subgroup analysis of those with cardiogenic shock (n = 280) showed an increased rate of death at 28 days in the dopamine group (*N Engl J Med 2010; 362:779–89*).
  - **Dobutamine** (see Table 5-4) is a synthetic analog of dopamine with predominantly β₁-adrenoreceptor activity. It increases cardiac output, lowers cardiac filling pressures, and generally has a neutral effect on systemic blood pressure. Dobutamine tolerance has been described, and several studies have demonstrated increased mortality in patients

TABLE 5-4	Inotropic Agents[a]		
Drug	**Dose**	**Mechanism**	**Effects/Side Effects**
Dopamine	1–3 μg/kg/min	Dopaminergic receptors	Splanchnic vasodilation
	2–8 μg/kg/min	β₁-receptor agonist	+Inotropic
	7–10 μg/kg/min	α-receptor agonist	↑ SVR
Dobutamine	2.5–15.0 μg/kg/min	β₁- > β₂- > α-receptor agonist	+Inotropic, ↓ SVR, tachycardia
Epinephrine	0.05–1 μg/kg/min; titrate to desired mean arterial pressure. May adjust dose every 10–15 min by 0.05–0.2 μg/kg/min to achieve desired blood pressure goal	β₁ > α₁ Low doses = β High doses = α	+Inotropic, ↑ SVR
Milrinone[b]	50-μg/kg bolus IV over 10 min, 0.375–0.75 μg/kg/min	↑ cAMP	+Inotropic, ↓ SVR

cAMP, cyclic adenosine monophosphate; SVR, systemic vascular resistance; ↑, increased; ↓, decreased.
[a]Increased risk of atrial and ventricular tachyarrhythmias.
[b]Needs dose adjustment for creatinine clearance.

treated with continuous dobutamine. Dobutamine has no significant role in the treatment of HF resulting from diastolic dysfunction or a high-output state.

○ **Phosphodiesterase inhibitors** increase myocardial contractility and produce vasodilation by increasing intracellular cyclic adenosine monophosphate (cAMP). **Milrinone** is currently available for clinical use and is indicated for treatment of refractory HF. Hypotension may develop in patients who receive vasodilator therapy or have intravascular volume contraction, or both. Milrinone may improve hemodynamics in patients who are treated concurrently with dobutamine or dopamine. Data suggest that in-hospital short-term milrinone administration in addition to standard medical therapy does not reduce the length of hospitalization or the 60-day mortality or rehospitalization rate when compared with placebo (*JAMA 2002;287:1541*).

Antiarrhythmic Therapy

• Suppression of asymptomatic ventricular premature beats or nonsustained ventricular tachycardia (NSVT) using antiarrhythmic drugs in patients with HF does not improve survival and may increase mortality as a result of the pro-arrhythmic effects of the drugs (*N Engl J Med 1989;321:406; N Engl J Med 1995;333:77; N Engl J Med 2005;352:225*).
• For patients with atrial fibrillation (AF) as a suspected cause of new-onset HF, a rhythm control strategy should be pursued. For patients with preexisting HF who develop AF, despite evidence suggesting improved symptom status in patients treated with rhythm control, the use of antiarrhythmic drug therapy for the maintenance of sinus rhythm has not been shown to improve mortality (*N Engl J Med 2008;358:2667–77*).
• Agents recommended for the maintenance of sinus rhythm in HF with reduced LVEF include dofetilide and amiodarone. Sotalol may also be considered in patients with mildly depressed LVEF. These agents require close monitoring of the QT interval.
• In patients with severe LV systolic dysfunction and HF, dronedarone should not be used (*N Engl J Med 2008;358:2678–87*).

Anticoagulant and Antiplatelet Therapy

• Although patients with HF are at relatively greater risk for thromboembolic events, the absolute risk is modest, and routine anticoagulation is not recommended in HF patients in the absence of AF, prior thromboembolism, or a prior cardioembolic source.
• In patients with AF, use of the CHADS2 or CHADS2-VASc risk score is recommended for determining when to use anticoagulant therapies.
• The novel anticoagulants dabigatran, rivaroxaban, and apixaban have been shown to be effective in HF patients with nonvalvular AF.
• There are insufficient data to support the routine use of aspirin in patients with HF who do not have coronary disease or atherosclerosis. Furthermore, certain data suggest that aspirin use may reduce the beneficial effects of ACE inhibitors (*Arch Intern Med 2003;163(13):1574*).

NONPHARMACOLOGIC THERAPIES FOR HEART FAILURE

• **Coronary revascularization** reduces ischemia and may improve systolic function in some patients with CAD.
○ Guidelines state that surgical or percutaneous revascularization is recommended in HF patients with angina and suitable anatomy (Class I recommendation) and may be considered in patients without angina who have suitable anatomy, whether in the presence of viable myocardium (Class IIa recommendation) or nonviable myocardium (Class IIb recommendation) (*Circulation 2013;128:e240–e327*).
○ In a large randomized trial of HF patients with CAD and LVEF <35% comparing medical therapy to medical therapy plus coronary artery bypass graft surgery (CABG),

there was no difference in the primary outcome of death from any cause (hazard ratio [HR] with CABG, 0.86; 95% confidence interval [CI], 0.72–1.04; $P = 0.12$). A prespecified secondary analysis of death from cardiovascular causes favored CABG over medical therapy alone (HR with CABG, 0.81; 95% CI, 0.66–1.00; $P = 0.05$) (*N Engl J Med 2011;364:1607–16*).

• **Cardiac resynchronization therapy (CRT)** or **biventricular pacing** (see Chapter 7, Cardiac Arrhythmias) can improve quality of life and reduce the risk of death in certain patients with an EF of ≤35%, NYHA class II–IV HF, and conduction abnormalities (left bundle branch block [LBBB] and atrioventricular delay) (*N Engl J Med 2005;352:1539*; *N Engl J Med 2010;363:2385–95*).
  ○ CRT can also be useful (Class IIA recommendation) in the following situations (*Circulation 2013;128:1810–52*):
    ▪ LVEF ≤35%, sinus rhythm, a non-LBBB pattern with a QRS ≥150 milliseconds, and NYHA class III/ambulatory class IV symptoms on GDMT
    ▪ LVEF ≤35%, sinus rhythm, LBBB with a QRS 120–149 milliseconds, and NYHA class II, III, or ambulatory IV symptoms on GDMT
    ▪ AF and LVEF ≤35% on GDMT if the patient requires ventricular pacing and atrioventricular nodal ablation or rate control allows near 100% ventricular pacing with CRT
    ▪ Patients on GDMT who have LVEF ≤35% and are undergoing new or replacement device implantation with anticipated frequent ventricular pacing (>40% of the time)
  ○ Factors most strongly favoring response to CRT include female sex, QRS duration ≥150 milliseconds, LBBB, body mass index <30 kg/m², nonischemic cardiomyopathy, and a small left atrium (*J Am Coll Cardiol 2012;59(25):2366–73*).
• **Implantable cardioverter-defibrillator (ICD)** placement is recommended for selected HF patients with a persistently reduced LVEF ≤35% for primary prevention of SCD. SCD occurs six to nine times more often in patients with HF compared to the general population and is the leading cause of death in ambulatory HF patients.
  ○ Multiple large randomized trials have demonstrated a survival benefit of 1–1.5% per year in patients with both ischemic and nonischemic cardiomyopathy (*N Engl J Med 2005;352:1539*; *Circulation 2013;128:e240–e327*).
  ○ Patients should receive at least 3–6 months of optimal GDMT prior to reassessment of EF and implantation of an ICD.
  ○ Following an acute MI or revascularization, EF should be assessed after 40 days of GDMT prior to ICD implantation.
  ○ ICD therapy should be reserved for patients expected to otherwise live >1 year with good functional capacity. ICD therapy should not be used in end-stage HF patients who are not candidates for transplantation or durable mechanical circulatory support.
• An **intra-aortic balloon pump (IABP)** can be considered for temporary hemodynamic support in patients who have failed pharmacologic therapies and have transient myocardial dysfunction or are awaiting a definitive procedure such as a LV assist device (LVAD) or transplantation. Severe aortoiliac atherosclerosis and moderate to severe aortic valve insufficiency are contraindications to IABP placement.
• **Percutaneous LVADs** are now available to provide short-term hemodynamic support for patients in cardiogenic shock. These devices have been shown to provide superior hemodynamic effects compared to IABP. However, use of percutaneous LVADs compared to IABP did not improve 30-day survival in critically ill patients (*Eur Heart J 2009;30:2102*).

SURGICAL MANAGEMENT

• **Surgical or nonsurgical replacement or repair** of the mitral valve in the setting of a reduced LVEF and severe MR is discussed elsewhere (see Chapter 6, Pericardial and Valvular Heart Disease).

- **Ventricular assist devices (VADs)** are surgically implanted devices that draw blood from the left ventricle, energize flow through a motor unit, and deliver the energized blood to the aorta, resulting in augmented cardiac output and lower intracardiac filling pressures. These devices may be temporary (CentriMag, percutaneous LVADs) or durable (Heart-mate II, HeartWare).
  - Temporary support is indicated for patients with severe HF after cardiac surgery or individuals with intractable cardiogenic shock after acute MI.
  - Durable support is indicated as a "bridge to transplantation" for patients awaiting heart transplantation or as "destination" therapy for select patients ineligible for transplant with refractory end-stage HF and HF-related life expectancy with therapy of <2 years (*Circulation 2013;128:e240–e327*).
  - Currently available devices vary with regard to degree of mechanical hemolysis, intensity of anticoagulation required, and difficulty of implantation.
  - The decision to institute mechanical circulatory support must be made in consultation with an HF cardiologist and a cardiac surgeon who have experience with this technology.
- **Cardiac transplantation** is an option for selected patients with severe end-stage HF that has become refractory to aggressive medical therapy and for whom no other conventional treatment options are available.
  - Only approximately 2200 heart transplants are performed each year in the United States.
  - Candidates considered for transplantation should generally be <65 years old (although selected older patients may also benefit), have advanced HF (NYHA class III–IV), have a strong psychosocial support system, have exhausted all other therapeutic options, and be free of irreversible extracardiac organ dysfunction that would limit functional recovery or predispose them to posttransplant complications (*J Heart Lung Transplant 2006;25:1024–42*).
  - Survival rates after heart transplant are approximately 90%, 70%, and 50% at 1, 5, and 10 years, respectively. Annual statistics can be found on the United Network for Organ Sharing website (*www.unos.org*).
  - In general, functional capacity and quality of life improve significantly after transplantation, although VO_2 does not reach levels of age- and gender-matched controls, improving by approximately 40% at 2 years (*Eur J Heart Fail 2007;9(3):310–6*).
  - **Posttransplant complications** may include acute or chronic rejection, typical and atypical infections, and adverse effects of immunosuppressive agents. Surgical complications and acute rejection are the major causes of death in the first posttransplant year. Cardiac allograft vasculopathy (CAD/chronic rejection) and malignancy are the leading causes of death after the first posttransplant year.

LIFESTYLE/RISK MODIFICATION

- Dietary counseling for sodium and fluid restriction should be provided. Daily intake of approximately 2 g of sodium per day is reasonable. Excessive restriction (<1.5 g/d of sodium) may be harmful.
- Smoking cessation should be strongly encouraged.
- Abstinence from alcohol is recommended in symptomatic HF patients with low EF.
- Exercise training is recommended in stable HF patients as an adjunct to pharmacologic treatment. Exercise training in patients with HF has been shown to improve exercise capacity (peak VO_2 max as well as 6-minute walk time), improve quality of life, and decrease neurohormonal activation (*JAMA 2009;301:1439; JAMA 2009;301:1451*). Treatment programs should be individualized and include a warm-up period, 20–30 minutes of exercise at the desired intensity, and a cool-down period (*Circulation 2003;107:1210*).
- Weight loss should be recommended in obese HF patients.

Special Considerations

- **Fluid and free water restriction** (<1.5 L/d) is especially important in the setting of hyponatremia (serum sodium <130 mEq/L) and volume overload.
- **Minimization of medications** with deleterious effects in HF should be attempted.
  - **Negative inotropes** (e.g., verapamil, diltiazem) should be avoided in patients with impaired ventricular contractility, as should over-the-counter β stimulants (e.g., compounds containing ephedra, pseudoephedrine hydrochloride).
  - **NSAIDs**, which antagonize the effect of ACE inhibitors and diuretic therapy, should be avoided if possible.
- **Administration of supplemental oxygen** may relieve dyspnea, improve oxygen delivery, reduce the work of breathing, and limit pulmonary vasoconstriction in patients with hypoxemia but is not routinely recommended in patients without hypoxemia.
- **Sleep apnea** has a prevalence as high as 37% in the HF population. Treatment with nocturnal positive airway pressure improves symptoms and EF (*Am J Respir Crit Care Med 2001;164:2147*; *N Engl J Med 2003;348:1233*).
- **Dialysis** or **ultrafiltration** may be beneficial in patients with severe HF and renal dysfunction who cannot respond adequately to fluid and sodium restriction and diuretics (*J Am Coll Cardiol 2007;49:675*) but is not superior to a scaled diuretic regimen in patients with acute HF and cardiorenal syndrome (*N Engl J Med 2012;367:2296–304*). Other mechanical methods of fluid removal such as therapeutic thoracentesis and paracentesis may provide temporary symptomatic relief of dyspnea. Care must be taken to avoid rapid fluid removal and hypotension.
- **End-of-life considerations** may be necessary in patients with advanced HF who are refractory to therapy. Discussions regarding the disease course, treatment options, survival, functional status, and advance directives should be addressed early in the treatment of the patient with HF. For those with end-stage disease (stage D, NYHA class IV) with multiple hospitalizations and severe decline in their functional status and quality of life, hospice and palliative care should be considered (*J Card Fail 2014;20(2):121–34*).

Acute Heart Failure and Cardiogenic Pulmonary Edema

GENERAL PRINCIPLES

Cardiogenic pulmonary edema (CPE) occurs when the pulmonary capillary pressure exceeds the forces that maintain fluid within the vascular space (serum oncotic pressure and interstitial hydrostatic pressure).
- Increased pulmonary capillary pressure may be caused by LV failure of any cause, obstruction to transmitral flow (e.g., mitral stenosis [MS], atrial myxoma), or rarely, pulmonary veno-occlusive disease.
- Alveolar flooding and impairment of gas exchange follow accumulation of fluid in the pulmonary interstitium.

DIAGNOSIS

Clinical Presentation

- Clinical manifestations of CPE may occur rapidly and include dyspnea, anxiety, cough, and restlessness.
- The patient may expectorate pink frothy fluid.
- Physical signs of decreased peripheral perfusion, pulmonary congestion, hypoxemia, use of accessory respiratory muscles, and wheezing are often present.

Diagnostic Testing

- Radiographic abnormalities include cardiomegaly, interstitial and perihilar vascular engorgement, Kerley B lines, and pleural effusions.
- The radiographic abnormalities may follow the development of symptoms by several hours, and their resolution may be out of phase with clinical improvement.

TREATMENT

- Placing the patient in a sitting position improves pulmonary function.
- Bed rest, pain control, and relief of anxiety can decrease cardiac workload.
- **Supplemental oxygen** should be administered initially to raise the arterial oxygen tension to >60 mm Hg.
- **Mechanical ventilation** is indicated if oxygenation is inadequate or hypercapnia occurs. Noninvasive positive-pressure ventilation is preferred and may have particularly favorable effects in the setting of pulmonary edema (*JAMA 2005;294(24):3124–30*).
- **Precipitating factors** should be identified and corrected, because resolution of pulmonary edema can often be accomplished with correction of the underlying process. The most common precipitants are:
  - Severe hypertension
  - MI or myocardial ischemia (particularly if associated with MR)
  - Acute valvular regurgitation
  - New-onset tachyarrhythmias or bradyarrhythmias
  - Volume overload in the setting of severe LV dysfunction

Medications

- **Morphine sulfate** reduces anxiety and dilates pulmonary and systemic veins; 2–4 mg can be given intravenously over several minutes and can be repeated every 10–25 minutes until an effect is seen.
- **Furosemide** is a venodilator that decreases pulmonary congestion within minutes of IV administration, well before its diuretic action begins. An initial dose of 20–80 mg IV should be given over several minutes and can be increased based on response to a maximum of 200 mg in subsequent doses.
- **Nitroglycerin** is a venodilator that can potentiate the effect of furosemide. IV administration is preferable to oral and transdermal forms because it can be rapidly titrated.
- **Nitroprusside** is an effective adjunct in the treatment of acute CPE and is useful when CPE is brought on by acute valvular regurgitation or hypertension (see Chapter 6, Pericardial and Valvular Heart Disease). Pulmonary and systemic arterial catheterization should be considered to guide titration of nitroprusside therapy.
- **Inotropic agents**, such as dobutamine or milrinone, may be helpful after initial treatment of CPE in patients with concomitant hypotension or shock.
- **Recombinant BNP (nesiritide)** is administered as an IV bolus followed by an IV infusion. Nesiritide reduces intracardiac filling pressures by producing vasodilation and indirectly increases the cardiac output. In conjunction with furosemide, nesiritide produces natriuresis and diuresis.

SPECIAL CONSIDERATIONS

- **Right heart catheterization** (e.g., Swan-Ganz catheter) may be helpful in cases where a prompt response to therapy does not occur by allowing differentiation between cardiogenic and noncardiogenic causes of pulmonary edema via measurement of central hemodynamics and cardiac output. It may then be used to guide subsequent therapy. The routine use of right heart catheterization in acute HF patients is not beneficial (*JAMA 2005;294(13):1625–33*).

• **Acute hemodialysis and ultrafiltration** may be required in the patient with significant renal dysfunction and diuretic resistance (*J Am Coll Cardiol 2007;49:675*; *Congest Heart Fail 2008;14:19*) but is not a first-line therapy.

CARDIOMYOPATHY

Dilated Cardiomyopathy

GENERAL PRINCIPLES

Definition

Dilated cardiomyopathy (DCM) is a disease of heart muscle characterized by dilation of the cardiac chambers and reduction in ventricular contractile function.

Epidemiology

DCM is the most common form of cardiomyopathy and is responsible for approximately 10,000 deaths and 46,000 hospitalizations each year. The lifetime incidence of DCM is about 30 cases per 100,000 persons.

Pathophysiology

• DCM may be secondary to progression of any process that affects the myocardium, and dilation is directly related to neurohormonal activation. The majority of cases are idiopathic (*Am J Cardiol 1992;69:1458*), although genetic causes are increasingly recognized (*J Am Coll Cardiol 2005;45(7):969*).
• Dilation of the cardiac chambers and varying degrees of hypertrophy are anatomic hallmarks. Tricuspid and mitral regurgitation are common due to the effect of chamber dilation on the valvular apparatus.
• **Atrial and ventricular arrhythmias** are present in as many as one-half of these patients and contribute to the high incidence of sudden death in this population.

DIAGNOSIS

Clinical Presentation

• Symptomatic HF (dyspnea, volume overload) is often present.
• A portion of patients with clinical disease may be asymptomatic.
• The ECG is usually abnormal, but changes are typically nonspecific.

Diagnostic Testing

Imaging
• Diagnosis of DCM can be confirmed with echocardiography or radionuclide ventriculography.
• Two-dimensional and Doppler echocardiography are helpful in differentiating this condition from HCM or restrictive cardiomyopathy (RCM), pericardial disease, and valvular disorders.

Diagnostic Procedures
Endomyocardial biopsy provides little information that affects treatment of patients with DCMs and is not routinely recommended (*Eur Heart J 2007;28:3076*; *Circulation 2013;128:e240–e327*). Settings where endomyocardial biopsy for DCM is recommended include:
• New-onset HF of <2 weeks in duration with normal-sized or dilated left ventricle and hemodynamic compromise.

- New-onset HF of 2 weeks to 3 months in duration associated with a dilated left ventricle and new ventricular arrhythmias, high-grade atrioventricular block (type II second-degree or third-degree), and failure to respond to usual care.
- Clinical scenarios that may result in the diagnosis of a treatable form of acute myocarditis, such as giant cell myocarditis or eosinophilic myocarditis.

TREATMENT

Medications

- The medical management of symptomatic patients is identical to that for HFrEF from other causes. This consists of controlling total body sodium and volume and pharmacotherapy including β-blockers, ACE inhibitors or ARBs, aldosterone antagonists, and vasodilator therapy.
- Immunizations against influenza and pneumococcal pneumonia are recommended.
- Immunosuppressive therapy with agents such as prednisone, azathioprine, and cyclosporine for biopsy-proven myocarditis has been advocated by some, but efficacy has not been established, with the possible exception of the very rare patient with giant cell myocarditis (*N Engl J Med 1995;333:269*; *Circulation 2013;128:e240–e327*).

Other Nonpharmacologic Therapies

Nonpharmacologic therapies for DCM are identical to those for HFrEF in general and, when indicated by practice guidelines, include ICD implantation, CRT, and temporary mechanical circulatory support.

Surgical Management

- Cardiac transplantation should be considered for selected patients with HF due to DCM that is refractory to medical therapy.
- LVAD placement may be necessary for stabilization of patients in whom cardiac transplantation is an option or in select patients who are not eligible for transplantation.

Heart Failure with Preserved Ejection Fraction

GENERAL PRINCIPLES

Definition

- HFpEF, also called diastolic HF, refers to the clinical syndrome of HF in the presence of preserved systolic function (LVEF >50%).
- Diastolic dysfunction refers to an abnormality in the mechanical function of the heart during the relaxation phase of the cardiac cycle, resulting in elevated filling pressures and impairment of ventricular filling.

Epidemiology

- Almost half of patients admitted to the hospital with HF have a normal or near-normal EF.
- HFpEF is most prevalent in older women, most of whom have hypertension and/or diabetes mellitus. Many of these patients also have CAD and/or AF.

Etiology

- The vast majority of patients with HFpEF have hypertension and LV hypertrophy.
- Myocardial disorders associated with HFpEF include RCM, obstructive and nonobstructive HCM, infiltrative cardiomyopathies, and constrictive pericarditis.

Pathophysiology

- Reduced ventricular compliance and elastance play a major role in the pathophysiology of HFpEF.
- Factors contributing to the clinical HFpEF syndrome include abnormal sodium handling by the kidneys, atrial dysfunction, autonomic dysfunction, increased arterial stiffness, pulmonary hypertension, sarcopenia, obesity, deconditioning, and other comorbidities.

DIAGNOSIS

- Differentiating between HFpEF and HFrEF cannot be reliably accomplished without assessment of LVEF, preferably with two-dimensional echocardiography.
- Diagnosis is based on echocardiographic criteria and Doppler findings of normal LVEF and impaired diastolic relaxation and elevated filling pressures. More sensitive echocardiographic parameters of systolic function, such as LV strain, may be abnormal in patients with HFpEF.

TREATMENT

No pharmacologic therapy has been shown in a randomized controlled trial to reduce mortality in HFpEF patients. Subgroup analysis indicates a possible modest benefit with respect to morbidity from the use of aldosterone receptor antagonists, ACE inhibitors/ARBs, and β-blockers. Practice guidelines for HFpEF emphasize blood pressure control, heart rate control or restoration of sinus rhythm in symptomatic patients, judicious diuretic use, and treatment of ischemic heart disease.

Hypertrophic Cardiomyopathy

GENERAL PRINCIPLES

Definition

HCM can be defined broadly as the presence of increased LV wall thickness that is not solely explained by abnormal loading conditions (*Eur Heart J 2014;35(39):2733–79*). More specifically, HCM is a genetically determined disease wherein sarcomere mutations lead to LV hypertrophy associated with nondilated ventricular chambers in the absence of another disease that would be capable of causing the magnitude of hypertrophy present in a given individual (*J Am Coll Cardiol 2011;58(25):e212–60*).

Epidemiology

- HCM is the most commonly inherited heart defect, occurring in 1 out of 500 individuals.
- Approximately 500,000 people have HCM in the United States, although many are unaware. An estimated 36% of young athletes who die suddenly have probable or definite HCM, making it the leading cause of SCD in young people in the United States, including trained athletes (*Circulation 2013;128:e240–e327*).

Pathophysiology

- HCM results from a mutation in a gene encoding one of the proteins involved in essential myocardial sarcomere functions, such as structural or contractile proteins, calcium handling proteins, or mitochondrial proteins.
  - There are currently at least 27 putative HCM susceptibility genes that lead to autosomal dominant transmission with variable phenotypic expression and penetrance.

- ○ The most common mutations involve myosin binding protein C (*MYBPC3*) and myosin heavy chain 7 (*MYH7*).
- ○ Over 50% of clinically affected patients have an identified mutation (*J Am Coll Cardiol 2009;54(3):201–11*).
- The histopathologic change in HCM consists of hypertrophied myocytes arranged in a disorganized manner with interstitial fibrosis.
- These changes lead grossly to myocardial hypertrophy that is typically predominant in the ventricular septum (asymmetric septal hypertrophy) but may involve any and all ventricular segments. HCM can be classified clinically according to the presence or absence of LV outflow tract (LVOT) obstruction. When present, it is termed **hypertrophic obstructive cardiomyopathy (HOCM)**.
- LVOT obstruction may occur at rest but is enhanced by factors that increase LV contractility (exercise), decrease ventricular volume (e.g., Valsalva maneuver, volume depletion, large meal), or decrease afterload (vasodilators).
- Delayed ventricular diastolic relaxation and decreased compliance are common and, along with MR, may lead to pulmonary congestion.
- Myocardial ischemia is common, secondary to a myocardial oxygen supply–demand mismatch.
- Systolic anterior motion (SAM) of the anterior leaflet of the mitral valve is often associated with MR and likely determines the severity of LVOT obstruction.

DIAGNOSIS

HCM is usually diagnosed by maximal LV wall thickness ≥15 mm in the absence of another disease that could account for the degree of hypertrophy, often accompanied by supporting information (family history of HCM or sudden death, SAM, genetic testing).

Clinical Presentation

- Presentation varies but may include exertional dyspnea, angina, fatigue, dizziness, syncope, palpitations, or sudden death.
- Sudden death is most common in children and young adults between the ages of 10 and 35 years and often occurs during or immediately after periods of strenuous exertion.

Physical Examination
- Coarse **systolic outflow murmur** localized along the left sternal border that is **accentuated by maneuvers that decrease preload** (e.g., standing, Valsalva maneuver) and may be associated with a forceful double or triple apical impulse.
- Bisferiens (double peak per cardiac cycle) carotid pulse (in the presence of obstruction).

Diagnostic Testing
Electrocardiography
The ECG of HCM is usually abnormal and invariably so in symptomatic patients with LVOT obstruction. The most common abnormalities are ST-segment and T-wave abnormalities, followed by evidence of LV hypertrophy (*Am J Cardiol 2002;90:1020*). The ECG in apical-variant HCM is characterized by large, inverted T waves across the precordial leads.

Imaging
- Two-dimensional echocardiography and Doppler flow studies can establish the presence of a significant LV outflow gradient at rest or with provocation.
- Additional risk stratification should be pursued with 24- to 48-hour Holter monitoring and exercise testing.
- Cardiac MRI is indicated in patients with suspected HCM in whom the diagnosis cannot be confirmed with echocardiography.

Genetic Testing

Genetic testing for HCM is commercially available. Roughly 50% of patients with HCM have a known pathogenic mutation. Genetic testing can be used to aid in diagnosis of HCM when the clinical presentation is unclear. Genetic testing is reasonable in an index patient to facilitate family screening to determine at-risk first-degree relatives (*J Am Coll Cardiol 2011;58(25):e212–60*).

TREATMENT

- Management is directed toward relief of symptoms and prevention of sudden death.
- Infective endocarditis prophylaxis remains controversial, and prophylactic antibiotics are no longer recommended by guidelines.
- Treatment in asymptomatic individuals is controversial, and no conclusive evidence has been found that medical therapy is beneficial.
- All individuals with HCM should avoid strenuous physical activity, including most competitive sports. Activity-specific recommendations are available (*Circulation 2004; 109:2807–16*).

Medications

- β-Blockers are generally the first-line agent to reduce symptoms of HCM by reducing myocardial contractility and heart rate.
- Nondihydropyridine calcium channel antagonists (verapamil and diltiazem) may improve the symptoms of HCM by reducing myocardial contractility and heart rate. Therapy should be initiated at low doses, with careful titration in patients with outflow obstruction. The dose should be increased gradually over several days to weeks if symptoms persist. Dihydropyridines should be avoided in patients with LVOT obstruction as a result of their vasodilatory properties.
- Disopyramide, a negative inotropic agent that results in lowering of the LVOT gradient, may be added for HCM patients who remain symptomatic despite the use of β-blockers and calcium channel blockers (alone or in combination). Use requires monitoring of the QT interval, and concomitant use of other antiarrhythmic drugs should be avoided.
- Diuretics may improve pulmonary congestive symptoms in patients with elevated pulmonary venous pressures. These agents should be used cautiously in patients with LVOT obstruction because excessive preload reduction worsens the obstruction.
- Nitrates and vasodilators should be avoided because of the risk of increasing the LVOT gradient.
- **Atrial and ventricular arrhythmias** occur commonly in patients with HCM. Supraventricular tachyarrhythmias are tolerated poorly and should be treated aggressively. Cardioversion is indicated if hemodynamic compromise develops.
  - **Digoxin is relatively contraindicated** because of its positive inotropic properties and potential for exacerbating ventricular outflow obstruction.
  - AF should be converted to sinus rhythm when possible, and anticoagulation is recommended if paroxysmal or chronic AF develops.
  - **Diltiazem, verapamil, or β-blockers** can be used to control the ventricular response before cardioversion. Procainamide, disopyramide, or amiodarone (see Chapter 7, Cardiac Arrhythmias) may be effective in the chronic suppression of AF.
  - ICD implantation is recommended for patients with HCM and prior cardiac arrest, ventricular fibrillation, or hemodynamically significant ventricular tachycardia.
  - ICD placement is reasonable in high-risk patients such as those with:
    - Recent unexplained syncope
    - LV hypertrophy with a maximal wall thickness >30 mm

- History of sudden death presumably caused by HCM in one or more first-degree relatives
- Multiple episodes of NSVT on Holter recordings (especially in patients <30 years old)
- Hypotensive response to exercise
  ○ Symptomatic ventricular arrhythmias should be treated as outlined in Chapter 7, Cardiac Arrhythmias.

Nonpharmacologic Therapies for HCM

Dual-chamber pacing (see Chapter 7, Cardiac Arrhythmias) improves symptoms in some patients with HCM. Alteration of the ventricular activation sequence via RV pacing may minimize LVOT obstruction secondary to asymmetric septal hypertrophy. Only 10% of patients with HCM meet the criteria for pacemaker implantation, and the effect on decreasing the LVOT gradient is only 25%. A subset of patients with HCM may derive symptomatic benefit from dual-chamber pacing without an effect on survival (*Heart 2010;96(5):352*).

Surgical Management

- Septal reduction therapy (surgical myectomy or catheter-based alcohol septal ablation) provides symptom relief without proven survival benefit in the treatment of medication-refractory HCM symptoms.
- Septal myectomy is the most commonly performed surgical intervention in HCM. In experienced centers, it is associated with symptom improvement in 95% of patients with <1% operative mortality (*J Am Coll Cardiol 2005;46:470–6*). Concomitant mitral valve intervention (mitral valve repair or replacement) is rarely required in experienced centers because MR generally responds well to septal reduction.
- Alcohol septal ablation, a catheter-based alternative to surgical myectomy, also provides relief of obstruction and symptomatic benefit with low procedural mortality, although it can be associated with heart block, requiring pacemaker placement in up to 20% of patients (*Circulation 2008;118:131–9*).
- Cardiac transplantation should be considered for patients with refractory end-stage HCM with symptomatic HF.

PATIENT EDUCATION

Genetic counseling and family screening are recommended for first-degree relatives of patients with HCM because it is transmitted as an autosomal dominant trait.

Restrictive Cardiomyopathy

GENERAL PRINCIPLES

Definition

- RCM is characterized by a rigid heart with poor ventricular filling but generally a nondilated LV and normal LVEF. Right heart failure symptoms often predominate.
- RCM may be primary, including conditions such as idiopathic RCM, endomyocardial fibrosis, and Löffler endocarditis, or secondary to either infiltrative conditions (amyloidosis, sarcoidosis, hypereosinophilic syndrome) or storage diseases (Fabry disease, hemochromatosis, and the glycogen storage diseases).
- Constrictive pericarditis may present similarly to RCM but is a disease wherein the pericardium limits diastolic filling. Constriction carries a different prognosis and therapy, and the distinction between constriction and RCM is essential.

Pathophysiology

- In amyloidosis, misfolded protein (amyloid) deposits in the cardiac interstitium, interrupting the normal myocardial contractile units and causing restriction.
- In sarcoidosis, granulomatous infiltration of the myocardium is often subclinical and more commonly presents with arrhythmias or conduction system disease; however, in up to 5% of sarcoidosis cases, restriction is manifested.
- In hemochromatosis, excess iron is deposited in the cardiomyocyte sarcoplasm, ultimately overcoming antioxidant capacity and resulting in lipid peroxidation and membrane permeability. Injury occurs initially in the epicardium and then later in the myocardium and endocardium, with systolic function initially preserved.
- Fabry disease, an X-linked genetic disorder, is characterized by deficient activity of the lysosomal enzyme α-galactosidase A, resulting in lysosomal accumulation of globotriaosylceramide in tissues, with more than half of patients manifesting cardiomyopathy, typically with LV hypertrophy and RCM.

DIAGNOSIS

Diagnostic Testing

Electrocardiography
The classic ECG finding in amyloidosis is low voltage (despite echocardiographically evident ventricular thickening) with poor R-wave progression. In sarcoidosis, conduction disease is often present.

Imaging
- In RCM, echocardiography with Doppler analysis often demonstrates thickened myocardium with normal or abnormal systolic function, abnormal diastolic filling patterns, and evidence of elevated intracardiac pressure. Compared with constrictive pericarditis, respiratory variation is less marked and tissue Doppler velocities are reduced.
- Cardiac MRI, position emission tomography (PET), and CT are emerging as useful diagnostic tools for patients with cardiac sarcoidosis because granulomas, inflammation, and edema may be seen, which appear to improve with therapy (*Am Heart J 2009;157:746*).

Diagnostic Procedures
- On cardiac catheterization, elevated and equalized RV and LV filling pressures are seen with a classic "dip-and-plateau" pattern in the RV and LV pressure tracing. Although pericardial constriction may produce similar findings, absence of ventricular interdependence identifies RCM as opposed to constriction (*J Am Coll Cardiol 2008;51(3):315–9*).
- RV endomyocardial biopsy may be diagnostic and should be considered in patients in whom a diagnosis is not established.

TREATMENT

- Specific therapy aimed at amelioration of the underlying cause should be initiated.
- Cardiac hemochromatosis may respond to reduction of total body iron stores via phlebotomy or chelation therapy with desferoxamine.
- Cardiac sarcoidosis may respond to glucocorticoid therapy, but prolongation of survival with this approach has not been established.
- Fabry disease may be treated with recombinant α-galactosidase A enzyme replacement therapy.
- In those with syncope and/or ventricular arrhythmias, placement of an ICD is indicated. Patients with high-grade conduction disease warrant pacemaker placement.
- No pharmacotherapy is known to be effective at reversing the progression of cardiac amyloidosis.

- Digoxin should be avoided in patients with cardiac amyloidosis because digoxin is bound extracellularly by amyloid fibrils and may cause hypersensitivity and toxicity (*Circulation 1981;63:1285*).

Peripartum Cardiomyopathy

GENERAL PRINCIPLES

Definition
- PPCM is defined as LV systolic dysfunction diagnosed in the last month of pregnancy up to 5 months postpartum.
- The incidence of PPCM is 1 in 3000 to 4000 pregnancies in the United States.

Etiology
- The etiology of PPCM remains unclear. There is evidence to support **viral triggers**, including coxsackievirus, parvovirus B19, adenovirus, and herpesvirus, which may replicate unchecked in the reduced immunologic state brought on by pregnancy.
- **Fetal microchimerism**, wherein fetal cells escape into the maternal circulation and induce an autoimmune myocarditis, has also been suggested as a cause (*Lancet 2006;368:687*).
- A cleavage product of **prolactin** has also been implicated in the development of PPCM (*Cell 2007;128:589*).

Risk Factors
Risk factors that predispose a woman to PPCM include advanced maternal age, multiparity, multiple pregnancies, preeclampsia, and gestational hypertension. There is a higher risk in African American women, but this may be confounded by the higher prevalence of hypertension in this population.

DIAGNOSIS

Clinical Presentation
- Clinically, women with PPCM present with the signs and symptoms of HF.
- Because dyspnea on exertion and lower extremity edema are common in late pregnancy, PPCM may be difficult to recognize. Cough, orthopnea, and paroxysmal nocturnal dyspnea are warning signs that PPCM may be present, as is the presence of a displaced apical impulse and a new MR murmur on exam.
- Most commonly, patients present with NYHA class III and IV HF, although mild cases and sudden cardiac arrest also occur.

Diagnostic Testing
Electrocardiography
On ECG, LV hypertrophy is often present, as are ST-T–wave abnormalities.

Imaging
Diagnosis requires an echocardiogram with a newly depressed EF and/or LV dilatation.

TREATMENT

Medications
- The mainstay of treatment is afterload and preload reduction.
- **ACE inhibitors** are used in the postpartum patient, whereas hydralazine is used in the patient who is still pregnant.

- **β-Blockers** are used to reduce tachycardia, arrhythmia, and risk of SCD and are relatively safe, although β_1-selective blockers are preferred because they avoid peripheral vasodilation and uterine relaxation.
- **Digoxin** is also safe during pregnancy and may be used to augment contractility and for rate control, although levels need to be closely monitored.
- **Diuretics** are used for preload reduction and symptom relief and are also safe.
- In those with thromboembolism, **heparin** is required, followed by **warfarin** after delivery.

OUTCOME/PROGNOSIS

- The prognosis in PPCM is better than that seen in other forms of nonischemic cardiomyopathy.
- The extent of ventricular recovery at 6 months after delivery can predict overall recovery, although continued improvement has been seen up to 2–3 years after diagnosis.
- Subsequent pregnancies in patients with PPCM may be associated with significant deterioration in LV function and can even result in death. Family planning counseling is essential after the diagnosis of PPCM is made, and women who do not recover their LV function should be encouraged to consider foregoing future pregnancy.

6 Pericardial and Valvular Heart Disease

Jacob S. Goldstein and Brian R. Lindman

PERICARDIAL DISEASE

Acute Pericarditis

GENERAL PRINCIPLES

Etiology

- The yield of standard diagnostic testing is relatively low.
- **Common:** neoplastic, autoimmune, viral, tuberculosis, bacterial (nontuberculous), uremia, post–cardiac surgery, idiopathic.
- **Less common:** trauma, post–myocardial infarction, drugs, dissecting aortic aneurysm.

Pathophysiology

The pericardium is a fibrous sac surrounding the heart consisting of two layers: a thin visceral layer attached to the pericardium and a thicker parietal layer. The pericardial space is normally filled with 15–50 mL of fluid, and the two layers slide smoothly against each other, allowing for normal expansion and contraction of the heart. Pericarditis occurs when these layers are inflamed.

DIAGNOSIS

Clinical Presentation

History
- The clinical presentation of acute pericarditis can vary depending on the underlying etiology. Patients with a known autoimmune diagnosis or malignancy can present with signs or symptoms specific to the underlying disorder. An infectious etiology can be preceded by, for example, a viral prodrome.
- Chest pain: typically sudden onset, anterior chest, sharp and pleuritic, improved by sitting up and leaning forward, made worse by inspiration, lying flat.

Physical Exam
Pericardial friction rub: highly specific for acute pericarditis. A scratchy or squeaking sound heard best over the left sternal border with the diaphragm of the stethoscope.

Differential Diagnosis

Must differentiate from other causes of acute chest pain: myocardial ischemia, aortic dissection, pulmonary embolism, musculoskeletal pain, gastroesophageal reflux disease.

Diagnostic Testing

- **ECG:** Diffuse ST-segment elevation and PR depression
- **CXR:** typically normal

- Echocardiogram: often normal, but may observe an associated pericardial effusion
- Other tests: complete blood count, troponin level, C-reactive protein, erythrocyte sedimentation rate, blood cultures (if febrile)

TREATMENT

- Tailor therapy to the etiology, as appropriate.
- NSAIDs: ibuprofen, aspirin, ketorolac.
- Colchicine: when added to conventional anti-inflammatory therapy, significantly reduces symptoms, recurrence rates, and hospitalizations.
- Glucocorticoids: reserved for cases refractory to standard therapy or in the setting of uremia, connective tissue disease, or immune-mediated pericarditis.

Constrictive Pericarditis

GENERAL PRINCIPLES

Constrictive pericarditis, as a cause of right-sided heart failure (HF), often goes undiagnosed. It is often difficult to distinguish from restrictive cardiomyopathies (RCMs). Multiple imaging modalities and invasive hemodynamics are often needed to confirm the diagnosis.

Etiology
- **Common**
  Idiopathic, viral pericarditis (chronic or recurrent), postcardiotomy, chest irradiation
- **Less common**
  Autoimmune connective tissue disorders, end-stage renal disease, uremia, malignancy (e.g., breast, lung, lymphoma), tuberculosis (most common cause in developing countries)

Pathophysiology
In the setting of chronic inflammation, the pericardial layers become thickened, scarred, and calcified; the pericardial space is obliterated, and the pericardium becomes noncompliant, which impairs ventricular filling and leads to an equalization of pressures in all four chambers and subsequent HF symptoms.

DIAGNOSIS

Clinical Presentation
History
The clinical presentation of constrictive pericarditis is insidious, with gradual development of fatigue, exercise intolerance, and venous congestion.

Physical Examination
- Features of right-sided HF
  Lower extremity edema, hepatomegaly, ascites, elevated jugular venous pressure (JVP)
- Features more specific for constriction
  ○ Increased JVP with prominent y descent
  ○ Kussmaul sign: lack of expected decrease or obvious increase of JVP on inspiration
  ○ Pericardial knock: early, loud, high-pitched S_3

Differential Diagnosis

- **Pericardial constriction**
  - Ventricular interdependence **present**
  - Abnormal pericardial features (thickened, adherent, and/or calcified)
  - Preserved (or increased) tissue Doppler velocities on echocardiography
  - Pulmonary hypertension (PH) mild or absent
  - Septal bounce seen on noninvasive imaging
  - Equalization of pressures in all cardiac chambers
  - B-type natriuretic peptide (BNP) usually low or mildly elevated
- **RCM**
  - Ventricular interdependence **absent**
  - Abnormal myocardial features (infiltration, thickened, fibrotic, conduction system disease)
  - Decreased tissue Doppler velocities on echocardiography
  - PH present
  - Normal septal motion
  - Left ventricular end-diastolic pressure (LVEDP) – right ventricular end-diastolic pressure (RVEDP) >5 mm Hg, RVEDP/right ventricular systolic pressure <1/3
  - BNP elevated

Diagnostic Testing

- **Echocardiogram**
  - First-line diagnostic test.
  - Helpful for distinguishing constriction from restriction (see earlier).
  - Ventricular systolic function is often normal and can lead to the false assessment that the heart function is "normal" and not a cause of the patient's symptoms.
  - Features suggestive of constriction include:
    - Thickened, echogenic pericardium
    - Tethering of the pericardium to the myocardium
    - Dilated, incompressible inferior vena cava (IVC)
    - Septal bounce
    - Inspiratory variation in mitral flow velocity curves
    - Expiratory reversal of hepatic vein flow
    - Preserved (or increased) tissue Doppler velocities of the mitral annulus
- **Cardiac catheterization**
  Often required to make the diagnosis of constriction and is the method of choice for an accurate hemodynamic assessment. Allows simultaneous measurement of RVEDP and LVEDP. Right atrial pressure will be very high, whereas pulmonary artery pressures will be near normal.
- **Cardiac CT and MRI**
  - Provide excellent anatomy of the pericardium (thickness and calcification).
  - An MRI and gated CT can show evidence of ventricular interdependence (septal bounce).
  - Can provide other anatomic information that may be helpful in making the diagnosis of constriction (i.e., engorgement of IVC and hepatic veins) and its etiology (i.e., lymph nodes, tumors).

TREATMENT

- Limited role for medical therapy: diuretics and low-salt diet to alleviate edema.
- Patients with constriction often have a resting sinus tachycardia. Due to limited stroke volume (SV), they are more dependent on heart rate for adequate cardiac output (CO). Avoid efforts to slow the heart rate.

Surgical Management

Surgical pericardiectomy is the only definitive treatment and should be pursued once the diagnosis is made. Operative mortality is 5–15%; more advanced congestive heart failure (CHF) symptoms confer higher operative risk. A significant majority experience a symptomatic benefit from surgery.

Cardiac Tamponade

GENERAL PRINCIPLES

Cardiac tamponade is a **clinical diagnosis** and is considered a medical emergency.

Etiology

- More likely to cause tamponade: procedural complications, infection, neoplasms, or idiopathic pericarditis
- Others: postcardiotomy, autoimmune connective tissue disorders, uremia, trauma, radiation, myocardial infarction (subacute), drugs (hydralazine, procainamide, isoniazid, phenytoin, minoxidil), hypothyroidism

Pathophysiology

Fluid accumulation in the pericardial space increases the pericardial pressure. The pressure depends on the amount of fluid, the rate of accumulation, and the compliance of the pericardium. Tamponade develops when the pressure in the pericardial space is sufficiently high to interfere with adequate cardiac filling, resulting in a decrease in CO.

DIAGNOSIS

Clinical Presentation

History

- The diagnosis of cardiac tamponade should be suspected in patients with elevated JVP, hypotension, and distant heart sounds (**Beck triad**).
- Symptoms can include dyspnea, fatigue, anxiety, presyncope, chest discomfort, abdominal fullness, lethargy, and a vague sense of being "uncomfortable"; patients often feel more comfortable sitting forward.

Physical Examination

- Pulsus paradoxus >10 mm Hg, jugular venous distention, and diminished heart sounds
- Tachycardia, hypotension, and signs of shock

Diagnostic Testing

- **ECG**
  Low voltage (more likely with larger effusions), tachycardia, electrical alternans (specific but not sensitive)
- **Transthoracic echocardiogram (TTE)**
  - First-line diagnostic test to diagnose an effusion and evaluate its hemodynamic significance.
  - Features suggestive of a hemodynamically significant effusion:
    - Dilated, incompressible IVC.
    - Significant respiratory variation of tricuspid and mitral inflow velocities.
    - Early diastolic collapse of the right ventricle and systolic collapse of the right atrium.
    - Usually the effusion is circumferential.

- **Transesophageal echocardiogram (TEE)**
Helpful when TTE images are poor or when there is a suspicion for a loculated effusion (particularly those that might develop posteriorly, adjacent to the atria, after cardiac surgery).
- **CT and MRI**
Can be helpful in assessing the anatomic location of the effusion (particularly if loculated). May be helpful in determining the etiology of the effusion and the content of the pericardial fluid. Should be avoided in an unstable patient.

TREATMENT

- Limited role for medical therapy. Goal is to maintain adequate filling pressures with IV fluids. Avoid diuretics, nitrates, and any other preload-reducing medications. Avoid efforts to slow sinus tachycardia; it compensates for a reduced SV to try to maintain adequate CO.
- If intubation is to be performed for respiratory distress before the fluid is drained, make sure volume status is replete and a pericardiocentesis needle is immediately available before any sedatives are given (a patient can arrest with the preload reduction from sedation).

Other Nonoperative Therapies

Percutaneous pericardiocentesis with echocardiographic guidance can be a relatively safe and effective way to drain the pericardial fluid; the approach should be guided by location of the fluid and is usually easiest when the effusion is anterior.

Surgical Management

- Open pericardiocentesis with the creation of a window is a minimally invasive procedure and is preferred for recurring effusions, loculated effusions, or those not safely accessible percutaneously.
- Allows pericardial biopsies to be taken, which may be helpful in making a diagnosis.

VALVULAR HEART DISEASE

The 2014 American Heart Association/American College of Cardiology (AHA/ACC) Guidelines describe different stages in the progression of valvular heart disease (VHD).
- Stage A (at risk): patients with risk factors for development of VHD
- Stage B (progressive): patients with progressive VHD (mild to moderate severity and asymptomatic)
- Stage C (asymptomatic severe): asymptomatic patients who meet criteria for severe VHD
  ○ C1: asymptomatic patients with a compensated left and right ventricle
  ○ C2: asymptomatic patients with decompensation of the left or right ventricle
- Stage D (symptomatic severe): patients who have developed symptoms as a result of VHD

Mitral Stenosis

GENERAL PRINCIPLES

- Mitral stenosis (MS) is characterized by incomplete opening of the mitral valve during diastole, which limits antegrade flow and yields a sustained diastolic pressure gradient between the left atrium (LA) and the left ventricle (LV).
- Due to the widespread use of antibiotics, the incidence of rheumatic heart disease (and MS) has decreased in the developed world.

Etiology

- **Rheumatic**
  - Predominant cause of MS; two-thirds of patients are females; may be associated with mitral regurgitation (MR).
  - Rheumatic fever can cause fibrosis, thickening, and calcification, leading to fusion of the commissures, leaflets, chordae, and/or papillary muscles.
- **Other causes:** systemic lupus erythematosus (SLE), rheumatoid arthritis, congenital, substantial mitral annular calcification, oversewn or small mitral annuloplasty ring; "functional MS" may occur with obstruction of the LA outflow due to tumor (particularly myxoma), LA thrombus, or endocarditis with a large vegetation.

Pathophysiology

Physiologic states that either increase the transvalvular flow (enhance CO) or decrease diastolic filling time (via tachycardia) can increase symptoms at any given valve area. Pregnancy, exercise, hyperthyroidism, atrial fibrillation (AF) with rapid ventricular response, and fever are examples in which either or both of these conditions occur. Symptoms are often first noticed at these times. MS causes increased pressure in the LA, which then dilates as a compensatory mechanism to minimize the increase in pressure. A dilated and fibrosed atrium develops, predisposing to atrial arrhythmias and clot formation. A sustained increase in pulmonary venous pressures is transmitted backward to cause PH and, with time, increased pulmonary vascular resistance and right ventricular pressure overload and dysfunction.

DIAGNOSIS

Clinical Presentation

History

After a prolonged asymptomatic period, patients may report any of the following: dyspnea, decreased functional capacity, orthopnea and/or paroxysmal nocturnal dyspnea, fatigue, palpitations (often due to AF), systemic embolism, hemoptysis, chest pain, and/or signs and symptoms of infective endocarditis.

Physical Examination

Findings on physical exam will depend on the severity of valve obstruction and the associated adaptations that developed; they may include:

- Opening snap (OS) caused by sudden tensing of the valve leaflets; the A_2-OS interval varies inversely with the severity of stenosis (shorter interval = more severe stenosis).
- Mid-diastolic rumble: low-pitched murmur heard best at the apex with the bell of the stethoscope; the severity of stenosis is related to the duration of the murmur, not intensity.
- Signs of right-sided HF and PH.

Diagnostic Testing

- **ECG**
  P mitrale (P-wave duration in lead II ≥0.12 seconds indicating LA enlargement [LAE]), AF, right ventricular hypertrophy
- **CXR**
  - LAE, enlarged right atrium/right ventricle and/or enlarged pulmonary arteries
  - Calcification of the mitral valve (MV) and/or annulus
- **TTE**
  - Assess etiology of MS.
  - Assess leaflets and subvalvular apparatus to determine candidacy for percutaneous mitral balloon commissurotomy (PMBC).

- ○ Determine MV area and mean transmitral gradient.
- ○ Estimate pulmonary artery systolic pressure and evaluate right ventricular size and function.
- **TEE**
  - ○ Assess presence or absence of clot and severity of MR in patients being considered for percutaneous mitral balloon valvuloplasty.
  - ○ Evaluate MV morphology and hemodynamics in patients with MS for whom TTE was suboptimal.
- **Cardiac catheterization**
  - ○ Indicated to determine severity of MS when clinical and echocardiography assessment are discordant
  - ○ Reasonable in patients with MS to assess the cause of severe PH when out of proportion to the severity of MS as determined by noninvasive testing; can also assess the reversibility of PH
- **Severe MS**
  - ○ Valve area ≤ 1.5 cm^2 (very severe MS ≤ 1.0 cm^2)
  - ○ Usually accompanied by LAE and often PH

TREATMENT

Medical Management
- Diuretics and low-salt diet for HF symptoms.
- Secondary prevention of rheumatic fever is indicated for rheumatic MS.
- **AF** (occurs in 30–40% of patients with severe MS).
  - ○ Therapy is mostly aimed at rate control (negative dromotropic agents) and prevention of thromboembolism; rhythm control is rarely successful.
  - ○ **AHA/ACC Guidelines—class I indications for anticoagulation** for prevention of systemic embolization in patients with MS:
    - MS and AF (paroxysmal, persistent, or permanent)
    - MS and a prior embolic event, even in sinus rhythm
    - MS with LA thrombus

Other Nonoperative Therapies
PMBC
- **AHA/ACC recommendations for intervention:**
  - ○ Symptomatic patients with severe MS (valve area ≤ 1.5 cm^2) (stage D) and favorable valve anatomy in the absence of an LA clot or moderate to severe MR (class I)
  - ○ Asymptomatic patients with very severe MS (valve area ≤ 1.0 cm^2) (stage C) and favorable valve anatomy in the absence of a LA clot or moderate to severe MR (class IIa)
  - ○ Asymptomatic patients with severe MS (stage C) and favorable valve anatomy in the absence of a LA clot or moderate to severe MR who have new-onset AF (class IIb)
- Balloon inflation separates the commissures and fractures some of the nodular calcium in the leaflets, yielding an increased valve area.
- It compares favorably with surgical mitral commissurotomy (open or closed) and is the procedure of choice in experienced centers in patients without contraindications.

Surgical Management
AHA/ACC recommendations for intervention (repair, commissurotomy, or replacement)
- Severely symptomatic patients (NYHA class III/IV) with severe MS (valve area < 1.5 cm^2; stage D) who are not high risk for surgery and who are not candidates for or failed previous PMBC (class I).
- Concomitant MV surgery is indicated for patients with severe MS (valve area < 1.5 cm^2; stage C or D) undergoing other cardiac surgery.

Aortic Stenosis

GENERAL PRINCIPLES

- **Aortic stenosis** (AS) is the most common cause of LV outflow tract obstruction.
- Other causes of obstruction occur above the valve (supravalvular) and below the valve (subvalvular), both fixed (i.e., subaortic membrane) and dynamic (i.e., hypertrophic cardiomyopathy with obstruction).
- **Aortic sclerosis** is thickening of the aortic valve leaflets that causes turbulent flow through the valve and a murmur but no significant gradient; over time, it can develop into AS.

Epidemiology
- **Calcific/degenerative**
  - Most common cause in United States.
  - Trileaflet calcific AS usually presents in the seventh to ninth decades (mean age, mid-70s).
  - Risk factors similar to coronary artery disease (CAD).
- **Bicuspid**
  - Occurs in 1–2% of population (congenital lesion).
  - Usually presents in the sixth to eighth decades (mean age, mid–late 60s).
  - Approximately 50% of patients needing aortic valve replacement (AVR) for AS have a bicuspid valve.
  - More prone to endocarditis than trileaflet valves.
  - Associated with aortopathies (i.e., dissection, aneurysm) in a significant proportion of patients.
- **Rheumatic**
  - More common cause worldwide; much less common in the United States.
  - Usually presents in the third to fifth decades.
  - Almost always accompanied by MV disease.

Pathophysiology
The pathophysiology for calcific AS involves both the valve and the ventricular adaptation to the stenosis. Within the valve (trileaflet and bicuspid), there is growing evidence for an active biologic process that begins much like the formation of an atherosclerotic plaque and eventually leads to calcified bone formation (Figure 6-1).

DIAGNOSIS

Clinical Presentation
History
- The classic triad of symptoms includes **angina, syncope, and HF**.
- Frequently, patients will gradually limit themselves in ways that mask the presence of symptoms but indicate a progressive and premature decline in functional capacity. In the setting of severe AS, these patients should be viewed as symptomatic.

Physical Examination
- Harsh systolic crescendo–decrescendo murmur heard best at the right upper sternal border and radiating to both carotids; time to peak intensity correlates with severity (later peak = more severe).
- Diminished or absent A_2 (soft S_2) suggests severe AS.
- An ejection click suggests bicuspid AS.
- Pulsus parvus et tardus: late-peaking and diminished carotid upstroke in severe AS.
- Gallavardin phenomenon is an AS murmur heard best at the apex (could be confused with MR).

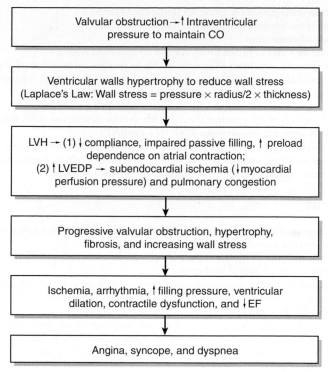

Figure 6-1. Pathophysiology of aortic stenosis. CO, cardiac output; EF, ejection fraction; LVEDP, left ventricular end-diastolic pressure; LVH, left ventricular hypertrophy.

Diagnostic Testing

- **ECG:** LAE and LV hypertrophy (LVH)
- **CXR:** LVH, cardiomegaly, and calcification of the aorta, aortic valve, and/or coronaries
- **TTE**
  - Leaflet number, morphology, and calcification
  - Calculate valve area using continuity equation and measure transvalvular mean and peak gradients
  - **Severe AS**
  Peak jet velocity >4.0 m/s, mean gradient >40 mm Hg, valve area <1.0 cm^2
- **Further evaluation in selected patients**
  - **TEE**
    - Clarify whether there is a bicuspid valve if unclear on TTE.
    - Occasionally needed to evaluate for other or additional causes of LV outflow tract obstruction.
  - **Exercise testing:** Performed in the patient presumed to be asymptomatic or in whom symptoms are unclear; evaluate for exercise capacity, abnormal blood pressure response (<20 mm Hg increase with exercise), or exercise-induced symptoms.
  - **Dobutamine stress echocardiography**
    - Useful to assess the patient with a reduced SV (which may occur with a reduced or preserved ejection fraction [EF]) with a small calculated valve area (suggesting severe AS) but a low (<30–40 mm Hg) mean transvalvular gradient (suggesting less severe AS)

- Can help distinguish truly severe AS from pseudo-severe AS
- Assess for the presence of contractile reserve
○ **Cardiac catheterization**
  - Evaluate for CAD in patients with AS and symptoms of angina.
  - Hemodynamic assessment of severity of AS in patients for whom noninvasive tests are inconclusive or when there is discrepancy between noninvasive tests and clinical findings regarding AS severity (utilizes the Gorlin formula).
○ **CT**
  When the severity of AS is unclear, the extent of valve calcification can clarify the diagnosis.
○ **BNP or N-terminal prohormone BNP (NT-proBNP)**
  May be useful in predicting symptom-free survival in a patient with severe asymptomatic AS or clarifying whether symptoms of shortness of breath are more related to the lungs or the valve in a patient with concomitant severe lung disease.

TREATMENT

- **Severe symptomatic AS is a surgical disease;** currently, there are no medical treatments proven to decrease mortality or to delay surgery.
- **Hypertension** should be treated in patients with AS because inadequately treated hypertension imposes an additional load on the LV.
- **Diuretics** may alleviate shortness of breath in patients with symptomatic AS and evidence of volume overload prior to definitive therapy with valve replacement.
- **Severe AS with decompensated HF**
  ○ Patients with severe AS and LV dysfunction may experience decompensated HF; depending on the clinical scenario, several options may help bridge the patient to definitive surgical management (e.g., AVR): Intra-aortic balloon pump (IABP) (contraindicated in patients with moderate to severe AR), sodium nitroprusside, balloon aortic valvuloplasty
  ○ Each of the above measures provides some degree of afterload reduction, either at the level of the valve (valvuloplasty) or systemic vascular resistance (IABP, sodium nitroprusside [Nipride]), which can facilitate forward flow.

Other Nonoperative Therapies
Percutaneous
- Balloon aortic valvuloplasty has a limited role in the treatment of patients with severe AS; the improvement in valve area is modest, and the clinical improvement that it provides usually lasts weeks to months.
- **Transcatheter aortic valve replacement (TAVR)**
  ○ Requires a team of cardiologists and cardiac surgeons using fluoroscopic and echocardiographic guidance to place a stented bioprosthetic valve within the stenotic valve. This can be performed via a transfemoral, transaortic, or transapical approach.
  ○ To date, clinical trials have demonstrated that in patients at prohibitive risk for surgery, TAVR reduces mortality compared to medical therapy; for high-risk patients, TAVR and surgical valve replacement have similar outcomes.
  ○ These less-invasive, catheter-based techniques for valve replacement are rapidly evolving and are being investigated in ongoing clinical trials and clinical registries.

Surgical Management
- Symptomatic severe AS is a deadly disease; AVR is the only currently effective treatment.
- **AHA/ACC recommendations for intervention**
  ○ Symptomatic with severe high-gradient AS (stage D1; class I)
  ○ Asymptomatic with severe AS and LVEF <50% (stage C2; class I)

- Patients with severe AS (stage C or D) undergoing other cardiac surgery (class I)
- Asymptomatic patients with very severe AS (stage C1) and low surgical risk (class IIa)
- Asymptomatic patients with severe AS (stage C1) and decreased exercise tolerance or fall in blood pressure on exercise testing (class IIa)

OUTCOME/PROGNOSIS

AS is a progressive disease typically characterized by an asymptomatic phase until the valve area reaches a minimum threshold, generally <1 cm². In the absence of symptoms, patients with AS have a good prognosis with a risk of sudden death estimated to be approximately 1% per year. Once patients experience symptoms, their average survival is 2–3 years with a high risk of sudden death.

Mitral Regurgitation

GENERAL PRINCIPLES

- Prevention of MR is dependent on the integrated and proper function of the MV (annulus and leaflets), subvalvular apparatus (chordae tendineae and papillary muscles), and LA and LV; abnormal function or size of any one of these components can lead to MR.
- **Primary MR**, or organic MR, refers to MR caused primarily by lesions to the valve leaflets and/or chordae tendineae (i.e., myxomatous degeneration, endocarditis, rheumatic).
- **Secondary MR**, or functional MR, refers to MR caused primarily by ventricular dysfunction usually with accompanying annular dilatation (i.e., dilated cardiomyopathy and ischemic MR).
- It is critical to define the mechanism of MR and the time course (acute vs. chronic) because these significantly impact clinical management.

Etiology
- **Primary MR**
  - **Degenerative** (overlap with MV prolapse syndrome)
    - Usually occurs as a primary condition (Barlow disease or fibroelastic deficiency) but has also been associated with heritable diseases affecting the connective tissue including Marfan syndrome, Ehlers-Danlos syndrome, osteogenesis imperfecta, etc.
    - May be familial or nonfamilial. Occurs in 1.0–2.5% of the population (based on stricter echocardiography criteria) in a female-to-male ratio of 2:1.
    - Most common reason for MV surgery.
    - Myxomatous proliferation and cartilage formation can occur in the leaflets, chordae tendineae, and/or annulus.
  - **Rheumatic**
    - May be pure MR or combined MR/MS.
    - Caused by thickening and/or calcification of the leaflets and chords.
  - **Infective endocarditis:** Usually caused by destruction of the leaflet tissue (i.e., perforation).
- **Secondary MR**
  - **Dilated cardiomyopathy**
    Mechanism of MR is due to both of the following:
    - Annular dilatation from ventricular enlargement.
    - Papillary muscle displacement due to ventricular enlargement and remodeling prevents adequate leaflet coaptation.
  - **Ischemic**
    - **Ischemic MR is mostly a misnomer**, because this is primarily postinfarction MR, not MR caused by active ischemia.

- Mechanism of MR usually involves one or both of the following:
  - Annular dilatation from ventricular enlargement.
  - Local LV remodeling with papillary muscle displacement (both the dilatation of the ventricle and the akinesis/dyskinesis of the wall to which the papillary muscle is attached can prevent adequate leaflet coaptation).
- Rarely, MR may develop acutely from papillary muscle rupture (more commonly of the posteromedial papillary muscle).
- **Other causes**
  Congenital, infiltrative diseases (i.e., amyloid), SLE (Libman-Sacks lesion), hypertrophic cardiomyopathy with obstruction, mitral annular calcification, paravalvular prosthetic leak, drug toxicity (e.g., Fen-phen)
- **Acute causes**
  Ruptured papillary muscle, ruptured chordae tendineae, infective endocarditis

Pathophysiology
- Acute MR (Figure 6-2)
- Chronic MR (Figure 6-3)

DIAGNOSIS

Clinical Presentation
History
- Acute MR
  Most prominent symptom is relatively rapid onset of significant shortness of breath, which may lead quickly to respiratory failure.

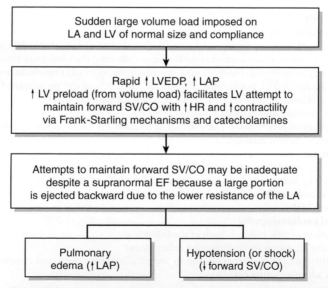

Figure 6-2. Acute mitral regurgitation. CO, cardiac output; EF, ejection fraction; HR, heart rate; LA, left atrium; LAP, left atrial pressure; LV, left ventricle; LVEDP, left ventricular end-diastolic pressure; SV, stroke volume.

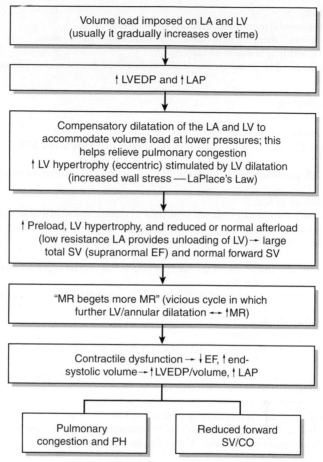

Figure 6-3. Chronic mitral regurgitation. CO, cardiac output; EF, ejection fraction; LA, left atrium; LAP, left atrial pressure; LV, left ventricle; LVEDP, left ventricular end-diastolic pressure; MR, mitral regurgitation; PH, pulmonary hypertension; SV, stroke volume.

- Chronic MR
  - The etiology of MR and the time at which the patient presents will influence the symptoms reported.
  - In primary MR (usually degenerative MR) that has gradually progressed, the patient may be asymptomatic even when the MR is severe. As compensatory mechanisms fail, patients may note dyspnea on exertion (may be due to PH and/or pulmonary edema), palpitations (from an atrial arrhythmia), fatigue, and volume overload.

Physical Examination
- Acute MR
  - Tachypnea with respiratory distress, tachycardia, relative hypotension (even shock)
  - Systolic murmur, usually at the apex (may not be holosystolic and may be absent)

- Chronic MR
  - Apical holosystolic murmur that radiates to the axilla.
  - In MV prolapse, there is a midsystolic click heard before the murmur.
  - S_2 may be widely split due to an early A_2.
  - Other signs of CHF (lower extremity edema, increased central venous pressure, crackles, etc.).

Diagnostic Testing

- **ECG**
  - LAE, LVH/LV enlargement, AF
  - Pathologic Q waves from previous myocardial infarction in ischemic MR
- **CXR**
  Enlarged LA, pulmonary edema, enlarged pulmonary arteries, and cardiomegaly
- **TTE**
  - Assess etiology of MR
  - LA size and LV dimensions (should be dilated in chronic severe MR of any etiology)
  - EF (LV dysfunction is present if EF ≤60%)
  - Qualitative and quantitative measures of MR severity
- **TEE**
  - Provides better visualization of the valve to help define anatomy, presence of endocarditis, and feasibility of repair
  - May help determine severity of MR when TTE is nondiagnostic, particularly in the setting of an eccentric jet
- **Cardiac catheterization**
  - Right heart catheterization
    - PH in patients with chronic severe MR, LA filling pressure in patients with unclear symptoms.
    - Giant "V" waves on pulmonary capillary wedge pressure tracing may suggest severe MR.
  - Left heart catheterization
    - May influence therapeutic strategy in ischemic MR
    - Evaluation of CAD in patients with risk factors undergoing MV surgery
  - Left ventriculogram can evaluate LV function and severity of MR.
- **MRI**
  - Assess EF in patients with severe MR but with an inadequate assessment of EF by echocardiography.
  - Assess quantitative measures of MR severity when echocardiography is nondiagnostic.
  - Viability assessment may play a role in considering therapeutic strategy in ischemic MR.
- **Nuclear**
  - Assess EF in patients with severe MR but with an inadequate assessment of EF by echocardiography.
  - Viability assessment may play a role in considering therapeutic strategy in ischemic MR.

TREATMENT

Acute MR

- While awaiting surgery, aggressive afterload reduction with IV nitroprusside or an IABP can diminish the amount of MR and stabilize the patient by promoting forward flow and reducing pulmonary edema.
- These patients are usually tachycardic, but attempts to slow their heart rate should be avoided because they are often heart rate dependent for an adequate forward CO.

Chronic MR

The role for medical therapy may differ depending on the etiology of the MR.

- **Primary MR**
  - In the asymptomatic patient with normal LV function and chronic severe MR due to leaflet prolapse, there is generally no accepted medical therapy.
  - In the absence of systemic hypertension, there is no established indication for vasodilating drugs.
  - Whether angiotensin-converting enzyme (ACE) inhibitors or β-blockers delay ventricular remodeling and the need for surgery is being investigated in prospective studies.
- **Secondary MR**
  - Treat as other patients with LV dysfunction.
  - ACE inhibitors and β-blockers are indicated and have been shown to reduce mortality and the severity of MR.
  - Some patients may also qualify for cardiac resynchronization therapy, which can favorably remodel the LV and reduce the severity of MR.

Other Nonoperative Therapies

Percutaneous

Currently, the most developed device may be the placement of a mitral clip, which pinches the leaflets together in an attempt to enhance coaptation (a percutaneous treatment analogous to the surgical Alfieri stitch), creating a figure-eight orifice.

This procedure is performed via femoral venous access, and a transseptal puncture is used to position the delivery system in the LA. Using fluoroscopy and TEE guidance, the clip is advanced and attempts are made to grasp the leaflet tips of the anterior and posterior MV leaflets and clip them together.

Surgical Management

AHA/ACC recommendations for intervention

- **Primary MR**
  - Symptomatic with chronic severe primary MR (stage D) and LVEF >30% (class I).
  - Asymptomatic with chronic severe primary MR with EF 30–60% or LV end-systolic dimension ≥40 mm) (stage C2; class I).
  - Chronic severe primary MR undergoing cardiac surgery for other indications (class I).
  - Repair is recommended over replacement (class I).
  - Asymptomatic patients with chronic severe primary MR (stage C1) in whom repair is highly likely (>95%) and operative mortality is low (<1%) or in the setting of new-onset AF or PH (class IIa).
- **Secondary MR** (benefits of surgery not well established)
  - Chronic severe secondary MR undergoing cardiac surgery for other indications (class IIa).
  - Severely symptomatic patients (NYHA III/IV) with chronic severe secondary MR (stage D; class IIb)
- Patients with AF should be considered for a concomitant surgical Maze procedure.

Aortic Regurgitation

GENERAL PRINCIPLES

- Aortic regurgitation (AR) may result from pathology of the aortic valve, the aortic root, or both; it is important that both the valve and the root are evaluated to determine the appropriate management and treatment.
- AR usually progresses insidiously with a long asymptomatic period; when it occurs acutely, patients are often very sick and must be managed aggressively.

Etiology

- **More common**
  Bicuspid aortic valve, rheumatic disease, calcific degeneration, infective endocarditis, idiopathic dilatation of the aorta, myxomatous degeneration, systemic hypertension, dissection of the ascending aorta, Marfan syndrome
- **Less common**
  Traumatic injury to the aortic valve, collagen vascular diseases (ankylosing spondylitis, rheumatoid arthritis, reactive arthritis, giant cell aortitis, and Whipple disease), syphilitic aortitis, discrete subaortic stenosis, ventricular septal defect with prolapse of an aortic cusp
- **Acute**
  Infective endocarditis, dissection of the ascending aorta, trauma

Pathophysiology

- Acute AR (Figure 6-4)
- Chronic AR (Figure 6-5)

DIAGNOSIS

Clinical Presentation

History

- **Acute:** Patients with acute AR may present with **symptoms of cardiogenic shock and severe dyspnea.** Other presenting symptoms may be related to the cause of acute AR.

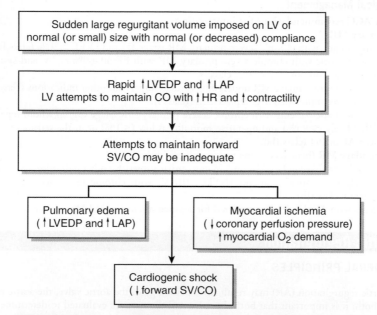

Figure 6-4. Acute aortic regurgitation. CO, cardiac output; HR, heart rate; LAP, left atrial pressure; LV, left ventricle; LVEDP, left ventricular end-diastolic pressure; SV, stroke volume.

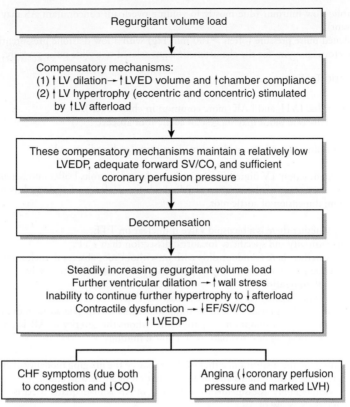

Figure 6-5. Chronic aortic regurgitation. CO, cardiac output; CHF, congestive heart failure; EF, ejection fraction; LV, left ventricle; LVED, left ventricular end-diastolic; LVEDP, left ventricular end-diastolic pressure; LVH, left ventricular hypertrophy; SV, stroke volume.

- **Chronic:** Symptoms depend on the presence of LV dysfunction and whether the patient is in the **compensated versus decompensated stage**. Compensated patients are typically asymptomatic, whereas those in the decompensated stage may note decreased exercise tolerance, dyspnea, fatigue, and/or angina.

Physical Examination
- Acute
  - **Tachycardia:** Wide pulse pressure may be present, but is often not present because forward SV (and therefore systolic blood pressure) is reduced; brief soft diastolic murmur heard best at third left intercostal space (often not heard); systolic flow murmur (due to volume overload and hyperdynamic LV).
  - Look for evidence of aortic dissection, infective endocarditis, and Marfanoid characteristics.
- Chronic
  - LV heave; point of maximal impulse is laterally displaced.
  - Diastolic decrescendo murmur heard best at left sternal border leaning forward at end-expiration (severity of AR correlates with duration, not intensity, of the murmur).

- Systolic flow murmur (due mostly to volume overload; concomitant AS may also be present).
- Widened pulse pressure (often >100 mm Hg) with a low diastolic pressure; there are numerous eponyms for the characteristic signs related to a wide pulse pressure.

Diagnostic Testing

- **ECG**
  - Tachycardia, LVH, and LAE (more common in chronic AR).
  - New conduction block may suggest an aortic root abscess.
- **CXR**
  Look for pulmonary edema, widened mediastinum, and cardiomegaly.
- **TTE**
  LV systolic function, LV dimensions at end systole and diastole, leaflet number and morphology, assessment of the severity of AR; look for evidence of endocarditis or aortic dissection; dimension of aortic root.
- **TEE**
  - Clarify whether there is a bicuspid valve if unclear on TTE.
  - Better sensitivity and specificity for aortic dissection than TTE.
  - Clarify whether there is endocarditis with or without root abscess if unclear on TTE.
  - Better visualization of aortic valve in patients with a prosthetic aortic valve.
- **Cardiac catheterization**
  - In patients undergoing AVR who are at risk for CAD.
  - Assessment of LV pressure, LV function, and severity of AR (via aortic root angiography) is indicated in symptomatic patients in whom the severity of AR is unclear on noninvasive imaging or discordant with clinical findings.
- **MRI/CT**
  - Depending on the institution, either of these may be the imaging modality of choice for evaluating aortic dimensions and/or for evaluation of aortic dissection.
  - If echocardiography assessment of the severity of AR is inadequate, MRI is useful for assessing the severity of AR.

TREATMENT

- **The role of medical therapy in patients with AR is limited**; there are currently no randomized, placebo-controlled data showing that vasodilator therapy delays the development of symptoms or LV dysfunction warranting surgery.
- **Vasodilator therapy (i.e., nifedipine, ACE inhibitor, hydralazine)** is indicated to reduce systolic blood pressure in hypertensive patients with AR.
- Retrospective data suggest that β-blocker use may be associated with a survival benefit in patients with severe AR, but prospective studies are needed.
- When endocarditis is suspected or confirmed, appropriate antibiotic coverage is critical.

Surgical Management

- **AHA/ACC recommendations for intervention**
  - Symptomatic patients with severe AR (stage D) regardless of LV systolic function (class I)
  - Asymptomatic patients with chronic severe AR and LV systolic dysfunction (EF ≤50%) (stage C2; class I)
  - Patients with severe AR (stage C or D) undergoing cardiac surgery for other indications (class I)
  - Asymptomatic patients with severe AR and normal LV systolic function (EF >50%) but with severe LV dilation (LV end-systolic dimension >50 mm) (stage C2; class IIa)

- Acute, severe AR is almost universally symptomatic and is treated surgically.
- If the aortic root is dilated, it may be repaired or replaced at the time of AVR. For patients with a bicuspid valve, Marfan syndrome, or a related genetically triggered aortopathy, surgery on the aorta should be considered at the time of AVR.

OUTCOME/PROGNOSIS

- Asymptomatic patients with normal LV systolic function
  - ○ Progression to symptoms and/or LV dysfunction <6% per year
  - ○ Progression to asymptomatic LV dysfunction <3.5% per year
  - ○ Sudden death <0.2% per year
- Asymptomatic patients with LV dysfunction
  Progression to cardiac symptoms >25% per year
- Symptomatic patients
  Mortality rate >10% per year

Prosthetic Heart Valves

GENERAL PRINCIPLES

The choice of valve prosthesis depends on many factors including the patient, surgeon, cardiologist, and clinical scenario. With improvements in bioprosthetic valves, the recommendation for a mechanical valve in patients <65 years of age is no longer as firm, and bioprosthetic valve use has increased in younger patients.

- **Mechanical**
  - ○ Ball-and-cage (Starr-Edwards): rarely, if ever, used today
  - ○ Bileaflet (i.e., St. Jude, Carbomedics): most commonly used
  - ○ Single tilting disk (i.e., Björk-Shiley, Medtronic Hall, Omnicarbon)
  - ○ **Advantages:** structurally stable, long lasting, relatively hemodynamically efficient (particularly bileaflet)
  - ○ **Disadvantages:** need for anticoagulation, risk of bleeding, risk of thrombosis/embolism despite anticoagulation, severe hemodynamic compromise if disk thrombosis or immobility occurs (single tilting disk), risk of endocarditis
- **Bioprosthetic**
  - ○ Porcine aortic valve tissue (i.e., Hancock, Carpentier-Edwards)
  - ○ Bovine pericardial tissue (i.e., Carpentier-Edwards Perimount)
  - ○ **Advantages:** no need for anticoagulation, low thromboembolism risk, low risk of catastrophic valve failure
  - ○ **Disadvantages:** structural valve deterioration, imperfect hemodynamic efficiency, risk of endocarditis, still a small risk (0.7% per year) of thromboembolism without anticoagulation
- **Homograft (cadaveric)**
  Rarely used for atrioventricular surgery; most commonly used to replace the pulmonic valve

TREATMENT

- **AHA/ACC recommendations for anticoagulation for prosthetic valves**
  - ○ Anticoagulation with a vitamin K antagonist and international normalized ratio (INR) monitoring is recommended in patients with a mechanical prosthetic valve (class I).
  - ○ Anticoagulation with a vitamin K antagonist to achieve an INR of 2.5 is recommended in patients with a mechanical/AVR (bileaflet or current-generation single tilting disk) and no risk factors for thromboembolism (class I).

- Anticoagulation with a vitamin K antagonist is indicated to achieve an INR of 3.0 in patients with a mechanical AVR and additional risk factors for thromboembolic events (AF, previous thromboembolism, LV dysfunction, or hypercoagulable conditions) or an older generation mechanical AVR (such as ball-in-cage) (class I).
  - Anticoagulation with a vitamin K antagonist is indicated to achieve an INR of 3.0 in patients with a mechanical MV replacement (class I).
  - Aspirin 75–100 mg daily is recommended in addition to anticoagulation with a vitamin K antagonist in patients with a mechanical valve prosthesis (class I).
  - Aspirin 75–100 mg daily is reasonable in all patients with a bioprosthetic aortic valve or MV (class IIa).
  - Anticoagulant therapy with oral direct thrombin inhibitors or anti-Xa agents should **not** be used in patients with mechanical valve prostheses (class III).
- **AHA/ACC recommendations for bridging therapy for prosthetic valves**
  - Continuation of vitamin K antagonist anticoagulation with a therapeutic INR is recommended in patients with mechanical heart valves undergoing minor procedures (i.e., dental extractions) where bleeding is easily controlled (class I).
  - Temporary interruption of vitamin K antagonist anticoagulation, without bridging agents while the INR is subtherapeutic, is recommended in patients with bileaflet mechanical AVR and no other risk factors for thrombosis who are undergoing invasive or surgical procedures (class I).
  - Bridging anticoagulation with either IV unfractionated heparin or SC low–molecular-weight heparin is recommended during the time interval when the INR is subtherapeutic preoperatively in patients who are undergoing invasive or surgical procedures with mechanical AVR and any thromboembolic risk factor, older generation mechanical AVR, or mechanical MV replacement (class I).

7 Cardiac Arrhythmias

Daniel H. Cooper and Mitchell N. Faddis

TACHYARRHYTHMIAS

Approach to Tachyarrhythmias

GENERAL PRINCIPLES

- Tachyarrhythmias are commonly encountered in the inpatient setting.
- Recognition and analysis of these rhythms in stepwise manner will facilitate initiation of appropriate therapy.
- Clinical decision making is guided by patient symptoms and signs of hemodynamic stability.

Definition

Cardiac rhythms whose ventricular rate exceeds **100 beats per minute** (bpm).

Classification

Tachyarrhythmias are broadly classified based on the width of the QRS complex on the ECG.
- Narrow-complex tachyarrhythmia (QRS <120 msec): Arrhythmia (supraventricular tachycardia) originates within the atria and rapidly activates the ventricles via the His-Purkinje system.
- Wide-complex tachyarrhythmia (QRS ≥120 msec): Arrhythmia originates outside the normal conduction system (ventricular tachycardia [VT]) or travels via an abnormal His-Purkinje system (supraventricular tachycardia with aberrancy) activating the ventricles in an abnormally slow manner.

Etiology

Mechanism divided into disorders of **impulse conduction** and **impulse formation**:
- **Disorders of impulse conduction:** Reentry is the most common mechanism of tachyarrhythmias. A reentrant mechanism can occur when differential refractory periods and conduction velocities allow for propagation of an activation wavefront in a unidirectional manner around a zone of scar or refractory cardiac tissue. Reentry of the activation wavefront around a myocardial circuit sustains the arrhythmia (e.g., VT).
- **Disorders of impulse formation: Enhanced automaticity** (e.g., accelerated junctional and accelerated idioventricular rhythm) **and triggered activity** (e.g., long QT syndrome and digitalis toxicity) are other less common mechanisms of tachyarrhythmias.

DIAGNOSIS

Clinical Presentation

- Tachyarrhythmias often produce symptoms that lead to patient presentation at an outpatient or acute care setting.
- They can be associated with systemic illnesses in patients who are being evaluated in the emergency department or are being treated in an inpatient setting.

185

History
- Symptoms generally guide clinical decision making.
- **Dyspnea, angina, lightheadedness or syncope, and decreased level of consciousness** are severe symptoms that mandate urgent treatment.
- Baseline symptoms that reflect **poor left ventricular (LV) function**, such as dyspnea on exertion (DOE), orthopnea, paroxysmal nocturnal dyspnea (PND), and lower extremity swelling, are critical to elucidate.
- **Palpitations:** Common symptom of tachyarrhythmias. The pattern of onset and termination is useful to suggest the presence of a primary arrhythmia.
  Sudden onset and termination is highly suggestive of a tachyarrhythmia.
- Termination of palpitations with breath holding or the Valsalva maneuver is suggestive of a supraventricular tachyarrhythmia.
- History of **organic heart disease** (i.e., ischemic, nonischemic, valvular cardiomyopathy) or **endocrinopathy** (i.e., thyroid disease, pheochromocytoma) should be sought.
- History of **familial or congenital causes of arrhythmias** such as hypertrophic cardiomyopathy (HCM), long QT syndrome, or other congenital heart disease should be addressed as well.
  ○ **Hypertrophic obstructive cardiomyopathy** (HOCM) is associated with atrial arrhythmias (atrial fibrillation [AF] in 20–25%), as well as malignant ventricular arrhythmias.
  ○ **Mitral valve prolapse** (MVP) is associated with supraventricular and ventricular arrhythmias.
- **Medications history should be carefully taken**, including over-the-counter and herbal medications, to assess a possible causal link.

Physical Examination
- Signs of clinical stability or instability, including vital signs, mental status, peripheral perfusion, etc., are critical in guiding initial decision making.
- If clinically stable, then physical exam should be focused on determining underlying cardiovascular abnormalities that may make certain rhythms more or less likely.
- Findings of **congestive heart failure (CHF)**, including elevated jugular venous pressure (JVP), pulmonary rales, peripheral edema, and S_3 gallop, make the diagnosis of malignant ventricular arrhythmias more likely.
- If arrhythmia is sustained, here are some special considerations during physical exam:
  ○ **Palpate the pulse** and assess for rate and regularity.
    ▪ If rate is about 150 bpm, suspect atrial flutter (AFl) with 2:1 block.
    ▪ If pulse is irregular with no pattern, suspect AF.
    ▪ Irregular pulse with a discernible pattern (group beating) suggests the presence of second-degree heart block.
  ○ **"Cannon" A waves:** Revealed on inspection of JVP reflect atrial contraction against a closed tricuspid valve. If irregular, then suggestive of underlying atrioventricular (AV) dissociation and possible presence of VT.
  ○ If regular in 1:1 ratio with peripheral pulse, then suggestive of AV nodal reentrant tachycardia (AVNRT), AV reentrant tachycardia (AVRT), or a junctional tachycardia, all leading to retrograde atrial activation occurring simultaneously with ventricular contraction.

Diagnostic Testing
Laboratories
Serum electrolytes, complete blood count (CBC), thyroid function tests, serum concentration of digoxin (when applicable), and a urine toxicology screen should be considered for all patients.

Electrocardiography
- **A 12-lead ECG, in the presence of the rhythm abnormality and in normal sinus rhythm,** is the most useful initial diagnostic test.
- If the patient is clinically stable, obtain a 12-lead ECG and a **continuous rhythm strip** with leads that best demonstrate atrial activation (e.g., V_1, II, III, aVF).
- Examine the ECG for evidence of conduction abnormalities, such as preexcitation or bundle branch block, or signs of structural heart disease such as prior myocardial infarction (MI).
- Comparison of the ECG obtained during arrhythmia with that at baseline can highlight subtle features of the QRS deflection that indicate the superposition of atrial and ventricular depolarization.
- Rhythm strip is very useful to document the response to interventions (e.g., vagal maneuvers, antiarrhythmic drug therapy, or electrical cardioversion).

Imaging
Chest radiographs and **transthoracic echocardiograms** can help provide evidence of structural heart disease that may make ventricular arrhythmias more likely.

Diagnostic Procedures
- **Continuous ambulatory ECG monitoring**
  - One or more days; useful for documenting symptomatic transient arrhythmias that occur with sufficient frequency.
  - Recording mode useful for assessment of patient's heart rate response to daily activities or antiarrhythmic drug treatment.
  - Correlation between patient-reported symptoms in a time-marked diary and heart rhythm recordings is the key to determining if symptoms are attributable to an arrhythmia.
- **In-hospital telemetry monitoring**
  Mainstay of surveillance monitoring during the course of hospitalization for cardiac arrhythmia patients who are seriously ill or are having life-threatening arrhythmias.
- **Event recorders**
  - Weeks to months; useful for documenting symptomatic transient arrhythmias that occur infrequently.
  - A "loop recorder" is worn by the patient and continuously records the ECG. When activated by the patient or via an autodetection feature, the ECG recording is saved with several minutes of preceding rhythm data.
  - An **implantable loop recorder or insertable loop recorder (ILR)** is a subcutaneous monitoring device used to provide an automated or patient-activated recording of significant arrhythmic events that occur very infrequently over many months or used for patients who are unable to activate external recorders.
- **Exercise ECG**
  Useful for studying exercise-induced arrhythmias or to assess the sinus node response to exercise.
- **Electrophysiology study (EPS)**
  - Invasive, catheter-based procedure that is used to study a patient's susceptibility to arrhythmias or to investigate the mechanism of a known arrhythmia.
  - EPS is also combined with catheter ablation for curative treatment of many arrhythmia mechanisms.
  - The efficacy of EPS to induce and study arrhythmias is highest for reentrant mechanisms.

TREATMENT

Please refer to the treatment of individual tachyarrhythmias for hemodynamically stable patients and advanced cardiac life support (ACLS) algorithm for tachycardias in Appendix C.

Supraventricular Tachyarrhythmias

GENERAL PRINCIPLES

- **Supraventricular tachyarrhythmias (SVTs)** are often recurrent, rarely persistent, and a frequent cause of visits to emergency departments and primary care physician offices.
- The evaluation of patients with SVT should always begin with prompt assessment of hemodynamic stability and clinical "substrate."
- The diagnostic and therapeutic discussion that follows is aimed at the hemodynamically stable patient. If a patient is deemed clinically unstable based on clinical signs and symptoms, one should immediately proceed to cardioversion per ACLS guidelines.

Definition

- Tachyarrhythmias that require atrial or AV nodal tissue, or both, for their initiation and maintenance are termed SVT.
- The QRS complex in most SVTs is narrow (QRS <120 msec). However, they can certainly present as a wide-complex tachycardia (QRS ≥120 msec) in SVT with aberrancy or an accessory pathway–mediated tachycardia.

Classification

- SVT is initially classified by ECG appearance in an effort to understand the likely underlying arrhythmia mechanism.
- A diagnostic approach, based on the ECG, is summarized in Figure 7-1.

Epidemiology

Published incidence data vary widely between studies, and the prevalence of asymptomatic episodes is not known.

DIAGNOSIS

A general understanding of the prevalence of various arrhythmia mechanisms is useful to guide evaluation of an individual patient.

- **AF** is the most common narrow-complex tachycardia seen in the inpatient setting. **AFl** can often accompany AF and is diagnosed one-tenth as often as AF but is twice as prevalent as the paroxysmal SVTs. The other atrial tachyarrhythmias are far less common.
- In one case series, **AVNRT** was reported as the most common diagnosis of the paroxysmal SVTs (60%), followed by AVRT (30%) (*Crit Care Med 2000;28(10 suppl):N129*).
- However, if the patient is younger than age 40, then AVRT, often in the context of Wolff-Parkinson-White (WPW) syndrome, is the most common arrhythmia mechanism.

Clinical Presentation

The clinical presentation for SVT is similar to tachyarrhythmias in general and has been previously outlined in this section.

Differential Diagnosis

- **AF**
  The most common sustained tachyarrhythmia and discussed as a separate topic in this section.
- **AFl**
  ○ AFl is the second most common atrial arrhythmia, with an estimated 200,000 new cases in the United States annually, and is associated with increasing age, underlying heart disease, and male gender (*J Am Coll Cardiol 2000;36:2242*).
  ○ AFl usually presents as a **regular rhythm** but can be **irregularly irregular** when associated with variable AV block (2:1 to 4:1 to 3:1, etc.).

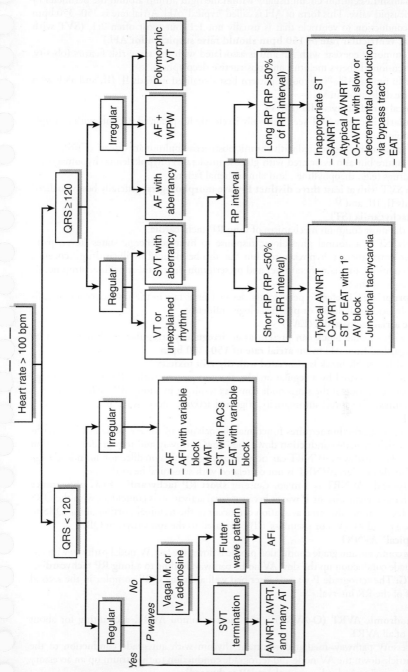

Figure 7-1. Diagnostic approach to tachyarrhythmias. AF, atrial fibrillation; AFl, atrial flutter; AV, atrioventricular; AVNRT, atrioventricular nodal reentrant tachycardia; AVRT, atrioventricular reentrant tachycardia; EAT, ectopic atrial tachycardia; MAT, multifocal atrial tachycardia; O-AVRT, orthodromic AVRT; PAC, premature atrial complex; SANRT, sinoatrial nodal reentrant tachycardia; ST, sinus tachycardia; SVT, supraventricular tachyarrhythmia; VT, ventricular tachycardia; WPW, Wolff-Parkinson-White; AT, atrial tachycardia.

- **Mechanism:** Reentrant circuit usually within the right atrium around the perimeter of the tricuspid valve. This form of AFl is called "typical" AFl. Atrial rate is 250–350 bpm with conduction to ventricle that is usually not 1:1, but most often 2:1. **(SVT with regular ventricular rate of 150 bpm should raise suspicion for AFl.)**
  - AFl commonly coexists with AF and is associated with the same risk factors (obesity, hypertension, diabetes mellitus, and obstructive sleep apnea).
  - **ECG:** In typical AFl, "saw tooth" pattern best visualized in leads II, III, and aVF with negative deflections in V_1.
- **Multifocal atrial tachycardia (MAT)**
  - **Irregularly irregular** SVT seen generally in elderly hospitalized patients with multiple comorbidities.
  - MAT is most often associated with chronic obstructive pulmonary disease (COPD) and heart failure but also associated with glucose intolerance, hypokalemia, hypomagnesemia, drugs (e.g., theophylline), and chronic renal failure.
  - **ECG:** SVT with at least **three distinct P-wave morphologies**, generally best visualized in leads II, III, and V_1.
- **Sinus tachycardia (ST)**
  - ST is the most common mechanism of **long RP tachycardia**.
  - Usually, ST is a normal physiologic response to hyperadrenergic states (fever, pain, hypovolemia, anemia, hypoxia, etc.) but can also be induced by illicit drugs (cocaine, amphetamines, methamphetamine) and prescription drugs (theophylline, atropine, β-adrenergic agonists).
  - **Inappropriate ST** refers to persistently elevated sinus rate in the absence of an identifiable physical, pathologic, or pharmacologic influence.
- **Ectopic atrial tachycardia (EAT)**
  - EAT with variable block can present as an **irregularly irregular** rhythm and can be distinguished from AFl by an **atrial rate of 150–200 bpm**.
  - EAT with variable block is associated with **digoxin toxicity**.
  - EAT is characterized by a regular atrial activation pattern with a P-wave morphology originating outside of the sinus node complex resulting in a **long RP tachycardia**.
  - **Mechanism:** Enhanced automaticity, triggered activity, and possibly microreentry.
- **AVNRT**
  - This reentrant rhythm requires functional dissociation of the AV node into two pathways with antegrade conduction down the "slow" pathway and retrograde conduction up the "fast" pathway. AVNRT can occur at any age, with a predilection for **middle age** and **female gender**. AVNRT is not correlated with structural heart disease.
    "Typical" AVNRT is a major cause of **short RP tachycardia. ECG appearance has characteristic absent P waves** because atrial activation is coincident with the QRS complex. Commonly, atrial activation can occur at the terminal portion of the QRS to create a pseudo-r' (V_1) or pseudo-s' (II) compared to the sinus rhythm QRS.
  - **"Atypical" AVNRT**
    - Less common; antegrade conduction proceeds down the fast AV nodal pathway with retrograde conduction up the slow AV nodal pathway, leading to a **long RP tachycardia**.
    - **ECG:** The retrograde P wave is inscribed well after the QRS complex in the second half of the RR interval.
- **AVRT**
  - **Orthodromic AVRT (O-AVRT)** is the most common AVRT, accounting for about 95% of all AVRT.
    - Accessory pathway–mediated reentrant rhythm with antegrade conduction to the ventricle down the AV node and retrograde conduction to the atrium up an accessory or "bypass" tract, leading to a **short RP tachycardia**.
    - **ECG:** Retrograde P waves are frequently seen after the QRS complex and are usually distinguishable from the QRS (i.e., separated by >70 msec).

- O-AVRT is the most common mechanism of SVT in patients with WPW syndrome who have preexcitation (defined by short PR and a delta wave on upstroke of QRS) present on sinus rhythm ECG.
- O-AVRT can occur without preexcitation when conduction through the bypass tract occurs only during tachycardia in a retrograde fashion ("concealed pathway").
- Less commonly, retrograde conduction over the accessory pathway to the atrium proceeds slowly enough for atrial activation to occur in the second half of the RR interval, leading to a **long RP tachycardia**. The associated incessant tachycardia can cause tachycardia-induced cardiomyopathy.
  ○ **Antidromic AVRT:** This reentrant form of SVT occurs when conduction to the ventricle is down an accessory bypass tract with retrograde conduction through the AV node or a second bypass tract.
    - **ECG:** The QRS seems consistent with VT; however, the presence of preexcitation on the baseline QRS should be diagnostic for WPW syndrome.
    - Antidromic AVRT is seen in <5% of patients with WPW syndrome.
- **Junctional tachycardia**
  ○ Due to enhanced automaticity of the AV junction. The electrical impulses conduct to the ventricle and atrium simultaneously, similar to typical AVNRT, so that the retrograde P waves are frequently concealed in the QRS complex.
  ○ Uncommon in adults.
  ○ Common in young children, particularly after cardiac surgery.
- **Sinoatrial nodal reentrant tachycardia (SANRT)**
  ○ Reentrant circuit is localized at least partially within the sinoatrial node.
  ○ Abrupt onset and termination, triggered by a premature atrial complex.
  ○ **ECG:** P-wave morphology and axis are identical to the native sinus P wave during normal sinus rhythm.

TREATMENT

- Please refer to Table 7-1 for general therapeutic approach to common SVTs.
- Acute treatment of symptomatic SVT should follow the **ACLS protocol** as outlined in Appendix C.
- Chronic treatment is guided by the severity of associated symptoms, the frequency, and the duration of recurrent events.
- Many SVTs can be terminated by **AV nodal blocking agents or techniques** (Table 7-2), whereas AF, AFl, and some atrial tachycardias will persist with a slowing of the ventricular rate due to partial AV nodal blockade.
- **Radiofrequency ablation (RFA):** Definitive cure with high success rates from 85–95% for many SVTs, including AVNRT, accessory bypass tract–mediated tachycardias, focal atrial tachycardia, and AFl. Complication risk is generally <1%. This risk includes major bleeding, cardiac perforation or tamponade, stroke, pulmonary embolism, and complete heart block requiring permanent pacemaker (PPM).
- There is limited evidence, but no large randomized trials with long-term follow-up, that suggests catheter ablation compared to antiarrhythmic therapy improves quality of life and is more cost-effective in the long term (*Am J Cardiol 1998;82:589*).

Atrial Fibrillation

GENERAL PRINCIPLES

The medical management of **AF** requires careful consideration of three issues: **rate control, prevention of thromboembolic events, and rhythm control**.

TABLE 7-1	Treatment of Common Supraventricular Tachyarrhythmias

Treatment Strategies

Atrial flutter (AFl)	Anticoagulation similar to AF; risk of thromboembolic complications is similar. Rate control with same agents as AF. If highly symptomatic or rate control difficult, electrical or chemical cardioversion is appropriate. If pacemaker present, overdrive atrial pacing can achieve cardioversion. Catheter ablation of typical right AFl with long-term success above 90% and rare complications.
Multifocal atrial tachycardia (MAT)	Therapy targeted at treatment of underlying pathophysiologic process. Maintain potassium and magnesium electrolyte balance. Antiarrhythmic, if symptomatic rapid ventricular response. Individualize β-adrenergic blockers vs. calcium channel blocker therapy. DC cardioversion is not effective.
Sinus tachycardia (ST)	Therapy targeted at treatment of underlying pathophysiologic process.
Ectopic atrial tachycardia (EAT)	**Acute therapy:** Identify and treat precipitating factors like digoxin toxicity; if hemodynamically stable, then β-blockers and calcium channel blockers. In rare cases, amiodarone, flecainide, or sotalol. **Chronic therapy:** Rate control with β-adrenergic blockers and calcium channel blockers. If unsuccessful, options include catheter ablation (86% success rate), flecainide, propafenone, sotalol, or amiodarone.
AV nodal reentrant tachycardia (AVNRT)	Catheter ablation highly successful (96%) but has to be individualized to each patient. If medical therapy more desirable—β-adrenergic blockers, calcium channel blockers, and digoxin; then consider propafenone, flecainide, etc.
Orthodromic AV reentrant tachycardia (O-AVRT)	**Acute therapy:** Vagal maneuvers, adenosine, calcium channel blockers. If ineffective, then procainamide or β-blockers. **Chronic suppressive therapy:** Catheter ablation highly successful (95%) but has to be individualized to each patient. If medical therapy more desirable for prevention, flecainide and procainamide are indicated.
Antidromic AV reentrant tachycardia (A-AVRT)	**Acute therapy:** Avoid adenosine or other AV node–specific blocking agents. Consider ibutilide, procainamide, or flecainide. **Chronic suppressive therapy:** Accessory pathway catheter ablation is preferred and successful (95%). If medical therapy desired, consider flecainide and propafenone.

AF, atrial fibrillation; AV, atrioventricular; DC, direct current.

From Blomström-Lundqvist C, Scheinman MM, Aliot EM, et al. ACC/AHA/ESC guidelines for the management of patients with supraventricular arrhythmias—Executive summary: A report of the American college of cardiology/American heart association task force on practice guidelines and the European society of cardiology committee for practice guidelines. *J Am Coll Cardiol* 2003;42:1493.

TABLE 7-2	Common Vagal Maneuvers and Adenosine					
	Patient Preparation[a]	Mechanism	Dose/Duration/Details	Toxicity	Contraindication	Potentiators/ Antagonists	Common Side Effects
Valsalva	Describe the procedure.	Vagal stimulation during relaxation phase.	Exhale forcefully against a closed airway for several seconds followed by relaxation.	Well tolerated.	Patient unable to follow commands.	—	—
Carotid sinus massage	Check for carotid bruits and history of CVA; then place in recumbent position with neck extended.	Vagal stimulation.	First, apply enough pressure to simply feel carotid pulse with index and middle fingers. If no effect, then use rotating motion for 3–5 s.	Well tolerated. Risk of embolizing carotid plaque. **Never massage both carotids.**	Recent TIA or stroke, or ipsilateral significant carotid artery stenosis or carotid artery bruit.	—	—
Adenosine	Explain the potential side effects to the patient.	AV nodal blocking agent. Short-acting (serum half-life 4–8 min).	Initial: 6 mg IV rapid bolus via antecubital vein, followed by 10–30 mL saline flush. If desired or effect not achieved, can repeat 12 mg followed by 12 mg after 1- to 2-min intervals. Central venous line: 3 mg IV initial dose.	Precipitate prolonged asystole in patients with sick sinus syndrome or second- or third-degree AV block.	Significant bronchospasm.	Potentiators: Dipyridamole and carbamazepine. **Effect pronounced in heart transplant recipients.** Antagonists: Caffeine and theophylline.	Facial flushing, palpitations, chest pain, hypotension, exacerbation of bronchospasm.

AV, atrioventricular; CVA, cerebrovascular accident; TIA, transient ischemic attack.
Atrioventricular nodal reentrant tachycardia, atrioventricular reentrant tachycardia, and many atrial tachycardias will terminate with vagal maneuvers or adenosine, and in atrial flutter, the appearance of flutter waveform will help diagnosis.
Water immersion, eyeball pressure, coughing, gagging, deep breathing, etc., are other alternative vagal maneuvers.
[a]Patients should be under continuous ECG monitoring for each of these procedures. To enhance diagnostic value of rhythm strip, use leads V_1 and II (atrial activity).

Definition

AF is an atrial tachyarrhythmia characterized by chaotic activation of the atria with loss of atrial mechanical function. AF has a pattern on 12-lead ECG characterized by the absence of consistent P waves. Instead, rapid, low-amplitude oscillations or fibrillatory waves are noted in the baseline of leads that best demonstrate atrial activation (V_1, II, III, aVF). The ventricular response to AF is characteristically irregular and often rapid in the presence of intact AV conduction. AF is the most common cardiac arrhythmia.

Classification

AF has been classified into four forms based on the clinical presentation: first occurrence, paroxysmal, persistent, and permanent forms.
- **First occurrence** may be symptomatic or asymptomatic. The spontaneous conversion rate is high, measured >60% in hospitalized patients.
- **Paroxysmal** AF describes a recurrent form of AF in which individual episodes are <7 days and usually <48 hours in duration.
- **Persistent** AF describes a recurrent form of AF in which individual episodes are >7 days in duration or require electrical cardioversion to terminate.
- **Longstanding persistent** AF describes the form of AF that has failed attempts at cardioversion, electrical or pharmacologic, or has been accepted due to contraindications for cardioversion or a lack of symptoms.

Epidemiology

- AF is the most common sustained tachyarrhythmia for which patients seek treatment and the most likely etiology for an irregularly irregular rhythm discovered on an inpatient ECG. AF is typically a disease of the elderly, affecting >10% of those >75 years old.
- Independent risk factors for AF, in addition to advanced age, include male sex, diabetes mellitus, cardiovascular disease such as CHF, valvular heart disease, hypertension (HTN), and previous MI (*JAMA 1994;271:840*). Below age 65, obesity and obstructive sleep apnea are important risk factors for new-onset AF (*J Am Coll Cardiol 2007;49(5):565*). Although clinical hyperthyroidism is associated with new-onset AF, the prevalence is low in a population of patients with AF (*J Epidemiol 2008;18(5):209*).
- Following cardiothoracic surgery, AF occurs in 20–50% of patients (*J Am Coll Cardiol 2006;48(4):8540*).

Pathophysiology

The precise mechanisms giving rise to AF are incompletely understood. The initiation of AF is commonly due to rapid, repetitive firing of an ectopic focus within the pulmonary veins with fibrillatory conduction to the bodies of the atria. The maintenance of persistent AF likely requires multiple reentrant circuits varying in location and timing to explain the self-perpetuating characteristic of AF. Structural and electrical remodeling of the left atrium associated with cardiovascular disease promotes ectopic activity and heterogeneous conduction patterns that provide the substrate for AF. AF, when present, also promotes structural and electrical remodeling in the atria that stabilizes the rhythm. Inflammation and fibrosis may play a major role in initiation and maintenance of AF. Inflammatory markers, such as interleukin-6 and C-reactive protein, are raised in AF and correlate with the duration of AF, success of cardioversion, and thrombogenesis.

Prevention

- Currently, there is a lack of prospective clinical trials that examine the value of primary prevention of non–postoperative AF through treatment of associated conditions or risk factor modification. Some analyses suggest that statins may reduce recurrent AF by 61%, independent of their lipid-lowering effect (*J Am Coll Cardiol 2008;51:828*). Angiotensin-converting enzyme (ACE) inhibitors and angiotensin receptor blockers (ARBs) have been shown to prevent atrial remodeling in animals via suppression of the renin–angiotensin system. A meta-analysis of patients with CHF and HTN treated with either ACEIs or ARBs demonstrated a reduction in new-onset AF by 20–30% (*J Am Coll Cardiol 2005;45:1832*).

- A number of pharmacologic and nonpharmacologic strategies have been evaluated to prevent postoperative AF. Perioperative continuation of β-adrenergic antagonists has been shown to reduce postoperative AF rates. **Amiodarone, sotalol, magnesium, and omega-3 fatty acids** used in the perioperative period have demonstrated a reduction in postoperative AF (*Ann Pharmacother 2007;41:587*).

DIAGNOSIS

AF is diagnosed by 12-lead ECG with a stereotypical pattern of an irregularly fluctuating baseline with an irregular, and often rapid, ventricular rate (>100 bpm). AF should be distinguished from other tachycardia mechanisms with an irregular ventricular response such as MAT and AFl with variable conduction.

Clinical Presentation

Symptoms associated with AF can range from severe (acute pulmonary edema, palpitations, angina, syncope) to nonspecific (fatigue) to none at all. Symptoms are usually secondary to the rapid ventricular response to AF rather than the loss of atrial systole. However, patients with significant ventricular systolic or diastolic dysfunction can have symptoms directly attributable to the loss of atrial systole. Prolonged episodes of tachycardia due to AF may lead to a **tachycardia-induced cardiomyopathy**.

TREATMENT

The medical management of AF is directed at three therapeutic goals: **rate control, prevention of thromboembolic events, and rhythm control** through maintenance of sinus rhythm. Previous studies have shown that there is no mortality advantage to a management strategy aimed at maintaining sinus rhythm (*N Engl J Med 2002;347:1825*). Therefore, rate control and management of thromboembolic risk are the preferred strategy in minimally symptomatic patients. Rhythm control is reserved for patients who remain symptomatic despite reasonable efforts at pharmacologic rate control.

Medications

Medical management begins with consideration of appropriate antithrombotic therapy. Warfarin has been shown to be consistently superior to aspirin (ASA) or ASA in combination with clopidogrel for prevention of thromboembolus. The novel oral anticoagulants (NOACs) dabigatran, rivaroxaban, apixaban, and edoxaban have been directly compared to warfarin in randomized prospective trials that documented a lower rate of stroke and systemic emboli compared to warfarin. Rate control of the ventricular response to AF is achieved with medications that limit conduction through the AV node such as **verapamil, diltiazem, β-adrenergic antagonists, and digoxin**. Rhythm control through maintenance of sinus rhythm can be attempted with selected antiarrhythmic drugs. Pharmacologic control with antiarrhythmic drugs is most effective at preventing recurrence of AF and less effective at chemical cardioversion of AF (Table 7-3).

First Line
- **Prevention of stroke and systemic emboli** is a central tenet of AF management guided by individual risk assessment in each patient. Systemic anticoagulation with warfarin or an NOAC will attenuate the risk of stroke or systemic emboli associated with AF; however, the use of any one of these agents requires a careful risk–benefit analysis to identify

TABLE 7-3	Pharmacologic Agents Used for Heart Rate Control in Atrial Fibrillation				
Drug	**Loading Dose**	**Onset of Action**	**Maintenance Dose**	**Major Side Effects**	**Recommendation**
Without evidence of accessory pathway					
Esmolol[a]	IV: 0.5 mg/kg over 1 min	5 min[b]	0.06–0.2 mg/kg/min	↓BP, ↓HR, HB, HF, bronchospasm	I
Metoprolol[a]	IV: 2.5–5.0 mg bolus over 2 min (up to three doses) PO: Same as maintenance	5 min	NA 25–100 mg bid	↓BP, ↓HR, HB, HF, bronchospasm	I
Propranolol[a]	IV: 0.15 mg/kg PO: Same as maintenance	4–6 h 5 min	NA 80–240 mg/d in divided doses	↓BP, ↓HR, HB, HF, bronchospasm	I
Diltiazem	IV: 0.25 mg/kg over 2 min PO: Same as maintenance	60–90 min 2–7 min 2–4 h	5–15 mg/h 120–360 mg/d in divided doses; slow release available	↓BP, HB, HF	I
Verapamil	IV: 0.075–0.15 mg/kg over 2 min PO: Same as maintenance	3–5 min 1–2 h	NA 120–360 mg/d in divided doses; slow release available	↓BP, HB, HF	I

With evidence of accessory pathway[c]

Amiodarone	IV: 150 mg over 10 min	Days	1 mg/min × 6 h, then 0.5 mg/min	See below	IIa

In patients with heart failure and without accessory pathway

Digoxin	IV: 0.25 mg q2h, up to 1.5 mg	60 min or more	0.125–0.375 mg/d IV or orally	Digoxin toxicity, HB, ↓HR	I
Amiodarone[d]	PO: 0.5 mg/d; IV: 150 mg over 10 min; PO: 800 mg/d for 1 wk, 600 mg/d for 1 wk, 400 mg/d for 1 wk,	2 days; Days; 1–3 wk	1 mg/min × 6 h, then 0.5 mg/min; 100–400 mg PO daily	↓BP, HB, ↓HR, warfarin interaction; see text for description of dermatologic, thyroid, pulmonary, corneal, and liver side effects	Acute setting: IIa (IV); Nonacute/chronic: IIb (PO)

↓BP, hypotension; ↓HR, bradycardia; HB, heart block; HF, heart failure; NA, not applicable.

[a]Only representative β-blockers are included in the table, but other similar agents could be used for this indication in appropriate doses.

[b]Onset is variable, and some effects occur earlier.

[c]Conversion to sinus rhythm and catheter ablation of the accessory pathway are generally recommended; pharmacologic therapy for rate control may be appropriate therapy in certain patients. See text for discussion of atrial fibrillation in setting of preexcitation/Wolff-Parkinson-White syndrome.

[d]Amiodarone can be useful to control the heart rate in patients with atrial fibrillation when other measures are unsuccessful or contraindicated.

Adapted from Fuster V, Ryden LE, Cannom DS, et al. ACC/AHA/ESC 2006 guidelines for the management of patients with atrial fibrillation: A report of the American College of Cardiology/American Heart Association Task Force on Practice Guidelines and the European Society of Cardiology Committee for Practice Guidelines (Writing Committee to Revise the 2001 Guidelines for the Management of Patients With Atrial Fibrillation). *Circulation* 2006;114:e257–e354.

patients who are at sufficient risk for thromboembolic events to outweigh the increased risk of hemorrhagic complications.

- ○ The **CHA$_2$DS$_2$-VASc score** is a validated, risk stratification tool in nonvalvular AF that predicts stroke or systemic embolus risk based on the presence of the following risk factors: CHF, HTN, age >65 or >75 years, diabetes mellitus, female sex, prior stroke/transient ischemic attacks (TIAs), and history of vascular disease (Table 7-4).
- ○ Antithrombotic therapy can be omitted in patients with a **CHA$_2$DS$_2$-VASc score = 0.**
- ○ In patients with a **CHA$_2$DS$_2$-VASc score of 1, no antithrombotic therapy or treatment with an oral anticoagulant or ASA may be considered.**
- ○ Systemic anticoagulation with warfarin or an NOAC is recommended for patients with a CHA$_2$DS$_2$-VASc risk of ≥2 and no contraindications for anticoagulation.
- ○ Measurement of renal function is critical to assess the safety and dosing of NOACs in patients with a **CHA$_2$DS$_2$-VASc score of ≥2 and chronic kidney disease.**
- ○ The role of antithrombotic therapy leading up to and after restoration of sinus rhythm is discussed in the following text in the context of cardioversion.
- • **Rate control** of AF can be achieved with drugs that prolong conduction through the AV node. These include the nondihydropyridine calcium channel blockers (diltiazem, verapamil), β-adrenergic blockers, and digoxin. Refer to Table 7-3 for loading and dosing recommendations.
  - ○ **Digoxin** is useful in controlling the resting ventricular rate in AF in the setting of LV dysfunction and CHF. Its utility in other clinical settings is limited by reduced efficacy of rate control during exertion. **Digitalis toxicity** is characterized by symptoms of **nausea, abdominal pain, vision changes, confusion, and delirium.** Patients with renal

TABLE 7-4	Annual Stroke Risk in Patients with Nonvalvular Atrial Fibrillation Not Treated with Anticoagulation According to the CHA$_2$DS$_2$-VASc Score
CHA$_2$DS$_2$-VASc Score	**Stroke Risk (%)[a]**
0	0
1	1.3
2	2.2
3	3.2
4	4.0
5	6.7
6	9.8
7	9.6
8	12.5
9	15.2

CHA$_2$DS$_2$-VASc, cardiac failure, hypertension, age 65–74 or age >74 (doubled), diabetes, female sex, stroke (doubled), and a history of vascular disease.
[a]The adjusted stroke rate was derived from multivariate analysis assuming no aspirin usage.
Adapted from Lip GY, Nieuwlaat R, Pisters R, Lane DA, Crijns HJ. Refining clinical risk stratification for predicting stroke and thromboembolism in atrial fibrillation using a novel risk factor-based approach: The Euro Heart Survey on atrial fibrillation. *Chest* 2010;137:263–72.

dysfunction are at high risk as are patients on agents known to increase digoxin levels (e.g., verapamil, diltiazem, erythromycin, cyclosporine). **Paroxysmal atrial tachycardia with varying degrees of AV block and bidirectional VT** are the most commonly seen arrhythmias in association with digitalis toxicity. Treatment is supportive, by withholding the drug, insertion of temporary pacemakers for AV block, and **IV phenytoin for bidirectional VT.**

○ **Nonpharmacologic rate control** of AF can be accomplished by AV nodal ablation in association with PPM implantation. This strategy should be reserved for patients who have failed pharmacologic rate control and in whom rhythm control is either ineffective or contraindicated.

Second Line

Rhythm control of AF is accomplished pharmacologically with antiarrhythmic drugs that modify impulse formation or propagation to prevent initiation of AF. Antiarrhythmic drugs are less effective at restoration of sinus rhythm through **pharmacologic cardioversion. The risk of thromboembolus associated with a pharmacologic cardioversion should be considered before beginning antiarrhythmic drug therapy.** Guidelines for anticoagulation are discussed in the following text:

• **Pharmacologic cardioversion** should be done in the hospital setting with continuous ECG monitoring because of a small risk of life-threatening tachyarrhythmias or bradyarrhythmias. **Ibutilide** is the only drug that is approved by the U.S. Food and Drug Administration for pharmacologic cardioversion. Clinical trials have shown a 45% conversion rate for AF and a 60% conversion rate for AFl. Ibutilide is associated with a 4–8% risk for torsades de pointes (TdP), especially in the first 2–4 hours after administration of the drug. Because of this risk, patients must be monitored on telemetry with an external defibrillator immediately available during ibutilide infusion and for at least 4 hours after the infusion. The risk for TdP is higher in patients with cardiomyopathy and CHF. Ibutilide is given via an IV, at a dosage of 1 mg (0.01 mg/kg if patient is <60 kg), **infused slowly over 10 minutes**. Faster administration can promote TdP. The efficacy of antiarrhythmics to achieve pharmacologic conversion drops sharply when AF is >7 days in duration. For shorter duration AF episodes, dofetilide, sotalol, flecainide, and propafenone have some efficacy, whereas amiodarone has limited efficacy to achieve pharmacologic cardioversion.

• **Maintenance of sinus rhythm** with antiarrhythmic agents is associated with a small risk for life-threatening proarrhythmia. As a result, antiarrhythmic therapy should be reserved for patients who have highly symptomatic AF despite adequate rate control. Commonly used antiarrhythmic agents, their major route of elimination, and dosing regimens are listed in Table 7-5. The most effective agents for maintenance of sinus rhythm are flecainide, propafenone, sotalol, dofetilide, amiodarone, and dronedarone.

○ **Flecainide** and **propafenone** can be considered for maintenance of sinus rhythm in patients with **structurally normal hearts**. In patients with structural heart disease, these agents are associated with an increased mortality rate (*N Engl J Med 1989;321:406*), and both agents are potent negative inotropes that can provoke or exacerbate heart failure. Both agents prolong the QRS duration as an early manifestation of toxicity. Toxicity increases with heart rate due to preferential blockade of active sodium channels. This property is described as **positive use dependence**. Exercise ECG can be used to give additional information about dose safety at higher heart rates. Flecainide should be used with caution without concomitant dosing with an AV nodal blocker because a paradoxical increase in the ventricular rate may occur due to drug-induced conversion of AF to AFl. Propafenone is less prone to this phenomenon due to intrinsic β-adrenergic antagonism.

○ **Sotalol** is useful for the maintenance of sinus rhythm. Sotalol is a mixture of stereoisomers (DL-); D-sotalol is a potassium channel blocker, whereas L-sotalol is a β-antagonist.

TABLE 7-5	Commonly Used Antiarrhythmic Drugs			
Class	Drug	Route of Administration (Elimination)	Initial/Loading Dose	Maintenance Dose	Major Adverse Effects[a]/ Comments
Ia	Procainamide	IV (R, H) PO (R, H)	15–18 mg/kg at 20 mg/min 50 mg/kg/24 h, Max: 5 g/24 h	1–4 mg/min IR: 250–500 mg q3–6h SR: 500 mg q6h Procanbid: 1000–2500 mg q12h	GI, CNS, +ANA/SLE-like syndrome, fever, hematologic, anticholinergic. Follow QT_c, serum procainamide (4–8 mg/L) and NAPA levels (<20 mg/mL)
	Quinidine	PO (H)	Sulfate, 200–400 mg q6h; gluconate, 324–972 mg q8–12h	NA	↑QT, TdP, ↓BP, thrombocytopenia, cinchonism, GI upset
	Disopyramide	PO (H, R)	300–400 mg	IR: 100–200 mg q6h SR: 200–400 mg q12h	Anticholinergic, HF
Ib	Lidocaine	IV (H)	1 mg/kg over 2 min (may repeat × 2 up to 3 mg/kg total)	1–4 mg/min	↓HR, CNS, GI; adjust dose in patients with hepatic failure, AMI, HF, or shock
	Mexiletine	PO (H)	400 mg one-time dose	200–300 mg q8h	GI, CNS
Ic	Flecainide	PO (H, R)	50 mg q12h	Increase by 50–100 mg/d every 4 days to max 400 mg/d	HF, GI, CNS, blurred vision
	Propafenone	PO (H)	IR: 150 mg q8h ER: 225 mg q12h	IR: Increase at 3- to 4-day intervals up to 300 mg q8h; ER: May increase at 5-day intervals, up to 425 mg q12h	GI, dizziness

III	Sotalol	PO (R)	80 mg q12h	May increase every 3 days up to 240–320 mg/d in two to three divided doses	↓HR, ↓BP, CHF, CNS Limit QT$_c$ prolongation to <550 ms
	Dofetilide	PO (R, H)	CrCl (mL/min): Dose (µg bid): >60: 500 40–60: 250 20–39: 125 <20: Contraindicated	Dose adjusted based on QT$_c$ 2–3 h after inpatient doses 1 through 5 Chronic therapy requires calculation of QT$_c$ and CrCl every 3 months with adjustment as necessary	↑QT, VT/TdP, HA, dizziness; see text for further details on initiating and monitoring treatment
	Ibutilide	IV (H)	1 mg (0.01 mg/kg if patient <60 kg) over 10 min; can repeat if no response 10 min after initial infusion	NA	↑QT, TdP, AV block, GI, HA
	Amiodarone	IV (H) PO (H)	IV: 150 mg over 10 min, then 1 mg/min × 6 h, then 0.5 mg/min PO: 800 mg/d for 1 wk, then 600 mg/d for 1 wk, then 400 mg/d for 1 wk	100–400 mg PO daily	↓BP, HB, ↓HR, warfarin interaction; see text for description of dermatologic, thyroid, pulmonary, corneal, and liver effects

AMI, acute myocardial infarction; ANA, antinuclear antibodies; ↓BP, hypotension; CNS, central nervous system; CHF, congestive heart failure; CrCl, creatinine clearance; ER, extended release; GI, gastrointestinal; H, hepatic; HA, headache; HB, heart block; HF, heart failure; ↓HR, bradycardia; IR, immediate release; NA, not applicable; NAPA, N-acetylprocainamide; R, renal; SLE, systemic lupus erythematosus; SR, sustained release; TdP, torsades de pointes; VT, ventricular tachycardia.

aEither common or life-threatening adverse effects of these medications are listed. This is not a comprehensive list of all possible adverse effects.

Side effects reflect both mechanisms of action. In addition to QT interval prolongation leading to TdP, DL-sotalol may result in sinus bradycardia or AV conduction abnormalities. Sotalol should not be used in patients with decompensated CHF (due to the negative inotropic effect) or with a prolonged QT interval. Initiation of sotalol should be done in an inpatient monitored setting.

○ **Dofetilide** is useful for the maintenance of sinus rhythm. Dofetilide is a pure potassium channel blocker. Initiation of dofetilide should be done in an inpatient, monitored setting.

○ QT prolongation with sotalol or dofetilide is intensified by bradycardia, a characteristic known as "**reverse use dependence.**" The main risk of dofetilide is TdP. Dofetilide is contraindicated in patients with a baseline corrected QT interval (QT_c) >440 msec, or >500 msec in patients with bundle branch block. Initial dosing of dofetilide is based on the creatinine clearance. A 12-lead ECG should be obtained before the first dose of dofetilide and 1–2 hours after each dose. If the QT_c interval after the first dose is prolonged by 15% of the baseline or exceeds 500 msec, a 50% dosage reduction is indicated. If the QT_c exceeds 500 msec after the second dose, dofetilide must be discontinued. Several medications block the renal secretion of dofetilide (verapamil, cimetidine, prochlorperazine, trimethoprim, megestrol, ketoconazole) and are contraindicated with dofetilide. The advantages of dofetilide are that it is not associated with increased CHF or mortality in patients with LV dysfunction (*N Engl J Med 1999;341:857*) and it does not cause sinus node dysfunction or conduction abnormalities.

○ **Dronedarone** is the newest antiarrhythmic agent approved for treatment of AF. Like amiodarone, from which it was derived, dronedarone shares properties with Vaughan Williams classes I–IV antiarrhythmic drugs. Dronedarone has been shown to be more effective than placebo at maintaining sinus rhythm after cardioversion but less effective than amiodarone at maintenance of sinus rhythm. The incidence of proarrhythmia is low with dronedarone, as is the incidence of organ toxicity. A trend toward increased mortality has been shown in patients with advanced heart failure symptoms, and it is contraindicated in this patient group. Dronedarone is metabolized in the liver and should not be used in patients with significant hepatic dysfunction. Dronedarone can be used in patients with significant renal dysfunction because clearance is predominantly in the feces.

○ **Amiodarone** is arguably the most effective antiarrhythmic agent for maintenance of sinus rhythm. **Because of the extensive toxicity profile of amiodarone, it should not be considered as a first-line agent for rhythm control of AF in patients in whom an alternative antiarrhythmic can be safely used.** IV amiodarone has a low efficacy for acute conversion of AF, although conversion after several days of IV amiodarone has been observed. Given its common use and relatively high incidence of side effects, a more detailed discussion of these effects is required.

  ▪ Adverse effects of oral amiodarone are partially dose dependent and may occur in up to 75% of patients treated at high doses for 5 years. At lower doses (200–300 mg/d), adverse effects that require discontinuation occur in approximately 5–10% of patients per year.

  ▪ **Pulmonary toxicity** occurs in 1–15% of treated patients but appears less likely in those who receive <300 mg/d (*Circulation 1990;82:580*). Patients characteristically have a dry cough and dyspnea associated with pulmonary infiltrates and rales. The process appears to be reversible if detected early, but undetected cases may result in a mortality rate of up to 10% of those affected. A CXR and pulmonary function tests should be obtained at baseline and every 12 months or when patients complain of shortness of breath. The presence of interstitial infiltrates on the chest radiograph and a decreased diffusing capacity raise concern of amiodarone pulmonary toxicity.

- **Photosensitivity** is a common adverse reaction, and in some patients, a violaceous skin discoloration develops in sun-exposed areas. The blue-gray discoloration may not resolve completely with discontinuation of therapy.
- **Thyroid dysfunction** is a common adverse effect. Hypothyroidism and hyperthyroidism have been reported, with an incidence of 2–5% per year. Thyroid-stimulating hormone should be obtained at baseline and monitored every 6 months. If hypothyroidism develops, concurrent treatment with levothyroxine may allow continued amiodarone use.
- **Corneal microdeposits**, detectable on slit-lamp examination, develop in virtually all patients. These deposits rarely interfere with vision and are not an indication for discontinuation of the drug. Optic neuritis, leading to blindness, is rare but has been reported in association with amiodarone.
- The most common **ECG changes** are lengthened PR intervals and bradycardia; however, high-grade AV block may occur in patients who have preexisting conduction abnormalities. Amiodarone may prolong QT intervals, although usually not extensively, and **TdP is rare**. Other agents that prolong the QT interval, however, should be avoided in patients who are taking amiodarone.
- **Liver dysfunction** usually manifests in an asymptomatic and transient rise in hepatic transaminases. If the increase exceeds three times normal or doubles in a patient with an elevated baseline level, amiodarone should be discontinued or the dose should be reduced. Aspartate transaminase (AST) and alanine transaminase (ALT) should be monitored every 6 months in patients who are receiving amiodarone.
- **Drug interactions.** Amiodarone may raise the blood levels of warfarin and digoxin; therefore, these drugs should be reduced routinely by one-half when amiodarone is started, and levels should be followed closely.

Other Nonpharmacologic Therapies

Nonpharmacologic methods of rhythm control include catheter or surgical ablation techniques that block the initiation and maintenance of AF.

- **Direct current cardioversion (DCCV)** is the safest and most effective method of acutely restoring sinus rhythm. Prior to cardioversion, consideration of thromboembolic risk and anticoagulation is critical, when possible, to minimize thromboembolic events triggered by the cardioversion process. AF with a rapid ventricular response in the setting of ongoing myocardial ischemia, MI, hypotension, or respiratory distress should receive prompt cardioversion regardless of the anticoagulation status.
  - If the duration of AF is documented to be **<48 hours**, cardioversion may proceed without anticoagulation. If AF has persisted for **>48 hours** (or for an unknown duration), patients should be anticoagulated for at least 3 weeks before cardioversion, and anticoagulation should be continued in the same therapeutic range following successful cardioversion.
  - An alternative to anticoagulation for 3 weeks before cardioversion is to perform a **transesophageal echocardiogram** to rule out left atrial appendage thrombus before cardioversion. This method is safe and has the advantage of a shorter time to cardioversion than 3 weeks of anticoagulation. Therapeutic anticoagulation is indicated after the cardioversion for a minimum of 4 weeks (*Am J Cardiol 1998;82:1545*).
  - When practical, sedation should be accomplished with midazolam (1–2 mg IV q2min to a maximum of 5 mg), methohexital (25–75 mg IV), etomidate (0.2–0.6 mg/kg IV), or propofol (initial dose, 5 mg/kg/h IV).
  - Proper synchronization of the DC shock to the QRS is critical to avoid induction of VT by a cardioversion shock delivered during a vulnerable period of the ventricle.
  - For cardioversion of atrial arrhythmias, the anterior patch electrode should be positioned just right of the sternum at the level of the third or fourth intercostal space, with

the second electrode positioned just below the left scapula posteriorly. **Care should be taken to position patch electrodes at least 6 cm from PPM or defibrillator generators.** If electrode paddles are used, firm pressure and conductive gel should be applied to minimize contact impedance. Direct contact with the patient or the bed should be avoided. Atropine (1 mg IV) should be readily available to treat prolonged pauses. Reports of serious arrhythmias, such as VT, ventricular fibrillation (VF), or asystole, are rare and are more likely in the setting of improperly synchronized cardioversions, digitalis toxicity, or concomitant antiarrhythmic drug therapy.

• **Curative catheter ablation of AF** has been shown to be highly effective in young patients with structurally normal hearts and a paroxysmal pattern of AF. Cure rates in this patient category are in the range of 70%. Cure rates are diminished in patients with structural heart disease, advanced age, and persistent AF. A significant fraction of patients require more than one ablation procedure to achieve cure. The goal of the catheter ablation procedure in paroxysmal AF patients is to achieve electrical isolation of the pulmonary veins. In patients with persistent AF, this goal is frequently combined with substrate modification strategies whereby regions of the atria are targeted for ablation to block reentry or the presence of focal drivers of AF. Because of potential complications and modest success, patients should undergo at least one trial of an antiarrhythmic drug for maintenance of sinus rhythm. If this trial is ineffective or poorly tolerated, curative catheter ablation can be contemplated.

Surgical Management

Surgical techniques for cure of AF have been evaluated since the 1980s. Of these techniques, the Cox-Maze procedure has the highest demonstrated efficacy and the most substantial published follow-up data documenting sustained efficacy. Including patients with persistent AF and structural heart disease, cure rates approach 90%. Because of its highly invasive nature, surgical treatment is usually reserved for patients who have failed a catheter ablation strategy or who have planned concomitant cardiac surgery.

Ventricular Tachyarrhythmias

GENERAL PRINCIPLES

• Ventricular tachyarrhythmias should be initially approached with the assumption that they will have a malignant course until proven otherwise.
• Characterization of the arrhythmia involves consideration of hemodynamic stability, duration, morphology, and presence or lack of underlying structural heart disease.
• Ultimately, this characterization will aid in determining the patient's risk for **sudden cardiac arrest** and need for device or ablation-based therapy.

Definitions

• **Nonsustained VT:** Three or more consecutive ventricular complexes (>100 bpm) that terminate spontaneously within 30 seconds.
• **Sustained monomorphic VT:** Tachycardia of ventricular origin with single QRS morphology that lasts longer than 30 seconds or requires cardioversion due to hemodynamic compromise.
• **Polymorphic VT:** VT characterized by an ever-changing QRS morphology. **TdP** is a variant of polymorphic VT that is typically preceded by a prolonged QT interval in sinus rhythm. Polymorphic VT is associated with hemodynamic collapse or instability.
• **VF** is associated with disorganized mechanical contraction, hemodynamic collapse, and sudden death. The ECG reveals irregular and rapid oscillations (250–400 bpm) of highly variable amplitude without uniquely identifiable QRS complexes or T waves.

- Ventricular arrhythmias are the major cause of **sudden cardiac death (SCD)**. **SCD** is defined as death that occurs within 1 hour of the onset of symptoms. In the United States, approximately 350,000 cases of SCD occur annually. Among patients with aborted SCD, ischemic heart disease is the most common associated cardiac structural abnormality. Most cardiac arrest survivors do not have evidence of an acute MI; however, >75% have evidence of previous infarcts. A nonischemic cardiomyopathy is also associated with an elevated risk for SCD.

Etiology

- **VT associated with structural heart disease**
  - Most ventricular arrhythmias are associated with structural heart disease, typically related to active ischemia or history of infarct.
    - Scar and the peri-infarct area provide the substrate for reentry that produces sustained monomorphic VT.
    - Polymorphic VT and VF are commonly associated with ischemia and are the presumed cause of most out-of-hospital SCDs.
  - Nonischemic cardiomyopathy typically involves progressive dilation and fibrosis of the ventricular myocardium, providing an arrhythmogenic substrate.
  - Infiltrative cardiomyopathies (sarcoid, hemochromatosis, amyloid) represent a smaller patient population that is at significant risk for ventricular arrhythmias whose management is less clearly defined.
  - Adults with prior repair of congenital heart disease are commonly afflicted with both VT and SVT.
  - Arrhythmogenic right ventricular (RV) dysplasia or cardiomyopathy is marked by fibrofatty replacement of the RV (and sometimes LV) myocardium that gives rise to left bundle branch block (LBBB) morphology VT and is associated with sudden death, particularly in young athletes.
  - Bundle branch reentry VT is a form of VT that uses the His-Purkinje system in a reentrant circuit and is typically associated with cardiomyopathy and an abnormal conduction system.
- **VT in the absence of structural heart disease**
  - Inherited ion channelopathies, such as those seen in Brugada and long QT syndromes, can lead to polymorphic VT and sudden death in patients without evidence of structural heart disease on imaging.
  - Catecholaminergic polymorphic VT involves familial, exercise-induced VT that is related to irregular calcium processing.
  - **Idiopathic VT** is a diagnosis of exclusion that requires the documented absence of structural heart disease, genetic disorders, and reversible etiologies (i.e., ischemia, electrolyte/metabolic abnormalities). Most idiopathic VTs originate from the RV outflow tract (RVOT) and are amenable to ablation. Less commonly, LV outflow tract (LVOT) VT or fascicular VT (using anterior and posterior divisions of the left bundle branch) may be discovered on EPS.

DIAGNOSIS

Clinical Presentation

- The evaluation of wide-complex tachyarrhythmias (WCTs) should always begin with prompt assessment of vital signs and clinical symptoms. If the arrhythmia is poorly tolerated, postpone further detailed evaluation and proceed to acute management per ACLS guidelines. If stable, there are several important questions to address that can guide one toward the most likely diagnosis. A common mistake is the assumption that hemodynamic stability supports the diagnosis of SVT over VT.

- VT represents the vast majority of WCT seen in the inpatient setting with reported prevalence upward of 80%. With that in mind, one can then proceed to elicit several historical points of emphasis and scrutinize ECG properties of the arrhythmia to further delineate the mechanism of the underlying rhythm disturbance. Begin with the following questions:
  - Does the patient have a history of structural heart disease?
    Patients with structural heart disease are much more likely to have VT rather than SVT as the etiology of a WCT. In one report, 98% of patients with WCT who had prior MI proved to have VT (*Am J Med 1988;84:53*).
  - Does the patient have a pacemaker, implantable cardioverter-defibrillator (ICD), or wide QRS at baseline?
    - The presence of either a pacemaker or an ICD should raise suspicion for a device-mediated WCT.
    - **Device-mediated WCT** can be due to ventricular pacing at a rapid rate either due to device tracking of an atrial tachyarrhythmia or an "endless loop tachycardia" created by tracking of the retrograde atrial impulses created by the preceding ventricular paced beat. In either case, the tachycardia rate is a clue to the mechanism because this is typically equal to the programmed upper rate limit (URL) of the device. A commonly programmed URL is 120 paces per minute (ppm). A tachycardia rate above the URL effectively excludes a device-mediated WCT.
    - Device can be confirmed by inspection of the chest wall (usually left chest for right-handed patients), chest radiograph (CXR), or the presence of pacing spikes seen on ECG.
    - Patients with known right bundle branch block (RBBB), LBBB, or intraventricular conduction delay (IVCD) at baseline who present with WCT will have a QRS morphology identical to baseline in the presence of SVT. In addition, some patients with a narrow QRS at baseline will manifest a WCT due to SVT when a rate-related bundle branch block is present (SVT with aberrancy).
  - What medications is the patient taking?
    - The medication list should be scanned for any medication with proarrhythmic side effects, especially those that can prolong the baseline QT interval. These medicines include many of the class I and III antiarrhythmics, certain antibiotics, antipsychotics, and many more.
    - Medications that can lead to electrolyte abnormalities, such as loop and potassium-sparing diuretics, ACEIs, ARBs, etc., should be ascertained. Also, digoxin toxicity is always an important consideration in the setting of any arrhythmia.

Differential Diagnosis

- WCT may be due to either SVT with aberrant conduction or VT. Differentiation between these mechanisms is of the utmost importance. **The pharmacologic agents used in the management of SVT (i.e., adenosine, β-blockers, calcium channel blockers) can cause hemodynamic instability if used in the setting of VT.** Therefore, all WCTs are considered to be ventricular in origin until proven otherwise.
    Other less common mechanisms of WCT include **antidromic AVRT, hyperkalemia-induced arrhythmia, or pacemaker-induced tachycardia**.
- **Telemetry artifact** due to poor lead contact or repetitive patient motion (tremor, shivering, brushing teeth, chest physical therapy, etc.) can mimic VT or VF.

Diagnostic Testing

Laboratories
Laboratory studies should include basic metabolic panel, magnesium, CBC, and serial troponins.

Electrocardiography
- **Differentiation of SVT with aberrancy from VT** based on ECG analysis is critical in the determination of appropriate acute and chronic therapy. Features that are diagnostic of VT are **AV dissociation**, **capture or fusion beats**, an absence of RS morphology in the precordial leads (V_1–V_6), and **LBBB morphology with right axis deviation**. In the absence of these features, examination of an RS complex in a precordial lead for an RS interval >100 msec is consistent with VT. In addition, characteristic QRS morphologies that are suggestive of VT may be sought, as shown in Figure 7-2.
- **ECG pearls**
  ○ **Classic Brugada pattern**
    ▪ Baseline: Pseudo-RBBB with ST-segment elevation and T-wave inversion in V_1, V_2
    ▪ May be unmasked by stress, illness, fever, illicit drug use, etc.
  ○ **Arrhythmogenic RV dysplasia**
    ▪ Baseline: Epsilon wave (late potential just after QRS), ± wide QRS, ± T-wave inversion (V_1, V_2)
    ▪ VT: Reflects RV origin, likely LBBB configuration; may present with polymorphic VT
  ○ **Bundle branch reentrant VT**
    ▪ Baseline: IVCD
    ▪ VT: LBBB morphology typically ("down" the right bundle; "up" the left bundle)
  ○ **Fascicular VT**
    VT: Superior axis, RBBB morphology
  ○ **Long QT syndrome**
    ▪ Baseline: QT >50% of the RR interval if HR 60–100 bpm; QT_c ≥440 msec
    ▪ VT: TdP degenerating into VF
  ○ **Outflow tract VT**
    VT: Inferior axis, LBBB morphology. R/S transition in the precordial leads can aid in localization. Early transition (V_1 or V_2) suggests an LVOT origin; later transition (V_4) suggests RVOT origin.

Imaging
- The presence or absence of structural heart disease should be initially evaluated by transthoracic echocardiography.
- Further imaging (cardiac MRI, noninvasive stress test, coronary angiogram, etc.) should be obtained based on suspected etiology.

TREATMENT

- **Differentiation of SVT with aberrancy from VT** based on analysis of the surface ECG is critical in the determination of appropriate acute and chronic therapy.
  ○ For acute therapy of SVT, IV medications such as adenosine, calcium channel blockers, or β-blockers are used. However, calcium channel blockers and β-blockers can produce hemodynamic instability in patients with VT.
  ○ Chronically, many SVTs are amenable to RFA, whereas most VTs are malignant and require an antiarrhythmic agent and/or ICD implantation.
- Immediate unsynchronized DCCV is the primary therapy for pulseless VT and VF.

Other Nonpharmacologic Therapies

- **ICDs** provide automatic recognition and treatment of ventricular arrhythmias. ICD implantation improves survival in patients resuscitated from ventricular arrhythmias (secondary prevention of SCD) and in individuals without prior symptoms who are at high risk for SCD (primary prevention of SCD).

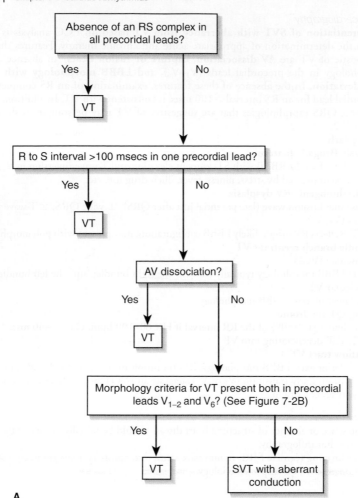

A

Figure 7-2. A and B. Brugada criteria for distinguishing ventricular tachycardia from supraventricular tachycardia with aberrancy in wide-complex tachycardias. LBBB, left bundle branch block; RBBB, right bundle branch block; SVT, supraventricular tachyarrhythmia; VT, ventricular tachycardia. (From Sharma S, Smith TW. Advanced electrocardiography: ECG 201. In: Cuculich PS, Kates AM, eds. *The Washington Manual Cardiology Subspecialty Consult.* 3rd ed. Philadelphia, PA: Wolters Kluwer Health; 2014.)

	LBBB		RBBB	
	VT	SVT	VT	SVT
Lead V1	In V1, V2 any of: (a) r ≥0.04 sec (b) Notched S downstroke (c) Delayed S nadir >0.06 sec	In V1, V2 absence of: (a) r ≥0.04 sec (b) Notched S downstroke (c) Delayed S nadir >0.06 sec	Taller left peak Biphasic RS or QR	Triphasic rsR' or rR'
Lead V6	Monophasic QS 		Biphasic rS 	Triphasic qRs

B

Figure 7-2. (*Continued*).

○ **Secondary prevention of SCD** with ICD implantation is indicated for most patients who survive SCD outside of the peri-MI setting. The superiority of ICD therapy to chronic antiarrhythmic drug therapy has been demonstrated (AVID trial; *N Engl J Med 1997;337:1576*).

○ **Primary prevention of SCD** with ICD implantation is indicated for patients who are at high risk of SCD. The efficacy of ICD implantation for primary prevention of SCD in the setting of cardiomyopathy has been established in multiple prospective clinical trials (see Multicenter Automatic Defibrillator Implantation Trial [**MADIT**], *N Engl J Med 1996;335:1933*; Multicenter Un-Sustained Tachycardia Trial [**MUSTT**], *N Engl J Med 1999;341:1882*; **MADIT II Trial**, *N Engl J Med 2002;346:877*; and **SCD-HeFT**, *N Engl J Med 2005;352(3):225*). Most patients with an LV ejection fraction of <35% for more than 3 months on optimal medical therapy meet current indications for prophylactic ICD implantation.

○ **Other indications for ICD**

  ▪ Phenotypes associated with **HCM, arrhythmogenic RV cardiomyopathy, congenital long QT syndrome, or Brugada syndrome have a higher risk of SCD.** ICD implantation is indicated if patients with one of these syndromes have had a resuscitated cardiac arrest or documented ventricular arrhythmia. Prophylactic ICD implantation is based on disease-specific risk factors.

- Patients who are awaiting cardiac transplantation are at high risk for SCD, especially if they are receiving an intravenous inotrope. Prophylactic ICD implantation is reasonable to protect against SCD prior to transplantation.

    ICDs are **contraindicated** in patients who have incessant VT, recent MI <40 days or revascularization <3 months in the case of primary prevention, significant psychiatric illnesses, or life expectancy of <12–24 months.

- **Radiofrequency catheter ablation of VT** is most successfully performed in patients with hemodynamically stable forms of idiopathic VT that is not associated with structural heart disease. Long-term cure rates in these patients are similar to those achieved for catheter ablation of SVT. In the presence of structural heart disease, catheter ablation has a lower efficacy and a higher morbidity but is an important treatment option, particularly in drug-refractory, symptomatic VT that is leading to ICD therapy.
    - **Idiopathic VT is usually associated with a structurally normal heart, but an associated tachycardia-mediated cardiomyopathy has been described.**
        - **Outflow tract VT** often presents as repetitive, nonsustained bursts of VT that originates most commonly from the RV (RVOT) and less commonly from the LV near the coronary cusps or aorto-mitral continuity. These can be responsive to β-adrenergic blockers, diltiazem, verapamil, and adenosine.
        - Both forms of idiopathic VT are thought to be benign in the absence of structural heart disease. Therefore, ICD implantation is not appropriate. All forms of idiopathic VT are amenable to treatment with RFA or drug therapy.
    - **VT associated with ischemic heart disease** can also be treated by catheter ablation by targeting the scar-based substrate. Emergent catheter ablation in the setting of frequent hemodynamically unstable VT requiring defibrillation (VT storm) can be life-saving. Ablation has been shown to be reduce ICD therapy and improve quality of life.
    - **Ablation of VT in nonischemic cardiomyopathy** is also reasonable, particularly in drug-refractory patients, but VT circuits may be intramyocardial or epicardial. As a result, success rates are typically lower than those associated with ischemic VT, and referral to a center that routinely performs both endocardial and epicardial ablations should be considered.

Medications

- VF that is resistant to external defibrillation requires the addition of IV antiarrhythmic agents.
    - IV lidocaine is frequently used; however, IV amiodarone appears to be more effective in increasing survival of VF when used in conjunction with defibrillation (*N Engl J Med 2002;346:884*).
    - After successful defibrillation, continuous IV infusion of effective antiarrhythmic therapy should be maintained until any reversible causes have been corrected.
- Chronic antiarrhythmic drug therapy is indicated for the treatment of recurrent symptomatic ventricular arrhythmias. In the setting of hemodynamically unstable ventricular arrhythmias treated with an ICD, antiarrhythmic drug therapy is often necessary to prevent frequent device discharges.

First Line

- **Amiodarone** is safe and well tolerated for the acute management of ventricular arrhythmias. Amiodarone has complex pharmacokinetics and is associated with significant toxicities arising from chronic therapy (*Am Heart J 1993;125:109*).

    After oral loading, amiodarone prevents the recurrence of sustained VT or VF in up to 60% of patients. A therapeutic latency of more than 5 days exists before beneficial antiarrhythmic effects are observed with oral dosing, and full suppression of arrhythmias may not occur for 4–6 weeks after therapy is initiated. Unfortunately, recurrence of ventricular arrhythmias during long-term follow-up is common.

- **Class II** agents, the β-adrenergic antagonists, are the only class of antiarrhythmic agents to have consistently shown improved survival in post-MI patients.
  - ○ β-Adrenergic blockers reduce postinfarction total mortality by 25–40% and SCD by 32–50% (*Lancet 1981;2:823*; *Lancet 1999;353:9*; *Lancet 1999;353:2001*; *N Engl J Med 2001;344:1651*; *Lancet 2001;357:1385*).
  - ○ After acute therapy of VT/VF and stabilization, β-adrenergic blockers should be initiated and titrated as blood pressure and heart rate allow.
- **ACEIs** have also been shown to reduce sudden death and overall mortality in patients with coronary artery disease (CAD) or CHF.

Second Line
- **Sotalol** is a **class III** agent indicated for the chronic treatment of VT/VF. Sotalol prevents the recurrence of sustained VT and VF in 70% of patients (*N Engl J Med 1993;329:452*) but must be used with caution in individuals with CHF.
- **Class I** agents in general have not been shown to reduce mortality in patients with VT/VF. In fact, the class Ic agents, **flecainide** and **propafenone**, are associated with increased mortality in patients with ventricular arrhythmias after MI (*N Engl J Med 1991;324:781*).
- **Lidocaine** is a **class Ib** agent available only in IV form with efficacy in the management of sustained and recurrent VT/VF. The prophylactic use of lidocaine for suppression of premature ventricular contractions and nonsustained VT in the otherwise uncomplicated post-MI setting should be avoided. Toxicities of lidocaine include central nervous system (CNS) effects (convulsions, confusion, stupor, and, rarely, respiratory arrest), all of which resolve with discontinuation of therapy. Serum levels should be followed during prolonged use.
- **Mexiletine** is similar to lidocaine but is available in oral form. **Mexiletine is most often used in combination with either amiodarone or sotalol for chronic treatment of refractory ventricular arrhythmias.** CNS toxicity includes tremor, dizziness, and blurred vision. Higher levels may result in dysarthria, diplopia, nystagmus, and an impaired level of consciousness. Nausea and vomiting are common.
- **Phenytoin** can be used in the treatment of **digitalis-induced ventricular arrhythmias**. It may have a limited role in the treatment of ventricular arrhythmias associated with congenital long QT syndromes and those with structural heart disease.

SPECIAL CONSIDERATIONS

- **Class IV** agents have no role in the chronic management of VT associated with structural heart disease.
- Primary therapy for VF that occurs secondary to ischemia in the setting of an MI is complete revascularization. In the absence of complete revascularization, the patient remains at high risk for recurrent VT/VF.
- In the case of **TdP associated with long QT syndrome**, acute therapy is immediate defibrillation.
- Bolus administration of magnesium sulfate in 1- to 2-g increments up to 4–6 g IV is effective.
- In cases of acquired long QT, identification and treatment of the underlying condition should be undertaken, if possible.
- Elimination of long–short triggering sequences and shortening of the QT interval can be achieved by increasing the heart rate to the range of 90–120 bpm by either IV isoproterenol infusion (initial rate at 1–2 μg/min) or temporary transvenous pacing.

BRADYARRHYTHMIAS

GENERAL PRINCIPLES

- Bradyarrhythmias are commonly encountered rhythms in the inpatient setting that result in a ventricular rate of <60 bpm.
- **Anatomy of the conduction system**
  - The **sinus node** is a collection of specialized pacemaker cells located in the high right atrium. Under normal conditions, it initiates a wave of depolarization that spreads inferiorly and leftward via atrial myocardium and intranodal tracts, producing atrial systole.
  - The wave of depolarization then reaches another grouping of specialized cells, the **AV node**, located in the right atrial side of the interatrial septum. Normally, the AV node should serve as the lone electrical connection between the atria and ventricles.
  - From the AV node, the wave of depolarization travels down the **His bundle**, located in the membranous septum, and into the **right and left bundle branches** before reaching the **Purkinje fibers** that depolarize the rest of the ventricular myocardium.

Etiology

Common causes of bradycardia are listed in Table 7-6.

TABLE 7-6	Causes of Bradycardia

Intrinsic

Congenital disease (may present later in life)
Idiopathic degeneration (aging)
Infarction or ischemia
Cardiomyopathy
Infiltrative disease: sarcoidosis, amyloidosis, hemochromatosis
Collagen vascular diseases: systemic lupus erythematosus, rheumatoid arthritis, scleroderma
Surgical trauma: valve surgery, transplantation
Infectious disease: endocarditis, Lyme disease, Chagas disease

Extrinsic

Autonomically mediated
Neurocardiogenic syncope
Carotid sinus hypersensitivity
Increased vagal tone: coughing, vomiting, micturition, defecation, intubation
Drugs: β-blockers, calcium channel blockers, digoxin, antiarrhythmic agents
Hypothyroidism
Hypothermia
Neurologic disorders: increased intracranial pressure
Electrolyte imbalances: hyperkalemia, hypermagnesemia
Hypercarbia/obstructive sleep apnea
Sepsis

From Fansler DR, Chen J. Bradyarrhythmias and permanent pacemakers. In: Cuculich PS, Kates AM, eds. *The Washington Manual Cardiology Subspecialty Consult*. 3rd ed. Philadelphia, PA: Wolters Kluwer Health; 2014.

DIAGNOSIS

Clinical Presentation

When evaluating a suspected bradyarrhythmia, one should efficiently use the history, physical exam, and available data to address stability, symptoms, reversibility, site of dysfunction, and need for pacing.

History and Physical Examination

- If the patient is demonstrating signs of poor perfusion (hypotension, confusion, decreased consciousness, cyanosis, etc.), immediate management per ACLS protocol should be initiated. The clinical manifestations of bradyarrhythmias are variable, ranging from asymptomatic to nonspecific (lightheadedness, fatigue, weakness, exercise intolerance) to overt (syncope).
- Emphasis should be placed on delineating **whether the presenting symptoms have a direct temporal relationship to underlying bradycardia.** Other historical points of emphasis include the following:
  - Ischemic heart disease, particularly involving the right-sided circulation, can precipitate a number of bradyarrhythmias. Therefore, symptoms of acute coronary syndrome should always be sought.
  - **Precipitating circumstances** (micturition, coughing, defecation, noxious smells) surrounding episodes may help identify a neurocardiogenic etiology.
  - **Tachyarrhythmias,** particularly in patients with underlying sinus node dysfunction, can be followed by long pauses due to sinus node suppression during tachycardia.
  - History of structural heart disease, hypothyroidism, obstructive sleep apnea, collagen vascular disease, infections (bacteremia, endocarditis, Lyme, Chagas), infiltrative diseases (amyloid, hemochromatosis, and sarcoid), neuromuscular diseases, and prior cardiac surgery (valve replacement, congenital repair) should be sought.
  - **Medications** should be reviewed with emphasis on those that affect the sinus and AV nodes (i.e., calcium channel blockers, β-adrenergic blockers, digoxin).
- After hemodynamic stability is confirmed, a more thorough examination with particular emphasis on the cardiovascular exam and any findings consistent with the above comorbidities is appropriate (Figure 7-3).

Diagnostic Testing

Laboratories

Laboratory studies should include serum electrolytes and thyroid function tests in most patients. Digoxin levels and serial troponins should be drawn when clinically appropriate.

Electrocardiography

- The **12-lead ECG** is the cornerstone for diagnosis in any workup where arrhythmia is suspected.
  - Rhythm strips from leads that provide the best view of atrial activity (II, III, aVF, or V_1) should be examined.
  - Emphasis should be placed on identifying evidence of **sinus node dysfunction** (P-wave intervals) or **AV conduction abnormalities** (PR interval).
  - Evidence of both old and acute manifestations of ischemic heart disease should be sought as well.
- **Sinus node dysfunction,** or sick sinus syndrome, represents the most common reason for pacemaker implantation in the United States. Manifestations of sick sinus syndrome include (Figure 7-4):
  - **Sinus bradycardia** is defined as a regular rhythm with QRS complexes preceded by "sinus" P waves (upright in II, III, aVF) at a rate <60 bpm. Young patients and athletes

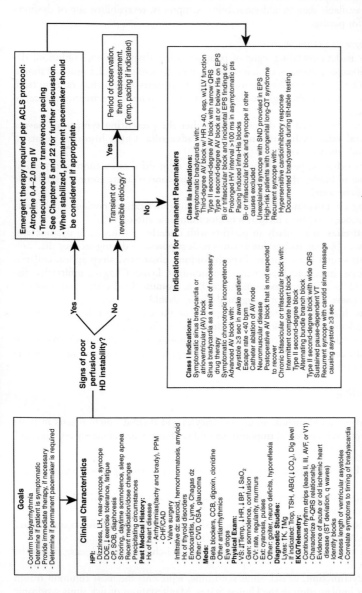

Figure 7-3. Approach to bradyarrhythmias. ABG, arterial blood gas; ACLS, advanced cardiac life support; ↓BP, hypotension; CCB, calcium channel blocker; CHF, congestive heart failure; CP, chest pain; CVD, cerebrovascular disease; DOE, dyspnea on exertion; dz, disease; EPS, electrophysiologic study; HD, hemodynamic; HPI, history of present illness; ↓HR, bradycardia; Hx, history; ↑K, hyperkalemia; LH, lightheadedness; ↑Mg, hypermagnesemia; OSA, obstructive sleep apnea; PPM, permanent pacemaker; ↓SaO₂, hypoxia; SND, sinus node dysfunction; SOB, shortness of breath; TSH, thyroid-stimulating hormone; VS, vital signs; VT, ventricular tachycardia. (From Fansler DR, Chen J. Bradyarrhythmias and permanent pacemakers. In: Cuculich PS, Kates AM, eds. *The Washington Manual Cardiology Subspecialty Consult*. 3rd ed. Philadelphia, PA: Wolters Kluwer Health; 2014.)

Sinus Bradycardia

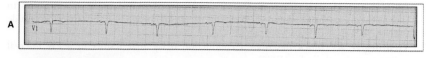

Sinoatrial Node Exit Block

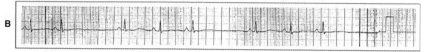

Sinus Rhythm with Blocked Premature Atrial Complexes

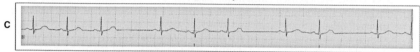

Tachy-Brady Syndrome with Prolonged Sinus Pause

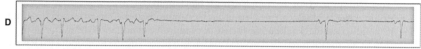

Figure 7-4. Examples of sinus node dysfunction. **A.** Sinus bradycardia. The sinus rate is approximately 45 bpm. **B.** Sinoatrial node exit block. Note that the PP interval in which the pause occurs is exactly twice that of the nonpaused PP interval. **C.** Blocked premature atrial complexes. This rhythm is often confused for sinus node dysfunction or atrioventricular block. Note the premature, nonconducted P waves inscribed in the T wave that resets the sinus node leading to the observed pauses. **D.** Tachy-brady syndrome. Note the termination of the irregular tachyarrhythmia followed by a prolonged 4.5-second pause prior to the first sinus beat. (From Fansler DR, Chen J. Bradyarrhythmias and permanent pacemakers. In: Cuculich PS, Kates AM, eds. *The Washington Manual Cardiology Subspecialty Consult.* 3rd ed. Philadelphia, PA: Wolters Kluwer Health; 2014.)

often have resting sinus bradycardia that is well tolerated. Nocturnal heart rates are lower in all patients, but the elderly tend to have higher resting heart rates and sinus bradycardia is a far less common normal variant.

- ○ **Sinus arrest** and **sinus pauses** refer to failure of the sinus node to depolarize, which manifest as periods of atrial asystole (no P waves). This may be accompanied by ventricular asystole or escape beats from junctional tissue or ventricular myocardium. Pauses of 2–3 seconds can be found in healthy, asymptomatic people, especially during sleep. Pauses >3 seconds, particularly during daytime hours, raise concern for significant sinus node dysfunction.
- ○ **Sinus exit block** represents the appropriate firing of the sinus node, but the wave of depolarization fails to traverse past the perinodal tissue. It is indistinguishable from sinus arrest on surface ECGs except that the R-R interval will be a multiple of the R-R preceding the bradycardia.
- ○ **Tachy-brady syndrome** occurs when tachyarrhythmias alternate with bradyarrhythmias, especially AF.
- ○ **Chronotropic incompetence** is the inability to increase the heart rate appropriately in response to metabolic need.
- **AV conduction disturbances**
  - ○ AV conduction can be **diverted** (fascicular or bundle branch blocks); **delayed** (first-degree AV block); **occasionally interrupted** (second-degree AV block); **frequently, but**

not always, interrupted (advanced or high-degree AV block); or **completely absent** (third-degree AV block). Assignment of the bradyarrhythmia under investigation to one of these categories allows one to better determine prognosis and, therefore, guide therapy.

○ **First-degree AV block** describes a conduction delay that results in a PR interval >200 msec on the surface ECG.

○ **Second-degree AV block** is present when there are periodic interruptions (i.e., "dropped beats") in AV conduction. Distinction between Mobitz I and II is important because they possess differing natural histories of progression to complete heart block.

■ **Mobitz type I block (Wenckebach)** is represented by a progressive delay in AV conduction with successive atrial impulses until an impulse fails to conduct. On surface ECG, classic Wenckebach block manifests as:

□ Progressive prolongation of the PR interval of each successive beat, before the dropped beat.

□ Shortening of each subsequent RR interval before the dropped beat.

□ A regularly irregular grouping of QRS complexes (group beating).

□ Type I block is usually within the AV node and portends a more benign natural history with progression to complete heart block unlikely.

■ **Mobitz type II block** carries a less favorable prognosis and is characterized by abrupt AV conduction block without evidence of progressive conduction delay.

□ On ECG, the PR intervals remained unchanged preceding the nonconducted P wave.

□ The presence of type II block, particularly if a bundle branch block is present, often antedates progression to complete heart block.

■ The presence of **AV 2:1 block** makes the differentiation between Mobitz type I or II mechanisms difficult. Diagnostic clues to the site of block include the following:

□ Concomitant first-degree AV block, periodic AV Wenckebach, or improved conduction (1:1) with enhanced sinus rates or sympathetic input suggests a more proximal interruption of conduction (i.e., Mobitz type I mechanism).

□ Concomitant bundle branch block, fascicular block, or worsened conduction (3:1, 4:1, etc.) with enhanced sympathetic input localizes the site of block more distally (Mobitz type II mechanism).

○ **Third-degree (complete) AV block** is present when all atrial impulses fail to conduct to the ventricles. There is complete dissociation between the atria and ventricles ("A > V" rates). This should be distinguished from dissociation with competition at the AV node ("V > A" rates).

○ **Advanced or high-degree AV block** is present when more than one consecutive atrial depolarization fails to conduct to the ventricles (i.e., 3:1 block or greater). On ECG, consecutive P waves will be seen without associated QRS complexes. However, there will be demonstrable P:QRS conduction somewhere on the record to avoid a "third-degree" designation (Figure 7-5).

Imaging

• The presence or absence of structural heart disease should be initially evaluated by transthoracic echocardiography.

• Further imaging should be obtained based on suspected etiology.

TREATMENT

Pharmacologic Therapy

• Bradyarrhythmias that lead to significant symptoms and hemodynamic instability should be managed emergently as outlined in ACLS guidelines (see Appendix C).

First-Degree AVB

A
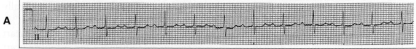

Second-Degree AVB-Mobitz type I (Wenckebach Block)

B
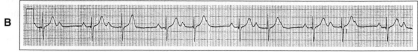

Second-Degree AVB-Mobitz type II

C
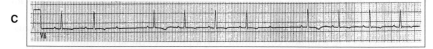

2:1 Second Degree AV Block

D
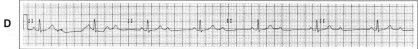

Third-Degree (Complete) AVB

E
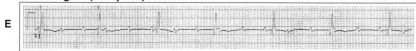

Figure 7-5. Examples of atrioventricular block (AVB). **A.** First-degree AVB. There are no dropped beats, and the PR interval is >200 msec. **B.** 3:2 Second-degree AVB-Mobitz I. Note the "group beating" and the prolonging PR interval prior to the dropped beat. The third P wave in the sequence is subtly inscribed in the T wave of the preceding beat. **C.** Second-degree AVB-Mobitz II. Note the abrupt atrioventricular conduction block without evidence of progressive conduction delay. **D.** 2:1 AVB. This pattern makes it difficult to distinguish between Mobitz I versus II type mechanisms of block. Note the narrow QRS complex, which supports a more proximal origin of block (type I mechanism). A wider QRS (concomitant bundle branch or fascicular block) would suggest a type II mechanism. **E.** Complete heart block. Note the independent regularity of both the atrial and ventricular rhythms (junctional escape) with no clear association with each other throughout the rhythm strip. (From Fansler DR, Chen J. Bradyarrhythmias and permanent pacemakers. In: Cuculich PS, Kates AM, eds. *The Washington Manual Cardiology Subspecialty Consult.* 3rd ed. Philadelphia, PA: Wolters Kluwer Health; 2014.)

- **Atropine**, an anticholinergic agent given in doses of 0.5–2.0 mg IV, is the cornerstone pharmacologic agent for emergent bradycardia treatment.
  ○ Dysfunction localized more proximally in the conduction system (i.e., symptomatic sinus bradycardia, first-degree AV block, Mobitz I second-degree AV block) tends to be responsive to atropine.
  ○ Distal disease is not responsive and can be worsened by atropine.
- Reversible causes of bradyarrhythmias should be identified, and any agents (digoxin, calcium channel blockers, β-adrenergic blockers) that caused or exacerbated the underlying dysrhythmia should be withheld.

Other Nonpharmacologic Therapies

- For bradyarrhythmias that have irreversible etiologies or that are secondary to medically necessary pharmacologic therapy, pacemaker therapy should be considered.
  - Temporary pacing is indicated for symptomatic second-degree or third-degree heart block caused by transient drug intoxication or electrolyte imbalance and complete heart block or Mobitz II second-degree AV block in the setting of an acute MI.
  - Sinus bradycardia, AF with a slow ventricular response, or Mobitz I second-degree AV block should be treated with temporary pacing only if significant symptoms or hemodynamic instability is present.
  - Temporary pacing is achieved preferably via insertion of a transvenous pacemaker. Transthoracic external pacing can be used, although the lack of reliability of capture and patient discomfort make this a second-line modality.
- Once hemodynamic stability has been established, attention turns to the indications for PPM placement.
  - In symptomatic patients, the key determinants include **potential reversibility of causative factors** and **temporal correlation of symptoms to the arrhythmia.**
  - In asymptomatic patients, the key determinant is based on whether the **discovered conduction abnormality has a natural history of progression to higher degrees of heart block** that portends a poor prognosis.
- **Permanent pacing**
  - Permanent pacing involves the placement of anchored, intracardiac pacing leads for the purpose of maintaining a heart rate sufficient to avoid symptoms and hemodynamic instability. Current devices, through maintenance of AV synchrony and rate-adaptive programming, more closely mimic normal physiologic heart rate behavior.
    - Class I (general agreement/evidence for benefit) and IIa (weight of conflicting opinion/evidence in favor of benefit) indications for permanent pacing are listed in Figure 7-3.
    - Pacemakers are designed to provide an electrical stimulus to the heart whenever the rate drops below a preprogrammed **lower rate limit.** Therefore, the ECG appearance of a PPM varies depending on the heart rate and state of AV conduction.
    - The pacing spikes produced by modern pacemakers are low amplitude, sharp, and immediately preceding the generated P wave or QRS complex indicating capture of the chamber. Figure 7-6 illustrates some common ECG appearances of normally and abnormally functioning pacemakers.
  - The pacemaker generator is commonly placed subcutaneously in the pectoral region on the side of the nondominant arm. The electronic lead(s) is placed in the cardiac chamber(s) via central veins. Complications of placement include **pneumothorax, device infection, bleeding, and rarely, cardiac perforation with tamponade.**
    - Before implantation, the patient must be free of any active infections, and anticoagulation issues must be carefully considered. Hematomas in the pacemaker pocket develop most commonly in patients who are receiving IV heparin or SC low–molecular-weight heparin. In severe cases, surgical evacuation is required.
    - Following implantation, **posteroanterior (PA) and lateral CXRs** are obtained to confirm appropriate lead placement. The pacemaker is interrogated at appropriate intervals—typically, before discharge, 2–6 weeks following discharge, and every 6–12 months thereafter.
  - **Pacing modes** are classified by a sequence of three to five letters. Most pacemakers are referred to by the three-letter code alone.
    - **Position I denotes the chamber that is paced:** A for atria, V for ventricle, or D for dual (A + V).
    - **Position II refers to the chamber that is sensed:** A for atria, V for ventricle, D for dual (A + V), or O for none.

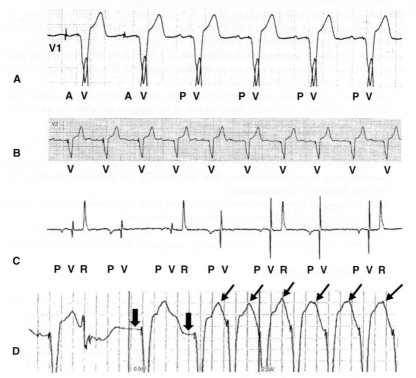

Figure 7-6. Pacemaker rhythms. **A.** Normal dual-chamber (DDD) pacing. First two complexes are atrioventricular (AV) sequential pacing, followed by sinus with atrial sensing and ventricular pacing. **B.** Normal single-chamber (VVI) pacing. The underlying rhythm is atrial fibrillation (no distinct P waves), with ventricular pacing at 60 bpm. **C.** Pacemaker malfunction. The underlying rhythm is sinus (P) at 80 bpm with 2:1 heart block and first-degree AV block (long PR). Ventricular pacing spikes are seen (V) after each P wave, demonstrating appropriate sensing and tracking of the P waves; however, there is failure to capture. **D.** Pacemaker-mediated tachycardia. A, paced atrial events; V, paced ventricular events; P, sensed atrial events; R, sensed ventricular events. (**D,** From Fansler DR, Chen J. Bradyarrhythmias and permanent pacemakers. In: Cuculich PS, Kates AM, eds. *The Washington Manual Cardiology Subspecialty Consult.* 3rd ed. Philadelphia, PA: Wolters Kluwer Health; 2014.)

- **Position III denotes the type of response the pacemaker will have to a sensed signal:** I for inhibition, T for triggering, D for dual (I + T), or O for none.
- **Position IV is used to signify the presence of rate-adaptive pacing (R)** in response to increased metabolic need.
  ○ The most common pacing systems used today include VVI, DDD, or AAI.
    - AAI systems should be used only for sinus node dysfunction in the absence of any AV conduction abnormalities.
    - The presence of AV nodal or His-Purkinje disease makes a dual-chamber device (i.e., DDD) more appropriate.
    - Patients in chronic AF warrant a single ventricular lead with VVI programming.
  ○ Modern-day pacemakers also have the capability of **mode switching**. This is useful in patients with DDD pacers who have paroxysmal tachyarrhythmias. When these

patients develop an atrial arrhythmia faster than a programmed mode switch rate, the device will switch to a mode (i.e., VVI) that does not track atrial signals. It will return to DDD when the tachyarrhythmia resolves.

○ Although infrequent, **pacemaker malfunction** is a potentially life-threatening situation, particularly for patients who are pacemaker dependent. The workup of suspected malfunction should begin with a 12-lead ECG.

  ▪ If no pacing activity is seen, one can place a magnet over the pacemaker to assess for output failure and ability to capture. **Application of the magnet switches the pacemaker to an asynchronous pacing mode.** For example, VVI mode becomes VOO (ventricular asynchronous pacing), and DDD mode becomes DOO (asynchronous AV pacing).

  ▪ If malfunction is obvious or if the ECG is unrevealing and malfunction is still suspected, then a formal interrogation of the device should be done. **Patients are given a card to carry upon implantation that will identify the make and model of the device to facilitate this evaluation.**

  ▪ **Chest radiograph (two views)** should also be obtained to assess for evidence of overt lead abnormalities (dislodgement, fracture, migration, etc.).

○ General categories of pacemaker malfunction include failure to pace (output failure), failure to capture, failure to sense (undersensing), and pacemaker-mediated dysrhythmias.

SPECIAL CONSIDERATIONS

• Often, episodes of bradycardia are transient and episodic; therefore, a baseline ECG may not be sufficient to capture the bradycardia. Some form of continuous monitoring is often required.
  ○ In the inpatient setting, **continuous central telemetry monitoring** can be used.
  ○ If further workup is done as an outpatient, **24- to 72-hour Holter monitoring** can be used if the episodes occur somewhat frequently. If infrequent, **an event recorder** or **ILR** should be considered.
  ○ Again, it is vital to correlate symptoms with the rhythm disturbances discovered via continuous monitoring—a task easily accomplished during inpatient care but more difficult as an outpatient. Therefore, the importance of accurate symptom diaries in the ambulatory setting should be emphasized to patients.
• To evaluate the sinus node's response to exertion (chronotropic competence), walking the patient in the hallway or up a flight of stairs under appropriate supervision is easy and inexpensive. A formal **exercise ECG** can be ordered if necessary.
• An **EPS** can also be used to assess sinus node function and AV conduction, but it is rarely necessary if the rhythm is already discovered via noninvasive modalities.

SYNCOPE

GENERAL PRINCIPLES

Syncope is a common clinical problem, and a primary goal of evaluation is to determine whether the patient is at increased risk of death.

Definition
Sudden, self-limited loss of consciousness and postural tone caused by transient global cerebral hypoperfusion and followed by spontaneous, complete, and prompt recovery.

Classification
Syncope can be classified into four major categories based on etiology:
• **Neurocardiogenic** (most common): vasovagal, carotid sinus hypersensitivity, and situational

- **Orthostatic hypotension:** hypovolemia, medication induced (iatrogenic), and autonomic dysfunction
- **Cardiovascular:**
  - **Arrhythmia:** sinus node dysfunction, AV block, pacemaker malfunction, VT/VF, SVT (rare)
  - **Mechanical:** HCM, valvular stenosis, aortic dissection, myxomas, pulmonary embolism, pulmonary HTN, acute MI, subclavian steal, etc.
- **Miscellaneous** (not true syncope): seizures, stroke/TIA, hypoglycemia, hypoxia, psychogenic, etc. Atherosclerotic cerebral artery disease is a rare cause of true syncope; the exception is severe obstructive four-vessel cerebrovascular disease (expect focal neurologic findings prior to syncope).

Epidemiology

- Common in the general population—**6% of medical admissions and 3% of emergency room visits**.
- Incidence is similar among men and women; one of the largest epidemiologic studies revealed an 11% incidence during an average follow-up of 17 years, with a sharp rise after age 70 years (*N Engl J Med 2002;347:878*).

Pathophysiology

- The two components of **neurocardiogenic syncope** are described as **cardioinhibitory**, in which bradycardia or asystole results from increased vagal outflow to the heart, and **vasodepression**, where peripheral vasodilation results from sympathetic withdrawal to peripheral arteries. Most patients have a combination of both components as the mechanism of their syncope.
- Specific stimuli may evoke a neurocardiogenic mechanism, leading to **situational syncope** (e.g., micturition, defecation, coughing, swallowing).

Risk Factors

Cardiovascular disease, history of **stroke or TIA**, and **HTN**. Also, low body mass index, increased alcohol intake, and diabetes are associated with syncope (*Am J Cardiol 2000;85:1189; N Engl J Med 2002;347:878*).

DIAGNOSIS

- A syncopal event may herald an otherwise unsuspected, potentially lethal cardiac condition, and therefore, a careful evaluation of the patient with syncope is warranted.
- A meticulous history and physical exam are key to an accurate diagnosis of the etiology of syncope. In 40% of episodes, the mechanism of syncope remains unexplained (*Ann Intern Med 1997;126:989*).

Clinical Presentation

History
Special attention should be focused on the **events or symptoms** that **precede and follow** the syncopal event, **eyewitness** accounts during the event, the **time course** of loss and resumption of consciousness (abrupt vs. gradual), and the patient's **medical history**.
- A characteristic prodrome of nausea, diaphoresis, visual changes, or flushing suggests neurocardiogenic syncope, as does the identification of a particular emotional or situational trigger and postepisode fatigue.
- Alternatively, an unusual sensory prodrome, incontinence, or a decreased level of consciousness that gradually clears suggests a seizure as a likely diagnosis.

- With transient ventricular arrhythmias, an abrupt loss of consciousness may occur with a rapid recovery.
- Syncope with exertion is a matter of concern for structural heart disease, pulmonary HTN, and CAD.

Physical Examination

The **cardiovascular** and **neurologic** exams should be the primary focus of initial evaluation.
- Orthostatic vital signs can reveal orthostatic hypotension. All patients should have blood pressure checked in both arms.
- Cardiac exam findings may help detect valvular heart disease, LV dysfunction, pulmonary HTN, etc.
- Neurologic findings are often absent but, if present, may point to a possible neurologic etiology of the syncopal event.
- Carotid sinus massage for 5–10 seconds with reproduction of symptoms and consequent ventricular pause >3 seconds is considered positive for carotid sinus hypersensitivity. It is critical to take proper precautions of telemetry monitoring, availability of bradycardia treatments, and avoiding the procedure in patients with known or suspected carotid disease.

Diagnostic Testing

- The presence of known **structural heart disease, abnormal ECG, age >65 years, focal neurologic findings**, and **severe orthostatic hypotension** suggest a potentially more ominous etiology. Therefore, these patients should be admitted for their workup to avoid delay and adverse outcomes.
- After the history and physical exam, the ECG is the most important diagnostic tool in the evaluation of the patient. It will be abnormal in 50% of cases but alone will yield a diagnosis in only 5% of these patients.
- If the patient has no history of heart disease or baseline ECG abnormalities, **tilt-table testing** has been used to evaluate a patient's hemodynamic response during transition from supine to upright state to precipitate a neurocardiogenic response. In an unselected population, the predictive value of this test is low.
- Please refer to Figure 7-7 for the diagnostic approach to syncope.

TREATMENT

In general, therapy is tailored to the underlying etiology of syncope with goals of preventing recurrence and reducing risk of injury or death.
- **Neurocardiogenic syncope:**
  - **Counsel** patients to take steps to avoid injury by being aware of prodromal symptoms and maintaining a **horizontal position** at those times.
  - Avoid known precipitants and maintain adequate **hydration**.
  - Employ **isometric muscle contraction** during prodrome to abort episode.
  - Evidence suggests that β-adrenergic blockers are probably unhelpful (*Circulation 2006;113:1164*); **selective serotonin reuptake inhibitor (SSRI) antidepressants** and **fludrocortisone** have a debatable effect; and **midodrine** (started at 5 mg PO tid and can be increased to 15 mg tid) is probably helpful in the treatment of neurocardiogenic syncope (*Am J Cardiol 2001;88:80; Heart Rhythm 2008;5:1609*).
  - In general, **PPMs** have no proven benefit (*JAMA 2003;289:2224*); however, permanent dual-chamber pacemakers with a hysteresis function (high-rate pacing in response to a detected sudden drop in heart rate) have been shown to be useful in highly selected patients with recurrent neurocardiogenic syncope with a prominent cardioinhibitory component (*J Am Coll Cardiol 1990;16:165*).

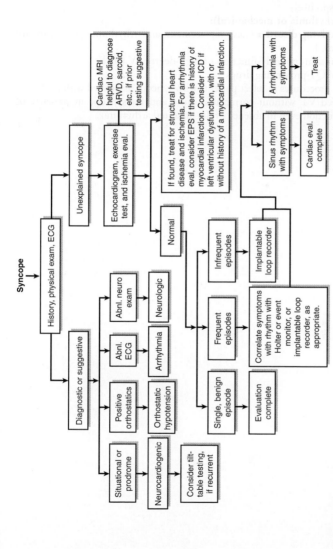

Figure 7-7. Algorithm for the evaluation of syncope. ARVD, arrhythmogenic right ventricular dysplasia; EPS, electrophysiology study; ICD, implantable cardioverter-defibrillator. (Data from Holley C. Evaluation of syncope. In: Cooper DH, et al., eds. *The Washington Manual of Medical Therapeutics.* 32nd ed. Philadelphia, PA: Lippincott Williams & Wilkins; 2007; and Strickberger SA, Benson DW, Biaggioni I, et al.; American Heart Association Councils on Clinical Cardiology, Cardiovascular Nursing, Cardiovascular Disease in the Young, and Stroke; Quality of Care and Outcomes Research Interdisciplinary Working Group; American College of Cardiology Foundation; Heart Rhythm Society; American Autonomic Society. AHA/ACCF Scientific Statement on the evaluation of syncope: From the American Heart Association Councils on Clinical Cardiology, Cardiovascular Nursing, Cardiovascular Disease in the Young, and Stroke, and the Quality of Care and Outcomes Research Interdisciplinary Working Group; and the American College of Cardiology Foundation: In collaboration with the Heart Rhythm Society: endorsed by the American Autonomic Society. *Circulation* 2006;113(2):316–27.)

- ○ **Cardiac pacing** for **carotid sinus hypersensitivity** is appropriate in syncopal patients.
- ○ In general, neurocardiogenic syncope is not associated with increased risk of mortality.
- **Orthostatic hypotension:**
  - ○ **Adequate hydration** and elimination of offending drugs.
  - ○ Salt supplementation, compressive stockings, and counseling on standing slowly.
  - ○ Midodrine and fludrocortisone can help by increasing systolic BP and expanding plasma volume, respectively.
- **Cardiovascular (arrhythmia or mechanical):**
  - ○ Treatment of **underlying disorder** (valve replacement, antiarrhythmic agent, coronary revascularization, etc.)
  - ○ **Cardiac pacing** for sinus node dysfunction or high-degree AV block
  - ○ Discontinuation of QT-prolonging drugs
  - ○ Catheter **ablation** procedures in select patients with syncope associated with SVT
- **ICD** for documented VT without correctable cause and for syncope in presence of significant LV dysfunction even in absence of documented arrhythmia.

8

Critical Care

Catherine Chen, Vladimir Despotovic, and
Marin H. Kollef

Respiratory Failure

GENERAL PRINCIPLES

Definitions

- **Hypercapnic respiratory failure:** Occurs with acute elevation of carbon dioxide (arterial carbon dioxide tension [$PaCO_2$] >45 mm Hg), producing a respiratory acidosis (pH <7.35).
- **Hypoxemic respiratory failure:** Occurs when normal gas exchange is seriously impaired, causing hypoxemia (arterial oxygen tension [PaO_2] <60 mm Hg or arterial oxygen saturation [SaO_2] <90%). Usually associated with tachypnea and hypocapnia; however, progression can lead to hypercapnia as well.
  - **Acute respiratory distress syndrome (ARDS)** is a form of hypoxemic respiratory failure caused by acute lung injury. The common end result is disruption of the alveolocapillary membrane, leading to increased vascular permeability and accumulation of inflammatory cells and protein-rich edema fluid within the alveolar space.
  - The ARDS Definition Task Force redefined ARDS as follows (*JAMA 2012;307:2526*):
    - Onset within 1 week of a known clinical insult or new or worsening respiratory symptoms;
    - Bilateral opacities not fully explained by effusions, lobar/lung collapse, or nodules;
    - Respiratory failure not fully explained by cardiac failure or volume overload; and
    - Impaired oxygenation with low PaO_2 to fraction of inspired oxygen (FIO_2) ratio ($PaO_2/FIO_2 \leq 300$ mm Hg)
  - Severity of ARDS stratified based on PaO_2/FIO_2:
    - Mild: 200 mm Hg < $PaO_2/FIO_2 \leq 300$ mm Hg with positive end-expiratory pressure (PEEP) ≥ 5 cm H_2O
    - Moderate: 100 mm Hg < $PaO_2/FIO_2 \leq 200$ mm Hg with PEEP ≥ 5 cm H_2O
    - Severe: $PaO_2/FIO_2 \leq 100$ mm Hg with PEEP ≥ 5 cm H_2O

Pathophysiology

- **Hypercapnic respiratory failure** primarily occurs due to ventilatory failure, resulting in an elevated $PaCO_2$:

$$PaCO_2 = \frac{\dot{V}CO_2}{\dot{V}_A} = \frac{\dot{V}CO_2}{\dot{V}_E - \dot{V}_D}$$

where $\dot{V}CO_2$ = CO_2 production, $\dot{V}_A$ = alveolar ventilation, $\dot{V}_E$ = expired total ventilation, and $\dot{V}_D$ = dead space ventilation. Rarely, increased carbon dioxide production may contribute to hypercapnia. The differential diagnosis for ventilator failure can be categorized as follows:
  - Central nervous system: Hypoventilation/apnea causing decreased respiratory rate ("won't breathe"); e.g., opiate overdose, central apnea/hypoventilation
  - Peripheral nervous system: Neuromuscular failure causing decreased tidal volume ("can't breathe"); e.g., Guillain-Barré, myasthenia gravis, amyotrophic lateral sclerosis
  - Intercostal muscles: Muscle weakness causing decreased tidal volume; e.g., muscular dystrophies, myopathies
  - Thoracic cavity: Anatomic abnormalities causing decreased tidal volume; e.g., scoliosis, thoracoplasty
  - Airways: Airway pathologies causing increased dead space; e.g., asthma, chronic obstructive pulmonary disease (COPD)

- **Hypoxemic respiratory failure** usually is the result of the lung's reduced ability to deliver oxygen across the alveolocapillary membrane. The severity of gas exchange impairment is determined by calculating the $P(A–a)O_2$ gradient using the alveolar gas equation:

$$PaO_2 = FIO_2 (P_{ATM} - P_{H_2O}) - \frac{PACO_2}{R}$$

where FIO_2 = the fraction of inspired oxygen, P_{ATM} = atmospheric pressure, P_{H_2O} = water vapor pressure, and R = the respiratory quotient. Hypoxemia is caused by:
  - **Ventilation–perfusion (V/Q) mismatch:** Occurs when perfusion does not compensate for a change in ventilation or vice versa (e.g., pulmonary embolism and emphysema). Administration of supplemental oxygen increases PaO_2, although it should be noted that oxygen administration paradoxically worsens V/Q matching in emphysema via reversing hypoxic vasoconstriction of pulmonary capillaries, leading to hypercarbia.
  - **Shunt:** An extreme of V/Q mismatch. Occurs when mixed venous blood bypasses lung units and enters systemic arterial circulation. Congenital shunts are due to developmental anomalies of the heart and great vessels. Acquired shunts are due to pus, water, blood, or atelectasis. Acquired cardiac and peripheral vascular shunts also can occur (Table 8-1). Shunts are associated with a widened $P(A–a)O_2$ gradient, and the resultant hypoxemia is resistant to correction with supplemental oxygen alone.

TABLE 8-1	Causes of Shunt
Cause	**Examples**
Pulmonary shunts	
Pus	Pneumonia
Water	Cardiogenic pulmonary edema
	Acute myocardial infarction
	Systolic or diastolic left ventricular failure
	Mitral regurgitation or stenosis
	Noncardiogenic pulmonary edema
	Primary acute respiratory distress syndrome
	Aspiration
	Inhalational injury
	Near drowning
	Secondary acute respiratory distress syndrome
	Sepsis
	Pancreatitis
	Reperfusion injury
	Upper airway obstruction pulmonary edema
	Neurogenic pulmonary edema
	High-altitude pulmonary edema
Blood	Diffuse alveolar hemorrhage
Atelectasis	Pleural effusion with atelectasis
	Mucous plugging with lobar collapse
Cardiac shunts	Patent foramen ovale
	Atrial septal defect
	Ventricular septal defect
Vascular shunts	Arteriovenous malformation

- ○ **Diffusion impairment:** Diseases that cause thickening of the interstitium, such as idiopathic pulmonary fibrosis, result in hypoxemia due to gas equilibration time exceeding red blood cell transit time. Hypoxemia usually responds to supplemental oxygen therapy.
- ○ **Hypoventilation:** A decrease in minute ventilation results in an increase in $PACO_2$, displacing oxygen. In pure hypoventilation, the $P(A-a)O_2$ gradient is normal. Primary treatment is directed at correcting the cause of hypoventilation.
- ○ **Low mixed venous oxygenation:** Normally, the lungs fully oxygenate pulmonary arterial blood, and mixed venous oxygen tension (PvO_2) does not affect PaO_2 significantly. However, a decreased PvO_2 can lower the PaO_2 significantly when either intrapulmonary shunting or V/Q mismatch is present. Factors that can contribute to low mixed venous oxygenation include anemia, hypoxemia, inadequate cardiac output (CO), and increased oxygen consumption. Improving oxygen delivery to tissues by increasing hemoglobin or CO usually decreases oxygen extraction and improves mixed venous oxygen saturation (SvO_2).
- ○ **Low inspired oxygen:** The partial pressure of inspired oxygen is reduced at high altitude secondary to decreased barometric pressure. Inhaled toxic gas decreases FIO_2.
- **Mixed respiratory failure:** Most patients who have respiratory failure have both hypoxemia and hypercarbia. Frequently seen in postoperative patients and patients with COPD exacerbations.

Noninvasive Oxygen Therapy

GENERAL PRINCIPLES

- **Nasal cannulas** are most commonly used, but the exact FIO_2 delivered is unknown because it is influenced by peak inspiratory flow demand. Each additional liter of flow increases FIO_2 by approximately 4%. Flow rates should be limited to ≤ 5 L/min.
- **Humidified high-flow nasal cannula** can deliver heated and humidified oxygen at higher flows and concentration—up to 50 L/min and 100% FIO_2—than traditional nasal prongs. Optiflow is the most commonly used system.
- **Venturi masks** allow the precise administration of oxygen. Usual FIO_2 values delivered are 24%, 28%, 31%, 35%, 40%, and 50%.
- **Nonrebreathing masks** achieve higher oxygen concentrations (80–90%). A one-way valve prevents exhaled gases from entering the reservoir bag, maximizing the FIO_2.
- **Noninvasive positive-pressure ventilation (NPPV):** Includes continuous positive airway pressure (CPAP) and bilevel positive airway pressure (BPAP) ventilation.
  - ○ Decreases the need for endotracheal intubation and mechanical ventilation in patients with neuromuscular disease, COPD, congestive heart failure, and postoperative respiratory insufficiency (*Crit Care Clin 2007;23:201*).
  - ○ Use limited to patients who are conscious, cooperative, able to protect their airway, and hemodynamically stable (*N Engl J Med 1998;339:429*).
  - ○ May be poorly tolerated due to claustrophobia or aerophagia, so **use should be limited to those with an anticipated short duration of respiratory failure** (e.g., cardiogenic pulmonary edema, COPD exacerbation).
  - ○ **Close monitoring is required during its use.**
  - ○ **CPAP** prevents alveolar collapse during expiration. Initially, 5 cm H_2O of pressure should be applied, and if hypoxemia persists, the level should be increased by 3–5 cm H_2O up to a level of 10–15 cm H_2O.
  - ○ **BPAP** supports both inspiration and expiration to decrease work of breathing. An inspiratory pressure of 5–10 cm H_2O and an expiratory pressure of 5 cm H_2O are reasonable starting points. Ventilation is determined by the difference between inspiratory and expiratory pressures (i.e., "drive pressure"), and inspiratory pressures can be uptitrated to achieve adequate tidal volumes and minute ventilation.

Airway Management and Tracheal Intubation

GENERAL PRINCIPLES

- **Airway management**
  - **Head and jaw positioning:** The oropharynx should be inspected, and all foreign bodies should be removed. If the patient is unresponsive, the head tilt–chin lift maneuver should be performed (see Airway Emergencies in Chapter 26, Medical Emergencies). If neck immobilization is required, jaw thrust should be performed.
  - **Oral and nasopharyngeal airways:** Used when head and jaw positioning fail to establish a patent airway. Initially inserted with the concave curve of the airway facing toward the roof of the mouth. The oral airway then is turned 180 degrees as it is inserted so that the concave curve of the airway follows the natural curve of the tongue. Careful monitoring of airway patency is required, as malpositioning can push the tongue posteriorly and result in oropharyngeal obstruction. Nasopharyngeal airways are made of soft plastic and are passed easily down one of the nasal passages to the posterior pharynx after topical nasal lubrication and anesthesia with viscous lidocaine jelly.
  - **Bag-valve-mask ventilation:** Ineffective respiratory efforts can be augmented with simple bag-valve-mask ventilation. Proper fitting and positioning of the mask using the "EC" hand position—thumb and index finger forming a "C" around the mask, and the remaining fingers forming an "E" to support the jaw—ensure a tight seal around the mouth and nose. Used in conjunction with proper positioning and airway adjuncts, e.g., oral airway.
  - **Laryngeal mask airway (LMA):** The LMA is a supraglottic airway device shaped like an endotracheal tube connected to an elliptical mask. It is designed to be inserted over the tongue and seated in the hypopharynx, covering the supraglottic structures and relatively isolating the trachea. It is a temporary airway and should not be used for prolonged ventilatory support.
- **Endotracheal intubation** (*Int Anesthesiol Clin 2000;38:1*)
  - **Indications:** Initiation of mechanical ventilation, airway protection, inadequate oxygenation with less invasive methods, prevention of aspiration, excessive pulmonary secretions, and hyperventilation as a treatment for increased intracranial pressure
  - **Before endotracheal tube intubation** is attempted:
    - Evaluate head and neck positioning: Oral, pharyngeal, and tracheal axes should be aligned by flexing the neck and extending the head, achieving the "sniffing" position.
    - Obese patients may require a shoulder roll or ramp.
    - Necessary equipment must be at the bedside: oxygen tubing, bag-valve-mask device, suction and tubing, endotracheal tube with stylet, 10-mL syringe, direct laryngoscope, direct laryngoscope blades (most commonly Macintosh or Miller size 3 or 4), and end-tidal carbon dioxide (CO_2) colorimeter.
    - Medications that may be used during intubation include neuromuscular blocking agents, opiates, and anxiolytics. Commonly used agents are listed in Table 8-2.
  - **Techniques** include:
    - Direct laryngoscopic orotracheal intubation: Most commonly used, requiring only a direct laryngoscope and light source. Procedure available in Table 8-3.
    - Video laryngoscopic orotracheal intubation: Allows for direct visual confirmation of intubation by a second observer via video monitoring.
    - Advanced techniques for specialists include blind nasotracheal intubation and flexible fiber optically guided orotracheal or nasotracheal intubation.
  - **Verification of correct endotracheal tube location and positioning:** Proper tube location must be ensured by:
    - Fiber optic inspection of the airways through the endotracheal tube; *or*
    - Direct visualization of the endotracheal tube passing through the vocal cords; *and*

- Use of an end-tidal CO_2 monitor; *and*
- CXR
- Clinical evaluation of the patient (i.e., listening for bilateral breath sounds over the chest and the absence of ventilation over the stomach) and radiographic evaluation alone are unreliable for establishing correct endotracheal tube location.
- The tip of the endotracheal tube should be 3–5 cm above the carina, depending on head and neck position.
  ○ **After successful intubation:**
    - Tracheal tube cuff pressures: Should be monitored at regular intervals and maintained below capillary filling pressure (25 mm Hg) to prevent ischemic mucosal injury.
    - Sedation: Anxiolytics and opiates are frequently used to facilitate endotracheal intubation and mechanical ventilation. Commonly used agents are listed in Table 8-2.
  ○ **Complications:** Improper endotracheal tube location or positioning is the most important immediate complication to be recognized and corrected.
    - Esophageal intubation should be suspected if no end-tidal CO_2 is detected after three to five breaths, hypoxemia persists or develops, there is a lack of breath sounds, or abdominal distention or regurgitation of stomach contents occurs.
    - Mainstem intubation should be suspected if peak airway pressures are elevated or there are unilateral breath sounds.
    - Other complications include dislodgment of teeth and upper airway trauma.
- **Surgical airways**
  ○ **Indications** for surgical airways in critical care:
    - Life-threatening upper airway obstruction (e.g., epiglottitis, angioedema, facial burns, laryngeal/vocal cord edema) preventing bag-valve-mask ventilation and endotracheal intubation cannot be performed.
    - Need for prolonged respiratory support.
  ○ **Needle cricothyrotomy:** Indicated in emergency settings when the patient cannot be ventilated noninvasively, standard endotracheal intubation is unsuccessful, and a surgical airway cannot be immediately performed. The steps of the procedure are listed in Table 8-3.
  ○ **Cricothyrotomy:** Indicated in emergency settings when the patient cannot be ventilated noninvasively and standard endotracheal intubation is unsuccessful. The steps of the procedure are listed in Table 8-3.
  ○ **Tracheostomy:** Most commonly performed due to need for prolonged respiratory support.
    - Recent review demonstrated no benefit of early (≤10 days) tracheostomy over late (>10 days) tracheostomy (*Br J Anaesth 2006 Jan;96(1):127–31*).
    - Tracheostomy should be considered if prolonged ventilatory support is anticipated after 10–14 days of endotracheal intubation.
    - **Complications:** Tracheostomy sites require at least 72 hours to mature, and tube dislodgment prior to maturation can lead to serious, life-threatening complications.
      □ A tracheostomy tube that has been dislodged prior to stoma maturation **should not be reinserted** due to the risk of creating a false tract.
      □ **Standard orotracheal intubation** should be performed if a tracheostomy tube is dislodged prior to stoma maturation.
      □ **Tracheo-innominate artery fistulas** are an uncommon but life-threatening complication of tracheostomy that most commonly occurs 7–14 days after the procedure but can occur up to 6 weeks after the procedure. Immediate management includes overinflation of the tracheostomy tube cuff, digital compression of the stoma, and surgical exploration (*Br J Anaesth 2006;96:127*).

TABLE 8-2 Drugs to Facilitate Endotracheal Intubation and Mechanical Ventilation

Drug	Bolus Dosages (IV)	Continuous-Infusion Dosages[a]	Onset	Duration After Single Dose
Succinylcholine[b]	0.3–1 mg/kg	—	45–60 s	2–10 min
Pancuronium	0.05–0.1 mg/kg	1–2 µg/kg/min	2–4 min	60–90 min
Vecuronium	0.08–0.1 mg/kg	0.3–1 µg/kg/min	2–4 min	30–45 min
Atracurium	0.2–0.6 mg/kg	5–15 µg/kg/min	2–4 min	20–35 min
Lorazepam[a]	0.03–0.1 mg/kg	0.01–0.1 mg/kg/h, titrate to effect	5–20 min	2–6 h[c]
Midazolam[a]	0.02–0.08 mg/kg	0.04–0.2 mg/kg/h, titrate to effect	1–5 min	30–60 min[c]
Morphine	0.01–0.15 mg/kg	0.1–0.5 mg/kg/h, titrate to effect	2–10 min	2–4 h[c]
Fentanyl	0.35–1.5 µg/kg	1–10 µg/kg/h, titrate to effect	30–60 s	30–60 min[c]
Etomidate[b]	0.3–0.4 mg/kg	—	10–20 s	4–10 min
Propofol	0.25–0.5 mg/kg	25–80 µg/kg/min	15–60 s	3–10 min[c]
Dexmedetomidine	1 µg/kg	0.2–0.7 µg/kg/h	10 min	30 min

[a]A continuous infusion should be started or titrated upward only after the desired level of sedation is achieved with bolus administration.
[b]Use only in the process of rapid sequence intubation.
[c]Duration is prolonged with continuous IV administration. Frequent titration to the minimum effective dose is required to prevent accumulation of drug.

TABLE 8-3	Procedure for Endotracheal Intubation, Needle Cricothyroid-otomy, and Cricothyrotomy

Endotracheal Intubation Using Direct Laryngoscopy

Equipment	Oxygen tubing, bag-valve-mask device, suction and tubing, oral airway, laryngoscope, laryngoscope blades, 7.0-mm inner diameter endotracheal tube with stylet, syringe, end-tidal carbon dioxide colorimeter
Technique	Step 1	Place the patient in the "sniffing" position, with neck flexed and head extended; obese patients will require shoulder roll or ramp.
	Step 2	Preoxygenate the patient with 100% oxygen through the bag-valve-mask device until saturations are maintained at >95% for 3–5 min, and suction oral secretions as necessary.
	Step 3	During preoxygenation, ensure that all equipment necessary is present and functional: check the endotracheal tube cuff with inflation and deflation, and that the light of the laryngoscope is functional.
	Step 4	Administer IV sedation; once the patient is appropriately sedated, open the mouth with the right hand and insert the laryngoscope blade into the right side of mouth with the left hand, sweeping the tongue to the left.
	Step 5	Advance the blade to the base of the tongue, then lift vertically to visualize the vocal cords; **do not tilt the laryngoscope.**
	Step 6	If vocal cords are visible, insert the endotracheal tube with the stylet with the right hand; once the cuff is past the vocal cords, remove stylet. **Do not attempt intubation if the vocal cords are not visible.**
	Step 7	Advance the endotracheal tube until it is at 21 cm at the gum/teeth for women and 22 cm for men, and inflate the cuff.
	Step 8	**Check tube location** with end-tidal carbon dioxide colorimeter, auscultation over the chest and abdomen, AND chest radiograph.

Needle Cricothyroidotomy (*Br J Hosp Med (Lond) 2009;70:M186*)

Equipment	Large-bore IV catheter with needle stylet, 3-mL Luer lock syringe with plunger removed, 7-mm inner diameter endotracheal tube adapter
Technique	Step 1	Extend the neck and identify the cricothyroid membrane, located inferior to the thyroid cartilage and superior to the thyroid gland.
	Step 2	Stabilize the thyroid cartilage with the nondominant hand and, using the dominant hand, introduce the IV catheter with the needle stylet at a 45-degree angle through the cricothyroid membrane into the trachea, aspirating air to confirm location.

(continued)

TABLE 8-3		Procedure for Endotracheal Intubation, Needle Cricothyroidotomy, and Cricothyrotomy (*Continued*)
	Step 3	Advance the catheter to the hub, and remove the needle stylet.
	Step 4	Attach the Luer lock syringe to the catheter, and then the endotracheal tube adapter to the syringe to allow for bag-valve ventilation.

Cricothyrotomy (*Principles of Critical Care, 3e. Chapter 34;2005*)

Equipment		Scalpel, Kelly forceps, 6-mm inner diameter or smaller endotracheal tube
Technique	Step 1	Extend the neck and identify the cricothyroid membrane, located inferior to the thyroid cartilage and superior to the thyroid gland.
	Step 2	Stabilize the thyroid cartilage with the nondominant hand and, using the dominant hand, make a 1-cm horizontal incision just above the superior border of the cricoid.
	Step 3	Using the Kelly forceps, dissect until the cricothyroid membrane is visualized, and then make a vertical incision through the midline of the membrane, being careful to not pass the blade too deeply.
	Step 4	Widen the incision with Kelly forceps until the endotracheal tube can be inserted, and then inflate the cuff.

Mechanical Ventilation

GENERAL PRINCIPLES

- **Basic modes of ventilation:** Determines how the ventilator initiates a breath (triggering), how the breath is delivered, how patient-initiated breaths are supported, and when to terminate the breath to allow expiration (cycling).
  - **Triggering a breath** occurs after a period of time has elapsed (time-triggered) or when the patient has generated sufficient negative airway pressure or inspiratory flow that exceeds a predetermined threshold (patient-triggered).
  - **Assist-control (AC):** Primary mode of ventilation used in respiratory failure Delivers a fully supported breath whether time- or patient-triggered
  - **Synchronized intermittent mandatory ventilation (SIMV):** Commonly used in surgical patients
    - Delivers a fully supported breath only when time-triggered.
    - Patient-triggered breaths are unassisted or minimally assisted; volumes determined by patient's effort and lung compliance.
  - **Pressure support ventilation (PSV):** A spontaneous mode of ventilation without a set respiratory rate. Delivers a practitioner-determined inspiratory pressure during patient-triggered breathing. **No respiratory rate is set, so no guaranteed minute ventilation.**
  - **Volume control (VC):** Delivers a practitioner-determined tidal volume (V_T) for each breath. Patient airflow is limited to constant or decelerating ramp pattern. When predetermined V_T is delivered, airflow is terminated and exhalation occurs.
  - **Pressure control (PC):** Delivers a practitioner-determined inspiratory pressure for a predetermined inspiratory time for each breath. Airflow is determined by the patient and limited by the inspiratory pressure. When inspiratory time has elapsed, inspiratory

pressure is terminated and exhalation occurs. **Does not deliver a guaranteed V_T and, therefore, minute ventilation.**

- **Basic ventilator settings:** Requires both a mode (AC vs. SIMV) and a control (VC vs. PC).
  - **Respiratory rate**, **FIO₂**, and **PEEP** must be set for all modes of ventilation.
  - For VC, the following must be entered:
    - **V_T:** 6–8 mL/kg ideal body weight (IBW) to prevent barotrauma.
      IBW: Male IBW = 50 kg + 2.3 kg/in × (Height in inches − 60) [imperial], 50 kg + 1.1 kg/cm × (Height in cm − 152.4) [metric]; Female IBW = 45.5 kg + 2.3 kg/in × (Height in inches − 60) [imperial], 45.5 kg + 1.1 kg/cm × (Height in cm − 152.4) [metric]
    - **Inspiratory flow rate:** May be constant (square wave) or ramp (decelerating). Recommend 60 L/min or greater; higher flow rates increase expiration time.
  - For PC, the following must be entered:
    - **Inspiratory pressure:** Should be sufficient to generate V_T of 6–8 mL/kg IBW. Should not exceed 35 cm H₂O due to risk of barotrauma.
    - **Inspiratory time:** Usually <1 second. Shorter inspiratory times increase expiration time.
  - For SIMV, patient-initiated breaths may be assisted with pressure support.
- **Basic ventilator terminology and management:** Flow-time and pressure-time tracings are demonstrated in Figure 8-1.
  - FIO₂: Initial FIO₂ when initiating mechanical ventilation should be 100%, and FIO₂ should be titrated to maintain SaO₂ >87% or PaO₂ >55 mm Hg.
  - **Minute ventilation:** Defined as the product of V_T and respiratory rate (V_T × RR). Normally between 5–10 L/min in resting adults, but may be much higher in high metabolic states, e.g., septic shock.
  - **Peak airway pressure:** Composed of pressures necessary to overcome inspiratory airflow resistance, chest wall recoil resistance, and alveolar opening resistance. Does not reflect alveolar pressure.
  - **Mean airway pressure:** Mean pressures applied during the inspiratory cycle. Approximates alveolar pressure until overdistention occurs.
  - **Plateau pressure:** Reflects alveolar pressure. Checked by performing an end-inspiratory hold maneuver to allow pressures through the tracheobronchial tree to equilibrate.
- **Mechanical ventilation for patients with ARDS:** Due to severe hypoxia associated with ARDS, oxygenation and prevention of barotrauma may have to be prioritized over ventilation, resulting in hypercapnia. Hypercapnia resulting in a pH of 7.20–7.35 may need to be tolerated in order to sufficiently oxygenate the patient ("**permissive hypercapnia**").
- Advanced modes of ventilation: Should be used only after discussion with higher-level practitioners.
  - Volume-assured PSV: Ventilator initially delivers practitioner-determined pressure support; if insufficient to achieve desired V_T within the breath, then ventilator will increase inspiratory pressure to achieve desired V_T.
  - Pressure-regulated VC ventilation: Ventilator determines after each breath if inspiratory pressure was sufficient to achieve targeted V_T; if insufficient or excessive, then ventilator will adjust inspiratory pressure to achieve desired V_T.
  - Inverse-ratio ventilation (IRV): A pressure-controlled method of ventilation most commonly used in ARDS. Inspiratory time exceeds expiratory time to improve oxygenation at the expense of ventilation; patients are permitted to become hypercapnic to pH 7.20. If obstructive lung disease is present, can cause auto-PEEP and excessive hypercapnia.
  - Airway pressure release ventilation (APRV): An extreme version of IRV. Inspiratory pressure (P_{high}) applied for a prolonged period of time (T_{high}) with a short expiratory time (T_{low}, or release time)—usually <1 second—to allow for ventilation. Like IRV, patients are permitted to be hypercapnic to pH 7.20.
    Bilevel ventilation: **Not to be confused with BPAP.** APRV with spontaneous breathing allowed during T_{high} to improve ventilation.

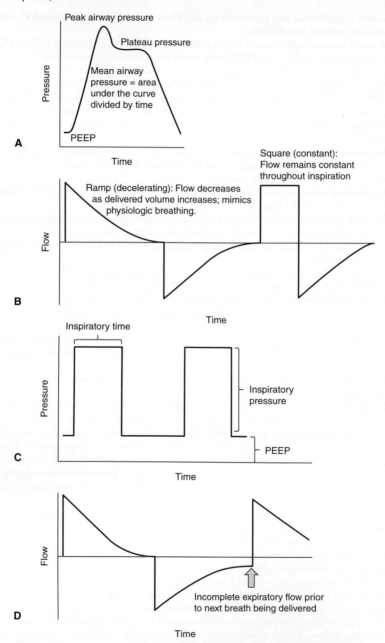

Figure 8-1. Flow-time and pressure-time tracings. **A.** Pressure-time curve for one breath. **B.** Flow-time curve for volume-control ventilation. Pressure varies throughout inspiratory time, depending on lung compliance. **C.** Pressure-time curve for pressure-control ventilation. Flow varies throughout inspiratory time, depending on lung compliance. **D.** Pressure-time curve demonstrating auto–positive end-expiratory pressure (auto-PEEP).

○ High-frequency oscillatory ventilation: A pressure-controlled form of ventilation. Mean airway pressure set at the mean airway pressure that was previously required to maintain oxygenation. Very small, rapidly delivered breaths at 3–15 Hz allow for CO_2 clearance. Power determines V_T of these very small breaths and should be set at a level that causes vibration of the mid-thigh. Patients must be paralyzed to tolerate this form of ventilation. Previously thought to potentially improve outcomes in ARDS (*BMJ 2010;340:c2327*), but **recent prospective randomized controlled trials demonstrate no reduction** (*N Engl J Med 2013;368:806*) **and possible increase in mortality** (*N Engl J Med 2013;368:795*).

ADJUNCTS TO MECHANICAL VENTILATION

• **Neuromuscular blockade:** Most commonly used in severe ARDS to decrease oxygen consumption from accessory inspiratory muscle use. Recent meta-analysis indicates that its use is associated with lower risk of barotrauma and lower mortality, but more investigation is needed (*Crit Care 2013;17:R43*).
• **Prone positioning:** Improves oxygenation in patients with ARDS by improving V/Q mismatching and decreasing shunt by decreasing amount of atelectatic lung. Early application is associated with improved mortality in ARDS (*N Engl J Med 2013;368:2159*).
  ○ Patients with moderate to severe ARDS (PaO_2/FIO_2 <150 mm Hg) should be considered.
  ○ Patients should receive neuromuscular blockade to tolerate proning.
  ○ Hemodynamic instability an **absolute contraindication**.
  ○ Morbid obesity a relative contraindication.
  ○ Patients should remain prone for at least 16 consecutive hours for benefit.
    Complete proning protocol available online at *New England Journal of Medicine. Available at http://www.nejm.org/action/showMediaPlayer?doi=10.1056%2FNEJMoa121410 3&aid=NEJMoa1214103_attach_1&area=*
• Inhaled prostacyclins: Used in ARDS. Theoretically, inhalation of prostacyclins—a class of vasodilators—improves oxygenation by preferential vasodilation of the capillary beds of ventilated lung.
  ○ Small studies have demonstrated transient improvement in oxygenation (*Pharmacotherapy 2014;34:279*).
  ○ **No studies have been performed to investigate whether mortality benefit exists.**
  ○ Has antiplatelet effects, so theoretical concern for worsening diffuse alveolar hemorrhage.
  ○ Expensive therapy: $150 per day (*J Thorac Cardiovasc Surg 2004;127:1058*).
• Nitric oxide: Used in ARDS. Like inhaled prostacyclins, improves oxygenation by preferential vasodilation of capillary beds of ventilated lung.
  ○ Transient (24-hour) improvement in oxygenation that resolves by 48 hours (*JAMA 2004;291:1603*)
  ○ **Does not improve mortality** (*Crit Care Med 2014;42:404*) **and may increase incidence of renal failure** (*Anesth Analg 2011;112:1411*)
  ○ Very expensive therapy: $3000 per day (*J Thorac Cardiovasc Surg 2004;127:1058*)
• **Helium-oxygen mixture (Heliox):** Used in asthma and severe bronchospasm. Usually, a mixture of 80% helium and 20% oxygen, although also available in other ratios. Theoretically decreases airway resistance due to its low density, thereby decreasing work of breathing. Studies have suggested benefit only in patients with more severe obstruction (*Cochrane Database Syst Rev 2006;(4):CD002884:1–28*).

COMPLICATIONS OF MECHANICAL VENTILATION

• **Airway malpositioning and occlusion:** See Airway Management and Tracheal Intubation section.
• **Troubleshooting ventilator alarms:** See Figure 8-2.

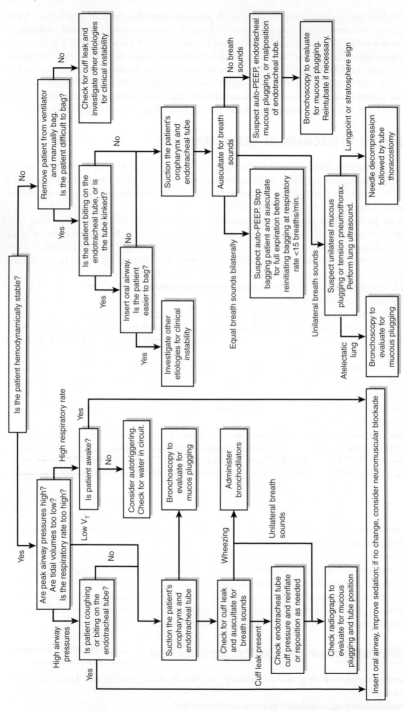

Figure 8-2. Troubleshooting ventilator alarms: what to do when the patient is hypoxic. Auto-PEEP, auto–positive end-expiratory pressure.

- **Auto-PEEP:** Occurs when inspiration is initiated before complete exhalation is complete. May be detected on physical exam by wheezing that does not terminate prior to the next breath. Demonstrated on ventilator flow-time loop by flow not returning to baseline prior to delivery of next breath (Figure 8-1). Excessive auto-PEEP can lead to cardiac decompensation due to tension pneumothorax–like physiology.
- **Barotrauma/volutrauma:** Occurs when excessive PEEP, inspiratory pressures, or tidal volumes are applied, resulting in alveolar rupture and dissection of air along interstitial tissues and causing pneumothorax, pneumomediastinum, pneumopericardium, or pneumoperitoneum. If undetected, can result in life-threatening cardiac decompensation.
- **Ventilator-associated events (VAE):** Encompasses a broad range of conditions and complications that occur in mechanically ventilated patients. Must have a baseline stability of >2 days, defined as stable or decreasing daily minimum PEEP or FIO_2 (*Centers for Disease Control and Prevention 2015 VAE*). Available at *http://www.cdc.gov/nhsn/PDFs/pscManual/10-VAE_FINAL.pdf*
  ○ **Ventilator-associated condition:** Patient develops worsening oxygenation, defined as requiring increased daily minimum PEEP ($\geq$3 cm H_2O above baseline) or FIO_2 ($\geq$20% above baseline) for $\geq$2 calendar days
  ○ **Infection-related ventilator-associated complication:** Within 2 calendar days of worsening oxygenation, **both** of the following criteria are met:
    ▪ Temperature >38°C or < 36°C **or** WBC count $\geq$12,000 or $\leq$4000 cells/μL
    ▪ At least one new antimicrobial agent is initiated and continued for $\geq$4 calendar days
  ○ **Ventilator-associated pneumonia (VAP):** On or after calendar day 3 of mechanical ventilation and within 2 calendar days before or after worsening oxygenation, one of the following criteria are met:
    ▪ **Positive culture** from endotracheal aspirate, bronchoalveolar lavage, lung tissue, or protected specimen brush that meets quantitative or semi-qualitative thresholds
    ▪ **Purulent respiratory secretions and positive culture** from one of the above specimens that does not meet quantitative threshold
    ▪ Positive pleural fluid culture; diagnostic test for *Legionella* species; diagnostic test on respiratory secretions for influenza virus, respiratory syncytial virus, adenovirus, parainfluenza virus, rhinovirus, human metapneumovirus, or coronavirus
    ▪ Lung histopathology demonstrating abscess formation, consolidation, parenchymal invasion by fungi, or evidence of infection of the viral pathogens listed above
  ○ Daily oral care with chlorhexidine mouthwash decreases risk of VAP.
- Stress-induced peptic ulcer disease: Traditionally thought to be a significant risk of prolonged critical illness and mechanical ventilation, requiring prophylaxis with proton pump inhibitor or H_2 receptor antagonists. However, concerns of increased risk of VAP and recent meta-analyses indicate that stress ulcer prophylaxis needs to be more closely examined (*J Intensive Care Med 2014;40:11*).
- Oxygen toxicity: Breathing high FIO_2 (>60%) for a prolonged period of time (>48 hours) can lead to excessive free radical generation, resulting in lung injury. However, hypoxemia is more dangerous than brief exposure to high FIO_2.

LIBERATION FROM MECHANICAL VENTILATION

- Readiness to wean: Daily assessment of readiness for extubation should begin once underlying disease process begins to resolve and minimal ventilator support is required.
  ○ Minimal ventilator support: FIO_2 $\leq$40%, PEEP 5 cm H_2O to maintain SpO_2 >90%.
  ○ Arterial blood gas: pH and $PaCO_2$ should be at the patient's baseline; particularly important for patients with chronic CO_2 retention.
  ○ Ventilation requirement: Minute ventilation should be <10 L/min and respiratory rate <30 breaths/min.

○ Mental status: Patient should be awake, alert, and cooperative.
○ Secretions: Secretions should be thin, scant in amount, and easily suctioned; patient should not require suctioning more frequently than every 4 hours prior to extubation.
○ Strength: Patient should have strong cough and be able to lift head off the bed and hold it in flexion for >5 seconds.
○ Breathing trial: Patient should be able to generate spontaneous V_T >5 mL/kg IBW.
○ Rapid shallow breathing index (RSBI): Defined as ratio of respiratory rate to V_T in liters (f/V_T). RSBI >105 accurately predicts weaning failure (*N Engl J Med 1991;23:1445*), but RSBI ≤105 is less accurate at predicting weaning success.
• Methods: **Protocol of daily sedation interruption and breathing trials** is most important predictor of timely liberation from mechanical ventilation (*Cochrane Database Syst Rev 2014;11:CD006904:1–61*), regardless of technique used. Trial times vary between 30 minutes and 2 hours.
○ PSV: No time-triggered breaths, but patient remains connected to the ventilator. PEEP is usually at 5 cm H_2O, with low levels of pressure support (5–10 cm H_2O) during spontaneous breathing.
○ T-piece/spontaneous breathing trial: Patient is removed from the ventilator but remains intubated. Endotracheal tube is connected to a heated, humidified circuit with minimal or no supplemental oxygen. End-tidal CO_2 monitoring may be used for additional safety.
○ SIMV: Used most frequently in surgical and neurosurgical patients. Set respiratory rate is gradually decreased over hours to days until patient is primarily breathing spontaneously. **Has the poorest weaning outcomes of all techniques** (*Chest 2001;120:474S*).
• Extubation: Should be performed early in the day, when full ancillary staff are available.
○ Laryngeal edema: In patients with concern for laryngeal edema (e.g., angioedema, traumatic intubation), cuff leak should be checked prior to extubation. **Absence of cuff leak should preclude extubation**, and patients should be treated with intravenous corticosteroids for 12–24 hours prior to extubation (*Cochrane Database Syst Rev 2009;(3):CD001000:1–24*).
  Cuff leak test is performed by recording the expired tidal volume when the cuff is inflated and then deflating the cuff and recording the expired tidal volume over the next six breaths. The mean of the three lowest tidal volumes is used to calculate the cuff leak volume: the difference between the expired tidal volume with the cuff inflated and expired tidal volume with the cuff deflated. A cuff leak volume <110 mL is predictive of postextubation stridor (*Chest 1996;110:4*).
○ Extubation to NPPV: In patients with COPD who are intubated for acute respiratory failure, extubation to NPPV is associated with a reduction in mortality and health care–associated pneumonia (*Cochrane Database Syst Rev 2013;12:CD004127:1–60*). Similar benefit has **not** been demonstrated in other etiologies of respiratory failure.
• Failure to wean: Defined as inability to liberate from mechanical ventilation 48–72 hours after resolution of underlying disease process. Factors that should be considered include the following:
○ Endotracheal tubes with smaller inner diameter increase airway resistance and may make breathing trials more difficult.
○ Use of neuromuscular blockade is associated with prolonged weakness, particularly when used with corticosteroids (*Curr Opin Crit Care 2004;10:47*).
○ Acid–base disturbances may make liberation from mechanical ventilation difficult.
  ▪ Non–anion gap metabolic acidosis causes compensatory increase in minute ventilation (respiratory alkalosis) to normalize pH, which can lead to tachypnea and respiratory fatigue upon extubation.
  ▪ Metabolic alkalosis causes blunting of ventilatory drive and decrease in minute ventilation (respiratory acidosis) to maintain normal pH, which can lead to hypercapnia upon extubation.

Shock

GENERAL PRINCIPLES

- A process in which blood flow and oxygen delivery to tissues are deranged, leading to tissue hypoxia and resultant compromise of cellular metabolic activity and organ function.
- Main goal of therapy is rapid cardiovascular resuscitation to reestablish tissue perfusion.
- Definitive treatment requires reversal of underlying processes.

Classifications of Shock

- **Distributive:** Shock caused by massive vasodilation and impaired distribution of blood flow, resulting in tissue hypoxia. Usually associated with hyperdynamic cardiac function, unless cardiac function is somehow impaired (see later discussion of cardiogenic shock).
  - **Primary etiologies** are septic shock and anaphylactic shock. Septic shock is most commonly seen in medical intensive care units and will be further discussed in the next section. Anaphylaxis is discussed in Chapter 11, Allergy and Immunology.
  - **Hemodynamic parameters** will demonstrate increased CO, decreased systemic vascular resistance (SVR) due to vasodilation, and elevated central venous oxygen saturation ($ScvO_2$) due to ineffective oxygen extraction by tissue.
  - Primary goals of therapy are:
    - Volume resuscitation: Due to massive peripheral vasodilation, patients have a functionally decreased oxygen-carrying capacity, requiring volume resuscitation. IV crystalloid fluids are primarily used.
    - Treatment of underlying infection: Inadequate initial antimicrobial therapy is an independent risk factor for in-hospital mortality in patients with septic shock (*Chest 1999;115:462*), so timely, effective antimicrobial therapy is a cornerstone of treatment.
    - Removal of offending agent in anaphylactic shock.
    - Cardiovascular support with vasoactive agents (e.g., norepinephrine, epinephrine). Vasoactive agents will be discussed in more detail in a later section.
- **Hypovolemic:** Shock caused by decrease in effective intravascular volume and decreased oxygen-carrying capacity.
  - **Primary etiologies** are hemorrhagic (e.g., trauma, gastrointestinal bleeding) or fluid depletion (e.g., diarrhea, vomiting).
  - **Hemodynamic parameters** will demonstrate an increased CO, increased SVR, and decreased $ScvO_2$ due to increased oxygen extraction by peripheral tissue.
  - Primary goals of therapy are:
    - Volume resuscitation: Traditionally, IV blood product and crystalloid were used for resuscitation of hemorrhagic and fluid depletion shock, respectively, with goal mean arterial pressure (MAP) of 60–65 mm Hg. However, recent studies indicate that over-resuscitation may be detrimental in hemorrhagic (*Air Med J 2014;33:172*) and patients without significant comorbidities may tolerate lower hemoglobin levels (7 g/dL) than previously believed. Further investigation of the appropriate fluid volume to give to patients is warranted.
    - Definitive treatment of underlying etiology of volume loss: For hemorrhagic shock, surgical intervention may be necessary for definitive treatment.
- **Obstructive:** Shock caused by obstruction of the heart or great vessels, resulting in decreased left ventricular filling and cardiovascular collapse.
  - **Primary etiology** is **pulmonary embolism** with resulting right ventricular failure.
  - **Hemodynamic parameters** will demonstrate decreased CO, normal to increased SVR, and normal to decreased $ScvO_2$.

TABLE 8-4	Hemodynamic Patterns Associated with Specific Shock States							
Type of Shock	CI	SVR	PVR	SvO₂	RAP	RVP	PAP	PAOP
Cardiogenic[a]	↓	↑	N	↓	↑	↑	↑	↑
Hypovolemic	↓	↑	N	↓	↓	↓	↓	↓
Distributive	N–↑	↓	N	N–↑	N–↓	N–↓	N–↓	N–↓
Obstructive	↓	↑–N	↑	N–↓	↑	↑	↑	N–↓

CI, cardiac index; N, normal; PAOP, pulmonary artery occlusion pressure; PAP, pulmonary artery pressure; PVR, pulmonary vascular resistance; RAP, right atrial pressure; RVP, right ventricular pressure; SvO₂, mixed venous oxygen saturation; SVR, systemic vascular resistance.
[a]Equalization of RAP, PAOP, diastolic PAP, and diastolic RVP establishes a diagnosis of cardiac tamponade.

○ Primary goals of therapy are:
  ▪ Supportive: Although patients are preload dependent, excessive fluid administration can lead to right ventricular overload, thereby worsening shock.
  ▪ In a carefully selected group of patients, **thrombolytic therapy** may be beneficial.
• **Cardiogenic:** Shock caused by left ventricular systolic failure, resulting in decreased CO and subsequent insufficient oxygen distribution.
  ○ **Primary etiologies** are myocardial infarction, acute mitral regurgitation, myocarditis, pericardial effusion with tamponade, and septal wall rupture.
  ○ **Hemodynamic parameters** will demonstrate decreased CO, increased SVR, and decreased ScvO₂.
  ○ Primary goals of therapy are:
    ▪ Mitigation of pulmonary edema: NPPV or endotracheal intubation with mechanical ventilation reduces afterload, thereby encouraging forward flow. Additionally, the application of positive pressure to the alveolar space causes pulmonary edema fluid to move to the interstitial space.
    ▪ Careful fluid management: Adequate preload to optimize ventricular function is important, but volume overload will worsen respiratory status, so careful fluid management is necessary.
    ▪ Definitive therapy for underlying cardiac disease: In the event of myocardial infarction, percutaneous revascularization should be performed in a timely fashion.
    ▪ Supportive: Inotropic agents such as dobutamine may be used to augment CO. Other inotropes are discussed in Pharmacologic Therapies. Mechanical circulatory assist devices, including **left ventricular assist devices** and **intra-aortic balloon pumps**, may be necessary in patients who do not respond to medical therapy.
• Hemodynamic patterns associated with the different shock states are listed in Table 8-4.

Septic Shock
• **Definition:** Presence of at least two systemic inflammatory response syndrome (SIRS) criteria, with evidence of infection, end-organ dysfunction, and refractory hypotension
  ○ SIRS criteria: Two of the following four findings must be present:
    ▪ Tachypnea: Respiratory rate >20 breaths/min or PaCO₂ <32 mm Hg
    ▪ White blood cell count <4000 cells/μL or >12,000 cells/μL
    ▪ Tachycardia: Pulse >90 bpm
    ▪ Hypo- or hyperthermia: Temperature >38.0°C or <36.0°C
  ○ End-organ dysfunction, including, but not limited to:
    ▪ Urine output ≤50 mL/kg/h
    ▪ Hepatic dysfunction, as evidenced by abnormal hepatic enzymes

- Altered mental status
- Platelet count ≤80,000/μL
- pH ≤7.30 and plasma lactate ≥4 mmol/L
  ○ Refractory hypotension defined as systolic blood pressure ≤90 mm Hg or MAP ≤70 mm Hg that does not improve following adequate fluid resuscitation of 30 mL/ kg IBW IV crystalloid fluid or requires vasopressors to maintain adequate MAP (*Crit Care Med 2013;31:580*).
- Caused by the systemic release of cytokines and other immunomodulatory mediators by circulating bacteria or bacterial byproducts, resulting in profound vasodilation and compensatory increased CO.
- Management of septic shock:
  ○ **Volume resuscitation:** Patients should initially receive **30 mL/kg IBW IV crystalloid fluid** within first hour of presentation, with additional volume administered if the patient remains volume responsive. Parameters to determine volume responsiveness (discussed in Hemodynamic Measurements section) should be closely monitored during volume resuscitation to prevent volume overload.
    - Conservative fluid management in acute lung injury is associated with shorter mechanical ventilation time (*N Engl J Med 2005;354:2564*).
    - There is weak evidence that volume overload may be associated with increased mortality in septic shock (*Chest 2000;117:1749*).
  ○ **Cardiovascular support:** Vasoactive medications may be necessary if volume resuscitation is insufficient to maintain MAP ≥65 mm Hg. **Norepinephrine** has become the first-line agent after it was demonstrated that dopamine has more adverse events (*N Engl J Med 2010;362:779*). Vasopressin is frequently used as a second-line agent. Mechanisms of action and other agents are discussed in Pharmacologic Therapies.
  ○ **Timely, effective antimicrobial administration:** Duration of hypotension before initiation of effective antimicrobial therapy is independently associated with in-hospital mortality (*Crit Care Med 2006;34:1589*).
  ○ **Source control:** If a specific anatomical source of infection is identified (e.g., necrotizing soft tissue infection), intervention for source control should be performed within the first 12 hours, if possible (*Crit Care Med 2013;41:580*).
- **Early goal-directed therapy:** Protocol for management of the **first 6 hours** of sepsis proposed by Rivers et al. in 2001 (*N Engl J Med 2001;345:1368*). Widely adapted in practice before recent multicenter, prospective, randomized controlled trials called its effectiveness into question (*N Engl J Med 2014;370:1683*; *N Engl J Med 2014;371:1496*); studies limited by practice changes in control group (Figure 8-3).
- **Lactate clearance:** Weak evidence demonstrating that early lactate clearance may be associated with improved outcome in septic shock (*Crit Care Med 2004;32:1637*), although recent multicenter randomized controlled trials did not demonstrate difference in in-hospital mortality (*JAMA 2010;303:739*). Most recent Surviving Sepsis Guidelines recommend targeting resuscitation to normalize lactate in patients with elevated lactate levels (*Crit Care Med 2013;41:580*).

Pharmacologic Therapies
Vasoconstrictive and Inotropic Agents
- **Norepinephrine:** Causes potent vasoconstriction via α_1- and β_1-adrenergic activity. Preferred agent in septic shock due to lack of concomitant tachycardia.
- **Vasopressin:** Causes vasoconstriction via three different G-peptide receptors. Primarily used as an adjunct to norepinephrine. Weak evidence that it may have mortality benefit over norepinephrine in less severe septic shock, defined as requiring treatment with norepinephrine 5–14 μg/min to maintain MAP ≥65 mm Hg (*N Engl J Med 358;9:877*). Standard dosage of vasopressin is 0.04 unit/min.

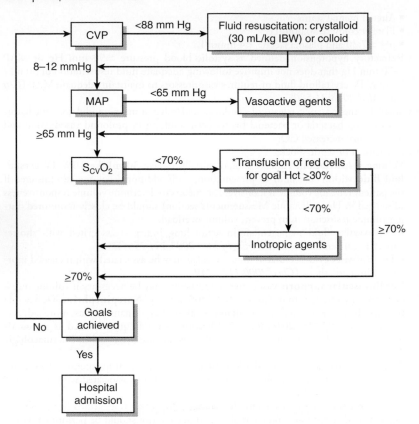

Figure 8-3. Early goal-directed therapy protocol (adapted from *N Engl J Med 2001;345:1368*). *Although included in the original early goal-directed therapy protocol, more recent trials have demonstrated a trend toward increased harm in patients who receive more transfusions; current Surviving Sepsis Guidelines do not recommend transfusing to achieve Hct of 30%. CVP, central venous pressure; Hct, hematocrit; IBW, ideal body weight; MAP, mean arterial pressure; $ScvO_2$, central venous oxygen saturation.

- **Epinephrine:** Has inotropic and vasoconstrictive properties in a dose-dependent fashion due to α_1- and β-adrenergic activity. At low doses ($\leq$0.05 μg/kg/min), it increases CO and slightly reduces SVR due to predominant β activity. At higher doses (>0.05 μg/kg/min), vasoconstriction predominates due to increased α_1 activity. Preferred agent for anaphylactic shock.
- **Phenylephrine:** Selective α_1-receptor agonist causing vasoconstriction of larger arterioles. Few studies supporting its use in septic shock. May be administered via peripheral intravenous catheters if central venous access has not yet been established.
- **Dobutamine:** Inotropic agent that reduces afterload and increases stroke volume and heart rate via β_1-agonist activity. Preferred agent for cardiogenic shock but increases risk of cardiac arrhythmias.
- **Dopamine:** Has inotropic, vasodilatory, and vasoconstrictive properties in a dose-dependent fashion due to action on peripheral α_1-receptors, cardiac β_1-receptors, and renal and splanchnic dopaminergic receptors. At doses <5 μg/kg/min, primarily behaves

as a vasodilator, increasing renal blood flow. At doses of 5–10 μg/kg/min, behaves as an inotrope. At doses >10 μg/kg/min, behaves as a vasopressor. Is associated with a higher rate of cardiac arrhythmias than norepinephrine (*N Engl J Med 2010;362:779*).
• **Milrinone:** Phosphodiesterase III inhibitor that has positive inotropic effect, causing increase in CO. Also causes systemic vasodilation, which can worsen hypotension.

Adjunctive Therapies
• **Corticosteroids:** Relative adrenal insufficiency may contribute to refractory hypotension during septic shock. High-dose steroids (methylprednisolone 30 mg/kg or dexamethasone 3–6 mg/kg) are associated with worse outcomes (*Am J Respir Crit Care Med 2012;185:133*), but "stress-dose" steroids (hydrocortisone 50 mg IV q6h) were associated with improved outcomes in one study (*Crit Care Med 2006;34:22*). Most recent Surviving Sepsis Guidelines recommend using hydrocortisone 200 mg IV daily in divided doses only if hypotension is refractory to fluid resuscitation and vasopressor therapy (*Crit Care Med 2013;41:580*).
• **Sodium bicarbonate:** No evidence supports the use of bicarbonate therapy in lactic acidemia from sepsis with pH ≥7.15. Effect of bicarbonate on hemodynamics and vasopressor requirements with more severe acidemia is unknown (*Crit Care Med 2013; 41:580*).
• **Methylene blue:** Selective guanylate cyclase inhibitor, thereby mitigating nitric oxide–mediated vasodilation. Observational studies have demonstrated beneficial effects on hemodynamic parameters, but effects on morbidity and mortality are unknown (*Pharmacotherapy 2010;30:702*).
• **Recombinant human activated protein C:** Previously recommended based on results from one study that demonstrated reduction in mortality (*Crit Care Med 2004;32:2207*), but subsequent studies demonstrated no benefit (*N Engl J Med 2012;366:2055*), and the drug was withdrawn from the market in 2011.
• **Immunoglobulins:** Not recommended due to a lack of benefit (*Crit Care Med 2013; 41:580*).

Hemodynamic Measurements and Critical Care Ultrasound

Although central venous pressure (CVP), MAP, and $SvO_2/ScvO_2$ are used as therapeutic endpoints in treating shock, there is evidence that these parameters do not reflect intravascular volume. There is a growing body of evidence that dynamic parameters, including pulse pressure variation and inferior vena cava (IVC) diameters, may better reflect intravascular volume, but it is unclear that these lead to improved outcomes.

Hemodynamic Measurements
Static Parameters
• **CVP:** An approximation of right atrial pressure and, therefore, preload. Should be measured from an internal jugular or subclavian venous catheter because readings from femoral catheters are influenced by intra-abdominal pressures and thus inaccurate. Poor relationship between CVP and blood volume (*Chest 2008;134:172*), but low values (<4 mm Hg) should lead to fluid resuscitation with careful monitoring (*Intensive Care Med 2007;33:575*).
• **$ScvO_2$:** Percentage of oxygen bound to hemoglobin in blood returning in the superior vena cava. **Not to be confused with SvO_2**; measured from an internal jugular or subclavian venous catheter. Low values indicate inadequate oxygen delivery, either due to inadequate intravascular volume or poor CO.
• **SvO_2:** Percentage of oxygen bound to hemoglobin in blood returning to the right side of the heart. **Not to be confused with $ScvO_2$; can only be measured with pulmonary artery catheter (PAC).** Low values indicate inadequate oxygen delivery, either due to inadequate intravascular volume or poor CO.

- **Pulmonary artery occlusive pressure or wedge pressure:** An approximation of left atrial pressure, which can be used to differentiate between cardiogenic and noncardiogenic pulmonary edema. Measured using PAC. Previously commonly used in the management of septic shock and ARDS, but did not affect mortality or morbidity (*JAMA 2003;290:2713*).
  - Insertion method: Following insertion into a central vein, distal balloon is inflated and PAC is advanced. Bedside waveform analysis or fluoroscopy is used to determine successful passage of the catheter through the right atrium, right ventricle, and into the pulmonary artery (PA).
  - Risks: Overwedging of a PAC can cause **PA rupture with resultant exsanguination** or pulmonary infarct.
- **PAC measurement of CO:** CO can be measured either via thermodilution or Fick principle with a PAC.
  - Thermodilution: An injectate of known volume and temperature is injected into the PAC, and the cooled blood traverses a thermistor at the distal end of the catheter. The CO is inversely proportional to the duration of transit of cooled blood (i.e., the longer the transit time, the lower the CO).
  - Fick principle: CO is the quotient of oxygen consumption and the arteriovenous oxygen difference. To calculate CO, arterial and mixed venous blood are drawn to determine the arteriovenous oxygen difference, and oxygen consumption is determined by respiratory gas analysis or indirect calorimetry.

Dynamic Parameters
- **Aortic Doppler monitoring:** Several systems are available that use Doppler ultrasonography to calculate **CO** and stroke volume. Correlates well with CO as measured by PAC (*Intensive Care Med 2004;30:2060*). **Reliably predicts volume responsiveness in critically ill, ventilated patients without spontaneous breathing** (*Intensive Care Med 2005;31:1195*).
  - Method: Doppler probe is inserted into the esophagus or placed at the suprasternal notch and rotated or tilted until a clear flow-velocity waveform is detected and displayed on the monitor. Aortic diameter is either measured by the system or based on an internally programmed height nomogram.
  - Output parameters: Blood velocity and flow time are measured and used to calculate stroke distance, stroke volume, and CO.
    - Stroke distance: Area under the curve of flow-velocity waveform
    - Stroke volume: Product of stroke distance and aortic cross-sectional area
    - CO: Product of stroke volume and heart rate
- **Pulse pressure variation (ΔPp):** Requires arterial line placement. Calculated as the difference between maximal and minimal systolic blood pressures measured over one respiratory cycle divided by the mean of those values. ΔPp of 13% was an accurate predictor of fluid responsiveness in mechanically ventilated patients without spontaneous breathing (*Am J Respir Crit Care Med 2000;162:134*).
- **IVC distensibility index (dIVC):** Calculated as the difference between maximal and minimal IVC diameter measured over one respiratory cycle divided by the minimal IVC diameter. dIVC of 18% discriminated between volume responders and nonresponders with 90% sensitivity and specificity in mechanically ventilated patients without spontaneous breathing in one study (*Intensive Care Med 2004;30:1740*), but more recent studies have not demonstrated similar reproducibility (*Emerg Med Australas 2012;24:534*).

Critical Care Ultrasound
The use of bedside ultrasonography has greatly expanded recently and is rapidly becoming standard of care in intensive care units. Courses in critical care ultrasonography are

becoming more readily available and are necessary for complete proficiency. This section is intended to serve as an overview of basic concepts only. **Critical care ultrasound is intended to be used as an adjunct to other clinical data.**

- Basic concepts: Air and calcified structures transmit sound waves poorly. Free-flowing fluids transmit sound waves well.
- Basic definitions (*Int J Shoulder Surg 2010;4:55*)
  - Echogenicity: The ability of an object to reflect sound waves.
  - Hyperechoic: Containing structures that reflect sound waves well; shows as white on ultrasound.
    Examples: Bone, pleura, lung
  - Hypoechoic: Containing structures that reflect sound waves poorly; shows as gray on ultrasound. Deeper structures are also more hypoechoic due to attenuation with distance.
    Examples: Lymph nodes, adipose tissue, muscle
  - Anechoic: Containing structures that allow sound waves to pass through freely; shows as black on ultrasound.
    Examples: Blood vessels, transudative pleural effusion
- Ultrasound to facilitate vascular access: More detailed instructions are available in the *Washington Manual of Critical Care*, Section XIX. Use of ultrasound to guide central venous access results in increased success and reduced complication rates.
  - Location: Ultrasound guidance is most commonly used for internal jugular and femoral venous access.
  - Prior to starting the procedure: Both internal jugular and femoral veins should be scanned to evaluate for aberrant anatomy or venous thrombosis. Lung ultrasound can be performed to rule out pneumothorax.
  - After applying the sterile field: The probe is positioned so that the needle is visualized for the entire duration of accessing the vessel.
  - During the procedure: Following insertion of the guidewire, the length of the vessel is scanned to ensure that the guidewire did not inadvertently enter any adjacent arteries.
  - After the procedure: Lung ultrasound is repeated to rule out pneumothorax.
- Cardiac ultrasound: Includes five standard views, reviewed below. Uses body transducer. Intended to facilitate assessment of volume responsiveness, global left and right ventricular systolic function, and valvular function, and indicated for imminently life-threatening causes of hemodynamic failure.
  - Parasternal long-axis view: Probe is placed adjacent to the sternum in the left third to fifth intercostal space with the orientation marker pointing toward the patient's right shoulder. The right ventricular outflow tract, left ventricular cavity, ascending aorta, mitral valve, and left atrium should be visualized. Assesses for pericardial effusion, left and right ventricular dysfunction, and valvular pathologies.
  - Parasternal short-axis view: Probe remains adjacent to the sternum in the left third to fifth intercostal space, but orientation marker is rotated 90 degrees clockwise to point at the patient's left shoulder. Cross-sectional view of the left and right ventricles at the level of the papillary muscles should be visualized. Assesses for pericardial effusion and left and right ventricular dysfunction.
  - Apical four-chamber view: Probe is placed between the midclavicular and midaxillary lines of the left lateral chest between the fifth and seventh intercostal spaces, underneath the left nipple, with the orientation marker pointed at 3 o'clock. The left and right ventricles and atria, as well as the tricuspid and mitral valves, should be visualized. Assesses left and right ventricular size and function.
  - Subcostal long-axis view: Probe is placed below the xiphoid process with the orientation marker pointed at 3 o'clock. The left and right ventricles and atria should be visualized. Assesses for pericardial effusion and left and right ventricular dysfunction. May be used for rapid assessment of cardiac function during performance of cardiopulmonary resuscitation.

- ○ IVC longitudinal view: Probe remains below the xiphoid process, but orientation marker is rotated 90 degrees counterclockwise to point at 12 o'clock. IVC in the longitudinal axis should be visualized. Assesses IVC diameter during the respiratory cycle to determine volume responsiveness.
- • Thoracic ultrasound: Includes four standard positions, performed bilaterally. Uses the body transducer on the abdominal setting to examine lung parenchyma; vascular transducer may be used for detailed examination of the pleura. Intended to facilitate the diagnosis of pleural effusion, pulmonary edema, pulmonary consolidation, and pneumothorax and to guide safe thoracentesis.
  - ○ Areas of investigation: BLUE protocol, intended for immediate diagnosis of acute respiratory failure, defines four areas for investigation (*Crit Ultrasound J 2011;3:109*). The orientation marker should be pointed toward the patient's head.
    - ▪ Upper BLUE point: Midclavicular line, second intercostal space
    - ▪ Lower BLUE point: Anterior axillary line, fourth or fifth intercostal space
    - ▪ Phrenic point: Midaxillary line, sixth or seventh intercostal space; location of the diaphragm
    - ▪ PLAPS point: Posterior to the posterior axillary line, fourth or fifth intercostal space
  - ○ Anatomic landmarks and ultrasound appearance: Knowledge of the normal sonographic appearance of thoracic anatomy is paramount to identifying key structures.
    - ▪ Chest wall: Hypoechoic, linear shadows of soft tissue density.
    - ▪ Ribs: Hyperechoic, curvilinear structures with a deep, hypoechoic, posterior acoustic shadow.
    - ▪ Pleura: Bright, hyperechoic, roughly horizontal line located approximately 0.5 cm below rib shadows.
    - ▪ Diaphragm: Curvilinear, hyperechoic line that moves caudally with inspiration. In a seated patient, it is located caudad to the ninth rib.
    - ▪ Splenorenal and hepatorenal recesses: Should be confirmed prior to any procedure because its curvilinear appearance is similar to that of the diaphragm. Identified by visualization of the liver or spleen and the kidney caudally.
    - ▪ Lung: Air-filled lung appears hyperechoic due to the poor echogenicity of air. Atelectatic or consolidated lung appears hypoechoic relative to normal lung.
  - ○ Sonographic artifacts and terminology: A number of sonographic artifacts are caused by air–tissue interfaces, and presence or absence of these artifacts is indicative of disease (*Crit Care Med 2007;35:S250*).
    - ▪ **Pleural line:** Brightly echogenic, roughly horizontal line; caused by parietopulmonary interface and indicating the lung surface.
    - ▪ **A-lines:** Brightly echogenic horizontal lines roughly parallel to the chest wall; caused by reverberations of the pleural line.
    - ▪ **B-lines:** Also called "**comet tails**"; a grouping within one intercostal space is called "**lung rockets**." Hyperechoic line arising perpendicularly from the pleural line that extends across the whole screen without fading, erasing A-lines; moves with lung slide. Caused by thickened interlobular septa or ground-glass areas; isolated B-lines are a normal variant.
    - ▪ **Lung slide:** "Twinkling" movement of the pleural line that occurs with the respiratory cycle; caused by movement of the lung along the craniocaudal axis during respiration. In M-mode, lung slide is visualized as the "**seashore sign**," with the chest wall generating the "waves," the aerated lung forming the "sand," and the pleural line as the interface.
    - ▪ **Lung pulse:** Pulsation of the pleural line due to transmission of the heartbeat through noninflated lung (*Ann Intensive Care 2014;4:1*).
  - ○ Ultrasonography of lung pathology (*Crit Care Med 2007;35:S250*)
    - ▪ **Pleural effusion:** A fluid collection bordered by the diaphragm, chest wall, and lung surface. Transudative effusions are typically anechoic; exudative effusions may have

some echogenicity. If the effusion is loculated, septations—visualized as hyperechoic, web-like structures—may be seen. Atelectatic lung may be seen in the effusion.

- **Pneumothorax:** Due to air's poor echogenicity, diagnosis of pneumothorax on ultrasound is made by artifact analysis.
  - □ The presence of **lung slide** or **lung pulse** effectively rules out pneumothorax **in the location being investigated**.
  - □ **Abolishment of lung slide** has a characteristic **stratosphere sign** in M-mode, with loss of the "sand," but is **neither sufficient nor specific for diagnosis of pneumothorax**.
  - □ **Lung point** is **pathognomonic** for pneumothorax, but has poor sensitivity. Occurs at the interface of the pneumothorax and aerated lung. Characterized by alternation between absent lung slide and present lung slide or B-lines in one location with respirations. In M-mode, will transition between seashore sign and stratosphere sign.
- **Pneumonia:** Can only be visualized when the consolidation abuts the pleura. A heterogeneous, hypoechoic area with irregular margins where aerated lung abuts the consolidated area. Air bronchograms should be seen to make the diagnosis of pneumonia (*Crit Care Med 2011;39:839*).
- **Pulmonary edema:** Presence of multiple B-lines within one intercostal space ("lung rockets") may indicate cardiogenic or noncardiogenic pulmonary edema. Corresponds to the Kerley B lines seen on chest radiograph. Isolated B-lines are a normal variant.

• Abdominal ultrasound: Abdominal ultrasound in critical care is limited and intended to evaluate for intra-abdominal fluid and assess the urinary tract and abdominal aorta.
  ○ Evaluating for intra-abdominal fluid: Standard evaluation of the trauma patient who may have intra-abdominal bleeding includes the focused assessment with sonography for trauma (FAST) examination. The patient is in the supine position, and four views are obtained:
  - Hepatorenal space: The probe is placed on the right in the tenth or eleventh intercostal space at the posterior axillary line with the orientation mark pointed cephalad.
  - Pelvis: The probe is placed in the suprapubic area with the orientation mark in the 3 o'clock position.
  - Perisplenic space: The probe is placed on the left in the tenth or eleventh space at or slightly posterior to the posterior axillary line with the orientation mark pointed cephalad.
  - Pericardial space: The probe is placed in the subxiphoid position with the orientation marker in the 3 o'clock position.
  ○ Paracentesis: Paracentesis should be performed under ultrasound guidance because there is evidence supporting a decrease in complications (*Ann Am Thorac Soc 2013;10:713*). More details can be found in the *Washington Manual for Critical Care*, Section XIX.
  ○ Assessment of the urinary tract: Bedside ultrasonography can identify bladder distention or hydronephrosis.
  - Bladder distention: The probe is placed in the suprapubic position with the orientation marker pointed cephalad for longitudinal dimensions and in the 3 o'clock position for transverse dimensions.
  - Hydronephrosis: The probe should be placed slightly caudad to the locations used for examination of the hepatorenal and perisplenic spaces in the FAST examination. Hydronephrosis is characterized by thinning of the renal cortex as the collecting system dilates.
  ○ Assessment of the abdominal aorta: The goal is to visualize the entire abdominal aorta to ensure that its diameter from outer wall to outer wall is <3 cm. The examination begins caudad to the xiphoid process, with the probe perpendicular to the abdominal wall and the orientation marker in the 3 o'clock position (*Ann Am Thorac Soc 2013;10:713*).

• Vascular diagnostic ultrasound: Bedside ultrasonography may be performed to evaluate for deep vein thrombosis when clinically indicated. The target vein is visualized in the transverse plane. A vessel with normal blood flow should appear internally anechoic and should be easily compressible. Organized thrombus appears as a discrete, echogenic structure within the venous lumen. A very recently formed thrombus may be anechoic, but the vessel will be incompressible.

9 Obstructive Lung Disease

Jeffrey J. Atkinson, Junfang Jiao, and Mario Castro

Chronic Obstructive Pulmonary Disease

GENERAL PRINCIPLES

Definition

Chronic obstructive pulmonary disease (COPD) is a mostly preventable and treatable disorder characterized by expiratory airflow limitation that is not fully reversible. The airflow limitation is often progressive and associated with an abnormal inflammatory response of the lungs to noxious particles or gases, principally cigarette smoke (*GOLD Global Strategy for the Diagnosis, Management, and Prevention of Chronic Obstructive Pulmonary Disease [Updated 2014]. Available at www.goldcopd.com*). **The airflow obstruction in COPD is caused by emphysema and airway disease.**

- Emphysema is defined pathologically as permanent enlargement of air spaces distal to the terminal bronchiole accompanied by destruction of the alveolar walls and absence of associated fibrosis.
- The airway disease in COPD occurs principally in small airways (i.e., those with an internal diameter of <2 mm). Chronic bronchitis is a common feature of COPD and is defined clinically as productive cough on most days for at least 3 consecutive months per year for at least 2 consecutive years, in the absence of other lung disease that could account for this symptom. Individuals with chronic bronchitis but without airflow obstruction do not have COPD.

Epidemiology

- Although the prevalence of COPD is difficult to determine, it is estimated to affect 10–24 million Americans.
- COPD and other chronic lower respiratory diseases represent the third leading cause of death in the United States (*Natl Vital Stat Rep 2015;64(10):8*).
- In the United States, the age-adjusted mortality rate remains higher among Caucasians compared with African Americans, Hispanics, or Pacific Islanders, but rate differences between men and women have closed.

Etiology

- Most cases of COPD are attributable to **cigarette smoking**. Although only a minority of cigarette smokers develop clinically significant COPD, a much higher proportion develop abnormal lung function (*Lancet 2011;378:991*).
- **Environmental (e.g., wood-burning stoves) and occupational dusts, fumes, gases, and chemicals** are other etiologic agents of COPD. Household indoor air pollution is a major cause of fatal COPD in underdeveloped countries (*Science 2011;334:180*).
- **α_1-Antitrypsin deficiency** is found in 1–2% of COPD patients. Clinical characteristics of affected patients may include a minimal smoking history, early-onset COPD (e.g., younger than 45 years of age), a family history of lung disease, or lower lobe-predominant emphysema. Despite its relative rarity, some authorities recommend diagnostic testing for this condition in all patients with COPD (*Am J Respir Crit Care Med 2003;168:818*).

Pathophysiology

- Processes in the lungs and airways important in the pathogenesis of COPD include inflammation, immune reactions, imbalance of proteinases and antiproteinases, turnover of extracellular matrix, oxidative stress, and apoptosis.
- Pathologic features include destruction of alveolar tissue and small airways, airway wall inflammation, edema and fibrosis, and intraluminal mucus.
- Pulmonary function changes include decreased maximal expiratory airflow, hyperinflation, air trapping, and alveolar gas exchange abnormalities.
- An increased incidence of osteoporosis, skeletal muscle dysfunction, and coronary artery disease occur in COPD, perhaps indicating a systemic component of inflammation (*Chest 2005;128:2640*).

Prevention

- **Abstinence from smoking is the most effective measure for preventing COPD.**
- In patients with COPD, smoking cessation may result in a reduction in the rate of lung function decline (*Am J Respir Crit Care Med 2002;166:675*) and improve survival (*Ann Intern Med 2005;142:233*).
- Tobacco dependence warrants repeated treatment until patients stop smoking (*N Engl J Med 2011;365:1222*). Most smokers fail initial attempts at smoking cessation, and relapse reflects the nature of the dependence and not the failure of the patient or the physician.
- A multimodality approach is recommended to optimize smoking quit rates.
  - Counseling on the preventable health risks of smoking, providing advice to stop smoking, and encouraging patients to make further attempts to stop smoking even after previous failures
  - Providing smoking cessation materials to patients
  - Prescribing pharmacotherapy (Table 9-1)
- Formal smoking cessation programs, often administered in a group setting, can more be effective than non–face-to-face methods (*Cochrane Database Syst Rev 2005;(2):CD001007*).
- The U.S. Department of Health and Human Services has developed a telephone-based support system (1-800-QUIT NOW) with an Internet analog (smokefree.gov).

DIAGNOSIS

Clinical Presentation

History

- Common symptoms of COPD are dyspnea on exertion, cough, sputum production, and wheezing.
- Typically, dyspnea on exertion progresses gradually over years.
- Significant nocturnal symptoms should lead to a search for comorbidities, such as gastroesophageal reflux, congestive heart failure, or sleep-disordered breathing.
- Clinicians should obtain a lifelong smoking history and quantify exposure to environmental and occupational risk factors.
- Careful assessment of severity of symptoms and frequency of COPD exacerbations is very important, as these will guide treatment choices.
- Some tools used to evaluate dyspnea and symptom severity in COPD include the COPD Assessment Tool (CAT; Table 9-2) and patient-oriented questionnaires like the Modified (British) Medical Research Council questionnaire (mMRC; Table 9-3).
- Weight loss often occurs in patients with end-stage COPD, but other etiologies, such as malignancy and depression, should be sought.
- Although dyspnea contributes predominantly to the morbidity of COPD, death in patients with COPD commonly results from cardiovascular disease, lung cancer, or non-lung cancers (*Chest 2005;128:2640; Ann Intern Med 2005;142:233*).

TABLE 9-1	Pharmacotherapy for Smoking Cessation	

Nicotine Replacement Therapy[a]

Product	Dosing	Side Effects/Precautions
Transdermal patch[b]	7, 14, or 21 mg/24 h Usual regimen = 21 mg/d = 6 wk, 14 mg/d × 2 wk, 7 mg/d × 2 wk	Headache, insomnia, nightmares, nausea, dizziness, blurred vision (applies to all nicotine products)
Chewing gum, lozenges	2–4 mg q1–8h Gradually taper use	
Inhaler	10 mg/cartridge (4 mg delivered dose) 6–16 cartridges/d	
Nasal spray	0.5 mg/spray 1–2 sprays in each nostril q1h	

Non-nicotine Pharmacotherapy

Bupropion ER (Zyban)	150 mg/d × 3 days, then bid × 7–12 wk Start 1 wk before quit date	Dizziness, headache, insomnia, nausea, xerostomia, hypertension, seizure Avoid monoamine oxidase inhibitors
Varenicline (Chantix)	0.5 mg/d × 3 days, bid × 4 days, then 1 mg bid × 12–24 wk Start 1 wk before quit date	Nausea, vomiting, headache, insomnia, abnormal dreams Worsening of underlying psychiatric illness

[a]Combination therapy is often used. A long-acting product (e.g., patch) is used for basal nicotine replacement, with a short-acting product (e.g., inhaler) used for breakthrough cravings.
[b]If patient smokes less than a half pack per day, start at 14-mg dose.
See also *N Engl J Med* 2011;365:1222 for strategies and approach.

Physical Examination
- Until significant reduction of lung function occurs (e.g., forced expiratory volume in 1 second [FEV_1] <50% predicted), physical signs of COPD are usually not present.
- Patients with severe COPD may exhibit prolonged (>6 seconds) breath sounds on a maximal forced exhalation, decreased breath sounds, use of accessory muscles of respiration, and hyperresonance to chest percussion. Expiratory wheezing may or may not be present.
- Signs of pulmonary hypertension (PH) and right heart failure may be present.
- **Clubbing is not a feature of COPD**, so its presence should prompt an evaluation for other conditions, especially lung cancer.

Differential Diagnosis

Airway tumors, asthma, bronchiectasis, chronic pulmonary thromboembolic disease, congestive heart failure, cystic fibrosis, constrictive bronchiolitis, diffuse panbronchiolitis, eosinophilic granuloma, ischemic heart disease, lymphangioleiomyomatosis, mycobacterial infection (tuberculous and nontuberculous), tracheobronchomalacia, and tracheal stenosis all must be considered as part of the differential in the workup of COPD.

TABLE 9-2	Chronic Obstructive Pulmonary Disease Assessment Tool (CAT)					
I never cough.	1	2	3	4	5	I cough all the time.
I have no phlegm or mucus in my chest.	1	2	3	4	5	My chest is completely full of mucus or phlegm.
My chest does not feel tight.	1	2	3	4	5	My chest feels tight.
When I walk up a hill or one flight of stairs, I am not breathless.	1	2	3	4	5	When I walk up a hill or one flight of stairs, I am very breathless.
I am not limited doing any activities at home.	1	2	3	4	5	I am limited doing activities at home.
I am confident leaving my home despite my lung condition.	1	2	3	4	5	I am not at all confident leaving my home because of my lung condition.
I sleep soundly.	1	2	3	4	5	I don't sleep soundly because of my lung condition.
I have lots of energy.	1	2	3	4	5	I have no energy at all.

Total score is sum of scores from individual question scales.
From Jones PW, Harding G, Berry P, et al. Development and first validation of the COPD Assessment Test. *Eur Respir J* 2009;34:648–54.

Diagnostic Testing

- Consider the diagnosis of COPD in any patient with chronic cough, dyspnea, or sputum production as well as any patient with a history of exposure to COPD risk factors, especially cigarette smoking (*GOLD Global Strategy for the Diagnosis, Management, and Prevention of Chronic Obstructive Pulmonary Disease [Updated 2014]. Available at www .goldcopd.com*).
- **Pulmonary function testing**
  - A definite diagnosis of COPD requires the presence of expiratory airflow limitation on spirometry, measured as the FEV_1/forced vital capacity (FVC) ratio. Although

TABLE 9-3	Modified British Medical Research Council Questionnaire (mMRC)
0	I only get breathless with strenuous exercise.
1	I get short of breath when hurrying on level ground or walking up a slight hill.
2	On level ground, I walk slower than people of the same age because of breathlessness, or have to stop for breath when walking at my own pace.
3	I stop for breath after walking about 100 yards or after a few minutes on level ground.
4	I am too breathless to leave the house or I am breathless when dressing.

From Launois C, Barbe Coralie, Bertin E, et al. The modified Medical Research Council scale for the assessment of dyspnea in daily living in obesity: A pilot study. *BMC Pulm Med* 2012;12:61.

TABLE 9-4	Classification of Severity of Airflow Limitation in Chronic Obstructive Pulmonary Disease (Based on Postbronchodilator FEV_1)

In patients with FEV_1/FVC <0.70:

GOLD 1	Mild	$FEV_1 \geq 80\%$ predicted
GOLD 2	Moderate	$50\% \leq FEV_1 < 80\%$ predicted
GOLD 3	Severe	$30\% \leq FEV_1 < 50\%$ predicted
GOLD 4	Very severe	$FEV_1 < 30\%$ predicted

FEV_1, forced expiratory volume in 1 second; FVC, forced vital capacity; GOLD, Global Initiative for Chronic Obstructive Lung Disease.
From the Global Strategy for Diagnosis, Management, and Prevention of COPD, 2015, © Global Initiative for Chronic Obstructive Lung Disease (GOLD), all rights reserved. Available from http://www.goldcopd.com.

0.7 is taken as the lower limit of normal for all adults, with advancing age, the ratio may decrease below 0.7 in individuals who are asymptomatic and have never smoked. Therefore, a reduced ratio should not be interpreted automatically as diagnostic of COPD. The FEV_1 is usually reduced.
- The FEV_1 relative to the predicted normal defines the severity of expiratory airflow obstruction (Table 9-4) and is a predictor of mortality.
- The FEV_1 is often used to assess the clinical course and response to therapy.
- Spirometry may assist in the evaluation of worsened symptoms of unclear etiology.
- The total lung capacity, functional residual capacity, and residual volume often increase to supernormal values in patients with COPD, indicating lung hyperinflation and air trapping.
- The diffusing capacity for carbon monoxide (DLCO) may be reduced.

Laboratories
- A baseline arterial blood gas (ABG) is recommended for patients with severe COPD to assess for the presence and severity of hypoxemia and hypercapnia. Annual monitoring may be considered.
- Elevated venous bicarbonate may signify chronic hypercapnia.
- Polycythemia may reflect a physiologic response to chronic hypoxemia and inadequate supplemental oxygen use.

Imaging
- CXRs are not sensitive for determining the presence of COPD, but they are useful for evaluating alternative diagnoses.
- Chest CT without contrast can detect emphysema and other conditions associated with tobacco smoking and COPD, especially lung cancer (see Complications section). However, routine diagnostic chest CT adds little to management and is not required to exclude many alternative diagnoses, unless historical or examination findings suggest occult thromboembolic or interstitial lung disease.
- With increasing severity of COPD, patients often develop radiographic signs of thoracic hyperinflation, including flattening of the diaphragm, increased retrosternal/retrocardiac air spaces, and lung hyperlucency with diminished vascular markings. Bullae may be visible. In severe disease, chest CT is used to determine candidacy for lung volume reduction surgery (LVRS) (see Treatment: Surgical Therapy section).

TREATMENT

- Long-term management of patients with COPD aims to improve quality of life, decrease the frequency and severity of acute exacerbations, slow the progression of disease, and prolong survival.
- Of all chronic medical therapies, **smoking cessation and the correction of hypoxemia with supplemental oxygen have the best evidence for improving survival** (*Ann Intern Med 2005;142:233*; *Cochrane Database Syst Rev 2005;(4):CD001744*). Among surgical interventions, LVRS improves survival only in select patients (*Am J Respir Crit Care Med 2011;184:763*).
- COPD should be treated in a stepwise approach based on the combined COPD assessment (Table 9-5) with attention to risk of future exacerbations and symptoms for targeting of therapies with known benefit (Table 9-6).

Medications

A pharmacologic treatment plan (Table 9-7) is based on a patient's disease severity, response to specific medications, frequency of exacerbations, drug availability and affordability, and patient compliance.

TABLE 9-5	Chronic Obstructive Pulmonary Disease Assessment Using Symptoms, Breathlessness, Spirometric Classification, and Risk of Exacerbations

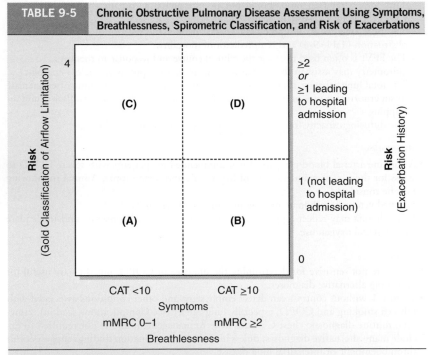

CAT, Chronic Obstructive Pulmonary Disease Assessment Tool; GOLD, Global Initiative for Chronic Obstructive Lung Disease.

From the Global Strategy for Diagnosis, Management, and Prevention of COPD, 2015, © Global Initiative for Chronic Obstructive Lung Disease (GOLD), all rights reserved. Available from http://www.goldcopd.com.

TABLE 9-6	GOLD Category–Based[a] Intervention Strategy
GOLD Category	**Intervention**
A	Smoking cessation Vaccinations (influenza, pneumococcus) Short-acting bronchodilator as needed
B	**All of the above plus:** Long-acting bronchodilator Consider fixed-dose combined long-acting bronchodilators
C	**All of the above plus:** Oxygen if needed Long-acting bronchodilators (or fixed-dose combined) Consider inhaled corticosteroid bronchodilator combination[a] Consider macrolide if frequent exacerbations not controlled Consider PDE4 inhibitor if chronic bronchitis and frequent exacerbations not controlled
D	**All of the above plus:** Pulmonary rehabilitation Consider surgical treatments

GOLD, Global Initiative for Chronic Obstructive Lung Disease; PDE4, phosphodiesterase-4.
[a]Intervention benefit based on exacerbation risk versus risk of pneumonia in individual patient.
Adapted from the Global Strategy for Diagnosis, Management, and Prevention of COPD, 2015,
© Global Initiative for Chronic Obstructive Lung Disease (GOLD), all rights reserved. Available
from http://www.goldcopd.com.

- **Inhaled bronchodilators**
  - Inhaled bronchodilators are the foundation of COPD pharmacotherapy. They work mainly by relaxing airway smooth muscle tone. This results in a reduction in expiratory airflow obstruction.
  - Proper use of a metered-dose inhaler (MDI) results in equally effective drug delivery as use of a nebulizer in most patients (*Health Technol Assess 2001;5(26):1–149*). Health care providers should routinely assess a patient's MDI technique and provide training.
  - Long-acting inhaled anticholinergic agents result in significant improvements in lung function, quality of life, and COPD exacerbations, although the rate of decline of FEV_1 is unaffected (*N Engl J Med 2008;359:1543*).
  - Long-acting β-adrenergic agonists (LABAs) offer improvements that are at least similar to long-acting anticholinergic agents and inhaled corticosteroids (ICSs) (*Cochrane Database Syst Rev 2011(12):CD004106*).
- **ICSs**
  - The rationale for using ICSs stems from the central role of inflammation in the pathogenesis of COPD.
  - ICSs may increase the FEV_1, reduce the frequency of COPD exacerbations, and improve quality of life. They do not slow the rate of decline of lung function over time (*N Engl J Med 1999;340:1948; BMJ 2000;320:1297; Eur Respir J 2003;21:68*).
- **Combination therapy:** Compared to single-agent therapy, a combination of medications may yield superior efficacy while reducing the potential for toxicity. Some examples follow:
  - The combination of an ICS and an LABA is effective in reducing the rate of COPD exacerbations, but this benefit must be balanced against an increased risk of pneumonia (*N Engl J Med 2007;356:775*).

TABLE 9-7	Inhalational Pharmacotherapy for Stable Chronic Obstructive Pulmonary Disease[a]

Short-Acting β-Agonists

Name	Dose	Side Effects[b]
Albuterol	MDI: two puffs q4–6h Nebulizer: 2.5 mg q6–8h	Palpitations, tremor, anxiety, nausea/vomiting, throat irritation, dyspepsia, tachycardia, arrhythmia, hypertension
Levalbuterol (Xopenex)	MDI: two puffs q4–6h Nebulizer: 0.63–1.25 mg q6–8h	Cardiovascular effects may be less common with levalbuterol

Long-Acting β-Agonists

Salmeterol (Serevent Diskus)	DPI: one inhalation (50 μg) bid	Headache, upper respiratory tract infection, cough, palpitations, fatigue, diarrhea
Formoterol (Foradil)	DPI: one capsule (12 μg) bid	
Arformoterol (Brovana)	Nebulizer: 15 μg bid	
Indacaterol[c] (Arcapta)	DPI: one capsule (75 μg) daily	

Anticholinergics[d]

Ipratropium (Atrovent)	MDI: two puffs q4–6h Nebulizer: 0.5 mg q6–8h	Xerostomia, cough, nausea/ vomiting, diarrhea, urinary retention
Tiotropium (Spiriva)	DPI: one puff (18 μg) daily	
Aclidinium (Tudorza)	DPI: one puff (400 μg) bid	

Fixed Combination Medications

| Albuterol/ Ipratropium (Combivent Respimat, DuoNeb) | Inhalational spray: one spray qid Nebulizer: one 3-mL vial qid (each vial contains 2.5 mg albuterol and 0.5 mg ipratropium) | As above for each individual medi- cation class (anticholinergic, β-agonist) |
| Fluticasone/ Salmeterol (Advair) | DPI: one puff bid Recommended dose is 250 μg fluticasone/ 50 μg salmeterol Reduced exacerba- tions seen with 500 μg/50 μg dose | As above, plus lower respiratory tract infection (pneumonia) and oral candidiasis |

(continued)

TABLE 9-7	Inhalational Pharmacotherapy for Stable Chronic Obstructive Pulmonary Disease[a] (Continued)	
Name	**Dose**	**Side Effects[b]**
	Fixed Combination Medications (Continued)	
Budesonide/ Formoterol (Symbicort)	DPI: two puffs bid 160 μg budesonide/ 4 μg formoterol	
Umeclidinium/ Vilanterol (Anoro)	DPI: one puff daily 62.5 μg umeclidinium/ 25 μg vilanterol	As above for each individual medication class

DPI, dry powder inhaler; MDI, metered-dose inhaler.
[a]Commonly used medications are listed. This table is not exhaustive.
[b]Only the most common side effects are listed.
[c]Indacaterol dosage approved in United States is lower than in other countries including Canada.
[d]Short-acting anticholinergic therapy (e.g., ipratropium) is usually discontinued with initiation of long-acting anticholinergic therapy (e.g., tiotropium), because minimal additional benefit is expected, side effects may increase, and use of two inhaled anticholinergic agents has had limited evaluation.

○ Combination therapy with a LABA and a long-acting anticholinergic agent sustains improved lung function compared to either agent alone (*Eur Respir J 2005;26:214*).
○ Fixed-dose, long-acting combination therapies improve lung function better than either preparation alone, but data on symptom and exacerbation reduction are limited (*Lancet Respir Med 2013;1:199*).
○ Questions remain regarding the value of the incremental gains of adding long-acting anticholinergic therapy to LABA/ICS combinations, suggesting a stepwise approach with individualized therapy based on symptoms, side effects, and exacerbation frequency (*Cochrane Database Syst Rev 2014(3):CD010844*).
• **Macrolide antibiotics** (e.g., azithromycin 250 mg daily)
○ May function as an anti-infective or direct anti-inflammatory in COPD.
○ In patients with previous exacerbations, the frequency of subsequent exacerbations decreased by 19%; however, improvement in clinical symptoms was modest (*N Engl J Med 2011;365:689*).
○ The benefit may be absent in current smokers and greater in older individuals (>65 years) and milder disease (FEV_1 >50%).
○ Hearing loss in the absence of tinnitus was reported, suggesting routine monitoring with audiometry should be considered with chronic therapy.
• **Phosphodiesterase-4 (PDE4) inhibitors** (e.g., roflumilast 500 μg daily)
○ U.S. Food and Drug Administration (FDA) approved for a relatively narrow indication of severe COPD (FEV_1 <50%) and chronic bronchitis with frequent exacerbations, demonstrating a 17% reduction in exacerbations (*Lancet 2009;374:685*).
○ Appears to be safe when used as additional therapy to chronic bronchodilators.
○ Did not result in improvements in clinical symptoms possibly due to a higher frequency of side effects, particularly gastrointestinal, that limit the dose tolerated.
○ Limited long-term data and the possibility of weight loss and increased psychiatric symptoms suggest close monitoring is indicated.
• **Theophylline**
○ Theophylline is a xanthine derivative with bronchodilator properties. Patients not responding adequately to inhaled bronchodilator therapy may benefit from the addition

of theophylline, but potential toxicities and lack of data regarding efficacy in patients already on long-acting inhaled combination therapies limit its use.

○ Sustained-release theophylline is dosed once or twice a day. Serum levels should be maintained between 8 and 12 μg/mL to avoid toxicity.

○ Side effects include anxiety, tremor, headache, insomnia, nausea, vomiting, dyspepsia, tachycardia, tachyarrhythmia, and seizure.

○ In the event of suspected toxicity, theophylline should be stopped and a serum level measured.

○ Patients with severe COPD may experience clinical deterioration with discontinuation of theophylline.

○ Theophylline clearance is increased in current smokers and reduced in the elderly and patients with liver disease or congestive heart failure.

• **Systemic corticosteroids** are not recommended for the long-term management of COPD due to an unfavorable side effect profile and limited efficacy. However, they are sometimes used in patients with severe disease who are not responding to other therapies. If used, chronic oral steroid therapy should be administered at the minimum effective dose and discontinued as soon as is feasible. Routine bone mineral density assessment to prevent complications of osteoporosis should be incorporated.

• **IV α_1-antitrypsin (A1AT)** augmentation therapy may benefit select patients with severe A1AT deficiency and COPD (*Am J Respir Crit Care Med 2012;185:246*). Weekly infusion of 60 mg/kg is the standard treatment.

• For the treatment of stable COPD, antibiotics, mucolytics, antioxidants, immunoregulators, antitussives, vasodilators, respiratory stimulants, narcotics, and leukotriene inhibitors have not shown significant benefit.

Other Nonpharmacologic Therapies

• **Supplemental oxygen** decreases mortality and improves physical and mental functioning in hypoxemic patients with COPD.

○ A room-air resting ABG is the gold standard test for determining the need for supplemental oxygen. Pulse oximetry may be useful for routine checks after a baseline oxyhemoglobin saturation is assessed and compared for accuracy with the measured arterial oxyhemoglobin saturation (SaO_2).

○ Oxygen therapy is indicated for patients with an arterial partial pressure of oxygen (PaO_2) ≤55 mm Hg or an SaO_2 ≤88%, or if a patient has a PaO_2 <60 mm Hg or an SaO_2 <90% and evidence of PH, polycythemia (hematocrit >55%), or heart failure.

○ Supplemental oxygen requirements are typically greatest during exertion and least at rest while awake. Patients who require supplemental oxygen during exertion often need it during sleep as well. Although the exact amount of supplemental oxygen required during sleep can be measured with pulse oximetry, it is reasonable to initially estimate the amount needed by setting the oxygen flow rate at 1 L/min greater than that required during rest while awake.

○ The oxygen prescription should include the delivery system (compressed gas, liquid, or concentrator) and the required oxygen flow rates (liters per minute) for rest, sleep, and exercise.

○ Patients receiving long-term oxygen therapy should undergo reevaluation to assess oxygen requirements at least once a year.

• **Pulmonary rehabilitation** is a multidisciplinary intervention that improves symptoms and quality of life and reduces the frequency of exacerbations in patients with COPD (*Am J Respir Crit Care Med 2006;173:1390*). Components of a rehabilitation program include exercise training, nutritional counseling, and psychosocial support. Pulmonary rehabilitation should be considered for all patients with moderate to severe COPD (*N Engl J Med 2009;360:1329*).

- **Vaccinations**
  - ○ Annual influenza vaccination reduces the incidence of influenza-related acute respiratory illnesses in COPD patients (*Chest 2004;125:2011*).
  - ○ Although pneumococcal vaccination has not been shown to significantly reduce morbidity and mortality in COPD patients, it is still reasonable to give this vaccination (*Cochrane Database Syst Rev 2006;(4):CD001390*).

Surgical Therapy

- **Lung transplantation** for severe COPD can improve quality of life and functional capacity. The data are conflicting regarding survival, and a consistent survival benefit has not been demonstrated.
  Selection criteria for transplantation for COPD patients include a BODE score (Table 9-8) (see Outcome/Prognosis section) of 7 to 10 or at least one of the following: history of hospitalization for a COPD exacerbation associated with acute hypercapnia (arterial partial pressure of carbon dioxide [$PaCO_2$] >50 mm Hg); PH, right heart failure, or both, despite supplemental oxygen therapy; FEV_1 <20%; and either a DLCO <20% or homogeneous distribution of emphysema (*J Heart Lung Transplant 2006;25:745*).
- **LVRS** may provide quality of life and survival benefits in a specific subset of patients with upper lobe–predominant emphysema and significantly reduced exercise capacity (*Am J Respir Crit Care Med 2011;184(7):763*).

SPECIAL CONSIDERATIONS

Acute Exacerbation of COPD

- A COPD exacerbation is defined as increased dyspnea, often accompanied by increased cough, sputum production, sputum purulence, wheezing, chest tightness, or other symptoms (and signs) of acutely worsened respiratory status, in the absence of an alternative explanation.
- Respiratory infections (viral and bacterial) and air pollution cause most exacerbations (*Thorax 2006;61:250*).
- The differential diagnosis includes pneumothorax, pneumonia, pleural effusion, congestive heart failure, cardiac ischemia, and pulmonary embolism.

TABLE 9-8	BODE Index			
Points on BODE Index[a]				
Variable	0	1	2	3
FEV_1 (% of predicted)	≥65	50–64	36–49	≤35
Distance walked in 6 min (meters)	≥350	250–349	150–249	≤149
mMRC dyspnea scale	0–1	2	3	4
Body mass index	>21	≤21		

FEV_1, forced expiratory volume in 1 second; mMRC, Modified British Medical Research Council Questionnaire (see Table 9-3).
[a]The total possible cumulative values range from 0–10.
From Celli BR, Cote CG, Marin JM, et al. The body-mass index, airflow obstruction, dyspnea, and exercise capacity index in chronic obstructive pulmonary disease. *N Engl J Med* 2004;350(10):1005–12.

- In addition to the history and physical examination, assessment of a patient with a suspected COPD exacerbation should include oxyhemoglobin saturation, ABG, electrocardiogram, and CXR.
- Criteria for hospital admission include a significant increase in symptom severity, severe underlying COPD, significant comorbidities, failure to respond to initial medical management, diagnostic uncertainty, and insufficient home support (*GOLD Global Strategy for the Diagnosis, Management, and Prevention of Chronic Obstructive Pulmonary Disease [Update 2014]. Available at www.goldcopd.com*).
- Criteria for admission to an intensive care unit include the need for invasive mechanical ventilation, hemodynamic instability, severe dyspnea that does not adequately respond to therapy, mental status changes, and persistent or worsening hypoxemia, hypercapnia, or respiratory acidosis despite supplemental oxygen and noninvasive ventilation (*GOLD Global Strategy for the Diagnosis, Management, and Prevention of Chronic Obstructive Pulmonary Disease [Update 2014]. Available at www.goldcopd.com*).
- **Pharmacotherapy** (Table 9-9)
  - **Short-acting β-agonists (SABAs) are the first-line therapy for COPD exacerbations.** Short-acting anticholinergic agents can be added in the event of inadequate response to SABAs.

TABLE 9-9	Pharmacotherapy for Acute Exacerbations of Chronic Obstructive Pulmonary Disease

Medication Name	Dose
Albuterol	MDI: two to four puffs q1–4h Nebulizer: 2.5 mg q1–4h
Ipratropium	MDI: two puffs q4h Nebulizer: 0.5 mg q4h
Prednisone	40 mg/d × 5 days

Antibiotics[a]

Patient Characteristics	Pathogens to Consider	Antibiotic[b] (One of the Following)
No risk factors for poor outcome or drug-resistant pathogen[c]	*Haemophilus influenzae* *Streptococcus pneumoniae* *Moraxella catarrhalis*	Macrolide, second- or third-generation cephalosporin, doxycycline, trimethoprim/sulfamethoxazole
Risk factors present	As above, plus gram-negative rods, including *Pseudomonas*	Antipseudomonal fluoroquinolone or β-lactam

MDI, metered-dose inhaler.
[a]Indicated for all inpatients and most outpatients. Dosing recommendation from the Global Strategy for Diagnosis, Management, and Prevention of COPD, 2015, © Global Initiative for Chronic Obstructive Lung Disease (GOLD), all rights reserved. Available from http://www.goldcopd.com.
[b]Treat for 3–7 days. If recent antibiotic exposure, select an agent from an alternative class. Take local resistance patterns into account.
[c]Risk factors: age >65 years, comorbid conditions (especially cardiac disease), forced expiratory volume in 1 second (FEV_1) <50%, more than three exacerbations/year, antibiotic therapy within the past 3 months (*Thorax 2006;61:337*).

- Many patients experiencing an acute exacerbation of COPD have difficulty performing optimal MDI technique. Therefore, numerous clinicians opt to deliver bronchodilators via nebulization.
- Due to the risk of serious side effects, clinicians typically avoid using methylxanthines (e.g., theophylline) for acute exacerbations. However, if a patient uses methylxanthines chronically, discontinuation during an exacerbation is discouraged due to the risk of decompensation.
- **Systemic corticosteroids** produce improvement in hospital length of stay, lung function, and the incidence of relapse. They are recommended for all inpatients and most outpatients experiencing an exacerbation of COPD (*N Engl J Med 2003;348:2618; N Engl J Med 1999;340:1941; Lancet 1999;354:456*). A prednisone dose of 40 mg for 5 days is recommended over longer regimens (*JAMA 2013;309:2223*).
- **Antibiotic therapy** is routinely administered but most often benefits patients with sputum purulence as well as patients with a need for mechanical ventilation (*Ann Intern Med 1987;106:196; Chest 2000;117:1638; Lancet 2001;358:2020*).
- **Supplemental oxygen** should be administered with a target oxygen saturation of 88–92%.
- **Thromboprophylactic measures** should be used given the increased risk of deep venous thrombosis in patients hospitalized for COPD exacerbation (*Chest 2009;135:786*).
- **Noninvasive ventilation** (Table 9-10) reduces intubation rate, improves respiratory acidosis, decreases respiratory rate, and decreases hospital length of stay (*BMJ 2003;326:185*).
- **Endotracheal intubation** and invasive mechanical ventilation are required in some patients (Table 9-11).
- Discharge criteria for patients with acute exacerbations of COPD include the need for inhaled bronchodilators less frequently than every 4 hours; clinical and ABG stability for at least 12–24 hours; the ability to eat, sleep, and ambulate fairly comfortably; adequate patient understanding of home therapy; and adequate home arrangements.

Prior to discharge from the hospital, chronic therapy issues should be readdressed, including supplemental oxygen requirements, vaccinations, smoking cessation, assessment of inhaler technique, and pulmonary rehabilitation.

TABLE 9-10	Indications and Contraindications for Noninvasive Ventilation in Acute Exacerbations of Chronic Obstructive Pulmonary Disease
Indications	**Contraindications**
Moderate-to-severe dyspnea with evidence of increased work of breathing	Respiratory arrest Hemodynamic instability Altered mental status, inability to cooperate
Acute respiratory acidosis with pH ≤7.35 and/or PaCO$_2$ >45 mm Hg (6.0 kPa)	High risk of aspiration Viscous or copious secretions Recent facial or gastroesophageal surgery
Respiratory rate >25	Craniofacial trauma Fixed nasopharyngeal abnormalities Burns Extreme obesity

Data from the Global Strategy for Diagnosis, Management, and Prevention of COPD, 2015, © Global Initiative for Chronic Obstructive Lung Disease (GOLD), all rights reserved. Available from http://www.goldcopd.com.

TABLE 9-11	Indications for Invasive Mechanical Ventilation in Acute Exacerbations of Chronic Obstructive Pulmonary Disease

Failure to improve with or not a candidate for noninvasive ventilation (see Table 9-10)
Severe dyspnea with evidence of increased work of breathing
Acute respiratory acidosis with pH <7.25 and/or $PaCO_2$ >60 mm Hg (8.0 kPa)
PaO_2 <40 mm Hg (5.3 kPa)
Respiratory rate >35
Coexisting conditions such as cardiovascular disease, metabolic abnormalities, sepsis, pneumonia, pulmonary embolism, pneumothorax, large pleural effusion

Data from the Global Strategy for Diagnosis, Management, and Prevention of COPD, 2015, © Global Initiative for Chronic Obstructive Lung Disease (GOLD), all rights reserved. Available from http://www.goldcopd.com.

COMPLICATIONS

- Patients with severe COPD and chronic hypoxemia may develop PH and right-sided heart failure.
- COPD patients are at increased risk for lung cancer, ischemic heart disease, pneumothorax, arrhythmias, osteoporosis, and psychiatric disorders such as anxiety and depression.
  - Annual low-dose CT screening of asymptomatic heavy smokers (age >55 years, >30 pack-year history) provides a 20% reduction in mortality from lung cancer. This must be balanced with the risk of invasive procedures from false-positive tests that were seen in approximately 40% of screened individuals (*N Engl J Med 2011;365:395*). In the largest screening trial, the majority of false-positive results could be resolved with repeat imaging.
  - Many patients with mild and moderate (Global Initiative for Chronic Obstructive Lung Disease [GOLD] stage I and II) COPD will die of cardiovascular disease. Therefore, cardioselective β-blockers should be used when indicated.
  - Osteoporosis and vitamin D deficiency are common in COPD and should be monitored and treated.
- Sleep disturbances are estimated to affect 50% of patients with COPD. Newer nonbenzodiazepine medications such as zolpidem appear to be safe in patients with less severe COPD (*Proc Am Thorac Soc 2008;5:536*).

OUTCOME/PROGNOSIS

The BODE index (see Table 9-8) is a composite of body mass index, airflow obstruction, dyspnea, and exercise tolerance that has been validated as a more accurate predictor of COPD mortality than FEV_1 alone (*N Engl J Med 2004;350:1005*).

Asthma

GENERAL PRINCIPLES

Definition

- Asthma is a heterogeneous airway disease characterized by chronic inflammation, hyperresponsiveness with exposure to a wide variety of stimuli, and variable airflow obstruction. As a consequence, patients have paroxysms of cough, dyspnea, chest tightness, and wheezing.
- **Asthma is a chronic disease with episodic acute exacerbations that are interspersed with symptom-free periods.** Exacerbations are characterized by a progressive increase in

asthma symptoms that can last minutes to hours. They are associated with viral infections, allergens, and occupational exposures, and occur when airway reactivity is increased and lung function becomes unstable.

Classification

- Asthma severity should be classified based on both level of impairment (symptoms, lung function, daily activities, and rescue medication use) and risk (exacerbations, lung function decline, and medication side effects).
- At the initial evaluation, this assessment will determine the level of severity in patients not on controller medications (Table 9-12). The level of severity is based on the most severe category in which any feature appears. On subsequent visits, or if the patient is on a controller medication, this assessment is based on the lowest step of therapy to maintain clinical control (Table 9-13). Control of asthma is based on the most severe impairment or risk category.
- During an exacerbation, the acute severity of the attack should be classified based on symptoms, signs, and objective measures of lung function (Table 9-14).
- Patients who have had two or more exacerbations requiring systemic corticosteroids in the past year may be considered in the same category as those who have persistent asthma, regardless of level of impairment.

Epidemiology

In the United States:
- Asthma is the leading chronic illness among children (20–30%) (*NCHS Data Brief 2012;1*).
- The prevalence of asthma and asthma-related mortality had been increasing from 1980 to the mid-1990s, but since the 2000s, a more gradual increase in prevalence and decrease in mortality have occurred. Currently, an estimated 300 million individuals are affected worldwide and 250,000 individuals worldwide die every year due to asthma.
- African Americans are more likely than Caucasians to have emergency department (ED) visits and hospitalizations and have a higher rate of mortality due to asthma.

Etiology

Possible factors for asthma development can be broadly divided into host, genetic, and environmental factors.
- There have been multiple genes, chromosomal regions, and epigenetic changes associated with the development of asthma. Racial and ethnic differences have also been reported in asthma and are likely the result of a complex interaction between genetic, socioeconomic, and environmental factors.
- There are multiple environmental factors that contribute to the development and persistence of asthma. Severe viral infections early in life, particularly respiratory syncytial virus (RSV) and rhinovirus, are associated with the development of asthma in childhood and play a role in its pathogenesis.
- Childhood exposure and sensitization to a variety of allergens and irritants (e.g., cigarette smoke, mold, pet dander, dust mites, cockroaches) may play a role in the development of asthma, but the exact nature of this relationship is not yet fully elucidated. By contrast, early-life exposure to indoor allergens together with certain bacteria (microbiome) may be protective for urban children. The prevalence of asthma in children raised in a rural setting is reduced, although the reason for this is not fully known.

Pathophysiology

Asthma is characterized by airway obstruction, hyperinflation, and airflow limitation resulting from multiple processes:
- Acute and chronic airway inflammation characterized by infiltration of the airway wall, mucosa, and lumen by activated eosinophils, mast cells, macrophages, and T lymphocytes.

TABLE 9-12	Classification of Asthma Severity on Initial Assessment			
	Intermittent	**Mild Persistent**	**Moderate Persistent**	**Severe Persistent**
Daytime symptoms	≤2 d/wk	≥2 d/wk but not daily	Daily	Throughout the day
Nighttime symptoms	≤2×/mo	3–4×/mo	≥1×/wk but not nightly	Nightly
Activity limitations	None	Minor	Some	Extreme
Reliever medicine use	≤2 da/wk	≥2 d/wk but not daily	Daily	Several times per day
FEV$_1$	≥80%	≥80%	60–80%	<60%
Exacerbations	0–1×/yr	≥2×/yr	≥2×/yr	≥2×/yr
Management	Step 1	Step 2	Step 3	Step 4	Step 5
Preferred	Low-dose ICS	Low-dose ICS	Low-dose ICS	Medium- or high-dose ICS + LABA	Add-on therapy: i.e., omalizumab, bronchial thermoplasty
Alternative	Low-dose ICS		LTRA, cromolyn, theophylline	High-dose ICS+LTRA or theophylline	Consider low-dose OCS

In 2–6 wk, evaluate level of asthma control and adjust therapy accordingly.

FEV$_1$, forced expiratory volume in 1 second; ICS, inhaled corticosteroids; LABA, long-acting β-adrenergic agonist; LTRA, leukotriene receptor antagonist; OCS, oral corticosteroids.
Data from the Global Strategy for Asthma Management and Prevention, Global Initiative for Asthma (GINA) 2014. Available from: http://www.ginasthma.org
National Asthma Education and Prevention Program. Expert Panel Report 3. http://www.nhlbi.nih.gov/guidelines/asthma/asthgdln.pdf, 2007.

TABLE 9-13	Assessment of Asthma Control		
	Well Controlled	Not Well Controlled	Very Poorly Controlled
Daytime symptoms	≤2 d/wk	>2 d/wk	Throughout the day
Nighttime symptoms	None	1–3×/wk	≥4×/wk
Activity limitations	None	Some	Extreme
Reliever medicine use	≤2×/wk	>2×/wk	Frequent
FEV$_1$ or PEF	≥80%	60–80%	<60%
Validated questionnaire	ACT ≥20 ACQ <0.75	ACT 16–19 ACQ >1.5	ACT ≤15
Exacerbations	0–1/yr	≥2×/yr	≥2×/yr
Management	Maintain at lowest step possible Consider step down if well controlled for ≥3 mo	Step up one step	Step up one to two steps and consider short-course OCS
Follow-up	1–6 mo	2–6 wk	2 wk

ACT, Asthma Control Test; ACQ, Asthma Control Questionnaire; FEV$_1$, forced expiratory volume in 1 second; OCS, oral corticosteroids PEF, peak expiratory flow.
Data from the Global Strategy for Asthma Management and Prevention, Global Initiative for Asthma (GINA) 2014. Available at: http://www.ginasthma.org. National Asthma Education and Prevention Program. Expert Panel Report 3. http://www.nhlbi.nih.gov/guidelines/asthma/asthgdln.pdf.

Components of innate immunity including natural killer T cells, neutrophils, and innate lymphoid lymphocytes are also implicated.
- Bronchial smooth muscle contraction resulting from mediators released by a variety of cell types including inflammatory, local neural, and epithelial cells.
- Epithelial damage manifested by denudation and desquamation of the epithelium leading to mucous plugs that obstruct the airway.
- Airway remodeling characterized by the following findings:
  ○ Subepithelial fibrosis, specifically thickening of the lamina reticularis from collagen deposition
  ○ Smooth muscle hypertrophy and hyperplasia
  ○ Goblet cell and submucosal gland hypertrophy and hyperplasia resulting in mucous hypersecretion
  ○ Airway angiogenesis
  ○ Airway wall thickening due to edema and cellular infiltration

Risk Factors

A number of factors increase airway hyperresponsiveness and can cause an acute and chronic increase in the severity of the disease:
- Allergens such as dust mites, cockroaches, pollens, molds, and pet dander in susceptible patients.
- Viral upper respiratory tract infections.

TABLE 9-14	Classification of Asthma Exacerbation Severity		
	Moderate	**Severe**	**Impending Respiratory Arrest**
FEV₁ or PEF predicted or personal best	40–69%	<40%	<25% or unable to measure
Symptoms	DOE or SOB with talking	SOB at rest	Severe SOB
Exam	Expiratory wheeze	Inspiratory and expiratory wheeze	Wheeze may become absent
	Some accessory muscle use	Increased accessory muscle use Chest retraction Agitation or confusion	Accessory muscle use with paradoxical thoracoabdominal movement Depressed mental status
Vitals	RR <28/min HR <110 bpm O₂sat >91% RA No pulsus paradoxus	RR >28/min HR >110 bpm O₂sat <91% RA Pulsus paradoxus >25 mm Hg	Same as severe but could develop respiratory depression and/or bradycardia
PaCO₂	Normal to hypocapnia	>42 mm Hg	Hypercapnia is a late sign

DOE, dyspnea on exertion; FEV_1, forced expiratory volume in 1 second; HR, heart rate; O₂sat, oxygen saturation; PEF, peak expiratory flow; RA, room air; RR, respiratory rate; SOB, shortness of breath.
Data from Global Initiative for Asthma. GINA report, global strategy for asthma management and prevention. http://www.ginasthma.org. 2011; National Asthma Education and Prevention Program. Expert Panel Report 3. http://www.nhlbi.nih.gov/guidelines/asthma/asthgdln.pdf, 2007.

- Many occupational allergens and irritants such as perfumes, cleaners, or detergents, even in small doses.
- Changes in weather (i.e., from warm to cold), strong emotional stimuli, and exercise.
- Indoor and outdoor pollutants, such as nitrogen dioxide (NO_2) and tobacco and wood smoke, can trigger acute bronchospasm and should be avoided by all patients.
- Obesity is associated with increased asthma severity.
- Medications such as β-blockers (including ophthalmic preparations), aspirin, and NSAIDs can cause the sudden onset of severe airway obstruction.

Prevention
- Strict compliance and appropriate follow-up can help prevent worsening of asthma control.
- Identification and avoidance of risk factors (allergens, irritants) that exacerbate symptoms play a key role in prevention.
- Recognition and management of comorbidities such as obesity, sinonasal diseases, gastroesophageal reflux disease (GERD), and psychiatric disorders are important.
- All patients with asthma should receive a yearly influenza vaccination.

Associated Conditions

- **Rhinosinusitis**, with or without nasal polyps, is frequently present and should be treated with intranasal or oral corticosteroids, saline rinses, and/or antihistamines. Antibiotics should be reserved for superimposed bacterial infections.
- **Vocal cord dysfunction (VCD)** can coexist with or masquerade severe, uncontrolled asthma. Treatment consists of speech and, if needed, behavioral therapy.
- Symptomatic **GERD** can cause cough and wheezing in some patients and may benefit from treatment with H_2 blockers or proton pump inhibitors. Empiric treatment of GERD in asymptomatic patients with uncontrolled asthma is not an effective strategy.
- **Obesity** is increasingly being recognized as a comorbid condition as well as possibly playing a role in worsening asthma control. This may be related to altered lung mechanics, altered respiratory patterns, or an increase in systemic inflammation. Obese patients should be strongly encouraged to focus on weight loss through diet and exercise.
- Smoking prevalence in patients with asthma is the same as the general population. Although no convincing evidence links tobacco use with developing asthma, it may make patients less responsive to ICSs and more difficult to control. Tobacco cessation should be encouraged in all patients.
- **Obstructive sleep apnea (OSA)** may make asthma more difficult to control and should be addressed with an overnight polysomnogram if suspected.

DIAGNOSIS

Clinical Presentation

History
- Recurring episodes of cough, dyspnea, chest tightness, and wheezing are suggestive of asthma. Symptoms are often worse at night or early morning, in the presence of potential triggers, and/or in a seasonal pattern.
- A personal or family history of atopy can increase the likelihood of asthma.
- Patients presenting for the first time over 50 years old, patients with >20 pack-years of smoking, and lack of response to asthma therapy are features that make asthma less likely as the sole cause of respiratory symptoms.

Physical Examination
- Auscultation of wheezing and a prolonged expiratory phase can be present on exam, but a normal chest exam does not exclude asthma.
- Signs of atopy, such as eczema, rhinitis, or nasal polyps, often coexist with asthma.
- During a suspected asthma exacerbation, a rapid assessment should be performed to identify patients who require immediate intervention (see Table 9-14).
  - Respiratory distress and/or peak expiratory flow (PEF) <25% of predicted.
  - The presence or intensity of wheezing is an unreliable indicator of the severity of an attack.
  - SC emphysema should alert the examiner to the presence of a pneumothorax or pneumomediastinum.

Diagnostic Criteria

- In general, the diagnosis is supported by the presence of symptoms consistent with asthma combined with demonstration of variable expiratory airflow obstruction.
- Adequate response to asthma treatment is a valid method to assist with making the diagnosis.

Differential Diagnosis

Other conditions may present with wheezing and must be considered, especially in patients who are not responsive to therapy (Table 9-15).

TABLE 9-15	Conditions that Can Present as Refractory Asthma
Upper airway obstruction Tumor Epiglottitis Vocal cord dysfunction Obstructive sleep apnea **Lower airway disease** Allergic bronchopulmonary aspergillosis Chronic obstructive pulmonary disease Cystic fibrosis α_1-Antitrypsin deficiency Bronchiectasis Bronchiolitis obliterans Tracheomalacia Endobronchial lesion Foreign body Herpetic tracheobronchitis	**Adverse drug reaction** Aspirin β-Adrenergic antagonist Angiotensin-converting enzyme inhibitors Inhaled pentamidine Congestive heart failure Gastroesophageal reflux Sinusitis Hypersensitivity pneumonitis Churg-Strauss syndrome Eosinophilic pneumonia Hyperventilation with panic attacks Dysfunctional breathlessness

Diagnostic Testing

Laboratories
- Routine laboratory tests are not indicated for the diagnosis of asthma and should not delay the initiation of treatment.
- During an exacerbation, monitor oxygen saturation. ABG measurement should be considered in patients in severe distress or with an FEV_1 of <40% of predicted values after initial treatment.
  - A PaO_2 <60 mm Hg is a sign of severe bronchoconstriction or of a complicating condition, such as pulmonary edema or pneumonia.
  - Initially, the $PaCO_2$ is low due to an increase in respiratory rate. With a prolonged attack, the $PaCO_2$ may rise as a result of severe airway obstruction, increased dead space ventilation, and respiratory muscle fatigue. **A normal or increased $PaCO_2$ is a sign of impending respiratory failure and necessitates hospitalization.**

Allergy Tests
- Allergy skin tests or immunoassays for allergen-specific IgE are helpful to identify sensitization to specific inhalant allergens when allergen exposure is concerned as a trigger.
- Results of allergy tests must correlate with history and clinical presentation.

Exhaled Nitric Oxide
- Fractional concentration of exhaled nitric oxide (FeNO) may be used as a marker of eosinophilic airway inflammation in asthma.
- An FeNO level >50 parts per billion (ppb) is associated with a good response to ICSs. However, it is generally recommended not to use FeNO to guide asthma therapy.

Imaging
- Obtaining a CXR is not routinely required and is performed only if a complicating pulmonary process, such as pneumonia or pneumothorax, is suspected or to rule out other causes of respiratory symptoms in patients being evaluated for asthma.
- CT of the chest can be considered in patients with severe asthma refractory to treatment to evaluate for alternative diagnosis.

Diagnostic Procedures
- **Pulmonary function tests (PFTs)** are essential to the diagnosis of asthma. In patients with asthma, PFTs demonstrate an obstructive pattern—the hallmark of which is a decrease in expiratory flow rates.
  - A reduction in FEV_1 and a proportionally smaller reduction in the FVC occur. This produces a decreased FEV_1/FVC ratio (generally <0.7 or the lower limit of normal value). With mild obstructive disease that involves only the small airways, the FEV_1/FVC ratio may be normal, with the only abnormality being a decrease in airflow at midlung volumes (forced expiratory flow 25–75%).
  - The clinical diagnosis of asthma is supported by an obstructive pattern that improves after bronchodilator therapy. **Improvement is defined as an increase in FEV_1 of >12% and 200 mL after two to four puffs of a short-acting bronchodilator.** Most patients will not demonstrate reversibility at each assessment.
  - In patients with chronic, severe asthma, the airflow obstruction may no longer be completely reversible. In these patients, the most effective way to establish the maximal degree of airway reversibility is to repeat PFTs after a course of oral corticosteroids (usually 40 mg/d for 10–14 days) and to use the same criteria as above for reversibility. The lack of demonstrable airway obstruction or reactivity does not rule out a diagnosis of asthma.
  - In cases in which spirometry is normal, the diagnosis can be made by showing heightened airway responsiveness to a **methacholine challenge**. A methacholine challenge is considered positive when a provocative concentration of 8 mg/mL or less causes a drop in FEV_1 of 20% (PC_{20}). A PC_{20} >16 mg/mL is considered a negative test.
- An objective measurement of airflow obstruction is essential to the evaluation of an exacerbation. The severity of the exacerbation should be classified as:
  - Mild (PEF or FEV_1 >70% of predicted or personal best)
  - Moderate (PEF or FEV_1 40–69%)
  - Severe (PEF or FEV_1 <40%)
  - Life-threatening/impending respiratory arrest (PEF or FEV_1 <25%)

TREATMENT

- Medical management involves chronic management and a plan for acute exacerbations, otherwise known as the **asthma action plan**. Most often, it includes the daily use of an anti-inflammatory, disease-modifying medication (long-term control medications), and as-needed use of a short-acting bronchodilator (quick-relief medications).
- The goals of daily management are to **avoid impairment** (lack of symptoms while maintaining normal activity and pulmonary function) and to **minimize risk** (preventing exacerbations, loss of lung function, and medication side effects). Successful management requires patient education, objective measurement of airflow obstruction, and a medication plan for daily use and for exacerbations.
- When initiating therapy for a patient not already on controller medicine, one should assess the patient's severity and assign the patient to the highest level in which any one feature has occurred over the previous 2–4 weeks (see Table 9-12).
- Assessment of control on subsequent visits is used to modify therapy when following patients already on controller medication (see Table 9-13).
- Address the following issues before stepping up the therapy when there is a poor response to controller medicine after 2–3 months of treatment.
  - Nonadherence to medications
  - Incorrect inhaler technique
  - Ongoing exposure to allergens and/or irritants
  - Comorbidities: obesity, sinonasal diseases, GERD, OSA, and depression
  - Alternative diagnoses (see Table 9-15)

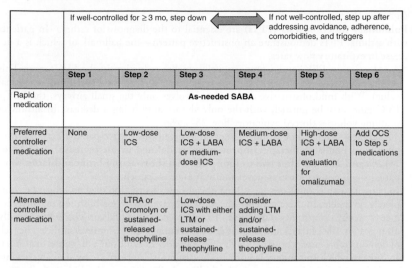

	Step 1	Step 2	Step 3	Step 4	Step 5	Step 6
	If well-controlled for ≥3 mo, step down ⟺ If not well-controlled, step up after addressing avoidance, adherence, comorbidities, and triggers					
Rapid medication	As-needed SABA					
Preferred controller medication	None	Low-dose ICS	Low-dose ICS + LABA or medium-dose ICS	Medium-dose ICS + LABA	High-dose ICS + LABA and evaluation for omalizumab	Add OCS to Step 5 medications
Alternate controller medication		LTRA or Cromolyn or sustained-released theophylline	Low-dose ICS with either LTM or sustained-release theophylline	Consider adding LTM and/or sustained-release theophylline		

Figure 9-1. Management algorithm based on level of control. ICS, inhaled corticosteroid; LABA, long-acting β$_2$-agonist; LTM, leukotriene modifier; LTRA, leukotriene receptor antagonist; OCS, oral corticosteroid; SABA, short-acting β$_2$-agonist. (From Global Initiative for Asthma. GINA Report, global strategy for asthma management and Prevention. http://www.ginasthma.org, 2011; National Asthma Education and Prevention Program. Expert panel report 3. http://www.nhlbi.nih.gov/guidelines/asthma/asthgdln.pdf, 2007.)

• The goal of the stepwise approach is to gain control of symptoms as quickly as possible. At the same time, level of control varies over time and, consequently, medication requirements as well, so therapy should be reviewed every 3 months to check whether stepwise reduction is possible (Figure 9-1).
• **Management of an exacerbation** requiring hospital-based care should follow a treatment algorithm to triage patients based on response to treatment (Figure 9-2).
  ○ The response to initial treatment (three treatments with a short-acting bronchodilator every 20 minutes for 60–90 minutes) can be a better predictor of the need for hospitalization than the severity of an exacerbation.
  ○ Patients at high risk of asthma-related death (see Outcome/Prognosis section) should be advised to seek medical attention early in the course of an exacerbation.
  ○ A low threshold for admission is appropriate for patients with recent hospitalization, a failure of aggressive outpatient management (with oral corticosteroids), or a previous life-threatening attack.

Medications

First Line
• **Short-acting bronchodilators**
  ○ Quick-relief medications used on an as-needed basis for long-term management of all severities of asthma as well as for rapid treatment of exacerbations given via either MDI or nebulization.
  ○ For long-term management, a **SABA** used on an as-needed basis (e.g., albuterol, two puffs q6h) is appropriate.
  ○ SABA is considered the drug of choice for preventing exercise-induced bronchoconstriction.

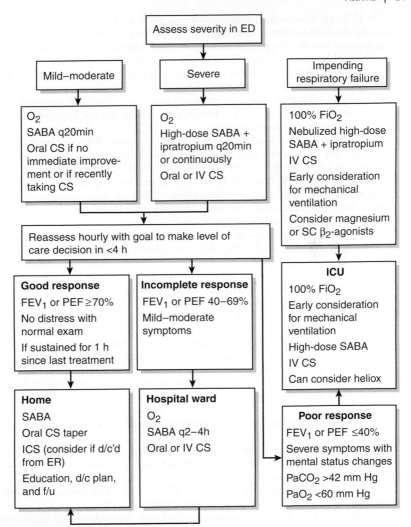

Figure 9-2. Treatment algorithm for asthma exacerbation. CS, corticosteroid; d/c, discharge; ED, emergency department; FEV$_1$, forced expiratory volume in 1 second; f/u, follow-up; ICS, inhaled corticosteroid; ICU, intensive care unit; PEF, peak expiratory flow; SABA, short-acting β$_2$-agonist. (From Global Initiative for Asthma. GINA Report, global strategy for asthma management and prevention. http://www.ginasthma.org, 2011; National Asthma Education and Prevention Program. Expert panel report 3. http://www.nhlbi.nih.gov/guidelines/asthma/asthgdln.pdf, 2007.)

○ During an exacerbation, reversal of airflow obstruction is achieved most effectively by frequent administration of an inhaled SABA.
- For a **mild-to-moderate exacerbation**, initial treatment starts with two to six puffs of albuterol via MDI with a spacer or 2.5 mg via nebulizer and is repeated q20min until improvement is obtained or toxicity is noted.
- For a **severe exacerbation**, albuterol 2.5–5.0 mg q20min with ipratropium bromide 0.5 mg q20min should be administered via nebulizer. Alternatively, albutero

10.0–15.0 mg, administered continuously over an hour, may be more effective in severely obstructed adults. If used, telemetry monitoring is necessary.

- Levalbuterol four to eight puffs or nebulized 1.25–2.5 mg q20min can be substituted for albuterol but has not been associated with fewer side effects in adults.
- The subsequent dosing schedule is adjusted according to the patient's symptoms and clinical presentation. Often, patients require a SABA q2–4h during an acute attack. The use of an MDI with a spacer device under supervision of trained personnel is as effective as aerosolized solution by nebulizer. Cooperation may not be possible in the patient with severe airflow obstruction.
- SC administration of a β_2-adrenergic agonist is unnecessary if inhaled medications can be administered quickly with an adequate response. In rare settings, aqueous epinephrine (0.3–0.5 mL of a 1:1000 solution SC q20min) or terbutaline (0.25 mg SC q20min) for up to three doses can be used. However, there has been no evidence to suggest their superiority over aerosolized therapy. Their use is contraindicated if the patient has had a myocardial infarction within the last 6 months or is having active angina. If used, ECG monitoring is necessary.
  - All SABAs now use hydrofluoroalkane (HFA) as a propellant. They should be primed with four puffs when first used and again if not used over 2 weeks.
- **ICSs**
  - ICSs are safe and effective for the treatment of persistent asthma. They are generally administered via a dry powder inhaler (DPI), MDI with a spacing device, or nebulized.
  - Dosing depends on assessment of severity and control (Table 9-16).
  - Once-daily dosing of ICS may be as effective as twice-daily dosing in the management of mild persistent asthma and may improve adherence.
  - Systemic corticosteroid absorption can occur in patients who use high doses of ICS. Consequently, prolonged therapy with high-dose ICS should be reserved for patients with severe disease or for those who otherwise require oral corticosteroids.
  - Attempts should be made to decrease the dose of ICS every 2–3 months to the lowest possible dose to maintain control.
- **LABAs**
  - Recommended for moderate and severe persistent asthma in patients not adequately controlled with ICS.
  - Salmeterol or the faster acting formoterol added to ICS has consistently been shown to improve lung function, improve both day and nighttime symptoms, reduce exacerbations, and minimize the required dose of ICS.
  - LABA should only be used in combination with ICS in patients with asthma (salmeterol/fluticasone, budesonide/formoterol, or mometasone/formoterol).
  - The benefits of adding LABAs are more substantial than those achieved by leukotriene modifiers (LTMs), theophylline, or increased doses of ICS.
- **Systemic corticosteroids**
  - May be necessary to gain control of disease quickly via either oral or IV route.
  - If chronic symptoms are severe and accompanied by nighttime awakening or PEF is <70% of predicted values, a short course of oral corticosteroid (prednisone 40–60 mg/d for 5–7 days) might be necessary.
  - Long-term therapy is occasionally necessary and should be started at low dose (≤10 mg/d prednisone or equivalent), and repeated attempts should be made to reduce the dose while patients are receiving high-dose ICS. Side effects associated with long-term therapy should be closely monitored. Osteoporosis prophylaxis may be necessary.
  - **During an exacerbation, systemic corticosteroids speed the resolution of exacerbations of asthma and should be administered promptly to all patients.**
    - The ideal dose of corticosteroid needed to speed recovery and limit symptoms is not well defined. A single or divided daily dose equivalent to prednisone 40–60 mg is

TABLE 9-16	Comparative Daily Adult Dosages for Inhaled Corticosteroids		
Drug	**Low Dose**	**Medium Dose**	**High Dose**
Triamcinolone HFA (75 µg/puff)	300–750 µg	>750–1500 µg	>1500 µg
Beclomethasone HFA (40 or 80 µg/puff)	80–240 µg	>240–480 µg	>480 µg
Budesonide DPI (90, 180, or 200 µg/dose)	180–600 µg	>600–1200 µg	>1200 µg
Budesonide nebulized respules (250, 500, or 1000 µg/respules)	250–500 µg	>500–1000 µg	>1000 µg
Ciclesonide HFA (80 or 160 µg/puff)	160–320 µg	>320–640 µg	>640 µg
Flunisolide HFA (80 µg/puff)	320 µg	>320–640 µg	>640 µg
Fluticasone HFA (44, 110, or 220 µg/puff)	88–264 µg	>264–440 µg	>440 µg
Fluticasone DPI (50, 100, or 250 µg/dose)	100–300 µg	>300–500 µg	>500 µg
Mometasone furoate DPI (110 or 220 µg/puff)	220 µg	440 µg	>440 µg
Combination agents			
Budesonide/formoterol (MDI: 80/4.5 or 160/4.5 µg/puff)	Two puffs bid: 80/4.5 µg/puff	Two puffs bid: 80/4.5 to 160/4.5 µg/puff	Two puffs bid: 160/4.5 µg/puff
Fluticasone/salmeterol (MDI: 45/21, 115/21, or 230/21 µg/puff) (DPI: 100/50, 250/50, or 500/50 µg/dose)	One inhalation bid: 100/50 µg	One inhalation bid: 250/50 µg	One inhalation bid: 500/50 µg
Mometasone/formoterol (MDI: 100/5 or 200/5 µg/puff)	Two inhalations bid: 100/5 µg/puff	Two inhalations bid: 100/5 µg/puff to 200/5 µg/puff	Two inhalations bid: 200/5 µg/puff

DPI, dry powder inhaler; MDI, metered-dose inhaler.
Data from Global Initiative for Asthma. GINA Report, global strategy for asthma management and prevention. http://www.ginasthma.org. 2011; National Asthma Education and Prevention Program. Expert panel report 3. http://www.nhlbi.nih.gov/guidelines/asthma/asthgdln.pdf, 2007.

usually adequate. Oral corticosteroid administration seems to be as effective as IV administration if given in equivalent doses.

- IV methylprednisolone, 125 mg, given on initial presentation, decreases the rate of return to the ED for patients who are discharged.
- For maximal therapeutic response, tapering of high-dose corticosteroids should not take place until objective evidence of clinical improvement is observed (usually 36–48 hours or when PEF >70%). Initially, patients are given a daily dose of oral prednisone, which is then reduced slowly.
- A 7- to 14-day tapering dose of prednisone is usually successful in combination with an ICS instituted at the beginning of the tapering schedule. In patients with severe disease or with a history of respiratory failure, a slower reduction in dose is appropriate.
- Patients discharged from the ED should receive oral corticosteroids. A dose of prednisone, 40 mg/d for 5–7 days, can be substituted for a tapering schedule in selected patients. Either regimen should be accompanied by the initiation of an ICS or an increase in the previous dose of ICS.

Second Line
- **LTMs**
  ○ **Montelukast** (10 mg PO daily) and **zafirlukast** (20 mg PO bid) are oral leukotriene receptor antagonists (LTRAs), and **zileuton** (extended-release 1200 mg bid) is an oral 5-lipoxygenase inhibitor. The LTRAs are recommended as an alternative first-line medication for mild persistent asthma and as an add-on to ICS for more severe forms of asthma.
  ○ As add-on therapy to ICS, these agents have been shown to improve lung function, lead to improved quality of life, and lead to fewer exacerbations. However, compared with ICS plus LABA, they are not as effective in improving asthma outcomes.
  ○ **A LTM should be strongly considered for patients with aspirin-sensitive asthma, exercise-induced bronchoconstriction, or concurrent allergic rhinitis, or individuals who cannot master the use of an inhaler.**
- **Anti-IgE therapy**
  ○ **Omalizumab** is a monoclonal antibody against IgE that is approved for the management of patients with moderate to severe persistent allergic asthma with a demonstrable sensitivity to a perennial aeroallergen and incomplete control with ICS.
  ○ Omalizumab can decrease airway inflammation through its effects on IgE. Treatment with omalizumab decreases eosinophil counts in sputum and biopsy specimens and attenuates lymphocyte proliferation and cytokine production.
  ○ Omalizumab is administered 150–375 mg SC q2–4wk and dosed based on the patient's baseline IgE level (if between 30–700 IU/mL) and weight.
  ○ Addition of omalizumab in adults and children 12 years of age or older has been shown to reduce exacerbation rates and need for corticosteroids in patients on a controller medication regimen. Rescue medication use is often reduced, and asthma-related quality of life is improved. Health care utilization (ED visits, hospital admissions) is decreased with omalizumab use in severe asthmatics. At least 16 weeks of treatment are needed to determine the efficacy of omalizumab.
  ○ Allergic rhinitis symptoms often improve with omalizumab therapy. In one controlled trial, omalizumab use reduced nasal symptom severity scores and rescue antihistamine use in a dose-dependent manner (*JAMA 2001;286(23):2956*).
- **Long-acting muscarinic antagonists:** Tiotropium bromide as add-on therapy to ICS with or without LABA is associated with improved lung functions, fewer symptoms, and reduced exacerbations in patients with inadequately controlled asthma (*N Engl J Med 2012;367:1198*)
- **Methylxanthines:** Sustained-release theophylline at low doses (300 mg/d) may be useful as adjuvant therapy to an anti-inflammatory agent in persistent asthma, especially for

controlling nighttime symptoms. Clinical use is limited due to the narrow therapeutic window.

- **IV magnesium sulfate:** During a severe exacerbation refractory to standard treatment over 1 hour, one dose of 2 g IV over 20 minutes in the ED should be considered. It has been shown to acutely improve lung function especially in those with severe, life-threatening exacerbations (*Ann Emerg Med 2000;36:181*).
- **Inhaled heliox:** During a severe exacerbation refractory to standard treatment over 1 hour, heliox-driven albuterol nebulization in a mixture with oxygen (70:30) should be considered. It has been shown to acutely improve lung function, especially in those with severe, life-threatening exacerbations (*Acad Emerg Med 2005;12:820*).
- **Antibiotics:** Antibiotic therapy has not been shown to have any benefit when used to treat exacerbations. Antibiotics can only be recommended as needed for treatment of comorbid conditions, such as pneumonia or bacterial sinusitis.
- **Bronchial thermoplasty:** Bronchial thermoplasty is a novel therapy for severe asthma in which a specialized radiofrequency catheter is introduced through a bronchoscope to deliver thermal energy to smaller airways in order to reduce smooth muscle mass surrounding the airways. Although asthma symptoms worsen immediately after the procedure, long-term (at least 5 years) asthma-related quality of life and health care utilization improve with bronchial thermoplasty (*J Allergy Clin Immunol 2013;132:1295*). Bronchial thermoplasty should be performed by experienced bronchoscopists in conjunction with an asthma specialist.

Other Nonpharmacologic Therapies

- **Supplemental oxygen** should be administered to the patient who is awaiting an assessment of arterial oxygen tension and should be continued to maintain an oxygen saturation >92% (95% in patients with coexisting cardiac disease or pregnancy).
- **Mechanical ventilation** may be required for respiratory failure.
  - General principles include use of a **large endotracheal tube (≥7.5 mm), low tidal volumes, prolonged expiratory time with high inspiratory flows, low respiratory rate, and low positive end-expiratory pressure (PEEP)**, and in some patients, **permissive hypercapnia**, with the goal to avoid dynamic hyperinflation. Patients with asthma who are intubated often have elevated plateau pressures and intrinsic PEEP.
  - Heavy sedation may be needed and should be maximized before the use of paralytics, given their adverse side effects.
  - Evidence is lacking to suggest modes of noninvasive ventilation are beneficial.
- SC **allergen immunotherapy (SCIT)** can be considered in allergic patients with mild to moderate disease with persistent symptoms despite adherence to allergen avoidance and medication. SCIT is relatively contraindicated in patients with severe or unstable asthma (chronic oral corticosteroid use or severe exacerbations requiring hospitalization or intubation in the previous 6 months).

Lifestyle/Risk Modification
Diet
There is no general diet that is known to improve asthma control. However, a small percentage of patients may have reproducible deterioration after exposure to dietary sulfites used to prevent discoloration in foods such as beer, wine, processed potatoes, and dried fruit, and therefore, these foods should be avoided in patients if they have had prior reactions to these foods.

Activity
Patients should be encouraged to lead an active lifestyle. If their asthma is well controlled, they should expect to be as physically active as they desire. If exercise is a trigger, patient

should be advised to continue physical activity after prophylactic use of an LTM (montelukast 10 mg 2 hours before exercise) or an inhaled β_2-adrenergic agonist (two to four puffs 15–20 minutes before exposure).

SPECIAL CONSIDERATIONS

- During pregnancy, patients should have more frequent follow-up because the severity of asthma often changes and requires medication adjustment. **There is more potential risk to the fetus with poorly controlled asthma than with exposure to asthma medications, most of which are generally considered safe.** A recent birth cohort study of ICSs in pregnant women with asthma confirmed their safety (*Am J Resp Crit Care Med 2012;185(5):557*).
- Occupational asthma requires a detailed history of occupational exposure to a sensitizing agent, lack of asthma symptoms prior to exposure, and a documented relationship with symptoms and the workplace. Beyond standard asthma medical treatment, exposure avoidance is crucial.
- Aspirin-exacerbated respiratory disease (AERD): Patients with aspirin sensitivity and chronic rhinosinusitis with nasal polyps typically have onset of asthma in the third or fourth decade of life. A precipitous onset of symptoms should raise the possibility of reaction to acute ingestion of aspirin or an NSAID. Aspirin desensitization may be considered in patients with corticosteroid-dependent asthma or those requiring daily aspirin/NSAID therapy for other medical conditions.

COMPLICATIONS

Medication Side Effects
- **SABA:** Sympathomimetic symptoms (tremor, anxiety, tachycardia), decrease in serum potassium and magnesium, mild lactic acidosis, prolonged QT_c
- **ICS**
  - Increased risk for systemic effects at high doses (equivalent >1000 μg/d of beclomethasone) including skin bruising, cataracts, elevated intraocular pressure, and accelerated loss of bone mass.
  - Pharyngeal and laryngeal effects are common, such as sore throat, hoarse voice, and oral candidiasis. **Patients should be instructed to rinse their mouth after each administration to reduce the possibility of thrush.** A change in the delivery method and/or use of a valved holding chamber/spacer may alleviate the other side effects.
- **LABA**
  - Fewer sympathomimetic-type side effects.
  - Associated with an increased risk of severe asthma exacerbations and asthma-related death when used without ICS based on the Salmeterol Multicenter Asthma Research Trial (SMART), which showed a very low but significant increase in asthma-related deaths in patients receiving salmeterol (0.01–0.04%) (*Chest 2006;129(1):15*).
  - Should only be used in combination with ICS. FDA recommends discontinuation of LABA once asthma control is achieved and maintained.
- **LTM**
  - Cases of newly diagnosed Churg-Strauss vasculitis after exposure to LTRA have been described, but it is unclear whether they are related to unmasking of a preexisting case with concurrent corticosteroid tapering or whether there is a causal relationship.
  - Zileuton can cause a reversible hepatitis, so it is recommended that hepatic function be monitored at initiation once a month during the first 3 months, every 3 months for the first year, and then periodically.

- **Omalizumab (anti-IgE) therapy:** Anaphylaxis occurs in 1–2 per 1000 patients, usually within 2 hours of the first dose. For this reason, patients should be medically observed 2 hours after the initial dose and then for 30 minutes after subsequent dosing. Patients should possess self-administered epinephrine to be used as needed for anaphylaxis. No association between omalizumab therapy and increased risks of malignancy and thromboembolic events has been identified.
- **Methylxanthines**
  - Theophylline has a narrow therapeutic range with significant toxicities, such as arrhythmias and seizures, as well as many potential drug interactions, especially with antibiotics.
  - Serum concentrations of theophylline should be monitored on a regular basis, aiming for a peak level of 5–10 μg/mL; however, at the lower doses used for asthma, toxicity is much less likely.

REFERRAL

Referral to a specialist should be considered in the following situations:
- Patients who require step 4 (see Figure 9-1) or higher treatment, or patients who have had a life-threatening asthma exacerbation
- Patients being considered for anti-IgE therapy, bronchial thermoplasty, or other alternative treatments
- Patients with atypical signs or symptoms that make the diagnosis uncertain
- Patients with comorbidities such as chronic sinusitis, nasal polyposis, allergic bronchopulmonary aspergillosis, VCD, severe GERD, severe rhinitis, or significant psychiatric or psychosocial difficulties interfering with treatment
- Patients requiring additional diagnostic testing, such as rhinoscopy or bronchoscopy, bronchoprovocation testing, or allergy skin testing
- Patients who need to be evaluated for allergen immunotherapy

PATIENT EDUCATION

- Patient education should focus on the chronic and inflammatory nature of asthma, with identification of factors that contribute to increased inflammation.
  - The consequences of ongoing exposure to chronic irritants or allergens and the rationale for therapy should be explained. Patients should be instructed to avoid factors that aggravate their disease, on how to manage their daily medications, and on how to recognize and deal with acute exacerbations (known as an asthma action plan).
  - Review the principles of asthma medications and skills of inhaler technique.
  - The use of a **written daily management plan** as part of the education strategy is recommended for all patients with persistent asthma.
- It is important for patients to recognize signs of poorly controlled disease.
  - These signs include an increased or daily need for bronchodilators, limitation of activity, waking at night because of asthma symptoms, and variability in the PEF.
  - Specific instructions about handling these symptoms, including criteria for seeking emergency care, should be provided.

MONITORING/FOLLOW-UP

- PEF monitoring provides an objective measurement of airflow obstruction and can be considered in patients with moderate to severe persistent asthma. However, symptom-based asthma action plans are equivalent to PEF-based plans in terms of overall self-management and control (*Respirology 2001;6(4):297*).

The patient must be able to demonstrate correct use of the peak flow meter. The personal best PEF (the highest PEF obtained when the disease is under control) is identified, and the PEF is checked when symptoms escalate or in the setting of an asthma trigger. This should be incorporated into an asthma action plan, setting 80–100% of personal best PEF as the "green" zone, 50–80% as the "yellow" zone, and <50% as the "red" zone.

- Patients should learn to anticipate situations that cause increased symptoms. For most individuals, monitoring symptoms instead of PEF is sufficient (symptom-based asthma action plan).
- Questionnaires can also provide objective monitoring of asthma control. The Asthma Control Test (ACT) and Asthma Control Questionnaire (ACQ) are useful instruments to rapidly assess patient-reported asthma control.

OUTCOME/PROGNOSIS

- Most patients with asthma can be effectively treated and achieve good control of their disease when following the stepwise treatment approach. Goals should include minimal use of reliever medication, freedom from troublesome symptoms, near-normal lung function, absence of serious attacks, and ability to lead a physically active life.
- Previous exacerbations that have required the use of oral corticosteroids or led to respiratory failure, as well as the use of more than two canisters per month of inhaled short-acting bronchodilator and seizures with asthma attacks, have been associated with severe and potentially fatal asthma.

10

Pulmonary Diseases

Murali Chakinala, Tonya D. Russell, Patrick Aguilar,
Adrian Shifren, Andrea Loiselle, Alexander Chen,
Ali Sadoughi, Allen Burks, Praveen Chenna, Brad Bemiss,
and Daniel B. Rosenbluth

Pulmonary Hypertension

GENERAL PRINCIPLES

Definition

Pulmonary hypertension (PH) is the sustained elevation of the mean pulmonary artery pressure (mPAP) (≥25 mm Hg at rest).

Classification

- PH is subcategorized into five major groups (Table 10-1):
  - Group I—**Pulmonary arterial hypertension (PAH)**
  - Group II—**PH due to left heart disease**
  - Group III—**PH due to lung diseases and/or hypoxemia**
  - Group IV—**Chronic thromboembolic pulmonary hypertension (CTEPH)**
  - Group V—**PH with unclear multifactorial mechanisms**
- **PAH** represents a specific group of disorders with similar pathologies and clinical presentation, with a propensity for right heart failure in the absence of elevated left-sided pressures.

Epidemiology

- PH is most often due to left heart disease (Group II) or parenchymal lung disease (Group III).
- **Idiopathic PAH (IPAH)** (Group I) is a rare disorder with an estimated prevalence of 6–9 cases per million compared to an overall PAH prevalence of 15–26 cases per million (*Am J Respir Crit Care Med 2006;173:1023*; *Eur Respir J 2007;30:104*). The average age of PAH patients in modern registries is approximately 50 years (*Am J Respir Crit Care Med 2006;173:1023*; *Eur Respir J 2007;30:1103*). IPAH patients tend to be even younger, with a mean age of approximately 35 years (*Ann Intern Med 1987;107:216*).
- Despite increased awareness, PAH continues to be diagnosed late in its course, with a reported delay of 27 months from symptom onset and the majority of patients in advanced World Health Organization (WHO) functional class III or IV (*Am J Respir Crit Care Med 2006;173:1023*).
- IPAH and PAH associated with systemic sclerosis are the most common subtypes of PAH (*Eur Respir J 2007;30:1103*).
- Incidence of **CTEPH** (Group IV) may be as high as 4% among survivors of acute pulmonary embolism (*N Engl J Med 2004;350:2257*).

Pathophysiology

- Complex origins of PAH include infectious/environmental insults or comorbid conditions that "trigger" the condition in individuals susceptible due to a genetic predisposition.
  - Mutations in the bone morphogenetic protein receptor II (*BMPR-II*) gene are the overwhelming cause of heritable PAH. Other susceptibility factors are speculated to exist but have not been identified.
  - A total of 70% of familial PAH and 10–40% of sporadic or anorexigen-associated cases are found to have mutations in *BMPR-II* (*Circulation 2010;122:156*).

TABLE 10-1	Clinical Classification of Pulmonary Hypertension: Dana Point (2008) Classification System of Pulmonary Hypertension

I. **Pulmonary arterial hypertension (PAH)**
  Idiopathic PAH
  Heritable:
    BMPR-II, ALK-1 (ACVR1), ENG, SMAD9, CAV1, KCNK3
    Unknown
  Drug and toxin induced
  Associated with:
    Connective tissue diseases
    HIV infection
    Portal hypertension
    Congenital heart diseases
    Schistosomiasis
  Pulmonary veno-occlusive disease and/or pulmonary capillary hemangiomatosis
  Persistent pulmonary hypertension of the newborn
II. **Pulmonary hypertension due to left heart disease**
  Left ventricular systolic dysfunction
  Left ventricular diastolic dysfunction
  Valvular disease
  Congenital/acquired left heart inflow/outflow tract obstruction and congenital
    cardiomyopathies
III. **Pulmonary hypertension due to lung diseases and/or hypoxemia**
  Chronic obstructive lung disease
  Interstitial lung disease
  Other pulmonary diseases with mixed obstructive and restrictive pattern
  Sleep-disordered breathing
  Alveolar hypoventilation disorders
  Chronic exposure to high altitude
  Developmental lung diseases
IV. **Chronic thromboembolic pulmonary hypertension (CTEPH)**
V. **Pulmonary hypertension with unclear multifactorial mechanisms**
  Hematologic disorders: *chronic hemolytic anemia, myeloproliferative disorders,*
    splenectomy
  Systemic diseases: *sarcoidosis, pulmonary Langerhans cell histiocytosis,*
    neurofibromatosis, lymphangioleiomyomatosis
  Metabolic disorders: *glycogen storage disease, Gaucher disease, thyroid disorders*
  Others: *tumoral obstruction, fibrosing mediastinitis, chronic renal failure on*
    hemodialysis

ALK1 (ACVR1), activin-like receptor kinase-1; *BMPR-II*, bone morphogenetic protein receptor II; *CAV1*, caveolin-1; *ENG*, endoglin; *KCNK3*, potassium channel super family K member-3. From Simonneau G, Gatzoulis MA, Adatia I, et al. Updated clinical classification of pulmonary hypertension. *J Am Coll Cardiol* 2013;62:D34–41.

- PAH involves a complex interplay of factors resulting in progressive vascular remodeling with endothelial cell and smooth muscle proliferation, vasoconstriction, and in situ thrombosis at an arteriolar level. Vessel wall changes and luminal narrowing restrict the flow of blood and lead to higher than normal pressure as blood flows through the vessels, which is quantifiable by an elevated pulmonary vascular resistance (PVR) (*Circulation 2009;119:2252*).
  - Elevated PVR results in increased afterload to the right ventricle (RV), which over time increases RV wall tension and work, ultimately impacting RV contractility.

○ Initially, cardiac output diminishes during strenuous exercise. As PH severity worsens, maximal cardiac output is achieved at progressively lower workloads; ultimately, resting cardiac output is reduced.

○ Unlike the left ventricle (LV), the RV has limited ability to hypertrophy and tolerates high afterload poorly, causing "vascular–ventricular uncoupling" and eventual RV failure, the most common cause of death.

○ In very advanced stages, pulmonary artery pressures decline as the failing RV cannot generate enough blood flow to maintain high pressures.

• Mechanisms of PH in Groups II–V vary and include high postcapillary pressures, hypoxemia-mediated vasoconstriction and remodeling, parenchymal destruction, thromboembolic narrowing or occlusion of large arteries, and compression of proximal vasculature.

Prevention

Yearly screening transthoracic echocardiogram (TTE) is indicated for high-risk groups including individuals with known *BMPR-II* mutation, scleroderma spectrum of disease, portal hypertension undergoing liver transplantation evaluation, and congenital systemic-to-pulmonary shunts (e.g., ventricular septal defects, patent ductus arteriosus).

DIAGNOSIS

Clinical Presentation

• **Symptoms** include **dyspnea** (most common), exercise intolerance, fatigue, palpitations, exertional dizziness, **syncope**, chest pain, lower extremity swelling, increased abdominal girth (ascites), and hoarseness (impingement of recurrent laryngeal nerve by enlarging pulmonary artery).

• Explore for underlying risk factors (i.e., anorectic drugs, methamphetamines) or associated conditions (e.g., connective tissue diseases, LV heart failure [congestive heart failure (CHF)], obstructive sleep apnea syndrome [OSAS], and venous thromboembolism [VTE]).

• Auscultatory signs of PH include **prominent second heart sound** (loud S_2) with loud P_2 component, RV S_3, tricuspid regurgitation, and pulmonary insufficiency murmurs.

• **Signs of right heart failure**
  ○ Elevated jugular venous pressure
  ○ Hepatomegaly
  ○ Pulsatile liver
  ○ Pedal edema
  ○ Ascites

• Physical examination should focus on identifying underlying conditions linked to PH: skin changes of scleroderma, stigmata of liver disease, clubbing (congenital heart disease), and abnormal breath sounds (parenchymal lung disease).

Diagnostic Testing

• **The purpose of diagnostic testing is to confirm clinical suspicion of PH, determine etiology of PH, and gauge severity of condition, which assists with treatment planning.**

• **Acute illnesses** (e.g., pulmonary edema, pulmonary embolism, pneumonia, adult respiratory distress syndrome) can cause **mild PH** (pulmonary artery systolic pressure [PASP] <50 mm Hg) or aggravate preexisting PH.

• Evaluation of **chronic PH** becomes necessary if pulmonary artery pressures remain elevated after resolution of the acute process.

• If chronic PH is considered based on clinical suspicion or during the evaluation of a vulnerable population (see Prevention section), **TTE should be the initial test.**

TTE with Doppler and Agitated Saline Injection

- **Estimate PASP** by Doppler interrogation of tricuspid valve regurgitant jet. The absence of tricuspid regurgitation does not exclude elevated pulmonary artery pressure. Sensitivity for PH is 80–100%, and correlation coefficient with invasive measurement is 0.6–0.9 (*Chest 2004;126:14S*). **Invasive measurement is recommended if suspicion remains despite a normal estimation by echocardiogram.**
- **Assess RV characteristics**, looking for pressure overload and dysfunction (e.g., RV hypertrophy and/or dilation, RV hypokinesis, displaced intraventricular septum, paradoxical septal motion, LV compression, and pericardial effusion from impaired pericardial drainage). Tricuspid annular plane systolic excursion <1.8 cm is associated with worse survival (*Am J Respir Crit Care Med 2006;174(9):1034*). Absence of any RV abnormalities makes moderate or severe PH unlikely.
- **Identify causes of PH** (e.g., LV systolic or **diastolic dysfunction**, left-sided valvular disease, left atrial structural anomalies, and congenital systemic-to-pulmonary shunts). Left atrial enlargement, elevated LV filling pressures, and diastolic dysfunction are important clues for LV diastolic heart disease that frequently leads to PH, especially in the elderly (*J Am Coll Cardiol 2009;53:1119*).
- Transesophageal echocardiogram is indicated to exclude intracardiac shunts suspected by TTE, although the majority of such shunts are a patent foramen ovale.
- Additional studies, as outlined in the following text and in Figure 10-1, should be completed if PH is unexplained by TTE or if PAH is still a consideration after echocardiography (*Chest 2004;126:14S*).

Laboratories

- Evaluate for causative conditions and gauge degree of cardiac impairment.
  - Complete blood counts (CBCs)
  - Blood urea nitrogen, serum creatinine

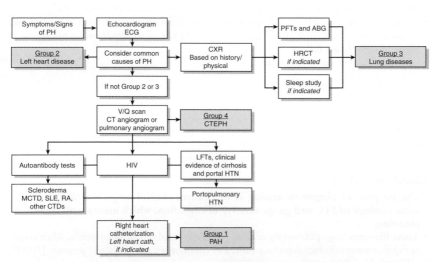

Figure 10-1. Algorithm for diagnostic workup of pulmonary hypertension. ABG, arterial blood gas; CTD, connective tissue disease; CTEPH, chronic thromboembolic pulmonary hypertension; HRCT, high-resolution CT; HTN, hypertension; LFT, liver function test; MCTD, mixed connective tissue disease; PAH, pulmonary arterial hypertension; PFT, pulmonary function test; PH, pulmonary hypertension; RA, rheumatoid arthritis; SLE, systemic lupus erythematosus; V/Q, ventilation–perfusion

- ○ Hepatic function tests
- ○ Brain natriuretic peptide (BNP)
- ○ HIV serology
- ○ Thyroid-stimulating hormone (TSH)
- ○ Antinuclear antibody (ANA), antitopoisomerase antibodies, anticentromere antibodies, extractable nuclear antigen antibody, and potentially other serologies of autoimmune disease
- • Additional laboratory studies, based on initial findings, include complete thyroid function studies, hepatitis B and C serologies, hemoglobin electrophoresis, antiphospholipid antibody, and lupus anticoagulant.

Electrocardiography
Signs of **right heart enlargement** include RV hypertrophy, right atrial enlargement, right bundle branch block, and RV strain pattern (S wave in lead I with Q wave and inverted T wave in lead III), but these findings have low sensitivity in milder PH.

Pulmonary Function Testing
- • **Spirometry and lung volumes** to assess for obstructive (e.g., **chronic obstructive lung disease**) or restrictive (e.g., interstitial lung disease [ILD]) ventilatory abnormalities.
- • **Diffusing capacity for carbon monoxide (DLCO)** is usually reduced with parenchymal lung diseases, but isolated mild to moderate reduction is often encountered in PAH.
- • **Arterial blood gas (ABG):** Elevated arterial partial pressure of carbon dioxide ($PaCO_2$) is an important clue for a hypoventilation syndrome.
- • **Six-minute walk (6MW) or simple exercise test**
  - ○ Unexplained exercise-induced desaturation could indicate PH.
  - ○ Distance walked correlates with WHO functional classification and provides intermediate prognosis (*Am J Respir Crit Care Med 2000;161:487*).
- • **Nocturnal oximetry:** Nocturnal desaturations could indicate OSAS. PH patients with symptoms of sleep-disordered breathing should undergo **polysomnography** (PSG). Nocturnal desaturations are common in PAH, even in the absence of OSAS, and should be treated with nocturnal supplemental oxygen (*Chest 2007;131:109*).

Imaging
- • General findings include enlarged central pulmonary arteries as well as RV enlargement with opacification of retrosternal space, seen best on lateral view.
- • Clues to specific PH diagnosis include:
  - ○ Decreased peripheral vascular markings or pruning (PAH)
  - ○ Very large pulmonary vasculature throughout lung fields (congenital-to-systemic shunt)
  - ○ Regional oligemia of pulmonary vasculature (chronic thromboembolic disease)
  - ○ Interstitial infiltrates (ILD)
  - ○ Hyperinflated lungs (chronic obstructive lung disease)
- • **Ventilation–perfusion (V/Q) lung scan**
  - ○ Critical for excluding chronic thromboembolic disease but could also be abnormal in pulmonary veno-occlusive disease and fibrosing mediastinitis.
  - ○ **Heterogeneous perfusion patterns** are associated with PAH.
  - ○ Presence of one or more segmental mismatches raises concern for chronic thromboembolic disease and should be investigated with computed tomography (CT) or pulmonary angiography (*N Engl J Med 2001;345:145*).
- • **Chest CT scan**
  - ○ Confirms suspicion of CTEPH, if initial screening V/Q scan suspicious
  - ○ Evaluates lung parenchyma and mediastinum
  - ○ High-resolution images to assess for interstitial or bronchiolar disease

- **Pulmonary angiography** can be done safely in the setting of severe PH.
  - Confirms CTEPH.
  - Determines surgical accessibility of thrombotic material.
  - Inferior vena cava filter can be deployed at the same time.
- **Cardiac MRI**
  - Investigates cardiac anomalies leading to the development of PAH, especially if trans-esophageal echocardiogram is contraindicated
  - Provides anatomic and functional information about the RV, including ventricular volumes, ejection fraction, and stroke volume index, which have prognostic value

Diagnostic Procedures
- **Lung biopsy**
  - Lung biopsy is rarely performed but useful if lung disease requires histologic confirmation (e.g., pulmonary vasculitis or veno-occlusive disease).
  - The risk of surgery is usually prohibitive in the setting of severe PH or RV dysfunction.
- **Right heart catheterization: Essential investigation if PAH is suspected and treatment is being considered.**
  - **Confirm noninvasive estimate of PASP**, because TTE can under- and overestimate PASP (*Am J Respir Crit Care Med 2009;179:615*).
  - **Measure cardiac output and mean right atrial pressure (RAP) to gauge severity of condition and predict future course.** Increased RAP is an indicator of RV dysfunction and has greatest odds ratio for predicting mortality (*Ann Intern Med 1987;107:216*).
  - **Investigate etiologies of PH**, including left heart disease (by measuring pulmonary artery wedge pressure [PAWP] manually at end-expiration) or missed systemic-to-pulmonary shunts (by noting "step-ups" in oxygen saturations).
  - Exercise hemodynamics can elicit PH occurring during exercise or also confirm suspicion of diastolic heart failure, but exercise protocols and methods of measurement are not standardized.
- **Acute vasodilator testing** is recommended if PAH is suspected.
  - Performed with a **short-acting vasodilator**, such as IV adenosine, IV epoprostenol, or inhaled nitric oxide. **Long-acting calcium channel blockers (CCBs) should not be used for initial vasodilator testing** due to risk of sustained systemic hypotension (*Chest 2004;26:35S*).
  - **Not recommended for patients in extreme right heart failure** (mean RAP >20 mm Hg).
  - Definition of a **responder** is **decline in mPAP of 10 mm Hg *and* concluding mPAP of 40 mm Hg with stable or improved cardiac output** (*Chest 2004;126:35S*).
  - Responders should undergo a CCB trial with pulmonary artery catheter in place. If vasoresponsiveness is recapitulated, chronic CCB therapy can be prescribed (see Treatment section).
- **Left heart catheterization** should be done to directly measure **LV end-diastolic pressure** if PAWP cannot reliably exclude left heart disease, especially in patients older than 65 years.

TREATMENT

- **Management of PH depends on the specific category of PH.**
  - Patients with PH due to left heart disease should receive appropriate therapy for the underlying causative condition with the goal of minimizing postcapillary pressures.
  - Patients with underlying lung diseases should be treated as appropriate for specific condition. Examples include bronchodilators (e.g., obstructive lung disease), immunomodulators (e.g., ILDs), noninvasive ventilation (e.g., OSAS), and supplemental oxygen.

- ○ CTEPH is often treated by **pulmonary thromboendarterectomy** at specialized centers and requires careful screening to determine resectability and expected hemodynamic response (*N Engl J Med 2001;345:1465*). Patients with inoperable CTEPH can benefit from riociguat, a soluble guanylate cyclase stimulator (*N Engl J Med 2013;369:319*).
- Regardless of PH diagnosis, normoxemia should be maintained to avoid hypoxic vasoconstriction and further aggravation of pulmonary artery pressures. **Supplemental oxygen** to maintain adequate arterial saturations (>89%) 24 hours a day is recommended. However, normoxemia may not be possible in the presence of a significant right-to-left shunt (e.g., intracardiac right-to-left shunt).
- **In-line filters** should be used to prevent paradoxical air emboli from IV catheters in PH patients with large right-to-left shunts.
- **Pneumovax and influenza vaccination** should be given to avoid respiratory tract infections.
- Patients with severe PH and RV dysfunction should **minimize behaviors** that can acutely decrease RV preload and/or increase RV afterload, which could cause circulatory collapse:
  - ○ **Deep Valsalva** maneuvers can raise intrathoracic pressure and induce syncope through diminished central venous return (e.g., vigorous exercise, severe coughing paroxysm, straining during defecation or micturition).
  - ○ **High altitudes** (>5000 ft) due to low inspired concentration of oxygen.
  - ○ **Cigarette smoking**, because of nicotine's vasoactive effects.
  - ○ **Pregnancy**, due to hemodynamic alterations that further strain the heart.
  - ○ Systemic **sympathomimetic** agents, such as decongestants and cocaine.

Medications

- **PAH patients are candidates for vasomodulator/vasodilator** therapy (Figure 10-2 and Table 10-2).
  - ○ There are four categories of PAH-specific therapies with unique mechanisms of action:
    - ▪ **Endothelin receptor antagonists** block the binding of endothelin-1 to its receptors on pulmonary artery smooth muscle cells, which would typically cause vasoconstriction and cellular hypertrophy/growth.
    - ▪ **Phosphodiesterase-5 inhibitors** block the enzyme that shuts down nitric oxide–mediated vasodilation and platelet inhibition.
    - ▪ **Soluble guanylate cyclase stimulator** activates the downstream signal of nitric oxide through stimulation of its intermediate messenger, soluble guanylate cyclase, and induces vasodilation and platelet inhibition.
    - ▪ **Prostanoids** induce vasodilation, inhibit cellular growth, and inhibit platelet aggregation.
  - ○ Initial choice of PAH-specific therapy should be individualized to the severity of one's condition (see Figure 10-2).
  - ○ **Predictors of poor prognosis** include (*Chest 2011;141:354*):
    - ▪ PAH subtype: scleroderma, portopulmonary hypertension, familial PAH
    - ▪ Men older than 60 years
    - ▪ Renal insufficiency
    - ▪ BNP >180 pg/mL
    - ▪ PVR >32 Wood units
    - ▪ RAP >20 mm Hg
    - ▪ DLCO ≤32%
    - ▪ Pericardial effusion
    - ▪ Systolic blood pressure <110 mm Hg
    - ▪ Resting heart rate >92 bpm

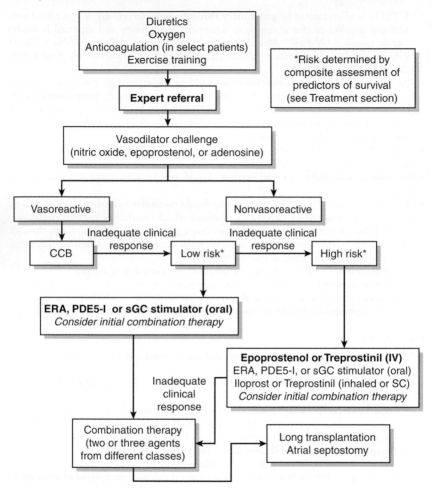

Figure 10-2. Algorithm for management of pulmonary arterial hypertension. CCB, calcium channel blocker; ERA, endothelin receptor antagonist; PDE-5 I, phosphodiesterase-5 inhibitor; sGC, soluble guanylate cyclase.

- New York Heart Association (NYHA) functional class IV
- 6MW distance <165 m
  - Due to the complexity of some therapies, an individual's comorbid conditions, cognitive abilities, and psychosocial makeup must also be heavily factored.
  - Combination therapy regimens, which include medications from more than one class of therapy, are quickly becoming common in the management of PAH.
  - Because current therapies for PAH are palliative and not curative, patients require close follow-up because deterioration often occurs, requiring alternative/additional medical and possibly surgical intervention (see Figure 10-2). Although there is no consensus on follow-up strategy, periodic functional (e.g., 6MW and WHO functional classification) and cardiac (e.g., TTE, MRI, or right heart catheterization) assessments provide the most sound strategy.

TABLE 10-2 Vasomodulator/Vasodilatory Therapy for Pulmonary Arterial Hypertension

Drug	Therapeutic Class	Route of Delivery	Dosing Range	Adverse Effects	Cautions
Nifedipine, amlodipine, diltiazem	Calcium channel blockers	PO	Varies by patient tolerance	Peripheral edema, hypotension, fatigue	**Use only in patients who are vaso-responsive during acute vasodila-tor challenge**: avoid if low cardiac output or decompensated right heart failure
Sildenafil, tadalafil	Phosphodiesterase-5 inhibitor	PO	20 mg tid/40 mg/d	Headache, hypotension, dyspepsia, myalgias, visual disturbances	Avoid using with **nitrates** or **protease inhibitors**
Riociguat	Soluble guanylate cyclase stimulator	PO	2.5 mg tid	Hypotension	Avoid using with **nitrates**; approved for PAH and inoperable CTEPH or PH persistent after endarterectomy
Bosentan	Endothelin receptor antagonist	PO	125 mg bid	Hepatotoxicity, teratogen, peripheral edema	**Monthly liver function monitoring;** avoid using with glyburide and glipizide
Ambrisentan	Endothelin receptor antagonist	PO	5–10 mg/d	Teratogen, peripheral edema, nasal congestion	**Monthly liver function monitoring;** avoid using with glyburide and glipizide.

(continued)

TABLE 10-2	Vasomodulator/Vasodilatory Therapy for Pulmonary Arterial Hypertension (Continued)				
Drug	Therapeutic Class	Route of Delivery	Dosing Range	Adverse Effects	Cautions
Macitentan	Endothelin receptor antagonist	PO	10 mg/d	Teratogen, peripheral edema, anemia	**Strong interaction with warfarin; monthly liver function monitoring**
Iloprost	Prostanoid	IH	2.5–5.0 μg 6–8×/d	Cough, flushing, headache, trismus	**Suboptimal adherence due to dosing frequency**: overnight drug holiday
Treprostinil	Prostanoid	SC, IV, or PO	Varies by patient tolerance	Headache, jaw pain, diarrhea, extremity pain	**With continuous parenteral use,** catheter-related complications (IV); **site pain/reaction (SC)**; GI distress with PO use
Epoprostenol	Prostanoid	IV	Varies by patient tolerance	Headache, jaw pain, diarrhea, extremity pain	**Continuous parenteral agent; very short half-life**; catheter-related complications (IV); **high-output state at higher doses**

CTEPH, chronic thromboembolic pulmonary hypertension; GI, gastrointestinal; IH, inhaled; PAH, pulmonary arterial hypertension; PH, pulmonary hypertension.

- **Diuretic therapy** (loop diuretic ± aldosterone antagonist ± thiazides)
  - Alleviates **right heart failure** and improves symptoms.
  - Overdiuresis or too rapid of a diuresis can be poorly tolerated due to **preload dependency** of the RV and limited ability of the cardiac output to compensate for systemic hypotension.
- **Anticoagulation**
  - Chronic anticoagulation improves survival, primarily in IPAH (*N Engl J Med 1992;327:76*; *Circulation 1984;70:580*). Use of anticoagulation in other types of PAH is controversial.
  - Warfarin is dosed to **target international normalized ratio (INR) of 1.5–2.5** (*Chest 2004;126:35S*).
  - Anticoagulant therapy is not urgent and can be stopped for invasive procedures or active bleeding.
- **Inotropic agents**
  - Modestly improve right heart function, cardiac output, and symptoms.
  - Dobutamine and milrinone are best suited for **short-term use** in extremely decompensated states.

Surgical Management

- **Lung transplantation or heart–lung transplantation**
  - Reserved for suitable patients with PAH who **remain in advanced functional class III–IV despite maximal medical therapy**.
  - The **Lung Allocation Score** (LAS), derived from multiple clinical variables, takes into consideration PH diagnosis and provides a mechanism for prioritizing PAH patients beyond their imputed LAS. This improves the likelihood for patients with IPAH to receive transplants; however, mortality on the waiting list is high compared to other diagnoses.
  - Because the RV recovers after isolated lung transplantation, heart–lung transplantation is usually reserved for complex congenital heart defects that cannot be repaired.
  - Median survival after lung transplantation is approximately 5 years, and **survival for IPAH patients at 5 years is approximately 50%** (*J Heart Lung Transplant 2005;24:956*).
- **Atrial septostomy**
  - Palliative procedure performed in cases of right heart failure (i.e., syncope, hepatic congestion, prerenal azotemia) refractory to medical therapy.
  - Percutaneous creation of a right-to-left shunt across the interatrial septum in patients whose RAPs are greater than left atrial pressures.
  - Despite arterial oxyhemoglobin desaturation and hypoxemia, oxygen delivery increases from improved LV filling and cardiac output.
- **Septal defect closure**
  - In select cases of intracardiac defects that still have significant left-to-right shunting, closure can be undertaken by **percutaneous or surgical** means.
  - Criteria for closure include net left-to-right shunt with flow ratio (pulmonary flow/systemic flow) ≥1.5, resistance ratio (PVR/systemic vascular resistance) ≤0.6 (*Circulation 2008;118:2395*), and PVR <4.6 Wood units (*J Am Coll Cardiol 2013; 62:D34*).

Prognosis

The 1-, 3-, and 5-year survival rates in PAH are 85%, 70%, and 55%, respectively, with median survival of 3.6 years (*Circulation 2010;122:156*; *Eur Respir J 2007; 30:1103*).

Obstructive Sleep Apnea–Hypopnea Syndrome

GENERAL PRINCIPLES

Definition

Obstructive sleep apnea–hypopnea syndrome (OSAHS) is a disorder in which patients experience apneas or hypopneas due to upper airway narrowing. It is associated with excessive daytime somnolence (*Sleep 1999;22:667*).

Classification

- **Apneas** represent complete cessation of airflow.
  - Obstructive events are associated with continued respiratory effort.
  - Central events are associated with no respiratory effort.
- **Hypopneas** represent diminished airflow associated with at least a 3–4% oxygen desaturation.
- **Respiratory effort–related arousals (RERAs)** represent changes in airflow that lead to an arousal but do not meet criteria for an apnea or hypopnea.
- All respiratory events must last at least 10 seconds to be counted.
- **Apnea-hypopnea index (AHI)** is the number of apneas and hypopneas per hour of sleep.
- **Respiratory disturbance index (RDI)** is the number of apneas, hypopneas, and RERAs per hour of sleep.

Epidemiology

- The prevalence of OSAHS in the general population is estimated to be about 4%, with men being twice as likely as women to be affected (*Eur Respir J 2009;33:907*; *JAMA 2004;291:2013*; *N Engl J Med 1993;328:1230*).
- Obesity is a significant risk factor for obstructive sleep apnea (OSA) (*N Engl J Med 1993;328:1230*).

Etiology

- **OSA:** Narrowing of the upper airway due to excessive soft tissue or structural abnormalities
- **Central sleep apnea:** Disturbance of central control of respiration during sleep

Pathophysiology

OSA occurs due to narrowing of the upper airway, which results in diminished airflow or cessation of airflow leading to arousals that fragment sleep.

Risk Factors

Risk factors for OSAHS include obesity, nasal obstruction, adenoidal or tonsillar hypertrophy, and mandibular size and positioning (*Otolaryngol Clin North Am 1990;23:727*). Potential risk factors also include family history and smoking (*JAMA 2004;291:2013*).

Prevention

- Weight loss
- Avoiding sedatives such as hypnotic medications or alcohol

Associated Conditions

- **Cardiovascular disease**, including systemic hypertension, heart failure, arrhythmia, myocardial infarction, and stroke (*Circulation 2008;118:1080*). OSA has been established as an independent risk factor for hypertension (*Eur Respir J 2007;29:156*).
- **Increased risk of death**, mainly due to cardiovascular events (*Sleep 2008;31:1071*; *Sleep 2008;31:1079*; *N Engl J Med 2005;353:2034*).

- Increased prevalence of **diabetes** has been noted in patients with OSAHS, independent of the effect of obesity (*Am J Respir Crit Care Med 2005;172:1590; J Clin Endocrinol Metab 2000;85:1151*).
- Higher risk of motor vehicle accidents (*Sleep 1997;20:608*).

DIAGNOSIS

Clinical Presentation

History
- **Habitual loud snoring** is the most common symptom of OSAHS, although not all people who snore have this syndrome. Patients with OSA may experience snore arousals along with a sensation of gasping or choking.
- Excessive daytime sleepiness (**hypersomnolence**) is a classic symptom of OSAHS (Table 10-3). Patients may describe falling asleep while driving or having difficulty concentrating at work.
- Patients may also complain of personality changes, intellectual deterioration, morning headaches, nocturnal angina, loss of libido, and chronic fatigue.

Physical Examination
- All patients should have a thorough nose and throat examination to detect sources of upper airway obstruction that are surgically correctable (e.g., septal deviation, enlarged tonsils), especially if continuous positive airway pressure (CPAP) is poorly tolerated.
- Increased severity of OSA has been associated with a higher **Mallampati class** (Table 10-4) (*Eur Respir J 2003;21:248*).

Diagnostic Criteria
A **polysomnogram** demonstrating obstructive events with an RDI >5 is diagnostic of OSA. If the RDI is between 5–15, a patient may qualify for CPAP if there is a comorbid condition such as hypertension, coronary artery disease, depression, or hypersomnolence. If there are no comorbid conditions, then the RDI has to be >15 in order for a patient to qualify for CPAP.

Differential Diagnosis
- In addition to OSAHS and sleep-related hypoventilation, the differential diagnosis for daytime sleepiness includes sleep deprivation, periodic limb movement disorder, narcolepsy, and medication side effects.

TABLE 10-3	Symptoms Associated with Obstructive Sleep Apnea–Hypopnea Syndrome

Excessive daytime sleepiness
Snoring
Nocturnal arousals
Nocturnal apneas
Nocturnal gasping, grunting, and choking
Nocturia
Enuresis
Awakening without feeling refreshed
Morning headaches
Impaired memory and concentration
Irritability and depression
Impotence

TABLE 10-4	Mallampati Airway Classification
Class	**Visible Structures with Mouth Maximally Open and Tongue Protruded**
I	Hard palate, soft palate, uvula, tonsillar pillars
II	Hard palate, soft palate, uvula
III	Hard palate, soft palate, base of uvula
IV	Hard palate

From Mallampati SR, Gatt SP, Gugino LD, et al. A clinical sign to predict difficult tracheal intubation: A prospective study. *Can Anaesth Soc J* 1985;32(4):429–34. With kind permission from Springer Science Business & Media B.V.

- Patients should also be evaluated for other medical conditions that may cause nighttime awakenings and dyspnea and thus mimic OSAHS, such as chronic lung disease, CHF, and gastroesophageal reflux disease.

Diagnostic Testing

- The gold standard for the diagnosis of OSAHS is **overnight PSG** ("sleep study") with direct observation by a qualified technician (*Am Rev Respir Dis 1989;139:559*). Sleep studies are typically performed in the outpatient setting.
- Typical indications for a sleep study include snoring with excessive daytime sleepiness, titration of optimal positive airway pressure therapy, and assessment of objective response to therapeutic interventions.
- PSG involves determination of sleep stages using electroencephalography, electromyography, and electro-oculography and assessment of respiratory airflow and effort, oxyhemoglobin saturation, cardiac electrical activity (e.g., ECG), and body position.
- Data are analyzed for sleep staging, the frequency of respiratory events, limb movements, and abnormal behaviors. Respiratory events are categorized as obstructive or central.
- Most sleep studies are performed as "split studies," where the first few hours of the study are diagnostic and the latter part of the study is used for CPAP titration if the AHI is consistent with moderate-to-severe OSA.
- Some patients only have significant events when lying in certain positions (usually supine) or during rapid eye movement (REM) sleep. These patients may require a complete overnight study for diagnosis and a second study for initiation of therapy.
- Recognizing the cost, required manpower, and limited availability of PSG, the American Academy of Sleep Medicine supports the use of unattended portable monitoring as an alternative to PSG for patients with a high pretest probability of moderate to severe OSA without significant comorbid medical conditions or other suspected sleep disorders. The portable device must record airflow, respiratory effort, and blood oxygenation, and results should be reviewed by a sleep specialist (*J Clin Sleep Med 2007;3:737*). Portable devices can underestimate the severity of OSA because the number of events per hour is calculated using total recording time rather than total sleep time.

TREATMENT

The therapeutic approach to OSAHS depends on the severity of the disease, comorbid medical conditions, and patient preference and expected compliance. Treatment must be highly individualized, with special attention paid to correcting potentially reversible exacerbating factors.

Medications

- No pharmacologic agent has sufficient efficacy to warrant replacement of positive airway pressure as the primary therapeutic modality for OSAHS.
- **Modafinil** may improve daytime sleepiness in patients with persistent symptoms despite adequate CPAP use (*Sleep 2006;29:31*).
- Medical treatment of conditions that may contribute to muscle hypotonia or weight gain, such as hypothyroidism, are of benefit.

Nonpharmacologic Therapies

- **Positive airway pressure**
  - ○ **CPAP** delivers air via a face mask at a constant pressure level throughout the respiratory cycle with the goal of pneumatically splinting open the upper airway, thus preventing collapse and airflow obstruction.
  - ○ The PSG determines the positive airway pressure (expressed in cm H_2O) required to optimize airflow. The pressure setting is gradually increased until obstructive events, snoring, and oxygen desaturations are minimized.
  - ○ The benefits of positive airway pressure include consolidated sleep and decreased daytime sleepiness. Hypertension, nocturia, peripheral edema, polycythemia, and PH may also improve. Additionally, CPAP is a highly cost-effective intervention (*Can J Physiol Pharmacol 2007;85:179*) that appears to reduce the risk of cardiovascular events (*Am J Respir Crit Care Med 2007;176:1274*) and may also improve the metabolic syndrome associated with OSA (*N Engl J Med 2011;365:2277*).
  - ○ **Nasal CPAP (nCPAP) is the current treatment of choice for most patients with OSAHS.**
    - ▪ The compliance rate with nCPAP is approximately 50%.
    - ▪ Compliance can be improved with education, instruction, follow-up, adjustment of the mask for fit and comfort, humidification of the air to decrease dryness, and treatment of nasal or sinus symptoms.
    - ▪ Use of a full face mask (oronasal) has not been shown to improve compliance compared to the use of nCPAP. However, full-face masks are frequently used in patients who "mouth breathe" or patients who require higher CPAP pressures, because they will often experience air leak through the mouth when using nCPAP.
  - ○ Autotitrating positive airway pressure machines use flow and pressure transducers to sense airflow patterns and then automatically adjust the pressure setting in response. Small studies have shown that autotitrating CPAP may be as effective as traditional CPAP and appears to be preferred by patients (*Respiration 2007;74:279*; *Chest 2006;129:638*).
  - ○ **Bilevel positive airway pressure** is typically used to treat OSA in the following settings: pressures >15–20 cm H_2O are required, intolerance of CPAP, or concern for concomitant hypoventilation.
  - ○ All noninvasive positive-pressure ventilation devices may induce dryness of the airway, nasal congestion, rhinorrhea, epistaxis, skin reactions to the mask, nasal bridge abrasions, and aerophagia. Some of these nasal symptoms may be treated with nasal saline, decongestants, and use of a humidifier.
  - ○ Some patients, such as those with coexisting chronic obstructive pulmonary disease, require supplemental oxygen to maintain adequate nocturnal oxygen saturations ($SaO_2 \geq 90\%$).
- **Oral appliances**
  - ○ Used for mild OSAHS, with aim to increase airway size to improve airflow. These devices, such as the mandibular advancement device, can be fixed or adjustable, and most require customized fitting. Many devices have not been well studied.
  - ○ Contraindications include temporomandibular joint disease, bruxism, full dentures, and inability to protrude the mandible.
- **Nasal expiratory resistance device**
  - ○ Nasal plugs increase resistance with expiration, creating a back pressure to stent open the upper airway.

○ Most effective for milder OSA. Should not be used in patients with significant comorbid conditions such as lung disease.
- **Upper airway stimulation device**
  ○ The U.S. Food and Drug Administration (FDA) has recently approved an upper airway stimulation device for use in patients with moderate to severe OSA who cannot tolerate CPAP.
  ○ Although AHI and daytime sleepiness improved with this device, there was residual mild OSA (*N Engl J Med 2014;370:139*).

Surgical Management

- **Tracheostomy**
  ○ Tracheostomy is very effective in treating OSAHS but is rarely used since the advent of positive airway pressure therapy.
  ○ Tracheostomy should be reserved for patients with life-threatening disease (cor pulmonale, arrhythmias, or severe hypoxemia) or significant alveolar hypoventilation that cannot be controlled with other measures.
- **Uvulopalatopharyngoplasty (UPPP)**
  ○ UPPP is the most common surgical treatment of mild-to-moderate OSAHS in patients who do not respond to medical therapy.
  ○ UPPP enlarges the airway by removing tissue from the tonsils, tonsillar pillars, uvula, and posterior palate. UPPP may be complicated by change in voice, nasopharyngeal stenosis, foreign body sensation, velopharyngeal insufficiency with associated nasal regurgitation during swallowing, and CPAP tolerance problems.
  ○ The success rate of UPPP for treatment of OSAHS is only approximately 50%, when defined as a 50% reduction of the AHI, and improvements related to UPPP may diminish over time (*Sleep 1996;19:156*). Thus, UPPP is considered a second-line treatment for patients with mild to moderate OSAHS who cannot successfully use CPAP and who have retropalatal obstruction.
- **Staged procedures**
  In experienced centers, other staged procedures for OSA can be performed, including mandibular osteotomy with genioglossus advancement, hyoid myotomy with suspension, and maxillomandibular advancement (MMA) (*Sleep Breath 2000;4:137*). Significant reductions in AHI have been reported with MMA, but more research is needed (*Sleep 2010;33:1396*).

Lifestyle/Risk Modification

- Weight reduction for the obese is recommended (*Chest 1987;92:631*).
- Weight loss, both surgical and through reduced caloric intake, has been shown to reduce the severity of OSA by reduction in AHI (*Am J Respir Crit Care Med 2009;179:320*; *Am J Med 2009;122:535*).
- OSAHS patients should avoid use of alcohol, tobacco, and sedatives.
- Clinicians should counsel patients with OSAHS regarding the increased risk of driving and operating dangerous equipment.

SPECIAL CONSIDERATIONS

Patients with a body mass index >40 kg/m^2 are at increased risk for concomitant sleep-related hypoventilation due to morbid obesity.

COMPLICATIONS

- When OSAHS is associated with disorders such as obesity and chronic lung disease, patients may develop hypoxemia, hypercapnia, polycythemia, PH, and cor pulmonale (*Mayo Clin Proc 1990;65:1087*).

- Patients with OSAHS are at greater risk for perioperative complications due to intubation difficulty and/or impaired arousal secondary to the effects of anesthetics, narcotics, and sedatives (*Otolaryngol Clin North Am 2007;40:877*).
- The risk of death, hypertension, and poor neuropsychological functioning rises with increasing severity of OSA.

REFERRAL

Patients with risk factors and symptoms or sequelae of OSAHS should be referred to a sleep specialist and sleep laboratory for further evaluation.

Interstitial Lung Disease

GENERAL PRINCIPLES

Definition
ILDs are a heterogeneous group of disorders, pathologically characterized by infiltration of the lung interstitium with cells, fluid, and/or connective tissue.

Classification
- ILD of known etiology
  - Medication (e.g., bleomycin, amiodarone, nitrofurantoin, methotrexate)
  - Connective tissue disease (e.g., rheumatoid arthritis, scleroderma, polymyositis/dermatomyositis)
  - Pneumoconiosis (e.g., coal worker's pneumoconiosis, silicosis, asbestosis)
  - Radiation
  - Lymphangitic carcinomatosis
- Idiopathic interstitial pneumonias
  - Usual interstitial pneumonia (UIP)
  - Nonspecific interstitial pneumonia (NSIP)
  - Desquamative interstitial pneumonia (DIP)
  - Respiratory bronchiolitis interstitial lung disease (RB-ILD)
  - Cryptogenic organizing pneumonia (COP)
  - Lymphocytic interstitial pneumonia
  - Acute interstitial pneumonia
- Granulomatous ILD
  - Sarcoidosis
  - Hypersensitivity pneumonitis (HP)
- Cystic lung disease
  - Lymphangioleiomyomatosis
  - Pulmonary Langerhans cell histiocytosis (LCH)
  - Genetic diseases (Birt-Hogg-Dubé, tuberous sclerosis)
  - Light chain deposition disease

DIAGNOSIS

Clinical Presentation
History
- Patients typically present with indolently progressive dyspnea and dry cough. History often reveals years of gradually worsening symptoms, although a subset (acute interstitial pneumonia, acute eosinophilic pneumonia) may present acutely.

- Careful questioning should focus on exposures (pharmacologic agents, asbestos exposure, exposure to industrial fumes or dusts, bird antigens, and mold) as well as symptoms of connective tissue disease.
- Clinical features of common ILDs are described in Table 10-5.

Physical Examination
Findings may include inspiratory crackles and digital clubbing. Close attention should be paid to extrapulmonary findings that point toward connective tissue diseases. Examples include sclerodactyly, mechanic's hands, Raynaud phenomenon, dry mucous membranes, and dermatologic findings such as telangiectasias, rash, or facial erythema.

Diagnostic Approach

Imaging
- Plain radiographs of the chest have variable appearance, with lung volume loss, interstitial thickening, and cystic changes being most common in ILD.
- If initial radiograph or clinical scenario is consistent with ILD, the patient should be referred for high-resolution CT (HRCT), which is the radiographic test of choice for patients with suspected ILD.
- The pattern of radiographic infiltrate is important in the differential diagnosis of ILD. Imaging patterns of common ILDs are described in Table 10-5. Notably, published guidelines exist for the definitive radiologic diagnosis of certain ILDs, specifically idiopathic pulmonary fibrosis (IPF)/UIP (*Am J Respir Crit Care Med 2011;183:788*).

Pulmonary Function Testing
- Spirometry typically demonstrates a restrictive ventilatory defect characterized by a symmetric reduction in forced vital capacity (FVC) and forced expiratory volume in 1 second (FEV_1). Definitive diagnosis of a restrictive ventilatory defect requires documentation of a reduction in total lung capacity to <80% predicted.
- In certain ILDs (e.g., sarcoidosis, LCH, HP), bronchiolar involvement may result in airflow obstruction, causing the FEV_1 to decrease disproportionately to the FVC. In this circumstance, a mixed obstructive and restrictive defect may be seen. This circumstance may also exist in cases of comorbid emphysema.
- DLCO is often significantly decreased in patients with ILD.

Laboratory Analysis
- Patients with a diagnosis of ILD should be evaluated for evidence of a connective tissue disease as a potential target for therapy. Some connective tissue diseases may manifest primarily with pulmonary symptoms. As an example, approximately 10–20% of patients with rheumatoid arthritis may have lung disease as their initial clinical presentation (*Proc Am Thorac Soc 2007;4(5):443*).
- ANA and rheumatoid factor (RF) should be tested in most patients, even patients with UIP on thoracic imaging. Cyclic citrullinated peptide should also be tested to evaluate for rheumatoid arthritis because the RF may be insufficiently sensitive and has a low positive predictive value.
- Aldolase and creatinine kinase should be tested to evaluate for evidence of myositis. In cases where suspicion is high for myositis, panels of muscle-specific antibodies should also be obtained.
- In any patient with evidence of scleroderma such as telangiectasis, esophageal dysmotility, or sclerodactyly, antibodies against topoisomerase I (anti-Scl-70) should be obtained.

Diagnostic Procedures
- Bronchoalveolar lavage has little role in ILD outside of evaluating for infection.
- Lung biopsy should be undertaken with the input of pulmonologists and thoracic surgeons with expertise in ILD.
  - Generally, biopsy should be reserved for circumstances where the diagnosis is uncertain and clarification would result in a significantly altered approach to management.

TABLE 10-5	Clinical and Radiologic Features of Interstitial Lung Diseases	
	Clinical Features	**HRCT findings**
UIP	• Forms the radiologic basis for diagnosing IPF in the absence of underlying cause • Insidious onset and progressive dyspnea • Dry cough • Poorly responsive to treatment, poor long-term survival • Variable course punctuated by intermittent exacerbations • Pattern can be associated with connective tissue disease	• Subpleural, basal predominant • Reticular interstitial thickening • Honeycombing with/ without traction bronchiectasis • Limited ground glass • May have atypical distribution in familial cases
NSIP	• Associated with younger patients and more common in females • Commonly associated with collagen vascular diseases, including scleroderma and myositis • Response to therapy is variable depending on etiology	• Interstitial thickening, often with a rim of peripheral subpleural sparing • Ground-glass infiltrates • Traction bronchiectasis more common than UIP • In end-stage disease, may develop fibrotic changes and "bronchiolectasis" that resembles UIP
RB-ILD	• May be asymptomatic • Associated with cigarette smoking • Generally responsive to smoking cessation	• Ground-glass micronodules with an upper lobe predominance
DIP	• Associated with cigarette smoking and occupational exposures • Generally responsive to smoking cessation • May be treated with corticosteroids	• Peripheral ground-glass opacities or consolidation • May have small, well-defined cysts
AIP	• Rapidly progressive ILD with progressive hypoxemia and high mortality • Clinically (and histologically) behaves similarly to "idiopathic ARDS"	• Ground-glass opacities admixed with consolidation in geographic pattern • Eventually progresses to fibrosis with architectural distortion and traction bronchiectasis
COP	• Subacute course, often presents as multiple treatment failures of bronchitis/pneumonia • Often associated with infections, drug exposures • Responsive to prolonged courses of corticosteroids • Often recurs if steroids are rapidly withdrawn	• Multifocal ground-glass opacities and consolidations • Usually lower lobe predominant • Infiltrates may be migratory • May have "reverse halo" or atoll sign

(continued)

TABLE 10-5	Clinical and Radiologic Features of Interstitial Lung Diseases *(Continued)*	
	Clinical Features	**HRCT findings**
CEP	• Presents as progressive dyspnea and cough • Patients may have a history of underlying asthma • Peripheral blood and BAL eosinophil counts usually highly elevated	• Peripheral consolidations described as the "reverse image of pulmonary edema" • Infiltrates may be migratory
Sarcoidosis	• Dyspnea, cough, and chest pain are common presenting symptoms • Systemic symptoms may be prominent • Approximately 1 in 20 cases are asymptomatic and incidentally detected on CXR • Almost any organ system may be affected	• Perilymphatic nodules • Patchy ground-glass opacities • Reticular infiltrates • Traction bronchiectasis • Progressive massive fibrosis • Hilar or mediastinal lymphadenopathy
Chronic HP	• Presents in a similar fashion to UIP/IPF • There may be a history of systemic symptoms (fever, myalgias)	• Reticular abnormality with an upper or mid-lung predominance • Micronodules • Mosaic attenuation/air trapping • Peribronchovascular predominance

AIP, acute interstitial pneumonia; ARDS, acute respiratory distress syndrome; BAL, bronchoalveolar lavage; CEP, chronic eosinophilic pneumonia; COP, cryptogenic organizing pneumonia; DIP, desquamative interstitial pneumonia; HP, hypersensitivity pneumonitis; HRCT, high-resolution CT; ILD, interstitial lung disease; IPF, idiopathic pulmonary fibrosis; NSIP, nonspecific interstitial pneumonia; RB-ILD, respiratory bronchiolitis interstitial lung disease; UIP, usual interstitial pneumonia.
Data from: *Curr Probl Diagn* Radiol 2015;44:15; *Am J Respir Crit Care Med* 2011;183:788; Webb RW. *Thoracic Imaging: Pulmonary and Cardiovascular Radiology.* 2005.

○ Transbronchial lung biopsy has the highest yield in bronchocentric ILDs, such as sarcoidosis, in which small biopsy samples may suffice for diagnosis (*Thorax 2008;63(Suppl 5):v1*).

○ Surgical lung biopsy can be performed by video-assisted thoracoscopic surgery (VATS) or open thoracotomy. HRCT is used to target areas of active disease and avoid lung regions with end-stage fibrosis.

○ Although many patients tolerate lung biopsy well, certain subgroups of patients are predisposed to complications, including decompensation of their ILD following lung biopsy (*Chest 2005;127:1600*). Patients with IPF in particular may develop disease exacerbations following lung biopsy, resulting in disease progression and even death.

SPECIFIC INTERSTITIAL LUNG DISEASES

Idiopathic Pulmonary Fibrosis (IPF)

- The incidence of IPF is estimated to be 4.6–16.3 cases per 100,000 population.
- Males are more frequently affected than females.
- Mutations in telomerase RNA component (*TERC*), telomerase reverse transcriptase (*TERT*), pulmonary surfactant protein C (*SFTPC*), surfactant protein A2 (*SFTPA2*), and mucin 5B (*MUC5B*) have been identified in individuals and families with IPF (*Am J Med Sci 2011;341:439*).
- Although the pathophysiology is incompletely understood, pulmonary epithelial cell injury and aberrant wound healing are thought to play a central role.
- Diagnosis is made by either a definite radiographic pattern for UIP on HRCT or UIP pattern on surgical lung biopsy in the absence of other known cause after thorough workup has been completed (*Am J Respir Crit Care Med 2011;183:788*).
- In the setting of a familial fibrotic lung disease, the CT pattern may be atypical, often lacking a basal predominance. Even histologically, strictly defined UIP is identified in less than half of familial fibrotic lung disease cases (*Arch Pathol Lab Med 2012;136:1366*).
- Disease-modifying treatment options are limited in IPF. Increased risks of death and hospitalization have been associated with combined use of *N*-acetylcysteine, azathioprine, and chronic prednisone (*N Engl J Med 2012;366:1968*).
- Pirfenidone, an oral antifibrotic agent, and nintedanib, an oral tyrosine kinase inhibitor, have both been shown to slow the rate of decline in lung function in patients with IPF (*N Engl J Med 2014;370:2083*; *N Engl J Med 2014;370:2071*).
- Pulmonary rehabilitation has been associated with improvements in 6MW distance and quality of life in IPF (*Cochrane Database Syst Rev 2014;10:CD006322*).
- Patients have a widely variable course, but those diagnosed with spirometrically mild, moderate, and severe disease have been reported to have median survivals of 55.6, 38.7, and 27.4 months, respectively (*Chest 2011;140:221*).
- Poor prognostic factors for IPF include a decline in FVC >10% over 6 months, a decrease in 6MW distance >150 m over 12 months, and a decrease in DLCO >15% over 6 months.
- Acute exacerbations of IPF are characterized by acute worsening of dyspnea or oxygenation with no evidence of infection, pulmonary embolus, or heart failure (*Am J Respir Crit Care Med 2011;183:788*). Exacerbations are typically treated with high-dose corticosteroids, although their benefit has not been systematically proven. Patients often do not return to their pre-exacerbation baseline after IPF exacerbations (*Chest 2007;132:1652*).
- Lung transplantation remains the ultimate therapy in patients with advanced IPF. Criteria for lung transplantation are listed in Table 10-6. Without lung transplantation, outcomes in IPF remain relatively poor. Patients should be referred for consideration of lung transplantation at time of diagnosis of IPF.

Nonspecific Interstitial Pneumonia (NSIP)

- NSIP is rarely idiopathic; there is typically an identifiable etiology. Idiopathic NSIP is a diagnosis of exclusion. Careful history and physical exam should be performed to guide laboratory testing in the search for an underlying etiology.
- Imaging demonstrates ground-glass opacities with reticular infiltrates in a peripheral distribution. There is often sparing of the immediate subpleural space from infiltration. Traction bronchiectasis can also be seen and may progress to "bronchiolectasis" in advanced disease. This can appear radiographically similar to UIP.
- Except in cases of advanced fibrosis, patients with NSIP fare better than those with IPF (*Am J Respir Crit Care Med 2008;177:1338*).

TABLE 10-6	Criteria for Lung Transplantation in Idiopathic Pulmonary Fibrosis and Sarcoidosis

IPF

Histologic or radiographic evidence of UIP and any of the following:
- DLCO <39% predicted
- ≥10% decrement in FVC during 6 months of follow-up
- SpO_2 <88% during a 6-minute walk test
- Honeycombing on HRCT

Sarcoidosis

NYHA functional class III or IV and any of the following:
- Hypoxemia at rest
- Pulmonary hypertension
- Right atrial pressure >15 mm Hg

DLCO, diffusing capacity of the lung for carbon monoxide; FVC, forced vital capacity; HRCT, high-resolution CT; IPF, idiopathic pulmonary fibrosis; NYHA, New York Heart Association; SpO_2, oxyhemoglobin saturation by pulse oximetry; UIP, usual interstitial pneumonia.
Modified from *J Heart Lung Transplant* 2006;25:745–55.

- Treatment of NSIP secondary to connective tissue diseases usually involves immunosuppression with steroids, in combination with agents such as mycophenolate, azathioprine, cyclophosphamide, or rituximab.
- Management of patients with connective tissue disease–related ILD should be undertaken in a multidisciplinary fashion with input from providers who are familiar and experienced with these conditions.
- The effects of treating idiopathic NSIP are not well known but are an area of active investigation. Treatment with mycophenolate mofetil in particular seems promising and has been associated with stable or improved pulmonary physiology (*J Rheumatol 2013;40:640*).

Hypersensitivity Pneumonitis (HP)

- HP is a complex syndrome caused by poorly understood immunologic processes resulting in symptoms of dyspnea and cough that may manifest acutely or progress indolently over time.
- Radiographically, HRCT will demonstrate diffuse nodularity with ground-glass opacities and evidence of air trapping. Findings will generally preferentially affect the upper lobes. In advanced disease, pulmonary fibrosis with architectural distortion may occur (*Semin Respir Crit Care Med 2012;33:543*).
- Innumerable antigenic stimuli have been associated with the development of HP. A careful exposure history should be taken and should include inquiry about exposure to birds or bird feathers (including down feather pillows and blankets), hot tubs (associated with mycobacterial exposure), air humidifiers, molds, animal furs, epoxies, plant matter, industrial dusts, and chemicals. Specific antibody measurements can be sent to specialized labs when indicated.
- HP is characterized by acute, subacute, and chronic phases, with most patients presenting in the chronic phase.
- Corticosteroid therapy has been the classic mainstay of treatment for HP. However, careful attention should be paid toward identification of the offending antigen because antigenic avoidance has been associated with significantly improved mortality (*Chest 2013;144(5):1644*).

Sarcoidosis

- Sarcoidosis is diagnosed by the presence of noncaseating granulomas on biopsy. Verifying absence of infectious etiology is of particular importance in patients with exposure to endemic fungi/mycobacteria.
- The incidence rate in the United States is 35.5/100,000 for blacks and 10.9/100,000 for whites (*Am J Respir Crit Care Med 1999;160:736*).
- The cause of sarcoidosis has not been identified, although there are likely environmental and genetic factors (*Am J Respir Crit Care Med 2011;183:573*).
- Patients frequently present for evaluation of progressive dyspnea and cough. Löfgren syndrome is defined as an acute presentation of sarcoidosis characterized by arthritis, erythema nodosum, and bilateral hilar lymphadenopathy (*Am J Respir Crit Care Med 2011;183:573*).
- CXR imaging varies from hilar adenopathy to diffuse pulmonary fibrosis and is used to stage the disease. Staging is reviewed in Table 10-7.
- On CT scan, air trapping may be present, and parenchymal nodules appear in at least 80% of patients, typically following a bronchovascular distribution with intermittent coalescence into larger opacities (*Eur Radiol 2014;24:807*).
- A granulomatous vasculitis may occur and dispose patients to the development of PH.
- Extrapulmonary manifestations are typical and most commonly include uveitis and skin manifestations such as erythema nodosum (raised, red, tender bumps or nodules on anterior legs) and lupus pernio (indurated plaques with associated discoloration of the nose, cheeks, lips, and ears).
- Central nervous system involvement can manifest as central lesions, mononeuritis multiplex, or a host of other neurologic anomalies. Patients with these findings should be referred to neurology specialists with experience in the treatment of this disorder.
- Myocardial involvement may result in cardiomyopathy, arrhythmia, and sudden cardiac death (*Am Heart J 2009;157:9*).
- Endocrine involvement can manifest as hypercalcemia and hypercalciuria secondary to dysregulated production of calcitriol (*Am J Respir Crit Care Med 1999;160:736*).
- Annual ophthalmology evaluation should be considered a standard part of sarcoidosis care to monitor for ocular involvement. Referral to other specialists may be necessary as other visceral symptoms develop.
- For early stage disease, symptoms and radiographic changes may remit in the absence of treatment. In the setting of symptomatic disease or disease progression, corticosteroid therapy is typically first line. Many patients can be treated with intermittent steroid therapy alone, although those with advanced disease may be transitioned to nonsteroid immunosuppression (*Respir Med 2010;104:717*).
- Prognosis is highly variable, ranging from indolent self-remitting disease to progressive fibrosis necessitating transplantation. Indications for transplantation are reviewed in Table 10-6.

TABLE 10-7	Staging of Sarcoidosis

CXR Findings

Stage 0: Normal
Stage 1: Hilar or mediastinal lymphadenopathy
Stage 2: Hilar or mediastinal lymphadenopathy with pulmonary infiltrates
Stage 3: Pulmonary infiltrates
Stage 4: End-stage fibrosis

Organizing Pneumonia

- Organizing pneumonia is radiographically represented by decreased lung volumes and multifocal patchy consolidation and ground-glass opacities.
- Pathologically, organizing pneumonia represents a response to a proinflammatory stimulus. This is often infectious in nature, although a wide variety of pharmacologic agents and environmental exposures have been implicated as well. Idiopathic cases known as COP do occur.
- The typical clinical scenario is a patient with multiple episodes of "pneumonia" treated with antibiotics with absence of complete recovery.
- COP is a diagnosis of exclusion, and a comprehensive search for infectious etiology should be undertaken. In the absence of infectious etiology, disease is typically responsive to steroid therapy. Recurrence, however, is common after steroid withdrawal, and long-term therapy (>6 months) is frequently necessary.

"Smoking-Related" ILD

- The risk of IPF is increased in smokers.
- RB-ILD presents in patients in the third to fifth decades of life with dyspnea, cough, and radiographic evidence of subtle upper lobe ground-glass nodules on HRCT. Prognosis is good with smoking cessation.
- DIP may represent a spectrum of disease along with RB-ILD. The predominant HRCT finding in DIP is ground-glass opacities, which may be peripheral, patchy, or diffuse in distribution. Small cystic spaces occasionally develop within the ground-glass opacities. Response to smoking cessation is generally good, although some patients require corticosteroid therapy. The disease occasionally persists despite therapy (*Eur Respir J 2001;17:122*). A more severe form of DIP may also be observed in occupational exposures, and a congenital form may be seen in children.
- LCH is a parenchymal cystic lung disease characterized by irregular cysts associated with parenchymal nodules, often with sparing of the lung bases. Response to smoking cessation and steroids is generally considered good, although some patients have persistent, treatment-unresponsive disease.

Pneumoconioses

- Pneumoconioses are diseases of the lung parenchyma that result from exposure to inorganic dusts.
- Asbestos-induced lung disease arises from exposure to asbestos. Radiographic findings may range from pleural thickening and plaques to changes similar to UIP. Presence of pleural plaques aids in differentiation from other ILDs, but asbestos-related fibrotic disease can exist in the absence of pleural manifestations. Treatment focuses on asbestos avoidance and supportive care. Prognosis is good in mild disease, although the risk of lung cancer is increased in the setting of concomitant cigarette use.
- Silicosis results from exposure to silica crystals, which are found in stone and sand. Foundry workers, construction workers, and glassblowers are at increased risk. CXRs demonstrate small nodules in the upper and mid zones with hilar adenopathy in a manner similar to sarcoidosis. Treatment is supportive, although close monitoring for development of tuberculosis (TB) is warranted because these patients are at increased risk (*Prim Care Respir J 2013;22:249*).
- Berylliosis is caused by exposure to beryllium and beryllium compounds. Exposure occurs in the aerospace industry, atomic industry, beryllium mining, and fluorescent light bulb manufacturing. It is clinically indistinguishable from sarcoidosis.

Cystic Lung Disease

- Lymphangioleiomyomatosis is a progressive cystic disease of the lung seen almost exclusively in young women. Imaging demonstrates diffuse, round, thin-walled cysts. Pneumothorax (from ruptured cyst) is a commonly described initial presentation.

Lymphangioleiomyomatosis is seen more frequently in patients with tuberous sclerosis. Extrapulmonary manifestations may include renal tumors, specifically angiomyolipomas. Sirolimus has been shown to reduce disease progression, but disease recurs once therapy is stopped, and long-term effects are uncertain at this point (*N Engl J Med 2011;364:1595*).

- LCH is described under the "Smoking-Related" ILD section.
- Amyloidosis and light chain deposition disease can be associated with cystic lung disease in the setting of underlying systemic amyloidosis, connective tissue disease, or myeloma. Cysts are variable in size and distribution. Treatment focuses on the underlying condition.
- Lymphocytic interstitial pneumonia is a rare disease, usually associated with connective tissue diseases. Imaging demonstrates irregular cysts, multifocal ground-glass opacities, nodularity, and septal thickening. Treatment and prognosis are variable depending on underlying condition.
- Birt-Hogg-Dubé syndrome is a rare cause of cystic disease associated with skin and renal neoplasms. Cysts are irregularly shaped and localized to the lung bases. Treatment is supportive, and progression is generally slow (*Front Med 2013;7:316*).

MANAGEMENT CONSIDERATIONS

- The medical management of selected ILDs is briefly reviewed in Table 10-8.
- All ILD patients should be monitored for the development of exertional hypoxemia. Supplemental oxygenation should be provided to maintain oxyhemoglobin saturation by pulse oximetry (SpO_2) ≥89% both with rest and exertion.

TABLE 10-8	Medical Treatment of Selected Interstitial Lung Diseases
ILD	**Potential Therapeutic Interventions[a]**
Medication-induced ILD	• Discontinue culprit medication • Corticosteroids
Connective tissue disease–associated ILD (UIP, NSIP, COP)	• Corticosteroids • Immunosuppressive therapy (e.g., cyclophosphamide, azathioprine, mycophenolate)
IPF	• Pirfenidone • Nintedanib • Consideration for participation in a clinical trial
DIP, RB-ILD	• Smoking cessation • Corticosteroids (likely of limited benefit)
Sarcoidosis	• Corticosteroids • Immunosuppressive therapy (e.g., methotrexate, azathioprine, hydroxychloroquine, TNF-α inhibitors)
Chronic HP	• Avoid offending antigens • Corticosteroids (likely of limited benefit) • Immunosuppressive therapy

COP, cryptogenic organizing pneumonia; DIP, desquamative interstitial pneumonia; HP, hypersensitivity pneumonitis; ILD, interstitial lung disease; IPF, idiopathic pulmonary fibrosis; NSIP, nonspecific interstitial pneumonia; RB-ILD, respiratory bronchiolitis-interstitial lung disease; TNF, tumor necrosis factor; UIP, usual interstitial pneumonia.
[a]Lung transplantation is a consideration for select patients with end-stage interstitial lung disease.

- Smoking cessation/avoidance should be strongly encouraged, and patients should avoid occupational/environmental triggers of their ILD, if identified.
- Pulmonary rehabilitation therapy should be prescribed for all patients if they meet eligibility criteria.
- Bone density assessment is recommended for patients receiving chronic systemic corticosteroid therapy, and periodic reassessment (e.g., every 1–2 years) should be performed.
- *Pneumocystis jirovecii* pneumonia prophylaxis should be considered in patients receiving chronic immunosuppressive therapy (*Mayo Clin Proc 1996;71:5*).
- Patients should receive vaccinations against pneumococcus and influenza.
- Those with advanced or idiopathic ILDs should be considered for referral to centers with expertise in the diagnosis and treatment of these conditions, with particular consideration for participation in ongoing clinical trials.
- ILD increases the risk of PH (*Am J Respir Crit Care Med 2011;45:1*). Patients with dyspnea out of proportion to their parenchymal lung disease or those with symptoms of right heart failure should be screened with TTE. Although the use of pulmonary vasodilators in this population remains controversial, other therapies targeted at maintenance of euvolemia and optimization of RV function can be helpful in controlling symptoms.
- Several of the ILDs are associated with an increased incidence of malignancy. Rapid weight loss or radiographic changes (e.g., new consolidation) should raise suspicion and prompt further workup.
- Goals of care should be made clear, particularly in patients who have advanced fibrotic lung diseases and are not candidates for transplantation. Open discussions of these issues in the clinical arena may prompt family discussions, which can be helpful during acute exacerbations or disease progression (*BMJ Support Palliat Care 2013;3:84*).

Solitary Pulmonary Nodule

GENERAL PRINCIPLES

- The goal of a careful evaluation of the solitary pulmonary nodule (SPN) is to determine if the lesion is more likely **malignant or benign**.
- **A lesion >3 cm has a high likelihood of malignancy and should be treated as such, whereas lesions <3 cm need more careful assessment.**
- Nodules with benign characteristics should be closely followed so that invasive procedures with associated risks can be avoided.
- Identifying early lung cancer is of the utmost importance because there is a >60% survival rate of patients who have a malignant SPN removed (*Chest 2013;145(5):e278S*).

Definition

An SPN is defined as a rounded lesion <3 cm in diameter. It is completely surrounded by lung parenchyma, unaccompanied by atelectasis, intrathoracic adenopathy, or pleural effusion. Pulmonary nodules <8 mm remain within this definition; however, there is evidence to suggest that these nodules have a lower overall malignancy risk (*Chest 2013;145(5):e278S*).

Epidemiology

- Approximately 150,000 SPNs are identified each year in the United States.
- It has been estimated that such a nodule is noted on 0.09–0.20% of all chest radiographs.

Etiology

- Although underlying etiologies for pulmonary nodules are varied, the most important designation clinically is deciphering between a malignant and a nonmalignant process.

- **Malignancy accounts for approximately 40% of SPNs, although this may vary geographically depending on the prevalence of nonmalignant processes such as histoplasmosis.**
- **Granulomas** (both infectious and noninfectious) account for 50% of undiagnosed SPNs.
- The remaining 10% are composed of **benign neoplasms**, such as **hamartomas** (5%) and a multitude of other causes.

Risk Factors

- **Smoking** is the most important associated risk factor for almost all malignant SPNs.
- For infectious etiologies, an immunocompromised state promotes an increased risk.

Lung Cancer Screening

Screening high-risk patients using low-dose chest CT resulted in a 20% relative reduction in mortality from lung cancer compared to screening with CXR (*N Engl J Med 2011;365:395*).

DIAGNOSIS

- Diagnosis of the SPN is made radiographically, usually via CXR or CT scan.
- Most frequently, the nodule is noted incidentally on a study performed for other reasons (e.g., chronic cough, chest pain).

Clinical Presentation

- As stated previously, the majority of SPNs are diagnosed incidentally by radiographic tests done for other reasons, so there may not be overt symptoms.
- There are instances when a nodule may precipitate cough, chest pain, hemoptysis, or sputum production depending on the etiology and location of the SPN.

History

- Ask typical screening questions for malignancy including **weight loss and night sweats**.
- **Hemoptysis** may indicate malignancy but may also prompt investigations for antineutrophil cytoplasmic antibody (ANCA)-associated vasculitis, TB, and hereditary hemorrhagic telangiectasia (HHT).
- Ask about arthritis and arthralgias for possible undiagnosed rheumatoid arthritis or sarcoidosis.
- Take an exposure history including recent travel history related to endemic mycoses (histoplasmosis, coccidioidomycosis, etc.) as well as possible TB exposures.
- A history of previous malignancies increases the risk of metastatic disease of the lung.
- Patients who are immunosuppressed from HIV, organ transplant, or chronic steroids have increased risk of infectious causes.
- Smoking is linked to 85% of lung cancers. A patient's risk of lung cancer decreases significantly 5 years after smoking cessation, but it never truly returns to normal.
- An occupational history is important including possible exposure to asbestosis (associated with not only mesothelioma, but also non–small-cell lung cancer), silica, beryllium, radon, and ionizing radiation, among others.

Physical Examination

- Although there are no specific physical exam findings related to SPNs, evidence for underlying etiologies may be discovered with a thorough exam.
- Note signs of weight loss or cachexia, suggestive of malignancy.
- Do a thorough lymph node exam. **A cervical lymph node might provide an easy diagnostic target to determine the etiology of an SPN.**

- Perform a breast exam in women and testicular exam in young men.
- A careful skin examination may reveal telangiectasias, erythema nodosum, rheumatoid nodules, or other findings that might suggest a cause.

Diagnostic Criteria

- As mentioned previously, an SPN is identified as a rounded lesion <3 cm in circumference. It is completely surrounded by lung parenchyma, unaccompanied by atelectasis, intrathoracic adenopathy, or pleural effusion.
- The first step in managing an SPN is to stratify the patient in terms of malignancy risk: low-, intermediate-, or high-risk categories (Table 10-9). Risk stratification can be accomplished either qualitatively via clinical judgment or quantitatively using validated risk assessment tools. These approaches appear to be complementary (*Ann Am Thorac Soc 2013;10(6):629*).
- Once the risk of malignancy has been established, further management can proceed, as outlined in Figure 10-3.

Differential Diagnosis

Pulmonary nodules are divided primarily into malignant or benign etiologies, with benign processes further divided into infectious or noninfectious causes (Table 10-10).

Diagnostic Testing

Laboratories
- Routine laboratory testing is seldom helpful unless the history and physical exam strongly suggest an etiology.
- If connective tissue diseases or vasculitides are suspected, perform appropriate testing.
- Hyponatremia may suggest syndrome of inappropriate antidiuretic hormone (SIADH) associated with primary lung cancer, as well as other pulmonary processes.
- Hypercalcemia might suggest lung cancer as well as sarcoidosis.
- Anemia may indicate chronic pulmonary hemorrhage (e.g., HHT) or a chronic inflammatory disease.
- Microbiologic studies, particularly sputum culture, may aid in the diagnosis of an infectious SPN.
- Sputum cytology has limited use, because yield is low for peripherally located, small lesions.

TABLE 10-9	Risk Stratification of a Solitary Pulmonary Nodule		
Variable	**Low Risk**	**Intermediate Risk**	**High Risk**
Lesion diameter (cm)	<1.5	1.5–2.2	>2.2
Patient age (years)	<45	45–60	>60
Smoking status	Never smoked or quit >7 yr ago	Current smoker of <20 cigarettes/d or quit <7 yr ago	Current smoker of >20 cigarettes/d
Lesion margin characteristics	Smooth and rounded	Scalloped	Spiculated or corona radiata
Densitometry in Hounsfield units (HU)	<15 HU	>15 HU	>15 HU

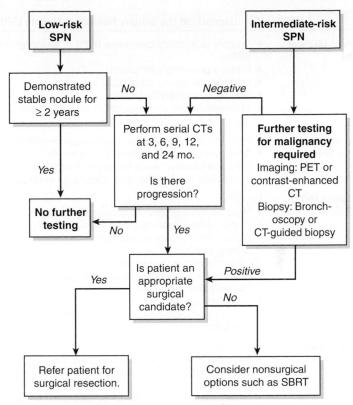

Figure 10-3. Diagnostic and therapeutic management of low- and intermediate-risk pulmonary nodules. PET, positron emission tomography; SBRT, stereotactic body radiation therapy; SPN, solitary pulmonary nodule.

Imaging

The mainstay of diagnostic evaluation of an SPN is via radiographic studies, primarily **CXR, chest CT, and positron emission tomography (PET) scan.**

- **CXR**
  - ○ A previous CXR is an important tool in the initial evaluation of an SPN.
  - ○ If an SPN has been present and unchanged on CXR for >2 years, then further evaluation may not be warranted. Ground-glass lesions may be followed for longer periods of time because the volume-doubling time may be extended in certain types of non–small-cell lung cancers.
  - ○ If an SPN appears on a new radiograph in <30 days, it is likely not malignant and most likely infectious or inflammatory.
  - ○ There are radiographic findings that make it more likely that a lesion is **benign (calcifications, a laminated appearance)**; or more likely **malignant (spiculated, irregular border)** (see Table 10-9).
  - ○ The CXR is easy to obtain and delivers a low dose of radiation; however, it has limitations in the initial characterization, and careful comparisons over time are required for SPN evaluation.

TABLE 10-10	Differential Diagnosis of the Solitary Pulmonary Nodule (SPN)
Malignant (40% of SPNs)	• Primary pulmonary carcinoma (80% of all malignant SPNs) • Primary pulmonary lymphoma • Primary pulmonary carcinoid • Solitary pulmonary metastasis • Melanoma, osteosarcoma, testicular, breast, prostate, colon, and renal cell carcinoma
Benign neoplasms (5% of SPNs)	• Hamartoma (accounts for most benign neoplastic SPNs) • Arteriovenous malformations (consider HHT) • Others, including neural tumors (schwannoma, neurofibroma), fibroma, and sclerosing hemangioma
Granulomas (50% of SPNs)	Infectious • Mycobacterial disease (most commonly tuberculosis) and fungal infections (histoplasmosis, coccidioidomycosis, blastomycosis, cryptococcosis, aspergillosis) Noninfectious granulomas associated with vasculitis • Granulomatosis with polyangiitis (Wegener granulomatosis), Churg-Strauss syndrome Noninfectious granulomas not associated with vasculitis • Sarcoid granulomatosis, hypersensitivity pneumonitis, and berylliosis
Other etiologies (5% of SPNs)	Infectious • Bacterial (nocardiosis, actinomycosis, round pneumonia), measles, abscess, septic embolus Noninfectious • Lipoid pneumonia, amyloidosis, subpleural lymph node, rheumatoid nodule, pulmonary scar or infarct, congenital malformations (bronchogenic cyst, sequestration), skin nodule, rib fracture, pleural thickening from mass or fluid

HHT, hereditary hemorrhagic telangiectasia.

- **Chest CT**
  - Chest CT is now considered the most important radiologic exam for SPN evaluation. With few exceptions, an SPN requires assessment by CT.
  - Accurate volumetric measurement of lesion size allows precise comparison to determine stability or growth.
  - Imaging allows a careful examination of mediastinal lymph nodes.
  - Thin cuts through the lesion are more sensitive than CXR for characterizing calcifications and lamination as well as the margins of the lesion.
- **PET scan**
  - 18-Fluorodeoxyglucose (FDG)-PET can help distinguish malignant and benign lesions because cancers are metabolically active and take up FDG avidly.
  - PET has a sensitivity of 80–100% and specificity of 79–100% for detecting malignancy.
  - **False negatives** can occur in bronchoalveolar carcinoma, carcinoid, and mucinous neoplasms, whereas **false positives** are common in nonmalignant "inflammatory" conditions (infectious and autoimmune processes).

- ○ Higher incidence of both false-positive and false-negative results occurs in nodules <10 mm, thus discouraging the use of PET scan in this situation (*Lung Cancer 2004;45:19*).
  - ○ PET scan is most commonly used in the evaluation of low- to moderate-risk indeterminate nodules for further risk stratification (see Figure 10-3).
- **Contrast-enhanced CT**
  - ○ Technique using contrast enhancement and measurement of Hounsfield units to risk stratify an SPN for malignancy.
  - ○ A multicenter analysis demonstrated high sensitivity but relatively low specificity for identifying malignant nodules (*Radiology 2000;214:73*).
  - ○ This method may be an important tool for risk assessment of an indeterminate SPN in centers that have experience with the technique.

Diagnostic Procedures
- **If a nodule is considered high risk and the patient is an appropriate surgical candidate, then the best approach is to forego biopsy and pursue resection.**
- Any change of an SPN on serial imaging warrants resection or invasive biopsy.
- If a lesion has low-risk characteristics, there is no indication to pursue biopsy and subjecting a patient to unneeded risk.
- **Biopsy** is most often pursued when there is discordance between clinical risk stratification and imaging tests. For example, when pretest suspicion for malignancy is significant but PET imaging is negative, biopsy may be indicated.
- Also, for patients in whom surgery represents significant risk secondary to comorbidities, using a less invasive biopsy strategy to determine the presence of malignancy is appropriate.
- There are primarily two options for biopsy of an SPN: transthoracic needle aspiration (TTNA) and fiber-optic flexible bronchoscopy.
  - ○ **TTNA**
    - ▪ This technique is usually performed under the guidance of fluoroscopy, ultrasound, or CT (more common).
    - ▪ This approach is most commonly used for nodules with a peripheral location and without anatomic impediment to a biopsy needle.
    - ▪ Sensitivity of TTNA for the diagnosis of lung cancer is 80–90% in selected patients.
    - ▪ Specificity for identifying malignancy is high with TTNA; however, there is a significant rate of nondiagnostic biopsies, and sensitivity depends on many factors, including nodule size and distance from the pleura.
    - ▪ A nondiagnostic biopsy does not rule out malignancy.
    - ▪ The main complication of TTNA is pneumothorax with 25% incidence of minor pneumothorax and 5% incidence of major pneumothorax requiring chest tube drainage.
  - ○ **Bronchoscopy**
    - ▪ Conventional flexible bronchoscopy is best suited for central airway lesions and has a sensitivity of 88% in malignancy. Advanced bronchoscopic techniques are recommended in the diagnosis of peripheral lesions where their diagnostic yield is superior to that of conventional bronchoscopy.
    - ▪ Advanced bronchoscopic modalities include radial probe endobronchial ultrasound and electromagnetic navigation, with sensitivities of 73% and 71%, respectively, for the detection of malignancy in peripheral nodules.
    - ▪ These techniques are currently recommended as potential alternatives to CT-guided TTNA by the American College of Chest Physicians for the diagnosis of pulmonary nodules.

TREATMENT

- Management of low- and intermediate-risk SPNs is outlined in Figure 10-3.
- Overall treatment strategy is to identify lesions with significant malignancy risk and pursue surgical resection when possible.

- If a nodule has low-risk characteristics and has demonstrated stability over a period of 2 years, then no further treatment is warranted. Further follow-up of subsolid and purely ground-glass lesions may be necessary, because their volume-doubling times may be prolonged.
- If a specific etiology for the SPN is diagnosed (e.g., a connective tissue disease or infection), then treatment is targeted toward the underlying process.

Other Nonpharmacologic Therapies

- Although **surgical resection is preferable in patients with either a high-risk lesion or biopsy-proven malignancy**, if surgical resection is not an option, there are other less effective therapies.
- **Stereotactic radiation** is currently the most widely used therapy in this clinical situation. This mode of external-beam therapy aims to decrease collateral radiation-induced damage to adjacent lung tissue.
- There are more experimental approaches, including brachytherapy and radiofrequency ablation, that are currently under development.

Surgical Management

- Surgical resection of an indeterminate SPN is indicated in the following situations:
  ○ The clinical probability of malignancy is moderate to high (>60%).
  ○ The nodule is hypermetabolic by PET imaging.
  ○ The nodule has been proven malignant by biopsy.
- A combination of surgical techniques, including VATS, mediastinoscopy, and thoracotomy, can lead to diagnosis (via intraoperative frozen section), staging, and potential cure during a single induction of anesthesia.

MONITORING/FOLLOW-UP

- For a low- or intermediate-risk pulmonary nodule for which resection is not warranted (see Figure 10-3), desired, or possible, routine follow-up with chest CT is standard practice.
- The typical practice for following an SPN is with serial chest CT performed at intervals of **3, 6, 12, 18, and 24 months** from initial detection, assessing for any evidence of growth.

Pleural Effusion

GENERAL PRINCIPLES

Definition
The accumulation of fluid in the pleural space.

Classification
Diagnosis and management are based on classifying a pleural effusion as either a **transudate or exudate**.

Etiology (*Thorax 2010;65(Suppl 2):ii4–ii17*)
- **Causes of transudative pleural effusions**
  ○ Common causes
    ▪ LV failure
    ▪ Liver cirrhosis
  ○ Less common causes
    ▪ Hypoalbuminemia
    ▪ Peritoneal dialysis
    ▪ Hypothyroidism

- Nephrotic syndrome
- Mitral stenosis
  - Rare causes
    - Constrictive pericarditis
    - Urinothorax
    - Meigs syndrome
- **Causes of exudative pleural effusions**
  - Common causes
    - Malignancy
    - Parapneumonic effusions
    - TB
  - Less common causes
    - Pulmonary embolism
    - Rheumatoid arthritis and other autoimmune pleuritis
    - Benign asbestos effusion
    - Pancreatitis
    - Post–myocardial infarction
    - Post–coronary artery bypass graft
  - Rare causes
    - Yellow nail syndrome (and other lymphatic disorders [e.g., lymphangioleiomyomatosis])
    - Drugs
    - Fungal infections

Pathophysiology

- **Normal pleural physiology**
  - Each pleural space produces and reabsorbs up to 15 mL of fluid per day and **contains about 10 mL of fluid at any one time** not apparent on imaging.
  - **Normal pleural fluid chemistries:** lactate dehydrogenase (LDH) <0.6 of serum, protein <0.5 of serum, glucose 0.6–0.8 of serum, pH 7.60.
- **Transudative effusion: alteration of hydrostatic and/or oncotic factors** that increase the formation and/or decrease reabsorption of pleural fluid.
  - CHF: increased venous pressures and lung edema
  - Hepatic cirrhosis and nephrotic syndrome: hypoalbuminemia
  - Malignancy: infiltration/obstruction of pleural capillaries and/or lymphatics (up to 10% of malignant effusions are transudative)
- **Exudative effusion:** either direct or cytokine-induced disruption of normal pleural membranes and/or vasculature leading to **increased capillary permeability**.
  - Infection/pneumonia
  - Malignancy
  - Inflammatory disease (i.e., systemic lupus erythematosus [SLE] or rheumatoid arthritis)
  - Trauma/surgery
  - Pulmonary embolus
- **Fluid markers of pleural infection, inflammation, and/or obstruction** often coexist.
  - **Low glucose and pH levels**
    - Byproducts of microorganism and/or inflammatory cell metabolism
    - Decreased acid removal due to pleural disruption from inflammation or malignancy
  - **High LDH level**
    Cell turnover and lysis

DIAGNOSIS

The clinical setting, combined with pleural fluid analysis, is crucial to establishing a proper diagnosis.

Clinical Presentation

Symptoms and signs may be directly related to the pleural effusion itself and/or to any underlying disease process.

History
- **Dyspnea** due to abnormal pulmonary mechanics: most common symptom, usually develops with >500–1000 mL of pleural fluid but may not correlate
- **Often asymptomatic**
- Pleurisy or referred chest/back/shoulder pain from pleural inflammation
- Should include survey of potential underlying causes

Physical Examination
- Vital signs: Assess for fever, hemodynamic instability, and hypoxemia.
- Chest exam: **Dullness to percussion, decreased breath sounds, and tactile fremitus.** These signs are more sensitive with larger effusions, but the chest exam is often unreliable and should not be used solely to diagnose and approximate size (*Cleve Clin J Med 2008;75:297*).
- A thorough system-based exam should evaluate for CHF, malignancy, pneumonia, hepatic cirrhosis, venous thrombosis, and other potential causes of pleural effusion.

Diagnostic Criteria

- **Analysis of pleural fluid obtained by thoracentesis** is the mainstay of diagnosing an etiology.
- **Transudate: Presence of *all* of Light's criteria** (*Ann Intern Med 1972;77:507*).
  - ○ Fluid:serum protein ratio <0.5
  - ○ Fluid:serum LDH ratio <0.6
  - ○ Pleural fluid LDH <0.67 of upper limit of normal for serum LDH
- **Exudate: Presence of *any* of Light's criteria** (*Ann Intern Med 1972;77:507*).
  - ○ Fluid:serum protein ratio >0.5
  - ○ Fluid:serum LDH ratio >0.6
  - ○ Pleural fluid LDH >0.67 of upper limit of normal for serum LDH
- **Pseudo-exudate:** An effusion that meets one or more of Light's criteria but is actually a transudate.
  - ○ **Usually due to diuretic-treated CHF,** cirrhosis, or nephrotic kidney disease.
  - ○ **Serum–to–pleural fluid albumin gradient >1.2.**
- **Simple parapneumonic effusion:** A sterile, small (encompassing less than one-half the hemithorax), free-flowing pleural effusion in the setting of pneumonia, with pH >7.20 and glucose >60 mg/dL.
- **Complicated parapneumonic effusion: *Any* one of the following** (*Chest 2000;118:1158*):
  - ○ Large (encompassing more than one-half of the hemithorax), free flowing
  - ○ Effusion of any size with loculations
  - ○ Thickened parietal pleura on chest CT
  - ○ Positive Gram stain or culture
  - ○ pH <7.20 or glucose <60 mg/dL
- **Empyema: Gross pus in the pleural space or positive Gram stain.** Positive culture is *not* required for diagnosis (high false-negative rate).

Differential Diagnosis
See Table 10-11.

Diagnostic Testing
- Pleural effusion is detected by chest imaging and characterized through sampling by thoracentesis.
- **All parapneumonic effusions and new, undiagnosed effusions should be sampled.**

TABLE 10-11	Clues to Diagnosing the Cause of a Pleural Effusion Based on Fluid Analysis

Gross appearance
- **Clear/serous/light yellow:** Transudate of any etiology (cardiac, liver, kidney disease), urinothorax (consider if smells like ammonia)
- **Bloody/serosanguineous:** Hemothorax (surgery/trauma), PE, malignancy
- **Purulent/turbid/brown:** Infectious/empyema; esophageal rupture
- **Putrid odor:** Anaerobic empyema
- **Milky:** Chylothorax/pseudochylothorax

Nucleated cells
- **Total >50,000, neutrophilia:** Infectious/empyema
- **Total <5000:** Transudate of any etiology, chronic malignant, tuberculous
- **Lymphocytosis (>85%):** Tuberculous, lymphoma, chronic rheumatoid, sarcoidosis, pseudo-exudates
- **Eosinophilia (>10%):** Pneumothorax, hemothorax, fungal, parasitic, medications, malignancy, benign asbestos effusion
- **Mesothelial cells (>5%):** Normal, transudate

Chemical analysis
- **Elevated protein:**
  - **>3 g/dL:** Most exudates; pseudo-exudates (serum-fluid albumin gradient >1.2 g/dL)
  - **>4 g/dL:** Tuberculous
  - **>7–8 g/dL:** Blood cell dyscrasias
- **Elevated LDH:**
  - **>1000 IU/L:** Empyema, rheumatoid, paragonimiasis, high burden malignant
  - **Fluid:serum ratio >1:** Pneumocystis or urinothorax
- **Glucose <60 mg/dL:** Infectious/empyema, rheumatoid, lupus, tuberculous, esophageal rupture, malignant
- **pH <7.3:** Infectious/empyema, rheumatoid, lupus, tuberculous, esophageal rupture, high burden malignant
- **Elevated amylase (> serum):** Pancreatitis, esophageal rupture, malignant
- **Adenosine deaminase >50 units/L:** Tuberculous (unlikely if level <40)
- **Triglycerides >110 mg/dL:** Chylothorax

LDH, lactate dehydrogenase; PE, pulmonary embolism.

Laboratories
- **Pleural fluid** (see Table 10-11):
  - Note color and consistency
  - Chemistries: Protein, albumin, LDH, glucose, pH
  - Cell count with differential
  - Hematocrit if suspicion for hemothorax (>0.5 of serum is diagnostic)
  - Microbiologic stains and culture per suspicion
  - Cytology (yield approximately 60%)
  - Consider triglyceride, amylase, adenosine deaminase as indicated
- Serum: CBC, comprehensive metabolic panel, LDH, urinalysis, coagulation studies, BNP
- Additional labs guided by suggestion of underlying illness

Electrocardiography

Assess for structural heart disease. Otherwise usually nonspecific and noncontributory.

Imaging

- Standard upright **posteroanterior/lateral CXR:**
  - Diagnostic for a suspected pleural effusion and approximates size (*Radiology: Diagnosis, Imaging, Intervention. Philadelphia: Lippincott, 2000:1*)
    - 75 mL obscures the posterior costophrenic sulcus.
    - 175 mL obscures the lateral costophrenic sulcus.
    - 500 mL obscures the entire diaphragmatic contour.
    - 1000 mL reaches the level of the anterior fourth rib.
  - Helps suggest associated conditions (CHF, pneumonia)
- **Lateral decubitus radiograph**
  - **Demonstrates fluidity**
  - Usually amenable for thoracentesis if fluid layers to >1 cm
- **Thoracic ultrasonography**
  - Accurate and practical in **detecting loculations**
  - Provides **real-time guidance for thoracentesis or thoracostomy tube placement**, reducing complication rates
- **Chest CT with contrast**
  - Helpful in distinguishing fluid from lung mass, atelectasis, pneumonia, or suggesting hemothorax
  - Defines and characterizes pleural loculations, thickening, nodularity, or other abnormalities

Diagnostic Procedures

- **Thoracentesis:** Can be performed safely at the bedside on effusions layering >1 cm on lateral decubitus CXR
  - **Complicated/organized effusions should be accessed using real-time ultrasound or CT guidance.**
  - **Optimize hemostasis:** prothrombin time/partial thromboplastin time <2× normal, platelets >25×10³/microliter, creatinine <6.0 mg/dL (*Transfusion 1991;31:164*).
  - **Microbiologic studies** of a parapneumonic effusion may be falsely negative after antibiotic administration.
  - **Cytology is positive for malignancy in up to 60% of cases**, and the sensitivity for diagnosis of pleural malignancy is dependent on the pleural fluid volume extracted during thoracentesis (*Chest 2010;137(1):68–73*). However, previous studies have shown that sending volumes >50 mL did not improve the diagnostic yield (*Chest 2009;135(4):999–1001*).
  - The yield from sending more than two specimens (taken on different occasions) is very low and should be avoided.
  - **Acid-fast bacteria (AFB) stain and culture sensitivity <30%** (*Chest 2007;131:880*).
- **Closed pleural biopsy:** Performed by transthoracic needle approach
  - **Indicated for the undiagnosed, suspected tuberculous or rheumatoid effusion. Sensitivity >80% when combined with pleural fluid AFB stain and culture** because tuberculous pleuritis is usually diffuse (*Chest 1997;112:702*).
  - This procedure is no longer commonly performed due to increasing evidence that "blind" pleural biopsy is less sensitive in the diagnosis of malignant pleural disease than CT-guided pleural biopsy or local anesthetic thoracoscopy (*Thorax 2010;65:ii54–ii60*).
- **Thoracoscopic pleural biopsy:** Performed under direct pleural visualization. **Semi-rigid thoracoscopy** is an efficacious and safe procedure in diagnosis of exudative pleural effusions. It has a diagnostic sensitivity and specificity of 91% and 100%, respectively, and is associated with negligible complications (*Chest 2013; 144(6):1857–67*).

TREATMENT

- **Transudates: Usually resolve with treatment of the underlying cause** (heart failure, hepatic disease, nephrotic syndrome)
  - ◦ Therapeutic thoracentesis as indicated for persistent larger effusions.
  - ◦ Uncommonly, more aggressive measures including pleurodesis, shunts, or placement of a chronic indwelling pleural catheter are indicated for comfort or palliation.
- **Simple/uncomplicated parapneumonic effusion:** Antibiotics and close observation
- **Complicated parapneumonic effusion and empyema** (Figure 10-4): Antibiotics and **early thoracostomy tube drainage** to avoid inflammatory adhesion and organization (*Chest 2000;118:1158*)
  - ◦ **Antibiotics should also target anaerobic organisms** because they often complicate empyema (*Lancet 1974;1:338; Chest 1993;103:1502*).
  - ◦ **Intrapleural tissue plasminogen activator (tPA)–DNase therapy** improves fluid drainage for loculated effusions in patients with pleural infection and reduces the frequency of surgical referral and the duration of the hospital stay. Treatment with DNase alone or tPA alone was shown to be ineffective (*N Engl J Med 2011;365:518–26*).

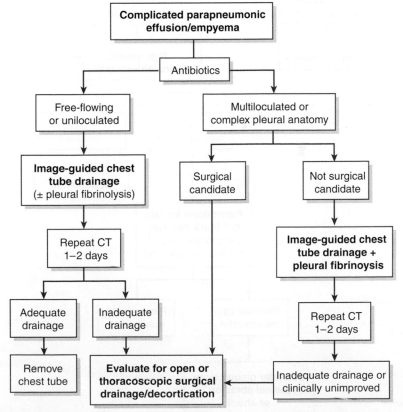

Figure 10-4. Suggested general approach to managing complicated parapneumonic effusions and empyema.

- ○ Chest tube can be removed when adequate drainage is accomplished (<50–100 mL output per day *and* resolution documented on follow-up imaging).
- ○ **Surgical decortication (thoracoscopic vs. open) may be required for effusions exhibiting complex anatomy** (extensive pleural thickening, fibrous organization, and/or multiple loculations) when unresponsive to chest tube drainage and/or intrapleural tPA-DNase therapy.
- **Malignant pleural effusion** (Figure 10-5): recurs in approximately 95% of cases, usually within a week
  - ○ Observation is appropriate in cases of small, asymptomatic, stable effusions.
  - ○ **Therapeutic (large-volume) thoracentesis** (LVT) for comfort.
    - ▪ Repeat thoracentesis is reasonable if effusion reaccumulates slowly.
    - ▪ **Reexpansion pulmonary edema is very rare** and is unlikely related to rate or volume of fluid removed (*Ann Thorac Surg 2007;84:1656*).

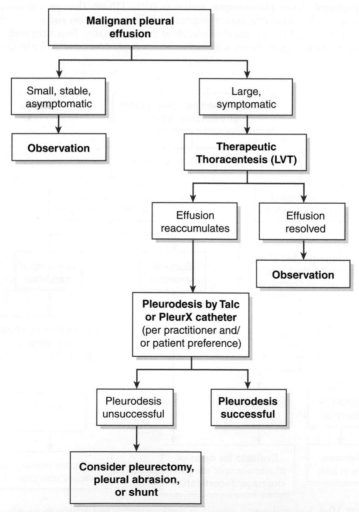

Figure 10-5. Suggested general approach to managing malignant pleural effusions. LVT, large-volume thoracentesis.

- **Removal of at least 1.5 L at a time is safe.** However, **LVT should be discontinued with development of chest discomfort**, which may be a surrogate marker for unsafe drop in pleural pressures (*Chest 2006;129:1556*).
- The correct treatment depends on several factors such as performance status, expected survival, presence of lung reexpansion following pleural drainage, and comorbidities. Among patients with malignant pleural effusion and no previous pleurodesis, there is no significant difference between indwelling pleural catheters and talc pleurodesis at relieving patient-reported dyspnea (*JAMA 2012;307(22):2383–89*).
  - **Chemical pleurodesis:** instillation of a pleural sclerosing agent such as talc or doxycycline (*Ann Intern Med 1994;120:56*).
    - Recommended when there is **rapid reaccumulation of fluid**.
    - **Talc**, instilled either as **"slurry"** through a thoracostomy tube or through insufflation during thoracoscopy (**"poudrage"**), is very effective and more comfortable than doxycycline (*Chest 2005;127:909*).
    - Less effective if lung reexpansion is incomplete after drainage ("trapped lung").
    - Often requires hospitalization for approximately 3–5 days.
  - **Chronic indwelling pleural catheter:** Practically, can be performed in the outpatient setting and maintained easily by the patient and caregiver.
    - A long-term indwelling pleural catheter could be a valid alternative to talc pleurodesis in selected patients with trapped lung syndrome (a lung that fails to reexpand after drainage of pleural effusion) and short life expectancy (*Am J Clin Oncol 2010;33:420*).
    - Spontaneous pleurodesis has been reported in 30–50% of patients with indwelling pleural catheters with repeated drainage, allowing for removal.
    - More successful at palliation than doxycycline pleurodesis (*Cancer 1999;86:1992*).
  - Pleurectomy, pleuroperitoneal shunt, chemotherapy/radiation therapy.

Surgical Management

- **Thoracic decortication:** in cases of complicated parapneumonic effusions that have complex pleural anatomy due to fibrous organization and/or are not amenable or responsive to pleural drainage
- **Pleurectomy or pleural abrasion:** for recurring malignant pleural effusion unresponsive to pleurodesis or chronic catheter drainage

REFERRAL

- Pulmonary (interventional, if available)
- Thoracic surgery as needed

OUTCOME/PROGNOSIS

Depends on etiology of the effusion and the extent of pleural disruption.
- **Transudate:** Depends on management and prognosis of the underlying cause but **generally a good outcome**.
- **Simple parapneumonic effusion: Low morbidity and mortality** if treated appropriately with antibiotics and close observation.
- **Complicated parapneumonic effusion and empyema: With delayed treatment, there is a significantly elevated risk for pleuropulmonary sequelae**, including need for intensive surgical decortication and possibly death.
- **Malignant pleural effusions** all indicate advanced malignant spread. The therapeutic options offered for these patients are usually successful in achieving desired palliation and add very little, if any, morbidity or mortality risk.

Hemoptysis

GENERAL PRINCIPLES

Hemoptysis should be considered a sign of an underlying pathologic process. It can be life threatening and, as such, requires rapid identification, workup, and treatment.

Definition

- **True hemoptysis** is expectoration of blood from the lower respiratory tree, below the glottis.
- **Massive hemoptysis/life-threatening hemoptysis:**
  - By volume: defined in the literature as from >100 mL in 16 hours to >1000 mL in 24 hours.
  - Most commonly defined as **>600 mL of blood expectorated per 24 hours** (*Arch Intern Med 1968;121:495; Ann Thorac Surg 1974;18:52; Ann Thorac Surg 1978;25:12; Am J Med Sci 1987;294,301; Flexible Bronchoscopy. 2nd ed. Hoboken: Wiley-Blackwell, 2004*).
  - Clinically: >100 mL in 24 hours is associated with gas exchange abnormality, airway obstruction, or hemodynamic instability.

Classification

The most clinically useful classification of hemoptysis is **massive/life threatening or not**, followed by the **anatomic location** of the bleeding.
- Massive/life threatening: >600 mL/24 h *or* >100 mL/24 h with gas exchange abnormality, airway obstruction, or hemodynamic instability.
- Anatomic location
  - Airway
  - Parenchyma
  - Vascular
  - Combination
- There are various other classifications in the literature based on characteristics (appearance, frequency, rate, volume, and potential for clinical consequences) that often suggest an underlying etiology and may predict outcome and thus help guide diagnostics and management. However, there is considerable overlap in clinical presentation within and among etiologies.

Epidemiology

The incidence of hemoptysis is dependent on the underlying diagnosis. Listed are the incidences of some of the most common causes of hemoptysis (*Arch Intern Med 1969;149:1667; Arch Intern Med 1991;151:2449; Chest 1997;112:2*).
- Bronchiectasis: 1–37%
- Bronchitis: 2–37%
- Malignancy: 2–24%
- TB/cavitary lung disease: 2–69% (incidence is much lower in the modern, Western world)
- Pneumonia: 1–16%
- Idiopathic: 2–22%

Etiology

It is generally most clinically useful to identify etiology according to anatomic location, because the more proximal the etiology, the more likely it is to require urgent intervention.
- Airway: **bronchitis/bronchiectasis**, **malignancy**, foreign body, trauma, pulmonary endometriosis, broncholithiasis
- Parenchyma/alveoli: **pneumonia, rheumatologic vasculitides, and pulmonary hemorrhage syndromes** (ANCA-positive vasculitis, Goodpasture syndrome, SLE, diffuse alveolar hemorrhage, acute respiratory distress syndrome)
- Vascular: **elevated pulmonary venous pressure** (LV failure, mitral stenosis), pulmonary embolism, arteriovenous malformation (AVM), pulmonary arterial trauma (i.e., pulmonary

arterial catheter balloon overinflation), varices/aneurysms, rheumatologic vasculitides, and pulmonary hemorrhage syndromes
- Etiologies potentially involving multiple anatomic locations: **cavitary lung disease** (TB, aspergilloma, lung abscess), thrombocytopenia, disseminated intravascular coagulation, anticoagulants, antiplatelets, cocaine, inhalants, lung biopsy, bronchovascular fistula, bronchopulmonary sequestration, Dieulafoy disease
- **Idiopathic/undiagnosed up to 25%:** prognosis usually favorable (*Ann Intern Med 1985;102:829*)

Pathophysiology

The pathogenesis of hemoptysis depends on the etiology and location of the underlying pathologic process.
- Hemoptysis due to bronchitis or bronchiectasis results from **inflammation/irritation of airway mucosa and its associated hyperplastic or otherwise abnormal vascular supply**.
- **The bronchial arterial circulation** (branching from the aorta) supplies high-pressure blood to the airways and, when disrupted (by a foreign body, tumor invasion, fungal invasion, or denuded airway mucosa), can result in massive, life-threatening hemoptysis.
- **The pulmonary arterial circulation** supplies the lung parenchyma (participates in gas exchange) and is under low pressure, but receives all of the cardiac output. Disruption can result in minor hemoptysis (via infections) or more life-threatening hemoptysis due to processes such as vasculitis, diffuse alveolar hemorrhage, pulmonary embolism, acute respiratory distress syndrome, AVM rupture, pulmonary artery catheter trauma, severe mitral stenosis, LV failure, or Rasmussen aneurysm (pulmonary artery aneurysm associated with TB).

DIAGNOSIS

Identifying and correcting the underlying disease is the basis of diagnosis and management of hemoptysis (Figure 10-6).

Clinical Presentation

Hemoptysis may be the only presenting sign or may accompany other manifestations of an underlying disorder (Table 10-12). The appearance, timing, and volume can provide important clues to narrowing the differential diagnosis.
- Appearance: grossly bloody, blood-tinged sputum, streaky, foamy
- Timing: first episode, recurrent episodes, chronic small amounts, acute large amounts
- Volume: submassive, massive

History
- Most important: amount of hemoptysis, age, smoking history, prior lung disease, previous malignancy, risk for coagulopathy, and prior episodes of hemoptysis.
- Review of systems should focus on symptoms suggesting cardiopulmonary disease, active infection, underlying malignancy, and systemic inflammatory disorders.

Physical Examination
- Most important: vital signs including oxygen saturation, general state of health, lung exam noting focal or diffuse abnormal findings such as bronchial breath sounds, crackles, inspiratory and/or expiratory wheezes.
- A thorough exam should always be performed, noting any manifestations suggesting underlying cardiopulmonary, infectious, immunologic, or malignant disease.

Differential Diagnosis

One must distinguish between **true hemoptysis** and **pseudohemoptysis**, which comes from the upper airway (above the glottis) or gastrointestinal tract that is expectorated. See Table 10-12 for most common diagnoses related to hemoptysis.

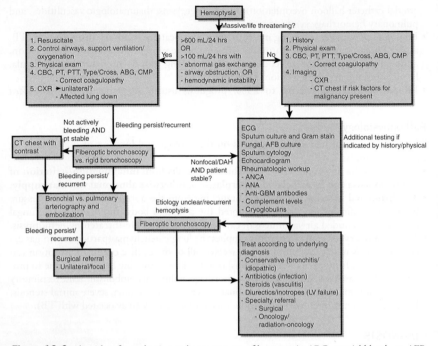

Figure 10-6. Algorithm for evaluation and management of hemoptysis. ABG, arterial blood gas; AFB, acid-fast bacteria; ANA, antinuclear antibody; ANCA, antineutrophil cytoplasmic antibody; CBC, complete blood count; CMP, comprehensive metabolic panel; DAH, diffuse alveolar hemorrhage; GBM, glomerular basement membrane; LV, left ventricle; PT, prothrombin time; PTT, partial thromboplastin time.

Diagnostic Testing

- A thorough **history and physical exam** is important to provide clues and guidance in additional testing.
- Additional testing is aimed at determining clinical stability, localizing the source, and identifying the underlying etiology.

Laboratories and Electrocardiography

- ECG to assess for underlying structural cardiac disease
- CBC, comprehensive metabolic panel, coagulation studies, urinalysis with microscopy
- Type and cross-match blood if hemoptysis massive
- ABG if indicated
- Sputum studies: routine Gram stain and culture, fungal, AFB, and cytology studies as indicated
- Specialized studies as suggested by clinical suspicion
  - CHF: BNP
  - Immunologic disease: ANA/ANCA screen, anti–glomerular basement membrane antibodies, complement levels, cryoglobulins, etc.

Imaging

- **Posteroanterior/lateral CXR** should be performed in all cases of hemoptysis.
  - **Normal or nonlocalizing in up to 50% of all cases** (*Chest 1988;92:70*; *Clin Radiol 1996;51:391*).
  - **Normal in up to 10% of cases caused by bronchogenic carcinoma** (*Chest 1988;92:70*).

TABLE 10-12	Clues to Diagnosing the Cause of Hemoptysis from the History and Physical Exam	
Cause of Hemoptysis	**Historical Clue**	**Physical Exam Finding**
Bronchogenic carcinoma	Smoker, age >40 yr; recurrent nonmassive hemoptysis, weight loss	Local chest wheezing
Chronic bronchitis/ bronchiectasis	Frequent, copious sputum production; frequent "pneumonias"	Scattered, bilateral, coarse chest crackles, wheezes; clubbing
TB, fungal lung disease, lung abscess	Subacute constitutional symptoms; travel and exposure history	Fever, focal coarse chest crackles, cachexia
Acute pneumonia	Acute fever, productive cough, pleurisy, rusty brown hemoptysis	Fever, focal coarse chest crackles, bronchial breath sounds
Vasculitis, hemorrhage syndrome	Subacute constitutional symptoms, hematuria, rash, arthralgias	Diffuse chest crackles, mucosal ulcers, rash
Heart failure	Orthopnea, lower extremity edema, history of valvular disease	Murmurs, diastolic rumble, S_3, loud S_1 or P_2, lower extremity edema
AVM/hereditary hemorrhagic telangiectasia	Platypnea, epistaxis, family history of similar signs and symptoms	Mucosal telangiectasias, orthodeoxia
Pulmonary embolus	Acute dyspnea, pleurisy	Hypoxemia, pleural rub, unilateral lower extremity edema

AVM, arteriovenous malformation; TB, tuberculosis.

- **Chest CT:** Indication often depends on clinical suspicion but should be performed if the diagnosis remains in doubt after initial clinical evaluation or if bronchoscopy is unrevealing (see Figure 10-6).
  - ○ Advantages:
    - ▪ Can visualize parenchyma, vasculature, and airways to varying extent.
    - ▪ **Especially useful for bronchiectasis, cavitary lung disease, masses, and vascular malformations** (*Chest 1994;105:1155*).
    - ▪ HRCT may visualize tumors with efficacy comparable to bronchoscopy (*Radiology 1993;189:677*).
  - ○ Disadvantages:
    - ▪ Less efficacious in recognizing subtle bronchial and mucosal lesions (*Chest 1994; 105:1155*)
    - ▪ Nonspecific in cases of parenchymal/alveolar hemorrhage
    - ▪ Delay in treatment is high risk in an unstable patient
- **Echocardiography** if suspect structural or valvular cardiac disease.

Diagnostic Procedures
- **Fiber-optic (flexible) bronchoscopy:** generally **localizes/lateralizes bleeding source** in over two-thirds of cases, depending on the setting (*Ann Thorac Surg 1989;48:272*)
  - **Indications**
    - If the source is unclear after initial evaluation and imaging or if hemoptysis persists/recurs
    - To rule out infection
    - If the clinical presentation suggests an airway abnormality
    - To obtain brushings/biopsy if CXR/imaging suggests malignancy or is nonlocalizing with the **presence of at least two risk factors for bronchogenic carcinoma:**
      - Male sex
      - Age >40 years
      - >40 pack-year smoking
      - Duration of hemoptysis >1 week
      - Volume expectorated >30 mL (*Chest 1985;87:142*; *Chest 1988;92:70*; *Ann Intern Med 1991;151:171*)
    - To identify potential anatomic area for arterial embolization
    - To rule out alveolar hemorrhage
  - Timing: Controversial, although increased yield when performed during or within 48 hours of bleeding (*Am Rev Respir Dis 1981;124:221*)
- **Bronchial and pulmonary arteriography:** perform in **persistent or recurring massive hemoptysis**
  - Advantage: Can be diagnostic and therapeutic via simultaneous **embolization** of the culprit vessel if localized
  - Disadvantages:
    - **Variable and inexact localization** of bleeding depending on clinical setting (*Ann Thorac Surg 1989;48:272*).
    - Anatomic variability.
    - Bleeding usually insufficient for contrast extravasation.
    - Diffuse lung diseases often have associated diffuse vascular abnormalities, making localization difficult (i.e., bronchiectasis).

TREATMENT

The general approach is primarily aimed at **distinguishing massive/life-threatening hemoptysis from nonmassive hemoptysis**. Three main goals: (1) stabilize, (2) diagnose and localize, and (3) decide on need and type of therapy.
- **Nonmassive hemoptysis:** usually treated conservatively and based on underlying disorder (see Figure 10-6).
  - Reverse coagulopathy
  - Antitussives and mild sedatives
  - Bronchoscopy if recurrent
  - Steroids for rheumatologic conditions
  - Antibiotics for infection (fungal, TB, pneumonia, etc.)
  - Diuretics and/or inotropes for heart disease (LV failure, mitral stenosis)
- **Massive hemoptysis:** requires urgent action, intensive monitoring, and an early multidisciplinary approach including an interventional pulmonologist and/or thoracic surgeon and an interventional radiologist (see Figure 10-6).
  - **Initial stabilization:**
    - **Airway management:** very low threshold for intubation, with a large (>8 French) endotracheal tube (*Chest 2000;118;5*)
      - Single-lumen main stem intubation for selective ventilation of unaffected lung.
      - Double-lumen endotracheal intubation for selective ventilation of unaffected lung. Should be performed and managed only under appropriately skilled supervision.

- **Lateral decubitus positioning** (affected lung down) to minimize aspiration into unaffected lung
  - **Bronchoscopy** with directed airway therapy:
    Rigid bronchoscopy is favored if available because it provides optimal airway access and ventilatory control, plus easier suctioning and manipulation of instruments.
    - **Direct tamponade with the distal end of the bronchoscope.**
    - **Balloon tamponade:** left in place for 1–2 days. Watch for ischemic mucosal injury or postobstructive pneumonitis (*Thorax 2003;58:814*).
    - Fogarty balloon, bronchial blocker, and pulmonary artery catheter balloons have all been described.
    - **Endobronchial electrocautery** (*Chest 2001;119:781*).
    - **Argon-plasma coagulation** (*Can Respir J 2004;11:305; Chest 2001;119:781*).
    - **Topical hemostatic agents:** cold saline, epinephrine, vasopressin, and thrombin (*Am Rev Respir Dis 1987;135:A108; Chest 1989;96:473; Thorax 1980; 35:901*).
- **Bronchial arteriography and embolization should be performed early** in massive or recurrent hemoptysis.
  - **Successful embolization (>85%)** with careful localization (*Chest 2002;121:789; Radiology 2004;233:741*).
  - Particularly useful in cystic fibrosis patients (*Am J Respir Crit Care Med 1998;157:1951; Chest 2002;121:796*).
  - **Early failure usually due to inadequate or incomplete source vessel identification.** Postembolization arteriography may identify additional systemic culprit vessels, most commonly from the intercostal and phrenic arteries (*Am J Roentgenol 2003; 180:1577*).
  - **Rebleeding common** (up to 20%) over 1 year (*Chest 1999;115:912; Respiration 2000;67:412*).
  - **Risks** include bronchial or partial pulmonary infarct/necrosis and, rarely, ischemic myelopathy due to inadvertent embolization of a spinal artery.

Medications

Systemic procoagulants: Use only in unstable massive hemoptysis as a temporizing measure or when conventional bronchoscopic, interventional, or surgical therapies are contraindicated and/or unavailable. Some examples are factor VII, vasopressin, and aminocaproic acid.

Surgical Management

Emergent surgery has high morbidity and mortality compared to elective surgery after stabilization (*Am J Med Sci 1987;294:301–9*).
- **Lobectomy/pneumonectomy offers definitive cure.**
- **Indications: persistent focal/unilateral massive hemoptysis despite other therapy**; particularly useful for stable patients with hemoptysis due to cavitary lung disease, localized bronchogenic carcinoma, AVM, or traumatic injuries (*Crit Care Med 2000;28:1642*).
- **Contraindications:** poor pulmonary reserve, advanced malignancy, active TB, diffuse lung disease, or diffuse alveolar hemorrhage.

REFERRAL

- Pulmonary (interventional for massive hemoptysis, if available)
- Thoracic surgery
- Interventional radiology

OUTCOME/PROGNOSIS

Mortality depends on etiology and amount (*Arch Intern Med 1983;143:1343*; *Am J Med Sci 1987;294:301*).

- Up to 80% with massive hemoptysis due to malignancy
- <10% with nonmassive hemoptysis
- <1% in bronchiectasis and lung infections

Cystic Fibrosis

GENERAL PRINCIPLES

Definition

Cystic fibrosis (CF) is an **autosomal recessive disorder** caused by mutations of the cystic fibrosis transmembrane conductance regulator gene (*CFTR*), located on chromosome 7, which results in multisystem exocrine organ dysfunction.

Epidemiology

- In the United States, approximately 30,000 people are affected by CF, with an incidence of 1 in 3500 live births (*Clin Chest Med 2007;28:279*).
- CF is the most common lethal genetic disease in Caucasians; however, the diagnosis should be considered in patients of diverse ethnic backgrounds as well.
- Patients are typically diagnosed via newborn screening or during childhood, but there is increasing recognition of milder variants that may not present until later in life.
- In 2013, approximately 50% of patients with CF were ≥18 years old.

Etiology

- CF is caused by **mutations in the *CFTR* gene**, a cyclic adenosine monophosphate (cAMP)-regulated chloride channel (*Science 1989;245:1073*).
- The most common mutation in the *CFTR* gene is F508del, the lack of a phenylalanine (F) amino acid at position 508. However, >1900 mutations have been identified.
- CFTR normally maintains hydration of exocrine organ secretions.
- Abnormal CFTR causes decreased chloride secretion and increased sodium absorption on the surface of epithelial cells with resulting thickened secretions in the airways, sinuses, pancreatic ducts, biliary tree, intestines, and reproductive tract.

Pathophysiology

- CFTR normally regulates transport of chloride ions across the epithelium (*Curr Opin Pulm Med 2003;9:486*).
- The primary pulmonary manifestations of disease are related to the malfunction of chloride transport across the airway epithelium, resulting in diminished airway surface liquid and impaired mucociliary clearance.
- Poor mucociliary clearance results in an impaired ability to clear infection. Recurrent infection begets an inflammatory cascade that results in bronchiectasis, chronic infection, and ultimately, premature death (*N Engl J Med 2005;352:1992*).
- Similarly, thickened secretions in the pancreatic and biliary ducts lead to maldigestion, malabsorption, and occasionally, liver disease and diabetes.

DIAGNOSIS

- The diagnosis of CF is typically made during childhood, but approximately 10% of patients are diagnosed after age 10 (*Cystic Fibrosis Foundation National Patient Registry Annual Data Report 2013. Bethesda, MD: Cystic Fibrosis Foundation, 2014*).

- Newborn screening has increased the frequency of early diagnosis (*J Pediatr 2002;141:804*). In 2013, 62% of new diagnoses were the result of newborn screening (*Cystic Fibrosis Foundation National Patient Registry Annual Data Report 2013. Bethesda, MD: Cystic Fibrosis Foundation, 2014*).
- **At least one criterion** from each set of features must be met to diagnose CF (*J Pediatr 2008;153:S1*):
  - ○ Compatible clinical features of CF (see clinical features), or
  - ○ A positive family history of CF, or
  - ○ A positive newborn screening test
    AND
  - ○ Elevated sweat chloride >60 mmol/L on two occasions, or
  - ○ Presence of two disease-causing mutations in *CFTR*, or
  - ○ Abnormal nasal transepithelial potential difference
- Atypical patients may lack classic symptoms and signs or have normal sweat tests (*Curr Opin Pulm Med 2003;9:498*).
- Although genotyping may assist in the diagnosis, it alone cannot establish or rule out the diagnosis of CF, and the initial test of choice remains the sweat test.

Clinical Presentation

- **Pulmonary manifestations**
  Cough with purulent sputum production, wheezing, hemoptysis, dyspnea, progressive airflow obstruction, bronchiectasis, and pneumothorax
- **Extrapulmonary manifestations**
  Chronic sinusitis, nasal polyposis, pancreatic insufficiency (vitamins A, D, E, and K deficiency), malnutrition, meconium ileus, distal intestinal obstruction syndrome, volvulus, intussusception, rectal prolapse, diabetes mellitus, liver cirrhosis, portal hypertension, cholelithiasis, cholecystitis, nephrolithiasis, male infertility (bilateral absence of the vas deferens), epididymitis, growth retardation, hypertrophic pulmonary osteoarthropathy, and osteopenia

History
Presenting symptoms may include (*J Pediatr 1993;122:1*):
- Cough with purulent sputum production (40%)
- Failure to thrive (29%)
- Malnutrition
- Steatorrhea
- Meconium ileus

Physical Examination
- Underweight
- Inspiratory crackles on lung exam typically anterior and in the apices
- Digital clubbing

Differential Diagnosis

- **Primary ciliary dyskinesia:** bronchiectasis, sinusitis, and infertility, but limited gastrointestinal symptoms and normal sweat chloride levels, occasionally seen with dextrocardia or situs inversus totalis (Kartagener syndrome)
- **Immunodeficiency (e.g., severe combined immunodeficiency, common variable immunodeficiency):** recurrent sinus and pulmonary infections but typically no gastrointestinal symptoms and normal sweat chloride levels
- **Shwachman-Diamond syndrome:** pancreatic insufficiency, cyclic neutropenia, and short stature, which may lead to lung disease, but normal sweat chloride levels (*Hematol Oncol Clin North Am 2009;23:233*)

- **Young syndrome:** bronchiectasis, sinusitis, and azoospermia, but mild respiratory symptoms, lack of gastrointestinal symptoms, and normal sweat chloride levels (*Thorax 1987;42:815*)
- **Idiopathic bronchiectasis**

Diagnostic Testing

- **Skin sweat testing** with a standardized quantitative pilocarpine iontophoresis method remains the **gold standard for the diagnosis of CF** (*Am J Respir Crit Care Med 2006;173:475*).
  - A sweat chloride concentration of ≥60 mmol/L on two separate occasions is consistent with the diagnosis of CF.
  - Borderline sweat test results (40–59 mmol/L sweat chloride) or nondiagnostic results in the setting of high clinical suspicion should lead to repeat sweat testing, nasal potential difference testing, genetic testing, or additional clinical evaluation.
  - Sweat testing should be performed at a CF care center to ensure reliability of results.
  - Abnormal sweat chloride concentrations are rarely detected in non-CF patients.
- **Genetic tests** have detected >1900 putative CF mutations.
  - Two recessive mutations on different alleles must be present to cause CF.
  - The most commonly encountered CF mutation is a deletion of the three nucleotides that code for phenylalanine (F) at amino acid 508 (F508del or **ΔF508**) of the CFTR protein. In the most recent Cystic Fibrosis Foundation Patient Registry, 86.4% of patients with CF carry this mutation (*Cystic Fibrosis Foundation National Patient Registry Annual Data Report 2013. Bethesda, MD: Cystic Fibrosis Foundation, 2014*).
  - Commercially available CF screens identify >90% of the abnormal genes in a Caucasian Northern European population, although they test for only a minority of the known CF genes. Full gene sequencing is commercially available, but interpretation may be complex. Information about specific mutations and reported clinical phenotype may be found at *http://www.cftr2.org/*.
- **Transepithelial nasal potential difference**
  - A test in which the voltage across the epithelial lining of the nose is measured at baseline, after inhibiting sodium channels with amiloride and after stimulating CFTR with a cAMP agonist (*J Pediatr 1986;108:517*; *Chest 2010;138:919*).
  - The test should be repeated on two separate days to confirm diagnosis and should be performed at specialized centers.
  - Results may be affected by nasal polyposis or mucosal inflammation.

Laboratories
- Sputum cultures typically identify multiple organisms, including *Staphylococcus aureus*, nontypeable *Haemophilus influenzae*, *Pseudomonas aeruginosa*, *Stenotrophomonas maltophilia*, and *Burkholderia cepacia*. Isolation of mucoid variants of *P. aeruginosa* from the respiratory tract occurs frequently. Use of special culture media to fastidious organisms is recommended.
- Nontuberculous mycobacteria are frequently isolated from the airways of persons with CF and may be pathogenic in some.
- **Testing for malabsorption** due to pancreatic exocrine insufficiency is often not formally performed because clinical evidence (the presence of foul-smelling, bulky, and loose stools; low fat-soluble vitamin levels [vitamins A, D, and E]; and a prolonged prothrombin time [vitamin K dependent]) and a clear response to pancreatic enzyme treatment are usually considered sufficient for the diagnosis. In atypical cases, low fecal elastase level or coefficient of fat absorption <85% on a formal 72-hour fecal fat collection may confirm pancreatic insufficiency.
- Tests that identify chronic sinusitis or infertility, especially obstructive azoospermia in men, also support the diagnosis of CF.

Testing
- CXR shows hyperinflation with cystic lung disease, bronchiectasis, and mucous plugging, especially in the upper lobes.
- HRCT scan may be helpful in evaluating patients with early or mild disease by detecting early changes in the airways.
- Pulmonary function tests demonstrate expiratory airflow obstruction with increased residual volume and total lung capacity.
- Impairment of alveolar gas exchange may be present later in the course of disease, progressing to hypoxemia and hypercapnia.

TREATMENT

- CF therapy aims to improve quality of life and functioning, decrease the number of exacerbations and hospitalizations, avoid complications associated with therapy, reduce the rate of decline in lung function, and decrease mortality.
- A comprehensive program addressing multiple organ system derangements, as provided at CF care centers, is recommended.
- **Pulmonary therapy** (*Am J Respir Crit Care Med 2007;176:957*): primarily focused on clearing pulmonary secretions and controlling infection.
  - **Inhaled bronchodilators:** β-Adrenergic agonists (albuterol metered-dose inhaler, two to four puffs bid–qid; salmeterol or formoterol, one dry powder inhalation bid). Used to treat the reversible components of airflow obstruction and facilitate mucus clearance
  - **Recombinant human deoxyribonuclease:** DNase, dornase-α, Pulmozyme (2.5 mg or one ampule per day inhaled using a jet nebulizer)
    - It digests extracellular DNA, decreasing the viscoelasticity of the sputum.
    - It improves pulmonary function and decreases the incidence of respiratory tract infections that require parenteral antibiotics (*N Engl J Med 1994;331(10):637–42*).
    - Adverse effects may include pharyngitis, laryngitis, rash, chest pain, and conjunctivitis.
  - **Hypertonic saline:** (4 mL of inhaled 7% saline twice daily)
    - Due to high osmolality, water is drawn from the airway epithelium and can rehydrate the pericilliary airway surface liquid.
    - Treatment results in fewer exacerbations and improvement in lung function (*N Engl J Med 2006;354:229*).
    - Inhaled bronchodilators should be administered prior to treatments to avoid treatment-induced bronchospasm.
  - **Antibiotics**
    - A combination of an antipseudomonal β-lactam and an aminoglycoside is typically recommended during acute exacerbations (*Am J Respir Crit Care Med 2009;180:802*).
    - Sputum culture and sensitivities should guide therapy. *P. aeruginosa* is the most frequent pulmonary pathogen.
    - The duration of antibiotic therapy is dictated by the clinical response. At least 14 days of antibiotics are typically needed to treat an exacerbation.
    - Home IV antibiotic therapy is common, but hospitalization may allow better access to comprehensive therapy and diagnostic testing. Oral antibiotics are recommended only for mild exacerbations.
    - The use of chronic or intermittent prophylactic antibiotics can be considered, especially in patients with frequent recurrent exacerbations, but antimicrobial resistance may develop.
    - In patients chronically infected with *P. aeruginosa*, the inhaled aerosolized antibiotics tobramycin (300 mg nebulized twice daily) and aztreonam lysinate (75 mg nebulized 3× daily) can be used via alternating 28 days on with 28 days off to

improve pulmonary function, decrease the density of *P. aeruginosa*, and decrease the risk of hospitalization. Voice alteration (13%) and tinnitus (3%) are potential adverse events associated with long-term inhaled tobramycin (*N Engl J Med 1999;340:23*), and pyrexia and airway irritation have been reported with inhaled aztreonam (*Chest 2009;135:1223*). More recently, continuous alternating inhaled antibiotic therapy has become the standard of care for many patients with chronic *Pseudomonas* infection and pulmonary impairment.

- Patients with CF have atypical pharmacokinetics and often require higher drug doses at more frequent intervals during an acute exacerbation. In adult patients with CF, for example, cefepime is often dosed at 2 g IV q8h, and tobramycin is often dosed at 8 mg/kg IV daily (aiming for peak levels of 20 μg/mL and trough levels of <2 μg/mL).
- Once-daily aminoglycoside dosing is preferred and should be guided by pharmacokinetic testing. Monitoring levels (peaks and troughs) of drugs such as aminoglycosides helps to ensure therapeutic levels and to decrease the risk of toxicity.

○ **Anti-inflammatory therapy**
- **Azithromycin** (500 mg oral 3×/week) used chronically shows mild improvement in lung function and reduces days in the hospital for treatment of respiratory exacerbations in patients who are chronically infected with *P. aeruginosa* (*JAMA 2003;290:1749*).
- **Glucocorticoids** used in short courses may be helpful to some patients with asthmalike symptoms, but long-term therapy should be avoided to minimize the side effects, which include glucose intolerance, osteopenia, and growth retardation.
- **Ibuprofen** used in high doses has been used as a chronic anti-inflammatory agent in children age 6–17 with mild impairment of lung function (*Chest 1999;124:689*).

○ **Restoration of CFTR function**
- **Ivacaftor** (150 mg orally twice daily) is a CFTR potentiator that improves lung function and decreases the risk of pulmonary exacerbations in patients with the **missense G551D mutation** (*N Engl J Med 2011;365:1663*). After 144 weeks of use, increases in lung function are maintained (*Lancet Respir Med 2014;2:902*). Only about 4% of the US CF population carries a G551D mutation. Since its initial release, the FDA has approved the use of ivacaftor in patients with the following mutations: G178R, S549N, S549R, G551S, G1244E, S1251N, S1255P, G1349D, and R117H. However, this only includes about 7% of the US CF population.
- **Lumacaftor** (a CFTR "corrector" or chaperone protein) combined with ivacaftor has been shown in two phase III trials to improve lung function and decrease the risk of pulmonary exacerbations in patients who are homozygous for the F508del mutation. This combination therapy is awaiting FDA approval (*Vertex Pharmaceuticals Inc. Two 24-Week Phase 3 Studies of Lumacaftor in Combination with Ivacaftor Met Primary Endpoint with Statistically Significant Improvements in Lung Function (FEV1) in People with Cystic Fibrosis who have Two Copies of the F508del Mutation, 2014*).
- Other CFTR corrector molecules, potentiators, and molecules that suppress *CFTR* nonsense mutations (premature stop codons) are in various phases of clinical development and testing.

○ **Mechanical airway clearance devices:** flutter valve, acapella device, high-frequency chest oscillation vests, low- and high-pressure positive expiratory pressure devices
- Can be used in combination with medical therapy to promote airway clearance.
- Other alternatives include postural drainage with chest percussion and vibration, and breathing and coughing exercises.

○ **Pulmonary rehabilitation**
When done with exercise rehabilitation may improve functional status and promote clearance of airway secretions

○ **Oxygen therapy**
  ▪ May be indicated based on standard recommendations used for the treatment of chronic obstructive pulmonary disease.
  ▪ Rest and exercise oxygen assessments should be performed as clinically indicated.
○ **Noninvasive ventilation**
  ▪ Used for chronic respiratory failure due to CF-related bronchiectasis
  ▪ Has not been clearly demonstrated to provide a survival benefit, although it may provide symptomatic relief or may be used as a bridge to transplantation
- **Extrapulmonary therapy**
○ **Pancreatic insufficiency**
  ▪ Primary management involves **pancreatic enzyme supplementation**.
  ▪ Enzyme dose should be titrated to achieve one to two semisolid stools per day and to maintain adequate growth and nutrition.
  ▪ Enzymes are taken immediately before meals and snacks.
  ▪ Dosing of pancreatic enzymes should be initiated at 500 units lipase/kg/meal and should not exceed 2500 units lipase/kg/meal.
  ▪ **High doses** (6000 units lipase/kg/meal) have been associated with **chronic intestinal strictures** (*N Engl J Med 1997;336:1283*).
  ▪ Gastric acid suppression may enhance enzyme activity.
○ **Vitamin deficiency**
  ▪ **Vitamins A, D, E, and K** can all be taken orally with meals and enzymes.
  ▪ Iron deficiency anemia requires iron supplementation.
○ **CF-related diabetes mellitus**
  ▪ Related to pancreatic insufficiency and managed with **insulin**.
  ▪ Typical diabetic dietary restrictions are liberalized (high-calorie diet with unrestricted fat) to meet the increased energy requirements of patients with CF and to encourage appropriate growth and weight maintenance.
○ **Bowel impaction**
  ▪ **Laxatives** such as senna, magnesium citrate, or polyethylene glycol can be tried initially.
  ▪ Refractory cases may require a Hypaque enema with visualization of clearance of the obstruction (*J Cyst Fibros 2011;10:S24*).
  ▪ Can be mistaken for appendicitis or gallbladder disease because the appendix can be enlarged in CF due to mucus inspissation and white blood cell counts and/or alkaline phosphatase elevations, which are common in CF.
  ▪ Narcotic use and/or significant dehydration and/or nonadherence with pancreatic enzyme supplementation can precipitate severe bowel obstruction, so prophylactic laxatives like daily polyethylene glycol (e.g., MiraLAX 17 g in 8 oz water) in postsurgical patients are often indicated.
○ **Osteopenia**
  Screening should be routinely performed on patients with CF, and if present, osteopenia may be managed with calcium, vitamin D supplementation, and bisphosphonate therapy as clinically indicated (*Am J Respir Crit Care Med 2004;169:77*).
○ **Chronic sinusitis**
  ▪ Many patients will benefit from chronic **nasal steroid** administration.
  ▪ Nasal saline washes may also be helpful.
  ▪ Patients whose symptoms cannot be controlled with medical management may benefit from functional endoscopic sinus surgery and nasal polypectomy.

Surgical Management

- **Massive hemoptysis**
  Treatment includes IV antibiotics and, in refractory cases, may require bronchial artery embolization. Surgical lung resection is rarely needed (*Am J Respir Crit Care Med 2010;182:298*).

- **Pneumothorax**
  Unless small, pneumothoraces are treated with chest tube placement. Surgical pleurodesis should be considered in cases of recurrent pneumothorax (*Am J Respir Crit Care Med 2010;182:298*).
- **Lung transplantation**
  ○ The majority of patients with CF die from pulmonary disease.
  ○ FEV$_1$ is a strong predictor of mortality and has been helpful in deciding when to refer patients for lung transplantation (*N Engl J Med 1992;326:1187*).
  ○ However, other factors such as marked alveolar gas exchange abnormalities (resting hypoxemia or hypercapnia), evidence of PH, or increased frequency or severity of pulmonary exacerbations should also be considered when deciding on referral for transplantation.

Lifestyle/Risk Modification

- **Avoidance of irritating inhaled fumes, dusts, or chemicals**, including second-hand smoke, is recommended.
- **Yearly influenza vaccination** (0.5 mL IM) decreases the incidence of infection and subsequent deterioration (*N Engl J Med 1984;311:1653*).
- **Pneumovax** (0.5 mL IM) may also provide benefit against invasive pneumococcal disease (*Ann Intern Med 1986;104:1*).
- People with CF should avoid contact with others with the disease, unless they are members of the same household, in order to reduce the risk of transmission of infection from one person to another (*Infect Control Hosp Epidemiol 2014;35:S1*).

Diet
A high-calorie diet with vitamin supplementation is typically recommended.

Activity
- CF patients should maintain as much activity as possible.
- Exercise is an excellent form of airway clearance.

SPECIAL CONSIDERATIONS

- When in a health care setting, all personnel should implement contact precautions, whether in the clinic or in the hospital (*Infect Control Hosp Epidemiol 2014;35:S1*).
- Patients with previous isolation of *Burkholderia* should be cared for in a separate area than those without this species.
- Although fertility may be decreased in women with CF secondary to thickened cervical mucus, many women with CF have tolerated pregnancy well (*N Engl J Med 1984;311:1653*).
- Maternal and fetal outcomes are good for women with adequate pulmonary reserve (FEV$_1$ >50% predicted) and good nutritional status, and pregnancy does not appear to affect their survival (*Chest 2000;118:85*).
- Pregnancies should be planned to optimize patient status and coordinate care with obstetrics. CF genetic screening should be offered to partners of patients with CF.

COMPLICATIONS

Other pulmonary complications of CF may include allergic bronchopulmonary aspergillosis, massive hemoptysis, acquisition of atypical mycobacterium, and pneumothorax.

REFERRAL

- CF patients or suspected CF patients should be referred to a national Cystic Fibrosis Foundation (CFF)-accredited care center.
- Tests such as sweat chloride testing and nasal potential difference are best done at specialized CF care centers.
- A team of CF specialists, including physicians, nutritionists, respiratory therapists, and social workers, aid in the routine care of these patients.

PATIENT EDUCATION

Information can be found at the CFF website (*www.cff.org*).

MONITORING/FOLLOW-UP

All persons with CF should be followed in an accredited CF care center. Patients should follow-up as an outpatient every 3 months with pulmonary function tests and yearly laboratories including vitamin levels and screening for CF-related diabetes.

OUTCOME/PROGNOSIS

- Predictors of increased mortality include age, female gender, low weight, low FEV_1, pancreatic insufficiency, diabetes mellitus, infection with *B. cepacia*, and the number of acute exacerbations (*JAMA 2001;286:2683*).
- With improved therapy, the median survival has been extended to approximately 40 years (*Cystic Fibrosis Foundation National Patient Registry Annual Data Report 2013. Bethesda, MD: Cystic Fibrosis Foundation, 2014*).

11

Allergy and Immunology

Sean Brady, Junfang Jiao, Jennifer M. Monroy, and
Andrew L. Kau

Adverse Drug Reactions

GENERAL PRINCIPLES

Definition

- An **adverse drug reaction** (ADR) is an undesired or unintended response that occurs when a drug is given for the appropriate purpose.
- The etiology of a drug reaction can be immunologic, toxic, or idiosyncratic in nature.
- An allergic drug reaction is due to an immune response that is mediated by immunoglobulin E (IgE) or T cells.

Classification

- *Type A* reactions are predictable, often dose dependent, and related to the pharmacokinetics of the drug.
- *Type B* reactions are unpredictable and are not related to the dose or the drug's pharmacokinetics. They account for 10–15% of all ADRs.
  - Immune-mediated adverse reactions can be from a variety of mechanisms. They usually occur upon reexposure to the offending drug.
  - **Pseudoallergic reactions**, formerly called anaphylactoid reactions, are caused by IgE-independent degranulation of mast cells.

Epidemiology

- From 1966–1996, 15.1% of hospitalized US patients experienced an ADR with an incidence of 3.1–6.2% of hospital admissions due to ADRs (*JAMA 1998;279:1200*).
- Mortality from ADRs is significant and ranges from 0.14–0.32% (*Curr Opin Allergy Clin Immunol 2005;5(4):309*).

Etiology

- **β-Lactam** antibiotics are most commonly associated with immunologically mediated drug reactions.
  - Anaphylaxis has been reported to occur in 1:100,000, with serious allergic reactions in 4.6 per 10,000 dispenses (*Drug Saf 2007;30(8):705*).
  - Hospitalized patients with a history of penicillin allergy have been shown to have a longer hospital stay with increased incidence of vancomycin-resistant *Enterococcus*, methicillin-resistant *Staphylococcus aureus*, and *Clostridium difficile* infections compared to patients without a reported penicillin allergy (*J Allergy Clin Immunol 2014;133(3):790–6*).
  - Typical reactions include rash, urticaria, fever, and bronchospasm.
  - The chemical structure of penicillins results in their high immunogenicity.
    - The core structure is composed of a reactive β-lactam ring that covalently binds with carrier proteins to form a hapten, which stimulates an immune response. The major determinant of immunogenicity of penicillin is the benzylpenicilloyl form seen in 93% of tissue-bound penicillin.
    - The minor antigenic determinants are all remaining penicillin conjugates. They are comprised of benzylpenicillin, benzylpenicilloate, and benzylpenilloate.
    - Most immediate reactions to penicillins are related to the major determinant. In other penicillins such as ampicillin, the side chain is the antigenic determinant.

- ○ Cross-reactivity of β-lactams.
  The cross-reactivity between β-lactam antibiotics is variable and largely determined by their side-chain structure attached to the β-lactam ring.
- ○ Prior to the 1980s, cephalosporins had a higher cross-reactivity to penicillin because they were contaminated with a small amount of penicillin (*J Allergy Clin Immunol 2010;125(2 suppl 2):S126*). Risk of a cross-reaction is 5.0–16.5% with first-generation cephalosporins, 4% with second-generation, and 1–3% with third- or fourth-generation (*J Allergy Clin Immunol 2006;117(2 suppl):S464*).
  - ▪ Although many of the reactions to second- and third-generation cephalosporins are directed at the side chains, skin testing to penicillin in these patients can be helpful because most severe anaphylactic reactions are directed against the reactive bicyclic core.
  - ▪ Patients with a history of a severe reaction to penicillin should be considered sensitive to cephalosporin unless they are skin test negative. Although patients with a history of a nonanaphylactic reaction to penicillin can often be given a second- or third-generation cephalosporin safely, it is advisable to precede the dose with an oral provocation challenge.
- ○ Skin test cross-reactivity has been documented between carbapenems and penicillins. Patients undergoing a graded carbapenem challenge with a positive penicillin skin test and a negative carbapenem skin test did not have any hypersensitivity reactions (*J Allergy Clin Immunol 2010;125(2 suppl 2):S126*).
- ○ The monobactam aztreonam rarely cross-reacts with penicillins. Ceftazidime does share an identical side chain to aztreonam and is highly cross-reactive (*Ann Pharmacother 2009;43(2):304*).
- • **Sulfonamide allergy**
  - ○ There is an increase in allergy to sulfonamides in patients with HIV compared to the general population. Trimethoprim-sulfamethoxazole hypersensitivity occurs in 60% of HIV-positive patients compared to 5% of HIV-negative patients (*Curr Opin Allergy Clin Immunol 2007;7(4):324*).
  - ○ The most frequently seen reaction is a maculopapular rash that develops 7–12 days after initiating the drug. Other reactions include urticaria and, less commonly, anaphylaxis, Stevens-Johnson syndrome (SJS), and toxic epidermal necrolysis (TEN).
  - ○ Cross-reactivity between antibiotic and nonantibiotic sulfa-containing medications is low.
- • **NSAIDs** (including aspirin) can induce pseudoallergic reactions through shunting of prostaglandin production to leukotriene synthesis in susceptible individuals. When NSAID administration results in respiratory symptoms, it is referred to as aspirin-exacerbated respiratory disease. Samter's triad is the combination of asthma, NSAID sensitivity, and nasal polyposis

Pathophysiology

The immunologic mechanisms for drug hypersensitivity are demonstrated in the Gell and Coombs classification of hypersensitivity (Table 11-1).

Risk Factors

Factors that increase a patient's risk of an ADR include size and structure of drug, route of exposure (cutaneous most immunogenic), dose, duration, frequency, gender (women > men), genetic factors (HLA type, history of atopy), prior drug reaction, coexisting medical illnesses, and concurrent medical therapy.

DIAGNOSIS

Clinical Presentation

- • A history is essential for making the diagnosis of an allergic drug reaction. Questions should be directed at establishing the following information: sign and symptoms, timing

TABLE 11-1	Immunologically Mediated Drug Reactions	
Type of Reaction	**Representative Examples**	**Mechanism**
Anaphylactic (type 1)	Anaphylaxis Urticaria Angioedema	IgE-mediated degranulation of mast cells with resultant mediator release
Cytotoxic (type 2)	Autoimmune hemolytic anemia Interstitial nephritis	IgG or IgM antibodies against cell antigens and complement activation
Immune complex (type 3)	Serum sickness Vasculitis	Immune complex deposition and subsequent complement activation
Cell mediated (type 4)	Contact dermatitis Photosensitivity dermatitis	Activated T cells against cell surface–bound antigens

of the reaction, purpose of the drug, other medications the patient is receiving, prior exposure to drug or related drug, and history of other allergic drug reactions.

- Urticaria, angioedema, wheezing, and anaphylaxis are all characteristics of IgE-mediated (type 1) reactions.
  - Symptoms do not typically occur on the first exposure to the medication unless the patient has been exposed to a structurally related medication. On reexposure, however, symptoms tend to manifest acutely (often <1 hour).
  - IgE-mediated reactions tend to worsen with repeated exposure to the offending medication.
  - Pseudoallergic reactions (non–IgE mediated) can be clinically indistinguishable from IgE-mediated reactions because the final common pathway for their reaction is mast cell degranulation.
- **Maculopapular exanthemas** are the most common cutaneous manifestation of drug allergy.
  - These reactions are mediated by T cells and typically delayed in onset, first occurring between 2–14 days of exposure to culprit medications. Lesions typically begin on the trunk, especially in dependent areas, and spread to the extremities.
  - Rarely, these rashes can progress to DRESS (**d**rug **r**eaction with **e**osinophilia and **s**ystemic **s**ymptoms) or SJS.
- **DRESS** or hypersensitivity syndrome is a serious ADR, often presenting with rash and fever (*Expert Opin Drug Saf 2005;4(3):571*).
  - Systemic involvement can manifest as hepatitis, eosinophilia, pneumonitis, lymphadenopathy, and nephritis.
  - Symptoms tend to present 2–6 weeks after introduction of medication.
  - First described with antiepileptic (carbamazepine) agents but has also been reported to occur with allopurinol, NSAIDs, some antibiotics, and β-blockers.
- **Erythema multiforme (EM), SJS, and TEN** are all serious drug reactions primarily involving the skin.
  - EM is characterized most typically by target lesions.
  - SJS and TEN manifest with varying degrees of sloughing of the skin and mucous membranes (<10% in SJS and >30% in TEN).
- Readministration or future skin testing with the offending drug is absolutely contraindicated.

PREVENTION AND TREATMENT

- **Discontinuation** of the suspected drug is the most important initial approach in managing an allergic drug reaction.

- **HLA testing may be indicated in susceptible populations for prevention of a severe ADR for some drugs such as abacavir and carbamazepine.**
- Other therapeutic maneuvers are directed at limiting further exacerbation of ADRs and may include management of anaphylaxis as well as other supportive measures.
- Future use of the drug in question should **always be avoided** unless there is no therapeutic alternative available.
- If use of the drug must be considered, a careful history of the reaction is helpful in defining the potential risk. Patients may lose their sensitivity to a drug over time, and determining the date of reaction is useful. Symptoms that occur with the start of a drug course are more likely to be IgE-mediated than symptoms that develop several days after the completion of a course.
- The types of symptoms are also important. Toxic reactions (e.g., nausea secondary to macrolide antibiotics or codeine) are not immunologic reactions and do not necessarily predict problems with other members in their respective class.
- If the patient is taking the drug for a life-threatening illness (e.g., meningitis with penicillin allergy) and the reaction is a mild skin reaction, it may be reasonable to continue the medication and treat the reaction symptomatically. **If the rash is progressive, however, the drug must be discontinued to avoid a desquamative process such as SJS.**

REFERRAL

- If no alternative drug is available and the patient has a history of an IgE-mediated reaction, the patient should be referred to an allergist for further evaluation.
- The allergist may perform one of several procedures if indicated depending on the medication, type of reaction, and availability of testing reagents.
  - **Skin testing** may be performed to assess for the presence of IgE to the medication.
    - Although skin testing may be performed to nearly any medication, sensitivity and specificity of the skin test results have been best established with penicillin. No case of penicillin-induced anaphylaxis has been reported in a patient who is skin test negative.
    - Results of testing to drugs other than penicillin must be interpreted within the clinical context of the case.
  - **Graded dose challenge** assesses how the patient tolerates progressively larger doses of medication (e.g., 1/1000, 1/10, and full dose given 20 minutes apart).
  - **Drug desensitization** is performed when the patient has an identified IgE-mediated reaction but still requires the medication.
    - The exact mechanism by which desensitization prevents anaphylaxis is unclear.
    - The drug must be taken daily at a specified dose to maintain the "desensitized state."
    - If a dose of drug is missed for a period >48 hours following a desensitization procedure, the patient will often need to undergo a repeat desensitization.
  - Successful desensitization or graded challenge does not preclude the development of a non–IgE-mediated, delayed reaction (e.g., rash).

Anaphylaxis

GENERAL PRINCIPLES

Definition

Anaphylaxis is a rapidly developing, life-threatening systemic reaction mediated by the release of mast cell and basophil-derived mediators into the circulation. The peak severity is seen usually within 5–30 minutes.

Classification

- **Immunologic anaphylaxis:**
  - Allergic IgE-mediated anaphylaxis (type 1 hypersensitivity)
  - IgG-mediated anaphylaxis (rare)
- **Nonimmunologic anaphylaxis**

Epidemiology

Incidence of anaphylaxis is approximately 50–2000 episodes per 100,000 person-years with a lifetime prevalence of 0.05–2%. Fatality is estimated at 0.7–2% per case of anaphylaxis.

Etiology

- **Immunologic causes**
  - Foods, especially peanuts, tree nuts, shellfish, finned fish, milk, and eggs
  - Insect stings (bees, wasps, and fire ants)
  - Medications
  - Latex rubber
  - Blood products
- **Nonimmunologic causes**
  - Radiocontrast media
  - Medications (i.e., NSAIDs, opiates, vancomycin, muscle relaxants, rarely ACE-inhibitors, and sulfating agents)
  - Hemodialysis
  - Physical factors (cold temperature or exercise)
  - Idiopathic

Pathophysiology

- Immunologic
  - Anaphylaxis is due to sensitization to an antigen and formation of specific IgE to that antigen. On reexposure, the IgE on mast cells and basophils binds the antigen and cross-links the IgE receptor, which causes activation of the cells with subsequent systemic release of preformed mediators, such as histamine.
  - The release of mediators ultimately causes capillary leakage, cellular edema, and smooth muscle contractions resulting in the constellation of physical symptoms.
- Nonimmunologic
  Non–IgE-mediated anaphylaxis is also mediated by direct degranulation of mast cells and basophils in the absence of immunoglobulins.

Risk Factors

- Immunologic anaphylaxis: IgE-mediated reactions
  - Asthma
  - Previous sensitization and formation of antigen-specific IgE with history of anaphylaxis
- Nonimmunologic anaphylaxis:
  Radiocontrast sensitivity reactions
  - Age >50 years.
  - Preexisting cardiovascular or renal disease.
  - History of allergy.
  - History of previous reaction to radiocontrast media.
  - **Sensitivity to seafood or iodine does not predispose to radiocontrast media reactions.**
- Individuals with **mastocytosis**, a disease characterized by a proliferation of mast cells, are at higher risk for severe anaphylaxis from both IgE- and non–IgE-mediated causes.

Prevention

- **For all types of anaphylaxis, recognition of potential triggers and avoidance are the best prevention.**
- **Self-injectable epinephrine and patient education for all patients with a history of anaphylaxis.**
- Radiocontrast sensitivity reactions
  - ○ Use of low-ionic contrast media is strongly suggested.
  - ○ Premedication before procedure.
    - Prednisone 50 mg PO given 13 hours, 7 hours, and 1 hour prior to procedure
    - Diphenhydramine 50 mg PO given 1 hour before procedure
    - H_2 blocker may also be given 1 hour before procedure
  - ○ **Premedication is not 100% effective, and appropriate precautions for handling a reaction should be taken.**
  - ○ Anaphylaxis can be a presenting sign of underlying mastocytosis.
- Red man's syndrome from vancomycin
  Symptoms can usually be prevented by slowing the rate of infusion and premedicating with diphenhydramine (50 mg PO) 30 minutes prior to start of the infusion.

DIAGNOSIS

Diagnosis is based primarily on history and physical examination and the documentation of the presence of a specific IgE to the suspected allergen (if the trigger is IgE mediated). Confirmation of anaphylaxis can, in some cases, be provided by the laboratory finding of an elevated serum tryptase level. However, the absence of an elevated tryptase level does not exclude anaphylaxis.

Clinical Presentation

- The clinical manifestations of allergic and nonallergic anaphylaxis are the same.
- Most serious reactions occur within minutes after exposure to the antigen, but in some circumstances, the reaction may be delayed for hours.
- Some patients experience a biphasic reaction characterized by a recurrence of symptoms after 4–8 hours. A few patients have a protracted course that requires several hours of continuous supportive treatment.
- Manifestations include pruritus, urticaria, angioedema, respiratory distress (due to laryngeal edema, laryngospasm, or bronchospasm), hypotension, uterine cramping, abdominal cramping, emesis, and diarrhea.

History
A thorough history is taken to help identify the potential trigger, such as new foods, medications, or other commonly known allergens. Also documenting the time of onset of symptoms—that is, minutes to hours or days after a suspected exposure—can help to classify the type of anaphylaxis.

Physical Examination
- Pay special attention to vital signs: Blood pressure, respiratory rate, and oxygen saturation.
- Airway and pulmonary: Assess for any evidence of laryngeal edema or angioedema. Auscultate lung fields to listen for evidence of wheezing. Continue to assess for need to protect the airway.
- Perform a focused cardiovascular exam.
- Skin: Urticaria or erythema.

Diagnostic Criteria

See Table 11-2 for diagnostic criteria for anaphylaxis.
Severity of anaphylactic reactions can be judged by the following:
- **Mild anaphylactic reactions:** Generalized erythema, urticaria, angioedema, or pruritus
- **Moderate anaphylactic reaction** (features suggesting respiratory, cardiovascular, or gastrointestinal involvement): Dyspnea, stridor, wheezing, nausea, vomiting, dizziness (presyncope), diaphoresis, chest or throat tightness, and abdominal pain in addition to cutaneous symptoms
- **Severe anaphylactic reaction** (hypoxia, hypotension, or neurologic compromise): May have cyanosis or partial pressure of arterial oxygen (PaO_2) $\leq 92\%$ at any stage, hypotension (systolic blood pressure <90 mm Hg), confusion, loss of consciousness, or neurologic compromise

Differential Diagnosis

- Anaphylaxis due to **preformed IgE and reexposure**: Medications, insect sting, and foods are the most common causes of anaphylaxis. Galactose-α-1,3-galactose allergy is thought to be triggered by tick bites and is a cause of delayed anaphylaxis to red meats including beef, pork, and lamb.
- Causes of **nonallergic anaphylaxis**:
  ○ **Radiocontrast sensitivity reactions** are thought to be from direct degranulation of mast cells in susceptible patients due to osmotic shifts. Reactions can occur in 5–10% of patients, with fatal reactions occurring in 1 in 40,000 procedures.
  ○ **Red man's syndrome** from vancomycin consists of pruritus and flushing of the face and neck.

TABLE 11-2	Anaphylaxis

Anaphylaxis is likely when one of the following three criteria occurs:

1. Acute skin and/or mucosal symptoms (e.g., hives, pruritus, flushing, lip/tongue/uvula swelling) and one of the following:
   - Respiratory symptoms (e.g., wheezing, stridor, shortness of breath, hypoxia)
   - Hypotension or associated end-organ dysfunction (e.g., hypotonia, syncope, incontinence)
2. Exposure to probable allergen for the patient and two or more of the following:
   - Skin/mucosal tissue involvement
   - Respiratory symptoms
   - Hypotension or end-organ dysfunction
   - Persistent gastrointestinal symptoms (e.g., emesis, abdominal pain)
3. Decreased blood pressure after exposure to known allergen for the patient:
   - Adults: Systolic blood pressure <90 mm Hg or $>30\%$ decrease in systolic blood pressure
   - Infants and children: Hypotension for age or $>30\%$ decrease in systolic blood pressure

Adapted from Sampson HA, Munoz-Furlong A, Campbell RL, et al. Second symposium on the definition and management of anaphylaxis: Summary report—Second National Institute of Allergy and Infectious Disease/Food Allergy and Anaphylaxis Network symposium. *J Allergy Clin Immunol* 2006;117:391–7.

- ○ **Mastocytosis** should be considered in patients with recurrent unexplained anaphylaxis or flushing, especially with previous reactions to nonspecific mast cell degranulators such as opiates and radiocontrast media.
- ○ **Ingestant-related reactions** can mimic anaphylaxis. This is usually due to sulfites or the presence of a histamine-like substance in spoiled fish (scombroidosis).
- ○ **Flushing syndromes** include flushing due to red man's syndrome, carcinoid, vasointestinal peptide (and other vasoactive intestinal peptide–secreting tumors), postmenopausal symptoms, and alcohol use.
- • Other forms of shock such as hypoglycemic, cardiogenic, septic, and hemorrhagic.
- • Miscellaneous syndromes such as hereditary angioedema (C1 esterase inhibitor [C1 INH] deficiency syndrome), pheochromocytoma, neurologic (seizure, stroke), and capillary leak syndrome.
- • Idiopathic.

Diagnostic Testing

- • Epicutaneous skin testing and serum specific IgE testing when available to identify trigger allergens.
- • Serum tryptase peaks at 1 hour after symptoms begin and may be present for up to 6 hours.

TREATMENT

- • Early recognition of signs and symptoms of anaphylaxis is a critical first step in treatment.
- • **Epinephrine is the medication of choice for treatment of anaphylaxis.**
- • **Maintain recumbent position while assessing and starting therapy.**
- • **Airway management is a priority.** Supplemental 100% oxygen therapy should be administered. Endotracheal intubation may be necessary. If laryngeal edema is not rapidly responsive to epinephrine, cricothyroidotomy or tracheotomy may be required.
- • **Volume expansion with IV fluids** may be necessary. An initial bolus of 500–1000 mL normal saline should be followed by an infusion at a rate that is titrated to blood pressure (BP) and urine output.

Medications

- • **Epinephrine** should be administered immediately. There are no absolute contraindications for treatment with epinephrine in anaphylaxis.
  - ○ Adult: 0.3–0.5 mg (0.3–0.5 mL of a 1:1000 solution) IM in the lateral thigh, repeated at 10- to 15-minute intervals if necessary.
  - ○ Child: 1:1000 dilution at 0.01 mg/kg or 0.1–0.3 mL administered IM in the lateral thigh, repeated at 10- to 15-minute intervals if necessary.
  - ○ 0.5 mL of 1:1000 solution sublingually in cases of major airway compromise or hypotension.
  - ○ 3–5 mL of 1:10,000 solution via central line.
  - ○ 3–5 mL of 1:10,000 solution diluted with 10 mL of normal saline via endotracheal tube.
  - ○ For protracted symptoms that require multiple doses of epinephrine, an IV epinephrine drip may be useful; the infusion is titrated to maintain adequate BP.
- • **Glucagon**, given as a 1-mg (one-ampule) bolus and followed by a drip of up to 1 mg/h can be used to provide inotropic support for patients who are taking β-adrenergic antagonists. β-Adrenergic antagonist therapy increases the risk of anaphylaxis and renders the reaction more difficult to treat (*Ann Intern Med 1991;115:270*).
- • **Inhaled β-adrenergic agonists** should be used to treat resistant bronchospasm.
- • **Glucocorticoids** have no significant immediate effect but may prevent biphasic reactions. Methylprednisolone 1–2 mg/kg daily for 1–2 days.

- **Antihistamines** relieve skin symptoms but have no immediate effect on the reaction. They may shorten the duration of the reaction.
  - Adult: Diphenhydramine 25–50 mg IM or IV
  - Child: Diphenhydramine 12.5–25.0 mg IM or IV

REFERRAL

Referrals to an allergist for further evaluation should be offered to all patients with a history of anaphylaxis. More importantly, patients with *Hymenoptera* sensitivity should be evaluated to determine eligibility for venom immunotherapy.

Eosinophilia

GENERAL PRINCIPLES

- Eosinophils are a blood granulocyte that can be involved in a variety of infectious, allergic, neoplastic, and idiopathic diseases.
- Eosinophil maturation is promoted by granulocyte-macrophage colony-stimulating hormone (GM-CSF), interleukin (IL)-3, and IL-5.
- Eosinophils are normally seen in peripheral tissue such as mucosal tissues in the gastrointestinal and respiratory tracts. They are recruited to sites of inflammation.

Definition

- The upper limit of normal varies for blood eosinophilia.
- A value >500 eosinophils/μL is abnormal in most cases.
- The extent of eosinophilia can be categorized as mild (500–1500 cells/μL), moderate (1500–5000 cells/μL), or severe (>5000 cells/μL).
- Degree of eosinophilia is *not* a reliable predictor of eosinophil-mediated organ damage.

Classification

- Peripheral eosinophilia can be divided into primary, secondary, or idiopathic.
  - Primary eosinophilia is seen with hematologic disorders where there may be a clonal expansion of eosinophils (chronic eosinophilic leukemia) or a clonal expansion of cells that stimulate eosinophil production (chronic myeloid or lymphocytic disorders).
  - Secondary eosinophilia has numerous causes such as parasites, allergic diseases, autoimmune disorders, toxins, medications, and endocrine disorders such as Addison disease.
  - Idiopathic eosinophilia is considered when primary and secondary causes are excluded.
- **Eosinophilia associated with atopic disease.**
  - In allergic rhinitis, increased nasal eosinophilia is more common than peripheral blood eosinophilia.
  - Nasal eosinophilia with or without blood eosinophilia may be seen in asthma, nasal polyposis, or nonallergic rhinitis with eosinophilia syndrome (NARES).
  - NARES is a syndrome of marked nasal eosinophilia and nasal polyps. These patients do not have a history of allergies, asthma, or aspirin sensitivity, and have negative skin tests and IgE levels.
  - Sputum eosinophilia is a common feature of asthma and suggests responsiveness to corticosteroid treatment.
- **Eosinophilia associated with pulmonary infiltrates.** This classification is inclusive of the pulmonary infiltrates with eosinophilia syndromes and the eosinophilic pneumonias.
  - **Allergic bronchopulmonary aspergillosis** (ABPA), an IgE-dependent immunologic reaction to *Aspergillus fumigatus* consisting of pulmonary infiltrates, proximal

bronchiectasis, elevated serum IgE, positive skin testing, presence of precipitins to *Aspergillus,* and peripheral eosinophilia in patients with asthma or cystic fibrosis.
- Disseminated coccidioidomycosis can lead to marked eosinophilia.
- **Eosinophilic pneumonias** consist of pulmonary infiltrates with lung eosinophilia and are only occasionally associated with blood eosinophilia.
  - Acute eosinophilic pneumonia is an idiopathic disease that presents with fever, cough, dyspnea, and hypoxemia occurring for days to weeks, typically in males and in individuals who have recently started to smoke tobacco.
  - Chronic eosinophilic pneumonia is an idiopathic disease that presents with fever, cough, dyspnea, and significant weight loss occurring for weeks to months, typically in females and nonsmokers. It is associated with peripheral blood eosinophilia. "The photographic negative of pulmonary edema" is a classic radiographic finding (radiographic pattern of predominately peripheral consolidation).
  - Löffler syndrome is combination of blood eosinophilia and transient pulmonary infiltrates due to passage of helminthic larvae, usually *Ascaris lumbricoides,* through the lungs.
  - Tropical pulmonary eosinophilia is a hypersensitivity response in the lung to lymphatic filariae. Peripheral blood microfilariae are usually not detected.
- **HIV.** Modest to marked eosinophilia of unknown cause can be seen occasionally in patients with HIV. The eosinophilia is usually due to reactions to medications, adrenal insufficiency due to cytomegalovirus with consequent eosinophilia, or eosinophilic folliculitis.
- **Eosinophilia associated with parasitic infection.** Various multicellular parasites or helminths such as *Ascaris,* hookworm, or *Strongyloides* can induce blood eosinophilia, whereas single-celled protozoan parasites such as *Giardia lamblia* do not. The level of eosinophilia reflects the degree of tissue invasion by the parasite. Eosinophilia is usually of the highest grade during the early phase of infection.
  - In cases of blood eosinophilia, ***Strongyloides stercoralis* infection must be excluded** because this helminth can set up a cycle of autoinfection leading to chronic infection with intermittent, sometimes marked, eosinophilia.
  - Tissue eosinophilia may not be accompanied by blood eosinophilia when the organism is sequestered within tissues (e.g., intact echinococcal cysts) or is limited to the intestinal lumen (e.g., *Ascaris* and tapeworms).
  - Among the helminths, the principal parasites that need to be evaluated are *S. stercoralis,* hookworm, and *Toxocara canis.* The diagnostic consideration can also vary according to geographic region.
  - There are some important caveats that need to be considered when evaluating patients for parasitic diseases and eosinophilia: *Strongyloides* can persist for decades without causing major symptoms and can elicit varying degrees of eosinophilia ranging from minimal to marked eosinophilia.
  - *T. canis* (visceral larva migrans) should be considered in children with a propensity to eat dirt contaminated by dog *Ascaris* eggs.
- **Eosinophilia associated with cutaneous disease.**
  - **Atopic dermatitis** is classically associated with blood and skin eosinophilia.
  - **Eosinophilic fasciitis (Shulman syndrome)** is characterized by acute erythema, swelling, and induration of the extremities progressing to symmetric induration of the skin that spares the fingers, feet, and face. It can be precipitated by exercise.
  - **Eosinophilic cellulitis (Wells syndrome)** presents with recurrent swelling of an extremity without tactile warmth and failure with antibiotic therapy.
  - **Eosinophilic pustular folliculitis** is a pruritic skin eruption that can be seen in patients with HIV.
  - **Episodic angioedema with eosinophilia** is a rare disease that leads to recurrent attacks of fever, angioedema, urticaria, weight gain, and blood eosinophilia without other organ damage.

○ **Angiolymphoid hyperplasia with eosinophilia:** Presents with eosinophilia and papules, plaques, and nodules on the head and neck.

○ **Kimura disease** presents with eosinophilia and large subcutaneous masses on the head or neck of Asian men.

• **Eosinophilia associated with multiorgan involvement.**

  ○ **Drug-induced eosinophilia.** Numerous drugs, herbal supplements, and cytokine therapies (e.g., GM-CSF and IL-2) can cause blood and/or tissue eosinophilia. Drug-induced eosinophilia typically responds to cessation of the culprit medication. Asymptomatic drug-induced eosinophilia does not necessitate cessation of therapy. However, end-organ involvement should always be investigated promptly.

  ○ **Eosinophilic granulomatosis with polyangiitis (EGPA), also known as Churg-Strauss syndrome,** is a small- and medium-vessel vasculitis with chronic rhinosinusitis, asthma, and peripheral blood eosinophilia (typically >1500 cells/μL). The onset of asthma and eosinophilia may precede the development of EGPA by several years.

    ▪ Noted to have intravascular and extravascular eosinophilic granuloma formation and lung involvement with transient infiltrates on chest radiograph. Other manifestations include mononeuropathy or polyneuropathy, subcutaneous nodules, rash, gastroenteritis, renal insufficiency, cardiac arrhythmias, and heart failure.

    ▪ Half of patients have antineutrophil cytoplasmic antibodies directed against myeloperoxidase (p-ANCA). Biopsy of affected tissue reveals a necrotizing vasculitis with extravascular granulomas and tissue eosinophilia.

    ▪ Initial treatment involves high-dose glucocorticoids with the addition of cyclophosphamide if necessary. Maintenance therapy with azathioprine is recommended after remission is achieved. Leukotriene modifiers, like all systemic steroid-sparing agents (including inhaled steroids and omalizumab), have been associated with unmasking of EGPA due to a decrease in systemic steroid therapy; however, no evidence exists that these drugs *cause* EGPA (*Chest 2000;117:708*).

  ○ **Mastocytosis.** Systemic mastocytosis is characterized by infiltration of mast cells into various organs including the skin, liver, lymph nodes, bone marrow, and spleen. Peripheral eosinophilia can be seen in up to 20% of cases of systemic mastocytosis, and bone marrow biopsies often show an excess number of eosinophils.

  ○ **Endocrine disorders.** Adrenal insufficiency (e.g., Addison disease) in critically ill patients is associated with low-grade eosinophilia.

  ○ **Hypereosinophilic syndrome** (HES) is a proliferative disorder of eosinophils characterized by sustained eosinophilia >1500 cells/μL for ≥1 month documented on two occasions with eosinophil-mediated damage to organs such as the heart, gastrointestinal tract, kidneys, brain, and lung. All other causes of eosinophilia should be excluded to make the diagnosis (*J Allergy Clin Immunol 2012;130:607*).

    ▪ HES occurs predominantly in men between the ages of 20–50 years and presents with insidious onset of fatigue, cough, and dyspnea.

    ▪ Myeloproliferative variants of HES (M-HES) are characterized by constitutive expression of *FIP1L1/PDGFRA* fusion protein and elevated serum vitamin B_{12} levels. Unusual IL-5–producing T cells are found in the lymphocytic variant of HES (L-HES).

    ▪ At presentation, patients typically are in the late thrombotic and fibrotic stages of eosinophil-mediated cardiac damage with signs of a restrictive cardiomyopathy and mitral regurgitation. An echocardiogram may detect intracardiac thrombi, endomyocardial fibrosis, or thickening of the posterior mitral valve leaflet. Neurologic manifestations range from peripheral neuropathy to stroke or encephalopathy. Bone marrow examination reveals increased eosinophil precursors.

  ○ **Acute eosinophilic leukemia** is a rare myeloproliferative disorder that is distinguished from HES by several factors: an increased number of immature eosinophils in the blood and/or marrow, >10% blast forms in the marrow, and symptoms and signs compatible with an acute leukemia. Treatment is similar to other leukemias.

○ **Lymphoma.** Eosinophilia can present in any T- or B-cell lymphoma. As many as 5% of patients with non-Hodgkin lymphoma and up to 15% of patients with Hodgkin lymphoma have modest peripheral blood eosinophilia. Eosinophilia in Hodgkin lymphoma has been correlated with IL-5 messenger RNA expression by Reed-Sternberg cells.

○ **Atheroembolic disease.** Cholesterol embolization can lead to eosinophilia, eosinophiluria, renal dysfunction, livedo reticularis, increased erythrocyte sedimentation rate (ESR), and purple toes.

○ **Immunodeficiency.** Hyper-IgE syndrome and Omenn syndrome can present with recurrent infections, dermatitis, and eosinophilia.

Epidemiology

In industrialized nations, peripheral blood eosinophilia is most often due to atopic disease, whereas helminthic infections are the most common cause of eosinophilia in the rest of the world.

Pathophysiology

Eosinophilic granules contain basic proteins, which bind to acidic dye. Once activated, eosinophils produce major basic protein, eosinophil cationic protein, eosinophil-derived neurotoxin, and eosinophil peroxidase, which are toxic to bacteria, helminths, and normal tissue.

DIAGNOSIS

There are two approaches that are useful for evaluating eosinophilia, either by associated clinical context (Table 11-3) or by degree of eosinophilia (Table 11-4).

Clinical Presentation

History

- A history is important in narrowing the differential diagnosis of eosinophilia. It is important to determine if the patient has symptoms of atopic disease (rhinitis, wheezing, rash) or cancer (weight loss, fatigue, fever, night sweats) and to evaluate for other specific organ involvement such as lung, heart, or nerves. Prior eosinophil count can help determine the duration and magnitude of eosinophilia.
- A complete medication list, including over-the-counter supplements, and a full travel, occupational, and dietary history should be obtained.
- Any pet contact should be ascertained for possible exposure to toxocariasis.

Physical Examination

Physical examination should be guided by the history, with a special focus on the skin, upper and lower respiratory tracts, and cardiovascular and neurologic systems.

Differential Diagnosis

- Various conditions can result in **eosinophilia associated with pulmonary infiltrates** (see Table 11-3). The presence of asthma should lead to consideration of ABPA or EGPA.
- The etiology of **eosinophilia associated with cutaneous lesions** (see Table 11-3) is guided by the appearance of the lesions and results of the skin biopsy. The diagnosis of EGPA cannot be made without a tissue biopsy showing infiltrating eosinophils and granulomas.
- When eosinophilia is marked and all other causes have been ruled out, the diagnosis of **HES** should be considered. Diagnosis requires a blood eosinophilia of >1500/μL on two occasions with associated organ involvement.

TABLE 11-3   Causes of Eosinophilia

Eosinophilia Associated with Atopic Disease

Allergic rhinitis
Asthma
Atopic dermatitis

Eosinophilia Associated with Pulmonary Infiltrates

Passage of larvae through the lung (Löffler syndrome)
Chronic eosinophilic pneumonia
Acute eosinophilic pneumonia
Tropical pulmonary eosinophilia
Allergic bronchopulmonary aspergillosis (ABPA)
Coccidioidomycosis

Eosinophilia Associated with Parasitic Infection

Helminths (*Ascaris lumbricoides, Strongyloides stercoralis, hookworm, Toxocara canis* or *Toxocara cati, Trichinella*)
Protozoa (*Dientamoeba fragilis, Sarcocystis,* and *Isospora belli*)

Eosinophilia Associated with Primary Cutaneous Disease

Atopic dermatitis
Eosinophilic fasciitis
Eosinophilic cellulitis
Eosinophilic folliculitis
Episodic angioedema with anaphylaxis

Eosinophilia Associated with Multiorgan Involvement

Drug-induced eosinophilia
Eosinophilic granulomatosis with polyangiitis (EGPA), or Churg-Strauss syndrome
Hypereosinophilic syndrome
Eosinophilic leukemia
Systemic mastocytosis
Lymphomas

Miscellaneous Causes

Eosinophilic gastroenteritis
Interstitial nephritis
Retroviral infections (HIV, human T-lymphotropic virus−1)
Eosinophilia myalgia syndrome
Transplant rejection
Atheroembolic disease
Adrenal insufficiency

Diagnostic Testing

Laboratories

- Initial laboratory evaluations generally include complete blood count (CBC) with differential and eosinophil count, liver function tests, serum chemistries and creatinine, markers of inflammation (e.g., ESR and/or C-reactive protein) and urinalysis. Further diagnostic studies are based on clinical presentations and initial findings. Mild **eosinophilia associated with symptoms of rhinitis or asthma** is indicative of underlying atopic disease, which can be confirmed by skin testing.
- Depending on the travel history, **stool examination** for ova and parasites should be done on three separate occasions. Because only small numbers of helminths may pass in the

TABLE 11-4	Classification of Eosinophilia Based on the Peripheral Blood Eosinophil Count	
Peripheral Blood Eosinophil Count (cells/μL)		
500–2000	**2000–5000**	**>5000**
Allergic rhinitis	Intrinsic asthma	Eosinophilia myalgia syndrome
Allergic asthma	Allergic bronchopulmonary aspergillosis	Hypereosinophilic syndrome
Food allergy	Helminthiasis	Episodic angioedema with eosinophilia
Urticaria	Eosinophilic granulomatosis with polyangiitis (EGPA), or Churg-Strauss syndrome	Leukemia
Addison disease	Drug reactions	
Pulmonary infiltrates with eosinophilia syndromes	Vascular neoplasms	
Solid neoplasms	Eosinophilic fasciitis	
Nasal polyposis	HIV	

stool and because tissue- or blood-dwelling helminths will not be found in the stool, **serologic tests** for antiparasite antibodies should also be sent. Such tests are available for strongyloidiasis, toxocariasis, and trichinellosis.

- Diagnosis at the time of presentation with Löffler syndrome can be made by detection of *Ascaris* larvae in respiratory secretions or gastric aspirates but not stool.
- Sinus CT, nerve conduction studies, and testing for p-ANCA may be helpful in the diagnosis of EGPA.
- Peripheral blood smear and flow cytometry of lymphocyte subpopulations can aid in the diagnosis of hematologic malignancy. Bone marrow biopsy for pathologic, cytogenetic, and molecular testing on bone marrow and/or peripheral blood (e.g., for *FIP1L1/PDGFRA* mutation) may be required. Serum vitamin B_{12} level may be elevated in hematologic causes of HES.
- Evaluation for idiopathic HES should also consist of troponin measurement, echocardiogram, and ECG.
- Immunoglobulin levels are helpful if concerned for an immunodeficiency. Elevated immunoglobulin levels can be found in L-HES.
- A tryptase level is necessary if mastocytosis is considered as a cause of eosinophilia.

Imaging
CXR findings may also help to narrow the differential diagnosis.
- Peripheral infiltrates with central clearing are indicative of chronic eosinophilic pneumonia.
- Diffuse infiltrates in an interstitial, alveolar, or mixed pattern may be seen in acute eosinophilic pneumonia as well as drug-induced eosinophilia with pulmonary involvement.
- Transient infiltrates may be seen in Löffler syndrome, EGPA, or ABPA.
- Central bronchiectasis is a major criterion in the diagnosis of ABPA.
- A diffuse miliary or nodular pattern, consolidation, or cavitation may be found in cases of tropical pulmonary eosinophilia.

Diagnostic Procedures
- If no other cause of pulmonary infiltrates has been identified, a **bronchoscopy** may be necessary for analysis of bronchoalveolar lavage (BAL) fluid and lung tissue. The presence of eosinophils in BAL fluid or sputum with eosinophilic infiltration of the parenchyma is most typical of acute or chronic eosinophilic pneumonia.
- Skin biopsy will aid in diagnosing the cutaneous eosinophilic diseases and EGPA.

TREATMENT

- Mild eosinophilia with no evidence of end-organ damage may not need treatment.
- Oral steroids are indicated when there is evidence of organ involvement. However, strongyloidiasis must be excluded prior to administration of steroids to prevent hyperinfection syndrome.
- When a drug reaction is suspected, discontinuation of the drug is both diagnostic and therapeutic. Other treatment options depend on the exact cause of eosinophilia because, with the exception of HES, eosinophilia is a manifestation of an underlying disease.
- **HES:** Patients with marked eosinophilia with no organ involvement may have a benign course. In contrast, those with organ involvement and *FIP1L1/PDGFRA*-associated disease may have an extremely aggressive course without treatment.
  - Monitoring and early initiation of high-dose glucocorticoids should be pursued in all patients except those who have the *FIP1L1/PDGFRA* fusion gene.
  - Patients with the *FIP1L1/PDGFRA* fusion mutation should be started on imatinib mesylate (Gleevec), a tyrosine kinase inhibitor. Treatment should be initiated promptly in these patients to prevent progression of cardiac disease and other end-organ damage. Imatinib has been shown to induce disease remission and halt progression (*Blood 2003;101:4714*).
  - Hydroxyurea has been the most frequently used effective second-line agent and/or steroid-sparing agent for HES. Interferon-α2b in combination with glucocorticoids has been used to treat L-HES. Hematopoietic cell transplantation may be considered in refractory HES.
  - Mepolizumab, a humanized anti–IL-5 antibody, has shown promising results in patients who do not have the *FIP1L1/PDGFRA* fusion protein (*N Engl J Med 2008; 358:1215*).
  - Alemtuzumab, an anti-CD52 antibody (CD52 is expressed on the surface of eosinophils), has been shown in a clinical trial to decrease eosinophils counts (*Clin Cancer Res 2009;15:368*).
- Primary eosinophilia disorders should be followed by a specialist; any cases of unresolved or unexplained eosinophilia warrant evaluation by an allergist/immunologist.

Urticaria and Angioedema

GENERAL PRINCIPLES

Definition

- **Urticaria** (hives) are raised, flat-topped, well-demarcated pruritic skin lesions with surrounding erythema. Central clearing can cause an annular lesion and is often seen after antihistamine use. An individual lesion usually lasts minutes to hours.
- **Angioedema** is swelling of the deep dermis and subcutaneous tissue. It is often painful rather than pruritic. It can be found anywhere on the body but most often involves the tongue, lips, eyelids, and/or genitals. When angioedema occurs without urticaria, specific diagnoses must be entertained (see Differential Diagnosis section).

Classification

- **Acute urticaria (with or without angioedema)** is defined as the occurrence of hives and/or angioedema lasting <6 weeks. It can be caused by an allergic reaction to a medication, food, insect sting, or exposure (contact or inhalation) to an allergen. Patients can develop a hypersensitivity to a food, medication, or self-care product that previously had been used without difficulty. In many cases of acute urticaria, no identifiable trigger can be found.
- **Chronic urticaria (with or without angioedema)** is defined as the occurrence of hives and/or angioedema for >6 weeks. There are many possible causes of chronic urticaria and angioedema, including medications, autoimmunity, self-care products, and physical triggers. However, the etiology remains unidentified in >80% of cases.

Epidemiology

- Urticaria is a common condition that affects 15–24% of the US population at some time in their life. Chronic idiopathic urticaria occurs in 0.1% of the US population, and there does not appear to be an increased risk in persons with atopy.
- Angioedema generally lasts 12–48 hours and occurs in 40–50% of patients with urticaria.

Etiology

- IgE-mediated: Drugs, foods, stinging and biting insects, latex, inhalant, or contact allergen
- Non–IgE-mediated: narcotics, muscle relaxants, radiocontrast, vancomycin, NSAIDs, ACE-inhibitors
- Transfusion reactions
- Infections (i.e., viral, bacterial, parasitic)
- Autoimmune diseases
- Malignancy
- Physical urticaria: Dermographism, cold, cholinergic, pressure, vibratory, solar, and aquagenic
- Mastocytosis
- Hereditary diseases
- Idiopathic

Pathophysiology

Most forms of urticaria and angioedema are caused by the degranulation of mast cells or basophils and the release of inflammatory mediators. Histamine is the primary mediator and elicits edema (wheal) and erythema (flare). Hereditary angioedema and related syndromes are mediated by the overproduction of bradykinin and are not responsive to antihistamines.

DIAGNOSIS

Diagnosis is based on complete history and physical examination, which should elicit identifiable triggers.

Clinical Presentation

- Patients with an acute urticaria episode present with history of pruritic, raised, erythematous lesions. Individual lesions resolve over a period of 1–24 hours.
- Angioedema usually presents with painful swelling without pruritus. The swelling can take up to 72 hours to resolve.

History
- A detailed history should elicit identifiable triggers and rule out any systemic causes. This also includes determining whether an individual lesion lasts >24 hours, in which case the diagnosis of urticarial vasculitis must be investigated by a skin biopsy.
- Any changes in environmental exposures, foods, medications, personal care products, etc., should be determined.
- It is important to differentiate from anaphylaxis, which affects organs other than the skin, as this will be treated differently (see Anaphylaxis section).

Physical Examination
- Complete examination of the affected and nonaffected skin.
- Urticaria appears as erythematous, raised lesions that blanch with pressure.
- Angioedema appears as swelling; can often involve the face, tongue, extremities, or genitalia; and may be asymmetric.

Differential Diagnosis
- IgE-mediated allergic reaction to drugs, foods, insects, inhalant, or contact allergen.
- Non–IgE-mediated drug and food reactions (i.e., medications including NSAIDs, vancomycin, radioactive iodine, opiates, muscle relaxants, foods including tomatoes and strawberries).
- Physical urticaria.
- Mast cell release syndromes (i.e., systemic mastocytosis, cutaneous mastocytosis including urticaria pigmentosa).
- Cutaneous small-vessel vasculitis (i.e., urticarial vasculitis, systemic lupus erythematosus).
- Toxic drug eruptions.
- EM.
- Allergic contact dermatitis (i.e., poison ivy, poison oak).
- **Angioedema without urticaria** should lead to consideration of specific entities.
  ○ Use of ACE-inhibitors or **angiotensin II receptor blockers** (ARBs) can be associated with angioedema at any point in the course of therapy.
  ○ **Hereditary angioedema (HAE), or C1 INH deficiency,** is inherited in an autosomal dominant pattern; 25% of cases arise from de novo mutations.
  ○ **Acquired C1 INH deficiency** presents similarly to HAE but is typically associated with an underlying lymphoproliferative disorder or connective tissue disease.

Diagnostic Testing
Epicutaneous skin testing and patch testing are only indicated when symptoms are associated with specific triggers.

Laboratories
- Routine laboratory testing in the absence of a clinical history is rarely helpful in determining an etiology in chronic urticaria.
- One can consider the following limited routine laboratory testing to evaluate for systemic disease that can lead to chronic urticaria: CBC with differential, ESR, thyroid-stimulating hormone, renal and liver profiles.
- Autologous serum skin testing, assays for basophil histamine release, and autoantibodies to IgE and the high-affinity IgE receptor are available, but the utility of these tests has not been established.
- All patients with **angioedema without urticaria should be screened with a C4 level, which is reduced during and between attacks of HAE.** If the C4 level is reduced, a quantitative and functional C1 INH assay should be performed. Measuring C1 INH levels alone is not sufficient because 15% of patients have normal levels of a dysfunctional C1 INH protein; therefore, it is important to also obtain the functional assay.

- Acquired C1 INH deficiency patients have reduced C1q, C1 INH, and C4 levels. Other patients with the acquired form have an autoantibody to C1 INH with low C4 and C1 INH levels but a normal C1 level.

Diagnostic Procedures
- A skin biopsy should be performed if individual lesions persist for >24 hours to rule out urticarial vasculitis.
  - Biopsy of acute urticarial lesions reveals dilation of small venules and capillaries located in the superficial dermis with widening of the dermal papillae, flattening of the rete pegs, and swelling of collagen fibers.
  - Chronic urticaria is characterized by a dense, nonnecrotizing, perivascular infiltrate consisting of T lymphocytes, mast cells, eosinophils, basophils, and neutrophils.
- Angioedema shows similar pathologic alterations in the deep, rather than superficial, dermis, and subcutaneous tissue.

TREATMENT

- The ideal treatment of acute urticaria with or without angioedema is identification and avoidance of specific causes. **All potential causes should be eliminated.** Most cases resolve within 1 week. In some instances, it is possible to reintroduce an agent cautiously if it is believed not to be the etiologic agent. This trial should be done in the presence of a physician with epinephrine readily available.
- Careful consideration should be given to the **elimination or substitution of each prescription or over-the-counter medication** or supplement. If a patient reacts to one medication in a class, the reaction likely will be triggered by all medications in that class. Exacerbating agents (e.g., NSAIDs, opiates, vancomycin, and alcohol) should be avoided because they may induce nonspecific mast cell degranulation and exacerbate urticaria caused by other agents.
- In patients presenting with hereditary and acquired angioedema, a prompt assessment of airway is critical, especially in those presenting with a laryngeal attack.

Medications
If acute urticaria is associated with additional systemic symptoms such as hypotension, laryngeal edema, or bronchospasm, treatment with epinephrine (0.3–0.5 mL of a 1:1000 solution IM) should be administered immediately. See Anaphylaxis section for additional information.

First Line
- **Acute urticaria and/or angioedema**
  - **Second-generation antihistamines** such as cetirizine, fexofenadine, or loratadine should be administered to patients until the hives have cleared. Higher than conventional, US Food and Drug Administration–approved doses may provide more efficacy. A first-generation antihistamine such as hydroxyzine may be added as an evening dose if needed to obtain control in refractory cases. H_2 antihistamines, such as ranitidine, may also be added to the above treatment.
  - **Oral corticosteroids** should be reserved for patients with moderate to severe symptoms. Corticosteroids will not have an immediate effect but may prevent relapse.
  - If a patient presents with systemic symptoms, self-administered epinephrine should be prescribed for use in the case of anaphylaxis.
- **Chronic urticaria**
  - A stepwise approach has been suggested for the treatment of chronic urticaria (*J Allergy Clin Immunol 2014;133(5):1270*).
  - Step 1: Monotherapy with a second-generation H_1 antihistamine.

- ○ Step 2: One or more of the following:
  - Dose advancement of the second-generation H_1 antihistamine, up to four times the conventional dose
  - Addition of another second-generation H_1 antihistamine
  - Addition of H_2 antihistamine
  - Addition of leukotriene receptor antagonist
  - Addition of first-generation H_1 antihistamine to be taken at bedtime
- ○ Step 3: Dose advancement of a potent antihistamine (i.e., doxepin, hydroxyzine) as tolerated. This is limited by sedation; use with caution in the elderly.
- ○ Step 4: Add an alternative agent.
  - Omalizumab: Proven safe and effective in several randomized clinical trials in patients with chronic urticaria not responsive to standard dose of H_1 antihistamines
  - Cyclosporine
  - Other anti-inflammatory agents, immunosuppressants, or biologics
- ○ **Optimal duration of therapy has not been established; tapering medications after 3–6 months of symptom control has been suggested.**
- **Hereditary and acquired angioedema (disorder of C1 inhibitor)**
  Laryngeal attacks or severe abdominal attacks: C1 inhibitor concentrate, icatibant, and ecallantide are first-line agents. If none of the first-line agents are available, fresh frozen plasma can be used. Also pursue symptomatic therapy and rehydration.

REFERRAL

All patients with chronic urticaria or a history of anaphylaxis should be referred to an allergy specialist for evaluation to identify potential allergic and autoimmune triggers.

Immunodeficiency

GENERAL PRINCIPLES

Definition
- Primary immunodeficiencies (PIDs) are disorders of the immune system that result in an increased susceptibility to infection.
- Secondary immunodeficiencies are also disorders of increased susceptibility to infection but are attributable to an external source.

Classification
PIDs can be organized by the defective immune components with considerable heterogeneity in each disorder.
- **Predominantly antibody deficiencies:** The defect is primarily in the ability to make antibodies.
  - ○ Common variable immune deficiency (CVID)
  - ○ X-linked (Bruton) agammaglobulinemia
  - ○ IgG subclass deficiency
  - ○ Specific antibody deficiency
  - ○ Selective IgA deficiency
- **Combined immunodeficiencies and syndromes:** The defect results in deficiencies in both cellular and humoral immune responses.
  - ○ Severe combined immunodeficiencies (SCIDs)
  - ○ DiGeorge syndrome
  - ○ Hyper-IgE (Job) syndrome

- ○ **Defects of innate immunity:** Defects in germline-encoded receptors and downstream signaling pathways
  - ○ Deficiency of Toll-like receptor (TLR) signaling
  - ○ Mendelian susceptibility to mycobacterial diseases (MSMD)
  - ○ Natural killer (NK) cell deficiency
  - ○ Phagocytic cell deficiencies
    Chronic granulomatous disease (CGD)
- • **Complement deficiencies.**
- • **Diseases of immune dysregulation:** Autoimmunity and lymphoproliferation are characteristic manifestations in these disorders.

Epidemiology

- • Secondary immunodeficiency syndromes, particularly HIV/AIDS, are the most common immunodeficiency disorders.
- • The estimated prevalence of PIDs is approximately 1 in 1200 live births.
- • Most PIDs presenting in adulthood are humoral immune defects.

Etiology

- • Predominantly antibody immune deficiencies are thought to be caused by defects in B-cell maturation. Combined immunodeficiencies are caused by defective T-cell–mediated immunity and associated antibody deficiency.
- • A variety of genetic mutations have been associated with specific PID syndromes.
- • Secondary immunodeficiencies can be caused by medications (chemotherapy, immunomodulatory agents, corticosteroids), infectious agents (e.g., HIV), malignancy, antibody loss (e.g., nephrotic syndrome, protein losing enteropathy, or consumption during a severe underlying infection), autoimmune disease (e.g., systemic lupus erythematosus, rheumatoid arthritis), malnutrition (vitamin D), and other underlying diseases (e.g., diabetes mellitus, cirrhosis, uremia).

DIAGNOSIS

Clinical Presentation

- • The hallmark of PID is recurrent infections. Clinical suspicion should be increased by recurrent sinopulmonary infection, deep-seated infections, opportunistic infections, or disseminated infections in an otherwise healthy patient.
- • Specific PIDs are often associated with particular types of pathogens (e.g., catalase-positive infections in CGD or MSMD).
- • Recurrent urinary tract infections are only rarely associated with PID.
- • Patients with PIDs may also present with autoimmunity, immune dysregulation, allergic diseases, and malignancies.
- • **Selective IgA deficiency** is the most common immune deficiency, with a prevalence of 1 in 300–500 people.
  - ○ Most patients are asymptomatic. Some may present with recurrent sinus and pulmonary infections. Therapy is directed at early treatment with antibiotics because IgA replacement is not available.
  - ○ Associated autoimmune diseases are observed in 20–30% of cases. Absolute IgA-deficient patients (i.e., <7 mg/dL) are at risk for developing a severe transfusion reaction to blood products including IV immunoglobulin (IVIG), because of the presence in some individuals of IgE anti-IgA antibodies; therefore, these patients should be transfused with washed red blood cells or receive blood products only from IgA-deficient donors.

- **CVID** is the most common symptomatic PID, occurring with a frequency of 1/10,000. It includes a heterogeneous group of disorders in which most patients present in the second to fourth decade of life with recurrent sinus and pulmonary infections and are discovered to have low and dysfunctional IgG, IgA, and/or IgM antibodies with poor response to immunizations.
  - B-cell numbers are often normal, but there is decreased ability to produce immunoglobulin due to the lack of isotype-switched memory B cells. Some patients may also exhibit T-cell dysfunction.
  - CVID is largely idiopathic, although there are molecular defects in the B-cell signaling and development pathways (e.g., TACI, ICOS, BAFF-R, and CD19) with some forms of the disorder.
  - Patients with CVID are particularly susceptible to infection with encapsulated organisms. Patients may have associated gastrointestinal disease or autoimmune abnormalities (most commonly autoimmune hemolytic anemia, idiopathic thrombocytopenic purpura, pernicious anemia, and rheumatoid arthritis).
  - There is an increased incidence of malignancy, especially lymphoid and gastrointestinal malignancy.
  - Therapy consists of IVIG or subcutaneous immunoglobulin (SCIG) replacement therapy as well as prompt treatment of infections with antibiotics.
- **Specific antibody deficiency** is defined as poor or absent antibody responses to polysaccharide antigens (i.e., 23-valent pneumococcus vaccine) in the setting of normal levels of immunoglobulins and IgG subclasses.
  - B-cell numbers and response to protein antigens (i.e., tetanus toxoid and diphtheria toxoid) are usually normal.
  - Patients have increased susceptibility to sinopulmonary infections. Allergic diseases are also common.
  - Therapeutic approaches include adequate antibiotic treatment for infections, pneumococcal conjugate vaccine, and sometimes immunoglobulin replacement.
- **X-linked (Bruton) agammaglobulinemia** clinically manifests very similarly to severe CVID and is typically diagnosed in childhood but can present in adulthood.
  - Patients usually have low levels of all immunoglobulin types and very low levels of B cells.
  - Specific genetic defect is in Bruton tyrosine kinase, which is involved in B-cell maturation.
- **Subclass deficiency.** Deficiencies of each of the IgG subclasses (IgG1, IgG2, IgG3, and IgG4) have been described.
  - These patients present with similar complaints as the CVID patients.
  - Total IgG levels may be normal. A strong association with IgA deficiency exists. There is disagreement as to whether this is a separate entity from CVID. In most cases, there is no need to evaluate IgG subclass levels.
  - Isolated subclass deficiency without recurrent infections is of unknown clinical significance.
- **Hyper-IgE syndrome (Job syndrome)** is characterized by recurrent pyogenic infections of the skin and lower respiratory tract. This syndrome can result in severe abscess and empyema formation. Some forms of the disease are associated with autosomal dominant mutation of *STAT3*.
  - The most common organism involved is *Staphylococcus aureus*, but other bacteria and fungi have been reported.
  - Patients present with recurrent infections and have associated pruritic dermatitis, coarse (lion-like) facies, growth retardation, scoliosis, retention of primary teeth, and hyperkeratotic nails.
  - Laboratory data reveal the presence of normal levels of IgG, IgA, and IgM but markedly elevated levels of IgE. A marked increase in tissue and blood eosinophils may also be observed.

- **Complement deficiencies** are a broad category of PID characterized by recurrent infections to a range of pathogens.
  - Recurrent disseminated neisserial infections are associated with a deficiency in the terminal complement system (C5–C9).
  - Systemic lupus-like disorders and recurrent infection with encapsulated organisms have been associated with deficiencies in other components of complement.
  - CH50 and AH50 are useful to screen for deficiencies of the classical pathway and alternative pathway, respectively.
- **CGD** is characterized by defective killing of intracellular pathogens by neutrophils.
  - Patients usually present with frequent infection, often with abscesses, from *S. aureus* and other catalase-positive organisms. *Aspergillus* is a particularly troublesome pathogen for patients with CGD.
  - Diagnosis is made by demonstration of defective respiratory burst with flow cytometry assay using dihydrorhodamine.
- **MSMD** is caused by defects in Th1 immunity and is associated with mutations in genes involved in interferon-γ and IL-12 signaling. Characteristic infections include mycobacterial infections (including typical and atypical *Mycobacterium*) and *Salmonella* infections.

Diagnostic Testing

- Frequent sinopulmonary infections, recurrent and invasive infections requiring IV antimicrobial agents, infections with unusual pathogens, and family history of PID are warning signs for PIDs.
- Initial evaluation should focus on identifying possible secondary causes of recurrent infection such as allergy, medications, and anatomic abnormalities. Workup begins with a CBC with differential, HIV test, quantitative immunoglobulin levels, and complement levels. Often the evaluation will need to include enumeration of lymphocytes by flow cytometry if B-, T-, or NK-cell defects are suspected. Other specialized tests including genetic testing may be needed to make a definitive diagnosis.
- If clinical suspicion is high for an underlying antibody-predominant PID, B-cell function can be assessed by measuring immunoglobulin response to vaccinations. Preimmunization and postimmunization titers for both a protein antigen (i.e., tetanus) and a polysaccharide antigen (i.e., Pneumovax, the unconjugated 23-valent vaccine) are measured because proteins and polysaccharide antigens are handled differently by the immune system.
- Titers of specific antibodies are measured before and at 4–8 weeks after immunization.

TREATMENT

- Killed or subcomponent vaccines are safe for most patients with PID, although some patients may not produce full response. Live attenuated vaccines may be contraindicated in some individuals with PID and their families.
- Prophylactic antibiotics may be considered in some PID syndromes to prevent infections.
- IgA deficiency: No specific treatment is available. However, these patients should be promptly treated at the first sign of infection with an antibiotic that covers *Streptococcus pneumoniae* or *Haemophilus influenzae*.
- CVID should be treated with immunoglobulin replacement in forms of IVIG or SCIG. Numerous preparations of immunoglobulin are available, all of which undergo viral inactivation steps.
  Possible side effects include myalgias, vomiting, chills, and lingering headache (due to immune complex–mediated aseptic meningitis).

REFERRAL

Patients in whom a PID is being seriously considered should undergo evaluation by an allergist/clinical immunologist with expertise in diagnosing and treating PID.

12 Fluid and Electrolyte Management

Anubha Mutneja, Steven Cheng, and Judy L. Jang

FLUID MANAGEMENT AND PERTURBATIONS IN VOLUME STATUS

- **Total body water (TBW).** Water comprises approximately 60% of lean body weight in men and 50% in women. TBW is distributed in two major compartments: two-thirds is **intracellular fluid** (ICF) and one-third is **extracellular fluid** (ECF). ECF is further subdivided into intravascular and interstitial spaces in a ratio of 1:4.
  - **Example:** For a healthy 70-kg man,

$$TBW = 0.6 \times 70 = 42 \text{ L}$$

  - ICF = 2/3 TBW = $0.66 \times 42 = 28$ L
  - ECF = 1/3 TBW = $0.33 \times 42 = 14$ L
  - Intravascular compartment = $0.25 \times 14 = 3.5$ L
  - Interstitial compartment = $0.75 \times 14 = 10.5$ L
  - The distribution of water between intravascular and interstitial spaces can also be affected by changes to the Starling balance of forces. Low oncotic pressure (i.e., low albumin states) and high hydrostatic pressure (i.e., Na^+-retentive states) increase the movement of fluid from vascular to interstitial compartments, which is an important step in the development of edema.
  - Because the majority of water is contained in the intracellular space, the loss of water alone (without Na^+) does not typically result in the hemodynamic changes associated with volume depletion. Instead, disturbances in TBW change serum **osmolality** and electrolyte concentrations.
  - The intact kidney adapts to changes in TBW by increasing water excretion or reabsorption. This is mediated by the **antidiuretic hormone (ADH; vasopressin)**, which permits water movement across the distal nephron. Although vasopressin release is predominately responsive to osmotic cues, volume contraction can cause a nonosmotic release of vasopressin, resulting in a reduction of renal water excretion.
- **Total body Na^+.** 85–90% of **total body Na^+** is extracellular and constitutes the predominate solute in the ECF. Changes to the body's total Na^+ content typically results from a loss or gain of this Na^+-rich fluid, leading to contraction or expansion of the ECF space. Clinically, this manifests as volume depletion (hypotension, tachycardia) and volume expansion (peripheral or pulmonary edema).
  - Na^+ *concentration* is distinct from Na^+ *content*. Na^+ concentration reflects the amount of Na^+ distributed in a fixed quantity of water. An increase in TBW can decrease the Na^+ concentration even if the body's total Na^+ content remains unchanged.
  - The intact kidney can respond to altered Na^+ content in the ECF space by increasing or decreasing Na^+ reabsorption. This response is mediated by cardiovascular, renal, hepatic, and central nervous system sensors of the effective circulating volume.

The Euvolemic Patient

- In a euvolemic patient, the goal of fluid and electrolyte administration is to maintain homeostasis. The best way to accomplish this is to allow free access to food and oral fluids.

Patients who are unable to tolerate oral input require maintenance fluids to replace renal, gastrointestinal (GI), and insensible fluid losses.

- The decision to provide maintenance IV fluid (IVF) should be thoughtfully considered and not administered by rote. Fluid administration should be reassessed *at least* daily. Patient weight, which may indicate net fluid balance, should be monitored carefully.
- Consider the **water** and **electrolyte** needs of the patient separately when prescribing IVF therapy.
  - Minimum **water** requirements for daily fluid balance can be approximated from the sum of the required urine output, stool water loss, and insensible losses.
    - The minimum urine output necessary to excrete the daily solute load is the amount of solute consumed each day (roughly 600–800 mOsm/d in an average individual) divided by the maximum amount of solute that can be excreted per liter of urine (maximum urine concentrating capacity is 1200 mOsm/L in healthy kidneys). The result is an obligate urine output of *at least* 0.5 L/d.
    - The water lost in stools is typically 200 mL/d.
    - **Insensible water losses** from the skin and respiratory tract amount to roughly 400–500 mL/d. The volume of water produced from endogenous metabolism (<250–350 mL/d) should be considered as well. The degree of insensible loss may vary tremendously depending on respiratory rate, metabolic state, and temperature (water losses increase by 100–150 mL/d for each degree of body temperature over 37°C).
    - Fluid from drain losses must be factored in as well.
    - After adding each of these components, the minimum amount of water needed to maintain homeostasis is roughly 1400 mL/d or 60 mL/h.
  - **Electrolytes** that are usually administered during maintenance fluid therapy are Na^+ and K^+ salts. Requirements depend on minimum obligatory and ongoing losses.
    - It is customary to provide **75–175 mEq Na^+/d** as NaCl. (A typical 2-g Na^+ diet provides 86 mEq Na^+/d.)
    - Generally, **20–60 mEq K^+/d** is included if renal function is normal.
    - Carbohydrate in the form of **dextrose, 100–150 g/d**, is given to minimize protein catabolism and prevent starvation ketoacidosis.
  - Table 12-1 provides a list of common IV solutions and their contents. By combining the necessary components, one can derive an appropriate maintenance fluid regimen tailored for each patient.
  - **Example:** A patient is admitted for a procedure and is made nothing by mouth (NPO). To maintain homeostasis, you must replace 2 L of water, 154 mEq Na^+, 40 mEq K^+, and 100 g dextrose over the next 24 hours (values are within **water** and **electrolyte** requirements described earlier).
    - 2 L of water: Dose fluid at 85 mL/h (2000 mL ÷ 24 hours)
    - 154 mEq of Na^+: Use 0.45% normal saline (NS) (77 mEq Na^+/L)
    - 40 mEq of K^+: Add 20 mEq/L KCl to each liter of IVF
    - 100 g dextrose: Use D5 (50 g of dextrose/L)
    - Order: **D5 0.45% NaCl with 20 mEq/L KCl at 85 mL/h**

The Hypovolemic Patient

GENERAL PRINCIPLES

- Volume depletion generally results from a deficit in **total body Na^+** content. This may result from **renal** or **extrarenal losses** of Na^+ from the ECF. **Water** losses alone can also

TABLE 12-1	Commonly Used Parenteral Solutions				
IV Solution	Osmolality (mOsm/L)	[Glucose] (g/L)	[Na$^+$] (mEq/L)	[Cl$^-$] (mEq/L)	HCO$_3^-$ Equivalents (mEq/L)
D5W	278	50	0	0	0
0.45% NaCl^a	154	—^{b}	77	77	0
0.9% NaCl^a	308	—^{b}	154	154	0
3% NaCl	1,026	—	513	513	0
Lactated Ringer's^c	274	—^{b}	130	109	28

D5W, 5% dextrose in water.
^{a}NaCl 0.45% and 0.9% are half-normal and normal saline, respectively.
^{b}Also available with 5% dextrose.
^{c}Also contains 4 mEq/L K$^+$, 1.5 mEq/L Ca^{2+}, and 28 mEq/L lactate.

cause volume depletion, but the quantity required to do so is large, as water is lost mainly from the ICF and not the ECF, where volume contraction can be assessed.

• **Renal losses** may be secondary to enhanced diuresis, salt-wasting nephropathies, mineralocorticoid deficiency, or resolution of obstructive renal disease.

• **Extrarenal losses** include fluid loss from the GI tract (vomiting, nasogastric suction, fistula drainage, diarrhea), respiratory losses, skin losses (especially with burns), hemorrhage, and severe third spacing of fluid in critically ill patients.

DIAGNOSIS

Clinical Presentation

• **Symptoms** include complaints of thirst, fatigue, weakness, muscle cramps, and postural dizziness. Sometimes, syncope and coma can result with severe volume depletion.

• **Signs** of hypovolemia include low jugular venous pressure, postural hypotension, postural tachycardia, and the absence of axillary sweat. Diminished skin turgor and dry mucous membranes are poor markers of decreased interstitial fluid. Mild degrees of volume depletion are often not clinically detectable, whereas larger fluid losses can lead to mental status changes, oliguria, and hypovolemic shock.

Diagnostic Testing

Laboratory studies are often helpful but must be used in conjunction with the clinical picture.

• **Urine sodium** is a marker for Na$^+$ avidity in the kidney.

  ○ Urine Na$^+$ <15 mEq is consistent with volume depletion, as is a fractional excretion of sodium (FeNa) <1%. The latter can be calculated as ([Urine Na$^+$ × Serum Cr] ÷ [Urine Cr × Serum Na$^+$]) × 100.

  ○ Concomitant metabolic alkalosis may increase urine Na$^+$ excretion despite volume depletion due to obligate excretion of Na$^+$ to accompany the bicarbonate anion. In such cases, a urine chloride of <20 mEq is often helpful to confirm volume contraction.

• **Urine osmolality** and **serum bicarbonate** levels may also be elevated.

• **Hematocrit** and **serum albumin** may be increased from hemoconcentration.

TREATMENT

- It is often difficult to estimate the **volume deficit** present, and thus, therapy is largely empiric, requiring frequent reassessments of volume status while resuscitation is under way.
- Mild volume contraction can usually be corrected via the oral route. However, the presence of hemodynamic instability, symptomatic fluid loss, or intolerance to oral administration requires IV therapy.
- The primary therapeutic goal is to protect hemodynamic stability and replenish **intravascular volume** with fluid that will preferentially expand the ECF compartment. This can be accomplished with Na^+-based solutions, because the Na^+ will be retained in the ECF.
  - ○ **Isotonic fluid**, such as NS (0.9% NaCl), contains a Na^+ content similar to that of plasma fluid in the ECF and thus remains entirely in the ECF space. It is the initial fluid of choice for replenishing **intravascular volume**.
    - The administration of solute-free water is largely ineffective, because the majority of water will distribute to the ICF space.
    - Half-normal saline (0.45% NS) has 77 mEq of Na^+ per liter, roughly half the Na^+ content of an equal volume in the ECF. Thus, half of this solution will stay in the ECF, and half will follow the predicted distribution of water.
  - ○ Fluids can be administered as a bolus or at a steady maintenance rate. In patients with symptomatic volume depletion, a 1- to 2-L bolus is often preferable to acutely expand the intravascular space. The bolus can be repeated if necessary, although close attention should be directed toward possible signs of volume overload. Smaller boluses should be used for patients with poor cardiac reserve or significant edema. Once the patient is stable, fluids can be administered at a maintenance rate to replace ongoing losses. In patients with hemorrhage or GI bleeding, **blood transfusion** can accomplish both volume expansion and concomitant correction of anemia.

The Hypervolemic Patient

The clinical manifestations of hypervolemia result from a surplus of **total body Na^+**. It can be caused by a primary disorder of renal Na^+ retention. Alternatively, it may be secondary to decreased **effective circulating volume**, as in heart failure, cirrhosis, or profound hypoalbuminemia.

DIAGNOSIS

Clinical Presentation

- Expansion of the **interstitial compartment** may result in peripheral edema, ascites, and pleural effusions. Expansion of the **intravascular compartment** may result in pulmonary rales, elevated jugular venous pressure, hepatojugular reflux, an S_3 gallop, and elevated blood pressures.
- Because overt signs of hypervolemia may not manifest until 3–4 L of fluid retention, a gradual rise in water weight is often the earliest indication of Na^+ retention.
- **Symptoms** may include dyspnea, abdominal distention, or swelling of extremities.

Diagnostic Testing

- Laboratory studies are generally not needed, and hypervolemia is primarily a bedside diagnosis.
- **The urine [Na^+]** may be low (<15 mEq/L) with decreased **effective circulating volume** reflecting renal sodium retention.
- A CXR may show pulmonary edema or pleural effusions, but clear lung fields do not exclude volume overload.

TREATMENT

Treatment must address not only the ECF volume excess but also the underlying pathologic process. Alleviating the Na^+ excess can be accomplished by the judicious use of diuretics and by limiting Na^+ intake.

Medications

- Diuretics enhance the renal excretion of Na^+ by blocking the various sites of Na^+ reabsorption along the nephron.
  - Thiazide diuretics block the NaCl transporters in the distal convoluted tubule. They are often used for mild states of chronic Na^+ retention. Because of their specific site of action, thiazide diuretics impair urinary dilutional capacity (the ability to excrete water) and often stimulate a responsive increase in proximal tubule reabsorption.
  - Loop diuretics block the Na^+-K^+-$2Cl^-$ transporter in the thick ascending loop of Henle. They are often used in circumstances requiring a brisk and immediate diuresis, such as acute volume overload. Loop diuretics impair urinary concentration (increase renal free water excretion) and enhance the excretion of divalent cations (Ca^{2+} and Mg^{2+}).
  - Potassium-sparing diuretics act by decreasing Na^+ reabsorption in the collecting duct. Although the overall diuretic effect of these agents is comparatively small, they serve as useful adjunctive agents. Furthermore, because aldosterone antagonists do not require tubular secretion, they can be particularly useful in those with decreased renal perfusion or impaired tubular function.
- Treatment of the underlying disease process is critical to prevent continued Na^+ reabsorption in the kidney. Nephrotic syndrome is discussed in Chapter 13, Renal Diseases. Treatment of heart failure is discussed in Chapter 5, Heart Failure and Cardiomyopathy, and cirrhosis is addressed in Chapter 19, Liver Diseases.

Disorders of Sodium Concentration

Hypernatremia and **hyponatremia** are primarily disorders of *water balance* or *water distribution*. The body is designed to withstand both drought and deluge with adaptations to renal water handling and the thirst mechanism. A persistent abnormality in $[Na^+]$ thus requires both an initial challenge to water balance as well as a disturbance of the adaptive response.

Hyponatremia

Hyponatremia is defined as a plasma $[Na^+]$ **<135 mEq/L.**

GENERAL PRINCIPLES

- To maintain a normal $[Na^+]$, the ingestion of water must be matched with an equal volume of water excretion. Any process that limits the elimination of water or expands the volume around a fixed Na^+ content may lead to a decrease in Na^+ concentration.
- Expansion of the space surrounding the Na^+ content can occur in a variety of ways:
  - **Pseudohyponatremia** refers to a laboratory phenomenon by which a high content of plasma proteins and lipids expands the nonaqueous portion of the plasma sample, leading to an errant report of a low ECF $[Na^+]$. This can be averted with Na^+-sensitive electrodes, and the normal ECF $[Na^+]$ can be confirmed with a normal serum osmolality.
  - **Hyperosmolar hyponatremia** refers to circumstances in which an osmotically active solute other than Na^+ accumulates in the ECF, drawing water into the ECF and

diluting the Na^+ content. This is most commonly caused by **hyperglycemia**, resulting in a fall in plasma $[Na^+]$ of 1.6–2.4 mEq/L for every 100 mg/dL rise in plasma glucose (*Am J Med 1999;106:399*). Other solutes, such as glycine, mannitol, or sorbitol, can be absorbed into the ECF during bladder irrigation, leading to the transient hypona-tremia seen in **post–transurethral resection of the prostate (post-TURP) syndrome**. Prompt renal excretion and metabolism of the absorbed fluid usually corrects the hypo-natremia rapidly, although symptomatic hyponatremia can occasionally be seen in the setting of renal insufficiency.

- ○ Rarely, the ECF water content rises simply because the ingested quantity of water ex-ceeds the physiologic capacity of water excretion in the kidney. This is seen in psy-chogenic polydipsia, water intoxication from poorly conceived drinking games, beer potomania, and the so-called "tea and toast" diet. Underlying each of these circum-stances is the fact that there is a limit to renal water clearance. Urine cannot be diluted to an osmolality less than approximately 50 mOsm/L, meaning that a small amount of solute is required in even the most dilute urine. Ingestion of a high volume of water can thus exceed the capacity for excretion, particularly in those with a solute-poor diet, because the solute load required to generate urinary water loss is quickly depleted. The excess water is retained, Na^+ concentrations falls, and hyponatremia results.
- Decreased clearance of water from the kidney can also occur through a variety of pro-cesses. As mentioned previously, renal water handling is largely controlled by ADH (or vasopressin). Nonosmotic stimulation of this hormone occurs with volume contrac-tion. Although this seems counterintuitive from an osmotic standpoint (it further reduces renal water clearance and increases water retention), it is an "appropriate" adaptive response to the threat of volume loss, tissue hypoperfusion, and impending hemodynamic col-lapse. Other conditions are characterized by secretion of ADH, which is "inappropriate," stimulated by neither osmotic nor volume-related changes.
- **"Appropriate"** ADH secretion occurs with a fall in effective circulating volume. In these conditions, thirst and water retention are stimulated, protecting volume status at the cost of the osmolar status. This category is classically subdivided based on the associated assessment of ECF status.
  - ○ **Hypovolemic hyponatremia** may result from **any** cause of net Na^+ loss, such as in thiazide use and cerebral salt wasting.
  - ○ **Hypervolemic hyponatremia** occurs in edematous states such as congestive heart failure (CHF), hepatic cirrhosis, and severe nephrotic syndrome. Despite the expanded interstitial space, the circulating volume is reduced. Alterations in Starling forces con-tribute to this apparent paradox, shifting fluid from the intravascular to interstitial space.
- **"Inappropriate"** secretion of ADH is characterized by the activation of water-conserving mechanisms despite the absence of osmotic- or volume-related stimuli. Because the renal response to volume expansion remains intact, these patients are typically **euvolemic**. However, because of the rise in TBW, serum concentrations of Na^+ are decreased.
  - ○ The most common form of this is the **syndrome of inappropriate ADH (SIADH)**. This disorder is caused by the nonphysiologic release of vasopressin from the posterior pitu-itary or an ectopic source. Common causes of SIADH include neuropsychiatric disorders (e.g., meningitis, encephalitis, acute psychosis, cerebrovascular accident, head trauma), pulmonary diseases (e.g., pneumonia, tuberculosis, positive-pressure ventilation, acute respiratory failure), and malignant tumors (most commonly, small-cell lung cancer).
    - ▪ **SIADH** is diagnosed by the following:
      - □ Hypo-osmotic hyponatremia
      - □ Urine osmolality >100 mOsm/L
      - □ Euvolemia
      - □ The absence of conditions that stimulate ADH secretion, including volume con-traction, nausea, adrenal dysfunction, and hypothyroidism

- **Pharmacologic agents** may also stimulate inappropriate ADH secretion. Common culprits include antidepressants (particularly selective serotonin reuptake inhibitors [SSRIs]), narcotics, antipsychotic agents, chlorpropamide, and NSAIDs.
  - **Reset osmostat** is a phenomenon in which the set point for plasma osmolality is reduced. Thus, ADH and thirst responses, although functional, maintain plasma osmolality at this new, lower level. This phenomenon occurs in almost all pregnant women (perhaps in response to changes in the hormonal milieu) and occasionally in those with a chronic decreased effective circulating volume.

DIAGNOSIS

Clinical Presentation

The clinical features of hyponatremia are related to the osmotic intracellular water shift leading to cerebral edema. Therefore, the symptoms are primarily neurologic, and their severity is dependent on both the magnitude and rapidity of decrease in plasma [Na$^+$]. In **acute hyponatremia** (i.e., developing in <2 days), patients may complain of nausea and malaise with [Na$^+$] of approximately 125 mEq/L. As the plasma [Na$^+$] falls further, symptoms may progress to include headache, lethargy, confusion, and obtundation. Stupor, seizures, and coma do not usually occur unless the plasma [Na$^+$] falls acutely below 115 mEq/L. In **chronic hyponatremia** (>3 days in duration), adaptive mechanisms designed to defend cell volume occur and tend to minimize the increase in ICF volume and its symptoms.

Diagnostic Testing

The underlying cause of hyponatremia can often be ascertained from an accurate history and physical examination, including an assessment of **ECF volume status** and the **effective circulating volume**.

Three laboratory analyses, when used with a clinical assessment of volume status, can narrow the differential diagnosis of hyponatremia: (a) the **plasma osmolality**, (b) the **urine osmolality**, and (c) the **urine [Na$^+$]** (Figure 12-1).

- **Plasma osmolality.** Most patients with hyponatremia have a low plasma osmolality (<275 mOsm/L). If the plasma osmolality is not low, **pseudohyponatremia** and **hyperosmolar hyponatremia** must be ruled out.
- **Urine osmolality.** The appropriate renal response to hypo-osmolality is to excrete a maximally dilute urine (urine osmolality <100 mOsm/L and specific gravity <1.003). A urine sample that is not dilute suggests impaired free water excretion due to appropriate or inappropriate secretion of the ADH.
- **Urine [Na$^+$]** adds laboratory corroboration to the bedside assessment of effective circulating volume and can discriminate between **extrarenal** and **renal losses** of Na$^+$. The appropriate response to decreased effective circulating volume is to enhance tubular Na$^+$ reabsorption such that urine [Na$^+$] is <10 mEq/L. A urine [Na$^+$] of >20 mEq/L suggests a normal effective circulating volume or a Na$^+$-wasting defect. Occasionally, the excretion of a nonreabsorbed anion obligates loss of the Na$^+$ cation despite volume depletion (ketonuria, bicarbonaturia).

TREATMENT

- Management requires one to determine **the rate of correction, the appropriate intervention**, and **the presence of other underlying disorders**.
- The **rate of correction** of hyponatremia depends on the acuity of its development and the presence of neurologic dysfunction.
- **Acute symptomatic hyponatremia.** Severe symptomatic hyponatremia, with evidence of neurologic dysfunction, should generally be treated promptly with hypertonic saline;

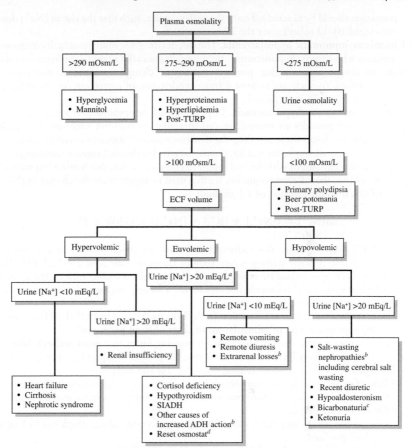

Figure 12-1. Algorithm depicting the diagnostic approach to hyponatremia. ADH, antidiuretic hormone; ECF, extracellular fluid; post-TURP, post–transurethral resection of the prostate syndrome; SIADH, syndrome of inappropriate antidiuretic hormone. [a]Urine [Na⁺] may be <20 mEq/L with low Na⁺ intake. [b]See text for details. [c]From vomiting-induced contraction alkalosis or proximal renal tubular acidosis. [d]Urine osmolality may be <100 mOsm/L after a water load.

however, any saline solution that is **hypertonic to the urine** (if the urine osmolality is known at the start of therapy) can increase the [Na+] when oral water intake is restricted.

○ The risks of correcting hyponatremia too rapidly are volume overload and the development of **central pontine myelinolysis** (CPM). CPM results from damage to neurons due to rapid osmotic shifts. In its most overt form, it is characterized by flaccid paralysis, dysarthria, and dysphagia, and in more subtle presentations, it can be confirmed by CT scan or MRI of the brain. The risk of precipitating CPM is increased with correction of the [Na⁺] by >12 mEq/L in a 24-hour period (*J Am Soc Nephrol 1994;4:1522*). In addition to overaggressive correction, other risk factors for developing CPM include preexisting hypokalemia, malnutrition, and alcoholism.

○ In patients with severe hyponatremia, in whom an immediate rise in [Na⁺] is necessary, [Na⁺] should be corrected 1–2 mEq/L/h for 3–4 hours. However, this initial rate of

correction should be tapered off once the patient is safe, such that the rise in [Na$^+$] does not exceed 10–12 mEq/L over the 24-hour period.
- **Chronic asymptomatic hyponatremia.** The risk of iatrogenic injury is actually increased in patients with chronic hyponatremia. Because cells gradually adapt to the hypo-osmolar state, an abrupt normalization presents a dramatic change from the accommodated osmotic milieu. As such, we suggest a more modest rate of correction on the order of 5–8 mEq/L over a 24-hour period.
- **Severe, symptomatic hyponatremia.** In patients with symptomatic hyponatremia, hypertonic saline provides an immediate and titratable intervention necessary to acutely raise serum Na$^+$ levels while avoiding the disastrous complications of overcorrection.
  - The most accurate way to correct hyponatremia entails a detailed registry matching total solute and water output with desired input. In clinical practice, this is often impractical.
  - In lieu of this, the following equation is often used to approximate the change in [Na$^+$] in mEq/L from the infusion of 1 L of fluid:

$$\Delta[Na^+] = ([Na^+{}_i] + [K^+{}_i] - [Na^+{}_s]) \div \{TBW + 1\}$$

  - [Na$^+{}_i$] and [K$^+{}_i$] are the sodium and potassium concentrations in the infused fluid, and [Na$^+{}_s$] is the starting serum sodium (*Intensive Care Med 1997;23:309*). Recall that TBW is estimated by multiplying the lean weight (in kilograms) by 0.6 in men (and 0.5 in women). This formula does not account for ongoing electrolyte or water losses and is only a rough guide.
  - Dividing the desired rate of correction (mEq/L/h) by Δ[Na$^+$] (mEq/L/L of fluid) gives you the appropriate **rate of administration (liter of fluid per hour)**.
  - Because this equation does not account for ongoing losses, one **must recheck laboratory data and adjust fluid rates** to make sure the patient is improving appropriately.
  - **Example:** An 80-kg woman is seizing. Her [Na$^+$] is 103 mEq/L.
    - **Rate of correction:** She has symptomatic hyponatremia requiring an acute correction (1–2 mEq/L/h for the first 3–4 hours) but no more than 12 mEq/L corrected over 24 hours.
    - **Means of correction:**
      □ Given the acuity, the patient should be given hypertonic saline, which has 513 mEq of Na$^+$ per liter.
      □ One liter of this fluid would increase [Na$^+$] by 10 mEq/L.

$$\Delta[Na^+] = (513 - 108) \div (80 \times 0.5 + 1) = 10 \text{ mEq/L}$$

      □ Dose hypertonic saline at 200 mL/h until symptoms improve.

$$\text{Rate} = (2 \text{ mEq/L/h}) \div (10 \text{ mEq/L per 1 L of saline})$$

    - To prevent a change of >10–12 mEq/L over 24 hours, no more than 1 L of fluid should be given.
- **Asymptomatic hyponatremia**
  - **Hypovolemic hyponatremia.** In patients with asymptomatic hypovolemic hyponatremia, **isotonic** saline can be used to restore the intravascular volume. Restoration of a euvolemic state will reduce the impetus toward renal water retention, leading to normalization of [Na$^+$]. If the duration of hyponatremia is unknown, the process described earlier can be used to calculate the expected change from 1 L of 0.9% NS, the rate of administration, and the maximal amount that can be given to avoid overcorrection.
  - **Hypervolemic hyponatremia.** Hyponatremia in CHF and cirrhosis often reflects the severity of the underlying disease. However, the hyponatremia itself is typically asymptomatic. Although *effective* circulating volume is decreased, the administration of fluid

may worsen the volume-overloaded state. Definitive treatment requires management of the underlying condition, although restriction of water intake and increasing water diuresis may help to attenuate the degree of hyponatremia.

- Oral fluid intake should be less than daily urine output.
- Urinary excretion of water can be promoted through the use of loop diuretics, which reduce the concentration gradient necessary to reabsorb water in the distal nephron. Vasopressin antagonists may also be helpful in both euvolemic (SIADH) and hypervolemic hyponatremia (particularly CHF). When using medications to promote water loss, laboratory data and volume status must be followed extremely closely, because the effect on water and electrolyte loss cannot be accurately predicted.

- **SIADH** should first be distinguished from the previously listed conditions that stimulate vasopressin secretion. The standard first-line therapy is water restriction and correction of any contributing factors (nausea, pneumonia, drugs, etc.). If this fails or if the patient is symptomatic, the following can be attempted to promote water excretion.
  - **Water restriction.** The amount of fluid restriction necessary depends on the extent of water elimination. A useful guide to the necessary degree of fluid restriction is as follows:
    - If (Urine Na^+ + Urine K^+)/Serum Na^+ <0.5, restrict to 1 L/d.
    - If (Urine Na^+ + Urine K^+)/Serum Na^+ is 0.5–1.0, restrict to 500 mL/d.
    - If (Urine Na^+ + Urine K^+)/Serum Na^+ is >1, the patient has a negative renal free water clearance and is actively reabsorbing water. Any amount of water given may be retained, and clinicians should consider the following options to enhance free water excretion.
  - **High dietary solute load.** The volume of water excreted as urine is governed by a relatively fixed urine osmolality. Thus, increasing solute intake with a high-salt, high-protein diet or administration of oral urea (30–60 g) may increase the capacity for water excretion and improve the hyponatremia.
  - Loop diuretics impair the urinary concentrating mechanism and can enhance free water excretion.
  - Vasopressin antagonists promote a water diuresis and may be useful in the therapy of SIADH. Both IV (conivaptan) and oral (tolvaptan) preparations are approved for the treatment of euvolemic hyponatremia. However, given the risks of overcorrection, these agents should be initiated in a closely monitored inpatient setting.
  - Lithium and demeclocycline interfere with the collecting tubule's ability to respond to ADH but are rarely used because of significant side effects. They should only be considered in severe hyponatremia that is unresponsive to more conservative measures.

Hypernatremia

GENERAL PRINCIPLES

- Hypernatremia is defined as a plasma $[Na^+]$ >**145 mEq/L** and represents a state of **hyperosmolality** (see Disorders of Sodium Concentration section).
- Hypernatremia may be caused by a primary **Na^+ gain** or a **water deficit**, the latter being much more common. Normally, this hyperosmolar state stimulates thirst and the excretion of a maximally concentrated urine. For hypernatremia to persist, one or both of these compensatory mechanisms must be impaired.
- **Impaired thirst response** may occur in situations where access to water is limited, often due to physical restrictions (institutionalized, handicapped, postoperative, or intubated patients) or mental impairment (delirium, dementia).
- **Hypernatremia due to water loss.** The loss of water must occur in excess of electrolyte losses in order to raise $[Na^+]$.
  - **Nonrenal water loss** may be due to evaporation from the skin and respiratory tract (insensible losses) or loss from the GI tract. Diarrhea is the most common GI cause of

hypernatremia. Osmotic diarrhea (induced by lactulose, sorbitol, or malabsorption of carbohydrate) and viral gastroenteritis, in particular, result in disproportional water loss.

○ **Renal water loss** results from either **osmotic diuresis** or **diabetes insipidus (DI)**.

■ **Osmotic diuresis** is frequently associated with glycosuria and high osmolar feeds. In addition, increased urea generation from accelerated catabolism, high-protein feeds, and stress-dose steroids can also result in an osmotic diuresis.

■ Hypernatremia secondary to nonosmotic urinary water loss is usually caused by impaired vasopressin secretion (**central diabetes insipidus [CDI]**) or resistance to the actions of vasopressin (**nephrogenic diabetes insipidus [NDI]**). Partial defects occur more commonly than complete defects in both types.

■ The most common cause of CDI is destruction of the neurohypophysis from trauma, neurosurgery, granulomatous disease, neoplasms, vascular accidents, or infection. In many cases, CDI is idiopathic.

■ NDI may either be inherited or acquired. The latter often results from a disruption to the renal concentrating mechanism due to drugs (lithium, demeclocycline, amphotericin), electrolyte disorders (hypercalcemia, hypokalemia), medullary washout (loop diuretics), and intrinsic renal diseases.

• **Hypernatremia due to primary Na$^+$ gain** occurs infrequently due to the kidney's capacity to excrete the retained Na$^+$. However, it can rarely occur after repetitive **hypertonic saline** administration or chronic **mineralocorticoid excess**.

• **Transcellular water shift** from ECF to ICF can occur in circumstances of transient intracellular hyperosmolality, as in seizures or rhabdomyolysis.

DIAGNOSIS

Clinical Presentation

• Hypernatremia results in contraction of brain cells as water shifts to attenuate the rising ECF osmolality. Thus, the most severe symptoms of hypernatremia are neurologic, including altered mental status, weakness, neuromuscular irritability, focal neurologic deficits, and, occasionally, coma or seizures. As with hyponatremia, the severity of the clinical manifestations is related to the *acuity* and *magnitude* of the rise in plasma [Na$^+$]. **Chronic hypernatremia** is generally less symptomatic as a result of adaptive mechanisms designed to defend cell volume.

• **CDI** and **NDI** generally present with complaints of polyuria and thirst. Signs of volume depletion or neurologic dysfunction are generally absent unless the patient has an associated thirst abnormality.

Diagnostic Testing

Urine osmolality and the **response to desmopressin acetate (DDAVP)** can help narrow the differential diagnosis for hypernatremia (Figure 12-2).

• The appropriate renal response to hypernatremia is a small volume of concentrated (urine osmolality >800 mOsm/L) urine. Submaximal **urine osmolality** (<800 mOsm/L) suggests a defect in renal water conservation.

○ A urine osmolality <300 mOsm/L in the setting of hypernatremia suggests complete forms of CDI and NDI.

○ Urine osmolality between 300–800 mOsm/L can occur from partial forms of DI as well as osmotic diuresis. The two can be differentiated by quantifying the daily solute excretion (estimated by the urine osmolality multiplied by urine volume in 24 hours). A daily solute excretion >900 mOsm/L defines an osmotic diuresis.

• **Response to DDAVP.** Complete forms of CDI and NDI can be distinguished by administering the vasopressin analog DDAVP (10 μg intranasally) after careful water restriction. The urine osmolality should increase by at least 50% in complete CDI and does not change in NDI. The diagnosis is sometimes difficult when partial defects are present.

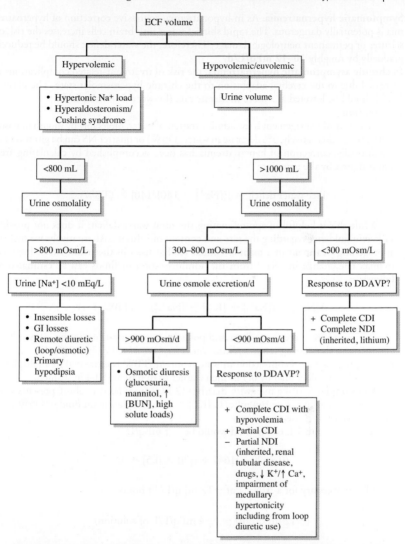

Figure 12-2. Algorithm depicting the diagnostic approach to hypernatremia. BUN, blood urea nitrogen; $\uparrow Ca^+$, hypercalcemia; CDI, central diabetes insipidus; DDAVP, desmopressin acetate; ECF, extracellular fluid; GI, gastrointestinal; NDI, nephrogenic diabetes insipidus; $\downarrow K^+$, hypokalemia; (+), conditions with increase in urine osmolality in response to desmopressin acetate; (−), conditions with little increase in urine osmolality in response to desmopressin acetate.

TREATMENT

- Management requires one to determine **the rate of correction**, **the appropriate intervention**, and **the presence of other underlying disorders**.
- The rate of correction of hypernatremia depends on the acuity of its development and the presence of neurologic dysfunction.

- **Symptomatic hypernatremia.** As in hyponatremia, aggressive correction of hypernatremia is potentially dangerous. The rapid shift of water into brain cells increases the risk of seizures or permanent neurologic damage. Therefore, the water deficit should be reduced gradually by roughly **10–12 mEq/L/d**.
- In **chronic asymptomatic hypernatremia**, the risk of treatment-related complications is increased due to the cerebral adaptation to the chronic hyperosmolar state. The plasma $[Na^+]$ should be lowered at a more moderate rate (between 5–8 mEq/L/d).
- **Intervention**
  ○ The mainstay of management is the administration of water, preferably by mouth or nasogastric tube. Alternatively, 5% dextrose in water (D5W) or quarter NS can be given via IV.
  ○ Traditionally, correction of hypernatremia has been accomplished by calculating **free water deficit** by the equation:

$$\text{Free water deficit} = \{([Na^+] - 140)/140\} \times (TBW)$$

While this is helpful in approximating the total water deficit, it does not provide sufficient guidance regarding the rate and content of infusate. Alternatively, we suggest approaching treatment in a manner similar to that used in the treatment of hyponatremia. The change in $[Na^+]$ from the administration of fluids can be estimated as follows:

$$\Delta[Na^+] = ([Na^+_i] + [K^+_i] - [Na^+_s]) \div (TBW + 1)$$

$[Na^+_i]$ and $[K^+_i]$ are the sodium and potassium concentrations in the infused fluid and $[Na^+_s]$ is the starting serum sodium (*Intensive Care Med 1997;23:309*). Because hypernatremia suggests a contraction in water content, TBW is estimated by multiplying lean weight (in kilograms) by 0.5 in men (rather than 0.6) and 0.4 in women.

An example: A 70-kg man with diarrhea (2 L/d) from laxative abuse presents with obtundation and $[Na^+] = 164$ mEq/L, $[K^+] = 3.0$. A replacement fluid of D5W with 20 mEq KCl/L is chosen.

- The $\Delta[Na^+]$ with 1 L of this fluid would be -4 mEq/L

$$(0 + 20 - 164) \div ([70 \times 0.5] + 1)$$

3 L are necessary for a $\Delta[Na^+]$ of -12 mEq/L/24 hours

$$(-12 \text{ mEq/L/d}) \div (-4 \text{ mEq/L/L of solution})$$

- The hourly rate of infusion is 125 mL/h (3 L/d ÷ 24 hours/day = 0.125 L/h). However, this should be followed closely because it does not account for ongoing GI or insensible losses, which may account for another 1.4 L/d of water required to keep $[Na^+]$ stable.
- **Specific therapies for the underlying cause**
  ○ **Hypovolemic hypernatremia.** In patients with mild volume depletion, Na^+-containing solutions, such as 0.45% NS, can be used to replenish the ECF as well as the water deficit. If patients have severe or symptomatic volume depletion, correction of volume status with **isotonic fluid** should take precedence over correction of the hyperosmolar state. Once the patient is hemodynamically stable, administration of hypotonic fluid can be given to replace the free water deficit.
  ○ **Hypernatremia from primary Na^+ gain** is unusual. Cessation of iatrogenic Na^+ is typically sufficient.

- ∘ **DI without hypernatremia.** DI is best treated by removing the underlying cause. Despite the renal water loss, DI should not result in hypernatremia if the thirst mechanism remains intact. Therefore, therapy, if required at all, is directed toward symptomatic polyuria.
  - ▪ **CDI.** Because the polyuria is the result of impaired secretion of vasopressin, treatment is best accomplished with the administration of DDAVP, a vasopressin analog.
  - ▪ **NDI.** A low-Na^+ diet combined with **thiazide** diuretics will decrease polyuria through inducing mild volume depletion. This enhances proximal reabsorption of salt and water, thus decreasing urinary free water loss. Decreasing protein intake will further decrease urine output by minimizing the solute load that must be excreted.

POTASSIUM

- Potassium is the major **intracellular** cation. Of the 3000–4000 mEq of K^+ found in the average human, 98% is sequestered within cells. Thus, although ECF [K^+] is normally 3.5–5.0 mEq/L, the intracellular concentration is roughly 150 mEq/L. This difference in ICF and ECF K^+ content is maintained by the **Na^+/K^+-adenosine triphosphatase pump**.
- The K^+ intake of individuals on an average Western diet is approximately 1 mEq/kg/d, 90% of which is absorbed by the GI tract. Maintenance of the steady state necessitates matching K^+ excretion with ingestion.
- The elimination of potassium occurs predominately through **renal excretion** at the distal nephron. K^+ secretion is enhanced by distal Na^+ reabsorption, which generates a **lumen-negative gradient** and **distal urine flow rate**.
- Renal potassium handling is responsive to **aldosterone**, which stimulates the expression of distal luminal Na^+ channels, and the **serum potassium concentration**. Aldosterone secretion is, in turn, responsive to angiotensin II and hyperkalemia.

Hypokalemia

GENERAL PRINCIPLES

- Hypokalemia is defined as a plasma [K^+] <3.5 mEq/L.
- **Spurious hypokalemia** may be seen in situations in which high numbers of metabolically active cells present in the blood sample absorb the ECF potassium.
- True hypokalemia may result from one or more of the following: (a) **decreased net intake**, (b) **shift into cells**, or (c) **increased net loss**.
  - ∘ **Diminished intake** is seldom the sole cause of K^+ depletion because urinary excretion can be effectively decreased to <15 mEq/d. However, dietary K^+ restriction may exacerbate the hypokalemia from GI or renal loss.
  - ∘ **Transcellular shift.** Movement of K^+ into cells may transiently decrease the plasma [K^+] without altering total body K^+ content. These shifts can result from alkalemia, insulin, and catecholamine release. **Periodic paralysis** is a rare disorder that predisposes patients to transcellular K^+ shifts that result in episodic muscle weakness. Both hyperkalemic and hypokalemic forms have been described and can be triggered after strenuous exercise. Unlike the hyperkalemic form, the hypokalemic form can be triggered after a carbohydrate-rich meal. In the hyperkalemic form, the potassium levels are usually mildly elevated during an attack. In both forms, a later onset proximal myopathy develops, most commonly affecting the pelvic girdle and the lower extremities.
  - ∘ **Nonrenal K^+ loss.** Hypokalemia may result from the loss of potassium-rich fluids from the lower GI tract. Hypokalemia from the loss of upper GI contents is typically more attributable to renal K^+ secretion from secondary hyperaldosteronism. Rarely, in excessive sweating, loss of K^+ through the integument can provoke hypokalemia.

- ○ **Renal K⁺ loss** accounts for most cases of *chronic* hypokalemia. This may be caused by factors that increase the lumen-negative gradient, thus enhancing K^+ secretion, or that augment distal urine flow rate.
  - **Augmented distal urine flow** occurs commonly with diuretic use and osmotic diuresis (e.g., glycosuria). Bartter and Gitelman syndromes mimic diuretic use and promote renal K^+ loss by the same mechanism.
  - A variety of disorders promote K^+ loss by increasing the **lumen-negative gradient**, which drives K^+ secretion. This can be achieved with the reabsorption of a cation (Na^+) or presence of a nonreabsorbed anion.
    - □ Distal Na^+ reabsorption is largely influenced by mineralocorticoid activity.
    - □ **Primary mineralocorticoid excess** can be seen in primary hyperaldosteronism due to an adrenal adenoma or adrenocortical hyperplasia.
    - □ Cortisol also has an affinity for mineralocorticoid receptors but is typically converted quickly to cortisone, which has markedly less mineralocorticoid activity. Still, if cortisol is present in abundance (Cushing syndrome) or fails to be converted to cortisone (syndrome of mineralocorticoid excess), it may mimic hyperaldosteronism.
    - □ **Secondary hyperaldosteronism** can be seen in any situation with a decreased effective circulating volume.
    - □ Constitutive activation of the distal renal epithelial Na^+ channel, independent of aldosterone, occurs in **Liddle syndrome**.
  - Increased distal delivery of a nonreabsorbable anion can also potentiate the lumen-negative gradient that drives K^+ secretion. Examples include bicarbonate (metabolic alkalosis or type 2 renal tubular acidosis [RTA]), ketones, and hippurate (from toluene intoxication or glue sniffing).

DIAGNOSIS

Clinical Presentation

- The clinical features of K^+ depletion vary greatly, and their severity depends in part on the degree of hypokalemia. Symptoms seldom occur unless the plasma $[K^+]$ is <3.0 mEq/L.
- Fatigue, myalgias, and muscular weakness or cramps of the lower extremities are common. Smooth muscle function may also be affected and may manifest with complaints of constipation or frank paralytic ileus. Severe hypokalemia may lead to complete paralysis, hypoventilation, or rhabdomyolysis.

Diagnostic Testing

When the etiology is not immediately apparent, **renal K⁺ excretion** and the **acid–base status** can help identify the cause.

- **Urine K⁺.** The appropriate response to hypokalemia is to excrete <25 mEq/d of K^+ in the urine. Urinary K^+ excretion can be measured with a 24-hour urine collection or estimated by multiplying the spot urine $[K^+]$ by the total daily urine output. A spot urine $[K^+]$ may be helpful (urine $[K^+]$ <15 mEq/L suggests appropriate K^+ conservation), but the results can be confounded by a variety of factors. Alternatively, the transtubular potassium gradient (TTKG), which estimates the potassium gradient between the urine and blood in the distal nephron, can be calculated as follows:

$$\text{TTKG} = (\text{Urine } K^+/\text{Serum } K^+) \div (\text{Urine Osmolality/Serum Osmolality})$$

A TTKG <2 suggests a nonrenal source, whereas a TTKG >4 suggests inappropriate renal K^+ secretion.

- **Acid–base status.** Intracellular shifting and renal excretion of K^+ are often closely linked with the acid–base status. Hypokalemia is generally associated with metabolic alkalosis and can play a critical role in the maintenance of metabolic alkalosis. The finding of metabolic acidosis in a patient with hypokalemia thus narrows the differential significantly, implying lower GI loss, distal RTA, or the excretion of a nonreabsorbable anion from an organic acid (diabetic ketoacidosis [DKA], hippurate from toluene intoxication).

• **ECG** changes associated with hypokalemia include flattening or inversion of the T wave, a prominent U wave, ST-segment depression, and a prolonged QU interval. Severe K^+ depletion may result in a prolonged PR interval, decreased voltage, and widening of the QRS complex.

TREATMENT

The **therapeutic goals** are to safely correct the K^+ deficit and to minimize ongoing losses through treatment of the underlying cause. Hypomagnesemia should also be sought in all hypokalemic patients and corrected to allow effective K^+ repletion.

• Correction of the K^+ deficit can be accomplished with either oral or IV therapy.

• **Oral therapy.** It is generally safer to correct the K^+ deficit via the oral route when hypokalemia is mild and the patient can tolerate oral administration. Oral doses of 40 mEq are generally well tolerated and can be given as often as every 4 hours. Traditionally, 10 mEq of potassium salts are given for each 0.10 mEq/L decrement in serum $[K^+]$. However, with increasing severity of hypokalemia, this grossly underestimates the K^+ necessary to normalize *total* K^+ content. Furthermore, as the K^+ shifts back to the intracellular space, it may appear as though K^+ supplementation is doing very little to correct ECF $[K^+]$. In such cases, potassium supplementation should be increased and continued until serum levels rise.

• **IV therapy.** Patients with imminently life-threatening hypokalemia and those who are unable to take anything by mouth require IV replacement therapy with KCl. The maximum concentration of administered K^+ should be no more than 40 mEq/L via a peripheral vein or 100 mEq/L via a central vein. The rate of infusion should not exceed 20 mEq/h unless paralysis or malignant ventricular arrhythmias are present. Ideally, KCl should be mixed in NS because dextrose solutions may initially exacerbate hypokalemia (as a result of insulin-mediated movement of K^+). Rapid IV administration of K^+ should be used judiciously and requires close observation.

Hyperkalemia

GENERAL PRINCIPLES

• Hyperkalemia is defined as a plasma $[K^+]$ **>5.0 mEq/L**.

• **Pseudohyperkalemia** represents an artificially elevated plasma $[K^+]$ due to K^+ movement out of cells immediately before or following venipuncture. Contributing factors include repeated fist clenching, hemolysis, and marked leukocytosis or thrombocytosis.

• True hyperkalemia occurs as a result of (a) **transcellular shift**, (b) **increased exposure to K^+**, and most commonly, (c) **decreased renal K^+ excretion**. Combinations of these mechanisms often underlie cases of hyperkalemia in clinical practice, and decreased renal excretion is nearly always some component of the pathophysiology.

  ○ **Transcellular shift.** Insulin deficiency, hyperosmolality, nonselective β-blockers, digitalis, metabolic acidosis (excluding those from organic acids), and depolarizing muscle relaxants, such as succinylcholine, release K^+ from predominate ICF stores into the ECF compartment. Exercise-induced hyperkalemia results from release of K^+ from muscles. Familial periodic paralysis, mentioned previously, is a rare cause of hyperkalemia. Massive cellular destruction, as seen in tumor lysis syndrome, also liberates cellular K^+ stores and releases them into the ECF.

  ○ **Increased exposure to K^+** is rarely the sole cause of hyperkalemia unless there is an impairment in renal excretion. Foods with a high content of K^+ include salt substitutes, dried fruits, nuts, tomatoes, potatoes, spinach, bananas, and oranges. Juices derived from these foods may be especially rich sources.

○ **Decreased renal K^+ excretion.** In the setting of hyperkalemia, the kidney is capable of generating a significant urinary excretion of K^+. This process can be impaired by a number of processes, including intrinsic renal disease, decreased delivery of filtrate to the distal nephron, adrenal insufficiency, and hyporeninemic hypoaldosteronism (type 4 RTA).

• **Drugs** may also be implicated in the genesis of hyperkalemia through a variety of mechanisms. Common culprits include angiotensin-converting enzyme inhibitors, angiotensin receptor blockers, potassium-sparing diuretics, NSAIDs, and cyclosporine. Heparin and ketoconazole can also contribute to hyperkalemia through the decreased production of aldosterone, although these agents alone are typically insufficient to sustain a clinically significant hyperkalemia.

DIAGNOSIS

Clinical Presentation

• The most serious effect of hyperkalemia is cardiac arrhythmogenesis secondary to potassium's pivotal role in membrane potentials. Patients may present with palpitations, syncope, or even sudden cardiac death.

• Severe hyperkalemia causes partial depolarization of the skeletal muscle cell membrane and may manifest as weakness, potentially progressing to flaccid paralysis and hypoventilation if the respiratory muscles are involved.

Diagnostic Testing

• If the etiology is not readily apparent and the patient is asymptomatic, **pseudohyperkalemia** should be excluded by rechecking laboratory data.

• An assessment of **renal $[K^+]$ excretion** and the **renin–angiotensin–aldosterone axis** can help narrow the differential diagnosis when the etiology is not immediately apparent.

○ Low aldosterone levels suggest either adrenal disease (renin levels elevated) or hyporeninemic hypoaldosteronism (renin levels low; occurs with type 4 RTA as well as chloride shunting or Gordon syndrome).

○ High aldosterone levels, typically accompanied by high renin levels, suggest aldosterone resistance (pseudohypoaldosteronism) but can also be seen in K^+-sparing diuretics.

• **ECG** changes include increased T-wave amplitude or peaked T waves. More severe degrees of hyperkalemia result in a prolonged PR interval and QRS duration, atrioventricular conduction delay, and loss of P waves. Progressive widening of the QRS complex and its merging with the T wave produce a sine wave pattern. The terminal event is usually ventricular fibrillation or asystole.

TREATMENT

Severe hyperkalemia with ECG changes is a medical emergency and requires immediate treatment directed at minimizing membrane depolarization and acutely reducing the ECF $[K^+]$. **Acute therapy** may consist of some or all of the following (the hypokalemic effect is additive).

• **Calcium gluconate** decreases membrane excitability but does not lower $[K^+]$. The usual dose is 10 mL of a 10% solution infused over 2–3 minutes. The effect begins within minutes but is short lived (30–60 minutes), and the dose can be repeated if no improvement in the ECG is seen after 5–10 minutes.

• **Insulin** causes K^+ to shift into cells and temporarily lowers the plasma $[K^+]$. A commonly used combination is 10–20 units of regular insulin and 25–50 g of glucose administered IV. Hyperglycemic patients should be given the insulin alone.

- **NaHCO₃** is effective for severe hyperkalemia associated with metabolic acidosis. In the acute setting, it can be given as an IV isotonic solution (three ampules of NaHCO₃ in 1 L of 5% dextrose).
- **β₂-Adrenergic agonists** promote cellular uptake of K⁺. The onset of action is 30 minutes, lowering the plasma [K⁺] by 0.5–1.5 mEq/L, and the effect lasts for 2–4 hours. Albuterol can be administered in a dose of 10–20 mg as a continuous nebulized treatment over 30–60 minutes.
- **Longer term** means for [K⁺] removal.
  ○ Increasing distal Na⁺ delivery in the kidney enhances renal K⁺ clearance. This can be achieved with the administration of saline in patients who appear volume depleted. Otherwise, diuretics can be used if renal function is adequate.
  ○ **Cation exchange resins**, such as sodium polystyrene sulfonate (Kayexalate), promote the exchange of Na⁺ for K⁺ in the GI tract. When given by mouth, the usual dose is 25–50 g mixed with 100 mL 20% sorbitol to prevent constipation. This generally lowers the plasma [K⁺] by 0.5–1.0 mEq/L within 1–2 hours and lasts for 4–6 hours. Sodium polystyrene sulfonate can also be administered as a retention enema consisting of 50 g resin in 150 mL tap water. Enemas should be avoided in postoperative patients because of the increased incidence of colonic necrosis, especially following renal transplantation. Newer agents such as sodium zirconium cyclosilicate are being studied and have shown improved safety profiles in preliminary studies.
- **Dialysis** should be reserved for patients with renal failure and those with severe life-threatening hyperkalemia who are unresponsive to more conservative measures.
- **Chronic therapy** may involve dietary modifications to avoid high K⁺ foods (see Potassium, Hyperkalemia, Etiology section), correction of metabolic acidosis with oral alkali, the promotion of kaliuresis with diuretics, and/or administration of exogenous mineralocorticoid in states of hypoaldosteronism.

CALCIUM

- Calcium is essential for bone formation and neuromuscular function.
- Approximately 99% of body calcium is in bone; most of the remaining 1% is in the ECF. Nearly 50% of serum calcium is ionized (free), whereas the remainder is complexed to albumin (40%) and anions such as phosphate (10%).
- **Calcium balance** is regulated by **parathyroid hormone** (PTH) and **calcitriol**.
  ○ **PTH** increases serum calcium by stimulating bone resorption, increasing calcium reclamation in the kidney, and promoting renal conversion of vitamin D to calcitriol. Serum calcium regulates PTH secretion by a negative feedback mechanism: Hypocalcemia stimulates and hypercalcemia suppresses PTH release.
  ○ **Calcitriol** [1,25-dihydroxycholecalciferol, 1,25-dihydroxyvitamin D₃, or 1,25(OH)₂D₃] is the active form of vitamin D. It stimulates intestinal absorption of calcium and is one of many factors that provide feedback to the parathyroid gland.

Hypercalcemia

GENERAL PRINCIPLES

- A serum calcium **>10.3 mg/dL** with a normal serum albumin or an ionized calcium **>5.2 mg/dL** defines hypercalcemia.
- Clinically significant hypercalcemia typically requires both an increase in ECF calcium and a decrease in renal calcium clearance. Underlying disturbances to calcium metabolism are thus often masked by compensatory mechanisms until the patient develops a

concomitant disorder, such as decreased renal clearance from volume depletion. More than 90% of cases are due to **primary hyperparathyroidism** or **malignancy**.

- **Primary hyperparathyroidism** causes most cases of hypercalcemia in *ambulatory* patients. It is a common disorder, especially in elderly women, in whom the annual incidence is approximately 2 in 1000. Nearly 85% of cases are due to an **adenoma** of a single gland, 15% to **hyperplasia** of all four glands, and 1% to **parathyroid carcinoma**.
- **Malignancy** is responsible for most cases of hypercalcemia among *hospitalized* patients. Patients usually have advanced, clinically obvious disease. In these patients, hypercalcemia may develop from stimulation of osteoclast bone resorption from tumor cell products, tumor derived **PTH-related peptides** (PTHrPs), and tumor calcitriol production.
- Less common causes account for about 10% of cases of hypercalcemia:
  ○ **Increased vitamin D activity** occurs with exogenous exposure to vitamin D or increased generation of calcitriol in chronic granulomatous diseases (e.g., sarcoidosis, tuberculosis).
  ○ The **milk-alkali syndrome** describes the acute or chronic development of hypercalcemia, alkalosis, and renal failure that may result from the ingestion of large quantities of calcium-containing antacids.
  ○ **Other.** Hyperthyroidism, adrenal insufficiency, prolonged immobilization, Paget disease, and acromegaly may be associated with hypercalcemia. **Familial hypocalciuric hypercalcemia** is a rare, autosomal dominant disorder of the calcium-sensing receptor, which is characterized by asymptomatic hypercalcemia from childhood and a family history of hypercalcemia.

DIAGNOSIS

Clinical Presentation

Clinical manifestations generally are present only if serum calcium exceeds 12 mg/dL and tend to be more severe if hypercalcemia develops rapidly. Most patients with **primary hyperparathyroidism** have asymptomatic hypercalcemia that is found incidentally.

- Renal manifestations include polyuria and nephrolithiasis. If serum calcium rises above 13 mg/dL, renal failure with nephrocalcinosis and ectopic soft tissue calcifications are possible.
- GI symptoms include anorexia, vomiting, constipation, and rarely, signs of pancreatitis.
- Neurologic findings include weakness, fatigue, confusion, stupor, and coma.
- Osteopenia and frequent fractures may occur from the disproportional resorption of bone in hyperparathyroidism. Rarely, **osteitis fibrosa cystica** can develop when hyperparathyroidism is profound and prolonged, resulting in "brown tumors" and marrow replacement.

Diagnostic Testing

- The history and physical examination should focus on (a) the duration of symptoms of hypercalcemia, (b) clinical evidence of any of the unusual causes of hypercalcemia, and (c) symptoms and signs of malignancy (which almost always precede **malignant hypercalcemia**). If hypercalcemia has been present for more than 6 months without an obvious etiology, primary hyperparathyroidism is almost certainly the cause.
- **Serum calcium** should be interpreted with knowledge of the serum albumin, or an ionized calcium should be measured. **Corrected $[Ca^{2+}]$** = $[Ca^{2+}]$ + {0.8 × (4.0 − [albumin])}. Many patients with primary hyperparathyroidism will have a calcium level that is chronically within the high-normal range.
- Intact **serum PTH** should be measured, because these assays are independent of renal function.
  ○ Elevations in ECF calcium typically result in suppression of PTH. Thus, the finding of a normal or elevated intact PTH in the setting of hypercalcemia is suggestive of primary hyperparathyroidism.

- ○ When the intact PTH is appropriately suppressed, **PTHrP** can be measured to investigate possible humoral hypercalcemia of malignancy.
- **1,25(OH)$_2$D$_3$** levels are elevated in granulomatous disorders, primary hyperparathyroidism, calcitriol overdose, and acromegaly. **25(OH)D$_3$** levels are elevated with noncalcitriol vitamin D intoxication.
- **Serum phosphorus** is often decreased in hyperparathyroidism due to stimulation of phosphaturia, whereas Paget disease and vitamin D intoxication both tend to have increased phosphorus levels.
- **Urine calcium** may be elevated in primary hyperparathyroidism due to a filtered load of calcium that exceeds the capacity for renal reabsorption. If the family history and clinical picture are suggestive, patients with **familial hypocalciuric hypercalcemia** can be distinguished from patients with primary hyperparathyroidism by documenting a low calcium clearance by 24-hour urine collection (<200 mg calcium per day) or fractional excretion of calcium (<1%).
- **ECG** may reveal a shortened QT interval and, with very severe hypercalcemia, variable degrees of atrioventricular block.

TREATMENT

- **Acute management** of hypercalcemia is warranted if severe symptoms are present or with serum calcium >12 mg/dL. The following regimen is presented in the order that therapy should be given.
  - ○ **Correction of hypovolemia** with 0.9% saline fluid is mandatory in patients who demonstrate volume depletion, because hypovolemia prevents effective calciuresis. Maintenance fluids can be continued after achieving euvolemia to sustain a urine output of 100–150 mL/h. The patient should be monitored closely for signs of volume overload.
  - ○ **Loop diuretics** can be used if signs of volume overload limit further saline administration while hypercalcemia persists. These agents reduce paracellular reabsorption of calcium in the loop of Henle and thus may slightly enhance calcium excretion. They should not be used in euvolemic or hypovolemic patients because they may further contract the ECF volume and prevent adequate restoration of the volume status.
  - ○ **IV bisphosphonates** can be used to decrease the liberation of calcium from bone in persistent hypercalcemia. Pamidronate 60 mg is infused over 2–4 hours; for severe hypercalcemia (>13.5 mg/dL), 90 mg can be given over the same duration. A hypocalcemic response is typically seen within 2 days and may persist for 2 weeks or longer. Treatment can be repeated after 7 days if hypercalcemia recurs. Zoledronate is a more potent bisphosphonate that is given as a 4-mg dose infused over at least 15 minutes. Hydration should precede bisphosphonate use. Renal insufficiency is a relative contraindication.
- Other options
  - ○ **Calcitonin** inhibits bone resorption and increases renal calcium excretion. Salmon calcitonin, 4–8 IU/kg IM or SC q6–12h, lowers serum calcium 1–2 mg/dL within several hours in 60–70% of patients. Although it is less potent than other inhibitors of bone resorption, it has no serious toxicity, is safe in renal failure, and may have an analgesic effect in patients with skeletal metastases.
  - ○ **Glucocorticoids** are effective in hypercalcemia due to hematologic malignancies and granulomatous production of calcitriol. The initial dose is 20–60 mg/d of prednisone or its equivalent. After serum calcium stabilizes, the dose should be gradually reduced to the minimum needed to control symptoms of hypercalcemia. Toxicity (see Chapter 25, Arthritis and Rheumatologic Diseases) limits the usefulness of glucocorticoids for long-term therapy.
  - ○ **Gallium nitrate** inhibits bone resorption as effectively as the IV bisphosphonates and has a similar delayed onset of 2 days. It is given as a 100- to 200-mg/m^2/d continuous infusion for up to 5 days, unless normocalcemia is achieved sooner. There is, however,

a significant risk of nephrotoxicity, and it is contraindicated if the serum creatinine is >2.5 mg/dL.

○ **Dialysis.** Hemodialysis and peritoneal dialysis using low calcium dialysate are effective for patients with very severe hypercalcemia (>16 mg/dL) and CHF or renal insufficiency.

• **Chronic management** of hypercalcemia

○ **Primary hyperparathyroidism.** In many patients, this disorder has a benign course, with minimal fluctuation in serum calcium concentration and no obvious clinical sequelae. Parathyroidectomy is indicated in patients with (a) corrected serum calcium >1.0 mg/dL above the upper limit of normal, (b) creatinine clearance <60 mL/min, (c) age <50 years, and (d) bone density at hip, lumbar spine, or distal radius >2.5 standard deviations below peak bone mass (T score <−2.5) and/or previous fragility fracture (*J Clin Endocrinol Metab 2009;94:335*). Surgical intervention typically has a high success rate (95%) with low morbidity and mortality.

○ **Medical therapy** may be a reasonable option in asymptomatic patients who are not surgical candidates. Management consists of liberal oral hydration with a high-salt diet, daily physical activity to lessen bone resorption, and avoidance of thiazide diuretics. Oral bisphosphonates and estrogen replacement therapy or raloxifene in postmenopausal women can be considered in the appropriate clinical context. Cinacalcet, an activator of the calcium-sensing receptor, has also been shown to reduce PTH secretion and serum calcium levels.

○ **Malignant hypercalcemia.** Bisphosphonate and glucocorticoid therapy with a calcium-restricted diet (<400 mg/d) can be tried, although these maneuvers rarely yield long-term success unless the malignancy responds to treatment. **Denosumab** may be used in patients with persistent hypercalcemia of malignancy in whom bisphosphonates may be contraindicated due to renal failure. It is given at a dose of 120 mg SC weekly for 4 weeks and then monthly.

Hypocalcemia

GENERAL PRINCIPLES

• A serum calcium **<8.4 mg/dL** with a normal serum albumin or an ionized calcium **<4.2 mg/dL** defines hypocalcemia.

• **Pseudohypocalcemia** describes the situation in which the total calcium is reduced due to hypoalbuminemia, but the **corrected [Ca^{2+}]** (see Calcium, Hypercalcemia, Diagnostic Testing section) and ionized calcium remain within the normal ranges.

• **Effective hypoparathyroidism.** Reduced PTH activity can result from decreased PTH release from autoimmune, infiltrative, or iatrogenic (e.g., postthyroidectomy) destruction of parathyroid tissue. In rare patients, hypoparathyroidism is congenital, as in DiGeorge syndrome or **familial hypocalcemia**. Release of PTH is also impaired with both hypomagnesemia (<1 mg/dL) and severe hypermagnesemia (>6 mg/dL).

• **Vitamin D deficiency** lowers total body calcium but does not usually affect serum calcium levels unless the deficiency is severe, because the resultant secondary hyperparathyroidism often corrects serum calcium levels. Significant vitamin D deficiency can occur in the elderly or those with limited sun exposure, in advanced liver disease (due to decreased synthesis of precursors), and in nephrotic syndrome. Reduced activity in vitamin D activation via 1-α-hydroxylase activity can be seen with vitamin D–dependent rickets and chronic renal insufficiency.

• Serum calcium levels may also be reduced by profound elevations in serum phosphorus, which binds with the calcium and deposits in a variety of tissues. Calcium can also be bound by citrate (during transfusion of citrate-containing blood products or with continual renal replacement using citrate anticoagulation) as well as by drugs such as foscarnet

and fluoroquinolones. Increased binding to albumin can also be seen in the context of alkalemia, which increases the exposure of negatively charged binding sites on albumin.
- **Other.** A low serum free calcium level is common in critically ill patients perhaps due to a cytokine-mediated decrease in PTH and calcitriol release with target organ resistance to their effects.

DIAGNOSIS

Clinical Presentation

- Clinical manifestations vary with the degree of hypocalcemia and rate of onset.
- Acute, severe hypocalcemia may cause laryngospasm, confusion, seizures, or vascular collapse with bradycardia and decompensated heart failure.
- Acute, moderate hypocalcemia may cause increased excitability of nerves and muscles, leading to circumoral or distal paresthesias and tetany.
- **Trousseau sign** is the development of carpal spasm when a blood pressure cuff is inflated above systolic pressure for 3 minutes. **Chvostek sign** refers to twitching of the facial muscles when the facial nerve is tapped anterior to the ear. The presence of these signs is known as **latent tetany**.
- Clues to the diagnosis may be provided by a bedside evaluation for (a) previous neck surgery (postoperative hypoparathyroidism), (b) systemic diseases (autoimmune, infiltrative disorders), (c) family history of hypocalcemia, (d) drug-induced hypocalcemia, and (e) conditions associated with vitamin D deficiency (e.g., uremia).

Diagnostic Testing

- Laboratory data should be used to evaluate the calcium–PTH axis as well as concurrent mineral abnormalities.
- **Albumin** should be measured any time there is an abnormality in serum calcium levels to rule out pseudohypocalcemia. As mentioned previously, calcium can be corrected by adding {0.8 × (4 − [albumin])} to the total serum calcium level.
- **Serum PTH** that is low or inappropriately normal in the setting of hypocalcemia is indicative of hypoparathyroidism. A high PTH is often found with vitamin D deficiency, PTH resistance, and hyperphosphatemia.
- **Serum phosphorus** is often helpful in identifying vitamin D deficiency (low calcium, low phosphorus) or intravascular chelation of calcium (low calcium, high phosphorus).
- **Vitamin D** stores are usually assessed by measuring only $25(OH)D_3$ because calcitriol $[1,25(OH)_2D_3]$ levels can be normalized through the compensatory increase of 1-α-hydroxylase activity.
- **Magnesium** deficiency should always be ruled out during management of hypocalcemia.
- **ECG** may show a prolonged QT interval and bradycardia.

TREATMENT

Acute management of symptomatic hypocalcemia requires prompt and aggressive therapy.
- **Phosphorus** must first be checked. In severe hyperphosphatemia (>6.5 mg/dL), administration of calcium will increase the calcium–phosphorus product and may exacerbate the formation of ectopic calcifications. In acute, symptomatic hypocalcemia with severe hyperphosphatemia, dialysis may be needed to acutely manage the mineral abnormalities. If the hypocalcemia is asymptomatic, a reduction of phosphorus should precede aggressive calcium supplementation.
- **Hypomagnesemia**, if present, must be treated first in order to effectively correct the hypocalcemia. Two grams of magnesium sulfate can be given IV over 15 minutes followed by an infusion (see Magnesium, Hypomagnesemia, Treatment section) and may even be given empirically if renal failure is not present.

- **Calcium supplementation.** IV calcium should be reserved for severe or symptomatic hypocalcemia and can be administered as calcium chloride or calcium gluconate. Calcium gluconate is typically favored due to reduced risk of tissue toxicity with extravasation. Calcium gluconate is often prepared as a 10% solution (100 mg of calcium gluconate per mL). One ampule (10 mL) of calcium gluconate thus contains 1000 mg of calcium gluconate and approximately 90 mg of elemental calcium.
  - When necessary to treat severe or symptomatic hypocalcemia, an initial dose of 90–180 mg of elemental calcium can be achieved with 1–2 g of **calcium gluconate** (equal to 10–20 mL or one to two ampules of 10% calcium gluconate) mixed in 50–100 mL of D5W administered over 10–20 minutes.
  - The effect of initial treatment is only *transient*, and maintenance of calcium levels typically requires a continuous infusion of 0.5–1.5 mg/kg/h of elemental calcium. A solution comprised of 1 L D5W with 100 mL of 10% calcium gluconate contains approximately 900 mg of elemental calcium per liter, approximating 1 mg of elemental calcium per milliliter of fluid. Infusion is typically begun at a rate of 50 mL/h (approximately 50 mg of elemental calcium per hour) and titrated up as needed.
- **Chronic management.** Treatment requires calcium supplements and vitamin D or its active metabolite to increase intestinal calcium absorption.
  - **Oral calcium supplements.** Calcium carbonate (40% elemental calcium) or calcium acetate (25% elemental calcium) can be given with the goal administration of 1–2 g of *elemental* calcium PO tid. Calcium supplementation should be given apart from meals to minimize binding with phosphorus and maximize enteric absorption. Serum levels should be checked once to twice per week to guide ongoing therapy.
  - **Vitamin D.** Simple dietary deficiency can be corrected by the use of ergocalciferol 400–1000 IU/d. However, in conjunction with other hypocalcemic disorders, larger doses may be required. A 6- to 8-week regimen of 50,000 IU should be dosed weekly in those with underlying impairments in vitamin D metabolism (i.e., renal insufficiency) and daily in patients with severe malnutrition or malabsorption.
  - In comparison, **calcitriol** has a much more rapid onset of action. The initial dosage is 0.25 μg daily, and most patients are maintained on 0.5–2.0 μg daily. The dose can be increased at 2- to 4-week intervals. Because calcitriol increases enteric absorption of phosphorus as well as calcium, phosphorus levels should be monitored and oral phosphate binders initiated if phosphorus exceeds the normal range.

COMPLICATIONS

Development of hypercalcemia. In the event that hypercalcemia develops, vitamin D and calcium supplements should be stopped. Once serum calcium falls to normal, both forms of supplementation should be restarted at lower doses. Hypercalcemia due to calcitriol usually resolves within 1 week.

PHOSPHORUS

- Phosphorus is critical for bone formation and cellular energy metabolism.
- Approximately 85% of **total body phosphorus** is in bone, and most of the remainder is within cells. Thus, serum phosphorus levels may not reflect total body phosphorus stores.
- **Phosphorus balance** is determined primarily by four factors:
  - **PTH** regulates the incorporation and release of minerals from bone stores and decreases proximal tubular reabsorption of phosphate, causing urinary wasting.
  - The **phosphate concentration** itself regulates renal proximal reabsorption.

○ **Insulin** lowers serum levels by shifting phosphate into cells.
○ **Calcitriol** [1,25(OH)$_2$D$_3$] increases serum phosphate by enhancing intestinal phosphorus absorption.

Hyperphosphatemia

GENERAL PRINCIPLES

- A serum phosphate **>4.5 mg/dL** defines hyperphosphatemia.
- **Hyperphosphatemia** is caused by (a) **transcellular shift**, (b) **increased intake**, and most commonly, (c) **decreased renal excretion**. In clinical practice, renal insufficiency is usually present and serves as the major predisposing factor toward the development of hyperphosphatemia.
- **Transcellular shift** occurs in rhabdomyolysis, tumor lysis syndrome, and massive hemolysis as phosphorus is released from cells into the ECF. Metabolic acidosis and hypoinsulinemia reduce phosphorus flux into cells and contribute to the hyperphosphatemia sometimes seen in DKA.
- **Increased intake** leading to hyperphosphatemia usually occurs in the setting of renal insufficiency, either with dietary indiscretion in chronic kidney disease or as an iatrogenic complication. The latter can be seen when Phospho-Soda enemas (e.g., Fleet) or active vitamin D analogs are given to patients with renal insufficiency.
- **Decreased renal excretion** occurs most commonly in the setting of renal failure. Occasionally, hypoparathyroidism and pseudohypoparathyroidism reduce renal phosphorus clearance as well.

DIAGNOSIS

Clinical Presentation

- Signs and symptoms are typically attributable to hypocalcemia and the metastatic calcification of soft tissues. Occasionally, skin deposition can result in severe pruritus. **Calciphylaxis** describes the tissue ischemia that may result from the calcification of smaller blood vessels and their subsequent thrombosis.
- Chronic hyperphosphatemia contributes to the development of renal osteodystrophy (see Chapter 13, Renal Diseases).

Diagnostic Testing

The elevated serum phosphorus can be accompanied by hypocalcemia as a result of **intravascular chelation** of calcium by phosphorus.

TREATMENT

- **Acute hyperphosphatemia** is treated by increasing renal excretion of phosphorus, and as such, treatment is limited when renal insufficiency is present.
  ○ **Recovery of renal function** will often correct the hyperphosphatemia in the patient within 12 hours. Saline and/or acetazolamide (15 mg/kg q4h) can be given to further encourage phosphaturia, if needed.
  ○ **Hemodialysis** may be required, especially if irreversible renal insufficiency or symptomatic hypocalcemia is present.
- **Chronic hyperphosphatemia** is almost always associated with chronic kidney disease. Its management consists of reducing phosphorus intake through dietary modification and the use of phosphate binders. This is discussed more fully in Chapter 13, Renal Diseases.

Hypophosphatemia

GENERAL PRINCIPLES

- A serum phosphate **<2.8 mg/dL** defines hypophosphatemia.
- Hypophosphatemia may be caused by (a) **impaired intestinal absorption**, (b) **increased renal excretion**, or (c) **transcellular shift** into cells. Often, there are several mechanisms that work in concert to lower serum phosphate.
  - **Impaired intestinal absorption** occurs with the malabsorption syndromes, the use of oral phosphate binders, or vitamin D deficiency from any cause (see Calcium, Hypocalcemia, Etiology section). Chronic alcoholism is often associated with poor intake of both phosphate and vitamin D, resulting in total body phosphorus depletion.
  - **Increased renal excretion** occurs with high levels of PTH, as seen in hyperparathyroidism. This can be particularly pronounced in patients with secondary or tertiary hyperparathyroidism who undergo renal transplantation, because the high PTH causes a profound phosphaturic effect on the functional allograft. Hypophosphatemia may also occur from osmotic diuresis and disorders of proximal tubular transport such as familial X-linked hypophosphatemic rickets and Fanconi syndrome.
  - **Transcellular shift** is stimulated by respiratory alkalosis as well as insulin. The latter is responsible for the paradoxical reduction in phosphorus during treatment of malnutrition with hyperalimentation (the refeeding syndrome). The endogenous increase in insulin during treatment shifts phosphorus intracellularly, further reducing serum phosphorus in the malnourished individual. Phosphorus can also be rapidly absorbed into bone following parathyroidectomy for severe hyperparathyroidism (hungry bone syndrome).

DIAGNOSIS

Clinical Presentation

Signs and symptoms typically occur only if total body phosphate depletion is present and the serum phosphorus level is <1 mg/dL. These end-organ effects are due to the inability to form adenosine triphosphate and the impaired tissue oxygen delivery that occurs with a decrease in red blood cell 2,3-diphosphoglycerate. These include muscle injury (rhabdomyolysis, impaired diaphragmatic function, and heart failure), neurologic abnormalities (paresthesias, dysarthria, confusion, stupor, seizures, and coma), and rarely, hemolysis and platelet dysfunction.

Diagnostic Testing

- The cause is usually apparent from the clinical situation in which the hypophosphatemia occurs. If not, measurement of **urine phosphorus excretion** helps define the mechanism. Renal excretion of >100 mg by 24-hour urine collection or a fractional excretion of phosphate >5% during hypophosphatemia indicates excessive renal loss.
- Low serum **25(OH)D$_3$** suggests dietary vitamin D deficiency or malabsorption. An elevated **intact PTH** may occur in primary or secondary hyperparathyroidism.

TREATMENT

- **Acute moderate hypophosphatemia** (1.0–2.5 mg/dL) is common in the hospitalized patient and is often due simply to **transcellular shifts**, requiring no treatment if asymptomatic, except correction of the underlying cause.
- **Acute severe hypophosphatemia** (<1.0 mg/dL) may require IV phosphate therapy when associated with serious clinical manifestations. IV preparations include potassium

phosphate (1.5 mEq potassium/mmol phosphate) and sodium phosphate (1.3 mEq sodium/mmol phosphate).

- ○ An infusion of phosphate, 0.08–0.16 mmol/kg in 500 mL 0.45% saline, is given via IV over 6 hours (1 mmol phosphate = 31 mg phosphorus). IV repletion should be stopped when the serum phosphorus level is >1.5 mg/dL and when the patient can tolerate oral therapy. Because of the need to replenish intracellular stores, 24–36 hours of phosphate administration may be required.
- ○ Extreme care must be used to avoid hyperphosphatemia, which may lead to hypocalcemia. If hypotension occurs, acute hypocalcemia should be suspected, and the infusion should be stopped or slowed. Further doses should be based on symptoms and on the serum calcium and phosphorus levels, which should be measured every 8 hours.
- **Chronic hypophosphatemia.** Vitamin D deficiency, if present, should be treated first (see Calcium, Hypocalcemia, Treatment section) followed by oral supplementation of 0.5–1.0 g elemental phosphorus PO bid to tid. Preparations include Neutra-Phos (250 mg elemental phosphorus and 7 mEq of Na^+ and K^+ per capsule) and Neutra-Phos K^+ (250 mg elemental phosphorus and 14 mEq K^+ per capsule). Contents of the capsules should be dissolved in water. Fleet Phospho-Soda (815 mg phosphorus and 33 mEq sodium per 5 mL) is an alternative oral agent. Limiting side effects include nausea and diarrhea.

MAGNESIUM

- **Magnesium** plays an important role in neuromuscular function.
- Approximately 60% of body magnesium is stored in bone, and most of the remainder is found in cells. Only 1% is in the ECF. As a result, the serum magnesium is a poor predictor of intracellular and total body stores and may grossly underestimate total magnesium deficits.
- The main determinant of magnesium balance is the **magnesium concentration** itself, which directly influences renal excretion. Hypomagnesemia stimulates tubular reabsorption of magnesium, whereas hypermagnesemia inhibits it.

Hypermagnesemia

GENERAL PRINCIPLES

- A serum magnesium **>2.2 mEq/L** defines hypermagnesemia.
- Most cases of clinically significant hypermagnesemia are **iatrogenic**, occurring with large doses of magnesium-containing antacids or laxatives and during treatment of preeclampsia with IV magnesium. Because renal excretion is the only means of lowering serum magnesium levels, the presence of significant renal insufficiency can lead to magnesium toxicity even with therapeutic doses of these antacids and laxatives.
- Mild, insignificant elevations in magnesium can occur in end-stage renal disease patients, theophylline intoxication, DKA, and tumor lysis syndrome.

DIAGNOSIS

Clinical Presentation

- Signs and symptoms are usually seen when the serum magnesium level is >4 mEq/L.
- Neuromuscular abnormalities usually include hyporeflexia (usually the first sign of magnesium toxicity), lethargy, and weakness that can progress to paralysis and diaphragmatic involvement, leading to respiratory failure.
- Cardiac findings include hypotension, bradycardia, and cardiac arrest.

Diagnostic Testing

The **ECG** may reveal bradycardia and prolonged PR, QRS, and QT intervals with magnesium levels of 5–10 mEq/L. Complete heart block or asystole may eventually ensue with levels >15 mEq/L.

TREATMENT

- **Prevention.** In the setting of significant renal insufficiency, the inadvertent administration of magnesium-containing medications (e.g., Maalox, magnesium citrate) should be avoided.
- **Asymptomatic hypermagnesemia.** In the setting of normal renal function, normal magnesium levels will quickly be attained with removal of the magnesium load.
- **Symptomatic hypermagnesemia**
  - Prompt supportive therapy is critical, including mechanical ventilation for respiratory failure and a temporary pacemaker for significant bradyarrhythmias.
  - The effects of hypermagnesemia can be antagonized quickly by the administration of 10% calcium gluconate 10–20 mL IV (1–2 g) over 10 minutes.
  - Renal excretion can be encouraged with saline administration.
  - With significant renal insufficiency, hemodialysis is required for definitive therapy.

Hypomagnesemia

GENERAL PRINCIPLES

- A serum magnesium **<1.3 mEq/L** defines hypomagnesemia.
- Hypomagnesemia is most commonly caused by impaired intestinal absorption and increased renal excretion.
  - **Decreased intestinal absorption** occurs in malnutrition, as is common in chronic alcoholics or any malabsorption syndrome. Magnesium can also be lost through prolonged diarrhea and nasogastric aspiration. Hypomagnesemia has been described with chronic use of proton pump inhibitors (PPIs), presumably due to impaired intestinal absorption.
  - **Increased renal excretion** of magnesium can occur from increased renal tubular flow (as occurs with osmotic diuresis) as well as impaired tubular function (as seen with resolving acute tubular necrosis [ATN], loop diuretics, and Bartter and Gitelman syndromes).
- **Drugs.** Several medications similarly induce defects in tubular magnesium transport including aminoglycosides, amphotericin B, cisplatin, pentamidine, and cyclosporine.

DIAGNOSIS

Clinical Presentation

- Neurologic manifestations include lethargy, confusion, tremor, fasciculations, ataxia, nystagmus, tetany, and seizures.
- Atrial and ventricular arrhythmias may occur, especially in patients treated with digoxin.

Diagnostic Testing

- Low serum $[Mg^{2+}]$ in conjunction with an appropriate clinical scenario is sufficient to establish the diagnosis of **magnesium deficiency**. However, due to the slow exchange of magnesium between the bone and intracellular pools (see Magnesium section), a normal serum level does not exclude total body **magnesium deficiency**.
- The etiology of hypomagnesemia usually is evident from the clinical context, but if there is uncertainty, measurement of **urine magnesium excretion** is helpful. A 24-hour urine magnesium of >2 mEq (or >24 mg) or a fractional excretion of magnesium of

>2% during hypomagnesemia suggests **increased renal excretion**. The fractional excretion of magnesium is calculated by

$$(\text{Urine Mg}^{2+}/\text{Urine Cr}) \div [(\text{Serum Mg}^{2+} \times 0.7)/\text{Serum Cr}] \times 100$$

- Hypocalcemia (see Calcium, Hypocalcemia, Etiology section) and/or hypokalemia (see Potassium, Hypokalemia, Etiology section) can often be found as a result of hypomagnesemia-induced derangements in mineral homeostasis.
- **ECG** abnormalities may include a prolonged PR and QT interval with a widened QRS. **Torsades de pointes** is the classically associated arrhythmia.

TREATMENT

- In patients with normal renal function, excess magnesium is readily excreted, and there is little risk of causing hypermagnesemia with recommended doses. However, *magnesium must be given with extreme care in the presence of renal insufficiency.*
- The route of magnesium administration depends on whether clinical manifestations from magnesium deficiency are present.
  - **Asymptomatic hypomagnesemia** can be treated orally. Numerous preparations exist, including Mag-Ox 400 (240 mg elemental magnesium per 400-mg tablet), UroMag (84 mg per 140-mg tablet), and sustained-release Slow-Mag (64 mg per tablet). Typically, approximately 240 mg of elemental magnesium is administered daily for mild deficiency, whereas more severe hypomagnesemia may require up to 720 mg/d of elemental magnesium. The major side effect is diarrhea. Normalization of serum magnesium levels can be deceiving, because the administered magnesium slowly shifts to replete intracellular and bone stores. Furthermore, abrupt increases in serum levels stimulate renal excretion. Thus, serum levels should be followed closely, and replacement should be maintained until patients demonstrate stable normalization of serum magnesium concentrations.
  - **Severe symptomatic hypomagnesemia** should be treated with 1–2 g magnesium sulfate (1 g magnesium sulfate = 96 mg elemental magnesium) IV over 15 minutes. To account for gradual redistribution to severely depleted intracellular stores, replacement therapy may need to be maintained, often for 3–7 days. Serum magnesium should be measured daily and the infusion rate adjusted to maintain a serum magnesium level of <2.5 mEq/L. Tendon reflexes should be tested frequently, because hyporeflexia suggests hypermagnesemia. Reduced doses and more frequent monitoring must be used even in mild renal insufficiency.

ACID–BASE DISTURBANCES

GENERAL PRINCIPLES

- The normal ECF **pH is 7.40 ± 0.03**. Perturbations in pH can occur with changes in the ratio of [HCO_3^-] to partial pressure of carbon dioxide (pCO_2) as described by the **Henderson-Hasselbalch equation:**

$$pH = 6.1 + \log([HCO_3^-] \div [pCO_2 \times 0.3])$$

- Maintenance of pH is essential for normal cellular function. Three general mechanisms exist to keep it within a narrow window:
  - **Chemical buffering** is mediated by HCO_3^- in the ECF and by protein and phosphate buffers in the ICF. The normal [HCO_3^-] is 24 ± 2 mEq/L.
  - **Alveolar ventilation** minimizes variations in the pH by altering the pCO_2. The normal pCO_2 is 40 ± 5 mm Hg.

- ○ **Renal H^+ handling** allows the kidney to adapt to changes in acid–base status via HCO_3^- reabsorption and excretion of titratable acid (e.g., $H_2PO_4^-$) and NH_4^+.
- **Acidemia** and **alkalemia** refer to processes that lower and raise pH regardless of mechanism. They can be caused by metabolic or respiratory disturbances:
  - ○ **Metabolic acidosis** is characterized by a decrease in the plasma $[HCO_3^-]$ due to either HCO_3^- loss or the accumulation of acid.
  - ○ **Metabolic alkalosis** is characterized by an elevation in the plasma $[HCO_3^-]$ due to either H^+ loss or HCO_3^- gain.
  - ○ **Respiratory acidosis** is characterized by an elevation in pCO_2 resulting from alveolar hypoventilation.
  - ○ **Respiratory alkalosis** is characterized by a decrease in pCO_2 resulting from hyperventilation.

DIAGNOSIS

Analysis should be systematic so that accurate conclusions are drawn and appropriate therapy initiated. Once the acid–base process is correctly identified, further diagnostic studies may be undertaken to determine the precise etiologies at play.
- **Step 1.** Check arterial blood gas. Acidemia is present when pH is <7.37 and alkalemia when pH >7.43.
- **Step 2.** Establish the primary disturbance by determining whether the change in $[HCO_3^-]$ or pCO_2 can account for the observed deflection in pH.
  - ○ In acidemia, a decreased $[HCO_3^-]$ suggests metabolic acidosis, and an elevated pCO_2 suggests respiratory acidosis. In alkalemia, an elevated $[HCO_3^-]$ suggests metabolic alkalosis, whereas a decreased pCO_2 suggests respiratory alkalosis.
  - ○ A **combined disorder** is present when pH is normal but the pCO_2 and $[HCO_3^-]$ are both abnormal. Changes in both pCO_2 and $[HCO_3^-]$ can cause the change in pH.
- **Step 3.** Determine whether compensation is appropriate.
  - ○ The **compensatory mechanism** is an adaptation to the primary acid–base disturbance intended to stabilize the changing pH. A respiratory process that shifts the pH in one direction will be compensated by a metabolic process that shifts the pH in the other and vice versa.
  - ○ The effect of compensation is to attenuate, *but not completely correct*, the primary change in pH.
  - ○ The expected compensations for the various primary acid–base derangements are given in Table 12-2.
  - ○ An inappropriate compensatory response suggests the presence of a combined disorder.
  - ○ Example: In a patient with metabolic acidosis, respiratory compensation attenuates the metabolic disturbance to pH by lowering pCO_2. However, if the pCO_2 is higher than expected, respiratory compensation is insufficient, revealing a respiratory acidosis with the primary metabolic acidosis. If pCO_2 is lower than expected, compensation is excessive, revealing a concomitant respiratory alkalosis.
- **Step 4.** Determine the **anion gap**.
  - ○ In normal individuals, the total serum cations are balanced with the total serum anions. Total cations are comprised of measured cations (MCs) and unmeasured cations (UCs), whereas total anions are comprised of measured anions (MAs) and unmeasured anions (UAs). Certain forms of acidosis are characterized by an increase in the pool of UAs. The **anion gap (AG)** is merely a way of demonstrating the accumulation of this UA.
  - ○ $AG = [Na^+] - ([Cl^-] + [HCO_3^-])$. The normal AG is 10 ± 2 mEq/L.

$$AG = \text{the excess of unmeasured anions (vs. unmeasured cations)}$$
$$= UA - UC$$

TABLE 12-2	Expected Compensatory Responses to Primary Acid–Base Disorders	
Disorder	**Primary Change**	**Compensatory Response**
Metabolic acidosis	↓ [HCO$_3$2]	↓ pCO$_2$ 1.2 mm Hg for every 1 mEq/L ↓ [HCO$_3$2] OR pCO$_2$ = last two digits of pH
Metabolic alkalosis	↑ [HCO$_3$2]	↑ pCO$_2$ 0.7 mm Hg for every 1 mEq/L ↑ [HCO$_3$2]
Respiratory acidosis	↑ pCO$_2$	
Acute		↑ [HCO$_3$2] 1.0 mEq/L for every 10 mm Hg ↑ pCO$_2$
Chronic		↑ [HCO$_3$2] 3.5 mEq/L for every 10 mm Hg ↑ pCO$_2$
Respiratory alkalosis	↓ pCO$_2$	
Acute		↓ [HCO$_3$2] 2.0 mEq/L for every 10 mm Hg ↓ pCO$_2$
Chronic		↓ [HCO$_3$2] 5.0 mEq/L for every 10 mm Hg ↓ pCO$_2$

Since total cations = total anions:

$$MC + UC = MA + UA$$

Rearranging the equation:

$$UA - UC = MC - MA$$

MCs are Na^+; MAs are Cl^- and HCO_3^-.

○ Because albumin is the principal UA, the AG should be corrected if there are gross changes in serum albumin levels.

$$\textbf{AG}_{\textbf{correct}} = \textbf{AG} + \{(4 - [\textbf{albumin}]) \times 2.5\}$$

○ An elevated AG suggests the presence of metabolic acidosis with a circulating anion (Table 12-3).
• **Step 5.** Assess the delta gap.
  ○ To maintain a stable total anion content, every increase in an UA should be met with a decrease in $[HCO_3^-]$. Comparing the change in the AG (ΔAG) with the change in the $[HCO_3^-]$ ($\Delta[HCO_3^-]$) is a simple way of making sure that each change in the AG is accounted for.
  ○ If the ΔAG = $\Delta[HCO_3^-]$, this is a simple AG metabolic acidosis.
  ○ If the ΔAG > $\Delta[HCO_3^-]$, the $[HCO_3^-]$ did not decrease as much as expected. This is a metabolic alkalosis **and** AG metabolic acidosis.
  Example: A patient with DKA has been vomiting prior to admission. He has an AG of 20 and an $[HCO_3^-]$ of 20. His ΔAG = 10 and $\Delta[HCO_3^-]$ = 4, revealing an AG metabolic acidosis (DKA) with a metabolic alkalosis (vomiting).
  ○ If the ΔAG < $\Delta[HCO_3^-]$, the $[HCO_3^-]$ decreased more than expected. This is a nongap metabolic acidosis **and** AG metabolic acidosis.
  Example: A patient is admitted with fevers and hypotension after a prolonged course of diarrhea. She has an AG of 15 and an $[HCO_3^-]$ of 12. Her ΔAG is 5 and her $\Delta[HCO_3^-]$ is 12, revealing a nongap metabolic acidosis (diarrhea) and an AG metabolic acidosis (lactic acidosis).

TABLE 12-3	The Four Primary Acid–Base Disorders and Their Common Etiologies	
	Acidosis	**Alkalosis**
Metabolic	Gap • Ketoacids (starvation, alcoholic, diabetic) • Exposures (methanol, ethylene glycol, salicylates) • Lactic acid (shock, drug related) • Profound uremia	Generation • Loss of H^+-rich fluids (GI loss) • Contraction alkalosis • Alkali administration
	Nongap • Nonrenal HCO_3^- loss (diarrhea) • Renal $HCO_3$2 loss (type 2 RTA) • ↓ H secretion (type 1 RTA) • Hypoaldosteronism (type 4 RTA)	Maintenance • Volume contraction • Chloride depletion • Hypokalemia

	Type 1 RTA	Type 2 RTA	Type 4 RTA
Serum [K]	↓ or nl	↓ or nl	↑
Serum [HCO_3]	<10	15–20	>15
Urine pH	>5.3	Varies	<5.3

Respiratory	Depression of respiratory center Neuromuscular failure Lung disease	CNS stimulation Hypoxemia Anxiety

CNS, central nervous system; GI, gastrointestinal; nl, normal; RTA, renal tubular acidosis.

Metabolic Acidosis

GENERAL PRINCIPLES

- The causes of a metabolic acidosis can be divided into those that cause an **elevated anion gap** and those with a **normal anion gap**. Many of the causes seen in clinical practice can be found in Table 12-3.
- AG acidosis results from exposure to acids, which contribute an unmeasured anion to the ECF. Common causes are DKA, lactic acidosis, and toxic alcohol ingestions.
- Non–anion gap acidosis can result from the loss of [HCO_3^-] from the GI tract. Renal causes due to renal excretion of [HCO_3^-] or disorders of renal acid handling are referred to collectively as **renal tubular acidoses (RTAs)**.
- Enteric [HCO_3^-] loss occurs most commonly in the setting of severe diarrhea.
- The three forms of RTA correlate with the three mechanisms that facilitate renal acid handling: proximal bicarbonate reabsorption, distal H^+ secretion, and generation of NH_3, the principle urinary buffer. Urinary buffers reduce the concentration of free H^+ in the filtrate, thus attenuating the back leak of H^+, which occurs at low urinary pH.
  - **Proximal (type 2) RTA** is caused by impaired proximal tubular HCO_3^- reabsorption. Causes include inherited mutations (cystinosis), heavy metals, drugs (tenofovir, ifosfamide, carbonic anhydrase inhibitors), and multiple myeloma and other monoclonal gammopathies.
  - **Distal (type 1) RTA** results from impaired distal H^+ secretion. This may occur due to impairment in H^+ secretion, as seen with a variety of autoimmune (Sjögren syndrome,

lupus, rheumatoid arthritis) or renal disorders. Hypercalciuria is another main cause of distal RTA in adults. It can also be caused by a back leak of H^+ due to increased membrane permeability, as seen with amphotericin B.

- **Distal hyperkalemic (type 4) RTA** may result from either low aldosterone levels or from aldosterone resistance. The resulting hyperkalemia reduces the availability of NH_3 to buffer urinary H^+. Hyporeninemic hypoaldosteronism is seen with some frequency in patients with diabetes. Certain drugs, including NSAIDs, β-blockers, and cyclosporine, have also been implicated.
- Occasionally, the kidney is unable to secrete sufficient H^+ due to an impaired luminal gradient. In these situations, poor filtrate delivery or impaired Na^+ reabsorption in the distal nephron is responsible for decreasing the voltage gradient, which augments H^+ secretion. This can be seen with marked volume depletion, urinary tract obstruction, sickle cell nephropathy, and amiloride or triamterene use.

DIAGNOSIS

The first step in narrowing the differential diagnosis for a metabolic acidosis is to calculate the **anion gap**.
- The specific cause of an **elevated anion gap** can usually be determined by clinical history. However, specific laboratory studies are available to identify certain anions such as lactate, acetoacetate, acetone, and β-hydroxybutyrate. (It should be noted that the use of nitroprusside to detect ketones may fail to identify ketoacidosis due to β-hydroxybutyrate.) The presence of an alcohol (methanol, ethanol, ethylene glycol) can also be determined with laboratory assays. Clinical suspicion for toxic alcohol ingestion is corroborated by an increased **osmolal gap**. This gap is the difference between measured and calculated serum osmolality:

$$[Osm]_{meas} - \{([Na^+] \times 2) + ([glucose] \div 18) + ([BUN] \div 2.8)\}$$

- If a **normal anion gap** is present, the GI HCO_3^- losses can be differentiated from RTAs via the **urine anion gap** (UAG). The **UAG** is the difference between the major measured anions and cations in urine: $[Na^+]_u + [K^+]_u - [Cl^-]_u$. Because NH_4^+ is the major unmeasured urinary cation, a negative UAG reflects high NH_4^+ excretion, an appropriate response to a metabolic acidosis. Conversely, a positive UAG signifies low NH_4^+ excretion, which in the face of a metabolic acidosis suggests a renal tubular defect.
- Serum $[K^+]$ and urine pH can be helpful in distinguishing between the RTAs.
  - Types 1 and 2 are typically associated with hypokalemia, whereas type 4 is characterized by hyperkalemia.
  - Urine pH is low (usually <5.3) in type 4 RTA because the defect is in the generation of the NH_3 buffer, and the mechanism for H^+ secretion is intact. In contrast, urine pH is inappropriately high in type 1 RTA (urine pH >5.3). In type 2 RTA, the urine pH is variable. It is elevated during the initial bicarbonaturia, when filtered bicarbonate exceeds the threshold for reabsorption, and low when the filtered load is below this threshold.

TREATMENT

- **Ketoacidosis** attributable to ethanol abuse and starvation can be corrected with the resumption of caloric intake through oral intake or dextrose-containing fluids and by correction of any volume depletion that may be present. The treatment of DKA is described in Chapter 23, Diabetes Mellitus and Related Disorders.
- **Lactic acidosis** will resolve once the underlying cause is treated and tissue perfusion is restored. Often, this involves aggressive therapeutic maneuvers for the treatment of shock as described in Chapter 8, Critical Care. The administration of alkali does not appear to have clear benefit

in lactic acidosis, and it may lead to a rebound metabolic alkalosis once the underlying cause is managed. Its use in dire circumstances or severe acidosis remains controversial.
- Management of toxic ingestions is described in Chapter 28, Toxicology.
- **Normal AG metabolic acidosis.** Treatment with $NaHCO_3$ is appropriate for patients with a normal AG metabolic acidosis. The HCO_3^- deficit can be calculated in mEq:

$$HCO_3^- \text{ deficit} = \{0.5 \times \text{lean weight} \times [24^- (HCO3^-)]\}$$

However, this assumes a volume of distribution equal to 50% of total body weight. In reality, the distribution of HCO_3^- increases with the severity of the acidosis and may exceed 100% of total body weight in very severe acidosis. It should be noted that the standard 650-mg tablet of oral $NaHCO_3$ provides only 7 mEq of HCO_3^-, whereas one ampule of IV $NaHCO_3$ contains 50 mEq. Still, parenteral $NaHCO_3$ should always be prescribed with caution because of the potential adverse effects, including pulmonary edema, hypokalemia, and hypocalcemia.
- **Treatment of the RTAs.** Correction of the chronic acidemia with alkali administration is warranted in order to prevent its catabolic effect on bone and muscle.
  ○ In *distal (type 1) RTA*, correction of the metabolic acidosis requires oral HCO_3^- replacement on the order of 1–2 mEq/kg/d with $NaHCO_3$ or sodium citrate. Potassium citrate replacement may be necessary for patients with hypokalemia, nephrolithiasis, or nephrocalcinosis. Underlying conditions should be sought and treated.
  ○ In *proximal (type 2) RTA*, much larger amounts of alkali (10–15 mEq/kg/d) are required to reverse the acidosis. Administration of potassium salts minimizes the degree of hypokalemia associated with alkali therapy.
  ○ Management of *type 4 RTA* requires correction of the underlying hyperkalemia. This consists of dietary K^+ restriction (40–60 mEq/d) and possibly a loop diuretic with or without oral $NaHCO_3$ (0.5–1 mEq/kg/d). Mineralocorticoid administration (fludrocortisone, 50–200 μg PO daily) should be used in patients with primary adrenal insufficiency and may be considered in other causes of hypoaldosteronism.

Metabolic Alkalosis

GENERAL PRINCIPLES

- Development of a persistent metabolic alkalosis requires both generation (an inciting cause) and maintenance (a persistent impairment of the corrective renal response).
- Generation often occurs with a primary increase in the plasma $[HCO_3^-]$ and may be due to either **HCO_3^- gain** from alkali administration or, more commonly, **excessive H^+ loss**. The latter may result from the loss of H^+-rich fluids, including upper GI secretions. **Contraction alkalosis** refers to the contraction of volume around a fixed content of bicarbonate.
- Maintenance requires a concomitant impairment in renal HCO_3^- excretion, because the kidney normally has a large capacity to excrete HCO_3^-. This occurs as a result of a **decreased glomerular filtration rate (GFR)** or enhanced tubular HCO_3^- reabsorption from **chloride depletion**, **volume contraction**, and **hypokalemia**. A decrease in filtered chloride is sensed by the macula densa and, as a result of tubuloglomerular feedback, reduces filtered HCO_3^- and stimulates aldosterone release. It also limits adaptive distal HCO_3^- secretion. Metabolic alkalosis is often described as being **chloride responsive** or **chloride unresponsive**.

DIAGNOSIS

Clinical Presentation

Because key causes of metabolic alkalosis are related to volume contraction, patients may present with signs of volume depletion. Occasionally, patients demonstrate hypertension or mild ECF expansion as a result of mineralocorticoid excess.

Diagnostic Testing

- The etiology of metabolic alkalosis is often obvious from the history. Common causes include loss of upper GI secretions through vomiting or excessive urinary H^+ loss from diuretics.
- Urine electrolytes are generally useful in identifying the etiology of a metabolic alkalosis when the history and physical are unrevealing.
  - A **urine [Cl⁻]** <20 mEq/L is consistent with **chloride-responsive** metabolic alkalosis and usually indicates volume depletion. A urine [Cl⁻] >20 mEq/L indicates a chloride-unresponsive cause (see Table 12-3).
  - Urine [Na⁺] is not reliable in predicting the effective circulating volume in these conditions, because *bicarbonaturia obligates renal Na⁺ loss* even in volume depletion.
- **Serum potassium** levels are often low in metabolic alkalosis due to transcellular shifts. Furthermore, hypokalemia contributes to alkalosis by increasing tubular H^+ secretion and Cl⁻ wasting.

TREATMENT

- **Chloride-responsive** metabolic alkaloses are most effectively treated with saline resuscitation until euvolemia is achieved. The increase in filtered chloride leads to improved renal handling of the bicarbonate load.
- **Chloride-unresponsive** metabolic alkaloses do not respond to saline administration and are often associated with a normal or expanded ECF volume.
  - Mineralocorticoid excess can be managed with a K^+-sparing diuretic (amiloride or spironolactone) and repletion of the K^+ deficit.
  - The alkalosis from excessive alkali administration will quickly resolve once the HCO_3^- load is withdrawn, assuming normal renal function.
  - Given that the presence of hypokalemia will continue to perpetuate some degree of alkalosis regardless of other interventions, potassium must be repleted in all cases of metabolic alkalosis.
  - Acetazolamide can be used if the alkalosis persists despite the above interventions or if saline administration is limited by a patient's volume overload. This therapy promotes bicarbonaturia, although renal K^+ loss is enhanced as well. Acetazolamide can be dosed at 250 mg q6h $\times$ 4 or as a single dose of 500 mg.
  - Severe alkalemia (pH >7.70) with ECF volume excess and/or renal failure can be treated with isotonic (150 mEq/L) HCl administered via a central vein. The amount of HCl required can be calculated as follows: $(0.5 \times \text{lean weight in kg}) \times ([HCO_3^-] - 24)$. Correction should occur over 8–24 hours.

Respiratory Acidosis

GENERAL PRINCIPLES

The causes of respiratory acidosis can be divided into hypoventilation from (a) **respiratory center depression**, (b) **neuromuscular failure**, (c) **decreased respiratory system compliance**, (d) **increased airway resistance**, and (e) **increased dead space** (see Table 12-3).

DIAGNOSIS

- Symptoms of respiratory acidosis result from changes in the cerebrospinal fluid (CSF) pH. A very severe hypercapnia may be well tolerated if it is accompanied by renal compensation and a relatively normal pH. Conversely, a modest rise in pCO_2 can be very symptomatic if acute.
- Initial symptoms and signs may include headache and restlessness, which may progress to generalized hyperreflexia/asterixis and coma.

TREATMENT

- Treatment is directed at correcting the underlying disorder and improving ventilation (see Chapter 10, Pulmonary Diseases).
- Administration of $NaHCO_3$ to improve the acidemia may *paradoxically worsen the pH* in situations of limited ventilation. The administered HCO_3^- will combine with H^+ in the tissues and form pCO_2 and water. If ventilation is fixed, this extra CO_2 generated cannot be blown off and worsening hypercapnia will result. Therefore, HCO_3^- should, in general, be avoided in *pure* respiratory acidoses.

Respiratory Alkalosis

GENERAL PRINCIPLES

The common causes of hyperventilation resulting in respiratory alkalosis are given in Table 12-3.

DIAGNOSIS

Clinical Presentation

- The rise in CSF pH that occurs with **acute respiratory alkalosis** is associated with a significant reduction in cerebral blood flow that may lead to light-headedness and impaired consciousness. Generalized membrane excitability can result in seizures and arrhythmias. Symptoms and signs of acute hypocalcemia (see Calcium, Hypocalcemia, Clinical Presentation section) may be evident from the abrupt fall in ionized calcium that can occur.
- **Chronic respiratory alkalosis** is usually asymptomatic because a normal pH is well defended by compensation.

Diagnostic Testing

The rise in pH from **acute respiratory alkalosis** can cause a reduced ionized calcium, a profound hypophosphatemia, and hypokalemia.

TREATMENT

- Treatment of respiratory alkalosis should focus on identifying and treating the underlying disease.
- In intensive care unit patients, this may involve changing the ventilator settings to decrease ventilation (see Chapter 8, Critical Care).

13 Renal Diseases

Rajesh Rajan, Seth Goldberg, and Daniel W. Coyne

Evaluation of the Patient with Renal Disease

DIAGNOSIS

Clinical Presentation

- Renal disease often is asymptomatic or presents with nonspecific complaints. Its presence is frequently first noted on abnormal routine laboratory data, generally as an elevated serum creatinine (Cr) level. An abnormal urinalysis or sediment, with proteinuria, hematuria, or pyuria, may also indicate renal disease.
- When the decline in renal function is acute or advanced, a variety of nonspecific symptoms may be present. Generalized malaise, worsening hypertension, dependent or generalized edema, or decreasing urine output may accompany more severe renal insufficiency.

Diagnostic Testing

The focus of the initial evaluation of the patient with renal disease is to determine the need for emergent dialysis. Then, investigations to identify the etiology are undertaken, while differentiating components of acute and chronic disease.

- **Basic diagnostic testing**
  - A basic evaluation includes electrolytes (with calcium and phosphorus), Cr, blood urea nitrogen (BUN), and albumin. When Cr is stable over days to weeks, it can be used to estimate glomerular filtration rate (GFR), which can be calculated by the Cockcroft-Gault formula for Cr clearance:

  $$[(140 - age) \text{ (ideal body weight in kg) } (0.85 \text{ for women})] / (72 \times \text{Cr in mg/dL})$$

  - However, as Cr is secreted by the tubules, particularly as renal function worsens, this formula has the tendency to overestimate the GFR.
  - The Modification of Diet in Renal Disease (MDRD) formulas can calculate the GFR and take into account BUN, albumin, and race in addition to age and gender (*http://mdrd.com*). When the MDRD GFR is >60 mL/min/1.73 m^2, chronic kidney disease (CKD) should not be diagnosed unless other evidence of renal damage (e.g., proteinuria) is present.
  - The Chronic Kidney Disease Epidemiology Collaboration (CKD-EPI) creatinine equation is based on the same variables as the MDRD equation but performs better and with less bias than the MDRD equation, especially in patients with higher GFR.
- **Urine studies**
  Routine urine studies include a urine dipstick (for protein, blood, glucose, leukocyte esterase, nitrites, pH, and specific gravity) as well as a freshly voided specimen for microscopic examination (looking for cells, casts, and crystals). The urine sample is centrifuged at 2100 rpm for 5 minutes, and then most of the supernatant is poured off. The pellet is resuspended by gently tapping the side of the tube.
  - **Proteinuria** can be estimated from a spot urine protein-to-creatinine ratio, where the serum Cr must be stable to ensure a steady state in the urine. A normal ratio is <250 mg of protein per gram of Cr. A 24-hour urine collection for protein can be obtained when the serum Cr is not at a stable baseline.

- ○ **Hematuria** (more than three red blood cells [RBCs] per high-power field) can represent an infectious, inflammatory, or malignant process anywhere along the urinary tract. Dysmorphic RBCs (with rounded protuberances) suggest a glomerular source of bleeding and can be accompanied by RBC casts formed within the tubules. The absence of RBCs in a patient with a positive dipstick for blood suggests hemolysis or rhabdomyolysis (forms of pigment nephropathy).
- ○ **White blood cells** (WBCs) in the urine represent an infectious or inflammatory process. This may be seen with a urinary tract infection (UTI), parenchymal infections such as pyelonephritis or abscess, or acute interstitial nephritis (AIN). Urine eosinophils can be identified with the Giemsa stain when evaluating for AIN, atheroembolic disease, or prostatitis, although the sensitivity of this test is low. WBC casts are consistent with AIN and pyelonephritis but can also be seen as part of an active sediment in inflammatory glomerular diseases.
- ○ **Additional biochemistry tests can be ordered to evaluate for specific etiologies and will be discussed in the individual sections below.**
- **Imaging**
  - ○ **Renal ultrasonography** can document the presence of two kidneys, assess size, and identify hydronephrosis or renal cysts. Small kidneys (<9 cm) generally reflect chronic disease, although kidneys may be large (generally >13 cm) in diabetes, HIV, deposition disorders, and polycystic kidney disease. A discrepancy in kidney size of >2 cm suggests unilateral renal artery stenosis with atrophy of the affected kidney. The presence of hydronephrosis suggests obstructive nephropathy. Retroperitoneal fibrosis can encase the ureters and prevent dilation despite the presence of an obstruction.
  - ○ **CT** has less utility in the evaluation of kidney disease because the iodinated contrast dye can be nephrotoxic and may cause worsening renal function. However, noncontrast helical CT scanning has become the test of choice in evaluating nephrolithiasis.
  - ○ **MRI** and magnetic resonance angiography (MRA) can be helpful in evaluating renal masses, detecting renal artery stenosis, and diagnosing renal vein thrombosis. Unlike standard arteriography, MRA does not require the administration of nephrotoxic contrast agents but does employ gadolinium-based contrast agents, which are associated with the development of nephrogenic systemic fibrosis (NSF) in patients with advanced renal failure or dialysis dependence (*Clin Radiol 2014;69:661*). Guidelines that limit the use of gadolinium in at-risk patients have decreased the incidence of NSF. The available contrast agents should be used with caution when necessary.
  - ○ **Radionuclide scanning** uses technetium isotopes to assess the contribution of each kidney to the overall renal function, providing important information if unilateral nephrectomy is being considered for malignancy or for living donation. Renal scanning is also useful in transplantation, where renal perfusion and excretion of the tracer can be followed.
- **Diagnostic procedures**
  - ○ **Kidney biopsy** can determine diagnosis, classify disease, guide therapy, and provide prognostic information in many settings, particularly in the evaluation of glomerular or deposition diseases. Biopsy of a native kidney may be indicated in adults with unexplained proteinuria, hematuria, or renal dysfunction. Biopsy of a renal transplant allograft may be necessary to distinguish acute rejection from medication toxicity and other causes of renal dysfunction. Shrunken fibrotic kidneys are unlikely to yield useful diagnostic information; they also have an increased risk of postprocedural bleeding, and biopsy should generally be avoided in these cases.
  - ○ Preparative measures for native kidney biopsy include avoiding aspirin and antiplatelet agents for 5–7 days and reversing anticoagulation before procedure,

ultrasonography (to document the presence of two kidneys and assess size and location), urinalysis or urine culture to exclude infection, blood pressure control, and correction of coagulation parameters. If uremic platelet dysfunction is suspected by an elevated bleeding time (>10 minutes) or abnormal platelet function assays, IV desmopressin acetate (DDAVP at 0.3 μg/kg) can be infused 30 minutes prior to biopsy. Patients on dialysis should not receive heparin immediately after the biopsy. If body habitus precludes a percutaneous approach, a transjugular renal biopsy can be performed.
○ Serial blood counts should be obtained at 6-hour intervals overnight. A hemoglobin drop of approximately 10% is common after the procedure. Difficulty voiding after the procedure may represent urethral clot obstructing the flow of urine.

Acute Kidney Injury

GENERAL PRINCIPLES

Definition

There is no precise definition for acute kidney injury (AKI). It may be characterized by an abrupt increase in serum Cr ≥0.3 mg/dL within 48 hours or a similar increase over a few weeks or months.

Classification

Renal failure can be classified as oliguric or nonoliguric based on the amount of urine output. Cutoffs of approximately 500 mL/d or 25 mL/h for 4 hours are frequently used in clinical practice.

Etiology

Etiologies of AKI are classically divided according to the anatomic location of the physiologic defect. **Prerenal** disease involves a disturbance of renal perfusion, whereas **postrenal** disease involves obstruction of the urinary collecting system. **Intrinsic** renal disease involves the glomeruli, microvasculature, tubules, or interstitium of the kidneys. Table 13-1 lists some of the common causes of AKI.

TABLE 13-1	Causes of Acute Renal Failure	
Prerenal	**Intrinsic**	**Postrenal**
Hypovolemia	Tubular: Ischemic ATN,	Urethral obstruction
Hypotension (including	toxic ATN (contrast,	Ureteral obstruction
sepsis)	pigment, uric acid)	(bilateral, or unilateral
Loss of autoregulation	Vascular: Glomerulone-	if solitary kidney)
(NSAIDs, RAAS blockers)	phritis, dysproteinemia,	
Abdominal compartment	thrombotic microan-	
syndrome	giopathy (HUS, TTP),	
Renal artery stenosis	atheroembolic disease	
Heart failure	Interstitial: Acute	
Hepatic cirrhosis	interstitial nephritis,	
	pyelonephritis	

ATN, acute tubular necrosis; HUS, hemolytic-uremic syndrome; RAAS, renin–angiotensin–aldosterone system; TTP, thrombotic thrombocytopenic purpura.

Prerenal

- The term **prerenal azotemia** implies preserved intrinsic renal function in the setting of renal hypoperfusion and reduced GFR. The effective circulating volume is decreased, resulting from intravascular volume depletion, low cardiac output, or disordered vasodilation (hepatic cirrhosis).
- When the cause is true volume depletion, presentation involves a history of excessive fluid loss, reduced intake, or orthostatic symptoms. The physical exam may reveal dry mucous membranes, poor skin turgor, and orthostatic vital signs (drop in blood pressure by at least 20/10 mm Hg or an increase in heart rate by 10 bpm after standing from a seated or lying position). The central venous pressure is typically <8 cm H_2O.
- Low cardiac output causes prerenal azotemia via a drop in the effective circulating volume, despite total body volume overload. In addition, sympathetic and neurohormonal systems are activated, leading to the stimulation of the renin–angiotensin–aldosterone system as well as antidiuretic hormone (ADH), promoting further salt and water retention. This can lead to increased reabsorption of urea nitrogen in relation to creatinine, and patients present with a prerenal pattern on laboratory investigations. In heart failure, diuresis may paradoxically improve the prerenal azotemia by unloading the ventricles and improving cardiac function (see Chapter 5, Heart Failure and Cardiomyopathy). The use of ultrafiltration was evaluated and found to be inferior to pharmacologic therapies; it resulted in more adverse events in the treatment of acute decompensated heart failure (*N Engl J Med 2012;367:2296–304*).
- Hepatic failure leads to splanchnic vasodilation and venous pooling, which diminishes the effective circulating volume and activates the renin–angiotensin–aldosterone system along with ADH secretion, despite total body volume overload. This can progress to the **hepatorenal syndrome** (HRS), which is characterized by a rise in serum creatinine of >1.5 mg/dL that is not reduced with administration of albumin (1 g/kg of body weight) and after a minimum of 2 days off diuretics. The diagnosis of HRS should be in the absence of shock, nephrotoxic agents, or findings of renal parenchymal disease (*N Engl J Med 2009;361:1279*). Spontaneous bacterial peritonitis, overdiuresis, gastrointestinal bleeding, or large-volume paracentesis can precipitate HRS in a cirrhotic patient. Management of the renal disease is supportive, and if definitive treatment of the liver disorder (either through recovery or via transplantation) can occur, renal recovery is common. Temporizing measures include treatment of the underlying precipitating factor (e.g., peritonitis, gastrointestinal bleeding) and withholding diuretics. Dialytic support can be used as a bridge to transplantation in appropriate candidates. Additional treatment options are discussed further in Chapter 19, Liver Diseases.
- In the volume-depleted patient, certain medications can block the ability of the kidney to autoregulate blood flow and GFR. NSAIDs inhibit the counterbalancing vasodilatory effects of prostaglandins and can induce AKI in volume-depleted patients. Angiotensin-converting enzyme (ACE) inhibitors and angiotensin receptor blockers (ARBs) can cause efferent arteriolar vasodilation and a drop in the GFR.
- Abdominal compartment syndrome, from intestinal ischemia, obstruction, or massive ascites, can compromise flow through the renal vasculature via increased intra-abdominal pressure (IAP). An IAP >20 mm Hg, measured via a pressure transducer attached to the bladder catheter, suggests the diagnosis.

Postrenal

- Postrenal failure occurs when the flow of urine is obstructed anywhere within the urinary collecting system. Common causes include **prostatic enlargement, bilateral kidney stones, or malignancy**. The increased intratubular hydrostatic pressure leads to the diminished GFR. Bilateral involvement (or unilateral obstruction to a solitary kidney) is required to produce a significant change in the Cr level. When the diagnosis is suspected, a renal ultrasound should be performed early to evaluate for hydronephrosis. However, hydronephrosis may be less pronounced when there is concomitant volume depletion or if retroperitoneal fibrosis has encased the ureters, preventing their expansion.

- Treatment depends on the level of obstruction. When urethral flow is impeded (usually by prostatic enlargement in men), placement of a bladder catheter can be both diagnostic and therapeutic; **a postvoid residual urine volume >300 mL** strongly suggests the diagnosis. When the upper urinary tract is involved, urologic or radiologic decompression is necessary, with stenting or placement of percutaneous nephrostomy tubes.
- Relief of bilateral obstruction is frequently followed by a **postobstructive diuresis**. Serum electrolytes need to be closely monitored if polyuria ensues, and replacement of approximately half of the urinary volume with 0.45% saline is recommended.
- Crystals may cause micro-obstructive uropathy within the tubules. IV acyclovir and the protease inhibitor indinavir can induce AKI by this mechanism. The urine may show evidence of crystals, although sometimes not until urine flow is reestablished. Treatment is typically supportive after the offending agent is discontinued. As with relief of other forms of obstructive uropathy, a polyuric phase may occur.

Intrinsic Renal

Causes of intrinsic renal failure can be divided anatomically into tubular, glomerular/vascular, and interstitial categories. Disease can be primarily renal in nature or part of a systemic process.

- **Tubular**
  - **Ischemic acute tubular necrosis (ATN)** is the most common cause of renal failure in the intensive care setting and is the end result of any process that leads to significant hypoperfusion of the kidneys, including sepsis, hemorrhage, or any prolonged prerenal insult.
    - The injury results in the sloughing of renal tubular cells, which can congeal with cellular debris in a matrix of Tamm–Horsfall protein to form granular casts. These have a "muddy brown" appearance and are strongly suggestive of ATN in the proper context. The fractional excretion of sodium (FE_{Na}) (>1%) and fractional excretion of urea (FE_{Urea}) (>35%) are typically elevated as the tubules lose their ability to concentrate the urine.
    - Management of ATN is supportive, with avoidance of further nephrotoxic insults. Fluid management is aimed at maintaining euvolemia. Volume deficits, if present, should be corrected. If volume overload and oliguria become evident, a diuretic challenge is reasonable, typically with IV furosemide (40–120 mg boluses or a continuous drip at 10–20 mg/h). This has not been shown to hasten recovery but can simplify overall management.
    - Recovery from ATN may take days to weeks to occur but can be expected in >85% of patients with a previously normal Cr. Dialysis may be necessary to bridge the time to recovery.
  - Toxic ATN can result from endogenous chemicals (e.g., hemoglobin, myoglobin) or exogenous medications (e.g., iodinated contrast, aminoglycosides). These forms share many of the diagnostic features of ischemic ATN.
    - **Iodinated contrast** is a potent renal vasoconstrictor and is toxic to renal tubules. When renal injury occurs, the Cr typically rises 24 hours after exposure and peaks in 3–5 days. Risk factors for contrast nephropathy include CKD, diabetes, volume depletion, heart failure, higher contrast volumes, and use of hyperosmolar contrast. Preventative measures include periprocedure hydration and discontinuation of diuretics. Isotonic saline at 1–2 mL/kg/h started 3–12 hours before the procedure along with a goal of postprocedural diuresis of 150 mL/h has been found to be beneficial in reducing contrast-induced injury in high-risk populations. Alternatively, sodium bicarbonate at 150 mEq/L (three ampules in 5% dextrose in water [D5W]) can be given at 3 mL/kg/h for 1 hour prior to exposure, then at 1 mL/kg/h for 6 hours

after the procedure (*Cardiology 2014;128:62*). Acetylcysteine has not been shown to reduce the incidence of contrast nephropathy.

- **Aminoglycoside nephrotoxicity** is typically nonoliguric, occurs from direct toxicity to the proximal tubules, and results in the renal wasting of potassium and magnesium. Replacement of these electrolytes may become necessary. A similar pattern of potassium and magnesium loss is seen in cisplatin toxicity. A prolonged exposure to the aminoglycoside of at least 5 days is required. Peak and trough levels correlate poorly with the risk of developing renal injury. Risk may be minimized by avoiding volume depletion and by using the extended-interval dosing method (see Chapter 15, Antimicrobials).

- **Pigment nephropathy** results from direct tubular toxicity by hemoglobin and myoglobin. Vasoconstriction may also play a role. The diagnosis may be suspected by a positive urine dipstick test for blood but an absence of RBCs on microscopic examination. In **rhabdomyolysis**, the creatine kinase (CK) level is elevated to at least 10 times the upper limit of normal with a disproportionate rise in Cr, potassium, and phosphorus. Aggressive IV fluid administration should be initiated immediately, and large volumes are required to replace the fluid lost into necrotic muscle tissue. If urine flow is established, alkalinization with sodium bicarbonate (150 mEq/L, three ampules) can increase the solubility of these pigments, although this maneuver may worsen the hypocalcemia.

- In **tumor lysis syndrome**, acute uric acid nephropathy can result. In addition to the elevated Cr, there is typically hyperuricemia, hyperphosphatemia, and hypocalcemia. A ratio of urine uric acid to urine Cr that is >1 is consistent with this diagnosis, as is the finding of uric acid crystals in the urine sediment. Prophylaxis with allopurinol 600 mg can decrease uric acid production. Rasburicase (15 mg/kg IV) is highly effective at depleting uric acid levels and can be given as prophylaxis or as treatment. Alkalinization of the urine should be avoided if hyperphosphatemia is present because this could increase the risk of calcium phosphate precipitation in the urine.

- **Glomerular/vascular**
  - The finding of **dysmorphic urinary RBCs, RBC casts, or proteinuria in the nephrotic range (>3.5 g/d)** strongly suggests the presence of a glomerular disease. Glomerular diseases are described individually in further detail later in this chapter.
  - A small subgroup of glomerular diseases can present with rapidly deteriorating renal function, termed **rapidly progressive glomerulonephritis** (RPGN). A nephritic picture is common, with RBC casts, edema, and hypertension. A renal biopsy may reveal the specific underlying disease, but crescent formation in >50% of glomeruli is usually present. For those deemed to have salvageable renal function, management is with high-dose pulse glucocorticoid therapy (IV methylprednisolone 7–15 mg/kg/d for 3 days) followed by a course of oral prednisone (1 mg/kg/d for 1 month, then tapered over the next 6–12 months). Cyclophosphamide is typically added to this regimen, with monthly IV doses (1 g/m^2) having less cumulative toxicity than the daily oral dosing strategy (2 mg/kg/d).
  - Thrombotic microangiopathy (TMA) includes both **hemolytic-uremic syndrome (HUS) and thrombotic thrombocytopenic purpura (TTP)**. Causes include diarrheal bacterial toxins and medications (mitomycin C, clopidogrel, cyclosporine, tacrolimus), and it may be associated with pregnancy or malignancies of the gastrointestinal tract. Atypical HUS has been described in patients with mutations in the genes coding for proteins that regulate the complement cascade, such as factor H and factor I. These patients have normal *ADAMTS13* activity and do not have Shiga toxin–associated diarrhea. Eculizumab has been found to be a safe and effective way of treating atypical HUS (*Pediatr Nephrol 2014;29:841*). Diagnosis and therapy are discussed in Chapter 20, Disorders of Hemostasis and Thrombosis.

○ **Atheroembolic disease** can be seen in patients with diffuse atherosclerosis after undergoing an invasive aortic or other large artery manipulation, including cardiac catheterization, coronary bypass surgery, aortic aneurysm repair, and placement of an intra-aortic balloon pump. Physical findings may include retinal arteriolar plaques, lower extremity livedo reticularis, and areas of digital necrosis. Eosinophilia, eosinophiluria, and hypocomplementemia may be present, and WBC casts may be found in the urine sediment. However, in many cases, the only laboratory abnormality is a rising Cr that follows a stepwise progression. Renal biopsy shows cholesterol clefts in the small arteries. Anticoagulation may worsen embolic disease and should be avoided if possible. No specific treatment is available. Many patients progress to CKD and even to end-stage renal disease (ESRD).

- **Interstitial**
  ○ **AIN** involves inflammation of the renal parenchyma, typically caused by medications or infections. The classic triad of **fever, rash, and eosinophilia** is seen in less than one-third of patients, and its absence does not exclude the diagnosis. Pyuria, WBC casts, and eosinophiluria are also suggestive of AIN. β-Lactam antibiotics are the most frequently cited causative agents, but nearly all antibiotics can be implicated. The time course typically requires exposure for at least 5–10 days before renal impairment occurs. Other medications, such as proton pump inhibitors and allopurinol, have been associated with AIN. NSAIDs can produce AIN with nephrotic range proteinuria. Streptococcal infections, leptospirosis, and sarcoidosis have all been implicated in AIN.
  ○ Treatment is principally the withdrawal of the offending agent. Renal recovery typically ensues, although the time course is variable, and temporary dialytic support may be necessary in severe cases. A short course of prednisone at 1 mg/kg/d may hasten recovery.
  ○ Parenchymal infections with **pyelonephritis or renal abscesses** are uncommon causes of AKI. Bilateral involvement is usually necessary to induce a rise in Cr. Urine findings include pyuria and WBC casts, and antibiotic therapy is guided by culture results.

DIAGNOSIS

- Uncovering the cause of AKI requires careful attention to the events preceding the rise in Cr. In the hospitalized patient, blood pressure patterns, hydration status, medications, and iodinated contrast use must be investigated. Antibiotic dose and duration as well as PRN medications should not be overlooked.
- Evidence of ongoing hypovolemia or hypoperfusion is suggestive of prerenal disease. Most causes of postrenal disease are identified on ultrasound by dilation of the collecting system or by massive urine output on placement of a bladder catheter. When promptly corrected, prerenal and postrenal disorders can show a rapid decrease in the serum Cr, and failure of this to occur can suggest an alternative diagnosis.
- **Urinary casts** point toward an intrinsic cause of AKI. Granular casts ("muddy brown") suggest ATN, WBC casts suggest an inflammatory or infectious interstitial process, and RBC casts strongly suggest glomerular disease. Identification of crystals in the urine sediment may be supportive of kidney disease related to intoxication of ethylene glycol, uric acid excretion, tumor lysis syndrome, or medications such as acyclovir and indinavir. This underscores the importance of examining fresh urinary sediment in the evaluation of AKI.

  Various laboratory parameters can be used to differentiate prerenal states from ATN in oliguric patients and are summarized in Table 13-2. The basis for these tests is to evaluate tubular integrity, which is preserved in prerenal disease and lost in ATN. In states of hypoperfusion, the kidneys should avidly reabsorb sodium, resulting in a low FE_{Na}: $FE_{Na} = [(U_{Na} \times P_{Cr})/(P_{Na} \times U_{Cr})] \times 100$, where U is urine and P is plasma.

TABLE 13-2	Laboratory Findings in Oliguric Acute Kidney Injury					
Diagnosis	BUN:Cr	FE_{Na} (%)	Urine Osmolality (mOsm/kg)	Urine Na	Urine SG	Sediment
Prerenal azotemia	>20:1	<1%	>500	<20	>1.020	Bland
Oliguric ATN	<20:1	>1%	<350	>40	Variable	Granular casts

ATN, acute tubular necrosis; BUN, blood urea nitrogen; Cr, creatinine; FE_{Na}, fractional excretion of sodium; SG, specific gravity.

- **A value <1% suggests renal hypoperfusion with intact tubular function.** Loop diuretics and metabolic alkalosis can induce natriuresis, increase the FE_{Na}, and mask the presence of renal hypoperfusion. The FE_{Urea} can instead be calculated in these settings, where a value of <35% suggests a prerenal process.
- Contrast and pigment nephropathy can result in a low FE_{Na} due to early vasoconstriction ("prerenal" drop in glomerular perfusion), as can glomerular diseases due to intact tubular function. The FE_{Na} also has limited utility when AKI is superimposed on CKD because the underlying tubular dysfunction makes the test difficult to interpret.
- With hypoperfusion, the urine is typically concentrated, containing an osmolality >500 mOsm/kg and a high specific gravity (>1.020). In ATN, concentrating ability is lost and the urine is usually isosmolar to the serum (isosthenuria). In the blood, the ratio of BUN to Cr is normally <20:1, and an elevation is consistent with hypovolemia.

TREATMENT

- Disease-specific therapies were covered earlier. In general, treatment of AKI is primarily supportive in nature. Volume status must be evaluated to correct for hypovolemia or hypervolemia. Volume deficits, if present, should be corrected, after which the goal of fluid management should be to keep input equal to output. In the oliguric volume-overloaded setting, a trial of diuretics (usually high-dose loop diuretics in a bolus or as a continuous drip) may simplify management, although it has not been shown to hasten recovery.
- Electrolyte imbalances should be corrected in the setting of AKI. Hyperkalemia, when mild (<6 mEq/L), may be treated with dietary potassium restriction and potassium-binding resins (e.g., sodium polystyrene sulfonate). When further elevated or accompanied by ECG abnormalities, immediate medical therapy is indicated, with calcium gluconate, insulin and glucose, inhaled β-agonists, and possibly bicarbonate (see Chapter 12, Fluid and Electrolyte Management). Severe hyperkalemia that is refractory to medical management is an indication for urgent dialysis.
- Mild **metabolic acidosis** can be treated with oral sodium bicarbonate, 650–1300 mg thrice daily. Severe acidosis (pH <7.2) can be temporized with IV sodium bicarbonate but requires monitoring for volume overload, rebound alkalosis, and hypocalcemia. Acidosis that is refractory to medical management is an indication for urgent dialysis.

SPECIAL CONSIDERATIONS

All patients with AKI require daily assessment to determine the need for renal replacement therapy. Severe acidosis, hyperkalemia, or volume overload refractory to medical management mandates the initiation of dialysis. Certain drug and alcohol intoxications (methanol, ethylene glycol, or salicylates) should be treated with hemodialysis. Uremic pericarditis (with a friction rub) or encephalopathy should also be treated promptly with renal replacement therapy. Patients suffering from acute oliguric renal failure who are not expected to recover promptly likely benefit from earlier initiation of dialysis.

Glomerulopathies

GENERAL PRINCIPLES

- The presentation of glomerular diseases can be thought of as existing on a continuum. On one end is the nephrotic syndrome, characterized by proteinuria >3.5 g/d and accompanied by hypoalbuminemia, hyperlipidemia, and edema, and on the other end of the spectrum is the nephritic syndrome, characterized by hematuria, hypertension, edema, and renal insufficiency. Most specific disease entities present somewhere in between and have overlapping features but with a tendency to produce one syndrome over the other.
- When a glomerular process is suspected, it may be useful to check antinuclear antibodies (ANA), complement levels (C3, C4), cryoglobulins, and viral (HIV, hepatitis B and C) serologies. A serum protein electrophoresis (SPEP) and urine immunofixation can be performed in proteinuric patients to evaluate for a monoclonal gammopathy and may be suspected by a large protein–albumin gap.
- When a nephritic process is suspected by the clinical presentation, testing for antiglomerular basement membrane (anti-GBM) antibodies, antineutrophil cytoplasmic antibodies (ANCA), and anti-streptolysin-O (ASO) titers may be helpful in narrowing the differential diagnosis.
- Biopsy findings also correlate with these syndromes. Nephrotic diseases typically show injury along the filtration barrier, with thickening of the GBM or fusion of the podocyte foot processes. By comparison, nephritic diseases generally show varying degrees of mesangial cell proliferation and mesangial deposition and, with more aggressive disease, may reveal crescent formation.
- Nephrotic diseases are more likely to be minimal change disease, membranous nephropathy, focal segmental glomerulosclerosis, diabetic nephropathy, and deposition dysproteinemias.
- Nephritic syndromes are more likely to be membranoproliferative glomerulonephropathy, IgA nephropathy/Henoch-Schönlein purpura, postinfectious glomerulonephritis, lupus nephritis, anti-GBM disease, and granulomatosis with polyangiitis.

TREATMENT

- Many disorders share the same features, and general therapeutic maneuvers can be addressed as a group. Specific therapies for individual glomerular diseases are discussed in the following text.
- Glomerular disease presenting with proteinuria should rely on treatment with **ACE inhibitors or ARBs** to reduce the intraglomerular pressure. Efficacy can be monitored by serial urine protein-to-Cr ratios. Electrolytes and Cr should be checked within 1–2 weeks of initiation of therapy or an increase in dose to document stability of renal function and potassium. Modest dietary protein restriction to 0.8 g/kg/d may slow progression, but this remains controversial.
- Edema and volume overload can usually be effectively managed with **diuretics** combined with **sodium restriction**. Aggressive treatment of hypertension can also slow progression of renal disease.

- The hyperlipidemia associated with the nephrotic syndrome responds to dietary modification and **statins (3-hydroxy-3-methylglutaryl–coenzyme A [HMG-CoA] reductase inhibitors)**.
- The nephrotic syndrome produces a hypercoagulable state and can predispose to thromboembolic complications. Deep venous thrombi and renal vein thrombosis may occur and should be treated with heparin anticoagulation followed by long-term warfarin therapy. Prophylactic anticoagulation is controversial and may be beneficial in severely nephrotic patients, particularly with membranous nephropathy (MN). Exact mechanisms of thrombosis remain controversial but likely include urinary loss of anticlotting proteins, increased synthesis of clotting factors, or local activation of the glomerular hemostasis system.
- When **immunosuppression** is considered, the risk of therapy should always be weighed against the potential benefit. Renal salvageability should be addressed, and patients with advanced disease on presentation who are unlikely to benefit from such treatment may be better served by avoiding the risks of high-dose immunosuppression. Cytotoxic agents (e.g., cyclophosphamide, chlorambucil) require close monitoring of WBC counts, checked at least weekly at the initiation of therapy. Dose adjustments may be needed to maintain the WBC count >3500 cells/μL. Rituximab, a monoclonal antibody directed against CD20, has shown promise in a variety of immune-mediated disorders, including severe lupus nephritis (LN), MN, and ANCA-positive vasculitis, where it has been given IV as four weekly doses of 375 mg/m^2 (*N Engl J Med 2010;363:221*).

Minimal Change Disease

GENERAL PRINCIPLES

Epidemiology

Minimal change disease (MCD) is the most common cause of the nephrotic syndrome in children but has a second peak in adults aged 50–60 years. Typically, there is sudden onset of proteinuria with hypertension and edema as well as the full nephrotic syndrome, although renal insufficiency is unusual.

Associated Conditions

Secondary forms of MCD may accompany certain malignancies (Hodgkin disease and solid tumors being the most common). A form of interstitial nephritis associated with NSAID use may also be associated with MCD.

DIAGNOSIS

The kidney biopsy reveals normal glomeruli on light microscopy and negative immunofluorescence. Electron microscopy shows effacement of the foot processes as the only histologic abnormality.

TREATMENT

- In adults, treatment with oral prednisone at 1 mg/kg/d may induce remission (decrease in proteinuria) in 8–16 weeks. Once in remission, the steroids can be tapered over 3 months and then discontinued. The urine protein excretion should be followed during this taper.
- Relapse may occur in up to 75% of adults. Reinstitution of prednisone is often effective. If the patient is steroid dependent or steroid resistant, cytotoxic agents may be needed, with cyclophosphamide 2 mg/kg/d or chlorambucil 0.2 mg/kg/d. Cyclosporine 5 mg/kg/d is an alternative therapy. Rituximab may be beneficial in frequently relapsing or glucocorticoid-dependent MCD (*Kidney Int 2013;83:511*).

Membranous Nephropathy

GENERAL PRINCIPLES

- MN usually presents with the nephrotic syndrome or heavy proteinuria, whereas renal function is often normal or near normal. Disease progression is variable, with one-third remitting spontaneously, one-third progressing to ESRD, and one-third with an intermediate course.
- Secondary forms of MN are associated with systemic lupus erythematosus (SLE; class V), viral hepatitis, syphilis, or solid organ malignancies. Medications such as gold and penicillamine can also induce this process.

DIAGNOSIS

Kidney biopsy shows thickening of the GBM on light microscopy, with "spikes" on silver stain, representing areas of normal basement membrane interposed between subepithelial deposits. These deposits correlate with IgG and C3 on immunofluorescence and are also seen on electron microscopy. Antibodies to the podocyte antigen phospholipase A_2 receptor have been implicated in 70% of adult idiopathic MN, although serologic testing is currently only used in the research setting.

TREATMENT

Because of the generally good prognosis, specific therapy should be reserved for patients at higher risk for progression (reduced GFR, male gender, age >50 years, hypertension) or heavy proteinuria. Treatment options include regimens with prednisone 0.5 mg/kg/d and cytotoxic agents (chlorambucil 0.2 mg/kg/d or cyclophosphamide 2.5 mg/kg/d) on alternating months for 6–12 months.

Focal Segmental Glomerulosclerosis

GENERAL PRINCIPLES

- Focal segmental glomerulosclerosis (FSGS) is not a single disease but rather a descriptive classification for diseases with shared histopathology. Presentation is with the nephrotic syndrome, hypertension, and renal insufficiency.
- Secondary forms of FSGS are associated with obesity, vesicoureteral reflux, and HIV infection (FSGS of the collapsing variant). HIV can also induce secondary forms of other glomerular diseases such as MN and membranoproliferative glomerulonephropathy.

DIAGNOSIS

The kidney biopsy reveals focal and segmental sclerosis of glomeruli under light microscopy. The degree of interstitial fibrosis and tubular atrophy (rather than glomerular scarring) correlates with prognosis. Immunofluorescence shows staining for C3 and IgM in areas of sclerosis, representing areas of trapped immune deposits. Electron microscopy shows effacement of the podocyte foot processes.

TREATMENT

For patients with nephrotic range proteinuria, a trial of prednisone 1 mg/kg/d can be attempted for 16 weeks. Patients who relapse after a period of apparent responsiveness may benefit from a repeat course of steroids. Nonresponders and relapsers may respond to treatment with cyclosporine 5 mg/kg/d. Cyclophosphamide and mycophenolate mofetil can also be used. Induction of a complete remission (<0.3 g/d of proteinuria) or a partial remission (50% reduction in proteinuria and <3.5 g/d) is associated with significantly slower loss of renal function.

Diabetic Nephropathy

GENERAL PRINCIPLES

Diabetic nephropathy (DN) is the most common cause of ESRD in the United States. Albuminuria correlates with the risk of progression and is classified as absent (<30 mg/g Cr), formerly microalbuminuria (30–300 mg/g Cr), or formerly macroalbuminuria (>300 mg/g Cr). Early disease has glomerular hyperfiltration with an elevated GFR, followed by a linear decline that may progress to ESRD.

DIAGNOSIS

Diagnostic Testing

Kidney biopsy is not usually performed, unless the rate of renal decline is more rapid than would be anticipated or other diagnoses are suspected. Histology for DN shows glomerular sclerosis with nodular mesangial expansion (Kimmelstiel-Wilson nodules) on light microscopy. Immunofluorescence does not reveal immune deposition. Electron microscopy may show GBM thickening.

TREATMENT

Treatment is centered on aggressive control of glucose and blood pressure. Specific hyperglycemic therapy is discussed further in Chapter 23, Diabetes Mellitus and Related Disorders. An ACE inhibitor or ARB is considered the first-line agent in the treatment of hypertension in diabetic patients and can offer better control of proteinuria. Studies combining ACE inhibitors with an ARB or the direct renin inhibitor aliskiren have shown worse renal and cardiovascular outcomes (*N Engl J Med 2008;358:1547*).

Deposition Disorders/Dysproteinemias

GENERAL PRINCIPLES

Dysproteinemias include **amyloidosis, light chain deposition disease (LCDD), heavy chain deposition disease (HCDD), fibrillary glomerulopathy, and immunotactoid glomerulopathy**. Multiple myeloma may be associated with amyloidosis or LCDD. These disorders can affect the kidney in a variety of ways, including glomerular or tubular deposition, formation of insoluble protein casts in the tubules (micro-obstructive cast nephropathy), or through hypercalcemia and volume depletion. Glomerular deposition is typically associated with heavy proteinuria due to overflow as well as disruption of filtration barrier integrity.

DIAGNOSIS

Diagnostic Testing

Diagnosis is suggested by an abnormal monoclonal protein found in the SPEP, urine protein electrophoresis, or serum free light chains. Immunoglobulin (Ig) chains are not detected by routine urine dipstick and may be missed unless glomerular involvement has led to general protein leakage. Rarely, these tests are negative, and only tissue biopsy can make the diagnosis.

Diagnostic Procedures
- Biopsy of the kidney can show characteristic deposits. For amyloidosis, this appears as Congo Red–positive β-pleated fibrils of 10 nm in diameter under electron microscopy. Immunofluorescence can identify the specific Ig chains for LCDD (more likely to occur with kappa light chains) and HCDD. Fibrillary and immunotactoid deposits are Congo Red negative. The fibrils of fibrillary glomerulopathy (12–20 nm) are typically thicker than those for amyloid, whereas the microtubules of immunotactoid glomerulopathy are even wider (20–60 nm) with a visible lumen in cross-section. Immunotactoid glomerulonephropathy has a strong association with myelodysplastic disorders.
- When cast nephropathy is implicated in a dysproteinemic disorder, the biopsy shows enlarged tubules filled with proteinaceous material. Immunofluorescence can identify the specific components of these casts.

TREATMENT

Melphalan and prednisone are beneficial in the treatment of amyloidosis and LCDD. Chemotherapy aimed at the underlying disease can be effective in reversing renal disease. When cast nephropathy is present on biopsy, a course of plasmapheresis in conjunction with treatment of the myeloma may stabilize renal function. There is no specific treatment for fibrillary or immunotactoid glomerulopathy, although addressing an underlying malignancy, if present, may slow progression in the latter.

Membranoproliferative Glomerulonephropathy

GENERAL PRINCIPLES

Primary idiopathic membranoproliferative glomerulonephropathy (MPGN) is uncommon. Hepatitis C accounts for most cases of secondary MPGN, frequently in association with cryoglobulinemia. Other secondary causes include HIV, SLE, chronic infections, and various malignancies.

DIAGNOSIS

Clinical Presentation

MPGN can present with the nephrotic syndrome, nephritic syndrome, or a combination of both. Classically, there are three defined subtypes of MPGN (I, II, and III). However, as the molecular basis for disease is elucidated, an alternate classification has been proposed (*N Engl J Med 2012;366:1119*).
- Types I and III are mediated through immune complex formation.
- Type II MPGN (also called dense-deposit disease) and the related disorder C3 glomerulonephritis (C3GN) depend on activation of the alternative complement pathway. Both C3 and C4 are usually low in the immune complex–mediated forms of MPGN, whereas only C3 is low in type II MPGN. The antibody C3 nephritic factor may be present in type II MPGN, stabilizing the C3-convertase and promoting complement consumption. Deficiencies of or antibodies against the complement regulators (factors H and I) may also activate the complement cascade.

Diagnostic Testing

Kidney biopsy shows mesangial proliferation and hypercellularity on light microscopy, with "lobulization" of the glomerular tuft. Accumulation of debris along the filtration barrier may lead to a damage–repair cycle that results in duplication of the GBM, giving a double-contour or "tram track" appearance on silver stain. Immunofluorescence can show granular mesangial and capillary wall deposits of Ig in the immune complex–mediated forms, whereas only the C3 staining is positive in type II MPGN or C3GN. Electron microscopy can show subendothelial (type I) or intramembranous (type II) deposits. Type III disease has subendothelial and subepithelial deposits.

TREATMENT

- In adult idiopathic MPGN, treatment with immunosuppression has not shown a consistent benefit, although this may have been a result of the lumping together of pathophysiologically dissimilar diseases under the older classification scheme.
- Treatment of the secondary forms is targeted at the underlying disease. If renal function is rapidly deteriorating in the presence of cryoglobulins, plasmapheresis may help stabilize disease. Case reports have demonstrated possible efficacy of eculizumab, an anti-C5 monoclonal antibody, in the treatment of type II MPGN (*N Engl J Med 2012;366:1161*).

IgA Nephropathy/Henoch-Schönlein Purpura

GENERAL PRINCIPLES

- IgA nephropathy is typically idiopathic, characterized by a nephritic picture with microscopic (and less commonly macroscopic) hematuria and mild nonnephrotic range proteinuria.
- Presentation is most commonly in the second or third decade of life, generally following a slowly progressive course. Some patients may exhibit a crescentic form with a rapid decline in renal function resulting in ESRD.
- Henoch-Schönlein purpura is a related disorder that may represent a systemic form of the same disease, with vasculitic involvement of the skin (palpable purpura of the lower trunk and extremities), gastrointestinal tract, and joints.

DIAGNOSIS

Diagnostic Testing

Kidney biopsy shows increased mesangial cellularity on light microscopy, with IgA and C3 deposition on immunofluorescence. Abnormally glycosylated IgA is thought to be responsible for immune complex formation and mesangial deposition. Although serum IgA levels do not correlate with disease activity, events that potentially lead to overproduction (concurrent upper respiratory infection) or decreased clearance (hepatic cirrhosis) may predispose to disease.

TREATMENT

Aggressiveness of therapy depends on severity of disease. For patients with a benign course, conservative management with ACE inhibitors, ARBs, or fish oil (omega-3 fatty acids) may prevent deterioration of renal function, although the benefit of fish oil remains controversial. Progressive disease may benefit from a course of prednisone 1 mg/kg/d with or without cytotoxic agents.

Postinfectious Glomerulonephropathy

GENERAL PRINCIPLES

- Postinfectious glomerulonephropathy classically presents with the nephritic syndrome, hematuria, hypertension, edema, and renal insufficiency. Proteinuria may be present and is usually in the subnephrotic range.
- It is classically associated with streptococcal infection, which typically affects children under the age of 10 years, after a latent period of 2–4 weeks from onset of pharyngitis or skin infection. However, bacterial endocarditis, visceral abscesses, and ventriculoperitoneal shunt infections can also lead to this immune complex–mediated disease.
- Low complement levels are usually seen. ASO titers may be elevated serially, as may anti-DNaseB antibodies in streptococcal-associated disease.

DIAGNOSIS

Kidney biopsy reveals subepithelial humps on light and electron microscopy corresponding to the deposits on immunofluorescence (IgG, C3). There is widespread mesangial proliferation as well as an infiltration of polymorphonuclear cells.

TREATMENT

Treatment is primarily supportive. Resolution of the underlying infection typically leads to renal recovery in 2–4 weeks, even in cases where dialytic support was needed. A brisk diuresis should be anticipated in the recovery period.

Lupus Nephritis

GENERAL PRINCIPLES

LN can manifest as proteinuria of varying degrees with dysmorphic RBCs and RBC casts and renal insufficiency. Positive lupus serology (e.g., ANA, anti–double-stranded DNA antibodies) and hypocomplementemia are often present during acute flares.

DIAGNOSIS

Renal biopsy can provides diagnostic and prognostic information. The World Health Organization classification has five major categories based on histologic appearance. Class I has normal glomeruli, classes II to IV have increasing degrees of mesangial proliferation, and class V has an appearance similar to MN. Immunofluorescence is usually positive for IgG, IgA, IgM, C1q, C3, and C4, for the "full-house" fluorescence pattern.

TREATMENT

Aggressiveness of therapy considers the renal and extrarenal manifestations of the disease.
- Classes I and II LN rarely require specific treatment, and therapy is directed at the extrarenal manifestations.
- Class III LN, when mild or moderate, can generally be treated with a short course of high-dose steroids (prednisone 1 mg/kg/d).

- Patients with severe class III LN, class IV and V LN, or severe nephritic syndrome should undergo pulse IV methylprednisolone (7–15 mg/kg/d for 3 days) followed by oral prednisone at 0.5–1.0 mg/kg/d. A second agent such as monthly IV cyclophosphamide 0.5–1.0 g/m² or oral mycophenolate mofetil 1000 mg thrice daily for a course of 6 months should be used. Remission can be maintained for several years with mycophenolate mofetil 1000 mg twice daily, which was shown to be superior to azathioprine 2 mg/kg/d in preventing relapse (*N Engl J Med 2011;365:1886*).

Pulmonary–Renal Syndromes

GENERAL PRINCIPLES

Several distinct clinical entities make up the pulmonary–renal syndromes where there is vasculitic involvement of the alveolar and glomerular capillaries. Typically, this results in rapidly progressive renal failure often with concurrent pulmonary involvement in the form of alveolar hemorrhage. A nephritic picture predominates, with dysmorphic RBCs and RBC casts in the urine. Arthralgias and fever may represent other systemic manifestations.

DIAGNOSIS

- In **anti-GBM antibody disease**, circulating antibody to the α-3 chain of type IV collagen is deposited in the basement membrane of alveoli and glomeruli, resulting in linear staining on immunofluorescence. **Goodpasture syndrome** includes pulmonary involvement and can present with life-threatening alveolar hemorrhage. The presence of anti-GBM antibody in the serum supports the diagnosis, and 10–30% of patients will have a positive ANCA serology as well.
- In **granulomatosis with polyangiitis** (GPA; formerly known as Wegener granulomatosis), vasculitic lesions involve the small vessels of the kidneys and may also involve the lungs, skin, and gastrointestinal tract. As in anti-GBM antibody disease, pulmonary hemorrhage may be life threatening. Biopsy findings include a small-vessel vasculitis with noncaseating granuloma formation in the kidneys, lungs, or sinuses.
  - GPA is part of a group of diseases known as *pauci-immune glomerulonephritis* (referring to the absence of immunostaining deposits), which includes Churg-Strauss syndrome (asthma and eosinophilia) and microscopic polyangiitis.
  - In GPA, there is a positive cytoplasmic ANCA directed against serine proteinase-3, whereas in microscopic polyangiitis and Churg-Strauss syndrome, there is a positive perinuclear ANCA directed against myeloperoxidase.

TREATMENT

- In **anti-GBM antibody disease**, the goal of therapy is to *clear the pathogenic antibody* while suppressing new production. Treatment is with daily total volume plasmapheresis for approximately 14 days in conjunction with cyclophosphamide 2 mg/kg/d and glucocorticoids (IV methylprednisolone 7–15 mg/kg/d for 3 days, followed by oral prednisone 1 mg/kg/d). Immunosuppression is tapered over 8 weeks. Serial measurement of the anti-GBM antibody level is useful to monitor therapy, with plasmapheresis and immunosuppression continuing until it is undetectable.

  Poor response to therapy is predicted by the presence of oliguria, Cr >5.7 mg/dL, or dialysis dependence on presentation. Even if the likelihood of renal recovery is low, evidence of pulmonary involvement warrants aggressive therapy.

- Treatment of **GPA** is with combined prednisone 1 mg/kg/d (with taper) and cyclophosphamide (IV at 1 g/m^2 monthly or orally at 2 mg/kg/d) for at least 3 months to induce remission. Therapy should then continue with oral steroids for 1 year to prevent relapse. More aggressive management with plasmapheresis and pulse IV steroids may be beneficial for patients presenting with pulmonary hemorrhage or dialysis dependence. Rituximab given IV as four weekly doses of 375 mg/m^2, in combination with steroids, has also been approved for treatment of GPA (*N Engl J Med 2010;363:221*).

  Double-strength sulfamethoxazole-trimethoprim given twice daily has been shown to reduce extrarenal relapses and to prevent *Pneumocystis (carinii) jirovecii* infection in patients on high-dose immunosuppression.

Polycystic Kidney Disease

GENERAL PRINCIPLES

- Autosomal dominant polycystic kidney disease (ADPKD) is a hereditary disorder resulting in cystic enlargement of the kidney and occurs in approximately 1 in 1000 persons. Approximately 20% of patients with ADPKD do not have a positive family history.
- There are two well-described mutations in the polycystin genes, *PKD1* and *PKD2*. *PKD1* is the most common and present in approximately 85% of ADPKD. *PKD2* is associated with a later onset of disease.
- The mechanism by which cysts form is unclear. The polycystin gene products primarily localize to the cilia of the tubular apical membrane. Disordered regulation of cell division may lead to overgrowth of the tubular segment, eventually pinching off from the rest of the collecting system. Cyst formation affects only a relatively small percentage of tubules, suggesting a "two-hit" hypothesis where a sporadic mutation of the wild-type allele results in local cystogenesis

DIAGNOSIS

Clinical Presentation

- Hypertension is an early feature of ADPKD. As the affected tubules enlarge, they impinge upon the blood flow to neighboring glomeruli, rendering them ischemic. This is turn activates the renin–angiotensin–aldosterone system, leading to systemic hypertension. Onset of kidney failure is highly variable, with half of patients reaching ESRD by the age of 60.
- Cerebral aneurysms, hepatic cysts, mitral valve prolapse, and colonic diverticula are found in association with ADPKD. As cysts enlarge, they may result in a palpable flank mass. Gross hematuria and pain may indicate cyst hemorrhage into the collecting system. Flank pain may also be caused by cyst infection or stretching of the renal capsule.

Diagnostic Testing

- Differentiation from other cystic diseases (acquired cystic disease, medullary sponge kidney, medullary cystic kidney disease) can be made by the presence of enlarged cystic kidneys rather than shrunken or normal-sized cystic kidneys. Acquired cystic disease is often seen in patients with CKD as well as patients on dialysis. The cysts are typically bilateral in atrophic kidneys.
- Ultrasonography reveals multiple cysts. In the setting of a positive family history, a diagnosis of ADPKD can be made from ultrasound findings, with criteria differing according to age. At least three cysts are required in patients under the age of 40 years. In patients aged 40–59 years, at least two cysts in each kidney are needed. For patients age 60 years and older, the diagnosis requires at least four cysts in each kidney.

- Patients with a family history of cerebral aneurysms or with symptoms attributable to a cerebral aneurysm should undergo evaluation with brain MRI/MRA.
- Genetic testing may be considered if patients have equivocal imaging results or if a definitive diagnosis is required.

TREATMENT

- There is currently no specific treatment to prevent cyst formation or slow cyst growth. Aggressive control of hypertension should be practiced, and blockade of the renin–angiotensin–aldosterone system with an ACE inhibitor or ARB is recommended as first-line therapy.
- Gross hematuria from cyst hemorrhage can usually be managed with bed rest, hydration, and analgesia. Resolution may take 5–7 days.
- Cyst infections are generally treated with antibiotics that achieve good penetration into the cysts. Sulfamethoxazole-trimethoprim and ciprofloxacin are the antibiotics of choice. The absence of bacterial growth in the urine does not rule out infection because the cystic fluid does not necessarily communicate with the rest of the collecting system.
- Pain that persists without an obvious hemorrhagic or infectious cause may respond to cyst reduction surgery, particularly if there is a culprit cyst that can be identified and targeted.
- As the underlying mechanism for cyst growth is clarified, newer treatment options are emerging. Past trials investigating the antimetabolites sirolimus and everolimus have been disappointing. A large study of tolvaptan in ADPKD showed a significant reduction in the cyst growth rate but with an uncertain benefit in long-term renal function coupled with signals of potential hepatotoxicity; formal approval awaits the results of further investigation (*N Engl J Med 2012;367:2407*).

Nephrolithiasis

GENERAL PRINCIPLES

- **Calcium-based stones** are the most common and appear predominantly as calcium oxalate or calcium phosphate salts. These stones are radiopaque. Calcium phosphate stones can appear as elongated, blunt crystals and form in alkaline urine. Calcium oxalate stones can be found in acidic or alkaline urine and can be dumbbell shaped or appear as paired pyramids (giving them an envelope appearance when viewed on end).
- **Uric acid stones** can be idiopathic or develop as part of hyperuricosuric states such as gout and myeloproliferative disorders. These stones are radiolucent and are found in acidic urine. Uric acid crystals exhibit a variety of shapes, with needles and rhomboid forms being the most common.
- **Struvite stones** contain magnesium, ammonium, and phosphate, and develop in alkaline urine associated with urea-splitting organisms (e.g., *Proteus*, *Klebsiella*). They are radiopaque and can extend to fill the renal pelvis, taking on a staghorn configuration. On microscopy, struvite crystals have a characteristic coffin-lid shape.
- **Cystine stones** are uncommon and can form as the result of an autosomal recessive disorder. These stones have an intermediate radiolucency and appear as hexagonal crystals in the urine.

DIAGNOSIS

Clinical Presentation

Patients often present with costovertebral angle or flank pain, which can radiate to the scrotum or labia. Hematuria with nondysmorphic RBCs may be noted. Oliguria and AKI are uncommon but can result if there is bilateral obstruction or if a solitary functioning kidney is affected.

Diagnostic Testing

- Basic laboratory investigation should include urine culture, pH, microscopy, and serum calcium, phosphate, parathyroid hormone, and uric acid levels. Urine should be strained and passed stones analyzed for composition.
- A plain abdominal film may reveal the radiopaque stones composed of calcium salts, struvite, or cystine; however, noncontrast CT scanning has replaced other imaging modalities as the study of choice for suspected nephrolithiasis.
- Recurrent stone formers should undergo a more extensive evaluation, with 24-hour urine collections for calcium, phosphate, uric acid, citrate, oxalate, and cystine. This collection should not be done during an acute episode in a hospitalized patient but rather reserved for when the patient is on his or her usual outpatient diet.

TREATMENT

- General treatment consists of **hydration** to increase urine output and analgesia. If the stone is obstructing outflow or is accompanied by infection, removal is indicated with urgent urologic or radiologic intervention.
- After passage of a stone, treatment is directed at **prevention of recurrent stone formation**. Regardless of stone type, the foundation of therapy is maintenance of high urine output (2–3 L/d) with oral hydration and a low-sodium diet (<2 g/d).
- For calcium oxalate stones, a low-calcium diet is no longer recommended given the risks of osteoporosis. Instead, patients should be on a normal-calcium diet with no added calcium supplements. Oxalate-rich foods (e.g., spinach, rhubarb) should be avoided. Thiazide diuretics may reduce calciuria, and potassium citrate may be added in patients with hypocitraturia.
- Uric acid stones can be prevented or reduced in size by allopurinol or urinary alkalinization with citrate, bicarbonate, or acetazolamide. A low-protein diet may also prevent these stones.
- Struvite calculi frequently require surgical intervention for their removal. Extracorporeal shock wave lithotripsy can be used as adjunctive therapy. Monthly urine cultures should be obtained, and if positive, aggressive antibiotic treatment is indicated.
- Cystine stones require extensive urinary alkalinization to a pH of 7.0–7.5 to induce solubility. D-penicillamine and mercaptopropionylglycine can further increase solubility through breakage and exchange of disulfide bonds. Side effects of D-penicillamine and mercaptopropionylglycine include fever, rash, arthritis, myelosuppression, hepatotoxicity, and vitamin B_6 deficiency.

Management of Chronic Kidney Disease

GENERAL PRINCIPLES

- CKD is divided into five stages based on the estimated GFR (Figure 13-1). To be classified as stage 1 or stage 2, *there must be an accompanying structural or functional defect* (e.g., proteinuria, hematuria) because the GFR is normal or near normal in these stages.
- Patients are usually asymptomatic until significant renal function is lost (late stage 4 and stage 5). However, *complications including hypertension, anemia, and mineral bone disorders* (renal osteodystrophy [ROD] and secondary hyperparathyroidism) often develop during stage 3 and thus must be investigated and addressed before patients become symptomatic.

Prognosis of CKD by GFR and albuminuria category

				Persistent albuminuria categories Description and range		
				A1	**A2**	**A3**
Prognosis of CKD by GFR and Albuminuria Categories: KDIGO 2012				Normal to mildly increased	Moderately increased	Severely increased
				<30 mg/g <3 mg/mmol	30–300 mg/g 3–30 mg/mmol	>300 mg/g >30 mg/mmol
GFR categories (ml/min/1.73 m²) Description and range	G1	Normal or high	≥90	Low	Moderate	High
	G2	Mildly decreased	60–89	Low	Moderate	High
	G3a	Mildly to moderately decreased	45–59	Moderate	High	Very high
	G3b	Moderately to severely decreased	30–44	High	Very high	Very high
	G4	Severely decreased	15–29	Very high	Very high	Very high
	G5	Kidney failure	<15			

Figure 13-1. Stages of chronic kidney disease. CKD, chronic kidney disease; GFR, glomerular filtration rate. (From KDIGO 2012 Clinical Practice Guideline for the Evaluation and Management of Chronic Kidney Disease. *Kidney Int* 2103;3[Suppl]:5–14.)

- The decline in GFR may be followed by plotting the reciprocal of Cr versus time, revealing a linear decrement. This can be useful in end-stage planning and in predicting when renal replacement therapy will be needed. A steeper than anticipated decline in GFR suggests a superimposed renal insult.
- Initiation of dialysis based solely on a target GFR has not shown a mortality benefit (*N Engl J Med 2010;363:609*). Dialysis should be started prior to the worsening of the patient's metabolic or nutritional status.

Risk Factors
- **Decreased renal perfusion** can lead to a decline in GFR. This can occur with true volume depletion or diminished effective circulating volume (e.g., congestive heart failure, hepatic cirrhosis). **NSAIDs** can be particularly deleterious in this setting because they block the renal autoregulatory mechanisms to preserve GFR. ACE inhibitors or ARBs also produce a reversible decrement in GFR.
- **Uncontrolled hypertension** leads to hyperfiltration, which may lead to worsening proteinuria and further damage to the glomeruli.
- **Albuminuria has also been identified as a risk factor for progression of renal disease. A prognostic scale has been developed incorporating both the GFR and degree of albuminuria to predict the likelihood to renal failure (see Figure 13-1).**
- **Nephrotoxic agents**, such as iodinated contrast agents and aminoglycosides, should be avoided when possible. Careful attention to drug dosing is mandatory, frequently

guided by the estimated GFR or CKD stage. Drug levels should be monitored where appropriate.

- Patients undergoing coronary angiography are at particular risk for worsening CKD. **Contrast nephropathy and atheroembolic disease** are potential complications, and the risks and benefits of the procedure must be weighed with the patient prior to proceeding.
- **UTI or obstruction** should be considered in all patients with an unexplained drop in renal function. Worsening renal artery stenosis may also lead to a more rapid decline in GFR as well as sudden worsening in previously controlled hypertension.
- **Renal vein thrombosis** may occur as a complication of the nephrotic syndrome and can exacerbate CKD. Hematuria and flank pain may be present.

TREATMENT

Treatment of CKD is focused on avoidance of risk factors (listed earlier), dietary modification, blood pressure control, adequate treatment of the associated conditions (listed in the following text), and ultimately, preparation for renal replacement therapy.

- **Dietary restrictions**
  - **Sodium restriction** to <3 g/d is usually adequate for most CKD patients. Restriction to <2 g/d should be used if heart failure or refractory hypertension is present. A 24-hour urine sodium level of 100 mEq roughly correlates with a 2 g/d diet.
  - Fluid restriction is generally not required in CKD patients and, if excessive, may lead to volume depletion and hypernatremia. Restriction is appropriate in patients with dilutional hyponatremia.
  - **Potassium should be restricted** to 60 mEq/d in individuals with hyperkalemia. Tomato-based products, bananas, potatoes, and citrus drinks are high in potassium and should be avoided in these patients.
  - **Dietary phosphate restriction** should be to 800–1000 mg/d. Dairy products, dark colas, and nuts should be avoided in hyperphosphatemia. Oral binders (calcium carbonate or acetate, lanthanum carbonate, sevelamer carbonate) can be used if dietary restrictions are unable to control phosphate levels.
- **Hypertension**
  - Uncontrolled hypertension accelerates the rate of decline of renal function. Blood pressure control to <140/90 mm Hg is recommended for patients with CKD (*JAMA 2014;311:507*).
  - **ACE inhibitors or ARBs** should be used preferentially in the CKD population. They lower intraglomerular pressure and possess renoprotective properties beyond the antihypertensive effect, particularly in proteinuric states. Due to their effects on intrarenal hemodynamics, a 30% rise in serum Cr should be anticipated and tolerated; a further rise should prompt a search for possible renal artery stenosis. The Cr and serum potassium should be checked approximately 1–2 weeks after a dose adjustment. Combined therapy with ACE inhibitors and ARBs is not recommended due to an increased risk of hyperkalemia and AKI without statistical benefit in mortality or long-term renal protection (*N Engl J Med 2013;369:1892*).
  - **Diuretics** are also beneficial in achieving euvolemia in hypertensive CKD patients. Thiazide diuretics become less effective as the GFR falls below 30 mL/min, whereas loop diuretics retain their efficacy, although higher doses may be required for the desired effect.
- **Anemia**
  - A normocytic anemia is common in CKD and should be searched for once the GFR falls below 60 mL/min (stage 3).
  - Alternate causes for an anemia should be entertained in the appropriate setting and iron stores assessed. If the transferrin saturation is <25% and there is no evidence of iron

overload (ferritin <1000 ng/mL), consideration should be given to iron repletion with 1 g of an IV preparation of iron dextran (1000 mg once with test dose of 25 mg), ferric gluconate (125 mg, eight doses), or iron sucrose (100 mg, 10 doses).

○ Erythropoiesis-stimulating agents (ESAs), such as epoetin and darbepoetin, can effectively reduce but do not prevent the need for RBC transfusions. ESA therapy increases the risk of stroke and thrombotic and cardiovascular events and worsens outcomes in patients with cancer. These agents should not be started in CKD unless the hemoglobin is <10 g/dL, other causes of anemia such as iron deficiency are addressed, and reduction in transfusions is a goal. The minimum dose that maintains the hemoglobin above the need for transfusion and *below 11 g/dL* should be used. Correction of iron deficiency frequently decreases the ESA dose requirement and may defer the need for ESA. Targeting the hemoglobin to higher levels has been associated with increased cardiovascular mortality, and this risk may be related to the higher doses of ESA (*N Engl J Med 2010;363:1146*).

• **Bone mineral disorders**
  ○ CKD bone mineral disorders increase in prevalence as the GFR declines through stage 3 and more advanced disease. They include disorders of bone turnover and secondary hyperparathyroidism.
  ○ **Osteitis fibrosa cystica** is commonly associated with secondary hyperparathyroidism and increased bone turnover, resulting in bone pain and fractures. Adynamic bone disease is a low-turnover state with suppressed parathyroid hormone (PTH) levels. Osteomalacia can involve deposition of aluminum into bone and is less commonly seen today with the decreased use of aluminum-based phosphate binders.
  ○ In CKD, starting in stage 3, vitamin D deficiency, low calcium, and elevated phosphate can all contribute to **secondary hyperparathyroidism**. The general goal of therapy is to suppress PTH toward normal while maintaining normal serum calcium and phosphate. This can be addressed in three steps: repletion of vitamin D stores (25-OH vitamin D), control of dietary phosphate with binders, and administration of active vitamin D (1,25-dihydroxyvitamin D or an analog).
    ▪ Deficient stores (25-OH vitamin D <30 ng/mL) should be corrected with oral ergocalciferol 50,000-IU capsule weekly or every other week or cholecalciferol 2000–4000 IU daily. The duration of treatment depends on severity of the deficiency, with levels <5 ng/dL warranting at least 12 weeks of treatment. Once at goal, maintenance therapy can rely on either monthly ergocalciferol 50,000 IU or daily cholecalciferol 1000–2000 IU.
    ▪ Phosphate control can be difficult as GFR declines, even with appropriate dietary restriction. Phosphate binders inhibit gastrointestinal absorption. Calcium-based binders are effective when given with meals as calcium carbonate (200 mg of elemental calcium per 500-mg tablet) or calcium acetate (169 mg of elemental calcium per 667-mg tablet). In general, the total daily elemental calcium administered should be <1500 mg. Lanthanum carbonate and sevelamer carbonate are non–calcium-based alternatives.
    ▪ Active vitamin D (1,25-dihydroxyvitamin D) and its synthetic analogs are potent suppressors of PTH and can be administered if serum PTH remains elevated. Options include daily calcitriol (0.25–1 μg), paricalcitol (1–5 μg), or doxercalciferol (1–5 μg). Calcium levels need to be monitored regularly and doses adjusted to avoid hypercalcemia.
    ▪ Cinacalcet is a calcimimetic that acts on the parathyroid gland to suppress PTH release. It should be used only in dialysis patients and usually in conjunction with active vitamin D, because it may induce significant hypocalcemia and is relatively ineffective as monotherapy.

• **Metabolic acidosis.** As renal function deteriorates, the kidney is unable to appropriately excrete sufficient acid, resulting in metabolic acidosis (mixed high and normal anion gap).

To compensate, alkaline buffer is released from the skeleton but can ultimately worsen bone mineral disease.

- ○ Treatment with **sodium bicarbonate** 650–1300 mg thrice daily can help maintain the serum bicarbonate level at 22 mEq/L. Such therapy, however, can increase the sodium load and contribute to edema or hypertension.
- ○ Citrate, another alkaline source, should not be used in the CKD or ESRD population because it can dramatically enhance gastrointestinal absorption of aluminum and lead to aluminum toxicity or osteomalacia.
- **Hyperlipidemia.** Therapy with statins combined with ezetimibe has shown improved cardiovascular outcomes with fewer major atherosclerotic events in patients with moderate to severe CKD and in the dialysis population, although the benefit in patients on dialysis was less (*Lancet 2011;377:2181*). Use of lipid-lowering therapy is appropriate in patients with atherosclerotic disease at all stages of CKD.
- **Preparation for renal replacement therapy**
- ○ Patients should be counseled at an early stage to determine preferences for renal replacement therapies, including hemodialysis, peritoneal dialysis (PD), and eligibility for renal transplantation.
- ○ In stage 4 CKD, preparation for the creation of a permanent vascular access for hemodialysis should be initiated by protecting the nondominant forearm from IV catheters and blood draws. Timely referral for vein mapping and to an access surgeon can facilitate the creation and maturation of an arteriovenous (AV) access.

RENAL REPLACEMENT THERAPIES

Approach to Dialysis

TREATMENT

- **Modalities**
- ○ Renal replacement therapy is indicated when conservative medical management is unable to control the metabolic derangements of kidney disease. This applies to the acute and chronic settings. Common acute indications include **hyperkalemia**, **metabolic acidosis**, and **volume overload** that are refractory to medical management. Uremic **encephalopathy** or **pericarditis**, as well as certain **intoxications** (methanol, ethylene glycol, or salicylates), can all be indications to initiate dialytic therapy acutely. In the chronic setting, renal replacement therapy is typically begun prior to the worsening of the metabolic or nutritional status of the patient.
- ○ Dialysis works by solute diffusion and water transport across a selectively permeable membrane. In hemodialysis, blood is pumped counter-currently to a dialysis solution within an extracorporeal membrane. This can be performed intermittently (3–4 hours during the day) or in a continuous 24-hour fashion depending on hemodynamic stability or goals of therapy. PD uses the patient's peritoneal membrane as the selective filter, and dialysis fluid is instilled into the peritoneal cavity.
- ○ Transplantation offers the best long-term survival and most completely replaces the filtrative and endocrine functions of the native kidney. However, it carries the risks that accompany long-term immunosuppression.
- **Diffusion**
The selectively permeable membrane contains pores that allow electrolytes and other small molecules to pass by diffusion while holding back larger molecules and cellular components of the blood. Movement relies on the molecular size and the concentration gradient, where Cr, urea, potassium, and other waste products of metabolism pass into the dialysis solution while alkaline buffers (bicarbonate or lactate) enter the blood from the dialysis solution.

- **Ultrafiltration/convection**
  - Removal of water is termed ultrafiltration (UF). It can be achieved in hemodialysis via a transmembrane hydrostatic pressure that removes excess fluid from the blood compartment. In PD, water follows its osmotic gradient into the relatively hyperosmolar dialysis solution (usually with dextrose providing the osmotic driving force).
  - As water is removed from the vascular compartment, it drags along solute. This is termed convective clearance. This usually accounts for only a small fraction of the total clearance but can be significantly increased if a physiologic "replacement fluid" is infused into the patient concurrently to prevent hypovolemia. This strategy is frequently employed by continuous hemodialysis modalities (see the following text).

Hemodialysis

GENERAL PRINCIPLES

- Hemodialysis is by far the most commonly used form of renal replacement therapy in the United States. Intermittent hemodialysis (IHD) typically runs for 3–4 hours per session and is performed three times weekly. Outpatient, in-center hemodialysis for ESRD generally uses this modality, although variations are available for patients undergoing home treatments.
- Continuous renal replacement therapy (CRRT) can be used in specialized circumstances, particularly when the patient's hemodynamic status would not tolerate the rapid fluid shifts of IHD. Although less efficient (with slower blood flows) and using slower UF rates, CRRT can achieve equivalent clearances of both solute and fluid compared to IHD due to its continuous, 24-hour nature. The slower blood flows usually necessitate anticoagulation (with systemic heparin or regional citrate) to prevent the filter from clotting. Continuous modalities require specialized nursing and an intensive care setting.
  - The most frequently employed form of CRRT is continuous venovenous hemodiafiltration (CVVHDF).
  - In CVVHDF, blood is slowly pumped counter-currently to a dialysis solution (diffusion), and a replacement fluid (a "cleansed" physiologic solution devoid of uremic toxins) is infused into the circuit to balance most of the ultrafiltrate (convection).
- Sustained low-efficiency dialysis (SLED) is essentially a hybrid form of IHD and CRRT used in an intensive care setting. Intermediate blood flows lower the clotting risk if anticoagulation is not used, while intermediate treatment lengths (8–10 hours) still allow for adequate clearances. Patients also spend a significant portion of the day off the machine to allow for nonbedside testing, procedures, and physical therapy.
- **Prescription and adequacy**
  - IHD typically runs for 3–4 hours and can ultrafilter 3–4 L safely in hemodynamically stable patients. In the chronic setting, IHD is generally performed three times weekly, although the longer interdialytic interval on the weekend has been associated with a heightened mortality risk (*N Engl J Med 2011;365:1099*). In the acute setting, the appropriate interval is not clearly known, although a thrice-weekly schedule is likely adequate; daily assessment should be performed to reevaluate dialytic needs.
  - Adequacy is assessed by calculating the clearance of BUN, which serves as a surrogate marker of the "uremic factors." The urea reduction ratio (URR) can be calculated by the following:

$$\text{URR} = [(\text{predialysis BUN} - \text{postdialysis BUN}) / (\text{predialysis BUN})] \times 100$$

A reduction rate of >65% is considered adequate in the chronic setting (*N Engl J Med 2002;347:2010*). An adequacy target is less well defined for AKI.

○ Intensive daily hemodialysis was not shown to be superior to standard thrice-weekly treatments (*N Engl J Med 2008;359:7*).

○ Clearance is measured differently in CRRT where dialytic therapy is taking place around the clock, effectively serving as an extracorporeal "GFR." Drug dosing needs to be adjusted accordingly. An estimate of this clearance can be calculated by the sum of the dialysis fluid and replacement fluid, and net UF rates are expressed as the number of milliliters per minute. For most circumstances, this approximates a clearance of 20–50 mL/min.

○ With CRRT, the net UF rate can be adjusted as needed, according to the patient's hemodynamic status. One must be vigilant in checking electrolyte levels (particularly ionized calcium and phosphorus) to ensure they remain within the desired ranges. Calcium levels are especially important to follow when regional citrate anticoagulation is being used.

○ Phosphate, which is predominantly intracellular, is generally poorly removed by IHD; however, in CRRT, there is continuous efflux of this anion, and significant hypophosphatemia can occur.

COMPLICATIONS

• Nontunneled catheters are typically placed in the internal jugular or femoral vein and carry the same risks as other central venous catheters (infection, bleeding, pneumothorax). They are almost exclusively used in the inpatient setting and are generally used for 1–2 weeks. Tunneled catheters have lower rates of infection and can be used for 6 months while a more definitive access is maturing (AV fistula or graft).

○ Fevers and rigors, particularly during dialysis, should prompt a search for an infectious cause, and empiric antibiotic coverage for staphylococci and gram-negative bacteria should be administered.

○ The catheter should then be replaced after a period of defervescence and sterilization of the blood (at least 48 hours). Documented bacteremia should be treated with antibiotics for at least 3 weeks.

• Thrombosis of an AV fistula or graft can frequently be recanalized by thrombolysis or thrombectomy. Stenotic regions can be evaluated by a fistulogram, and treatment may encompass angioplasty or stent deployment.

• Intradialytic hypotension is most commonly due to intravascular volume depletion from rapid UF. Antihypertensive medications may also contribute. Infectious causes should be sought in the appropriate setting. Acute treatment of the drop in blood pressure includes infusion of normal saline (as 200-mL boluses) and reduction of the UF rate.

• Dialysis disequilibrium is an uncommon syndrome that may occur in severely uremic patients undergoing their first few treatments. Rapid clearance of toxins is thought to induce cerebral edema by osmolar shifts and can present as nausea, emesis, headache, confusion, or seizures. Occurrence can be prevented or ameliorated by initiating patients on dialysis with slower blood flows and shorter treatments.

Peritoneal Dialysis

GENERAL PRINCIPLES

• Historically, PD has been used in the acute setting for hemodynamically unstable patients. However, with the development and availability of safe and effective continuous hemodialysis, use of PD in the treatment of AKI in adults has been mostly abandoned in the United States. Currently, its use is primarily in the treatment of ESRD.

- There are two modalities in use: manual exchanges and automated cycler exchanges.
  - The manual modality, also called continuous ambulatory peritoneal dialysis (CAPD), has the patient instill dialysis fluid into the peritoneum for a specified length of time, after which the dialysate is drained and replaced by another dwell.
  - The automated modality, also called continuous cycling peritoneal dialysis (CCPD), typically operates overnight where a machine runs a preprogrammed set of exchanges while the patient sleeps. A final fill usually remains in the peritoneum and is carried during the daytime for continued solute exchange.
- Both PD modalities require strict adherence to sterile technique, and careful patient selection is necessary. Generally, PD should not be used if there is a history of recent abdominal surgery or if multiple peritoneal adhesions are present.
- **Prescription and adequacy**
  - The choice between CAPD and CCPD usually depends on patient preference and on the transport characteristics of the peritoneal membrane. Manual exchanges (i.e., CAPD) can be used as a backup modality, particularly in the hospital where nurse staffing or machine availability may be limited.
  - In writing PD orders, the following variables must be specified: dwell volume, dwell time, number of exchanges, and dextrose concentration of the dialysis solution. The dwell volume is typically between 2–3 L. The dextrose concentration can be 1.50%, 2.50%, or 4.25%, providing the osmotic gradient for fluid removal. Higher dextrose concentrations allow for greater UF but also lead to more glucose absorption and worsening control of diabetes. Icodextrin is a glucose polymer preparation that can be used in longer dwell because it is minimally absorbed and thus maintains an effective osmotic gradient up to 18 hours. Commercially available PD solutions may have color-coded tabs, and patients may know these better than the actual concentrations (yellow for 1.50%, green for 2.50%, red for 4.25%). A sample order set for manual CAPD would be 2.5 L, four exchanges, 6 hours each, with 2.5% dextrose.
  - PD is less efficient than conventional hemodialysis. However, given its continuous nature, solute clearance and UF can approximate that of other modalities. Larger volumes and more frequent exchanges can assist with solute exchange. Increasing the concentration of dextrose can promote greater UF in volume-overloaded patients.
  - *Residual renal function is very important in the PD population, and avoidance of nephrotoxins should be practiced (J Am Soc Nephrol 2002;13:1307).*

COMPLICATIONS

- **Peritonitis** typically presents with diffuse abdominal pain and cloudy peritoneal fluid. A sample should be sent for cell count, differential, Gram stain, and culture. A WBC count of >100 cells/μL, of which at least 50% are neutrophils, supports the diagnosis.
  - Empiric therapy should cover for both gram-positive and gram-negative organisms, with a first-generation cephalosporin (cefazolin or cephalothin) and ceftazidime at 15–20 mg/kg of each in the longest dwell of the day (*Perit Dial Int 2005;25:107*). If a methicillin-resistant organism is suspected, use vancomycin (30 mg/kg every 5–7 days) for gram-positive coverage and a third-generation cephalosporin for gram-negative coverage, including *Pseudomonas*.
  - The intraperitoneal route is the preferred method of administration, unless the patient is overtly septic, in which case IV antibiotics should be used. Antibiotics can be tailored once culture results are known and should be continued for 2–3 weeks. Multiple organisms, particularly if gram negative, should prompt a search for intestinal perforation.
- Tunnel or exit site infections may present with local erythema, tenderness, or purulent drainage, although crusting at the exit site alone does not necessarily indicate infection. Treatment can be with oral cephalosporins (gram positive) or fluoroquinolones (gram

negative). However, infections can be difficult to eradicate, and catheter removal may be required with a temporary transition to hemodialysis.

- Failure of PD fluid to drain is termed outflow failure. This may result from kinking of the catheter, constipation, or plugging of the catheter with fibrin strands. Conservative treatment should aim at resolving constipation if present and instilling heparin into the PD fluid at 500 units/L.
- Small hernias are at particularly high risk for incarceration and should be corrected surgically while the patient is temporarily treated with hemodialysis. Fluid leaks can lead to abdominal wall and genital edema and typically result from anatomic defects. Hydrothorax usually occurs on the right side and can be diagnosed by a markedly elevated glucose concentration in the pleural fluid. Pleurodesis can eliminate the potential space and permit continuation of PD.
- **Sclerosing encapsulating peritonitis** is a complication of long-term PD. The peritoneal membrane becomes thickened and entraps loops of bowel, leading to symptoms of bowel obstruction. A bloody drainage may be present. Treatment is supportive with the focus on bowel rest and surgical lysis of adhesions. A trial of immunosuppression with prednisone 10–40 mg/d may have limited benefit.
- Hyperglycemia results from the systemic absorption of glucose from the dialysis fluid. Because peritoneal uptake of insulin is unpredictable, treatment with subcutaneous insulin is preferred.
- Hyperlipidemia is common in the PD population, and treatment should be reserved for those with specific cardiac indications.
- Unlike hemodialysis, patients on PD tend to experience hypokalemia, likely due to a continuous potassium exodus in the dialysate as well as from an intracellular shift from the increased endogenous insulin production. Oral replacement is usually sufficient, either with relaxation of prior dietary restrictions or with low-dose supplementation (10–20 mEq/d of potassium chloride).
- Protein loss can be high, and the dietary protein intake should be 1.2–1.3 g/kg/d. Episodes of peritonitis can make the membrane even more susceptible to protein losses.

Transplantation

GENERAL PRINCIPLES

- Renal transplantation offers patients an improved quality of life and survival as compared to other renal replacement modalities.
- Pretransplant evaluation focuses on cardiopulmonary status, vascular sufficiency, and human lymphocyte antigen typing. Structural abnormalities of the urinary tract need to be addressed. Contraindications include most malignancies, active infection, or significant cardiopulmonary disease.
- In adult recipients, the renal allograft is placed in the extraperitoneal space, in the anterior lower abdomen. Vascular anastomosis is typically to the iliac vessels, whereas the ureter is attached to the bladder through a muscular tunnel to approximate sphincter function.
- Immunosuppression protocols vary among institutions. A typical regimen would include prednisone along with a combination of a calcineurin inhibitor (cyclosporine or tacrolimus) and an antimetabolite (mycophenolate derivative, azathioprine, or rapamycin).
- Evaluation of allograft dysfunction frequently requires kidney biopsy. Current laboratory and radiologic tests cannot reliably distinguish acute rejection from drug toxicity, the two most common causes of a rising Cr in the transplant population. Posttransplant lymphoproliferative disease, interstitial nephritis, and infections such as cytomegalovirus, *Polyomavirus* (BK virus), and pyelonephritis may present similarly to acute allograft dysfunction and should be excluded.
- Complications and long-term management of transplant recipients are discussed further in Chapter 17, Solid Organ Transplant Medicine.

14 Treatment of Infectious Diseases

Allison L. Nazinitsky, Stephen Y. Liang, and Nigar Kirmani

Principles of Therapy

GENERAL PRINCIPLES

Infections may be caused by bacteria, viruses, fungi, and parasites and can involve any organ system. When antimicrobial therapy is indicated, a number of factors reviewed in this chapter should be considered. Infectious disease consultation may assist with diagnostics, therapeutics, and long-term monitoring of side effects and drug–drug interactions. Stewardship to avoid indiscriminate use of antibiotics may combat drug resistance, avoid adverse effects, and curb excess costs.

DIAGNOSIS

- **The history and physical exam** are important, especially for diagnostic dilemmas and fever of unknown origin (FUO) cases. Eliciting exposures, travel history, and hobbies will broaden the differential diagnosis to assist with workup.
- **Gram stains** from potentially infected specimens may permit a rapid presumptive diagnosis and guide empiric antibiotic selection.
- **Aerobic, anaerobic, fungal, or acid-fast bacilli (AFB) cultures** may be performed on specimens. The microbiology laboratory should be consulted if organisms with special growth requirements are suspected to ensure appropriate transport and processing of cultures.
- **Susceptibility testing** of cultures facilitates selection of antimicrobial agents.
- **Rapid diagnostic testing**, such as polymerase chain reaction (PCR) and antigen detection, may also provide early confirmation of an infectious etiologic agent.

TREATMENT

- **Choice of initial antimicrobial therapy**
  Empiric therapy should be directed against the most likely pathogens and possess the narrowest spectrum.
- **Local susceptibility patterns** must be considered in selecting empiric therapy because of wide variability among communities and individual hospitals.
- Drug allergies, previous cultures, and prior antibiotic exposure should guide selection.
- **Timing for the initiation of antimicrobial therapy**
  - In acute clinical scenarios, empiric therapy should begin immediately and ideally after appropriate cultures have been obtained. Urgent therapy is indicated in febrile patients who are neutropenic or asplenic. Sepsis, meningitis, and rapidly progressive necrotizing infections should also be treated promptly with antimicrobials.
  - In clinically stable patients, one may consider withholding empiric antimicrobials, pending workup, to allow for more targeted therapy and avoid unnecessary drugs.

- **Route of administration**
  - Patients with serious infections should be given IV antimicrobial agents.
  - Oral therapy is acceptable in less urgent circumstances if adequate drug concentrations can be achieved at the site of infection.
  - IM therapy can be considered in patients without IV access or when single doses of therapy are indicated.
- **Type of therapy**
  - Bactericidal therapy is preferred over bacteriostatic regimens, especially in patients with life-threatening infection, immunologic compromise, endocarditis, meningitis, and osteomyelitis.
  - Renal and hepatic function guide antimicrobial dosing regimens.
  - Drug interactions should always be assessed before starting treatment and may impact effectiveness of therapy.
- **Assessment of outcomes on antimicrobial therapy.** If there is concern for potential treatment failure, consider the following questions:
  - Is the isolated organism the etiologic agent?
  - Has an appropriate antimicrobial regimen been selected to cover the organism?
  - Is the concentration of antimicrobial agent adequate at the site of infection?
  - Have resistant pathogens emerged?
  - Is a persistent fever due to underlying disease, abscess formation, iatrogenic complication, drug reaction, or another process?
- **Duration of therapy**
  - Duration of therapy depends on the nature and severity of infection. Therapy should be modified in accordance with the patient's clinical course and culture results.
  - Treatment of acute uncomplicated infections should be continued until the patient has been afebrile and clinically well, usually for a minimum of 72 hours.
  - Infections at certain sites (e.g., endocarditis, septic arthritis, osteomyelitis) require prolonged therapy.

SPECIAL CONSIDERATIONS

- **Immunosuppressed hosts**
  - Examples include patients with HIV/AIDS, transplant recipients (solid organ and hematopoietic stem cell), patients undergoing chemotherapy, and patients on steroids or other immune-modulating agents for treatment of rheumatologic diseases.
  - Consider a more extensive differential diagnosis including opportunistic infections and broader empiric antimicrobial coverage.
- **Pregnancy and the postpartum patient**
  - Although no antimicrobial agent is known to be completely safe in pregnancy, the penicillins and cephalosporins are most often used. **Tetracyclines and fluoroquinolones are contraindicated.** Sulfonamides and aminoglycosides should not be used if alternative agents are available.
  - Many antibiotics can be excreted in breast milk. Caution should be used in prescribing antimicrobials to breast-feeding women.

TOXIN-MEDIATED INFECTIONS

Clostridium difficile Infection

GENERAL PRINCIPLES

Frequently seen after systemic antimicrobial therapy.

DIAGNOSIS

Clinical Presentation

- Symptoms may range from mild or moderate watery diarrhea to severe and potentially fatal pseudomembranous colitis. Abdominal pain, cramping, low-grade fever, and leukocytosis are often present.
- Fulminant disease can manifest as colonic ileus or toxic megacolon leading to bowel perforation.

Differential Diagnosis

Antibiotic-associated osmotic diarrhea without *Clostridium difficile* infection should be considered and will resolve after withdrawal of the antibiotic.

Diagnostic Testing

- Diagnosis is made by detection of *C. difficile* toxin in diarrheal stool through PCR or enzyme immunoassay (EIA) or detection of *C. difficile* organisms through EIA or culture.
- Visualization of pseudomembranes on colonoscopy or sigmoidoscopy with biopsy can also be diagnostic for *C. difficile* infection.

TREATMENT

- For **mild to moderate disease**, treatment should consist of metronidazole 500 mg PO (preferred over IV) tid for 10–14 days and discontinuation of the offending antibiotic if possible (*Am J Gastroenterol 2013;108:478*; *Infect Control Hosp Epidemiol 2010; 31:431*).
- In **severe disease**, vancomycin 125–500 mg PO q6h (IV is not effective) is preferred (*Clin Infect Dis 2007;45:302*). Vancomycin should also be considered for mild to moderate disease that has failed to respond to metronidazole after 5–7 days of therapy.
- For infections complicated by ileus, toxic megacolon, or shock, surgery consultation should be obtained and the addition of IV metronidazole and intracolonic vancomycin is recommended (*Clin Infect Dis 2002;35:690*). In some cases, colectomy may be necessary.
- Endpoint of therapy is cessation of diarrhea; **do not retest stool for toxin clearance**.
- Avoid antimotility agents in severe disease.
- Recurrence is common and is treated with metronidazole or vancomycin in extended duration, pulsed, or tapered regimens. Adjunctive therapy with oral rifaximin is sometimes used (*Clin Infect Dis 2007;44:846*).
- Fidaxomicin may have an evolving role in the treatment and prevention of recurrent *C. difficile* infection (*N Engl J Med 2011;364:422*). Fecal microbiota transplantation (FMT) may also be considered given the appropriate clinical scenario at experienced centers (*J Clin Gastroenterol 2014;48:693*).

Tetanus

GENERAL PRINCIPLES

- Caused by *Clostridium tetani* toxin from wound contamination with spores.
- Tetanus is best prevented by immunization. For high-risk wounds, prophylaxis with human tetanus immunoglobulin 250 units IM is recommended (*MMWR Morb Mortal Wkly Rep 2006;55(No. RR-17):1*).

DIAGNOSIS

Classically presents with intensely painful muscle spasms and rigidity, followed by autonomic dysfunction. Symptoms often begin in the face (trismus, risus sardonicus) and neck muscles. Delirium and high fever are usually absent. Diagnosis is clinical.

TREATMENT

- Passive immunization with human tetanus immunoglobulin 3000–5000 units IM (in divided doses) to neutralize unbound toxin is warranted. Active immunization with tetanus toxoid should be given at a separate site.
- Surgical debridement of the wound is critical.
- Antibiotic therapy, usually consisting of metronidazole 500 mg IV q6–8h or penicillin G 2–4 million units IV q4–6h, for 7–10 days is recommended.
- Benzodiazepines or neuromuscular blocking agents may be used to control spasms.

TOXIC SHOCK SYNDROME

Toxic shock syndrome (TSS) is a life-threatening systemic disease caused by exotoxin superantigens produced by *Staphylococcus aureus* or group A β-hemolytic *Streptococcus* (GABHS) tissue infections (Table 14-1).

TABLE 14-1	Treatment of Toxic Shock Syndromes		
Etiology	**Antibiotic Therapy**	**Adjunctive Therapy**	**Notes**
Group A β-hemolytic *Streptococcus* (GABHS)	Penicillin G 4 million units IV q4h + clindamycin 900 mg IV q8h for 10–14 d	IVIG 1 g/kg on day 1, then 0.5 g/kg on days 2 and 3 (*Clin Infect Dis 2003;37:333*)	Surgical debridement is almost always indicated for necrotizing infections. Clindamycin is added to decrease toxin production.
Staphylococcus	Oxacillin 2 g IV q4h or vancomycin 1 g IV q12h + clindamycin 900 mg IV q8h for 10–14 d	IVIG as per GABHS may be useful in severe cases, but higher doses may be needed (*Clin Infect Dis 2004;38:836*)	Surgical debridement may be necessary for wounds. Tampons and other foreign bodies should be removed and avoided in future, especially if TSST-1 antibody titers are negative.

IVIG, intravenous immunoglobulin; TSST-1, toxic shock syndrome toxin-1.

Staphylococcal Toxic Shock Syndrome

GENERAL PRINCIPLES

Most often associated with colonization of surgical wounds, burns, vaginitis, or tampon use in young women. Cases are also seen after nasal packing for epistaxis. Mortality is low (<3%) in menstrual cases.

DIAGNOSIS

Clinical Presentation

Typical findings are fever, hypotension, and a macular desquamating erythroderma of the palms and soles. Vomiting, diarrhea, myalgias, weakness, shortness of breath, and altered mental status may be early signs of multiorgan failure.

Diagnostic Testing

- Blood cultures are usually negative. Creatine phosphokinase (CPK) is often elevated.
- Staphylococcal isolates can be tested for toxin production, including toxic shock syndrome toxin-1 (TSST-1) and staphylococcal enterotoxin B and C, although results are not clinically relevant. Serum antibodies against TSST-1 may protect against future recurrences (*Clin Microbiol Rev 2013;26:422*).

TREATMENT

See Table 14-1.

Streptococcal Toxic Shock Syndrome

GENERAL PRINCIPLES

Associated with invasive GABHS infections, particularly necrotizing fasciitis or myositis (80% of cases). Mortality is much higher (30–70%) compared to staphylococcal TSS.

DIAGNOSIS

Clinical Presentation

Initial presentation is typically abrupt onset of severe diffuse or localized pain. The systemic manifestations are otherwise similar to staphylococcal TSS, but the desquamating erythroderma is much less common.

Diagnostic Testing

Blood cultures are usually positive, and antistreptolysin O (ASO) titers are elevated.

TREATMENT

See Table 14-1.

SKIN, SOFT TISSUE, AND BONE INFECTIONS

The increased incidence of community-associated methicillin-resistant *S. aureus* (CA-MRSA) has altered the approach to management of skin and soft tissue infections (SSTIs) (*Clin Infect Dis 2014;59:e10*).

Purulent Skin and Soft Tissue Infections (Furuncles, Carbuncles, and Abscesses)

GENERAL PRINCIPLES

MRSA and methicillin-sensitive *S. aureus* (MSSA) account for 25–50% of cases.

TREATMENT

- Incision and drainage (I&D) alone is usually adequate, especially for abscesses measuring <5 cm.
- Antibiotic therapy is needed for extensive disease; systemic illness; rapid progression with associated cellulitis; comorbid diseases (diabetes mellitus); immunosuppression, location on face, hand, or genitalia; or lack of response to I&D.
- Empiric antibiotic therapy should cover CA-MRSA. Oral antibiotics include clindamycin 300–450 mg tid, trimethoprim-sulfamethoxazole (TMP-SMX) 1–2 double-strength tablets bid, doxycycline 100 mg bid, and linezolid 600 mg q12h.
- Duration of antibiotic therapy is usually 5–7 days.

Nonpurulent Skin and Soft Tissue Infections (Erysipelas and Cellulitis)

Erysipelas

GENERAL PRINCIPLES

Erysipelas appears as a painful, superficial, erythematous, sharply demarcated lesion that is usually found on lower extremities. In normal hosts, GABHS is responsible for this infection.

TREATMENT

Penicillin V 250–1000 mg PO q6h or penicillin G 1.0–2.0 million units IV q6h, depending on the severity of illness. In patients who are penicillin allergic, macrolides and clindamycin are alternatives.

Cellulitis

GENERAL PRINCIPLES

- Common organisms include β-hemolytic streptococci and *S. aureus* (MSSA and MRSA).
- Severe cellulitis is sometimes seen after exposure to fresh (*Aeromonas hydrophila*) or salt (*Vibrio vulnificus*) water.

TREATMENT

- If streptococci or MSSA are suspected, a β-lactam antibiotic (cephalexin or dicloxacillin 500 mg PO q6h) or clindamycin can be used.
- If there is a strong concern for CA-MRSA, empiric antibiotic coverage may consist of clindamycin or linezolid. TMP-SMX can also be used in combination with a β-lactam antibiotic (e.g., cephalexin) to provide streptococcal coverage.

• Coverage for waterborne pathogens should initially consist of ceftazidime 2 g IV q8h, cefepime 2 g IV q8h, or ciprofloxacin 750 mg PO bid in combination with doxycycline 100 mg IV/PO q12h.

Complicated Skin and Soft Tissue Infections

GENERAL PRINCIPLES

Deep soft tissue infections, surgical and traumatic wound infections, large abscesses, complicated cellulitis, and infected ulcers and burns fall under this classification.

DIAGNOSIS

Cultures of abscesses and surgical debridement specimens should be obtained to guide antibiotic therapy.

TREATMENT

Patients should be hospitalized to receive IV antibiotics and undergo surgical intervention as necessary. Vancomycin 15–20 mg/kg IV q12h, linezolid 600 mg PO/IV q12h, daptomycin 4 mg/kg IV daily, clindamycin 900 mg IV q8h, and ceftaroline 600 mg IV q12h are all acceptable antibiotic options.

Infected Decubitus Ulcers and Limb-Threatening Diabetic Foot Ulcers

GENERAL PRINCIPLES

• Infections are usually polymicrobial. **Superficial swab cultures are unreliable.** Instead, deep tissue cultures obtained after wound debridement are preferred.
• Osteomyelitis is a frequent complication and should be excluded.

TREATMENT

• Wound care and debridement are important first-line therapies.
• **Mild diabetic foot infections** are usually due to *S. aureus* and streptococci, and can be treated with cephalexin or amoxicillin-clavulanate (875 mg/125 mg PO bid) (*Clin Infect Dis 2012;54:132*). If MRSA is suspected, either TMP-SMX or doxycycline is recommended.
• **Moderate to severe infections** require systemic antibiotics covering *S. aureus* (including MRSA), anaerobes, and enteric gram-negative organisms. Options include vancomycin plus a β-lactam/β-lactamase inhibitor combination, a carbapenem (ertapenem, doripenem, or meropenem), or vancomycin with metronidazole combined with either ciprofloxacin or a third-generation cephalosporin.

Necrotizing Fasciitis

GENERAL PRINCIPLES

• This is an infectious disease emergency with high mortality manifested by extensive soft tissue infection and thrombosis of the microcirculation with resulting necrosis (*Crit Care*

Med 2011;39:2156). Infection spreads quickly along fascial planes and may be associated with sepsis or TSS. Fournier gangrene is necrotizing fasciitis of the perineum.
* Bacterial etiology is either mixed (aerobic and anaerobic organisms) or monomicrobial (GABHS or *S. aureus*, including CA-MRSA).

DIAGNOSIS

Clinical Presentation
May present initially like simple cellulitis rapidly progressing to necrosis with dusky, hypo-esthetic skin and bulla formation in association with severe pain. Pain out of proportion to exam should raise concern for necrotizing fasciitis.

Diagnostic Testing
* Diagnosis is clinical. High suspicion should prompt **immediate surgical exploration** where lack of resistance to probing is diagnostic.
* Cultures of operative specimens and blood should be obtained. CPK may be elevated.
* CT and plain films may demonstrate gas and fascial edema early in the disease process.

TREATMENT

* Aggressive surgical debridement is critical, along with IV antibiotics and volume support.
* Initial empiric antibiotic therapy should be broad spectrum and consist of a β-lactam/β-lactamase inhibitor, high-dose penicillin, carbapenem, or fluoroquinolone in combination with clindamycin. Vancomycin should also be added until MRSA can be excluded.
* Adjunctive hyperbaric oxygen may be useful.

Anaerobic Myonecrosis (Gas Gangrene)

GENERAL PRINCIPLES

Usually due to *Clostridium perfringens*, *Clostridium septicum*, *S. aureus*, GABHS, or other anaerobes. Distinguishing this condition from necrotizing fasciitis requires gross inspection of the involved muscle at the time of surgery.

TREATMENT

Treatment requires prompt surgical debridement and combination antimicrobial therapy with IV penicillin plus clindamycin. A third-generation cephalosporin, cip-rofloxacin, or an aminoglycoside should be added until a gram-negative infection can be excluded.

Osteomyelitis

GENERAL PRINCIPLES

* Osteomyelitis is an inflammatory process caused by an infecting organism that can lead to bone destruction. It should be considered when skin or soft tissue infections overlie bone and when localized bone pain accompanies fever or sepsis.
* See Table 14-2.

TABLE 14-2	Treatment of Osteomyelitis	
Etiology of Osteomyelitis	**Organism**	**Treatment considerations**
Acute hematogenous	• *Staphylococcus aureus*	• Antibiotic therapy alone may be sufficient if no foreign body present.
Vertebral	• *S. aureus* • Gram-negative bacilli • *Mycobacterium tuber-culosis*	• Biopsy off antibiotics (preferred) to guide therapy. • Antibiotic therapy alone may be sufficient.
Associated with a contiguous focus of infection	• *S. aureus* • Gram-negative bacilli • Coagulase-negative staphylococci (surgical site infections) • Anaerobes/polymicro-bial (infected sacral decubitus ulcers, diabetics)	• Diabetics and patients with peripheral vascular disease seldom are cured with antibiotics alone. Revascu-larization, debridement, or amputation is often required. • Long-term, suppressive antimicrobial therapy can be used if surgery is not feasible. • Hyperbaric oxygen may be a useful adjunct.
Presence of an orthopedic device	• *S. aureus* • Coagulase-negative *Staphylococcus* species	• Rarely eradicated by antimi-crobials alone, and typically requires removal of the device. • If removal is impossible, the addition of rifampin 300 mg PO tid is recommended, and long-term, suppressive antimicrobial therapy may be needed.
Associated with hemoglobinopathies	• *S. aureus* • *Salmonella* species	
Chronic osteomyelitis	• Gram-negative pathogens (necrotic sequestrum) • *S. aureus*	• Surgical removal of seques-trum is recommended in addition to antibiotics.
Culture-negative osteomyelitis	• Review above pathogens	• Empiric therapy should cover *S. aureus* and all other likely pathogens.

DIAGNOSIS

• Diagnosis is made by detection of exposed bone through a skin ulcer or by imag-ing with plain films, bone scintigraphy, or MRI (*Clin Infect Dis 2008;47:519*; *JAMA 2008;299:806*).

• Biopsy and cultures of the affected bone should be performed (prior to initiation of anti-microbials when possible) for pathogen-directed therapy.

- Erythrocyte sedimentation rate (ESR) and C-reactive protein (CRP) are usually markedly elevated and can be used to monitor the response to therapy.

TREATMENT

- See Table 14-2.
- Parenteral β-lactam antibiotics (oxacillin, cefazolin) are effective against MSSA. Vancomycin, daptomycin, and linezolid are used to treat MRSA osteomyelitis. Oral agents capable of achieving reasonable bone levels include TMP-SMX, clindamycin, and doxycycline.
- Gram-negative osteomyelitis can be treated with parenteral or oral fluoroquinolones, which have excellent bone penetration and bioavailability, or with a third-generation cephalosporin.
- Cure typically requires at least 4–6 weeks of high-dose antimicrobial therapy. Parenteral therapy should be given initially; oral regimens may be considered after 2–3 weeks if the pathogen is susceptible and adequate bactericidal levels can be achieved (*Clin Infect Dis 2012;54:403*).
- If peripheral vascular disease is present, revascularization may be helpful.

CENTRAL NERVOUS SYSTEM INFECTIONS

Meningitis

GENERAL PRINCIPLES

- Meningitis (inflammation of the meninges) can be caused by bacterial, fungal, or viral infections or by noninfectious causes such as medications.
- Bacterial meningitis is a medical emergency. Therapy should not be delayed for diagnostic measures because prognosis hinges on rapid initiation of antimicrobial treatment.
- *Streptococcus pneumoniae* is the most common bacterial etiology in adults of all ages, followed by *Neisseria meningitidis*, group B *Streptococcus*, and *Haemophilus influenzae*. *Listeria monocytogenes* is more frequent in the elderly and in immunocompromised hosts (*N Engl J Med 2011;364:2016*).
- Health care–associated meningitis (after neurosurgical procedures or head trauma) is caused by staphylococci and gram-negative bacilli.

DIAGNOSIS

Clinical Presentation

- Meningitis should be considered in any patient with fever and stiff neck or neurologic symptoms, especially if another concurrent infection or head trauma is present.
- **Aseptic meningitis** (meningitis with negative bacterial cultures) is usually milder than bacterial meningitis and may be preceded by upper respiratory symptoms or pharyngitis. Viruses, especially enteroviruses, are common causes, as is drug-induced inflammation (e.g., NSAIDs, TMP-SMX).
- Distinction between bacterial, viral, and noninfectious etiologies cannot be made clinically.

Diagnostic Testing

- Diagnosis requires a lumbar puncture with measurement of opening pressure; examination of cerebrospinal fluid (CSF) protein, glucose, and cell count with differential; and Gram stain with culture (Table 14-3). Blood cultures should always be obtained. A head CT scan before lumbar puncture is controversial but is generally not required

TABLE 14-3	Typical Cerebrospinal Fluid Findings in Meningitis				
	Opening Pressure (mm H$_2$O)	White Cells (/μL)	Glucose (mg/dL)	Protein (mg/dL)	Laboratory Diagnosis
Normal	<180	0–5	50–75	15–40	None
Bacterial meningitis	↑	100–5000 neutrophils	<40	100–500	Gram stain, culture
Tuberculous meningitis	↑	50–300 lymphocytes	<45	50–300	Acid-fast bacilli smear, culture, polymerase chain reaction (PCR) for *Mycobacterium tuberculosis*
Cryptococcal meningitis	↑↑	20–500 lymphocytes	<40	>45	Cryptococcal antigen, India ink stain, fungal culture
Viral meningitis	↑	10–1000 lymphocytes	Normal	50–100	Virus-specific PCR

Adapted from Tunkel A. Approach to the patient with central nervous system infection. In: Bennett JE, Dolan R, Blaser MJ, eds. *Mandell, Douglas and Bennett's Principles and Practice of Infectious Diseases*. 8th ed. New York: Elsevier Churchill Livingston; 2015:1091–6.

for immunocompetent patients who present without focal neurologic abnormalities, seizures, or diminished level of consciousness (*Clin Infect Dis 2004;39:1267*).
• Typical CSF findings in **bacterial meningitis** include a neutrophilic pleocytosis, markedly elevated CSF protein, and decreased glucose level.
• In **aseptic meningitis**, a lymphocytic CSF pleocytosis is common (although neutrophils may predominate very early in the disease course). CSF PCR can detect enteroviruses, herpes simplex virus (HSV), and HIV. CSF lymphocytosis and decreased glucose level should prompt a workup for TB or fungal meningitis.
• Depending on the clinical scenario, other potentially useful CSF studies include Venereal Disease Research Laboratory (VDRL), acid-fast stain and culture, cryptococcal antigen and fungal culture, and arbovirus antibodies.

TREATMENT

• Treatment consists of supportive measures and antimicrobial therapy (*Clin Infect Dis 2004;39:1267*). Whenever acute bacterial meningitis is suspected, high-dose parenteral antimicrobial therapy should be started **immediately after lumbar puncture** (without delay for imaging). Until the etiology of the meningitis is known, an empiric regimen should be based on patient risk factors and Gram stain of the CSF.
• **If no organisms are seen**, high-dose third-generation cephalosporins (ceftriaxone 2 g IV q12h) and vancomycin 15–20 mg/kg IV q8–12h are recommended while culture results are pending.
• Ampicillin 2 g IV q4h should be added for **immunocompromised and older patients (>50 years old)** to cover *L. monocytogenes*.

- In the **postneurosurgical setting or after head or spinal trauma**, broad-spectrum coverage with high-dose vancomycin and ceftazidime or cefepime 2 g IV q8h is indicated. Empiric broad-spectrum regimens should be narrowed once culture and sensitivity data are known.
- **Dexamethasone** 0.15 mg/kg IV q6h started just prior to or with initial antibiotics and continued for 4 days reduces the risk of a poor neurologic outcome in patients with meningitis caused by *S. pneumoniae*. Steroids have not proven to be of benefit for bacterial meningitis caused by other organisms and should be discontinued if a different pathogen is isolated (*Cochrane Database Syst Rev 2013;6:CD004405*).
- **Therapy for specific infections**
  - For *S. pneumoniae*, initial therapy consists of ceftriaxone plus vancomycin. Vancomycin should be discontinued if the isolate is susceptible to ceftriaxone (minimum inhibitory concentration [MIC] <1.0 μg/mL). For penicillin-sensitive isolates (MIC <0.1 μg/mL), IV penicillin G 4 million units q4h can be used. Dexamethasone can be a valuable adjunct if given early in treatment.
  - For *N. meningitidis*, high-dose ceftriaxone or cefotaxime is used. If the isolate is susceptible, penicillin can be used. Alternatives are meropenem and chloramphenicol. Patients should be placed in droplet isolation for at least the first 24 hours of treatment. Close contacts (e.g., persons living in the same household and health care workers having close contact with secretions, such as intubation) should receive prophylaxis with either ciprofloxacin 500 mg PO once; rifampin, 600 mg PO bid for 2 days; or ceftriaxone 250 mg IM. Terminal component complement deficiency (C5 through C9) should be ruled out in patients with recurrent meningococcal infections.
  - *L. monocytogenes* meningitis is seen in immunosuppressed adults, pregnant women, and the elderly. Treatment is with ampicillin 2 g IV q4h for at least 3 weeks. TMP-SMX (TMP 5 mg/kg IV q6h) or meropenem (2 g IV q8h) is an alternative for the penicillin-allergic patient.
  - **Gram-negative bacillary meningitis** is usually a complication of head trauma or neurosurgical procedures. High-dose ceftazidime or cefepime 2 g IV q8h is used for most pathogens, including *Pseudomonas aeruginosa*. High-dose ceftriaxone or cefotaxime may be used for susceptible pathogens. Alternatives include meropenem and ciprofloxacin.
  - *S. aureus* meningitis is usually a result of high-grade bacteremia, direct extension from a parameningeal focus, or recent neurosurgical procedure. Vancomycin should be used initially in penicillin-allergic patients and for methicillin-resistant isolates. Oxacillin and nafcillin 2 g IV q4h are the drugs of choice for MSSA. Ceftriaxone is an alternative for MSSA. Avoid first-generation cephalosporins because they do not penetrate into the CSF.
  - For **enteroviral** meningitis, the treatment is supportive care. Acyclovir, 10 mg/kg IV q8h, is used for moderate to severe **HSV meningitis**.

Encephalitis

GENERAL PRINCIPLES

Encephalitis is inflammation of the brain parenchyma, usually associated with viral infections. **HSV-1** is the most common and most important cause of sporadic infectious encephalitis. Other causes include arboviruses such as West Nile virus (WNV), enteroviruses, other herpesviruses, and rabies. Nonviral causes include *Mycobacterium tuberculosis*, syphilis, fungi, *Mycoplasma pneumoniae*, and *Bartonella henselae*. In the summer months, tick-borne illness (e.g., *Ehrlichia*, Rocky Mountain spotted fever, Lyme disease) should be considered. Noninfectious causes include vasculitis, collagen vascular disease, paraneoplastic syndromes, and acute disseminated encephalomyelitis, which can occur after an infection or immunization.

DIAGNOSIS

Clinical Presentation

Presenting complaints include fever, altered mental status, and neurologic abnormalities, particularly with personality change or seizures, usually without meningeal signs.

Diagnostic Testing

CSF analysis is important and should include PCR testing for HSV and enteroviruses and measurement of CSF and serum arbovirus antibodies. A positive PCR for HSV-1 confirms the diagnosis, but a negative PCR does not rule out HSV encephalitis. Other PCR tests (*Ehrlichia, Bartonella, Mycoplasma*, varicella-zoster virus, cytomegalovirus) may be sent, depending on clinical suspicion. The diagnosis of WNV is made by detecting IgM antibodies in the CSF. MRI is the most sensitive neuroimaging and may show temporal lobe enhancement in HSV encephalitis.

TREATMENT

Acyclovir 10 mg/kg IV q8h should be started on all patients with suspected encephalitis and continued for 14–21 days, unless HSV is definitively ruled out. Delayed initiation of therapy greatly increases the risk of poor neurologic outcomes. Treatment of other viral causes is mainly supportive. Antibiotic therapy for presumed bacterial meningitis (see above) should be initiated if clinically indicated and discontinued once CSF cultures are negative. Doxycycline 100 mg q12h should be added if there is suspicion for tick-borne illness (*Clin Infect Dis 2008;47:303*).

Brain Abscess

GENERAL PRINCIPLES

Brain abscess in the immunocompetent host is usually bacterial in origin and a result of spread from a contiguous focus (mastoiditis, sinusitis, dental infection) or from septic emboli from endocarditis or bacteremia or related to trauma or surgery. Infection is often polymicrobial, with viridans streptococci, *S. aureus*, and anaerobes being the most common pathogens; staphylococci and gram-negative bacilli predominate after surgery. In immunocompromised hosts, etiologies include invasive fungal infection, *Nocardia*, and TB; in HIV-infected patients, toxoplasmosis is a leading consideration (*N Engl J Med 2014;371:447*).

DIAGNOSIS

- Diagnosis is radiographic, with ring-enhancing lesions seen on MRI or contrast-enhanced CT scan.
- A microbiologic etiology must be determined by aspiration, by biopsy, or at the time of surgery.

TREATMENT

Empiric therapy should cover the most likely pathogens based on the primary infection site. When no preceding infection can be found, a third-generation cephalosporin (ceftriaxone) combined with metronidazole and vancomycin is a reasonable regimen in immunocompetent hosts until culture data are available. Cefepime or ceftazidime should be substituted for ceftriaxone after neurosurgical procedures or with penetrating head trauma.

Neurosurgical consultation is imperative for drainage; cultures must be sent to enable pathogen-directed therapy. A prolonged course of antibiotic therapy is often needed, with follow-up imaging to assess improvement.

Neurocysticercosis

Neurocysticercosis should be suspected in patients from Mexico and Central and South America who present with seizures. Ingested eggs of *Taenia solium* differentiate into larvae, which disseminate to brain and other tissues and form cysts. Brain imaging reveals characteristic multiple unilocular cysts that eventually calcify. Treatment consists of anticonvulsants, albendazole or praziquantel (with steroids to decrease the inflammatory response), and/or surgery (*Lancet Neurol 2014;13:1202*).

CARDIOVASCULAR INFECTIONS

Infective Endocarditis

GENERAL PRINCIPLES

Epidemiology

- The incidence of acute bacterial endocarditis (ABE) and health care–associated endocarditis (related to IV catheters and invasive procedures) is rising (*Arch Intern Med 2009;109:463*).
- **Prosthetic valve endocarditis (PVE)** occurs in 1–4% of patients with prosthetic heart valves.

Etiology

- **Infective endocarditis (IE)** is usually caused by gram-positive cocci. *S. aureus* is the most common pathogen followed by viridans streptococci, enterococci, and coagulase-negative staphylococci.
- *Enterococcus* species cause 5–20% of cases of **subacute bacterial endocarditis (SBE)**.
- Gram-negative and fungal IE occur infrequently and are usually associated with injection drug use or prosthetic heart valves.
- Dental procedures and bacteremia from distant foci of infection are frequent seeding events.
- Early PVE (within 2 months of surgery) is typically caused by *S. aureus*, coagulase-negative staphylococci, gram-negative bacilli, and *Candida* species.
- Late-onset PVE is typically caused by *S. aureus*, coagulase-negative staphylococci, enterococci, and viridans streptococci.

Risk Factors

Structural heart disease, IV drug use, prosthetic heart valves, intravascular devices, chronic hemodialysis, and a prior history of endocarditis are predisposing factors for endocarditis.

DIAGNOSIS

The modified Duke criteria (Tables 14-4 and 14-5) for diagnosis of IE, incorporating microbiologic, pathologic, echocardiographic, and clinical findings, are widely used (*Clin Infect Dis 2000;30:633*).

Clinical Presentation

- Patients with **ABE** may present within 3–10 days of onset of infection with critical illness.
- **SBE** may present over weeks to months with constitutional symptoms (fever, malaise, anorexia), immune complex disease (nephritis, arthralgias, Osler nodes), and embolic phenomenon (renal, splenic, and cerebral infarcts; petechiae; Janeway lesions).
- **PVE** must be considered in any patient with persistent bacteremia after heart valve surgery.

TABLE 14-4	Modified Duke Criteria for the Diagnosis of Infective Endocarditis

Major Criteria

Positive blood cultures for IE

1. Two separate blood cultures with viridans streptococci, *Streptococcus gallolyticus* (formerly *bovis*), *Staphylococcus aureus*, HACEK group, or community-acquired enterococci (no primary focus)
2. Persistently positive blood cultures drawn more than 12 hours apart **OR** all of three or a majority of four separate blood cultures, drawn 1 hour apart
3. Single positive blood culture for *Coxiella burnetii*

Evidence of endocardial involvement

Positive echocardiogram for IE, such as:
1. Oscillating intracardiac mass on a valve or supporting structure, in the path of regurgitant jets, or on implanted materials in the absence of another anatomic explanation
2. Abscess
3. New partial dehiscence of a prosthetic valve
4. New valvular regurgitation (change in preexisting murmur not sufficient)

Minor Criteria

1. Predisposing heart condition or IV drug use
2. Fever ≥38°C (100.4°F)
3. Vascular phenomena: Arterial emboli, septic pulmonary infarcts, mycotic aneurysm, intracranial or conjunctival hemorrhage, Janeway lesions
4. Immunologic phenomena: Glomerulonephritis, Osler nodes, Roth spots, rheumatoid factor
5. Microbiologic evidence: Positive blood culture but not meeting major criteria **OR** serologic evidence of infection with an organism consistent with IE

HACEK, *Haemophilus, Aggregatibacter, Cardiobacterium, Eikenella, Kingella*; IE, infective endocarditis.

Diagnostic Testing

- The most reliable diagnostic criterion for IE is persistent bacteremia in a compatible clinical setting. Three blood cultures should be taken from separate sites over at least a 1-hour period prior to empiric antimicrobial therapy. Blood cultures are positive in at least 90% of patients but can be negative if the patient has already received antibiotics.
- Echocardiography plays an important role in establishing the diagnosis of IE and determining the need for surgical intervention.
- Patients with IE and vegetations seen by transthoracic echocardiography (TTE) are at higher risk of embolism, heart failure, and valvular disruption. However, a negative TTE cannot rule out IE.
- When clinical evidence of IE exists, **transesophageal echocardiography (TEE)** improves the sensitivity of the Duke criteria, especially in patients with prosthetic heart valves.
- **Culture-negative IE** is usually encountered when prior antimicrobial therapy has been given, or rarely, with fastidious pathogens, such as nutritionally deficient streptococci (now *Abiotrophia* and *Granulicatella*), HACEK organisms, *Coxiella burnetii* (Q fever), *Bartonella, Brucella, Tropheryma whipplei* (Whipple disease), and fungi. Empiric therapy can be initiated despite negative cultures (Table 14-6).

TABLE 14-5	Classification of Infective Endocarditis (IE) by Modified Duke Criteria

Definite IE

Pathologic criteria:

Vegetation or intracardiac abscess confirmed by histology showing active endocarditis **AND** an associated microorganism demonstrated by culture or histology

Clinical criteria:

    Two major criteria **OR**
    One major and three minor criteria **OR**
    Five minor criteria

Possible IE

    One major and one minor criteria **OR**
    Three minor criteria

Rejected IE

    Firm alternative diagnosis **OR**
    Resolution of manifestations with therapy for ≤4 days **OR**
    No pathologic evidence at surgery or autopsy after antibiotic therapy ≤4 days

Adapted from Li JS, Sexton DJ, Mick N, et al. Proposed modifications to the Duke Criteria for the diagnosis of infective endocarditis. *Clin Infect Dis* 2000;30:633–8.

- **HACEK** is an acronym for a group of fastidious, slow-growing, gram-negative bacteria (*Haemophilus*, *Actinobacillus* [now *Aggregatibacter*], *Cardiobacterium*, *Eikenella*, and *Kingella* species) that have a predilection for infecting heart valves.

TREATMENT

- **High doses of IV antimicrobials for extended periods (generally 4–6 weeks) are required.**
- Quantitative antimicrobial susceptibility testing of the causative organism is essential for optimal treatment.
- **ABE** often requires empiric antimicrobial treatment before culture results become available. Initial treatment for *S. aureus* should consist of vancomycin 15 mg/kg IV q12h. Therapy should then be modified based on culture and susceptibility data. For methicillin-sensitive isolates, oxacillin 2 g IV q4h is superior to vancomycin.
- **SBE** caused by susceptible organisms should be treated with penicillin, because this typically results in cure rates of >90%. Therapy can usually be delayed until culture data and susceptibilities are available.
- **PVE** requires aggressive combination therapy for at least 6 weeks or longer because of the increased risk for treatment failure and relapse. Indications for valve replacement are detailed in the following text. Initial empiric therapy pending culture data includes the addition of rifampin to vancomycin and gentamicin to improve biofilm penetration. Oxacillin should be substituted for vancomycin if sensitive. Treatment failure or relapse is common.
- Baseline audiometry is recommended for patients who will receive 7 or more days of aminoglycoside therapy, with repeat testing weekly while on treatment or if symptoms develop.

TABLE 14-6 Treatment of Endocarditis Caused by Specific Organisms[a]

Organism	Antibiotic Regimen	Duration	Notes
Viridans streptococci			
MIC <0.12 µg/mL	• Penicillin G (12–18 million units IV q24h) or ceftriaxone +/– gentamicin (3 mg/kg IV in two or three divided doses) • Vancomycin (15 mg/kg IV q12h) if PCN allergic	• 4 wk without gentamicin (2 wk total if used in combination)	• 2-wk course not indicated for prosthetic valves, major embolic or extended symptoms • Gentamicin may be ototoxic and nephrotoxic • Vancomycin monotherapy in allergic patients
MIC 0.12–0.5 µg/mL	• Penicillin G (4 million units IV q4h) or ceftriaxone + gentamicin • Vancomycin if PCN allergic and unable to desensitize to PCN	• 4 wk total with 2 wk of gentamicin	
MIC >0.5 µg/mL	• Treat as enterococcal endocarditis	• 4–6 wk	
Enterococcus species			
Penicillin susceptible	• Ampicillin 2 g IV q4h + gentamicin • Vancomycin + gentamicin	• 4–6 wk	• If high-level gentamicin resistance, substitute streptomycin (15 mg/kg IV q24h IV in two divided doses based on ideal body weight) or ceftriaxone (4 g IV q24h in two divided doses)
Penicillin resistant	• *β-lactamase:* Ampicillin/sulbactam 3 g IV q6h + gentamicin • *Intrinsically resistant:* Vancomycin + gentamicin	• 6 wk	
Vancomycin (VRE) and ampicillin resistant	• Linezolid (600 mg [IV or PO] q12h) or daptomycin • Quinupristin/dalfopristin ± doxycycline	• ≥8 wk	• Consult infectious diseases specialist because VRE IE is difficult to treat

Staphylococcus species

Native valve, MSSA
(*Clin Infect Dis* 2009;48:713; *Medicine (Baltimore)* 2003;82:333)

- Oxacillin or nafcillin (2 g IV q4h)
- Cefazolin 2 g IV q8h if penicillin allergy without anaphylaxis

• 6 wk

- Initial 3–5 d gentamicin for synergy may not be beneficial. Penicillins are superior to vancomycin, and desensitization is preferred when possible.

Tricuspid valve, MSSA (IV drug user)

- Oxacillin + gentamicin

• 2 wk

- Avoid vancomycin

Native valve, MRSA

- Vancomycin or daptomycin (6 mg/kg IV q24h) (also for MSSA if anaphylactic allergy)

• 6 wk

- Linezolid used with some success

Staphylococcus species (prosthetic valve)

MSSA/MSSE

- Oxacillin + rifampin (300 mg PO q8h) + gentamicin

• ≥6 wk total (2 wk of gentamicin)

MRSA/MRSE

- Vancomycin + rifampin + gentamicin

• ≥6 wk total (2 wk of gentamicin)

HACEK organisms and culture-negative IE

- Ceftriaxone (2g IV q24h) or ampicillin-sulbactam (3 g IV q6h) or ciprofloxacin (400 mg IV q12h)

• 4 wk

- HACEK stands for *Haemophilus, Aggregatibacter, Cardiobacterium, Eikenella, Kingella.*

IE, infective endocarditis; MIC, minimum inhibitory concentration; MRSA, methicillin-resistant *Staphylococcus aureus*; MRSE, methicillin-resistant *Staphylococcus epidermidis*; MSSA, methicillin-sensitive *Staphylococcus aureus*; MSSE, methicillin-sensitive *Staphylococcus epidermidis*; PCN, penicillin; VRE, vancomycin-resistant *Enterococcus*.

Baseline and weekly audiometry recommended for patients receiving aminoglycosides for >7 days. Monitor aminoglycoside and vancomycin levels. Goal vancomycin trough levels are near 15–20 μg/mL.

[a]See *Circulation* 2005;111:e393.

- **Antibiotic therapy for specific organisms** (see Table 14-6)
  - *Streptococcus pyogenes* and *S. pneumoniae* should be treated with penicillin G 2–4 million units IV q4h for 4–6 weeks. Penicillin-resistant pneumococci should be treated with ceftriaxone 2 g IV q24h for 4–6 weeks. *Streptococcus bovis* bacteremia and endocarditis are associated with lower gastrointestinal (GI) tract disease, including neoplasms. Groups B and G streptococcal endocarditis may also be associated with lower intestinal pathology.
  - **Culture-negative IE** can be treated with empiric antibiotics (see Table 14-6).
  - **Coagulase-negative *Staphylococcus*** (e.g., ***Staphylococcus epidermidis***) IE primarily occurs in patients with prosthetic heart valves, although native valve endocarditis is increasing, particularly in health care settings. *Staphylococcus lugdunensis* IE is associated with a high rate of perivalvular extension and metastatic spread. A β-lactam antibiotic or vancomycin is used for treatment.
- **Response to antimicrobial therapy**
  - Clinical improvement is frequently seen within 3–10 days of initiating therapy.
  - Blood cultures should be obtained daily until clearance of bacteremia has been documented.
  - Persistent or recurrent fever usually represents extensive cardiac infection but also may be due to septic emboli, drug hypersensitivity, or subsequent nosocomial infection (*Circulation 2005;111:e393*).

Surgical Management

- For native valve endocarditis, indications for surgery include refractory heart failure; aortic or mitral regurgitation with hemodynamic evidence of elevated left ventricular end-diastolic pressure; complications such as heart block, annular or aortic abscess, fistula, or perforation; and infection with fungi or other highly resistant organisms. Recurrent emboli and sustained bacteremia on appropriate therapy are other indications.
- For PVE, indications include heart failure, valve dehiscence, increasing valve obstruction or worsening regurgitation, complications such as abscess formation, persistent bacteremia or recurrent emboli, resistant organisms, and relapsing infection (*J Am Coll Cardiol 2006;48:e1*).

SPECIAL CONSIDERATIONS

The American Heart Association recommendations for prophylaxis for IE are outlined in Table 14-7.

Myocarditis

GENERAL PRINCIPLES

- When the heart is involved in an inflammatory process, the cause is often an infectious agent. Myocarditis may occur during and after viral, rickettsial, bacterial, fungal, and parasitic infections.
- Viruses are the most frequent cause and include enteroviruses (Coxsackie B and echovirus), adenovirus, human herpesvirus 6, parvovirus B-19, and many others. Myocarditis can also be a rare complication of smallpox vaccination.

DIAGNOSIS

- Nasopharyngeal swab testing and serology to detect viral infections are rarely helpful.
- Endomyocardial biopsy for histopathology and viral PCR is the "gold standard" but is not routinely done.

TABLE 14-7	Endocarditis Prophylaxis[a]

I. Endocarditis prophylaxis is recommended for the following cardiac conditions: prosthetic valves; previous endocarditis; unrepaired congenital heart disease, including palliative shunts or conduits, repaired congenital heart disease with prosthetic material during the first 6 months after procedure, or with residual defects at or adjacent to the site of the prosthetic device; and cardiac valvulopathy in transplant recipients.

II. Regimens for dental, oral, or respiratory tract procedures (including dental extractions, periodontal or endodontic procedures, professional teeth cleaning, bronchoscopy with biopsy, rigid bronchoscopy, surgery on respiratory mucosa, tonsillectomy):

Clinical Scenario	Drug and Dosage
Standard prophylaxis	Amoxicillin 2 g PO 1 h before procedure
Unable to take PO	Ampicillin 2 g IM or IV, or cefazolin or ceftriaxone 1 g IM or IV within 30 min before procedure
Penicillin-allergic patient	Clindamycin 600 mg PO, or cephalexin 2 g PO, or clarithromycin or azithromycin 500 mg PO 1 h before procedure
Penicillin allergic and unable to take PO	Clindamycin 600 mg IV, or cefazolin or ceftriaxone 1 g IV within 30 min before procedure

III. Gastrointestinal and genitourinary procedures do not require routine use of prophylaxis. High-risk patients infected or colonized with enterococci should receive amoxicillin, ampicillin, or vancomycin to eradicate the organism prior to urinary tract manipulation.

IV. Prophylaxis is recommended for procedures on infected skin, skin structures, or musculoskeletal tissue ONLY for patients with cardiac conditions outlined above. An antistaphylococcal penicillin or cephalosporin should be used.

[a]See *Circulation* 2007;116:1736.

TREATMENT

Supportive care is the mainstay of treatment. Nonsteroidal agents (NSAIDs) should be avoided. The role of IV immunoglobulin and antiviral agents in viral-mediated myocarditis remains anecdotal.

Pericarditis

GENERAL PRINCIPLES

Acute pericarditis is a syndrome caused by inflammation of the pericardium and characterized by chest pain, a pericardial friction rub, and diffuse ST-segment elevations on ECG. Viruses are the most common infectious etiology. Staphylococci, *S. pneumonia*, TB, and histoplasmosis are occasional causes (see the Tuberculosis section).

TREATMENT

The role of antiviral therapies in viral pericarditis remains unclear. NSAIDs may be used for pain. If an etiology is identified, specific treatment can be initiated.

UPPER RESPIRATORY TRACT INFECTIONS

Pharyngitis

GENERAL PRINCIPLES

Pharyngitis is commonly (>50%) caused by viruses, with infections due to group A streptococci (GABHS) and other bacteria responsible to a lesser extent. Unfortunately, 60% of adults with pharyngitis receive antibiotics (*JAMA Intern Med 2014;174:138*).

DIAGNOSIS

Clinical Presentation

Fever, cervical lymphadenopathy, tonsillar exudates, and lack of cough may or may not be present in addition to throat pain. Distinguishing bacterial from viral pharyngitis on clinical grounds alone is difficult.

Differential Diagnosis

- **Acute HIV infection** should be considered in the setting of pharyngitis with atypical lymphocytosis and negative *Streptococcus* and Epstein-Barr virus testing.
- **Epiglottitis** should be considered in the febrile patient with severe throat pain, odynophagia, new-onset drooling, and dysphagia (see Epiglottitis section)
- Suppurative complications including **peritonsillar or retropharyngeal abscess** should be considered in the patient with severe unilateral pain, muffled voice, trismus, and dysphagia.

Diagnostic Testing

- Diagnostic testing is usually reserved for symptomatic patients with exposure to a case of streptococcal pharyngitis, those with signs of significant infection (fever, tonsillar exudates, and cervical adenopathy), patients whose symptoms persist despite symptomatic therapy, and patients with a history of rheumatic fever.
- Rapid antigen detection testing (RADT) is useful for identifying **GABHS**, which requires therapy to prevent suppurative complications and rheumatic fever. A negative test does not reliably exclude GABHS, making throat culture necessary if clinical suspicion is high.
- Serology for **Epstein-Barr virus** (e.g., heterophile agglutinin or monospot) and examination of a peripheral blood smear for atypical lymphocytes should be performed when infectious mononucleosis is suspected.

TREATMENT

- Most cases of pharyngitis are self-limited and do not require antimicrobial therapy.
- Treatment for **GABHS** is indicated with a positive culture or RADT, if the patient is at high risk for development of rheumatic fever, or if the diagnosis is strongly suspected, pending culture results. Treatment options include penicillin V 250 mg PO qid or 500 mg PO bid for 10 days, clindamycin 300–450 mg PO q6–8h for 5 days, azithromycin 500 mg PO on day 1 followed by 250 mg on days 2–5, or benzathine penicillin G 1.2 million units IM as a one-time dose (*Clin Infect Dis 2012;55:1279*).

- Gonococcal pharyngitis is treated with ceftriaxone 250 mg IM as a single dose, plus azithromycin or doxycycline.

Epiglottitis

GENERAL PRINCIPLES

H. influenzae type B, *S. pneumoniae*, *S. aureus*, and GABHS are common bacterial causes of epiglottitis, although viral and fungal pathogens may also be implicated.

DIAGNOSIS

Clinical Presentation

Fever, sore throat, odynophagia, drooling, muffled voice, and dysphagia in a patient with a normal oropharyngeal examination should prompt a clinical diagnosis of epiglottitis. Inspiratory stridor is a sign of impending respiratory compromise.

Diagnostic Testing

- Throat and blood cultures are useful in determining the etiology.
- Soft tissue lateral radiographs of the neck may show the "thumb print" sign.
- Definitive diagnosis is made by visualization of the epiglottis.

TREATMENT

Prompt treatment including hospitalization, and otolaryngologic consultation for airway management is recommended in all suspected cases. Antimicrobial therapy should include an agent that is active against *H. influenzae*, such as ceftriaxone 2 g IV q24h or cefotaxime 2 g IV q6–8h. Vancomycin or clindamycin should be added if there is concern for MRSA.

Rhinosinusitis

GENERAL PRINCIPLES

- **Acute rhinosinusitis** is most frequently caused by upper respiratory viruses. Bacterial pathogens, such as *S. pneumoniae*, *H. influenzae*, *Moraxella catarrhalis*, and anaerobes are involved in <2% of cases and should be considered only if symptoms persist for >10 days.
- **Chronic rhinosinusitis** may be caused by any of the etiologic agents responsible for acute sinusitis, as well as *S. aureus*, *Corynebacterium diphtheriae*, and many anaerobes (e.g., *Prevotella* spp., *Veillonella* spp.). Possible contributing factors include asthma, nasal polyps, allergies, or immunodeficiency.

DIAGNOSIS

Clinical Presentation

- **Acute rhinosinusitis** presents with purulent nasal discharge, nasal obstruction, facial or dental pain, and sinus tenderness with or without fever, lasting <4 weeks.
- **Chronic rhinosinusitis** is defined by symptoms lasting >12 weeks including mucopurulent drainage, nasal obstruction, facial pain or pressure, and decreased sense of smell with documented signs of inflammation.

Diagnostic Testing

- Diagnosis requires objective evidence of mucosal disease, usually with rhinoscopy and nasal endoscopy or a sinus CT. Plain films are not recommended.
- Sinus cultures can be obtained from nasal endoscopy or sinus puncture. Nasal swabs are not helpful.

TREATMENT

- The goals of medical therapy for acute and chronic rhinosinusitis are to control infection, reduce tissue edema, facilitate drainage, maintain patency of the sinus ostia, and break the pathologic cycle that leads to chronic sinusitis.
- **Acute rhinosinusitis**
  - **Symptomatic treatment** is the mainstay of therapy, including oral decongestants and analgesics with or without a short course of topical decongestant or intranasal glucocorticoid (*Otolaryngol Head Neck Surg 2007;137:S1*).
  - **Empiric antibiotic therapy** is indicated only for severe persistent symptoms (≥10 days) or failure of symptomatic therapy. First-line therapy should consist of a 5- to 7-day course of amoxicillin-clavulanate 875 mg/125 mg PO bid. Doxycycline or a respiratory fluoroquinolone (e.g., moxifloxacin, levofloxacin) may be used as alternative therapy in case of β-lactam allergy or primary treatment failure. TMP-SMX and macrolides are not recommended for empiric therapy due to high rates of resistance (*Clin Infect Dis 2012;54:e72*).
- **Chronic rhinosinusitis.** Treatment usually includes topical and/or systemic glucocorticoids; the role of antimicrobial agents is unclear. If they are used, amoxicillin-clavulanate is the first-line treatment, with clindamycin for penicillin-allergic patients. Some chronic cases may require endoscopic surgery.

Influenza Virus Infection

GENERAL PRINCIPLES

Influenza is readily transmissible and associated with outbreaks of varying severity during the winter months.

DIAGNOSIS

Clinical Presentation

Influenza virus infection causes an acute, self-limited febrile illness marked with headache, myalgias, cough, coryza, and malaise.

Diagnostic Testing

Diagnosis is usually made clinically during influenza season, with confirmation by nasopharyngeal swab for rapid antigen testing, PCR, or direct fluorescent antibody test and culture.

TREATMENT

- Treatment is usually symptomatic.
- Antiviral medications may shorten the duration of illness but must be initiated within 24–48 hours of the onset of symptoms to be effective in immunocompetent patients (*MMWR Morb Mortal Wkly Rep 2011;60(1):1*). Antiviral therapy should not be withheld

from patients presenting >48 hours after symptom onset requiring hospitalization or at high risk for complications (see Complications section).
- ○ The **neuraminidase inhibitors** (oseltamivir 75 mg PO bid or zanamivir 10 mg inhaled twice a day, each for 5 days) are used in treatment and prophylaxis of influenza A and B. Peramivir, 600 mg single dose IV, has recently been approved by the U.S. Food and Drug Administration.
- ○ **Adamantanes** (amantadine and rimantadine, each 100 mg PO bid) are not recommended due to high rates of resistance.
- ○ Circulating strains change annually with varying resistance patterns to both classes of antivirals. **Treatment decisions must be based on annual resistance data**, available from the Centers for Disease Control and Preventions (CDC; *http://www.cdc.gov*).
- • **Vaccination** is the most reliable prevention strategy. Annual vaccination is recommended for all individuals 6 months of age and older (*MMWR Morb Mortal Wkly Rep 2011;60(33):1128*).

COMPLICATIONS

- • Adults >65 years old, residents of nursing homes and other long-term care facilities, pregnant women (and those up to 2 weeks postpartum), and patients with chronic medical conditions (e.g., pulmonary disease, cardiovascular disease, active malignancy, diabetes mellitus, chronic renal insufficiency, chronic liver disease, immunosuppression including HIV and transplantation, morbid obesity) are at greater risk of complications.
- • Influenza pneumonia and secondary bacterial pneumonia are the most common complications of influenza infection.
- • Viral antigenic drift and shift can cause emergence of strains with enhanced virulence or the potential for pandemic spread, requiring modified therapy or heightened infection control measures.

LOWER RESPIRATORY TRACT INFECTIONS

Acute Bronchitis

GENERAL PRINCIPLES

Acute bronchitis involves inflammation of the bronchi, most often caused by viruses such as coronavirus, rhinovirus, influenza, or parainfluenza. Uncommon causes include *M. pneumoniae*, *Chlamydophila pneumoniae*, and *Bordetella pertussis*. Unfortunately, 60–90% of patients with acute bronchitis are given antibiotics (*JAMA 2014;311:2020*).

DIAGNOSIS

Clinical Presentation
Symptoms include cough with or without sputum production lasting >5 days and may be indistinguishable from an upper respiratory tract infection early on. Fever is uncommon.

Diagnostic Testing
- • Diagnosis is made clinically. Sputum cultures are not recommended.
- • In febrile, systemically ill, or older patients with abnormal vital signs, pneumonia should be ruled out clinically or radiographically, and diagnostic tests for influenza should be performed depending on the season and local disease trends.
- • Cough lasting >2 weeks in an adult should be evaluated for pertussis with a nasopharyngeal swab for culture or PCR.

TREATMENT

- Treatment is symptomatic and should be directed toward controlling cough (dextromethorphan 15 mg PO q6h).
- Routine antimicrobial use is **not** recommended unless pertussis has been diagnosed (*Cochrane Database Syst Rev 2014;3:CD000245*).
- **Pertussis** treatment consists of clarithromycin 500 mg PO bid for 14 days or azithromycin 500 mg PO single dose followed by 250 mg PO daily for 4 more days.
- Pertussis cases should be reported to the local health department for contact tracing and administration of postexposure prophylaxis with azithromycin when indicated.

Community-Acquired Pneumonia

GENERAL PRINCIPLES

- The predominant organism involved is *S. pneumoniae*; other bacterial etiologies are *H. influenzae* and *M. catarrhalis*. Pneumonia caused by atypical agents, such as *Legionella pneumophila*, *C. pneumoniae*, or *M. pneumoniae*, cannot be reliably distinguished clinically. Influenza and other respiratory viruses may also cause pneumonia in adults.
- CA-MRSA is an important cause of severe, necrotizing pneumonia.
- Health care–associated pneumonia (HCAP; seen in nursing home residents, clinic and hemodialysis patients seen within 30 days, and patients hospitalized within prior 90 days) is more likely to involve multidrug-resistant organisms and should be distinguished from community-acquired pneumonia (CAP).

DIAGNOSIS

Clinical Presentation

- Fever and respiratory symptoms, including cough with sputum production, dyspnea, and pleuritic chest pain, are common presenting features in immunocompetent patients. Signs include tachypnea, rales, or signs of consolidation on auscultation.
- CAP presents acutely, over a matter of hours to days. If a patient has symptoms for more than 2–3 weeks, particularly if accompanied by weight loss or night sweats, this should raise the question of an alternate diagnosis, such as mycobacterial or fungal infection.

Diagnostic Testing

- Sputum Gram stain and culture of an adequate sample and blood cultures prior to antibiotic therapy should be obtained.
- In selected patients, urine *Legionella* or pneumococcal antigen, nasopharyngeal swab for influenza or other virus detection by PCR, and respiratory samples for atypical pathogens should be sent. If there is suspicion for TB, sputum for acid-fast staining and culture should be obtained, and the patient should be placed on airborne isolation.
- CXR should be performed and may reveal lobar consolidation, interstitial infiltrates, or cavitary lesions, confirming the diagnosis.
- Fiberoptic bronchoscopy may be used for detection of less common organisms, especially in immunocompromised patients, or if the patient is not responding to adequate therapy.

TREATMENT

- All patients should be assessed for hospitalization and evaluated for severity of illness, comorbid factors, and oxygenation. Guidelines giving detailed empiric treatment regimens have been published, with an emphasis on targeting the most likely pathogens within specific risk groups (*Clin Infect Dis 2007;44:S27*). Antibiotics should be given as soon as CAP is diagnosed because delay leads to higher patient mortality. Antibiotic therapy should be narrowed once a specific microbiologic etiology has been identified.

- **Immunocompetent outpatients** with no recent antibiotic exposure and no comorbidities should receive a macrolide, such as azithromycin 500 mg PO single dose followed by 250 mg PO daily for 4 more days, or doxycycline 100 mg PO for at least 5 days.
- **Outpatients with recent antibiotic exposure or comorbidities** should receive respiratory fluoroquinolone (e.g., moxifloxacin) monotherapy or a macrolide (azithromycin or clarithromycin) with high-dose amoxicillin 1 g PO q8h for at least 5 days.
- **Hospitalized patients** should be treated with ceftriaxone 1 g IV daily or cefotaxime 1 g IV q8h PLUS a macrolide (azithromycin or clarithromycin), OR monotherapy with a respiratory fluoroquinolone. Duration of therapy should be at least 5 days but is typically longer, because the patient should be afebrile for >48 hours with clinical improvement prior to discontinuation.
- In **critically ill patients**, the addition of azithromycin or a respiratory fluoroquinolone to a β-lactam (ceftriaxone, cefotaxime, ampicillin-sulbactam) is necessary to provide coverage for *L. pneumophila*. CA-MRSA coverage with vancomycin or linezolid should also be considered. If *P. aeruginosa* is a concern, an antipseudomonal β-lactam (cefepime, piperacillin-tazobactam, meropenem, imipenem) in combination with an antipseudomonal fluoroquinolone (ciprofloxacin, levofloxacin) is recommended. Once *Pseudomonas* has been isolated and antibiotic susceptibilities are available, monotherapy is an option.
- **Thoracentesis** of pleural effusions should be performed, with analysis of pH, cell count, Gram stain and bacterial culture, protein, and lactate dehydrogenase (see Chapter 10, Pulmonary Diseases). Empyemas should be drained.

Lung Abscess

GENERAL PRINCIPLES

Lung abscess typically results from aspiration of oral flora. Polymicrobial infections are common and involve oral anaerobes (*Prevotella* spp., *Peptostreptococcus*, *Fusobacterium*, *Bacteroides* spp., and *Actinomyces* spp.) (*Clin Infect Dis 2005;40:923*). Microaerophilic streptococci (*Streptococcus milleri*), enteric gram-negative bacilli (*Klebsiella pneumoniae*), and *S. aureu*s, including CA-MRSA, are less frequent causes. Risk factors include periodontal disease and conditions that predispose patients to aspiration of oropharyngeal contents (alcohol intoxication, seizures, stroke).

DIAGNOSIS

Clinical Presentation

Infections are indolent and may be reminiscent of pulmonary TB, with dyspnea, fever, chills, night sweats, weight loss, and cough productive of putrid or blood-streaked sputum for several weeks.

Diagnostic Testing

CXR is sensitive and typically reveals infiltrates with cavitation and air–fluid levels in dependent areas of the lung, such as the lower lobes or the posterior segments of the upper lobes. Chest CT can provide additional anatomic detail. Respiratory isolation and sputum testing for TB should be performed on all patients with cavitary lung lesions.

TREATMENT

- Antibiotic therapy should consist of clindamycin or a β-lactam/β-lactamase inhibitor (ampicillin-sulbactam, piperacillin-tazobactam, amoxicillin-clavulanate) or a carbapenem (ertapenem). For MRSA cavitary lung lesions, linezolid or vancomycin should be used. Metronidazole monotherapy is ineffective and should be combined with penicillin.
- Percutaneous drainage or surgical resection is rarely necessary and should be reserved for antibiotic-refractory disease, usually involving large abscesses (>6 cm) or infections with resistant organisms.

Tuberculosis

GENERAL PRINCIPLES

- TB infects >2 billion people and is a leading infectious cause of deaths worldwide. In the United States, cases fell to 3.0 per 100,000 in 2013. Most US cases occur in foreign-born individuals and result from reactivation of prior infection (*MMWR Morb Mortal Wkly Rep 2014;63:229*). Multidrug-resistant TB has increased among immigrants from Southeast Asia, sub-Saharan Africa, the Indian subcontinent, and Central America. Extensively drug-resistant TB is becoming increasingly prevalent in sub-Saharan Africa.
- High risk of TB exposure occurs in household contacts, prisoners, the homeless, IV drug abusers, and immigrants from high-prevalence countries. Persons at highest risk for progression include those with impaired immunity, such as HIV infection, silicosis, diabetes mellitus, chronic renal insufficiency, malignancy, malnutrition, and immunosuppressive medications, including therapy with tumor necrosis factor (TNF) antagonists (*Ann Rheum Dis 2013; 72:37*).
- Latent TB infection (LTBI) occurs when someone has been exposed to TB but has no signs, symptoms, or radiographic evidence of current active disease. Untreated, approximately 5% of persons with LTBI develop active TB disease within 2 years of infection. TB disease develops in an additional 5% of persons with LTBI over their remaining life span. Adequate treatment of LTBI can substantially reduce the risk of disease (*Am J Respir Crit Care Med 2014;190:1044*).

DIAGNOSIS

Clinical Presentation

- The most frequent clinical presentation is pulmonary disease. Symptoms are often indolent and may include cough, hemoptysis, dyspnea, fever, night sweats, weight loss, or fatigue. Misdiagnosis and treatment with a fluoroquinolone for presumed CAP can lead to treatment delay and fluoroquinolone resistance (*Int J Infect Dis 2011;15(3):e211*).
- Extrapulmonary disease can present as cervical lymphadenopathy, genitourinary disease, osteomyelitis, miliary dissemination, meningitis, peritonitis, or pericarditis.

Diagnostic Testing

- CXR may reveal focal infiltrates, nodules, cavitary lesions, miliary disease, pleural effusions, or hilar/mediastinal lymphadenopathy. Reactivation disease classically involves the upper lobes.
- Three sputum specimens should be sent for AFB smears and cultures. A diagnosis of active TB is made with a positive AFB smear along with a positive nucleic acid amplification (NAA) test for *M. tuberculosis* complex, which is confirmed on culture. Nontuberculous mycobacteria (NTM) may be positive on smear but negative on NAA test.

- *M. tuberculosis* can take several weeks to grow in culture, so if the clinical suspicion is high, presumptive therapy even with negative smears may be indicated until cultures are negative.
- Drug susceptibility testing should be performed on all initial isolates and on isolates obtained from patients who do not respond to standard therapy. Rapid detection of rifampin resistance, which correlates with multidrug-resistant TB, is possible with molecular techniques (Cepheid Gene Xpert MTB/RIF). Genetic testing on direct specimens is also available for selected cases through the CDC (molecular detection of drug resistance).
- Latent TB may be diagnosed by a positive tuberculin skin test (TST) or interferon-γ release assay. Criteria for a **positive TST** are based on the **maximum diameter of induration** (not erythema):
  ○ **5-mm induration** is considered positive in patients with HIV infection, close contacts of a known case of TB, patients with CXRs indicative of healed TB, and individuals with organ transplantation or other immunosuppression (TNF-α inhibitors, chemotherapy, steroids).
  ○ **10-mm induration** is considered positive in immigrants from high-prevalence areas (Asia, Africa, Latin America, Eastern Europe), prisoners, the homeless, IV drug users, nursing home residents, patients with chronic medical illnesses (silicosis, diabetes, hemodialysis, leukemia, lymphoma, malnutrition), and those who have frequent contact with these groups (e.g., health care workers, prison guards).
  ○ **15-mm induration** is considered positive for otherwise healthy individuals at low risk for TB.

TREATMENT

Active Tuberculosis

- If a patient is hospitalized, he or she should be put on airborne isolation in a **negative-pressure room** with use of N95 masks (*MMWR Morb Mortal Wkly Rep 2003;52(RR-11):1*).
- The local health department should be notified of all cases of TB so that contacts can be identified and directly observed therapy (DOT) administered when the patient is discharged. DOT is essential to ensure adherence and prevent emergence of drug resistance.
- **Multidrug anti-TB treatment regimens** are required because drug resistance develops when a single drug is administered. Extended therapy is necessary because of the prolonged generation time of mycobacteria.
- **Initial therapy** (the first 8 weeks) of uncomplicated pulmonary TB should consist of four drugs (RIPE): **rifampin** (**RIF**, 10 mg/kg; maximum, 600 mg PO daily), **isoniazid** (**INH** 5 mg/kg; maximum, 300 mg PO daily), **pyrazinamide** (**PZA**, 15–25 mg/kg; maximum, 2 g PO daily), and **ethambutol** (**EMB**, 15–25 mg/kg PO daily). Pyridoxine (vitamin B$_6$) 25–50 mg PO daily should be used with INH to prevent sensory neuropathy. If the isolate proves to be **fully susceptible** to INH and RIF, then EMB can be dropped and INH, RIF, and PZA continued to complete this initial phase.
- **Continuation therapy** consists of 16 weeks of INH and RIF to reach a standard total of 6 months of therapy for pulmonary TB. Patients at high risk for relapse (cavitary pulmonary disease or positive TB cultures after 2 months of therapy) should be treated for an additional 28 weeks beyond the 8-week initial phase, for a total of 9 months.
- After at least 2 weeks of daily therapy, intermittent drug administration (two or three times per week at adjusted doses) is effective and facilitates DOT.
- Patients with HIV with CD4 counts <100/μL must receive therapy at least three times weekly.
- If **INH resistance** is documented, INH should be discontinued and RIF, PZA, and EMB continued for the remaining duration of therapy. Organisms resistant only to INH can be effectively treated with a 6-month regimen if the standard four-drug regimen was started initially.

- Therapy for **multidrug-resistant TB** has been less well studied, and consultation with an expert in the treatment of TB is strongly recommended.
- **Extrapulmonary disease** in adults can be treated in the same manner as pulmonary disease, with 6- to 9-month regimens. Central nervous system (CNS) TB should be treated for 12 months.
- **Pregnant women** should not receive PZA and should be treated with a 9-month regimen. INH, RIF, and EMB, with pyridoxine, should be administered during the initial 8-week phase, until susceptibilities are known, with continuation of INH and RIF for the remainder of therapy.
- **Glucocorticoids** remain controversial in the management of TB but have been used in combination with antituberculous drugs to treat life-threatening complications such as pericarditis (*Circulation 2005;112:3608*) and meningitis (*N Engl J Med 2004;351:1741*). Prednisone 1 mg/kg (maximum, 60 mg) PO daily or dexamethasone 12 mg IV daily is tapered over several weeks.

Latent Tuberculosis

- Chemoprophylaxis for LTBI should be administered only after active disease has been ruled out by clinical assessment, CXR, and sputum collection.
- Risk factors for progression include a TST conversion within 2 years of a previously negative TST; a history of untreated TB or CXR evidence of previous fibrotic disease (calcified granulomas in the absence of fibrosis do not confer increased risk); patients with HIV infection, diabetes mellitus, end-stage renal disease, hematologic or lymphoreticular malignancy, chronic malnutrition, or silicosis or who are receiving immunosuppressive therapy; and household members and other close contacts of patients with active disease who have a reactive TST.
- Persons with advanced **HIV** infection or other severely immunocompromised states (e.g., transplant) who have had known contact with a patient with active TB should be treated for LTBI regardless of the TST.
- INH 300 mg PO daily for 9 months should be administered to persons with LTBI who have risk factors for progression to active TB disease, regardless of age.
- INH 900 mg PO plus rifapentine 900 mg PO (with dose adjustment for patients <50 kg) once weekly for 12 weeks is a newer regimen of shorter duration. It should be given by DOT to ensure compliance and monitor adverse effects (*N Engl J Med 2011;365:2155*).

Monitoring

- **Response to therapy.** Patients with initial positive sputum AFB smears should submit sputum for AFB smear and culture every 1–2 weeks until AFB smears become negative. Sputum should then be obtained monthly until two consecutive negative cultures are documented. Conversion of cultures from positive to negative is the most reliable indicator of response to treatment. Continued symptoms or persistently positive cultures after 3 months of treatment should raise the suspicion of drug resistance or nonadherence and prompt referral to an expert in the treatment of TB.
- **Adverse reactions.** Most patients should have a baseline laboratory evaluation at the start of therapy that includes hepatic enzymes, bilirubin, complete blood count (CBC), and serum creatinine. Routine laboratory monitoring for patients with normal baseline values is probably unnecessary except in the setting of HIV (particularly if receiving concurrent antiretroviral therapy), alcohol abuse, chronic liver disease, or pregnancy. Monthly clinical evaluations with specific inquiries about symptoms of drug toxicity are essential. Patients taking EMB should be tested monthly for visual acuity and red–green color perception.
- Referral to the public health department is recommended to ensure adherence by DOT and to monitor for medication-related complications.

GASTROINTESTINAL AND ABDOMINAL INFECTIONS

- Intra-abdominal infections can be classified as uncomplicated or complicated. Uncomplicated intra-abdominal infections include acute uncomplicated diverticulitis or colitis; involvement is limited to intramural inflammation. Complicated intra-abdominal infections extend beyond the initial organ, causing peritonitis or abscess formation.
- Iatrogenic infections may be complicated due to presence of multidrug-resistant organisms.
- Infections are typically polymicrobial with enteric gram-negative bacilli (e.g., *Escherichia coli*, *Klebsiella* spp.), *Enterococcus* spp., and anaerobes such as *Bacteroides* spp.
- Empiric antibiotic therapy should consist of a β-lactam/β-lactamase inhibitor, fluoroquinolone, or third-generation cephalosporin plus metronidazole (Table 14-8).
- A carbapenem should be considered in severe disease or if extended-spectrum β-lactamase–producing organisms are suspected.
- Empiric antifungal coverage is usually not indicated unless yeast is seen on Gram stain or grown in culture.
- Abscess drainage or surgical resection may be necessary for source control (*Clin Infect Dis 2010;50:133*).

Peritonitis

GENERAL PRINCIPLES

- **Primary** or **spontaneous bacterial peritonitis (SBP)** is a common complication of cirrhosis and ascites. *M. tuberculosis* and *Neisseria gonorrhoeae* (Fitz-Hugh–Curtis syndrome in women)

TABLE 14-8	Empiric Therapy Examples for Intra-Abdominal Infections

Oral Regimens
- Amoxicillin/clavulanate 875 mg/125 mg PO q12h
- Ciprofloxacin 500–750 mg PO q12h + metronidazole 500 mg PO q8h
- Moxifloxacin 400 mg PO q24h

Parenteral Regimens
No concern for *Pseudomonas aeruginosa*
- Ampicillin/sulbactam 3 g IV q6h
- Ceftriaxone 1–2 g IV q24h + metronidazole 500 mg IV q8h
- Ertapenem 1 g IV q24h
- Tigecycline 100 mg IV × 1 dose then 50 mg IV q12h
Confirmed or concern for *P. aeruginosa*
- Piperacillin/tazobactam 4.5 g IV q6h
- Cefepime 1–2 g IV q8h + metronidazole 500 mg IV q8h
- Ciprofloxacin 400 mg IV q8–12h + metronidazole 500 mg IV q8h
- Meropenem or imipenem

Concern for vancomycin-resistant *Enterococcus spp.*
- Add linezolid 600 mg PO/IV q12h or daptomycin 6–8 mg/kg IV q24h to above regimens

Concern for yeast
- Add echinocandin (e.g., micafungin 100 mg IV q24h) or fluconazole 400 mg PO/IV q24h to above regimens

also occasionally cause primary peritonitis (see Chapter 16, Sexually Transmitted Infections, Human Immunodeficiency Syndrome, and Acquired Immunodeficiency Syndrome).

• **Secondary peritonitis** may be caused by a perforated viscus in the GI or genitourinary (GU) tract or contiguous spread from a visceral infection, usually resulting in an *acute* surgical abdomen.

• Peritonitis related to **peritoneal dialysis** is addressed in Chapter 13, Renal Diseases.

DIAGNOSIS

Clinical Presentation

SBP may present without signs or symptoms typical for infection. SBP should be ruled out with a diagnostic paracentesis in patients admitted with cirrhosis and ascites presenting with GI bleeding, encephalopathy, acute kidney injury, or other decompensation of liver disease (*Gut 2012;61:297*). Patients with secondary peritonitis may appear acutely ill with abdominal tenderness and peritoneal signs.

Diagnostic Testing

• Send ascites fluid for culture (directly inoculate culture bottles at bedside), cell count, and differential. **SBP** is diagnosed when ascites fluid has >250 neutrophils.

• Diagnosis of **secondary peritonitis** is made clinically, supplemented by blood culture (positive 20–30%) and imaging to evaluate for free air (perforation) or other source of infection.

TREATMENT

• SBP treatment duration is 7 days but should be extended to 2 weeks if bacteremia is present. First-line treatment typically includes either a third-generation cephalosporin (e.g., cefotaxime 2 g IV q8h) or a fluoroquinolone (e.g., ciprofloxacin 400 mg IV q12h). Administration of IV albumin on days 1 and 3 of treatment may improve survival (*N Engl J Med 1999;341(6):403*). If a repeat paracentesis reveals <250 polymorphonuclear leukocytes (PMNs) and cultures remain negative, treatment may be shortened to 5 days. **SBP prophylaxis** should be initiated after the first episode of SBP or after variceal bleeding.

• **Secondary peritonitis** may require surgical intervention in the setting of perforation or intra-abdominal abscess formation. Percutaneous drainage of abscess may be preferable to surgical drainage. Antibiotics are often continued until imaging demonstrates resolution of the abscess.

• Treatment of chronic TB peritonitis is the same as that of pulmonary TB.

Hepatobiliary Infections

GENERAL PRINCIPLES

• **Acute cholecystitis** is typically preceded by biliary colic associated with cholelithiasis and characteristically presents with fever, right upper quadrant (RUQ) tenderness with Murphy sign, and vomiting. Acalculous cholecystitis occurs in 5–10% of cases. Organisms usually consist of normal gut flora. Leukocytosis and mild elevations of bilirubin, transaminases, and alkaline phosphatase are possible.

• **Ascending cholangitis** is a sometimes fulminant infectious complication of an obstructed common bile duct, often following pancreatitis or cholecystitis.

DIAGNOSIS

Clinical Presentation

Tenderness and guarding of the RUQ is a common sign of a hepatobiliary infection. **Murphy sign** can be elicited on physical exam to evaluate for cholecystitis. Ascending cholangitis presents as the **Charcot triad** of fever, RUQ pain, and jaundice. **Reynolds pentad** adds symptoms of confusion and hypotension and warrants rapid intervention. Bacteremia and shock are common.

Diagnostic Testing

- Liver function test (LFT) abnormalities are often severe.
- Diagnosis of biliary tract infections is usually made by imaging, with ultrasonography being the primary modality. Technetium-99m-hydroxy iminodiacetic acid scanning and CT scanning may also be useful (*N Engl J Med 2008;358(26):2804*).
- Endoscopic retrograde cholangiopancreatography (ERCP) allows for diagnosis as well as therapeutic intervention in the case of common bile duct obstruction and should be considered in patients with common bile duct dilation, jaundice, or LFT abnormalities.

TREATMENT

- Management of **acute cholecystitis** includes parenteral fluids, restricted PO intake, analgesia, and surgery. Advanced age, severe disease, or complications such as gallbladder ischemia or perforation, peritonitis, or bacteremia mandate broad-spectrum antibiotics (see Table 14-8). Immediate surgery is usually necessary for severe disease, but surgery may be delayed up to 6 weeks if there is an initial response to medical therapy (*Br J Surg 2010;97(2):141–50*). After cholecystectomy, perioperative antibiotics may be discontinued (*JAMA 2014;312(2):145–54*).
- The mainstay of therapy for **ascending cholangitis** is aggressive supportive care, including broad-spectrum antibiotics (see Table 14-8) and surgical or endoscopic decompression and drainage. Development of an abscess is a complication requiring surgical drainage.

OTHER INFECTIONS

- **Infectious diarrhea** (see Chapter 18, Gastrointestinal Diseases)
- **Viral hepatitis** (see Chapter 19, Liver Diseases)
- *Helicobacter pylori*–associated disease (see Chapter 18, Gastrointestinal Diseases)

GENITOURINARY INFECTIONS

- The spectrum of GU tract infections varies from uncomplicated to complicated depending on host factors and underlying conditions. Diagnostic and therapeutic approaches to adult GU infections are determined by gender-specific anatomic differences, prior antimicrobial exposures, and the presence of medical devices. Infections are primarily caused by Enterobacteriaceae (*E. coli, Proteus mirabilis,* and *K. pneumoniae*) and *Staphylococcus saprophyticus*.
- Workup typically includes a urinalysis and microscopic examination of a fresh, unspun, clean-voided or catheterized urine specimen. Pyuria (positive leukocyte esterase or more than eight leukocytes per high-power field) or bacteriuria (positive nitrites or more than one organism per oil-immersion field) suggests active infection. A urine Gram stain can be helpful in guiding initial antimicrobial choices. Quantitative culture often yields $>10^5$ bacteria/mL, but colony counts as low as $10^2–10^4$ bacteria/mL may indicate infection in women with acute dysuria.

Asymptomatic bacteriuria

- Asymptomatic bacteriuria is defined as the isolation of a specified quantitative count of bacteria in an appropriately collected urine specimen obtained from a person without symptoms or signs referable to urinary infection.
- **Asymptomatic bacteriuria is of limited clinical significance except in pregnant women or patients undergoing urologic surgery.** Pregnant women should have screening urine culture near the end of the first trimester and be treated if positive. Treatment is not recommended for asymptomatic bacteriuria in elderly, institutionalized patients, spinal cord injury patients, or catheterized patients when the catheter remains in place (*Clin Infect Dis 2005;40:643–54*).

Cystitis

Uncomplicated cystitis is defined as infection of the bladder or lower urinary tract in otherwise healthy, nonpregnant adult women. Complicated cystitis is defined based on several risk factors including anatomic abnormality, immunosuppression, pregnancy, indwelling catheters, or unusual pathogens. Recurrent cystitis may be seen in women and is usually due to reinfection rather than recurrence.

DIAGNOSIS

Clinical Presentation

- Lower urinary tract infection (UTI) is diagnosed based on clinical history of dysuria, urgency, or urinary frequency associated with urinalysis abnormalities of pyuria and bacteriuria and urine culture. Fever is more likely to be seen if there is associated pyelonephritis.
- Dysuria without pyuria in sexually active patients warrants consideration of sexually transmitted infection.

Diagnostic Testing

- **Acute uncomplicated cystitis in women.** A pretreatment urine culture is recommended for diabetics, patients who are symptomatic for >7 days, individuals with recurrent UTI, women who use a contraceptive diaphragm, and individuals older than 65 years.
- **Sterile pyuria.** Patients who have taken antimicrobials may have negative cultures. Differential diagnosis includes chronic interstitial nephritis, interstitial cystitis, or infection with atypical organisms including *Chlamydia trachomatis*, *Ureaplasma urealyticum*, or less frequently, *N. gonorrhoeae*. Specific cultures of the endocervix for sexually transmitted infections should be performed. Rare cases of TB can present with sterile pyuria as well.

TREATMENT

- See Tables 14-9 and 14-10 for details.
- **Acute uncomplicated cystitis in women.** A 3-day course of empiric antibiotic therapy is recommended for symptomatic women with pyuria. Therapy should be extended to 7 days in pregnant patients and diabetics. Posttreatment urine culture may be indicated in certain circumstances. Foreign bodies including stents and catheters should be removed (*JAMA 2014;312(16):1677–84*).
- **Recurrent cystitis in women** may be challenging to manage. Risk factors include frequency of intercourse and spermicide use in young women and urologic abnormalities like incontinence and cystocele in older women (*JAMA 2014;311(8):844–54*). Relapses with the original infecting organism that occur within 2 weeks of cessation of therapy should be treated for 2 weeks and may indicate a urologic abnormality.

TABLE 14-9	Empiric Therapy for Urinary Tract Infections

Disease	Empiric Therapy	Notes
Simple cystitis Women (*Clin Infect Dis 2011;* *52:e103*; *JAMA* *2014;312(16):1677*; *Cochrane Database* *Syst Rev 2011;19:* *CD002256*)	*First line:* • TMP-SMX • Nitrofurantoin • Fosfomycin *Alternative:* • FQ *Pregnancy:* • Nitrofurantoin • Cephalexin • Cefuroxime axetil	• Choose antibiotics based on local susceptibility patterns. • Usually treat for 3 d. Extend therapy to 7 d for diabetics and older patients. • Fosfomycin and β-lactams have lower efficacy than other agents; avoid if early pyelonephritis is suspected. • Treat asymptomatic bacteriuria in pregnancy.
Men (*J Antimicrob Chemother 2000;46* *(suppl 1):23*)	*First line:* • TMP-SMX • FQ	• Treat 7–14 days. • Avoid nitrofurantoin and β-lactam in men due to low tissue concentrations. • Consider urologic evaluation for recurrent disease or pyelonephritis.
Pyelonephritis, **complicated UTI** (*Clin Infect Dis* *2011;52:e103*)	*Outpatient, mild-moderate* *illness:* • FQ *Inpatient, severe illness:* • FQ • Aminoglycoside • β-lactam/β-lactamase inhibitor[a] • Third- or fourth-generation cephalosporin[b]	• Consider IV until afebrile followed by outpatient oral therapy in stable patients to complete 10–14 d. • Can consider shortening if complicating factor is resolved (i.e., removal of stone). • Do not use FQ in pregnancy.
Recurrent cystitis (*JAMA 2014;* *311(8):844*; *Clin Infect Dis* *2014;58:147*)	*Postcoital prophylaxis:* TMP-SMX SS × 1 or ciprofloxacin 250 mg × 1 or nitrofurantoin 100 mg × 1 *Continuous prophylaxis:* TMP-SMX 0.5 SS qday or every other day × 6 months or nitrofurantoin 50–100 mg qhs × 6 months *Intermittent self-treatment:* TMP-SMX DS PO bid × 3 d or ciprofloxacin 250 mg PO bid × 3 d	• Cranberry juice, topical vaginal estrogen in postmenopausal women, and methenamine hippurate may have a role in preventing recurrent UTI.

(continued)

TABLE 14-9	Empiric Therapy for Urinary Tract Infections *(Continued)*	
Disease	**Empiric Therapy**	**Notes**
Candiduria (*Clin Infect Dis* *2004;38:161*)	*Candida albicans:* • Fluconazole 100–200 mg PO qday *Critically ill or nonalbicans* *species:* • Amphotericin B	• Remove catheter if present. • Consider treatment if symptoms with pyuria, hardware, pregnancy, neutropenia, renal allografts, prior to GU surgery, or risk of dissemination.

DS, double strength; FQ, fluoroquinolone; GU, genitourinary; SS, single strength; TMP, trimethoprim; TMP-SMX, trimethoprim-sulfamethoxazole; UTI, urinary tract infection.
[a]β-lactam/β-lactamase inhibitors: ampicillin/sulbactam 1.5–3 g IV q6h, piperacillin/tazobactam 3.75–4.5 g IV q6h.
[b]Third- or fourth-generation cephalosporins include ceftriaxone 1–2 g IV q24h (third-generation) or cefepime 1 g IV q8h (fourth-generation).

TABLE 14-10	Dosing Examples for Urinary Tract Infections	
Class	**Oral (less severe)**	**Parenteral (more severe)**

Folate inhibitors	• TMP-SMX DS 160 mg/
	   800 mg PO q12h
	• Trimethoprim 100 mg PO
	   q12h
		N/A

Fluoroquino-
lone
	• Ciprofloxacin 250–500 mg
	   PO q12h
	• Levofloxacin 250–750 mg
	   PO daily
		• Ciprofloxacin 400 mg
		   IV q12h
		• Levofloxacin 250–750 mg
		   IV qday

β-Lactam/
β-lactamase
inhibitor
	• Amoxicillin-clavulanate
	   500 mg/125 mg PO
	   bid-tid
		• Ampicillin-sulbactam
		   1.5–3 g IV q6h
		• Piperacillin-tazobactam
		   3.375–4.5 g IV q6h

Cephalosporins	• Cephalexin 200–500 mg
	   PO qid
	• Cefpodoxime-proxetil
	   100 mg PO bid
		• Cefazolin 1 g IV q8h
		• Ceftriaxone 1 g IV qday
		• Cefepime 1 g IV q8h

Carbapenems	N/A	• Ertapenem 1 g IV q8h • Imipenem 500 mg IV q6h • Meropenem 1 g IV q8h
Aminoglycoside	N/A	• Gentamicin 5 mg/kg qday
Fosfomycin[a]	• Fosfomycin 3 g PO once	N/A
Nitrofurantoin[a]	• Nitrofurantoin 100 mg PO bid	N/A

DS, double strength; N/A, not applicable; TMP-SMX, trimethoprim-sulfamethoxazole.
[a]Uncomplicated cystitis.

- Prophylaxis may be considered for patients with frequent reinfection using continuous, postcoital, or self-initiated antibiotics. Cranberry pills and estrogen therapy may also have a role in prevention (*Clin Infect Dis 2014;58:147–60*).
- Dysuria without pyuria in sexually active patients warrants consideration of sexually transmitted infection. Consider **empiric treatment** for *C. trachomatis* and *U. urealyticum* with doxycycline 100 mg PO bid for 7 days or azithromycin 1 g PO in a single dose.

Genitourinary Infections in Men

CYSTITIS

Cystitis is uncommon in young men. Risk factors include urologic abnormality, anal intercourse, and lack of circumcision. Pyuria may be present due to sexually transmitted infections. Urologic studies are appropriate when no underlying risk factor is identified, when treatment fails, in the event of recurrent infections, or when pyelonephritis occurs.

PROSTATITIS

- **Acute prostatitis** is often a severe systemic illness characterized by fever, chills, dysuria, and a boggy, tender prostate on examination. Diagnosis is usually obvious by physical exam and urine Gram stain and culture. Prostatic massage is not necessary or recommended to diagnose acute prostatitis. Enteric gram-negative organisms are the usual causative organisms.
- **Chronic prostatitis** can manifest vaguely as low back pain; perineal, testicular, or penile pain; dysuria; ejaculatory pain; recurrent UTIs with the same organism; or hematospermia. Physical exam is usually unrevealing. Prostatitis is frequently abacterial; diagnosis requires identification of organisms by quantitative urine cultures before and after prostatic massage (*Tech Urol 1997;3:38*). Causative organisms are the same as for acute prostatitis. Transrectal ultrasound is only helpful if abscess is suspected.

Treatment

- **Acute bacterial prostatitis** should be treated with a 2- to 4-week course of either ciprofloxacin 500 mg PO bid or TMP-SMX 160 mg/800 mg (double-strength) PO bid.
- Culture-positive **chronic bacterial prostatitis** should receive prolonged therapy (for at least 6 weeks with a fluoroquinolone or 3 months with TMP-SMX).

EPIDIDYMITIS

Epididymitis presents as a unilateral scrotal ache with swollen and tender epididymis on exam. Causative organisms are usually *N. gonorrhoeae* or *C. trachomatis* in sexually active young men and gram-negative enteric organisms in older men. Diagnosis and therapy should be directed according to this epidemiology, with ceftriaxone and doxycycline in young men and TMP-SMX or ciprofloxacin in men older than 35 years.

Catheter-Associated Urinary Tract Infection

- Pyuria and bacteriuria are inevitable in patients with chronic indwelling catheters and should not be treated in absence of symptoms (unless there are complicating factors, as mentioned previously). Aseptic technique during insertion of a catheter is of utmost importance for prevention as well as prompt removal of the catheter when no longer needed.

- Symptomatic catheter-associated UTIs should be managed with removal or exchange of the catheter, collection of blood and urine cultures, and treatment with 7–10 days of antibiotic therapy (*Clin Infect Dis 2010;50:625*).
- Candiduria should be initially treated with catheter removal and should not be treated unless the patient is immunocompromised and at high risk for candidemia.

Pyelonephritis

DIAGNOSIS

Clinical Presentation

Patients present with fever, flank pain, and lower UTI symptoms due to ascending infection from the lower urinary tract.

Diagnostic Testing

- Urine specimens characteristically demonstrate significant bacteriuria, pyuria, red blood cells (RBCs), and occasional leukocyte casts.
- Diagnosis should include urine culture in all patients. Blood cultures should be obtained in those who are hospitalized because bacteremia may be present in 15–20% of cases. The causative agents are typically Enterobacteriaceae such as *E. coli* or *Proteus* spp. No further tests are usually needed for initial workup, but the presence of other organisms may suggest an anatomic abnormality or immune compromise.

TREATMENT

- See Tables 14-9 and 14-10 for details.
- Patients with **mild to moderate illness** who are able to take oral medication can typically be treated in the outpatient setting. Patients with more **severe illness** and pregnant patients should be treated initially with IV therapy. Nausea and vomiting may necessitate IV antibiotics until the patient can tolerate PO antibiotics.

SPECIAL CONSIDERATIONS

Evaluation for anatomic abnormalities should be done for patients who do not respond to initial empiric treatment within 48 hours. Ultrasonography, CT scan, or IV pyelogram may show presence of a renal abscess or renal calculi, which may require more invasive management for source control.

SYSTEMIC MYCOSES AND ATYPICALS

- Clinical presentations are protean and not pathogen specific. The systemic mycoses should be considered in normal hosts with unexplained chronic pulmonary pathology, chronic meningitis, lytic bone lesions, chronic skin lesions, FUO, or cytopenias. In immunocompromised patients, the development of new pulmonary, cutaneous, funduscopic, or head and neck signs and symptoms or persistent unexplained fever should prompt consideration of these pathogens
- The mycoses can often be identified by taking into account epidemiologic clues (many are geographically restricted), site of infection, inflammatory response, and microscopic fungal appearance. These infections can be complex and difficult to treat, and infectious disease consultation is recommended. Antifungal agents have variable doses depending on severity of infection and may vary based on renal and hepatic function. There are

significant drug–drug interactions between azole antifungals and many medications including antirejection drugs. Loading doses of azole antifungals may be recommended in certain circumstances. Because treatment may be prolonged for weeks to months, it is recommended to check therapeutic levels of several antifungals to minimize toxicity. Levels may be checked for flucytosine, itraconazole, posaconazole, and voriconazole. For details on treatment of fungal pathogens, *Nocardia*, and *Actinomyces*, see Table 14-11.

Candidiasis

GENERAL PRINCIPLES

Candida species are the most common cause of invasive fungal infections in humans. Infections ranging from uncomplicated mucosal disease to life-threatening invasive disease affecting any organ can occur (*Clin Infect Dis 2009;48:503*). Infections are often associated with concurrent antibiotic use, contraceptive use, immunosuppressant and cytotoxic therapy, and indwelling foreign bodies. Mucocutaneous disease may resolve after elimination of the causative condition (e.g., antibiotic therapy) or may persist and progress in the setting of immunosuppressive conditions. Serious complications, such as candidemia leading to skin lesions, ocular disease, endocarditis, and osteomyelitis, can occur.

DIAGNOSIS

Diagnosis of **mucocutaneous candidiasis** is usually based on clinical findings but can be confirmed by a potassium hydroxide preparation of exudates. Cultures can be obtained in refractory cases to exclude the presence of non–*Candida albicans* species. **Invasive candidiasis** is diagnosed by positive cultures of blood or tissue.

TREATMENT

- See Table 14-11.
- Also see the Catheter-Related Bloodstream Infections section under Health Care–Associated Infections.

Cryptococcosis

GENERAL PRINCIPLES

Cryptococcus neoformans is a ubiquitous yeast associated with soil and pigeon excrement. Disease is principally meningeal (headache and mental status changes) and pulmonary (ranging from asymptomatic nodular disease to fulminant respiratory failure). Skin lesions can also be seen. Significant infections are usually opportunistic.

DIAGNOSIS

Diagnosis requires detection of encapsulated yeast in tissue or body fluids (India ink stain) with confirmation by culture. The latex agglutination test for cryptococcal antigen in serum or CSF is helpful, and a positive serum antigen titer is highly suggestive of disseminated disease. Lumbar puncture is necessary in persons with systemic disease to exclude coexistent CNS involvement. Always measure opening pressure, because elevated opening pressure (>25 cm H_2O) has poor prognostic implications and must be managed, usually with serial lumbar punctures or with a lumbar drain.

TABLE 14-11 Treatment of Fungal Infections, *Nocardia*, and *Actinomyces*

Pathogen and Therapy	Additional Comments
Candida spp. (*Clin Infect Dis 2009;48:503*)	• *Prophylaxis:* May be beneficial in select patients with solid organ transplant, chemotherapy-induced neutropenia, or stem cell transplants.
Mucosal	
• Thrush: Clotrimazole troche or nystatin suspension × 7–14 d	• *Candidemia:* Treat from first negative blood culture. Perform ophthalmologic exam to rule out endophthalmitis. Catheters must be removed.
• Esophageal: Fluc 14–21 d	
• Vaginal: Topical azole × 3–7 d or Fluc 150 mg PO once	• *Complicated infection:* Duration may be extended if metastatic foci present or continued neutropenia.
• Frequent recurrence: Fluc 150 mg/wk × 6 mo	
Invasive	
• *Candida albicans* candidemia: Fluc × 14 d	
• Nonalbicans species: Echinocandin or Ampho × 14 d	
• Osteomyelitis: Fluc × 6–12 mo	
Cryptococcus neoformans (*Clin Infect Dis 2010;50:291*)	• Perform LP to rule out meningitis.
Nonmeningeal or Mild-Moderate Disease	• HIV: Initiate HAART 2–10 wk after starting Tx. Continue Fluc 200 mg PO qd for at least 12 mo and until CD4 count ≥100 for 6 mo.
• Immunocompetent/immunosuppressed: Fluc 400 mg PO/IV q24h × 6–12 mo	
Meningitis or Moderate-Severe Disease	• Check baseline CSF opening pressure. If ≥25 cm of CSF, reduce by 50% (up to 30 mL). Perform daily serial LPs if pressure elevated.
• Immunosuppressed: Ampho + 5-FC × 2 wk, then Fluc 400 mg PO q24h × 8 wk, then Fluc 200 mg q24h × 6–12 mo	
• Immunocompetent: Same as immunosuppressed except induction for 4–6 wk	
Histoplasma capsulatum (*Clin Infect Dis 2007;45:807*)	• Steroids may be considered for respiratory distress, hypoxemia, or severe mediastinal lymphadenitis.
Pulmonary	• HIV: Itra 200 mg PO qday ppx in areas of high endemicity if CD4 count <150.
• Acute, mild-moderate: Observation. May Tx if symptoms >1 mo	
• Acute, moderately severe to severe: Ampho for 1–2 wk or until clinically improved, then Itra for 12 wk	• PDH: Check urine antigen levels during/after Tx to monitor for relapse.
• Chronic cavitary: Itra for 12–24 mo	
Progressive disseminated histoplasmosis (PDH)	
• Mild-moderate: Itra for 12 mo	
• Moderately severe to severe: Ampho for 1–2 wk or until clinically improved, then Itra for 12 mo	

Blastomyces dermatitidis (*Clin Infect Dis 2008;46:1801*)

Pulmonary or Disseminated Extrapulmonary

- Mild to moderate: Itra for 6–12 mo
- Moderately severe to severe: Ampho for 1–2 wk or until clinically improved, then Itra for 6–12 mo
- Immunosuppressed: Treat as severe disease for 12 mo

Suppression: Itra lifelong if continued immunosuppression

CNS: Ampho for 4–6 wk then Fluc 800 mg PO q24h for 12 mo

- For CNS disease, Itra or Vori can be used instead of Fluc.

Coccidioides immitis (*Clin Infect Dis 2005;41:1217*)

Pulmonary

- Uncomplicated pneumonia, asymptomatic pulmonary nodule: May not need Tx. If Tx, Fluc 400 mg PO q24h for 3–6 mo
- Diffuse pneumonia: Ampho for 1–2 wk or until clinically improved, then Fluc 400 mg PO qday for 12 mo

Disseminated/Extrapulmonary

- Nonmeningeal: Fluc 400–800 mg IV/PO q24h
- Meningeal: Fluc +/– intrathecal Ampho; continue Fluc lifelong

- Can follow serum CF titers during/after treatment. Rising titers suggest recurrence.
- Consider surgery if pulmonary cavitary disease >2 yr or rupture.
- HIV: Continue Tx until CD4 count ≥250, lifelong if meningitis.
- Hydrocephalus may require shunt for decompression.

Sporothrix (*Clin Infect Dis 2007;45:1255*)

Lymphocutaneous/Cutaneous: Itra × 3–6 mo

Severe Systemic

- Pulmonary/disseminated/osteoarticular: Ampho for 1–2 wk or until clinically improved, then Itra for 12 mo
- Meningeal: Ampho for 4–6 wk then Itra for 12 mo

- If no initial response, can use higher doses of Itra or add topical saturated solution of potassium iodide.

(continued)

TABLE 14-11 Treatment of Fungal Infections, *Nocardia*, and *Actinomyces* (*Continued*)

Pathogen and Therapy	Additional Comments
Aspergillus (*Clin Infect Dis 2008;46:327; N Engl J Med 2009;360:1870*) *Pulmonary Aspergilloma:* Surgical resection or arterial embolization in cases of severe hemoptysis *Invasive Pulmonary Aspergillosis:* Vori for at least 6–12 wk until lesions resolve and immunosuppression resolves *Invasive Sinonasal Aspergillosis:* Ampho or Vori. Surgical debridement may be adjunctive for cure *Allergic Bronchopulmonary Aspergillosis:* Itra or intermittent steroids may decrease exacerbations. *Prophylaxis:* Posa in high-risk patients may be considered	• Ampho to cover mucormycosis as initial therapy for sinus disease pending confirmation of diagnosis. • If immunosuppression recurs, may need to restart ppx or Tx.
Mucormycosis (*Clin Infect Dis 2012;54:1629*) *Cutaneous, Rhinocerebral:* Aggressive surgical resection and debridement with clean margins followed by Ampho at upper dose range until improvement *Pulmonary:* Ampho	• Mortality is very high in immunosuppressed patients with disseminated disease. • Echinocandins may be beneficial when added to Ampho for initial induction therapy.
Nocardia (*Clin Infect Dis 2007;44:1307; Clin Infect Dis 1996;6:891*) *Cutaneous:* TMP-SMX *Severe Infection (including CNS):* Induction regimen typically includes two or three drugs including TMP-SMX or imipenem for 4–6 wk with stepdown to oral therapy for 6–12 mo *Suppression/prophylaxis:* TMP-SMX	• TMP-SMX is drug of choice but typically combined with other agents depending on disease manifestation. • Await susceptibility results to narrow treatment.
Actinomyces Penicillin G 18–24 million units IV per day × 4–6 wk then penicillin VK 1 g PO tid × 6–12 mo	• Surgery or drainage may be helpful in some cases. • Clindamycin or doxycycline can be used if penicillin allergy

5-FC, flucytosine; Ampho, amphotericin; CF, complement fixation; CNS, central nervous system; CSF, cerebrospinal fluid; Fluc, fluconazole; HAART, highly active antiretroviral therapy; Itra, itraconazole; LP, lumbar puncture; Posa, posaconazole; ppx, prophylaxis; TMP-SMX, trimethoprim-sulfamethoxazole; Tx, treatment: Vori, voriconazole.

TREATMENT

Treatment is dependent on the patient's immune function and site of infection (see Table 14-11). **Management of elevated intracranial pressure is critical.**

Histoplasmosis

GENERAL PRINCIPLES

Histoplasma capsulatum is more prevalent in the Ohio and Mississippi River Valleys of the United States and in Latin America and grows in soil contaminated by bat or bird droppings.

DIAGNOSIS

- Clinical manifestations are extremely varied, including acute flu-like or chronic granulomatous pulmonary disease or fulminant multiorgan failure in the immunocompromised patient.
- Diagnosis is based on culture or histopathology, antigen assay (urine, blood, or CSF), or complement fixation (CF) assay (≥1:16 or fourfold rise). Urine antigen assay is good for detecting disseminated disease and is helpful in following response to therapy.

TREATMENT

See Table 14-11.

Blastomycosis

GENERAL PRINCIPLES

Blastomyces dermatitidis is endemic in the upper midwestern, south central, and southeastern United States. This organism commonly disseminates, even in immunocompetent patients, and tends to affect the lungs, skin, bone, and GU tract. Aggressive pulmonary and CNS disease can occur in both immunocompromised and immunocompetent patients.

DIAGNOSIS

Diagnosis is based on culture, histopathology, or antigen assay. Serologic studies cross-react with tests for *Histoplasma* and *Cryptococcus* species and are unreliable for diagnosis but can be used to assess early response to therapy when positive.

TREATMENT

See Table 14-11.

Coccidioidomycosis

GENERAL PRINCIPLES

- *Coccidioides immitis* is endemic to the southwestern United States and Central America.
- Disease is usually a self-limited pulmonary syndrome. Less common manifestations are chronic pulmonary illness and disseminated disease, which can affect the meninges, bones, joints, and skin. Risk factors for development of severe or disseminated disease include immunocompromising conditions, African American or Filipino ethnicity, diabetes, and pregnancy.

DIAGNOSIS

- Diagnosis requires culture, histopathology, or positive CF serology.
- Serum CF titer of 1:16 or greater suggests extrathoracic dissemination.
- **Lumbar puncture** should be performed for culture and CF to rule out CNS involvement in persons with severe, rapidly progressive, or disseminated disease.
- **Skin testing** should only be used for epidemiologic purposes to evaluate exposure.

TREATMENT

See Table 14-11.

Aspergillosis

GENERAL PRINCIPLES

- *Aspergillus* species are ubiquitous environmental fungi that cause a broad spectrum of disease, usually affecting the respiratory system and sinuses.
- **Pulmonary aspergilloma.** Pulmonary aspergilloma occurs in the setting of preexisting bullous lung disease and can be easily recognized by characteristic radiographic presentation and *Aspergillus* serology.
- **Invasive aspergillosis (IA).** IA is a serious condition associated with vascular invasion, thrombosis, and ischemic infarction of involved tissues and progressive disease after hematogenous dissemination. IA is usually seen in severely immunocompromised patients, and clinical features vary by predisposing host characteristics.
- **Allergic bronchopulmonary aspergillosis (ABPA).** ABPA is a chronic relapsing and remitting respiratory syndrome associated with colonization with *Aspergillus*.

DIAGNOSIS

- Diagnosis can be very difficult given the varied manifestations of IA, and a high index of suspicion should be applied to patients with prolonged severe immunosuppression.
- Radiographic findings can be highly suggestive, if not diagnostic, of pulmonary IA, particularly the halo-crescent sign on CT in immunosuppressed patients.
- The diagnosis can be confirmed with characteristic histologic evidence of involved tissue. Fungal culture has a low yield.
- The galactomannan assay can support a diagnosis of IA and can be followed prospectively in at-risk patients (*Clin Infect Dis 2004;39:797*). Sensitivity is higher when performed on respiratory secretions as compared to serum (*Am J Respir Crit Care Med 2008;177:27*).

TREATMENT

See Table 14-11.

Sporotrichosis

GENERAL PRINCIPLES

Sporothrix schenckii is a globally endemic fungus that causes disease following traumatic inoculation with soil or plant material; most cases are vocational. Infection can also be associated with spread from infected cats or other digging animals (*Clin Infect Dis 2007;45:1255*).

DIAGNOSIS

Clinical Presentation

Lymphocutaneous disease is the usual manifestation with localization to skin and soft tissues. Pulmonary and disseminated forms of the infection are rarely seen from inhalation of the fungus.

Diagnostic Testing

Diagnosis requires culture or histopathologic demonstration of yeast in tissue or body fluids.

TREATMENT

See Table 14-11.

Mucormycosis

GENERAL PRINCIPLES

The Zygomycetes are a class of fungi that includes Mucorales, Mortierellales, and Entomophthorales. The Mucorales order contains the genera most commonly involved in human disease. These include *Mucor* spp., *Rhizopus* spp., and *Cunninghamella* spp. Disease manifestations may vary from head and neck, pulmonary, GI, and cutaneous disease to disseminated infection with angioinvasion and multiorgan infarction. Risk factors include immunosuppression, iron overload, high-dose glucocorticoid therapy, and diabetes with or without ketoacidosis.

DIAGNOSIS

- Clinical manifestations vary depending on which organ is affected. Invasive mucormycosis is devastating with rapid development of tissue necrosis from vascular invasion and thrombosis (*Lancet Infect Dis 2011;11:301*).
- Diagnosis requires tissue culture and silver stain with care to avoid disrupting fungal architecture.
- Head CT or MRI is helpful in head and neck disease to identify involved structures.
- Sinus endoscopy should be performed if there is concern for invasive fungal sinusitis.

TREATMENT

See Table 14-11.

Nocardiosis

GENERAL PRINCIPLES

Nocardia is a ubiquitous group of aerobic gram-positive branching filamentous bacteria that causes severe local and disseminated disease in the setting of impaired cell-mediated immunity (*Clin Infect Dis 2007;44:1307*). Typical infection tends to be pulmonary infiltrate, abscess, or empyema, but dissemination is common and tends to favor CNS infection, causing abscess.

DIAGNOSIS

- Clinical presentation can be acute, subacute, or chronic pneumonia.
- Chest imaging can reveal a variety of findings such as infiltrates, nodules, pleural effusions, or cavities (*Infection 2010;38:89*).
- Diagnosis requires sputum or tissue Gram stain and culture (including AFB), often needing multiple samples because yields are low.
- Look for CNS disease with brain MRI in patients with pulmonary disease.

TREATMENT

See Table 14-11.

Actinomycosis

GENERAL PRINCIPLES

Actinomyces is a microaerophilic gram-positive bacillus that usually causes oropharyngeal, pulmonary, and GI disease. Classic infections are chronic, indurated soft tissue lesions associated with draining fistulae that pass through tissue planes. Unlike *Nocardia*, infection is not limited to immunocompromised hosts.

DIAGNOSIS

Clinical presentation varies depending on what site is affected. Orocervicofacial infection is the most common form. Rare sites include the CNS and bones. Diagnosis is made by histopathology or observation of "sulfur granules" in drainage (*BMJ 2011; 343:d6099*).

TREATMENT

See Table 14-11.

Atypical (Nontuberculous) Mycobacteria

- NTM are ubiquitous environmental organisms that cause a spectrum of disease involving the lungs, skin, soft tissue, and lymph nodes. Susceptibility testing and infectious disease consultation are recommended to guide treatment.
- *Mycobacterium avium*, *Mycobacterium kansasii* (see Chapter 16, Sexually Transmitted Infections, Human Immunodeficiency Virus, and Acquired Immunodeficiency Syndrome).
- *Mycobacterium fortuitum*, *Mycobacterium marinum*, *Mycobacterium ulcerans*, *Mycobacterium haemophilum*, and *Mycobacterium scrofulaceum* cause a spectrum of chronic progressive disease of soft tissue and bone.
- *Mycobacterium leprae* is typically classified separately from the other NTM because of its potential for human-to-human transmission.

TICK-BORNE INFECTIONS

Tick-borne infections (TBIs) are common during the summer months in many areas of the United States; prevalence of specific diseases depends on the local population of vector ticks and animal reservoirs. Coinfection with multiple TBIs can occur and should be considered when patients present with overlapping syndromes. Risk should be assessed by outdoor activity in endemic regions rather than the report of a tick bite, which often goes unnoticed.

Lyme Borreliosis (Lyme Disease)

GENERAL PRINCIPLES

Lyme borreliosis is the most common vector-borne disease in the United States and is a systemic illness of variable severity caused by the spirochete *Borrelia burgdorferi*. It is seen in endemic regions, including northeastern coastal states, the upper Midwest, and northern California. Prophylactic doxycycline 200 mg PO (single dose) may reduce the risk of Lyme disease in endemic areas following a bite by a nymph-stage deer tick (*N Engl J Med 2001;345:79*).

DIAGNOSIS

Clinical Presentation

Lyme disease has three distinct clinical stages, which start after an incubation period of 7–10 days:
- Stage 1 (early local disease) is characterized by erythema migrans, a slowly expanding macular rash >5 cm in diameter, often with central clearing, and by mild constitutional symptoms.
- Stage 2 (early disseminated disease) occurs within several weeks to months and includes multiple erythema migrans lesions, neurologic symptoms (e.g., seventh cranial nerve palsy, meningoencephalitis), cardiac symptoms (atrioventricular block, myopericarditis), and asymmetric oligoarticular arthritis.
- Stage 3 (late disease) occurs after months to years and includes chronic dermatitis, neurologic disease, and asymmetric monoarticular or oligoarticular arthritis. Chronic fatigue is not seen more frequently in patients with Lyme borreliosis than in control subjects.

Diagnostic Testing

Diagnosis rests on clinical suspicion in the appropriate setting but can be supported by two-tiered serologic testing (screening enzyme-linked immunosorbent assay [ELISA] followed by Western blot) with acute and convalescent serologies.

TREATMENT

- Treatment depends on stage and severity of disease (*Clin Infect Dis 2006;43:1089*). Oral therapy (doxycycline 100 mg PO bid, amoxicillin 500 mg PO tid, or cefuroxime axetil 500 mg PO bid for 10–21 days) is used for early localized or disseminated disease without neurologic or cardiac involvement. The same agents, given for 28 days, are recommended for late Lyme disease. Doxycycline has the added benefit of covering potential coinfection with ehrlichiosis.
- Parenteral therapy (e.g., ceftriaxone 2 g IV daily, cefotaxime 2 g IV q8h, penicillin G 3–4 million units IV q4h) for 14–28 days should be used for severe neurologic or cardiac disease, regardless of stage.

Rocky Mountain Spotted Fever

GENERAL PRINCIPLES

Rocky Mountain spotted fever is caused by *Rickettsia rickettsii* after a tick bite. Endemic regions are east of the Rocky Mountains.

DIAGNOSIS

Clinical signs include fever, headache, and myalgias, followed 1–5 days later by a petechial rash starting on the distal extremities that may be faint and difficult to detect. Initial diagnosis leading to presumptive treatment should be based on the clinical syndrome, but skin biopsy and acute and convalescent serologies can provide additional support.

TREATMENT

Antibiotic treatment of choice is doxycycline 100 mg q12h IV or PO for 7 days or until afebrile for 2 days. Chloramphenicol is an alternative (*Lancet Infect Dis 2007;7:724*).

OUTCOME/PROGNOSIS

Death can occur when treatment is delayed.

Ehrlichiosis and Anaplasmosis

GENERAL PRINCIPLES

Ehrlichiosis and anaplasmosis are systemic TBIs caused by intracellular pathogens of the closely related *Ehrlichia* and *Anaplasma* genera. Two similar syndromes are recognized:
- **Human monocytic ehrlichiosis** (HME), caused by *Ehrlichia chaffeensis*, is endemic in south and south central United States.
- **Human granulocytic anaplasmosis** (HGA, formerly HGE), caused by *Anaplasma phagocytophilum*, is found in the same regions as Lyme borreliosis due to a shared tick vector.

DIAGNOSIS

Clinical Presentation

Clinical onset of illness usually occurs 1 week after tick exposure with fever, headache, and myalgias. Rash is only occasionally seen. Severe disease can result in respiratory failure, renal insufficiency, and neurologic decompensation. Leukopenia, thrombocytopenia, and elevated liver transaminases are the hallmarks of moderately severe disease.

Diagnostic Testing

- Diagnosis can be made by identification of morulae in circulating monocytes (HME) or granulocytes (HGA), which is uncommon but diagnostic in the appropriate clinical setting. Confirmation is by acute and convalescent serologies.
- PCR of blood or other fluids is rapidly becoming the test of choice (*Clin Infect Dis 2007;45:S45*).

TREATMENT

Prompt initiation of treatment with antimicrobials is likely to improve prognosis in severe disease. The drugs of choice are doxycycline 100 mg PO or IV q12h or tetracycline 25 mg/kg/d PO divided qid for 7–14 days. Rifampin dosed at 300 mg PO q12h for 7–10 days is an alternative treatment and is recommended only for patients with contraindications to doxycycline or tetracycline therapy (*Clin Infect Dis 2007;45:S45*).

Tularemia

GENERAL PRINCIPLES

Tularemia is caused by the gram-negative bacteria *Francisella tularensis* and is endemic to south central United States. It is transmitted by tick bite, by exposure to infected animals (particularly rabbits), or by exposure to infectious aerosol. *F. tularensis* is one of the most infectious pathogenic bacteria known. Inoculation or inhalation of as little as 10 organisms is adequate to cause disease. It is considered to be a dangerous potential biologic weapon due to its extreme infectivity, ease of dissemination, and capacity to cause illness and subsequent death (*JAMA 2001;285:2763*).

DIAGNOSIS

Clinical Presentation

Fever and malaise occur 2–5 days after exposure. The clinical presentation depends on the inoculation site and route of exposure. Painful regional lymphadenitis with (ulceroglandular) or without (glandular) a skin ulcer is the most common finding. Oculoglandular disease can occur. Systemic (typhoidal) and pneumonic diseases are more likely to be severe, with high mortality if not treated promptly.

Diagnostic Testing

Diagnosis can be confirmed by culture of blood, sputum, or pleural fluid but can lack sensitivity. The microbiology laboratory must be alerted promptly of culture specimens from patients with suspected tularemia to allow for use of advanced biohazard precautions. Acute and convalescent serologic studies provide a retrospective diagnosis.

TREATMENT

Treatment of choice is streptomycin 1 g IM q12h for 10 days; however, gentamicin 5 mg/kg IV divided q8h is nearly as effective and easier to administer. Doxycycline 100 mg PO/IV q12h for 14–21 days is an oral alternative but is more likely to result in relapse. Ciprofloxacin 500–750 mg PO bid for 14–21 days may also be effective (*JAMA 2001;285:2763*).

Babesiosis

GENERAL PRINCIPLES

Babesiosis is a malaria-like illness and is caused by the intraerythrocytic parasite *Babesia microti* after a tick bite. It is endemic in the same regions as Lyme borreliosis, with which patients may be co-infected.

DIAGNOSIS

- Clinical disease ranges from subclinical to severe, with fever, chills, myalgias, and headache. Hemolytic anemia may also be present.
- Diagnosis is made by visualization of the parasite in erythrocytes on thin blood smears. Serology and PCR may be available in certain laboratories.

TREATMENT

- Treatment may be necessary for moderate or severe disease, especially in asplenic patients.
- Atovaquone 750 mg PO bid plus azithromycin 500 mg PO on day 1, then 250 mg daily for 7–10 days, is the first choice for immunocompetent hosts. Clindamycin 600 mg IV q8h plus quinine 650 mg PO q8h for 7–10 days should be considered for life-threatening disease. Exchange transfusions may also be needed.
- Longer duration of therapy may be necessary in patients with persistent symptoms or until parasitemia has cleared (*Clin Infect Dis 2006;43:1089*).

MOSQUITO-BORNE INFECTIONS

Arboviral Meningoencephalitis

GENERAL PRINCIPLES

Arboviral meningoencephalitis can be caused by multiple viral agents, which vary by geographic area (e.g., WNV, Eastern and Western equine encephalitis, La Crosse encephalitis, St. Louis encephalitis). In addition to mosquitoes, transmission can occur from blood transfusion, organ transplant, and breast feeding. Infections usually occur in the summer months, and most are subclinical.

DIAGNOSIS

Clinical Presentation

Symptomatic cases of WNV infection range from a mild febrile illness to aseptic meningitis, fulminant encephalitis, or a poliomyelitis-like presentation with flaccid paralysis. Long-term neurologic sequelae are common with severe disease.

Diagnostic Testing

Diagnosis is usually clinical or by acute and convalescent serologic studies. Specific IgM antibody detection in CSF is diagnostic for acute WNV.

TREATMENT

Treatment for arboviral meningoencephalitides is mostly supportive. Interferon α-2b may reduce neurologic sequelae in cases of St. Louis encephalitis (*Clin Infect Dis 2008; 47:303*).

Malaria

GENERAL PRINCIPLES

- Malaria is a systemic parasitic disease that is endemic to most of the tropical and subtropical world. Several species of the parasite exist.
- Travel advice and appropriate chemoprophylaxis regimens are available from the CDC at *http://www.cdc.gov/travel/*.

DIAGNOSIS

Clinical Presentation

The onset of illness may occur within weeks or up to 6–12 months after infection with fever, headache, myalgias, and fatigue. Malaria is sometimes characterized by triphasic, periodic (every 48 hours for *Plasmodium ovale* and *Plasmodium vivax*) paroxysms of rigors followed by high fever with headache, cough, and nausea, then culminating in profuse sweating. *Plasmodium falciparum* malaria, the most severe form, is a potential medical emergency. Complicated, or severe, falciparum malaria is diagnosed in the setting of hyperparasitemia (>5%), cerebral malaria, hypoglycemia, lactic acidosis, renal failure, acute respiratory distress syndrome, or coagulopathy.

Diagnostic Testing

- Malaria should be suspected and excluded in all persons with fever who have traveled to an endemic area within the previous year.
- Diagnosis is made by visualization of parasites on Giemsa-stained thick blood smears. Smears should be obtained during febrile episodes to maximize parasite yield.
- Rapid diagnostic tests targeting antigens common to all *Plasmodium* species as well those specific to *P. falciparum* are available but should be confirmed with microscopy.

TREATMENT

- Treatment is dependent on the type of malaria, severity, and risk of chloroquine resistance where the infection was acquired. Updated information on geographic locations of chloroquine resistance and recommended treatment regimens from the CDC can be found at *http://www.cdc.gov/travel/* and *http://www.cdc.gov/malaria*.
- **Uncomplicated malaria (*P. falciparum, P. ovale, P. vivax, Plasmodium malariae, and Plasmodium knowlesi*) from chloroquine-sensitive areas:** Chloroquine 600 mg base PO single dose followed by 300 mg base PO at 6 hours, 24 hours, and 48 hours.
- **Uncomplicated *P. falciparum* from chloroquine-resistant areas and *P. vivax* from Australia, Indonesia, or South America:** Quinine sulfate 542 mg base PO tid plus doxycycline 100 mg PO bid for 7 days. Alternatively, can use atovaquone-proguanil (250 mg atovaquone/100 mg proguanil) four tablets daily for 3 days.
- ***P. ovale* or *P. vivax*:** Add primaquine phosphate 30 mg base PO daily for 14 days to above regimens to prevent relapse. Rule out glucose-6-phosphate dehydrogenase deficiency before initiating primaquine.
- **Complicated severe malaria (most commonly *P. falciparum*):** Quinidine gluconate 6.25 mg base/kg loading dose IV over 1–2 hours followed by 0.0125 base/kg/min as a continuous infusion plus doxycycline 100 mg PO/IV every 12 hours for at least 24 hours or until parasitemia is <1%, at which time complete treatment with oral quinine sulfate and doxycycline as previously described. IV artesunate is available in the United States on emergency request through the CDC Malaria Branch (*http://www.cdc.gov/malaria/*). Exchange transfusion may also be considered when *P. falciparum* parasitemia exceeds 15%, although the benefit has not been proven.

ZOONOSES

Avian and Swine Influenza (see the Emerging Infections and Bioterrorism section)
Anthrax (see the Emerging Infections and Bioterrorism section)
Plague (see the Emerging Infections and Bioterrorism section)

Cat-Scratch Disease (Bartonellosis)

GENERAL PRINCIPLES

Bartonellosis is caused by the bacterium *B. henselae*. It is usually self-limiting.

DIAGNOSIS

Clinical presentation usually consists of a few papulopustular lesions appearing 3–30 days after a cat bite or scratch, followed by regional lymphadenitis (usually cervical or axillary) and mild constitutional symptoms. Atypical presentations include oculoglandular disease, encephalopathy, arthritis, FUO, and culture-negative endocarditis. Diagnosis is made by exclusion of other causes of lymphadenitis and by detection of antibodies to *B. henselae* or PCR of infected tissue, skin, or pus.

TREATMENT

Localized disease spontaneously resolves in 2–4 months without treatment. If antimicrobial therapy is prescribed, azithromycin 500 mg PO single dose followed by 250 mg PO for 4 more days is recommended. Needle aspiration of suppurative lymph nodes may provide symptomatic relief. Culture-negative endocarditis has been discussed in the Cardiovascular Infections section (*Clin Infect Dis 2005;41:1373*).

Leptospirosis

GENERAL PRINCIPLES

- Leptospirosis is an acute febrile illness with varying presentations caused by *Leptospira interrogans*, a ubiquitous pathogen of wild and domestic mammals, reptiles, and amphibians. Symptom onset is 5–14 days after contact with infected animals or water contaminated with their urine.
- **Anicteric leptospirosis**, which accounts for most cases, is a biphasic illness that starts with influenza-like symptoms and proceeds to conjunctival suffusion and aseptic meningitis after a brief defervescent period.
- A minority of cases progress directly to **Weil disease (icteric leptospirosis)**, with multiorgan failure manifested by severe jaundice, uremia, and hemorrhagic pneumonitis.

DIAGNOSIS

Diagnosis is confirmed by specific cultures of urine or blood, PCR, or paired serologic studies.

TREATMENT

Therapy for anicteric disease, which can shorten the duration of illness, is doxycycline 100 mg PO bid or amoxicillin 500 mg PO q6h for 7 days. Penicillin G 1.5 million units IV q4–6h or a third-generation cephalosporin is used for treatment of severe disease, during which a Jarisch-Herxheimer reaction is possible (*Clin Microbiol Rev 2001;14:296*).

Brucellosis

GENERAL PRINCIPLES

Brucellosis is a protean systemic infection caused by members of the *Brucella* genus of gram-negative coccobacilli. Infection is usually preceded by direct contact with body fluids of livestock animals, by eating unpasteurized dairy foods, or by inhalation of infected aerosolized particles.

DIAGNOSIS

Clinical Presentation

Symptoms are initially nonspecific but usually include constitutional symptoms such as fever and perspiration. Fever can be spiking and accompanied by rigors but can also be relapsing and protracted. Malodorous perspiration is almost pathognomonic. Physical exam may be nonrevealing, although lymphadenopathy, hepatomegaly, or splenomegaly may be present. Complications within every organ system can occur (e.g., diarrhea, arthritis, meningitis, endocarditis, pneumonia, hepatitis).

Diagnostic Testing

Diagnosis is confirmed by isolation of the organism from blood or tissue culture. Serology may also be used, but cross-reactivity may exist with other bacteria.

TREATMENT

Antimicrobial treatment is doxycycline 100 mg PO bid for 6 weeks with streptomycin 15 mg/kg IM for 2–3 weeks. Gentamicin for 5–7 days or rifampin for 6 weeks may be alternatives to streptomycin (*N Engl J Med 2005;352:2325*).

BITE WOUNDS

Animal Bites

GENERAL PRINCIPLES

Management includes copious irrigation, culturing visibly infected wounds, and obtaining imaging to exclude fracture, foreign body, or joint space involvement. Most wounds should not be sutured unless they are on the face and have been thoroughly irrigated. Wound elevation should be encouraged.

TREATMENT

- Antimicrobial therapy is given to treat overt infection and as prophylaxis for high-risk bite wounds based on severity (e.g., moderate to severe), location (e.g., hands, genitalia, near joints), bite source (e.g., cats), immune status (e.g., diabetes mellitus, asplenia, immunosuppression), and type of injury (e.g., puncture, crush injury). Tetanus toxoid should be administered if the patient has been previously vaccinated but has not received a booster in the last 5 years.
- Prophylactic antibiotic therapy with amoxicillin-clavulanate 875 mg/125 mg PO bid for 3–5 days should usually be administered, unless the bite is trivial. Antibiotics are most

effective for patients presenting >8 hours after the injury (*Arch Emerg Med 1989;6:251*; *Lancet Infect Dis 2009;9:439*).

SPECIAL CONSIDERATIONS

- **Dog bites:** Normal oral flora includes *Pasteurella multocida*, streptococci, staphylococci, and *Capnocytophaga canimorsus*. Dog bites comprise 80% of animal bites, but only 5% of such bites become infected. For infected dog bite wounds, amoxicillin-clavulanate, or clindamycin plus ciprofloxacin, is effective.
- **Cat bites:** Normal oral flora includes *P. multocida* and *S. aureus*. Because more than 80% of cat bites become infected, prophylaxis with amoxicillin-clavulanate should be routinely provided. Cephalosporins should not be used. Bartonellosis can also develop after a cat bite.
- **Wild animal bites:** The need for rabies vaccination should be determined (see the following text). For most animal bites, amoxicillin-clavulanate is a good choice for prophylaxis and empiric treatment. Monkey bites should be treated with acyclovir because of the risk of *Herpesvirus simiae* (B virus).
- **Rabies**
  - Rabies causes an invariably fatal neurologic disease classically manifesting with hydrophobia, aerophobia, pharyngeal spasm, seizures, and coma.
  - The need for rabies vaccination and immunoglobulin prophylaxis (see Appendix A, Immunizations and Postexposure Therapies) should be determined after any animal bite. Risk of rabies depends on the animal species and geographic location. In the United States, most recent indigenous cases have been associated with bats, whereas dog bites account for the vast majority of human cases in the developing world.
  - Regardless of species, if the animal is rabid or suspected to be rabid, the human diploid vaccine and rabies immunoglobulin should be administered immediately. Bites by domestic animals rarely require prophylaxis unless the condition of the animal is unknown. Public health authorities should be consulted to determine whether prophylaxis is recommended for other types of animal bites.
  - A single case of survival after symptom onset using an aggressive coma-inducing regimen has been reported (*N Engl J Med 2005;352:2508*).

Human Bites

- Human bites, particularly clenched-fist injuries, are prone to infection and other complications. The normal oral flora of humans includes viridans streptococci, staphylococci, *Bacteroides* spp., *Fusobacterium* spp., peptostreptococci, and *Eikenella corrodens*.
- **Prophylaxis** with amoxicillin-clavulanate 875 mg/125 mg PO bid for 5 days is recommended for uninfected wounds.
- Infected wounds may require **parenteral therapy**, such as ampicillin-sulbactam 1.5 g IV q6h, cefoxitin 2 g IV q8h, or ticarcillin-clavulanate 3.1 g IV q6h for 1–2 weeks. Therapy should be extended to 4–6 weeks if osteomyelitis is present.

HEALTH CARE–ASSOCIATED INFECTIONS

Health care–associated infections (HAIs) substantially contribute to morbidity, mortality, and excess health care costs. Efforts to control and prevent the spread of HAIs require an institutional assessment of resources, priorities, and commitment to infection control practices (see Appendix B, Infection Control and Isolation Recommendations).

Catheter-Related Bloodstream Infections

GENERAL PRINCIPLES

- *S. aureus, S. epidermidis* (coagulase-negative staphylococci), aerobic gram-negative species, and *Candida* spp. are the most common organisms associated with catheter-related bloodstream infections (CRBSIs) (*Clin Infect Dis 2009;49:1*).
- Subclavian central venous catheters (CVCs) are associated with lower CRBSI rates than internal jugular CVCs, whereas femoral CVCs have the highest rates and should be removed within 72 hours of placement.
- Strategies for decreasing the incidence of CRBSIs include proper hand hygiene, skin antisepsis using an alcohol-based chlorhexidine solution, maximal sterile barrier precautions during insertion, strict adherence to aseptic technique, and removal of nonessential CVCs as soon as possible (*Infect Control Hosp Epidemiol 2014;35:753*). Subcutaneous tunneling and use of antiseptic-impregnated CVCs may further reduce the incidence of CRBSIs. Routine exchange of CVCs over guide wire is not recommended.

DIAGNOSIS

Clinical Presentation
CRBSIs should be suspected in any febrile patient with a CVC. Clinical findings that increase the suspicion of CRBSIs include local inflammation or phlebitis at the CVC insertion site, sepsis, endophthalmitis, lack of another source of bacteremia, and resolution of fever after catheter removal.

Diagnostic Testing
- Diagnosis is established by obtaining two or more blood cultures from both the CVC and a peripheral vein prior to initiation of antibiotics.
- Repeat blood cultures should be obtained after starting antibiotic therapy to demonstrate clearance of bacteremia.
- TEE is recommended to rule out endocarditis if the patient has an implantable cardiac pacemaker or defibrillator, a prosthetic heart valve, persistent bacteremia or fungemia, or persistent fever >3 days after initiation of appropriate antibiotic therapy and catheter removal, or if *S. aureus* is involved and <4 weeks of therapy is being considered.

TREATMENT

- Host factors, including comorbidities, severity of illness, multidrug-resistant colonization, prior infections, and current antimicrobial agents, are important considerations when selecting an antimicrobial regimen. Management guidelines are available from the Infectious Diseases Society of America (*Clin Infect Dis 2009;49:1*).
- **Empiric therapy**
  - Vancomycin 15–20 mg/kg IV q12h is appropriate for empiric therapy because a majority of CRBSIs are caused by staphylococci. The dose should be adjusted to achieve a vancomycin trough between 15–20 μg/mL.
  - Gram-negative bacilli, including *Pseudomonas*, should be covered broadly until species identification and susceptibilities are known. Fourth-generation cephalosporins (e.g., cefepime), carbapenems, or a β-lactam/β-lactamase inhibitor combined with or without an aminoglycoside are potential options.
  - The recommended duration of therapy depends on whether the infection is complicated or uncomplicated, beginning from the date of the first negative blood culture or removal of the infected CVC, whichever came later.

- **Pathogen-specific therapy:** Once the pathogen has been identified, antimicrobial therapy should be narrowed to the most effective regimen.
  - *S. aureus*: **MSSA** CRBSIs should be treated with oxacillin 2 g IV q4h or cefazolin 1–2 g IV q8h. First-line therapy for **MRSA** is vancomycin 15–20 mg/kg IV q12h with a target vancomycin trough between 15–20 μg/mL. Linezolid 600 mg PO or IV q12h or daptomycin 6 mg/kg IV daily are alternatives. Routine use of gentamicin for synergy in *S. aureus* bacteremia is not recommended (*Clin Infect Dis 2009;48:722*). TEE should be considered to evaluate for endocarditis. The recommended duration of therapy is generally 4–6 weeks. A 2-week course is acceptable for uncomplicated MRSA bacteremia, as defined by a negative TEE, negative blood cultures, and defervescence within 72 hours of starting effective therapy, absence of prosthetic material (e.g., pacemaker, valve), and no evidence of metastatic infection (*Clin Infect Dis 2011;52:1*).
  - *S. epidermidis* **(coagulase-negative staphylococci)** CRBSI is treated similarly to MRSA, with vancomycin being the drug of choice in most cases. Duration of therapy is 7 days after CVC removal or 14 days if the CVC is retained.
  - Sensitive ***Enterococcus*** CRBSI should be treated with ampicillin. Vancomycin should be used in the setting of ampicillin resistance. Vancomycin-resistant enterococci may require therapy with daptomycin or linezolid. Duration of treatment should be 7–14 days.
  - Therapy against **gram-negative bacilli** should be guided by antibiotic susceptibility testing. Duration may range from 7–14 days.
  - **Candidemia** should be treated with an echinocandin (e.g., micafungin 100 mg IV daily) in cases of moderate to severe illness pending species identification, after which therapy can be tailored. Fluconazole 400 mg IV or PO daily may be appropriate for stable patients who have not had any recent azole exposure. Duration of antifungal treatment should be for 14 days after the last positive blood culture (*Clin Infect Dis 2009;48:503*). A dilated ophthalmologic examination is advised to look for *Candida* endophthalmitis.
- **CVC removal** is always preferable. At a minimum, it is recommended that CVCs be removed in the following situations:
  - Any CRBSI involving *S. aureus*, most gram-negative bacilli, or *Candida* spp.
  - Insertion site or tunnel site infection (pus or significant inflammation at the site)
  - Immunocompromised patients with fever, neutropenia, and hemodynamic instability (e.g., sepsis)
- Antibiotic lock therapy in combination with an extended course of antibiotics may be an option in certain situations where CVC salvage is absolutely necessary.

Hospital- and Ventilator-Associated Pneumonia

GENERAL PRINCIPLES

The most frequent pathogens are gram-negative bacilli and *S. aureus*.

DIAGNOSIS

Clinical Presentation

- Hospital-acquired pneumonia (HAP) is defined as pneumonia occurring ≥48 hours after admission that was not incubating at the time of admission.
- Ventilator-associated pneumonia (VAP) is defined as HAP developing after >48–72 hours of endotracheal intubation and mechanical ventilation.
- In addition to new or progressive pulmonary infiltrate, patients may present with fever, purulent respiratory secretions, tachypnea, and hypoxia.

Diagnostic Testing

Diagnosis is made by clinical criteria as well as microbiologic testing. Optimal specimens are uncontaminated sterile body fluids (pleural or blood), bronchoscopy aspirates (cultured quantitatively), or aspirates from endotracheal tubes. Fiberoptic bronchoscopy may be diagnostic (quantitative cultures) and therapeutic (reexpansion of lung segment).

TREATMENT

* Initial empiric antimicrobial therapy should cover common health care–acquired pathogens, particularly *P. aeruginosa* and MRSA. Targeted therapy should be based on culture results and in vitro sensitivity testing (*Am J Respir Crit Care Med 2005;171:388*; *Clin Infect Dis 2010;51(S1):S42*).
* Empyemas require drainage.

Methicillin-Resistant *Staphylococcus aureus* Infections

GENERAL PRINCIPLES

MRSA infection should be distinguished from MRSA colonization, especially when isolated from nonsterile sites such as sputum. Contact precautions are indicated.

TREATMENT

* First-line therapy for most MRSA infections is vancomycin (dosed to therapeutic trough levels). Alternative agents include linezolid 600 mg IV or PO q12h, daptomycin 6 mg/kg IV q24h, ceftaroline, and telavancin. Daptomycin should not be used to treat pneumonia due to inactivation by pulmonary surfactant.
* Eradication of MRSA nasal carriage can sometimes be achieved with a 5-day course of twice-daily intranasal mupirocin. Other regimens include chlorhexidine soap products, bleach baths, and oral antibiotic treatment with TMP-SMX with or without rifampin. However, mupirocin resistance can develop, and carriage often recurs. Eradication efforts should target patients with recurrent MRSA infections.

Vancomycin-Resistant *Enterococcus* Infections

GENERAL PRINCIPLES

Vancomycin-resistant *Enterococcus* (VRE) infection should be distinguished from VRE colonization. Most VRE-related lower UTIs can be treated with nitrofurantoin, ampicillin, ciprofloxacin, or other agents that achieve high urinary concentrations. Contact precautions are indicated. Eradication of enteric VRE colonization has been attempted without success.

TREATMENT

The majority of patients with VRE bloodstream infections are treated with linezolid, daptomycin, or quinupristin/dalfopristin.

Multidrug-Resistant Gram-Negative Infections

GENERAL PRINCIPLES

Highly resistant gram-negative organisms (e.g., *Acinetobacter*, *Klebsiella*, and *Pseudomonas* species) have become increasingly common causes of HAI. Contact precautions are indicated.

TREATMENT

Antimicrobial choices are often limited. Options include broad-spectrum agents such as β-lactam/β-lactamase inhibitor combinations, carbapenems, tigecycline, and polymyxins. Infectious disease consultation is recommended for complicated multidrug-resistant infections.

EMERGING INFECTIONS AND BIOTERRORISM

- Changing patterns in human behavior and demographics, natural phenomena, and microbial evolution continually introduce new pathogens to human contact, leading to the introduction and spread of new or previously rare diseases. Included in this category are several highly fatal and easily produced microorganisms, which have the potential to be used as agents of bioterrorism and produce substantial illness in large populations via an aerosol route of exposure. Most of the likely diseases are rare, so a high index of suspicion is necessary to identify the first few cases.
- A bioterrorism-related outbreak should be considered if an unusually large number of patients present simultaneously with a respiratory, GI, or febrile rash syndrome; if several otherwise healthy patients present with unusually severe disease; or if an unusual pathogen for the region is isolated.

Anthrax

GENERAL PRINCIPLES

Spores from the gram-positive *Bacillus anthracis* germinate at the site of entry into the body, causing cutaneous, GI, or inhalational anthrax.

DIAGNOSIS

Clinical Presentation

- Natural transmission can occur through butchering and eating infected animals, usually resulting in cutaneous or GI disease.
- **Cutaneous anthrax** ("woolsorter's disease") is characterized by a painless black eschar with surrounding tissue edema.
- **GI anthrax** can present with nausea, vomiting, abdominal pain, ascites, and hemorrhage related to necrotic mucosal ulcers.
- **Inhalational anthrax** (45% case-fatality rate) may result from inadvertent aerosolization of spores from contaminated animal products (e.g., wool or animal hides) or an intentional release (*JAMA 2001;286:2549*). Infection presents initially with an influenza-like illness, GI symptoms, or both, followed by fulminant respiratory distress and multiorgan failure.

Diagnostic Testing

Diagnosis of inhalational disease is suggested by a widened mediastinum without infiltrates on CXR and confirmed by blood culture and PCR. Notify local infection control and public health department immediately for confirmed cases.

TREATMENT

- Treatment with immediate antibiotic initiation on first suspicion of inhalational anthrax reduces mortality. Empiric therapy is ciprofloxacin 400 mg IV q12h *or* doxycycline 100 mg IV q12h *and* one or two other antibiotics that are active against *B. anthracis* (e.g., penicillin, clindamycin, vancomycin) (*JAMA 2002;287:2236*). Oral therapy with

ciprofloxacin 500 mg PO bid *or* doxycycline 100 mg PO bid *and* one other active agent should be started after improvement and continued for 60 days to reduce the risk of delayed spore germination.
- Uncomplicated cutaneous anthrax can be treated with oral ciprofloxacin 500 mg bid *or* doxycycline 100 mg bid for the same duration. GI anthrax should be treated the same as inhalational disease.
- Postexposure prophylaxis for individuals at risk for inhalational anthrax consists of oral ciprofloxacin 500 mg bid for 60 days after exposure. Doxycycline and amoxicillin are alternatives if the strain proves susceptible.

Smallpox

GENERAL PRINCIPLES

- The variola virus that causes smallpox is easily transmitted person to person through respiratory droplets and carries a case-fatality rate of 25–30%.
- Smallpox, as a naturally occurring disease, was declared eradicated in 1979. However, remaining viral stocks pose a potential bioterrorism threat to unimmunized populations.

DIAGNOSIS

Clinical Presentation
High fever, myalgias, low back pain, and headache appear 7–17 days after exposure, followed by a distinctive rash 3–5 days later. Lesions progress through stages of macules, deep vesicles, pustules, scabs, and permanent pitting scars. The rash starts on the face and distal extremities, including palms and soles, with relative sparing of the trunk, and all lesions in one area are in the same stage of development. These features help to distinguish smallpox from chickenpox (varicella).

Diagnostic Testing
Diagnosis is primarily clinical but can be confirmed by electron microscopy and PCR of pustule fluid at reference laboratories. Notify local infection control, public health departments, and the CDC immediately. Treat all diagnostic samples as highly infectious.

TREATMENT

- Treatment consists of supportive care. No specific antiviral treatment is currently available, although several investigational drugs are in development.
- All suspected cases must be placed in contact and airborne isolation; patients remain infectious until all scabs have separated from the skin.
- Postexposure prophylaxis with live vaccinia virus vaccine within 3 days of exposure offers near-complete protection for responders but is associated with uncommon severe adverse reactions. Progressive vaccinia, eczema vaccinatum, and severe cases of generalized vaccinia can be treated with vaccinia immunoglobulin.

Plague

GENERAL PRINCIPLES

- Plague is caused by the gram-negative bacillus *Yersinia pestis.*
- Naturally acquired plague occurs rarely in the southwestern United States after exposure to infected animals (e.g., through scratches, bites, direct handling, inhalation of aerosolized respiratory secretions) and via rodent flea bites.

DIAGNOSIS

Clinical Presentation

There are three forms of plague.

- **Bubonic:** Local painful lymphadenitis (bubo) and fever (14% case-fatality rate).
- **Septicemic:** Can cause peripheral necrosis and disseminated intravascular coagulation (DIC) ("black death"). Usually from progression of bubonic disease (30–50% case-fatality rate).
- **Pneumonic:** Severe pneumonia with hemoptysis preceded by initial influenza-like illness (57% case-fatality rate, nearing 100% when treatment is delayed). Pneumonic disease can be transmitted from person to person and would be expected after inhalation of aerosolized *Y. pestis*.

Diagnostic Testing

Diagnosis is confirmed by isolation of *Y. pestis* from blood, sputum, or CSF. Treat all diagnostic samples as highly infectious. Notify local infection control and public health departments immediately.

TREATMENT

- Treatment should start at first suspicion of plague because rapid initiation of antibiotics improves survival. Agents of choice are streptomycin 1 g IM q12h; gentamicin 5 mg/kg IV/IM q24h *or* a 2 mg/kg loading dose and then 1.7 mg/kg IV/IM q8h, with appropriate monitoring of drug levels; or doxycycline 100 mg PO/IV bid. Alternatives include ciprofloxacin and chloramphenicol. Oral therapy can be started after clinical improvement, for a total course of 10–14 days.
- Postexposure prophylaxis is indicated after unprotected face-to-face contact with patients with known or suspected pneumonic plague and consists of doxycycline 100 mg PO bid or ciprofloxacin 500 mg PO bid for 7 days.

Botulism

GENERAL PRINCIPLES

- Botulism results from intoxication with botulinum toxin, produced by the anaerobic gram-positive bacillus *Clostridium botulinum*.
- Modes of acquisition include ingestion of the neurotoxin from improperly canned food and contamination of wounds with *C. botulinum* from the soil. Inhalational botulism could result from an intentional release of aerosolized toxin.
- Mortality is low when botulism is recognized early but may be very high in the setting of mass exposure and limited access to mechanical ventilation equipment.

DIAGNOSIS

- The classic triad consists of an absence of fever, clear sensorium, and symmetric descending flaccid paralysis with cranial nerve involvement, beginning with ptosis, diplopia, and dysarthria, and progressing to loss of gag reflex and diaphragmatic function with respiratory failure, followed by diffuse skeletal muscle paralysis. Sensation remains intact. Paralysis can last from weeks to months.
- Diagnosis is confirmed by detection of toxin in serum. Notify local infection control and public health departments.

TREATMENT

- Treatment is primarily supportive and may require mechanical ventilation in the setting of respiratory failure. Wound botulism requires extensive surgical debridement.
- Further progression of paralysis can be halted by early administration of botulinum antitoxin, available through the state public health department or the CDC. Antitoxin is reserved only for cases where there is a high suspicion for botulism based on clinical presentation and exposure history. Routine postexposure prophylaxis with antitoxin is not recommended because of the high incidence (10%) of hypersensitivity reactions and limited supply.

Viral Hemorrhagic Fever

GENERAL PRINCIPLES

- This syndrome is caused by many different RNA viruses, including filoviruses (Ebola and Marburg), flaviviruses (dengue, yellow fever), bunyaviruses (hantaviruses, Congo-Crimean hemorrhagic fever [CCHF], Rift Valley fever [RVF]), and arenaviruses (South American hemorrhagic fevers, Lassa fever).
- All of these viruses cause sporadic disease in endemic areas, and most can be transmitted as an aerosol or contact with infected body fluids. A recent multinational epidemic of Ebola virus disease (EVD) in West Africa demonstrates that sustained human-to-human transmission is also possible in vulnerable populations (*N Engl J Med 2014;371:1481*).
- Case-fatality rates are variable but can be as high as 90% for EVD in resource-limited settings.

DIAGNOSIS

Clinical Presentation

- Early symptoms include fevers, myalgias, and malaise, with varying severity and symptomatology depending on the virus, but all can severely disrupt vascular permeability and cause DIC. Thrombocytopenia, leukopenia, and hepatitis are common.
- Vomiting and severe diarrhea leading to significant dehydration and mortality, as evidenced by the West African EVD epidemic, can also be a prominent feature (*N Engl J Med 2014;371:2092; N Engl J Med 2015;372:40*).

Diagnostic Testing

- Diagnosis requires consideration of epidemiology and patient risk factors, especially travel to endemic areas.
- Serology performed by reference laboratories can confirm diagnosis. Notify local infection control and public health departments immediately.

TREATMENT

- Treatment is primarily supportive with attention to infection control.
- Ribavirin (2 g IV × 1, then 1 g q6h × 4 d, then 500 mg q8h × 6 d) has been used for CCHF, Lassa, and RVF (*JAMA 2002;287:2391; J Antimicrob Chemother 2011; 66:1215*).
- Exposed contacts should monitor temperature twice daily for 3 weeks. Postexposure prophylaxis with oral ribavirin can be administered to febrile CCHF, Lassa, and RVF contacts.

Severe Acute Respiratory Syndrome

GENERAL PRINCIPLES

- Severe acute respiratory syndrome (SARS) is a fulminant febrile influenza-like respiratory illness that progresses to pneumonia and acute respiratory distress syndrome (ARDS) (*JAMA 2003;290:374*) and is caused by SARS-associated coronavirus (SARS-CoV).
- SARS should be considered in clusters of cases of undiagnosed febrile illness, particularly in the setting of travel to mainland China, Hong Kong, or Taiwan within 10 days of symptom onset.

DIAGNOSIS

Diagnosis is confirmed by acute or convalescent SARS-CoV serum antibodies or PCR of clinical specimens (e.g., respiratory tract, stool, serum) by the CDC.

TREATMENT

Treatment is primarily supportive. Interferon and high-dose steroids have also been used.

Middle East Respiratory Syndrome

GENERAL PRINCIPLES

- Middle East respiratory syndrome (MERS) manifests primarily as a febrile respiratory illness with pneumonia and ARDS (*Ann Intern Med 2014;160:389*) and is caused by MERS coronavirus (MERS-CoV). Milder and asymptomatic infections are also possible (*Lancet Infect Dis 2013;13:752*; *N Engl J Med 2015;372:846*).
- Most cases have been reported in countries in and near the Arabian Peninsula. MERS should be considered in individuals with febrile respiratory illness who have traveled to this region within the past 14 days.

DIAGNOSIS

Diagnosis is confirmed by PCR of clinical specimens obtained from the lower respiratory tract, nasopharynx, or serum by the CDC.

TREATMENT

Treatment is primarily supportive. Interferon and ribavirin have also been used.

Pandemic, Avian, and Swine Influenza

- Genetic reassortment can result in influenza strains that were previously confined to avian and swine hosts gaining human infectivity, causing severe disease and/or rapid spread through human populations.
- Infection control measures and close communication with public health authorities are critical when pandemic strains are circulating. Each new strain may have different virulence, affected age ranges, clinical presentation, and antiviral susceptibilities. Following updated, local data during an outbreak is essential.

Chikungunya

GENERAL PRINCIPLES

- Chikungunya virus is an arthropod-borne alphavirus that is transmitted to humans by the bite of an infected *Aedes* mosquito. It is endemic to West Africa, but infections have been reported in Europe, the Caribbean, and North America (*Clin Infect Dis 2009;49:942*).
- The only way to prevent the virus is to minimize mosquito exposure. No vaccine is currently available.

DIAGNOSIS

Clinical Presentation

Fever and malaise are the earliest symptoms progressing to polyarthralgia that begins about 2–5 days after the onset of the fever. Multiple joints are involved and typically include the joints of the hands, wrists, and ankles. Pain may be disabling and can cause immobilization. Maculopapular rash may appear. Following acute illness, some patients may experience relapsing joint pain even 6 months after the infection.

Diagnostic Testing

Serology is the primary tool for diagnosis. PCR has high sensitivity and specificity within the first 5 days of symptoms.

TREATMENT

Supportive care with anti-inflammatory agents.

15 Antimicrobials

David J. Ritchie, Matthew P. Crotty, and Nigar Kirmani

Empiric antimicrobial therapy should be initiated based on expected pathogens for a given infection. As microbial resistance is increasing among many pathogens, a review of institutional as well as local, regional, national, and global susceptibility trends can assist in the development of empiric therapy regimens. Antimicrobial therapy should be modified, if possible, based on results of culture and sensitivity testing to agent(s) that have the narrowest spectrum possible. In some cases, shorter durations of therapy have been shown to be as effective as traditionally longer courses. Attention should be paid to the possibility of switching from parenteral to oral therapy where possible, as many oral agents have excellent bioavailability. Several antibiotics have major drug interactions or require alternate dosing in renal or hepatic insufficiency, or both. For antiretroviral, antiparasitic, and antihepatitis agents, see Chapter 16, Sexually Transmitted Infections, Human Immunodeficiency Virus, and Acquired Immunodeficiency Syndrome; Chapter 14, Treatment of Infectious Diseases; and Chapter 19, Liver Diseases, respectively.

ANTIBACTERIAL AGENTS

Penicillins

GENERAL PRINCIPLES

- Penicillins (PCNs) irreversibly bind PCN-binding proteins in the bacterial cell wall, causing osmotic rupture and death. These agents have a diminished role today because of acquired resistance in many bacterial species through alterations in PCN-binding proteins or expression of hydrolytic enzymes.
- PCNs remain among the drugs of choice for syphilis and infections caused by PCN-sensitive streptococci, methicillin-sensitive *Staphylococcus aureus* (MSSA), *Listeria monocytogenes*, *Pasteurella multocida*, and *Actinomyces*.

TREATMENT

- **Aqueous PCN G** (2–5 million units IV q4h or 12–30 million units daily by continuous infusion) is the IV preparation of PCN G and the drug of choice for most PCN-susceptible streptococcal infections and neurosyphilis.
- **Procaine PCN G** is an IM repository form of PCN G that can be used as an alternative treatment for neurosyphilis at a dose of 2.4 million units IM daily in combination with probenecid 500 mg PO qid for 10–14 days.
- **Benzathine PCN** is a long-acting IM repository form of PCN G that is commonly used for treating early latent syphilis (<1 year duration [one dose, 2.4 million units IM]) and late latent syphilis (unknown duration or >1 year [2.4 million units IM weekly for three doses]). It is occasionally given for group A streptococcal pharyngitis and prophylaxis after acute rheumatic fever.
- **PCN V** (250–500 mg PO q6h) is an oral formulation of PCN that is typically used to treat group A streptococcal pharyngitis.
- **Ampicillin** (1–3 g IV q4–6h) is the drug of choice for treatment of infections caused by susceptible *Enterococcus* species or *L. monocytogenes*. Oral ampicillin (250–500 mg PO q6h)

may be used for uncomplicated sinusitis, pharyngitis, otitis media, and urinary tract infections (UTIs), but amoxicillin is generally preferred.

- **Ampicillin/sulbactam** (1.5–3.0 g IV q6h) combines ampicillin with the β-lactamase inhibitor sulbactam, thereby extending the spectrum to include MSSA, anaerobes, and many Enterobacteriaceae. The sulbactam component also has unique activity against some strains of *Acinetobacter*. The agent is effective for upper and lower respiratory tract infections; genitourinary tract infections; and abdominal, pelvic, and polymicrobial soft tissue infections, including those due to human or animal bites.
- **Amoxicillin** (250–1000 mg PO q8h, 875 mg PO q12h, or 775 mg extended-release q24h) is an oral antibiotic similar to ampicillin that is commonly used for uncomplicated sinusitis, pharyngitis, otitis media, community-acquired pneumonia, and UTIs.
- **Amoxicillin/clavulanic acid** (875 mg PO q12h, 500 mg PO q8h, 90 mg/kg/d divided q12h [Augmentin ES-600 suspension], or 2000 mg PO q12h [Augmentin XR]) is an oral antibiotic similar to ampicillin/sulbactam that combines amoxicillin with the β-lactamase inhibitor clavulanate. It is useful for treating complicated sinusitis and otitis media and for prophylaxis of human or animal bites after appropriate local treatment.
- **Nafcillin and oxacillin** (1–2 g IV q4–6h) are penicillinase-resistant synthetic PCNs that are drugs of choice for treating MSSA infections. Dose reduction should be considered in decompensated liver disease.
- **Dicloxacillin** (250–500 mg PO q6h) is an oral antibiotic with a spectrum of activity similar to that of nafcillin and oxacillin, which is typically used to treat localized skin infections.
- **Piperacillin/tazobactam** (3.375 g IV q6h or the higher dose of 4.5 g IV q6h for *Pseudomonas*) combines piperacillin with the β-lactamase inhibitor tazobactam. This combination is active against most Enterobacteriaceae, Pseudomonas, MSSA, ampicillin-sensitive enterococci, and anaerobes, making it useful for intra-abdominal and complicated polymicrobial soft tissue infections. The addition of an aminoglycoside should be considered for treatment of serious infections caused by *Pseudomonas aeruginosa* or for nosocomial pneumonia.

SPECIAL CONSIDERATIONS

Adverse events: All PCN derivatives have been rarely associated with anaphylaxis, interstitial nephritis, anemia, and leukopenia. Prolonged high-dose therapy (>2 weeks) is typically monitored with weekly serum creatinine and complete blood count (CBC). Liver function tests (LFTs) are also monitored with oxacillin/nafcillin, as these agents can cause hepatitis. All patients should be asked about PCN, cephalosporin, or carbapenem allergies. These agents should not be used in patients with a reported serious PCN allergy without prior skin testing or desensitization, or both.

Cephalosporins

GENERAL PRINCIPLES

- Cephalosporins exert their bactericidal effect by interfering with cell wall synthesis by the same mechanism as PCNs.
- These agents are clinically useful because of their broad spectrum of activity and low toxicity profile. All cephalosporins are devoid of clinically significant activity against enterococci when used alone. Within this class, only ceftaroline is active against methicillin-resistant *S. aureus* (MRSA).

TREATMENT

- **First-generation cephalosporins** have activity against staphylococci, streptococci, *Escherichia coli*, and many *Klebsiella* and *Proteus* species. These agents have limited activity against other enteric gram-negative bacilli and anaerobes. **Cefazolin** (1–2 g IV/IM q8h) is the most commonly used parenteral preparation, and **cephalexin** (250–500 mg PO q6h) and **cefadroxil** (500 mg to 1 g PO q12h) are oral preparations. These agents are commonly used for treating skin/soft tissue infections, UTIs, and minor MSSA infections and for surgical prophylaxis (cefazolin).
- **Second-generation cephalosporins** have expanded coverage against enteric gram-negative rods and can be divided into above-the-diaphragm and below-the-diaphragm agents.
  - **Cefuroxime** (1.5 g IV/IM q8h) is useful for treatment of infections above the diaphragm. This agent has reasonable antistaphylococcal and antistreptococcal activity in addition to an extended spectrum against gram-negative aerobes and can be used for skin/soft tissue infections, complicated UTIs, and some community-acquired respiratory tract infections. It does not reliably cover *Bacteroides fragilis*.
  - **Cefuroxime axetil** (250–500 mg PO q12h), **cefprozil** (250–500 mg PO q12h), and **cefaclor** (250–500 mg PO q12h) are oral second-generation cephalosporins typically used for bronchitis, sinusitis, otitis media, UTIs, local soft tissue infections, and oral step-down therapy for pneumonia or cellulitis responsive to parenteral cephalosporins.
  - **Cefoxitin** (1–2 g IV q4–8h) and **cefotetan** (1–2 g IV q12h) are useful for treatment of infections below the diaphragm. These agents have reasonable activity against gram negatives and anaerobes, including *B. fragilis*, and are commonly used for intra-abdominal or gynecologic surgical prophylaxis and infections, including diverticulitis and pelvic inflammatory disease.
- **Third-generation cephalosporins** have broad coverage against aerobic gram-negative bacilli and retain significant activity against streptococci and MSSA. They have moderate anaerobic activity, but generally not against *B. fragilis*. Ceftazidime is the only third-generation cephalosporin that is useful for treating serious *P. aeruginosa* infections. Some of these agents have substantial central nervous system (CNS) penetration and are useful in treating meningitis (see Chapter 14, Treatment of Infectious Diseases). Third-generation cephalosporins are not reliable for the treatment of serious infections caused by organisms producing AmpC β-lactamases regardless of the results of susceptibility testing. These pathogens should be treated empirically with carbapenems, cefepime, or fluoroquinolones.
  - **Ceftriaxone** (1–2 g IV/IM q12–24h) and **cefotaxime** (1–2 g IV/IM q4–12h) are very similar in spectrum and efficacy. They can be used as empiric therapy for pyelonephritis, urosepsis, pneumonia, intra-abdominal infections (combined with metronidazole), gonorrhea, and meningitis. They can also be used for osteomyelitis, septic arthritis, endocarditis, and soft tissue infections caused by susceptible organisms. An emerging therapy is **ceftriaxone** 2 g IV q12h in combination with ampicillin IV for treatment of ampicillin-sensitive *Enterococcus faecalis* endocarditis when aminoglycosides need to be avoided.
  - **Cefpodoxime proxetil** (100–400 mg PO q12h), **cefdinir** (300 mg PO q12h), **ceftibuten** (400 mg PO q24h), and **cefditoren pivoxil** (200–400 mg PO q12h) are oral third-generation cephalosporins useful for the treatment of bronchitis and complicated sinusitis, otitis media, and UTIs. These agents can also be used as step-down therapy for community-acquired pneumonia. **Cefixime** (400 mg PO once) is no longer recommended as a first-line therapy for gonorrhea but may be used as alternative therapy for gonorrhea with close 7-day test-of-cure follow-up.
  - **Ceftazidime** (1–2 g IV/IM q8h) may be used for treatment of infections caused by susceptible strains of *P. aeruginosa*.

- **The fourth-generation cephalosporin cefepime** (500 mg to 2 g IV/IM q8–12h) has excellent aerobic gram-negative coverage, including *P. aeruginosa* and other bacteria producing AmpC β-lactamases. Its gram-positive activity is similar to that of ceftriaxone and cefotaxime. **Cefepime** is routinely used for empiric therapy in febrile neutropenic patients. It also has a prominent role in treating infections caused by antibiotic-resistant gram-negative bacteria and some infections involving both gram-negative and gram-positive aerobes in most sites. Anti-anaerobic coverage should be added where anaerobes are suspected.

- **Ceftaroline** (600 mg IV q12h) is a cephalosporin with anti-MRSA activity that is US Food and Drug Administration (FDA) approved for acute bacterial skin and skin structure infections and community-acquired bacterial pneumonia. **Ceftaroline's** unique MRSA activity is due to its affinity for PCN binding protein 2a (PBP2a), the same cell wall component that renders MRSA resistant to all other β-lactams. **Ceftaroline** has similar activity to ceftriaxone against gram-negative pathogens, with virtually no activity against *Pseudomonas* spp., *Acinetobacter*, and other organisms producing AmpC β-lactamase, extended-spectrum β-lactamase (ESBL), or *Klebsiella pneumoniae* carbapenemase (KPC). Like all other cephalosporins, it is relatively inactive against *Enterococcus* spp.

- **Ceftolozane-tazobactam** (1 g ceftolozane/0.5 g tazobactam IV q8 h) is a combination product consisting of a cephalosporin and a β-lactamase inhibitor. This agent is FDA approved for treatment of complicated intra-abdominal infections and complicated UTIs (cUTIs), including pyelonephritis. Ceftolozane-tazobactam has activity against many gram-negative bacteria, including some *P. aeruginosa* that are resistant to antipseudomonal carbapenems, antipseudomonal cephalosporins, and piperacillin-tazobactam. Ceftolozane-tazobactam is also active against some ESBL-producing organisms.

- **Ceftazidime-avibactam** (2 g ceftazidime/0.5 g avibactam IV q8h) is a combination product consisting of ceftazidime plus the novel β-lactamase inhibitor avibactam. This agent is FDA approved for treatment of cUTIs and complicated intra-abdominal infections. Ceftazidime-avibactam is active against gram-negative bacteria, including some *P. aeruginosa* that are resistant to other antipseudomonal β-lactams. This agent is also active against ESBL- and AmpC-producing strains and possesses unique activity against KPC-producing Enterobacteriaceae (but not against metallo-β-lactamases).

SPECIAL CONSIDERATIONS

Adverse events: All cephalosporins have been rarely associated with anaphylaxis, interstitial nephritis, anemia, and leukopenia. **PCN-allergic patients have a 5–10% incidence of a cross-hypersensitivity reaction to cephalosporins.** These agents should not be used in a patient with a reported severe PCN allergy (i.e., anaphylaxis, hives) without prior skin testing or desensitization, or both. Prolonged therapy (>2 weeks) is typically monitored with a weekly serum creatinine and CBC. Due to its biliary elimination, ceftriaxone may cause biliary sludging. Cefepime has been associated with CNS side effects, including delirium and seizures.

Monobactams

GENERAL PRINCIPLES

- **Aztreonam** (1–2 g IV/IM q6–12h) is a monobactam that is active only against aerobic gram-negative bacteria, including *P. aeruginosa*.
- It is useful in patients with known serious β-lactam allergy because there is no apparent cross-reactivity.

• Aztreonam is also available in an inhalational dosage form (75 mg inhaled q8h for 28 days) to improve respiratory symptoms in cystic fibrosis patients infected with *P. aeruginosa.*

Carbapenems

GENERAL PRINCIPLES

• **Imipenem** (500 mg to 1 g IV/IM q6–8h), **meropenem** (1–2 g IV q8h or 500 mg IV q6h), **doripenem** (500 mg IV q8h), and **ertapenem** (1 g IV q24h) are the currently available carbapenems.
• Carbapenems exert their bactericidal effect by interfering with cell wall synthesis, similar to PCNs and cephalosporins, and are active against most gram-positive and gram-negative bacteria, including anaerobes. They are among the antibiotics of choice for infections caused by organisms producing AmpC or ESBLs.

TREATMENT

• Carbapenems are important agents for treatment of many antibiotic-resistant bacterial infections at most body sites. These agents are commonly used for severe polymicrobial infections, including Fournier's gangrene, intra-abdominal catastrophes, and sepsis in immunocompromised hosts.
• Notable bacteria that are **resistant** to carbapenems include ampicillin-resistant enterococci, MRSA, *Stenotrophomonas*, and KPC- and metallo-β-lactamase-producing gram-negative organisms. In addition, ertapenem does not provide reliable coverage against *P. aeruginosa*, *Acinetobacter*, or enterococci; therefore, imipenem, doripenem, or meropenem would be preferred for empiric treatment of nosocomial infections when these pathogens are suspected. **Meropenem** is the preferred carbapenem for treatment of CNS infections.

SPECIAL CONSIDERATIONS

• **Adverse events:** Carbapenems can precipitate seizure activity, especially in older patients, individuals with renal insufficiency, and patients with preexisting seizure disorders or other CNS pathology. Carbapenems should be avoided in these patients unless no reasonable alternative therapy is available. Like cephalosporins, carbapenems have been rarely associated with anaphylaxis, interstitial nephritis, anemia, and leukopenia.
• **Patients who are allergic to PCNs/cephalosporins may have a cross-hypersensitivity reaction to carbapenems**, and these agents should not be used in a patient with a reported severe PCN allergy without prior skin testing, desensitization, or both. Prolonged therapy (>2 weeks) is typically monitored with a weekly serum creatinine, LFTs, and CBC.

Aminoglycosides

GENERAL PRINCIPLES

• Aminoglycosides exert their bactericidal effect by binding to the bacterial ribosome, causing misreading during translation of bacterial messenger RNA into proteins. These drugs are often used in combination with cell wall–active agents (i.e., β-lactams and vancomycin) for treatment of severe infections caused by gram-positive and gram-negative aerobes.

- Aminoglycosides tend to be synergistic with cell wall–active antibiotics such as PCNs, cephalosporins, and vancomycin. However, they do not have activity against anaerobes, and their activity is impaired in the low pH/low oxygen environment of abscesses. Cross-resistance among aminoglycosides is common, and in cases of serious infections, susceptibility testing with each aminoglycoside is recommended. Use of these antibiotics is limited by significant nephrotoxicity and ototoxicity.

TREATMENT

- Traditional dosing of aminoglycosides involves daily divided dosing with the upper end of the dosing range reserved for life-threatening infections. Peak and trough concentrations should be obtained with the third or fourth dose and then every 3–4 days, along with regular serum creatinine monitoring. **Increasing serum creatinine or peak/troughs out of the acceptable range requires immediate attention.**
- **Extended-interval dosing of aminoglycosides** is an alternative method of administration and is more convenient than traditional dosing for most indications. Extended-interval doses are provided in the following specific drug sections. A drug concentration is obtained 6–14 hours after the first dose, and a nomogram (Figure 15-1) is consulted to determine the subsequent dosing interval. Monitoring includes obtaining a drug concentration 6–14 hours after the dosage at least every week and a serum creatinine at least three times a week. In patients who are not responding to therapy, a 12-hour concentration should be checked, and if that concentration is undetectable, extended-interval dosing should be abandoned in favor of traditional dosing.
- For **obese patients** (actual weight >20% above ideal body weight [IBW]), an obese dosing weight (IBW + 0.4 × [actual body weight − IBW]) should be used for determining doses for both traditional and extended-interval methods. Traditional dosing, rather than extended-interval dosing, should be used for patients with endocarditis, burns that cover more than 20% of the body, anasarca, and creatinine clearance (CrCl) of <30 mL/min.
- **Gentamicin and tobramycin** traditional dosing is administered with an initial loading dose of 2 mg/kg IV (2–3 mg/kg in the critically ill), followed by 1.0–1.7 mg/kg IV q8h (peak, 4–10 μg/mL; trough, <1–2 μg/mL). Extended-interval dosing is administered with an initial loading dose of 5 mg/kg, with the subsequent dosing interval determined by a nomogram (see Figure 15-1). Tobramycin is also available as an inhaled agent for adjunctive therapy for patients with cystic fibrosis or bronchiectasis complicated by *P. aeruginosa* infection (300 mg inhalation q12h).
- **Amikacin** has an additional unique role for mycobacterial and *Nocardia* infections. Traditional dosing is an initial loading dose of 5.0–7.5 mg/kg IV (7.5–9.0 mg/kg in the critically ill), followed by 5 mg/kg IV q8h or 7.5 mg/kg IV q12h (peak, 20–35 μg/mL; trough, <10 μg/mL). Extended-interval dosing is 15 mg/kg, with the subsequent dosing interval determined by a nomogram (see Figure 15-1).

SPECIAL CONSIDERATIONS

- **Nephrotoxicity** is the major adverse effect of aminoglycosides. Nephrotoxicity is reversible when detected early but can be permanent, especially in patients with tenuous renal function due to other medical conditions. Aminoglycosides should be used cautiously or avoided, if possible, in patients with decompensated kidney disease. Concomitant administration of aminoglycosides with other known nephrotoxic agents (i.e., amphotericin B formulations, foscarnet, NSAIDs, pentamidine, polymyxins, cidofovir, and cisplatin) should be avoided if possible.

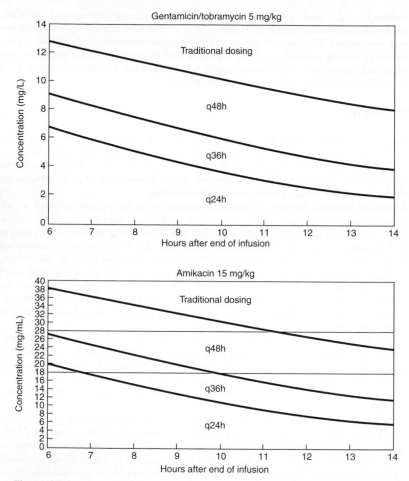

Figure 15-1. Nomograms for extended-interval aminoglycoside dosing. (Adapted from Bailey TC, Little JR, Littenberg B, et al. A meta-analysis of extended-interval dosing versus multiple daily dosing of aminoglycosides. *Clin Infect Dis* 1997;24:786–95.)

- **Ototoxicity** (vestibular or cochlear) is another possible adverse event that necessitates baseline and weekly hearing tests with extended therapy (>14 days).

Vancomycin

GENERAL PRINCIPLES

- **Vancomycin** (15 mg/kg IV q12h; up to 30 mg/kg IV q12h for meningitis) is a glycopeptide antibiotic that interferes with cell wall synthesis by binding to D-alanyl-D-alanine precursors that are critical for peptidoglycan cross-linking in most gram-positive bacterial cell walls. Vancomycin is bactericidal for staphylococci but bacteriostatic for enterococci.

• Vancomycin-resistant *Enterococcus faecium* (VRE) and vancomycin intermediately resistant *S. aureus* (VISA) present increasing treatment challenges for clinicians. Vancomycin-resistant *S. aureus* has been reported but remains rare.

TREATMENT

• Indications for use are listed in Table 15-1.
• The **goal trough** concentration is 15–20 µg/mL for treatment of serious infections.

SPECIAL CONSIDERATIONS

• Vancomycin is typically administered by slow IV infusion over at least 1 hour per gram dose. More rapid infusion rates can cause the **red man syndrome**, which is a histamine-mediated reaction that is typically manifested by flushing and redness of the upper body.
• **Adverse events.** Nephrotoxicity, neutropenia, thrombocytopenia, and rash may also occur.

Fluoroquinolones

GENERAL PRINCIPLES

• Fluoroquinolones exert their bactericidal effect by inhibiting bacterial DNA gyrase and topoisomerase function, which are critical for DNA replication. In general, these antibiotics are well absorbed orally, with serum concentrations that approach those of parenteral administration.
• Concomitant administration with aluminum- or magnesium-containing antacids, sucralfate, bismuth, oral iron, oral calcium, and oral zinc preparations can markedly impair absorption of all orally administered fluoroquinolones.

TREATMENT

• **Ciprofloxacin** (250–750 mg PO q12h. 500 mg PO q24h [Cipro XR], or 200–400 mg IV q8–12h) and **ofloxacin** (200–400 mg IV or PO q12h) are active against gram-negative aerobes including many AmpC β-lactamase–producing pathogens. These agents are commonly used for UTIs, pyelonephritis, infectious diarrhea, prostatitis, and intra-abdominal infections (with metronidazole). Ciprofloxacin is the most active quinolone against *P. aeruginosa* and is the quinolone of choice for serious infections with

TABLE 15-1	Indications for Vancomycin Use

Treatment of serious infections caused by documented or suspected methicillin-resistant *Staphylococcus aureus* (MRSA)
Treatment of serious infections caused by ampicillin-resistant, vancomycin-sensitive enterococci
Treatment of serious infections caused by gram-positive bacteria in patients who are allergic to other appropriate therapies
Oral treatment of severe *Clostridium difficile* colitis
Surgical prophylaxis for placement of prosthetic devices at institutions with known high rates of MRSA or in patients who are known to be colonized with MRSA
Empiric use in suspected gram-positive meningitis until an organism has been identified and sensitivities confirmed

that pathogen. However, ciprofloxacin has relatively poor activity against gram-positive pathogens and anaerobes and should not be used as empiric monotherapy for community-acquired pneumonia, skin and soft tissue infections, or intra-abdominal infections. Oral and IV ciprofloxacin give similar maximum serum levels at their respective doses, thus, oral therapy is appropriate unless contraindicated.

• **Levofloxacin** (250–750 mg PO or IV q24h), **moxifloxacin** (400 mg PO/IV q24h daily), and **gemifloxacin** (320 mg PO q24h daily) have improved coverage of streptococci but generally less gram-negative activity than ciprofloxacin (except levofloxacin, which does cover *P. aeruginosa*). Moxifloxacin may be used as monotherapy of intra-abdominal or skin and soft tissue infections due to its anti-anaerobic activity, although resistance among *B. fragilis* is increasing. Each of these agents is useful for treatment of sinusitis, bronchitis, community-acquired pneumonia, and UTIs (except moxifloxacin, which is only minimally eliminated in the urine). Some of these agents have activity against mycobacteria and have a potential role in treating drug-resistant TB and atypical mycobacterial infections. Levofloxacin may be used as an alternative for treatment of chlamydial urethritis.

SPECIAL CONSIDERATIONS

• **Adverse events** include nausea, CNS disturbances (headache, restlessness, and dizziness, especially in the elderly), rash, and phototoxicity. These agents can cause prolongation of the QT_c interval and should not be used in patients who are receiving class I or class III antiarrhythmics, in patients with known electrolyte or conduction abnormalities, or in those who are taking other medications that prolong the QT_c interval or induce bradycardia. These agents should also be used with caution in the elderly, in whom asymptomatic conduction disturbances are more common. Fluoroquinolones should not be routinely used in patients younger than 18 years or in pregnant or lactating women due to the risk of arthropathy in pediatric patients. They may also cause tendinitis or tendon rupture, especially of the Achilles tendon, particularly in elderly. An increase in the international normalized ratio (INR) may occur when used concurrently with warfarin.
• **This class of antimicrobials has major drug interactions.** Before initiating use of these agents, it is necessary to review concomitant medications.

Macrolide and Lincosamide Antibiotics

GENERAL PRINCIPLES

• Macrolide and lincosamide antibiotics are bacteriostatic agents that block protein synthesis in bacteria by binding to the 50S subunit of the bacterial ribosome.
• This class of antibiotics has activity against gram-positive cocci, including streptococci and staphylococci, and some upper respiratory gram-negative bacteria, but minimal activity against enteric gram-negative rods.

TREATMENT

• Macrolides are commonly used to treat pharyngitis, otitis media, sinusitis, and bronchitis, especially in PCN-allergic patients, and are among the drugs of choice for treating *Legionella*, *Chlamydia*, and *Mycoplasma* infections. Azithromycin and clarithromycin can be used as monotherapy for outpatient community-acquired pneumonia and have a unique role in the treatment and prophylaxis against *Mycobacterium avium* complex (MAC) infections. Many PCN-resistant strains of pneumococci are also resistant to macrolides.

- **Clarithromycin** (250–500 mg PO q12h or 1000 mg XL PO q24h) has enhanced activity against some respiratory pathogens (especially *Haemophilus*). It is commonly used to treat bronchitis, sinusitis, otitis media, pharyngitis, soft tissue infections, and community-acquired pneumonia. It has a prominent role in treating MAC infection and is an important component of regimens used to eradicate *Helicobacter pylori* (see Chapter 18, Gastrointestinal Diseases).

- **Azithromycin** (500 mg PO for 1 day, then 250 mg PO q24h for 4 days; 500 mg PO q24h for 3 days; 2000-mg microspheres PO for one dose; 500 mg IV q24h) has a similar spectrum of activity as clarithromycin and is commonly used to treat bronchitis, sinusitis, otitis media, pharyngitis, soft tissue infections, and community-acquired pneumonia. It has a prominent role in MAC prophylaxis (1200 mg PO every week) and treatment (500–600 mg PO q24h) in HIV patients. It is also commonly used to treat *Chlamydia trachomatis* infections (1 g PO single dose). A major advantage of azithromycin is that it does not have the numerous drug interactions seen with erythromycin and clarithromycin.

- **Clindamycin** (150–450 mg PO q6–8h or 600–900 mg IV q8h) is chemically classified as a lincosamide (related to macrolides), with activity against staphylococci and streptococci, as well as anaerobes, including *B. fragilis*. It has excellent oral bioavailability (90%) and penetrates well into the bone and abscess cavities. It is also used for treatment of aspiration pneumonia and lung abscesses. Clindamycin has activity against most community-associated strains of MRSA and has emerged as a treatment option for skin and soft tissue infections caused by this organism. Clindamycin may be used as a second agent in combination therapy for invasive streptococcal and clostridial infections to decrease toxin production. It may also be used for treatment of suspected anaerobic infections of the head and neck (peritonsillar or retropharyngeal abscesses, necrotizing fasciitis), although metronidazole is used more commonly for intra-abdominal infections (clindamycin has less reliable activity against *B. fragilis*). Clindamycin has additional uses, including treatment of babesiosis (in combination with quinine), toxoplasmosis (in combination with pyrimethamine), and *Pneumocystis jirovecii* pneumonia (in combination with primaquine).

SPECIAL CONSIDERATIONS

Adverse events: Macrolides and clindamycin are associated with nausea, abdominal cramping, and LFT abnormalities. Liver function profiles should be checked intermittently during extended therapy. Hypersensitivity reactions with prominent skin rash are more common with clindamycin, as is pseudomembranous colitis secondary to *Clostridium difficile*. Clarithromycin and azithromycin may cause QT_c interval prolongation. **Clarithromycin has major drug interactions** caused by inhibition of the cytochrome P450 system.

Sulfonamides and Trimethoprim

GENERAL PRINCIPLES

Sulfadiazine, sulfamethoxazole, and trimethoprim slowly kill bacteria by inhibiting folic acid metabolism. This class of antibiotics is most commonly used for uncomplicated UTIs, sinusitis, and otitis media. Some sulfonamide-containing agents also have unique roles in the treatment of *P. jirovecii, Nocardia, Toxoplasma*, and *Stenotrophomonas* infections.

TREATMENT

- **Trimethoprim** (100 mg PO q12h) is occasionally used as monotherapy for treatment of UTIs. Trimethoprim is more often used in the combination preparations/regimens outlined in the following sections. Trimethoprim in combination with dapsone is an alternate therapy for mild *P. jirovecii* pneumonia.

- **Trimethoprim/sulfamethoxazole** is a combination antibiotic (IV or PO) with a 1:5 ratio of trimethoprim to sulfamethoxazole. The IV preparation is dosed at 5 mg/kg IV q8h (based on the trimethoprim component) for serious infections. The oral preparations (160 mg trimethoprim/800 mg sulfamethoxazole per double-strength [DS] tablet) are extensively bioavailable, with similar drug concentrations obtained with IV and PO formulations. Both components have excellent tissue penetration, including bone, prostate, and CNS. The combination has a broad spectrum of activity but typically does not inhibit *P. aeruginosa*, anaerobes, or group A streptococci. It is the therapy of choice for *P. jirovecii* pneumonia, *Stenotrophomonas maltophilia*, *Tropheryma whipplei*, and *Nocardia* infections. It is commonly used for treating sinusitis, otitis media, bronchitis, prostatitis, and UTIs (one DS tab PO q12h). Trimethoprim/sulfamethoxazole is active against the majority of community-associated strains of MRSA and is widely used for uncomplicated cases of skin and soft tissue infections caused by this organism (often two DS tabs PO q12h). It is used as *P. jirovecii* pneumonia prophylaxis (one DS tab PO twice a week, three times a week, or single-strength or DS daily) in HIV-infected patients, solid organ transplant patients, bone marrow transplant patients, and patients receiving fludarabine. IV therapy is routinely converted to the PO equivalent for patients who require prolonged therapy.
- For serious infections, such as *Nocardia* brain abscesses, it may be useful to monitor drug levels with sulfamethoxazole peaks (100–150 µg/mL) and troughs (50–100 µg/mL) occasionally during the course of therapy and adjust the dose accordingly. In patients with renal insufficiency, doses can be adjusted by following trimethoprim peaks (5–10 µg/mL). Prolonged therapy can cause bone marrow suppression, possibly requiring treatment with leucovorin (5–10 mg PO q24h) until cell counts normalize.
- **Sulfadiazine** (1.0–1.5 g PO q6h) in combination with pyrimethamine (200 mg PO followed by 50–75 mg PO q24h) and leucovorin (10–20 mg PO q24h) is the regimen of choice for toxoplasmosis. Sulfadiazine is also occasionally used to treat *Nocardia* infections.

SPECIAL CONSIDERATIONS

Adverse events: These drugs are associated with cholestatic jaundice, bone marrow suppression, hyperkalemia (with trimethoprim/sulfamethoxazole), interstitial nephritis, "false" elevations in serum creatinine, and severe hypersensitivity reactions (Stevens-Johnson syndrome/erythema multiforme). Nausea is common with higher doses. **All patients should be asked whether they are allergic to "sulfa drugs,"** and specific commercial names should be mentioned (e.g., Bactrim or Septra).

Tetracyclines

GENERAL PRINCIPLES

- Tetracyclines are bacteriostatic antibiotics that bind to the 30S ribosomal subunit and block protein synthesis.
- These agents have unique roles in the treatment of *Rickettsia*, *Ehrlichia*, *Chlamydia*, and *Mycoplasma* infections. They are used as therapy for most tick-borne infections and Lyme disease–related arthritis, alternate therapy for syphilis, and therapy for *P. multocida* infections in PCN-allergic patients. Minocycline and doxycycline also have activity against some multidrug-resistant gram-negative pathogens and may be used in this setting based on results of susceptibility testing.

TREATMENT

- **Tetracycline** (250–500 mg PO q6h) is commonly used for severe acne and in some *H. pylori* eradication regimens. It can also be used for treatment of acute Lyme borreliosis,

Rocky Mountain spotted fever, ehrlichiosis, psittacosis, *Mycoplasma* pneumonia, *Chlamydia* pneumonia, and chlamydial infections of the eye or genitourinary tract, but these infections are generally treated with doxycycline or other antibiotics. Aluminum- and magnesium-containing antacids and preparations that contain oral calcium, oral iron, or other cations can significantly impair oral absorption of tetracycline and should be avoided within 2 hours of each dose.

- **Doxycycline** (100 mg PO/IV q12h) is the most commonly used tetracycline and is standard therapy for *C. trachomatis*, Rocky Mountain spotted fever, ehrlichiosis, and psittacosis. This agent also has a role for malaria prophylaxis and for treatment of community-acquired pneumonia. It also has utility in the treatment of uncomplicated skin and skin structure infections caused by community-associated MRSA.
- **Minocycline** (200 mg IV/PO, then 100 mg IV/PO q12h) is similar to doxycycline in its spectrum of activity and clinical indications. Among the tetracyclines, minocycline is most likely to provide coverage against *Acinetobacter*. Minocycline is second-line therapy for pulmonary nocardiosis and cervicofacial actinomycosis.

SPECIAL CONSIDERATIONS

Adverse events: Nausea and photosensitivity are common side effects, so patients should be warned about direct sun exposure. Rarely, these medications are associated with pseudotumor cerebri. **They should not routinely be given to children or to pregnant or lactating women** because they can cause tooth enamel discoloration in the developing fetus and young children. Minocycline is associated with vestibular disturbances.

ANTIMICROBIAL AGENTS, MISCELLANEOUS

Colistin and Polymyxin B

GENERAL PRINCIPLES

- **Colistimethate sodium** (colistin; 2.5–5 mg/kg/d IV divided q12h) and **polymyxin B** (15,000–25,000 units/kg/d IV divided q12h) are bactericidal polypeptide antibiotics that kill gram-negative bacteria by disrupting the cell membrane. These drugs have roles in the treatment of multidrug-resistant gram-negative bacilli but are inactive against *Proteus*, *Providencia*, and *Serratia*.
- **These medications should only be given under the guidance of an experienced clinician**, because parenteral therapy has significant CNS side effects and potential nephrotoxicity. Inhaled colistin (75–150 mg q12h given by nebulizer) is better tolerated than the IV formulation, generally causing only mild upper airway irritation, and has some efficacy as adjunctive therapy for *P. aeruginosa* or *Acinetobacter* pulmonary infections.

SPECIAL CONSIDERATIONS

Adverse events with parenteral therapy include paresthesias, slurred speech, peripheral numbness, tingling, and significant dose-dependent nephrotoxicity. The dosage should be carefully reduced in patients with renal insufficiency, because overdosage in this setting can result in neuromuscular blockade and apnea. Serum creatinine should be monitored daily early in therapy and then at a regular interval for the duration of therapy. **Concomitant use with aminoglycosides, other known nephrotoxins, or neuromuscular blockers should be avoided if at all possible.**

Dalbavancin

GENERAL PRINCIPLES

Dalbavancin (1000 mg IV on day 1 and 500 mg IV on day 8 to complete the course of therapy) is a long-acting lipoglycopeptide (terminal half-life of 346 hours) that inhibits cell wall biosynthesis and demonstrates concentration-dependent bactericidal activity. Dalbavancin has activity against many gram-positive aerobic bacteria, including staphylococci (including MRSA) and streptococci, and is FDA approved for acute bacterial skin and skin structure infections.

SPECIAL CONSIDERATIONS

Adverse events include nausea, diarrhea, vomiting, headache, insomnia, dizziness, and pruritus. In clinical trials, more dalbavancin-treated patients had alanine aminotransferase elevation greater than three times the upper limit of normal than patients treated with a comparative agent. Abnormalities in other liver tests occurred with a similar frequency in both groups.

Daptomycin

GENERAL PRINCIPLES

Daptomycin (4 mg/kg IV q24h for skin and skin structure infections; 6–8 mg/kg IV q24h for bloodstream infections) is a cyclic lipopeptide. The drug exhibits rapid bactericidal activity against a wide variety of gram-positive bacteria, including enterococci, staphylococci, and streptococci. Daptomycin is FDA approved for treatment of complicated skin and skin structure infections as well as *S. aureus* bacteremia and right-sided endocarditis. The drug should not be used to treat primary lung infections due to its decreased activity in the presence of pulmonary surfactant. Nonsusceptibility to daptomycin can develop, making it imperative that susceptibility of isolates be verified.

SPECIAL CONSIDERATIONS

Adverse events include gastrointestinal (GI) disturbances, injection site reactions, elevated LFTs, eosinophilic pneumonitis, and elevated creatine phosphokinase. Serum creatine phosphokinase should be monitored at baseline and weekly, because daptomycin has been associated with skeletal muscle effects, including rhabdomyolysis. Patients should also be monitored for signs of muscle weakness and pain, and the drug should be discontinued if these symptoms develop in conjunction with marked creatine phosphokinase elevations (5–10 times the upper limit of normal with symptoms or 10 times the upper limit of normal without symptoms). Consideration should also be given to avoiding concomitant use of daptomycin and 5-hydroxy-3-methylglutaryl–coenzyme A (HMG-CoA) reductase inhibitors due to the potential increased risk of myopathy.

Fosfomycin

GENERAL PRINCIPLES

• **Fosfomycin** (3-g sachet dissolved in cold water PO once) is a bactericidal oral antibiotic that kills bacteria by inhibiting an early step in cell wall synthesis. It has a spectrum of

activity that includes most urinary tract pathogens, including *P. aeruginosa, Enterobacter* spp., and enterococci (including VRE), and some multidrug-resistant gram-negative bacteria.
- It is most useful for treating uncomplicated UTIs in women with susceptible strains of *E. coli* or *E. faecalis*. The single-dose sachet formulation should not be routinely used to treat pyelonephritis or systemic infections.

SPECIAL CONSIDERATIONS

Adverse events include diarrhea. It should not be taken with metoclopramide, which interferes with fosfomycin absorption.

Oxazolidinones

GENERAL PRINCIPLES

- Oxazolidinones block assembly of bacterial ribosomes and inhibit protein synthesis.
- **Linezolid** (600 mg IV/PO q12h) IV and oral formulations produce equivalent serum concentrations, and the drug has potent activity against gram-positive bacteria, including drug-resistant enterococci, staphylococci, and streptococci. However, it has no meaningful activity against Enterobacteriaceae.
- Linezolid is useful for serious infections with VRE, as an alternative to vancomycin for treatment of MRSA infections, for patients with an indication for vancomycin therapy who are intolerant of that medication, and as oral therapy of MRSA infections when IV access is unavailable. Linezolid is not FDA approved for catheter-related bloodstream or catheter-site infections. Resistance can develop to this antibiotic, and it is imperative that organism susceptibility is verified.
- **Tedizolid** (200 mg PO/IV q24h) is an oxazolidinone antibiotic that is FDA approved for treating acute bacterial skin and skin structure infections. Tedizolid phosphate is a prodrug that is rapidly converted in vivo to the active moiety, tedizolid, which inhibits bacterial protein synthesis. Tedizolid has activity against staphylococci (including MRSA), streptococci, and enterococci (including some strains resistant to vancomycin).

SPECIAL CONSIDERATIONS

- **Adverse events** associated with linezolid include diarrhea, nausea, and headache. Thrombocytopenia occurs frequently in patients who receive more than 2 weeks of therapy, and serial platelet count monitoring is indicated. A CBC should be checked every week during prolonged therapy with this agent. Prolonged therapy has also been associated with peripheral and optic neuropathy. Lactic acidosis may also rarely occur.
- Linezolid has **several important drug interactions**. It is a mild monoamine oxidase inhibitor, and patients should be advised not to take selective serotonin reuptake inhibitors or other antidepressants, fentanyl, or meperidine while on linezolid to avoid the serotonin syndrome. Ideally, patients should be off antidepressants for at least a week before initiating linezolid. Over-the-counter cold remedies that contain pseudoephedrine or phenylpropanolamine should also be avoided, because coadministration with linezolid can elevate blood pressure. Linezolid does not require dose adjustments for renal or hepatic dysfunction.
- **Adverse events** associated with tedizolid include nausea, diarrhea, vomiting, headache, and dizziness. Tedizolid phosphate has primarily been studied as a 6-day regimen. Whether tedizolid is less prone to adverse effects characteristic of linezolid, such as

hematologic disturbances and peripheral and optic neuropathy, if used beyond 6 days, is uncertain. Tedizolid phosphate appears less likely to inhibit monoamine oxidase as compared to linezolid; however, patients on serotonergic agents were excluded from tedizolid phase III acute bacterial skin and skin structure infection clinical trials.

Metronidazole

GENERAL PRINCIPLES

- Metronidazole (250–750 mg PO/IV q6–12h) is only active against anaerobic bacteria and some protozoa. The drug exerts its bactericidal effect through accumulation of toxic metabolites that interfere with multiple biologic processes. It has excellent tissue penetration, including abscess cavities, bone, and the CNS.
- It has greater activity against gram-negative than gram-positive anaerobes but is active against *Clostridium perfringens* and *C. difficile*. It is the treatment of choice as monotherapy for mild to moderate *C. difficile* colitis as well as bacterial vaginosis and can be used in combination with other antibiotics to treat intra-abdominal infections and brain abscesses. Protozoal infections that are routinely treated with metronidazole include *Giardia*, *Entamoeba histolytica*, and *Trichomonas vaginalis*. A dose reduction may be warranted for patients with decompensated liver disease.

SPECIAL CONSIDERATIONS

Adverse events include nausea, dysgeusia, disulfiram-like reactions to alcohol, and mild CNS disturbances (headache, restlessness). Rarely, metronidazole causes peripheral neuropathy and seizures.

Nitrofurantoin

GENERAL PRINCIPLES

- **Nitrofurantoin** (50–100 mg PO macrocrystals q6h or 100 mg PO dual-release formulation q12h for 5–7 days) is a bactericidal oral antibiotic that is useful for uncomplicated UTIs except those caused by *Proteus*, *P. aeruginosa*, or *Serratia*. The drug is metabolized by bacteria into toxic intermediates that inhibit multiple bacterial processes. It has had a modest resurgence in use, as it is frequently effective for uncomplicated VRE UTIs.
- Although it was commonly used in the past for UTI prophylaxis, this practice should be avoided, because prolonged therapy is associated with chronic pulmonary syndromes that can be fatal. Nitrofurantoin should not be used for pyelonephritis or any other systemic infections and should be avoided in patients with renal dysfunction.

SPECIAL CONSIDERATIONS

Adverse events: Nausea is the most common adverse effect, and the drug should be taken with food to minimize this problem. Patients should be warned that their urine may become brown secondary to the medication. Neurotoxicity, hepatotoxicity, and pulmonary fibrosis may also rarely occur with nitrofurantoin. Furthermore, it should not be used in patients with CrCl <60 mL/min because the risk for development of treatment-associated adverse effects is increased. It should not be given with probenecid, because this combination decreases the concentration of nitrofurantoin in the urine.

Oritavancin

GENERAL PRINCIPLES

Oritavancin (1200 mg IV administered once to complete therapy) is a long-acting lipoglycopeptide (terminal half-life, 245 hours) that inhibits cell wall biosynthesis through multiple mechanisms and demonstrates concentration-dependent bactericidal activity. Oritavancin has activity against many gram-positive aerobic bacteria, including staphylococci (including MRSA) and streptococci, as well as some enterococci (including some strains resistant to vancomycin).

SPECIAL CONSIDERATIONS

Adverse events include nausea, diarrhea, vomiting, headache, insomnia, dizziness, and pruritus. Elevations of hepatic enzymes did not occur significantly more frequently in patients treated with oritavancin compared to vancomycin in phase III trials.

Quinupristin/Dalfopristin

GENERAL PRINCIPLES

- **Quinupristin/dalfopristin** (7.5 mg/kg IV q8h) is the first FDA-approved drug in the streptogramin class.
- This agent has activity against antibiotic-resistant gram-positive organisms, especially VRE, MRSA, and antibiotic-resistant strains of *Streptococcus pneumoniae*. It has some activity against gram-negative upper respiratory pathogens (*Haemophilus* and *Moraxella*) and anaerobes, but more appropriate antibiotics are available to treat these infections. Quinupristin/dalfopristin is bacteriostatic for enterococci and can be used for treatment of serious infections with VRE (only *E. faecium* because it is inactive against *E. faecalis*).

SPECIAL CONSIDERATIONS

Adverse events include arthralgias and myalgias, which occur frequently and can necessitate discontinuation of therapy. IV site pain and thrombophlebitis are common when the drug is administered through a peripheral vein. It has also been associated with elevated LFTs and, because it is primarily cleared by hepatic metabolism, patients with significant hepatic impairment require a dose adjustment. Quinupristin/dalfopristin is similar to clarithromycin with regard to drug interactions.

Telavancin

GENERAL PRINCIPLES

Telavancin (7.5–10 mg/kg q24–48h, based on CrCl) is a new lipoglycopeptide antibiotic that is FDA approved for treatment of hospital-acquired and ventilator-associated bacterial pneumonia caused by *S. aureus* and for complicated skin and skin structure infections. Telavancin is broadly active against gram-positive bacteria, including MRSA, VISA, heteroresistant VISA (hVISA), daptomycin- and linezolid-resistant *S. aureus*, streptococci, vancomycin-sensitive enterococci, and some gram-positive anaerobes. The agent is not active against gram-negative bacteria, vancomycin-resistant *S. aureus*, and VRE.

SPECIAL CONSIDERATIONS

Adverse events include nausea, vomiting, metallic or soapy taste, foamy urine, and nephrotoxicity (which necessitates serial monitoring of serum creatinine). Prehydration with normal saline may mitigate the nephrotoxicity observed with the use of this drug. Telavancin can also cause a minor prolongation of the QT_c interval. Women of childbearing potential require a negative serum pregnancy test prior to receiving telavancin due to teratogenic effects noted in animals.

Tigecycline

GENERAL PRINCIPLES

Tigecycline (100 mg IV loading dose, then 50 mg IV q12h) is the only FDA-approved antibiotic in the class of glycylcyclines. Its mechanism of action is similar to that of tetracyclines by inhibiting the translation of bacterial proteins through binding to the 30S ribosome. The addition of the glycyl side chain expands its activity against bacterial pathogens that are normally resistant to tetracycline and minocycline. It has a broad spectrum of bactericidal activity against gram-positive, gram-negative, and anaerobic bacteria except *P. aeruginosa* and some *Proteus* isolates. It is currently FDA approved for treatment of complicated skin and skin structure infections, complicated intra-abdominal infections, and community-acquired pneumonia. Additionally, it may be used for treatment of some other tissue infections due to susceptible strains of VRE and some multidrug-resistant gram-negative bacteria. Due to low achievable blood concentrations, tigecycline should not be used to treat primary bacteremia.

SPECIAL CONSIDERATIONS

Adverse events: Nausea and vomiting are the most common adverse events. Tigecycline has not been studied in patients younger than 18 years and is contraindicated in pregnant and lactating women. Because it has a similar structure to tetracyclines, photosensitivity, tooth discoloration, and, rarely, pseudotumor cerebri may occur. Pancreatitis may also occur.

ANTIMYCOBACTERIAL AGENTS

Effective therapy of *Mycobacterium tuberculosis* (MTB) infections requires combination chemotherapy designed to prevent the emergence of resistant organisms and maximize efficacy. Increased resistance to conventional antituberculous agents has led to the use of more complex regimens and has made susceptibility testing an integral part of TB management (see Chapter 14, Treatment of Infectious Diseases).

Isoniazid

GENERAL PRINCIPLES

Isoniazid (INH; 300 mg PO q24h) exerts bactericidal effects on susceptible mycobacteria by interfering with the synthesis of lipid components of the mycobacterial cell wall. INH is a component of nearly all treatment regimens and can be given twice a week in directly observed therapy (15 mg/kg/dose; 900 mg maximum). INH remains the drug of choice for treatment of latent TB infection (300 mg PO q24h for 9 months).

SPECIAL CONSIDERATIONS

Adverse events include elevations in liver transaminases (20%). This effect can be idiosyncratic but is usually seen in the setting of advanced age, underlying liver disease, or concomitant consumption of alcohol, and may be potentiated by rifampin. Transaminase elevations to greater than threefold the upper limit of the normal range necessitate holding therapy. Patients with known liver dysfunction should have weekly LFTs during the initial stage of therapy. INH also antagonizes vitamin B_6 metabolism and potentially can cause a peripheral neuropathy. This can be avoided or minimized by coadministration of pyridoxine, 25–50 mg PO daily, especially in the elderly, in pregnant women, and in patients with diabetes, renal failure, alcoholism, and seizure disorders.

Rifamycins

GENERAL PRINCIPLES

Rifamycins exert bactericidal activity on susceptible mycobacteria by inhibiting DNA-dependent RNA polymerase, thereby halting transcription.

- **Rifampin** (600 mg PO q24h or twice a week) is an integral component of most TB treatment regimens. It is also active against many gram-positive and gram-negative bacteria. Rifampin is used as adjunctive therapy in staphylococcal prosthetic valve endocarditis (300 mg PO q8h), for prophylaxis of close contacts of patients with infection caused by *Neisseria meningitidis* (600 mg PO q12h), and as adjunctive treatment of bone and joint infections associated with prosthetic material or devices. The drug is well absorbed orally and is widely distributed throughout the body including the cerebrospinal fluid (CSF).
- **Rifabutin** (300 mg PO q24h) is primarily used to treat TB and MAC infections in HIV-positive patients who are receiving highly active antiretroviral therapy, because it has fewer drug–drug interactions and less deleterious effects on protease inhibitor metabolism than does rifampin (see Chapter 16, Sexually Transmitted Infections, Human Immunodeficiency Virus, and Acquired Immunodeficiency Syndrome).

SPECIAL CONSIDERATIONS

Adverse events: Patients should be warned about reddish-orange discoloration of body fluids, and contact lenses should not be worn during treatment. Rash, GI disturbances, hematologic disturbances, hepatitis, and interstitial nephritis can occur. Uveitis has also been associated with rifabutin. **This class of antibiotics has major drug interactions.**

Pyrazinamide

GENERAL PRINCIPLES

- **Pyrazinamide** (15–30 mg/kg PO q24h [maximum, 2 g] or 50–75 mg/kg PO twice a week [maximum, 4 g/dose]) kills mycobacteria replicating in macrophages by an unknown disruption of membrane transport.
- It is well absorbed orally and widely distributed throughout the body, including the CSF. Pyrazinamide is typically used for the first 2 months of therapy.

SPECIAL CONSIDERATIONS

Adverse events include hyperuricemia and hepatitis.

Ethambutol

GENERAL PRINCIPLES

- **Ethambutol** (15–25 mg/kg PO q24h or 50–75 mg/kg PO twice a week; maximum, 2.4 g/dose) is bacteriostatic and inhibits arabinosyl transferase (involved in cell wall synthesis).
- Doses should be reduced in the presence of renal dysfunction.

SPECIAL CONSIDERATIONS

Adverse events may include optic neuritis, which manifests as decreased red-green color perception, decreased visual acuity, or visual field deficits. Baseline and monthly visual examinations should be performed during therapy. Renal function should also be carefully monitored because drug accumulation in the setting of renal insufficiency can increase risk of ocular effects.

Streptomycin

Streptomycin is an aminoglycoside that can be used as a substitute for ethambutol and for drug-resistant MTB. It does not adequately penetrate the CNS and should not be used for TB meningitis.

ANTIVIRAL AGENTS

Current antiviral agents only suppress viral replication. Viral containment or elimination requires an intact host immune response. Anti-HIV agents will be discussed in Chapter 16, Sexually Transmitted Infections, Human Immunodeficiency Virus, and Acquired Immunodeficiency Syndrome.

Anti-Influenza Agents (Neuraminidase Inhibitors)

Zanamivir, oseltamivir, and peramivir block influenza A and B neuraminidases. Neuraminidase activity is necessary for successful viral egress and release from infected cells. These drugs have shown modest activity in clinical trials, with a 1- to 2-day improvement in symptoms in patients who are treated within 48 hours of the onset of influenza symptoms. At the onset of each influenza season, a consultation with local health department officials is recommended to determine the most effective antiviral agent. Although oseltamivir and zanamivir are effective for prophylaxis of influenza, annual influenza vaccination remains the most effective method for prophylaxis in all high-risk patients and health care workers (see Appendix A, Immunizations and Postexposure Therapies).
- **Zanamivir** (10 mg [two inhalations] q12h for 5 days, started within 48 hours of the onset of symptoms) is an inhaled neuraminidase inhibitor that is active against influenza A and B. It is indicated for treatment of uncomplicated acute influenza infection in adults and children 7 years of age or older who have been symptomatic for <48 hours. The drug is also indicated for influenza prophylaxis in patients age 5 years and older.
  Adverse events. Headache, GI disturbances, dizziness, and upper respiratory symptoms are sometimes reported. Bronchospasms or declines in lung function, or both, may occur in patients with underlying respiratory disorders and may require a rapid-acting bronchodilator for control.
- **Oseltamivir** (75 mg PO q12h for 5 days) is an orally administered neuraminidase inhibitor that is active against influenza A and B. It is indicated for treatment of uncomplicated

acute influenza in adults and children 1 year of age or older who have been symptomatic for up to 2 days. This agent is also indicated for prophylaxis of influenza A and B in adults and children 1 year of age or older.

Adverse events include nausea, vomiting, and diarrhea. Dizziness and headache may also occur.

• **Peramivir** (600 mg IV single-dose therapy) is an IV neuraminidase inhibitor that is active against influenza A and B. It is FDA approved for single-dose treatment of acute, uncomplicated influenza in adults who have been symptomatic for up to 2 days. The agent has not been proven to be effective for serious influenza requiring hospitalization.

Adverse events include diarrhea and rare cases of skin reactions, behavioral disturbances, neutrophils <1000/μL, hyperglycemia, creatine phosphokinase elevation, and elevation of hepatic transaminases.

Antiherpetic Agents

GENERAL PRINCIPLES

Antiherpetic agents are nucleotide analogs that inhibit viral DNA synthesis.

• **Acyclovir** is active against herpes simplex virus (HSV) and varicella-zoster virus (VZV) (400 mg PO q8h for HSV, 800 mg PO five times a day for localized VZV infections, 5–10 mg/kg IV q8h for severe HSV infections, and 10 mg/kg IV q8h for severe VZV infections and HSV encephalitis).
  ○ It is indicated for treatment of primary and recurrent genital herpes, severe herpetic stomatitis, and herpes simplex encephalitis. It can be used as prophylaxis in patients who have frequent HSV recurrences (400 mg PO q12h). It is also used for herpes zoster ophthalmicus, disseminated primary VZV in adults (significant morbidity compared to the childhood illness), and severe disseminated primary VZV in children.
  ○ **Adverse events.** Reversible crystalline nephropathy may occur; preexisting renal failure, dehydration, and IV bolus dosing increase the risk of this effect. Rare cases of CNS disturbances, including delirium, tremors, and seizures, may also occur, particularly with high doses, in patients with renal failure and in the elderly.
• **Valacyclovir** (1000 mg PO q8h for herpes zoster, 1000 mg PO q12h for initial episode of genital HSV infection, and 500 mg PO q12h or 1000 mg PO q24h for recurrent episodes of HSV) is an orally administered prodrug of acyclovir used for the treatment of acute herpes zoster infections and for treatment or suppression of genital HSV infection. It is converted to acyclovir in the body. An advantage over oral acyclovir is less frequent dosing.

  The most common **adverse effect** is nausea. Valacyclovir can rarely cause CNS disturbances, and high doses (8 g/d) have been associated with development of hemolytic-uremic syndrome/thrombotic thrombocytopenic purpura in immunocompromised patients, including those with HIV and bone marrow and solid organ transplants.
• **Famciclovir** (500 mg PO q8h for herpes zoster, 250 mg PO q8h for the initial episode of genital HSV infection, and 125 mg PO q12h for recurrent episodes of genital HSV infection) is an orally administered antiviral agent used for the treatment of acute herpes zoster reactivation and for treatment or suppression of genital HSV infections.

  Adverse events include headache, nausea, and diarrhea.

Anticytomegalovirus Agents

• **Ganciclovir** (5 mg/kg IV q12h for 14–21 days for induction therapy of cytomegalovirus [CMV] retinitis, followed by 6 mg/kg IV for 5 days every week or 5 mg/kg IV q24h; the oral dose is 1000 mg PO q8h with food) is used to treat CMV.

- ○ It has activity against HSV and VZV, but safer drugs are available to treat those infections. The drug is widely distributed in the body, including the CSF.
- ○ It is indicated for treatment of CMV retinitis and other serious CMV infections in immunocompromised patients (e.g., transplant and AIDS patients). Chronic maintenance therapy is generally required to suppress CMV disease in patients with AIDS.
- ○ **Adverse events.** Neutropenia, which may require treatment with granulocyte colony-stimulating factor for management (300 μg SC daily to weekly), is the main therapy-limiting adverse effect. Thrombocytopenia, rash, confusion, headache, nephrotoxicity, and GI disturbances may also occur. Blood counts and electrolytes should be monitored weekly while the patient is receiving therapy. Other agents with nephrotoxic or bone marrow suppressive effects may enhance the adverse effects of ganciclovir.
- **Valganciclovir** (900 mg PO q12–24h) is the oral prodrug of ganciclovir. This agent has excellent bioavailability and can be used for treatment of CMV retinitis and, thus, has supplanted the use of oral ganciclovir, which has poor oral bioavailability. Adverse events are the same as those for ganciclovir.
- **Foscarnet** (60 mg/kg IV q8h or 90 mg/kg IV q12h for 14–21 days as induction therapy, followed by 90–120 mg/kg IV q24h as maintenance therapy for CMV; 40 mg/kg IV q8h for acyclovir-resistant HSV and VZV) is used to treat CMV retinitis in patients with AIDS. It is typically considered for use in patients who are not tolerating or not responding to ganciclovir.
- ○ Foscarnet is used for CMV disease in bone marrow transplant patients to avoid the bone marrow–suppressive effects of ganciclovir. It is also used for treatment of acyclovir-resistant HSV/VZV infections and ganciclovir-resistant CMV infections.
- ○ **Adverse events.** Risk for nephrotoxicity is a major concern. CrCl should be determined at baseline, and electrolytes (PO_4, Ca^{2+}, Mg^{2+}, and K^+) and serum creatinine should be checked at least twice a week. Normal saline (500–1000 mL) should be given before and during infusions to minimize nephrotoxicity. Foscarnet should be avoided in patients with a serum creatinine of >2.8 mg/dL or baseline CrCl of <50 mL/min. Concomitant use of other nephrotoxins (e.g., amphotericin, aminoglycosides, pentamidine, NSAIDs, cisplatin, or cidofovir) should also be avoided. Foscarnet chelates divalent cations and can cause tetany even with normal serum calcium levels. Use of foscarnet with pentamidine can cause severe hypocalcemia. Other side effects include seizures, phlebitis, rash, and genital ulcers. **Prolonged therapy with foscarnet should be monitored by physicians who are experienced with administration of home IV therapy and can systematically monitor patients' laboratory results.**
- **Cidofovir** (5 mg/kg IV qwk for 2 weeks as induction therapy, followed by 5 mg/kg IV q14d chronically as maintenance therapy) is used primarily to treat CMV retinitis in patients with AIDS. It can be administered through a peripheral IV line.
- ○ **Adverse events.** The most common adverse event is nephrotoxicity. It should be avoided in patients with a CrCl of <55 mL/min, a serum creatinine >1.5 mg/dL, significant proteinuria, or a recent history of receipt of other nephrotoxic medications.
- ○ **Each cidofovir dose should be administered with probenecid** (2 g PO 3 hours before the infusion and then 1 g at 2 and 8 hours after the infusion) along with 1 L normal saline IV 1–2 hours before the infusion to minimize nephrotoxicity. Patients should have a serum creatinine and urine protein check before each dose of cidofovir is given. These patients should be followed by a physician regularly, because administration of this drug requires systematic monitoring of laboratory studies.

ANTIFUNGAL AGENTS

Amphotericin B

GENERAL PRINCIPLES

- **Amphotericin B** is fungicidal by interacting with ergosterol and disrupting the fungal cell membrane. Reformulation of this agent in various lipid vehicles has decreased some of its adverse side effects. Amphotericin B formulations are not effective for *Pseudallescheria boydii*, *Candida lusitaniae*, or *Aspergillus terreus* infections.
- **Amphotericin B deoxycholate** (0.3–1.5 mg/kg q24h as a single infusion over 2–6 hours) was once the mainstay of antifungal therapy but has now been supplanted by lipid-based formulations of the drug as a result of their improved tolerability.
- **Lipid complexed preparations** of amphotericin B, including liposomal amphotericin B (3–6 mg/kg IV q24h), amphotericin B lipid complex (5 mg/kg IV q24h), and amphotericin B colloidal dispersion (3–4 mg/kg IV q24h), have decreased nephrotoxicity and are generally associated with fewer infusion-related reactions than amphotericin B deoxycholate. Liposomal amphotericin B has the most FDA-approved uses and also appears to be the best tolerated lipid amphotericin B formulation.

SPECIAL CONSIDERATIONS

- The major **adverse event** of all amphotericin B formulations, including the lipid formulations, is **nephrotoxicity**. Patients should receive 500 mL of normal saline before and after each infusion to minimize nephrotoxicity. Irreversible renal failure appears to be related to cumulative doses. Therefore, concomitant administration of other known nephrotoxins should be avoided if possible.
- Common **infusion-related effects** include fever/chills, nausea, headache, and myalgias. Premedication with 500–1000 mg of acetaminophen and 50 mg of diphenhydramine may control many of these symptoms. More severe reactions may be prevented by premedication with hydrocortisone 25–50 mg IV. Intolerable infusion-related chills can be managed with meperidine 25–50 mg IV.
- Amphotericin B therapy is associated with **potassium and magnesium wasting** that generally requires supplementation. Serum creatinine and electrolytes (including Mg^{2+} and K^+) should be monitored at least two to three times a week.

Azoles

GENERAL PRINCIPLES

Azoles are fungistatic agents that inhibit ergosterol synthesis.

- **Fluconazole** (100–800 mg PO/IV q24h) is the drug of choice for many localized candidal infections, such as UTIs, thrush, vaginal candidiasis (150-mg single dose), esophagitis, peritonitis, and hepatosplenic infection. It is also a viable agent for severe disseminated candidal infections (e.g., candidemia) and the treatment of choice for consolidation therapy of cryptococcal meningitis following an initial 14-day course of an amphotericin B product, or as a second-line agent for primary treatment of cryptococcal meningitis (400–800 mg PO q24h for 8 weeks, followed by 200 mg PO q24h thereafter for chronic maintenance treatment).
  - Fluconazole does not have activity against *Aspergillus* spp. or *Candida krusei* and, therefore, should not be used for treatment of those infections. *Candida glabrata* may also be resistant to fluconazole. Its absorption is not dependent on gastric acid.

- **Itraconazole** (200–400 mg PO q24h) is a triazole with broad-spectrum antifungal activity.
  - It is commonly used to treat the endemic mycoses like coccidioidomycosis, histoplasmosis, blastomycosis, and sporotrichosis.
  - It is an alternative therapy for *Aspergillus* and can also be used to treat infections caused by dermatophytes, including onychomycosis of the toenails (200 mg PO q24h for 12 weeks) and fingernails (200 mg PO q12h for 1 week, with a 3-week interruption, and then a second course of 200 mg PO q12h for 1 week).
  - The capsules require adequate gastric acidity for absorption and, therefore, should be taken with food or carbonated beverage, whereas the liquid formulation is not significantly affected by gastric acidity and is better absorbed on an empty stomach. As a result, the liquid formulation is preferred for most patients.
- **Posaconazole** (delayed-release tablet and IV doses are 300 mg PO/IV q12h on day 1, followed by 300 mg PO/IV q24h; oral suspension dose is 200 mg PO q8h for prophylaxis and 100–400 mg PO q12–24h for oropharyngeal candidiasis treatment) is an oral azole agent that is FDA approved for prophylaxis of invasive aspergillosis and candidiasis in hematopoietic stem cell transplant patients with graft-versus-host disease or in patients with hematologic malignancies experiencing prolonged neutropenia from chemotherapy as well as treatment of oropharyngeal candidiasis. This drug has also shown some benefit for treatment of mucormycosis, although it is not approved by the FDA for this use.
  - Each suspension dose should be administered with a full meal, liquid supplement, or acidic carbonated beverage (e.g., ginger ale). Acid-suppressive therapy may significantly reduce absorption of the oral suspension, but not the delayed-release tablets.
  - Rifabutin, phenytoin, and cimetidine significantly reduce posaconazole concentrations and should not routinely be used concomitantly.
  - Posaconazole significantly increases bioavailability of cyclosporine, tacrolimus, and midazolam, necessitating dosage reductions of these agents when used with posaconazole. Dosage reduction of vinca alkaloids, statins, and calcium channel blockers should also be considered.
  - Terfenadine, astemizole, pimozide, cisapride, quinidine, and ergot alkaloids are contraindicated with posaconazole.
- **Voriconazole** (loading dose of 6 mg/kg IV [two doses 12 hours apart], followed by a maintenance dose of 4 mg/kg IV q12h or 200 mg PO q12h [100 mg PO q12h if <40 kg]) is a triazole antifungal with a spectrum of activity against a wide range of pathogenic fungi. It has enhanced in vitro activity against all clinically important species of *Aspergillus*, as well as *Candida* (including most nonalbicans), *Scedosporium apiospermum*, and *Fusarium* spp.
  - It is the treatment of choice for most forms of invasive aspergillosis, for which it demonstrates typical response rates of 40–50% and superiority over conventional amphotericin B. It is also effective in treating candidemia, esophageal candidiasis, and *Scedosporium* and *Fusarium* infections.
  - An advantage of voriconazole is the easy transition from IV to PO therapy because of excellent bioavailability. For refractory fungal infections, a dose increase of 50% may be useful. The maintenance dose is reduced by 50% for patients with moderate hepatic failure.
  - Because of its metabolism through the **cytochrome P450 system** (enzymes 2C19, 2C9, and 3A4), there are several **clinically significant drug interactions** that must be considered. Rifampin, rifabutin, carbamazepine (markedly reduced voriconazole levels), sirolimus (increased drug concentrations), and astemizole (prolonged QT_c) are contraindicated with voriconazole. Concomitantly administered cyclosporine, tacrolimus, and warfarin require more careful monitoring.
- **Isavuconazonium sulfate, the prodrug of isavuconazole** (372 mg isavuconazonium sulfate [equivalent to 200 mg isavuconazole] PO/IV q8h for 48 hours, then 372 mg

isavuconazonium sulfate [equivalent to 200 mg isavuconazole] PO/IV q24h), is an azole with broad-spectrum antifungal activity that is FDA approved for treatment of invasive aspergillosis and invasive mucormycosis.
- The oral formulation has a 98% oral bioavailability that is unaffected by food.
- The IV formulation does not contain a cyclodextrin-based solubilizing vehicle and can be safely used in patients with CrCl $\leq$50 mL/min.
- It is not associated with QT_c prolongation, but rather a minor QT_c shortening.
- Rifampin, carbamazepine, long-acting barbiturates, and St. John's wort significantly reduce isavuconazole concentrations and are contraindicated with isavuconazole.
- High-dose ritonavir and ketoconazole can significantly increase isavuconazole concentrations and are contraindicated with isavuconazole.

SPECIAL CONSIDERATIONS

Nausea, diarrhea, and rash are mild side effects of the azoles. Hepatitis is a rare but serious complication. Therapy must be monitored closely in the setting of compromised liver function, and LFTs should be monitored regularly with chronic use. These agents may also cause prolongation of the QT_c interval. Itraconazole levels should be checked after 1 week of therapy to confirm absorption. Serum level monitoring is also advisable with use of oral formulations of posaconazole and voriconazole. The IV formulations of voriconazole and posaconazole should not be used routinely in patients with a CrCl of <50 mL/min because of the potential for accumulation and toxicity from the cyclodextrin vehicle. Transient visual disturbance is a common adverse effect (30%) of voriconazole. **This class of antibiotics has major drug interactions.**

Echinocandins

This class of antifungals inhibits the enzyme $(1,3)$-β-D-glucan synthase that is essential in fungal cell wall synthesis.
- **Caspofungin acetate** (70 mg IV loading dose, followed by 50 mg IV q24h) has fungicidal activity against most *Aspergillus* and *Candida* spp., including azole-resistant *Candida* strains. However, *Candida guilliermondii* and *Candida parapsilosis* may be less susceptible. Caspofungin does not have appreciable activity against *Cryptococcus, Histoplasma, Blastomyces, Coccidioides,* or *Mucor* spp. It is FDA approved for treatment of candidemia and refractory invasive aspergillosis and as empiric therapy in febrile neutropenia.
  - Metabolism is primarily hepatic, although the cytochrome P450 system is not significantly involved. An increased maintenance dosage is necessary with the use of drugs that induce hepatic metabolism (e.g., efavirenz, nelfinavir, phenytoin, rifampin, carbamazepine, dexamethasone). The maintenance dose should be reduced to 35 mg for patients with moderate hepatic impairment; however, no dose adjustment is necessary for renal failure.
  - In vitro and limited clinical data suggest a synergistic effect when caspofungin is given in conjunction with itraconazole, voriconazole, or amphotericin B for *Aspergillus* infections.
  - **Adverse events:** Fever, rash, nausea, and phlebitis at the injection site are infrequent.
- **Micafungin sodium** is used for candidemia (100 mg IV q24h), esophageal candidiasis (150 mg IV q24h), and as fungal prophylaxis for patients undergoing hematopoietic stem cell transplantation (50 mg IV q24h). The spectrum of activity is similar to that of anidulafungin and caspofungin. Although micafungin increases serum concentrations of sirolimus and nifedipine, these increases may not be clinically significant. Micafungin may increase cyclosporine concentrations in about 20% of patients. No change in dosing is necessary in renal or hepatic dysfunction.
  Adverse events include elevated LFTs and rare cases of rash and delirium.

• **Anidulafungin** (200 mg IV loading dose, followed by 100 mg IV q24h) is useful for treatment of candidemia and other systemic *Candida* infections (intra-abdominal abscess and peritonitis) as well as esophageal candidiasis (100-mg loading dose, followed by 50 mg daily). The spectrum of activity is similar to that of caspofungin and micafungin. Anidulafungin is not a substrate inhibitor or inducer of cytochrome P450 isoenzymes and does not have clinically relevant drug interactions. No dosage change is necessary in renal or hepatic insufficiency.

    Adverse events include possible histamine-mediated reactions, elevations in LFTs, and, rarely, hypokalemia.

Miscellaneous

• **Flucytosine** (25 mg/kg PO q6h) exerts its fungicidal effects on susceptible *Candida* and *Cryptococcus* spp. by interfering with DNA synthesis.
    ○ Main clinical uses are in the treatment of cryptococcal meningitis and severe *Candida* infections in combination with amphotericin B. This agent should not be used alone due to risk for rapid emergence of resistance.
    ○ **Adverse events** include dose-related bone marrow suppression and bloody diarrhea due to intestinal flora conversion of flucytosine to 5-fluorouracil.
    ○ Peak drug concentrations should be kept between 50–100 μg/mL. Close monitoring of serum concentrations and dose adjustments are critical in the setting of renal insufficiency. LFTs should be obtained at least once a week.
• **Terbinafine** (250 mg PO q24h for 6–12 weeks) is an allylamine antifungal agent that kills fungi by inhibiting ergosterol synthesis. It is FDA approved for the treatment of onychomycosis of the fingernails (6 weeks of treatment) or toenails (12 weeks of treatment). It is not generally used for systemic infections.

    Adverse events include headache, GI disturbances, rash, LFT abnormalities, and taste disturbances. This drug should not be used in patients with hepatic cirrhosis or a CrCl of <50 mL/min because of inadequate data. It has only moderate affinity for cytochrome P450 hepatic enzymes and does not significantly inhibit the metabolism of cyclosporine (15% decrease) or warfarin.

16 Sexually Transmitted Infections, Human Immunodeficiency Virus, and Acquired Immunodeficiency Syndrome

Caline Mattar, Rachel Presti, and Hilary E. L. Reno

SEXUALLY TRANSMITTED INFECTIONS, ULCERATIVE DISEASES

- Current sexually transmitted infection (STI) treatment guidelines are found at *www.cdc .gov/std/*.
- Treatment options for each infection can be found in Table 16-1.

Genital Herpes

GENERAL PRINCIPLES

Genital herpes is caused by **herpes simplex virus (HSV)**, types 1 and 2, usually type 2. The proportion of herpes caused by HSV-1 continues to increase.

DIAGNOSIS

- Infection is characterized by painful grouped vesicles in the genital and perianal regions that rapidly ulcerate and form shallow tender lesions.
- The initial episode may be associated with inguinal adenopathy, fever, headache, myalgias, and aseptic meningitis; recurrences are usually less severe. Asymptomatic shedding of virus is frequent and leads to transmission.
- Confirmation of HSV infection requires culture or polymerase chain reaction (PCR); however, clinical presentation is often adequate for diagnosis.

Syphilis

GENERAL PRINCIPLES

- Syphilis is caused by the spirochete *Treponema pallidum*.
- There is a high degree of HIV co-infection in patients with syphilis, from 40–70%, and HIV infection should be excluded with appropriate testing (*JAMA 2003;290(11):1510*).
- Syphilis can have an atypical course in HIV-infected patients; treatment failures and progression to neurosyphilis are more frequent in this population.

503

TABLE 16-1   Treatment of Sexually Transmitted Infections

Infection	Recommended Regimen(s)	Alternative Regimens and Notes
Genital ulcer disease		
Herpes simplex		
First episode	• Acyclovir 400 mg PO three times a day × 7–10 d or 200 mg PO five times daily × 7–10 d • Valacyclovir 1 g PO two times a day × 7–10 d • Famciclovir 250 mg PO three times a day × 7–10 d	
Recurrent episodes	• Acyclovir 400 mg PO three times a day × 5 d or 800 mg two times a day × 5 d or 800 mg PO three times a day × 2 d • Valacyclovir 1 g PO once a day × 5 d or 500 mg PO two times a day × 3 d • Famciclovir 1 g PO two times a day × 1 d or 125 mg PO two times a day × 5 d or 500 mg once, then 250 mg two times a day × 2 d	In patients with HIV: • Acyclovir 400 mg PO three times a day × 5–10 d • Valacyclovir 1 g PO twice a day × 5–10 d • Famciclovir 500 mg PO twice a day × 5–10 d
Suppressive therapy	• Acyclovir 400 mg PO twice a day • Valacyclovir 500 mg or 1 g PO once daily • Famciclovir 250 mg PO twice daily	In patients with HIV: • Acyclovir 400–800 mg PO twice to three times a day • Valacyclovir 500 mg PO twice a day • Famciclovir 500 mg PO twice a day
Syphilis		
Primary, secondary, or early latent <1 yr	• Benzathine penicillin G 2.4 million units IM single dose	Penicillin-allergic: • Doxycycline 100 mg PO twice daily × 14 d • Tetracycline 500 mg PO four times daily × 14 d
Latent >1 yr, latent unknown duration	• Benzathine penicillin G 2.4 million units IM once weekly × 3 doses	• Doxycycline 100 mg PO twice daily × 28 d • Tetracycline 500 mg PO four times daily × 28 d

(continued)

TABLE 16-1	Treatment of Sexually Transmitted Infections *(Continued)*	
Infection	**Recommended Regimen(s)**	**Alternative Regimens and Notes**
Neurosyphilis	• Aqueous crystalline penicillin G 18–24 million U/d × 10–14 d	• Procaine penicillin 2.4 million units IM once daily + probenecid 500 mg PO four times daily × 10–14 d
Pregnancy	• Penicillin is the recommended treatment—desensitize if necessary	
Chancroid	• Azithromycin 1 g PO single dose • Ceftriaxone 250 mg IM single dose	• Ciprofloxacin 500 mg PO twice daily × 3 d • Erythromycin base 500 mg PO twice daily × 7 d • Some resistance has been reported for these regimens.
Lymphogranuloma venereum	• Doxycycline 100 mg PO twice daily × 21 d	• Erythromycin 500 mg PO four times a day × 21 d
Urethritis/cervicitis		
Gonorrhea	• Ceftriaxone 250 mg IM once + azithromycin 1 g PO once even if testing for *Chlamydia trachomatis* is negative • Given concern for antibiotic resistance, dual treatment is recommended.	• Cefotaxime 500 mg IM × 1 or cefoxitin 2 g IM + probenecid 1 g PO × 1 • Oral cephalosporin treatment is not recommended as long as ceftriaxone is available.
Disseminated gonococcal infection	• Ceftriaxone 1 g IV daily or cefotaxime 1 g IV every 8 h × 7 d	
Chlamydia	• Azithromycin 1 g PO single dose • Doxycycline 100 mg PO twice daily × 7 d	• Erythromycin base 500 mg PO four times a day × 7 d • Retesting is recommended in 3 months.
Pelvic inflammatory disease		
Outpatient	• Ceftriaxone 250 mg IM once + doxycycline 100 mg PO twice daily × 14 d + consider metronidazole 500 mg orally twice daily × 14 d	• Cefoxitin 2 g IM + probenecid 1 g PO once can be substituted for ceftriaxone

(continued)

TABLE 16-1	Treatment of Sexually Transmitted Infections *(Continued)*

Infection	Recommended Regimen(s)	Alternative Regimens and Notes
Inpatient	• (Cefoxitin 2 g IV every 6 h or cefotetan 2 g IV every 12 h) + doxycycline 100 mg PO twice daily × 14 d + consider metronidazole 500 mg PO twice daily × 14 d	• Clindamycin 900 mg IV every 8 h + gentamicin 2 mg/kg loading dose, then 1.5 mg/kg every 8 h + doxycycline 100 mg PO twice daily × 14 d • Ampicillin-sulbactam 3 g IV every 6 h + doxycycline 100 mg PO twice daily × 14 d
Vaginitis/vaginosis		
Trichomonas	• Metronidazole 2 g PO single dose • Tinidazole 2 g PO single dose	Metronidazole 500 mg PO twice daily × 7 d
Pregnancy	• Metronidazole 2 g PO × 1 (not teratogenic)	
Bacterial vaginosis	• Metronidazole 500 mg PO twice daily × 7 d • Clindamycin cream 2% intravaginal at bedtime × 7 d • Metronidazole gel 0.75% intravaginal once a day for 5 d	• Tinidazole 2 g PO once daily × 2 d or 1 g PO once daily × 5 d • Clindamycin 300 mg PO twice daily × 7 d • Clindamycin ovules 100 mg intravaginal × 3 d
Candidiasis	• Intravaginal azoles in variety of strengths for 1–7 d • Fluconazole 150 mg PO × 1	
Severe candidiasis	• Fluconazole 150 mg PO every 72 h × 2–3 doses	• Intravaginal azoles for 7–14 d • Culture and sensitivities maybe helpful
Recurrent candidiasis	• Fluconazole 100, 150, or 200 mg PO once weekly × 6 mo	

See *cdc.gov/std/* for the current sexually transmitted infection treatment guidelines.

DIAGNOSIS

Clinical Presentation

• **Primary syphilis** develops within several weeks of exposure and manifests as one or more painless, indurated, superficial ulcerations (chancre).
• **Secondary syphilis** develops 2–10 weeks after the chancre resolves and may produce a rash, mucocutaneous lesions, adenopathy, and constitutional symptoms.

- **Tertiary syphilis** follows between 1–20 years after infection and includes cardiovascular, gummatous, and neurologic disease (general paresis, tabes dorsalis, or meningovascular syphilis).

Diagnostic Testing

- In **primary syphilis**, dark-field microscopy of lesion exudates, when available, may reveal spirochetes. A nontreponemal serologic test (e.g., rapid plasma reagin [RPR] or Venereal Disease Research Laboratory [VDRL]) should be confirmed with a treponemal-specific test (e.g., fluorescent treponemal antibody absorption or *T. pallidum* particle agglutination).
- Diagnosis of **secondary syphilis** is made on the basis of positive serologic studies and the presence of a compatible clinical illness.
- **Latent syphilis** is a serologic diagnosis in the absence of symptoms—early latent syphilis is serologically positive for <1 year, and late latent syphilis is serologically positive for >1 year.
- To exclude **neurosyphilis**, a lumbar puncture should be performed in all patients with neurologic, ophthalmic, or auditory signs or symptoms. Additionally, some experts recommend lumbar puncture in HIV-infected patients with evidence of tertiary disease, treatment failure, or late latent syphilis (*Clin Infect Dis 2007;44:1222*). VDRL should be performed on cerebrospinal fluid (CSF).
- Response to treatment should be monitored with nontreponemal serologic tests at 3, 6, and 12 months after treatment. In patients with HIV, tests should be checked every 3 months after treatment for 1 year.

Chancroid

GENERAL PRINCIPLES

Chancroid is caused by *Haemophilus ducreyi*.

DIAGNOSIS

- Chancroid produces a painful genital ulcer and tender suppurative inguinal lymphadenopathy.
- Identification of the organism is difficult and requires special culture media.

Lymphogranuloma Venereum

GENERAL PRINCIPLES

Lymphogranuloma venereum (LGV) is caused by *Chlamydia trachomatis* (serovars L_1, L_2, or L_3).

DIAGNOSIS

- Manifests as a painless genital ulcer, followed by heaped up, matted inguinal lymphadenopathy. Proctocolitis with pain and discharge can occur with anal infection (*Clin Infect Dis 2007;44:26*).
- Diagnosis is based on clinical suspicion and *C. trachomatis* nucleic acid and antibody testing, if available.

SEXUALLY TRANSMITTED INFECTIONS, VAGINITIS, AND VAGINOSIS

Trichomoniasis

DIAGNOSIS

Clinical Presentation

- Clinical symptoms of infection by *Trichomonas vaginalis* include malodorous purulent vaginal discharge, dysuria, and genital inflammation.
- Examination reveals profuse frothy discharge and cervical petechiae.
- *T. vaginalis* is often asymptomatic, especially in males.

Diagnostic Testing

- Nucleic acid amplification tests (NAATs) and antigen detection tests are available to detect *T. vaginalis* and offer improved sensitivity over the traditional visualization of motile trichomonads on a saline wet mount of vaginal discharge.
- Elevated vaginal pH (≥4.5) may be seen.

Bacterial Vaginosis

GENERAL PRINCIPLES

The replacement of normal lactobacilli with anaerobic bacteria in the vagina leads to bacterial vaginosis.

DIAGNOSIS

Three of the following criteria are needed to make the diagnosis:
- Homogenous, thin, white discharge
- Presence of clue cells on microscopic examination
- Elevated vaginal pH (≥4.5)
- Fishy odor associated with vaginal discharge before or after addition of 10% potassium hydroxide (KOH) (whiff test)

Vulvovaginal Candidiasis

GENERAL PRINCIPLES

Vulvovaginal candidiasis is not generally considered an STI but commonly develops in the setting of oral contraceptive use or antibiotic therapy. Recurrent infections may be a presenting manifestation of unrecognized HIV infection.

DIAGNOSIS

- Thick, cottage cheese–like vaginal discharge in conjunction with intense vulvar inflammation, pruritus, and dysuria is often present.
- Definitive diagnosis requires visualization of fungal elements on a KOH preparation of the vaginal discharge.

TREATMENT

- Therapy is often initiated on the basis of the clinical presentation.
- Fluconazole failure may indicate the presence of a **non–*Candida albicans* species**.

Cervicitis/Urethritis

GENERAL PRINCIPLES

Cervicitis and urethritis are frequent presentations of infection with *Neisseria gonorrhoeae* or *C. trachomatis*, and occasionally *Mycoplasma genitalium*, *Ureaplasma urealyticum*, and *T. vaginalis*. These infections often coexist, and clinical presentations can be identical.

DIAGNOSIS

Clinical Presentation

- Women with urethritis, cervicitis, or both complain of mucopurulent vaginal discharge, dyspareunia, and dysuria.
- Men with urethritis may have dysuria and purulent penile discharge.
- Most infections with these STIs are asymptomatic.
- Disseminated gonococcal infection (DGI) can present with fever, tenosynovitis, vesicopustular skin lesions, and polyarthralgias. DGI may also manifest solely as septic arthritis of the knee, wrist, or ankle (see Chapter 25, Arthritis and Rheumatologic Diseases).

Diagnostic Testing

- A positive NAAT performed on endocervical, vaginal, urethral (men), urine, or extragenital samples is recommended to make the diagnosis of *C. trachomatis* or *N. gonorrhoeae* infection. In the case of *N. gonorrhoeae*, a Gram stain of endocervical or urethral discharge with gram-negative intracellular diplococci can rapidly establish the diagnosis. Culture can be performed on urethral or endocervical swab specimens.
- Recommendations for testing include NAAT testing at extragenital sites of sexual contact (pharynx, rectum), especially in men who have sex with men (MSM).
- In addition to NAAT studies, patients with suspected DGI should have blood cultures drawn. In the setting of septic arthritis, synovial fluid analysis and culture is indicated.

TREATMENT

Because of increasing resistance concerns, treatment options for *N. gonorrhoeae* infection are reduced (see Table 16-1).

Pelvic Inflammatory Disease

GENERAL PRINCIPLES

Pelvic inflammatory disease (PID) is an upper genital tract infection in women, usually preceded by cervicitis. Long-term consequences of untreated PID include chronic pain, increased risk of ectopic pregnancy, and infertility.

DIAGNOSIS

Clinical Presentation

Symptoms can range from mild pelvic discomfort and dyspareunia to severe abdominal pain with fever, which may signal complicating perihepatitis (Fitz-Hugh-Curtis syndrome) or tubo-ovarian abscess.

Diagnostic Testing

- Cervical motion tenderness or uterine or adnexal tenderness, vaginal discharge or friability, and the presence of many white blood cells per low-power field on a saline preparation of vaginal or endocervical fluid are consistent with a diagnosis of PID.
- NAATs or culture of endocervical specimens should be obtained to identify *C. trachomatis* or *N. gonorrhoeae* infection.
- All women diagnosed with PID should be screened for HIV infection.

TREATMENT

Severely ill, pregnant, and HIV-infected women with PID should be hospitalized. Patients unable to tolerate oral antibiotics also warrant admission.

HIV TYPE 1

GENERAL PRINCIPLES

Definition

HIV type 1 is a retrovirus that predominantly infects lymphocytes that bear the CD4 surface protein, as well as coreceptors belonging to the chemokine receptor family (CCR5 or CXCR4), and causes AIDS.

Classification

Diagnosis of AIDS by the Centers for Disease Control and Prevention (CDC) classification is made on the basis of CD4 cell count <200 cells/μL, CD4 percentage <14%, or development of one of the 25 AIDS-defining conditions (*MMWR Recomm Rep 1992;41 (RR-17):1*).

Epidemiology

- HIV type 1 is common throughout the world. By the most recent estimates, over 34 million people worldwide are living with HIV or AIDS, with a significant burden of disease in sub-Saharan Africa (*http://www.who.int/hiv/data/en/index.html*).
- In the United States, 1.3 million people are estimated to be infected with HIV with one-fifth of these people unaware of their infection. The CDC estimates that as many as 70% of the 50,000 new annual infections in the United States are transmitted by persons who are unaware of their HIV status.
- Despite comprising only 14% of the population in the United States, African Americans account for nearly 44% of all new cases of HIV in this country. Hispanics are also disproportionately affected by HIV. Women comprise approximately 24% of the US epidemic (*http://www.cdc.gov/hiv/topics/women*).
- MSM remain the population most heavily affected by HIV in the United States. Of all new HIV infections in 2009, 61% were MSM (*http://www.cdc.gov/nchhstp/newsroom/docs/ HIV-Infections-2006-2009.pdf*).
- **HIV type 2** is endemic to regions in West Africa. It is characterized by much slower progression to AIDS and resistance to nonnucleoside reverse transcriptase inhibitors (NNRTIs).

Pathophysiology

- After entering the host cell, viral RNA is reverse transcribed into DNA using the HIV **reverse transcriptase**. This viral DNA is inserted into the host genome through the activity of the viral **integrase**. The host cell machinery is then used to produce the relevant viral proteins, which are appropriately truncated by a viral **protease**. Infectious viral particles bud away to infect other CD4 lymphocytes.
- Most infected cells are killed by the host CD8 T-cell response.
- Long-lived latently infected cells persist, especially memory T cells.
- Infection usually leads to CD4 T-cell depletion and **impaired cell-mediated immunity** over a period of 8–10 years.
- Without treatment, >90% of infected patients will progress to AIDS, which is characterized by the development of opportunistic infections (OIs), wasting, and viral-associated malignancies.

Risk Factors

- The virus is primarily transmitted sexually but also via parenteral and perinatal exposure.
- The highest risk of transmission is through blood transfusions (9250 per 10,000 exposures). Sharing needles or needlestick injuries result in transmission in 50 per 10,000 exposures.
- Among sexual practices, unprotected anal receptive intercourse carries the highest risk of transmission (138 per 10,000 exposures), followed by insertive anal intercourse, vaginal receptive intercourse, and vaginal insertive intercourse. Oral intercourse carries a lower risk of transmission.

Prevention

- HIV transmission can be prevented by safe sex practices, which include condom use (male or female) for vaginal, oral, and anal intercourse, decreasing the number of sexual partners, and avoiding needle sharing.
- Postexposure prophylaxis (PEP), or the provision of antiretroviral therapy (ART) after needlestick injury or high-risk sexual exposure, can prevent infection.
- Preexposure prophylaxis (PrEP), or continuous ART in HIV-negative patients, has proven to decrease the rate of HIV transmission. The current guidelines recommend the use of PrEP for the following high-risk groups (*http://www.cdc.gov/hiv/pdf/guidelines/ PrEPguidelines2014.pdf*):
  - MSM
  - Heterosexual HIV-discordant couples
  - Those with multiple sexual partners with inconsistent condom use
  - Commercial sex workers
  - IV drug users
- A combination of emtricitabine-tenofovir is the approved regimen for PrEP. Prior to starting PrEP, it is essential to document a negative HIV test, no signs or symptoms of acute HIV infection, hepatitis B status, and normal renal function. These patients should be followed every 3 months for repeat HIV testing as well as STI screening, risk reduction counseling, and monitoring of renal and hepatic function.

DIAGNOSIS

Clinical Presentation

- Acute retroviral syndrome is experienced by up to 75% of patients and is similar to other acute viral illnesses such as infectious mononucleosis due to Epstein-Barr virus (EBV) or cytomegalovirus (CMV) infection. Common presenting symptoms of acute retroviral syndrome are fever, sore throat, nonspecific rash, myalgias, headache, and fatigue.

- As the acute illness resolves spontaneously, many people present to care only after OIs (see later section for clinical presentations) occur late in infection once significant immune compromise has occurred (CD4 count <200 cells/μL). Late presentation can be avoided by routine screening.

History

Initial evaluation of persons with a confirmed HIV infection should include the following measures:
- Complete history with emphasis on previous OIs, viral co-infections, and other complications.
- Psychological and psychiatric history. Depression and substance use are common and should be identified and treated as necessary.
- Family and social support assessment.
- Assessment of knowledge and perceptions regarding HIV is also crucial to initiate ongoing education regarding the nature and ramifications of HIV infection.

Physical Examination

A complete physical exam is important to evaluate for manifestations of immune compromise. Initial findings may include the following:
- Oral findings: thrush (oral candidiasis), hairy leukoplakia, aphthous ulcers
- Lymphatic system: generalized lymphadenopathy
- Skin: psoriasis, eosinophilic folliculitis, Kaposi sarcoma, molluscum contagiosum, *Cryptococcus*
- Abdominal exam: evidence of hepatosplenomegaly
- Genital exam: presence of ulcers, genital warts, vaginal discharge, and rectal discharge
- Neurologic exam: note presence of sensory deficits and cognitive testing

Diagnostic Criteria

- The updated CDC guidelines for screening published in June of 2014 recommend the use of the fourth-generation assay, an antigen/antibody test that involves the detection of the p24 antigen as well as antibodies to HIV-1 and HIV-2. The p24 antigen is a viral capsid protein that can be detected as early as 4–10 days from acute infection, up to 2 weeks earlier than the antibody tests alone. An eclipse phase of infection, during which no testing is positive, still exists for up to 7 days after exposure.
- If the fourth-generation assay is positive, then a differentiation test for HIV-1 and HIV-2 antibodies is performed.
- If the HIV-1 and HIV-2 antibody differentiation test is negative for both HIV-1 and HIV-2, then nucleic acid testing (NAT) of HIV-1 RNA via PCR should be performed (Figure 16-1). If the NAT is positive, this indicates acute infection. Viral loads during acute infection are typically in the range of several million copies per milliliter, so a viral load <1000 should be repeated to confirm infection.

Diagnostic Testing

The CDC recommends that **all persons age 13–64 years be offered HIV testing in all health care settings using an opt-out format** (*MMWR Recomm Rep 2006;55:1–17*).
- These recommendations are based on the following considerations: significant individual health benefits if highly active ART (HAART) is initiated earlier in the course of illness, significant public health benefits with knowledge of HIV status leading to changes in risk behaviors, and the availability of inexpensive, reliable, and rapid testing technology.
- **Persons at high risk should be screened for HIV infection at least annually. High-risk groups include** IV drug users, MSM, sexual partners of a known HIV patient, persons involved in sex trading and their sexual partners, persons with STIs, persons who have multiple sexual partners or who engage in unprotected intercourse,

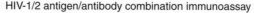

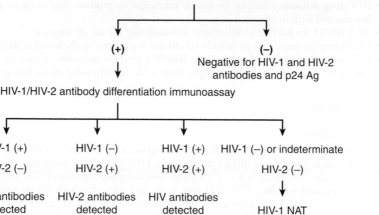

Figure 16-1. Recommended laboratory HIV testing algorithm for serum or plasma specimens. (From Centers for Disease Control and Prevention. National HIV Testing Day and new testing recommendations. *MMWR Morb Mortal Wkly Rep* 2014;63(25):537. Available at: http://www.cdc.gov/hiv/pdf/testingHIValgorithmQuickRef.pdf.)

persons who consider themselves at risk, and persons with findings that are suggestive of HIV infection.
- Other groups for whom HIV testing is indicated
  ○ Pregnant women (opt-out screening)
  ○ Patients with active TB
  ○ Donors of blood, semen, and organs
  ○ Persons with occupational exposures (e.g., needlesticks) and source patients of the exposures

Laboratories
- **Complete blood cell** (CBC) count and **comprehensive metabolic panel** (CMP) with assessment of liver and kidney parameters, as well as **urinalysis** to evaluate for proteinuria and glycosuria.
- **CD4 cell count** (normal range, 600–1500 cells/μL) and CD4 percentage. Significant immune deficiency requiring prophylactic antibiotics occurs with CD4 <200 cells/μL.
- **Virologic markers:** Plasma HIV RNA predicts the rate of disease progression.
- **Fasting lipid panel.** HIV is associated with an increased risk of metabolic syndrome and cardiovascular disease. Lipids can be affected by several antiretrovirals.
- **TB testing by interferon-γ release assay.**
- **RPR test for syphilis screening, confirmed by fluorescent treponemal antibody assay.**
- *Toxoplasma* and hepatitis A, B (HBsAg, HBsAb, HBcAb), and C serologies.
- **Chlamydia/gonococcal urine/cervical probe** for all patients. If patients report receptive anal sex, **rectal probes for gonorrhea and *Chlamydia*** are recommended. For those reporting receptive oral sex, **pharyngeal sample for gonorrhea** should be obtained (*Clin Infect Dis 2009;49:651*). NAAT is preferred.

- **Cervical Papanicolaou smear** (most commonly using the thin prep method).
- **HIV drug resistance testing** for reverse transcriptase, protease, and integrase genes at baseline and with treatment failure.
- **HLA B5701** for patients in whom one is considering the use of abacavir.
- **CCR5** tropism testing for patients in whom one is considering the use of maraviroc.
- **Glucose-6-phosphate dehydrogenase (G6PD) level** on initiation of care or prior to starting therapy with an oxidant drug in those with a predisposing ethnic background.

TREATMENT

Immunizations

- From "Primary Care Guidelines for the Management of Persons Infected with Human Immunodeficiency Virus: 2013 Update by the HIV Medicine Association of the Infectious Diseases Society of America" (*http://www.idsociety.org/Organism/#HIV/AIDS*).
- **Pneumococcal vaccine:** HIV infection is an indication for both the pneumococcal conjugate (Prevnar) and polysaccharide (Pneumovax) vaccines. If naïve, the conjugate vaccine should be given initially, then the polysaccharide vaccine after 6 months. Some experts recommend deferring the vaccine until the CD4 cell counts are >200 cells/μL because responses are poor when vaccination occurs with low CD4 cell counts. A single booster Pneumovax after 5 years is recommended.
- **Hepatitis A and B virus (HAV and HBV):** Vaccination for HAV and HBV is recommended if seronegative. Antibody response to these vaccines is improved with undetectable HIV viral load and higher CD4 count.
- **Influenza:** Annual inactivated influenza vaccination is recommended for all HIV-infected patients regardless of CD4 cell count. Use of the intranasally administered, live, attenuated vaccine is not currently recommended for HIV-infected persons.
- **Varicella:** The live, attenuated varicella vaccine (chickenpox, Varivax) can be safely given to persons with CD4 cell counts >200 cells/mL but is contraindicated for persons with CD4 counts <200 cells/mL. There is currently no recommendation to give the zoster vaccine (Zostavax), although recently presented data demonstrated that it was safe and induces effective immune responses in HIV-infected adults with CD4 counts >200 cells/mL. The Advisory Committee on Immunization Practices (ACIP) is expected to revise recommendations based on these study findings.
- **Measles/mumps/rubella (MMR):** MMR is a vaccine that can be safely given to persons with CD4 cell counts >200 cells/μL but is contraindicated for persons with CD4 counts <200 cells/μL.
- **Tetanus/diphtheria/pertussis:** All adults should receive tetanus/diphtheria (Td) booster every 10 years with a one-time substitution with tetanus/diphtheria/acellular pertussis vaccine (Tdap).
- **Human papillomavirus (HPV) vaccine:** HPV-associated malignancies are common in HIV-infected patients. The three-dose vaccine series is safe and effective in HIV-positive subjects and is currently recommended for females age 11–26 years and males age 12–26 years.

Medications
ART

- **Current recommendations from the International AIDS Society-USA (IAS-USA)** (*http://www.iasusa.org/guidelines/*) for the initiation of ART are to treat everyone infected with HIV, although the strength of that recommendation varies with CD4 count and the presence of co-infections or symptoms.
- Treatment decisions should be individualized by patient readiness, drug interactions, adherence issues, drug toxicities, comorbidities, and the level of risk indicated by CD4 T-cell counts.

- Women, especially if pregnant, should receive optimal ART to reduce the risk of vertical transmission.
- Maximal and durable suppression of HIV replication is the goal of therapy once it is initiated. **HAART** should be individualized and closely monitored by measuring plasma HIV viral load. Reductions in plasma viremia correlate with increased CD4 cell counts and prolonged AIDS-free survival. Isolated viral "blips" are not indicative of virologic failure, but confirmed virologic rebound should trigger an evaluation of adherence, drug interactions, and viral resistance.
- Any change in ART increases future therapeutic constraints and potential drug resistance.
- **Antiretroviral drugs:** Approved antiretroviral drugs are grouped into five categories. Experts currently recommend using three active drugs from two different classes to maximally and durably suppress HIV viremia.
  - **Nucleotide and nucleoside reverse transcriptase inhibitors (NRTIs)** constrain HIV replication by incorporating into the elongating strand of DNA, causing chain termination. All nucleoside analogs have been associated with **lactic acidosis**, presumably related to mitochondrial toxicity, although current recommended NRTIs have low incidence.
  - **Non-nucleoside reverse transcriptase inhibitors (NNRTIs)** inhibit HIV by binding noncompetitively to the reverse transcriptase. A single dosage of nevirapine at the time of labor has been shown to decrease perinatal transmission of the virus. Side effects of NNRTIs include rash, hepatotoxicity, and Stevens-Johnson syndrome (more likely with nevirapine). Central nervous system (CNS) side effects are commonly experienced with the use of efavirenz.
  - **Integrase strand transfer inhibitors (INSTIs)** target DNA strand transfer and integration into a human genome. They tend to have better safety and tolerability profiles than other classes and are associated with a rapid decrease in viral load after initiation. Elvitegravir requires coadministration of the pharmacologic booster, cobicistat, which leads to increased incidence of gastrointestinal (GI) intolerance. Due to its interaction with the cytochrome P450 system, **cobicistat has important drug interactions** that should be evaluated. Few drug interactions exist with the other INSTIs, raltegravir and dolutegravir.
  - **Protease inhibitors (PIs)** block the action of the viral protease required for protein processing late in the viral cycle. GI intolerance is one of the most commonly encountered adverse effects. All PIs can produce increased bleeding in hemophiliacs. These agents have also been associated with metabolic abnormalities such as glucose intolerance, increased cholesterol and triglycerides, and body fat redistribution. Boosting with ritonavir is a common practice to achieve better therapeutic concentrations. Due to its metabolism via cytochrome P450, **boosted PIs have important drug interactions**, and concomitant medications should be reviewed carefully.
  - **HIV entry inhibitors** target different stages of the HIV entry process. Two drugs are available in this class. **Enfuvirtide (T-20)** is a fusion inhibitor that prevents the fusion of the virus into the host cell. T-20 is only available for use as an SC injection, 90 mg bid. The most frequent side effect for T-20 is a significant local site reaction after the injection. **Maraviroc** is a CCR5 receptor blocker. Initiation of CCR5 inhibitor requires baseline determination of HIV coreceptor tropism (CCR5 or CXCR4).
- **Initial therapy:** ART should be started in an outpatient setting by a physician with expertise in the management of HIV infection. Adherence is the key factor for success. Treatment should be individualized and adapted to the patient's lifestyle and comorbidities. Any treatment decision influences future therapeutic options because of the possibility of drug cross-resistance. **Potent initial ART generally consists of a combination of two NRTIs, usually plus an NNRTI, an INSTI, or a boosted PI. It should be noted that many of the first-line regimens are co-formulated as single-tablet daily regimens. Current first-line regimens are listed below:**
  - **Atripla:** co-formulated tenofovir disoproxil fumarate (TDF) with emtricitabine (FTC) and efavirenz (NNRTI-based regimen)

- ○ **Complera:** co-formulated TDF/FTC and rilpivirine (NNRTI-based regimen, recommended for those with initial viral loads <100,000 copies/mL)
- ○ **Stribild:** co-formulated TDF/FTC, elvitegravir, and cobicistat (INSTI based)
- ○ **Triumeq:** co-formulated abacavir, epivir, and dolutegravir (INSTI based)
- ○ **TDF/FTC with ritonavir-boosted atazanavir (PI based)**
- ○ **TDF/FTC with ritonavir-boosted darunavir (PI based)**
- **Treatment monitoring:** After starting or changing ART, the viral load should be checked at 4–6 weeks with an expected 10-fold reduction (1.0 $\log_{10}$) and suppression to <50 copies/mL by 24 weeks of therapy. The regimen should then be reassessed if response to treatment is inadequate. When the HIV RNA becomes undetectable and the patient is on a stable regimen, monitoring can be done every 3–6 months.
- **Treatment failure** is defined as less than a log (10-fold) reduction of the viral load 4–6 weeks after starting a new antiretroviral regimen; failure to reach an undetectable viral load after 6 months of treatment; detection of the virus after initial complete suppression of viral load, which suggests development of resistance; or persistent decline of CD4 cell count or clinical deterioration. Confirmed treatment failure should prompt changes in HAART based on results of genotype testing. In this situation, at least two of the drugs should be substituted with other drugs that have no expected cross-resistance. **HIV resistance testing** at this stage may help determine a salvage regimen in patients with prior ART. The importance of adherence should be stressed. Referral to an HIV specialist is highly recommended in this situation.
- **Drug interactions:** Antiretroviral medications, especially PIs, have multiple drug interactions. **PIs and cobicistat both inhibit and induce the P450 system**, and thus interactions are frequent with other inhibitors of the P450 system, including macrolides (erythromycin, clarithromycin) and antifungals (ketoconazole, itraconazole), as well as other inducers such as rifamycins (rifampin, rifabutin) and anticonvulsants (phenobarbital, phenytoin, carbamazepine). **Drugs with narrow therapeutic indices that should be avoided or used with extreme caution** include antihistamines (although loratadine is safe), antiarrhythmics (flecainide, encainide, quinidine), long-acting opiates (fentanyl, meperidine), long-acting benzodiazepines (midazolam, triazolam), warfarin, 3-hydroxy-3-methylglutaryl–coenzyme A (HMG-CoA) reductase inhibitors (pravastatin is the safest), and oral contraceptives. Sildenafil concentrations are increased, whereas methadone and theophylline concentrations are decreased with concomitant administration of certain PIs and NNRTIs.

COMPLICATIONS

Complications of ART: The long-term use of antiretrovirals has been associated with toxicity, the pathogenesis of which is only partially understood at this time.
- **Hyperlipidemia**, especially hypertriglyceridemia, is associated mainly with PIs (especially ritonavir). Improvement has been seen after treatment with atorvastatin, pravastatin, and/or gemfibrozil.
- **Peripheral insulin resistance, impaired glucose tolerance, and hyperglycemia** have been associated with the use of PI-based regimens, mainly indinavir and ritonavir. Lifestyle changes or changing ART can be considered in these cases.
- **Osteopenia and osteoporosis** are well described in HIV-infected individuals. The pathogenic mechanism of this problem is likely related to the inflammatory milieu of HIV itself, although the use of TDF may contribute.
- **Osteonecrosis**, particularly of the hip, has been increasingly associated with HIV disease.
- **Lipodystrophy syndrome** is an alteration in body fat distribution and can be stigmatizing to individuals. Changes consist of the accumulation of visceral fat in the abdomen, neck (buffalo hump), and pelvic areas, and/or the depletion of SC fat, causing facial or

peripheral wasting. Lipodystrophy has been associated in particular with older PIs and NRTIs and is uncommon with currently recommended regimens
- **Lactic acidosis** with liver steatosis is a rare but sometimes fatal complication associated with NRTIs. The mechanism appears to be part of mitochondrial toxicity. Higher rates of lactic acidosis have been reported with the use of the older drugs stavudine and didanosine.

SPECIAL POPULATIONS

Pregnancy
- Maximally suppressive ART during pregnancy is critical in preventing mother-to-child transmission.
- Current guidelines (*http://aidsinfo.nih.gov/guidelines/html/3/perinatal-guidelines/0*) recommend that all HIV-infected partners in a couple planning pregnancy should attain virologic suppression before attempting conception.
     Periconception PrEP for the HIV-uninfected partner may provide additional protection to reduce the risk of sexual transmission and should be discussed with the couple.
- If a pregnant woman is already suppressed on ART and is tolerating that regimen, she should be maintained on her current ART regardless of the agents (including efavirenz).
- ART-naïve pregnant women should be started on a combination regimen of TDF/FTC with boosted atazanavir, boosted lopinavir, or raltegravir. Nevirapine has been associated with hepatotoxicity and should be avoided in those with preexisting liver disease or high CD4 count.
- Intrapartum IV zidovudine should be given to women during labor, although it is not required for women with consistent undetectable viral loads in late pregnancy.
- Cesarean delivery should be scheduled for women with HIV viral loads >1000 in late pregnancy.
- ART should be continued after delivery, consistent with current guidelines to treat everyone to prevent disease progression and HIV transmission.
- Neonatal zidovudine prophylaxis should be given for 4 weeks if the mother has maintained virologic suppression. Neonatal prophylaxis using zidovudine and nevirapine should be offered if the mother did not receive antepartum suppressive ART.

Acute HIV Infection
ART given immediately after diagnosing acute infection may provide additional benefits.
- The initiation of early ART in acute infection will suppress the extraordinarily high viral loads seen at this time and reduce further transmission of HIV.
- Early ART may reduce the reservoir of latent virus.
- Early ART maintains immune function and may allow for immunologic control of HIV off ART in some settings.

Hepatitis
- High rates of coinfection with HBV and hepatitis C virus (HCV) occur in HIV-infected patients.
- Several HIV ART medications (tenofovir, emtricitabine, and lamivudine) also have activity against HBV. Any plan to treat HBV in co-infected patients should ensure that the regimen is fully active against both HIV and HBV. Discontinuation of ART that has been suppressing unrecognized HBV disease can result in reactivation of HBV with resultant acute, and sometimes fatal, HBV infection.
- HCV therapy is rapidly evolving, and a complete delineation of treatment is available in Chapter 19, Liver Diseases.
- Older interferon-based therapy had a minor effect on HIV viral load, with approximately one or two log-reductions in HIV while on therapy. It was not well tolerated and worked

poorly in HIV-infected patients, with most studies showing only 15% of patients with sustained virologic response.
- Newer directly acting HCV agents appear to be as effective in HIV-infected patients as in monoinfected HCV patients; however, there are significant drug–drug interactions that should be considered, particularly with PI-based therapy, efavirenz, and therapy using the boosting agent cobicistat.

Aging
- With the success of ART, HIV-related mortality is decreasing and HIV-infected persons are experiencing prolonged survival.
- The CDC estimates that, in 2015, one-half of all HIV-infected persons will be over the age of 50 years.
- HIV infection is associated with premature end-organ disease, and thus many of the comorbidities associated with aging may be exacerbated in this growing population, including cardiovascular disease, insulin resistance and diabetes, osteoporosis, neurocognitive impairment, and physical frailty.
- Certain non–AIDS-defining cancers are more common in HIV-infected patients, including anal cancer, lung cancer, and hepatocellular carcinoma. The extent to which this is due to HIV infection versus other risk factors like smoking and hepatitis co-infection is unclear.
- The role of long-term HIV infection and ART use in these comorbidities is poorly understood, although the use of NNRTI and PI drug classes is associated with lipid profiles that may exacerbate cardiovascular disease (*AIDS 2003;17:1179*). Higher rates of smoking and alcohol use also exacerbate these comorbidities.

REFERRAL

- All HIV positive patients should be referred to a HIV specialist, if possible.
- Counseling regarding contraception, safer sex practices, medication adherence, and proper health maintenance is essential.
- Social work referral is important to ensure adequate social support system including housing, mental health assistance, and substance abuse treatment

OUTCOME/PROGNOSIS

With the advent of potent HAART, which causes durable virologic suppression and reconstitution of the immune system, the mortality among HIV-infected persons continues to decline. In the modern era of HAART, noninfectious conditions start to play a much more important role in the mortality among persons with HIV (*AIDS 2007;21(15):2093*).

Opportunistic Infections

GENERAL PRINCIPLES

- Potent ART has decreased the incidence, changed the manifestations, and improved the outcome of OIs.
- A clinical syndrome associated with the immune enhancement induced by potent ART, **immune reconstitution syndrome (IRIS)**, generally presents as local inflammatory reactions. Examples include recurrent symptoms of cryptococcal meningitis, paradoxical reactions with TB reactivation, localized *Mycobacterium avium* complex (MAC) adenitis, aggravation of hepatitis viral infection, and CMV vitreitis immediately after the initiation of potent ART.
- In the case of IRIS, ART is usually continued, and the addition of low-dose steroids might decrease the degree of inflammation. TB and cryptococcal meningitis are the only OIs for which delay of ART is recommended to prevent IRIS.

• Additional details with updates may be found in the Guidelines for the Prevention and Treatment of Opportunistic Infections in HIV-Infected Adults and Adolescents (*http://aidsinfo.nih.gov/contentfiles/lvguidelines/adult_oi.pdf*).

TREATMENT

• **Prophylaxis for OIs** can be divided into primary and secondary prophylaxis.
• **Primary prophylaxis** is established before an episode of OI occurs. Institution of primary prophylaxis depends on the level of immunosuppression as judged by the patient's CD4 cell count and percentage (Table 16-2).
• **Secondary prophylaxis** is instituted after an episode of infection has been adequately treated. Most OIs will require extended therapy.
• **Withdrawal of prophylaxis:** Recommendations suggest withdrawing primary and secondary prophylaxis for most OIs if sustained immunologic recovery has occurred (CD4 cell counts consistently >150–200 cells/µL) (*MMWR Recomm Rep 2009;58(RR-4):1*).

PULMONARY SYNDROMES

Pneumocystis jirovecii Pneumonia
General Principles
Pneumocystis jirovecii pneumonia (PCP) is the most common infection in patients with AIDS and is the leading cause of death in this population.

Diagnosis
Positive direct immunofluorescent stain from induced sputum samples or bronchoalveolar lavage fluid. Alternatively, histopathologic demonstration of organisms in tissue is also adequate for diagnosis.

TABLE 16-2	Opportunistic Infection Prophylaxis	
Opportunistic Infection	**Indications for Prophylaxis**	**Medications**
PCP	CD4 <200 cells/µL	TMP-SMX DS PO daily or three times per week one tablet daily, is the preferred regimen Alternatives: dapsone[a], atovaquone, aerosolized pentamidine
Toxoplasmosis[b]	CD4 <100 cells/µL,	TMP-SMX DS PO daily Alternatives: combination of dapsone + pyrimethamine and leucovorin; atovaquone
Mycobacterium avium complex prophylaxis	CD4 cell count <50 cells/µL	Azithromycin 1200 mg PO weekly Alternatives: clarithromycin or rifabutin

DS, double strength; PCP, *Pneumocystis jirovecii* pneumonia; TMP-SMX, trimethoprim-sulfamethoxazole.
[a]Glucose-6-phosphate dehydrogenase (G6PD) testing should be done for dapsone.
[b]If toxoplasmosis IgG is positive.

Treatment
- **Trimethoprim-sulfamethoxazole (TMP-SMX)** is the treatment of choice. The dosage is 15–20 mg/kg of the TMP component IV daily, divided q6–8h for severe cases, with a switch to oral therapy when the patient's condition improves. Total duration of therapy is 21 days. Prednisone should be added with severe disease as defined below. For patients who cannot receive TMP-SMX, the following alternatives are available:
  - For mild to moderately severe disease (arterial oxygen tension [PaO_2] >70 mm Hg or alveolar arterial oxygen gradient [$P(A–a)O_2$] <35 mm Hg):
    - TMP, 5 mg/kg PO q8h, and dapsone, 100 mg PO daily. G6PD deficiency should be ruled out before dapsone is used.
    - Clindamycin, 600 mg IV or PO q8h, plus primaquine, 30 mg PO daily. G6PD deficiency should be ruled out before primaquine is used.
    - Atovaquone, 750 mg PO q8h. This drug should be administered with meals to increase absorption.
  - For severe disease (PaO_2 <70 mm Hg or $P[A–a]O_2$ >35 mm Hg):
    - Prednisone taper should be added. The most frequently prescribed prednisone regimen is 40 mg PO bid on days 1–5 and 40 mg daily on days 6–10, followed by 20 mg on days 11–21.
    - IV pentamidine is used in cases when all other options are exhausted and requires close monitoring for side effects.
- Primary prophylaxis is indicated (see Table 16-2). Secondary PCP prophylaxis can be discontinued if the CD4 count is >200 cells/μL for more than 3 months as a result of ART.

Mycobacterium tuberculosis
General Principles
M. tuberculosis is more frequent among HIV-infected patients, particularly IV drug abusers. Primary or reactivated disease is common (*MMWR Recomm Rep 2009;58(RR-4):1*).

Diagnosis
- Clinical manifestations depend on the level of immunosuppression. Patients with higher CD4 cell counts tend to exhibit classic presentations with **apical cavitary disease**.
- Profoundly immunosuppressed patients may demonstrate atypical presentations that can resemble disseminated primary infection, with diffuse or localized pulmonary infiltrates and hilar lymphadenopathy.
- Extrapulmonary dissemination is more common in patients with HIV.

Treatment
- For treatment recommendations, see Chapter 14, Treatment of Infectious Diseases.
- Current recommendations suggest the **substitution of rifabutin for rifampin** in patients who are receiving concomitant ART, especially PIs. The dosage for rifabutin needs readjustment due to many significant interactions (*http://www.hivmedicationguide.com/*). In subjects who are ART naïve, ART can be delayed for a few weeks after TB-specific therapy is started.

FEBRILE SYNDROMES

M. avium Complex Infection
General Principles
MAC infection is the most commonly occurring mycobacterial infection in AIDS patients and is responsible for significant morbidity in patients with advanced disease (CD4 cell count <100 cells/μL).

Diagnosis

Clinical Presentation
- Disseminated infection with fever, weight loss, and night sweats is the most frequent presentation.
- MAC infection can result in bacteremia in AIDS patients.

Diagnostic Testing
- Anemia and an elevated alkaline phosphatase level are the usual laboratory abnormalities.
- Mycobacterial blood cultures should be sent in suspected cases.

Treatment
- Initial therapy should include a **macrolide** (i.e., clarithromycin, 500 mg PO bid) and **ethambutol**, 15 mg/kg PO daily.
- Rifabutin, 300 mg PO daily, or a fluoroquinolone can be added in severe cases and based on sensitivities.
- Secondary prophylaxis for disseminated MAC can be discontinued if the CD4 count has a sustained increase >100 cells/μL for 6 months or longer in response to ART, and if 12 months of therapy for MAC is completed and there are no symptoms or signs attributable to MAC.

Histoplasma capsulatum Infections

General Principles
- The severity of infection depends on the degree of the patient's immunosuppression.
- Histoplasmosis often occurs in AIDS patients who live in endemic areas such as the Mississippi and Ohio River Valleys.
- Such infections are usually disseminated at the time of diagnosis.

Diagnosis
- Suspect histoplasmosis in patients with fever, hepatosplenomegaly, and weight loss.
- Pancytopenia develops due to bone marrow involvement.
- Diagnosis is made by a positive culture or biopsy demonstrating 2–4 μm budding yeast, but the urine and serum *Histoplasma* antigens can also be used for diagnosis and to monitor treatment.

Treatment
- Disseminated disease is treated with **liposomal amphotericin B**, 3 mg/kg IV daily for 2 weeks or until the patient clinically improves, followed by **itraconazole**, 200 mg PO bid indefinitely.
- CNS disease is initially treated with **liposomal amphotericin B**, 5 mg/kg IV daily for 4–6 weeks, before starting itraconazole.
- Itraconazole absorption should be documented by a serum drug level.
- Discontinuation of itraconazole is possible if sustained increase in CD4 count is observed >100–200 cells/μL for more than 6 months.

Other Causes of Febrile Illness
- Bacterial infection and sepsis are more common in HIV-infected patients.
- Bacterial pneumonia, especially due to pneumococcus.
- Other disseminated fungal infections, depending on local incidence, including *Cryptococcus*, *Penicillium*, and *Coccidioides*.
- CMV and other disseminated herpes viral infections.

CENTRAL NERVOUS SYSTEM AND RETINAL DISEASE

Cryptococcus neoformans

General Principles
- The severity of infection depends on the degree of the patient's immunosuppression.
- **Cryptococcal meningitis** is the most frequent CNS fungal infection in AIDS patients.

Diagnosis
- Patients with CNS infection usually present with headaches, fever, and possibly mental status changes, but presentation can be more subtle.
- Cryptococcal infection can also present as pulmonary or cutaneous disease.
- Diagnosis is based on **lumbar puncture** results and on the determination of latex cryptococcal antigen, which is usually positive in the serum and in the CSF.
- **CSF opening pressure** should always be measured to assess the possibility of elevated intracranial pressure.

Treatment
- Initial treatment is with a lipid preparation of **amphotericin** dosed at 3–4 mg/kg/d IV, and **5-flucytosine**, 25 mg/kg PO q6h for at least 2 weeks, followed by **fluconazole**, 400 mg PO daily for at least 8 weeks and then 200 mg PO daily, either lifelong or until immune reconstitution occurs. Fluconazole can be discontinued in those who are asymptomatic with regard to signs and symptoms of cryptococcosis and have a sustained increase (>6 months) in their CD4+ counts to ≥200 cells/μL.
- The 5-flucytosine level should be monitored during therapy to avoid toxicity.
- Alternative initial therapy is with amphotericin B, 0.7 mg/kg/d IV, and flucytosine, 25 mg/kg PO q6h. Repeat lumbar punctures (removing up to 30 mL CSF until the pressure is <20–25 cm H_2O) may be required to relieve elevated intracranial pressure.
- In persons who have persistent elevation of intracranial pressure, a temporary lumbar drain is indicated.

Toxoplasma gondii

Diagnosis
Toxoplasmosis typically causes multiple CNS lesions and presents with encephalopathy and focal neurologic findings.

Diagnostic Testing
Laboratories
Disease represents reactivation of a previous infection, and the serologic workup is usually positive.
Imaging
- MRI of the brain is the best radiographic technique for diagnosis.
- Often the diagnosis relies on response to empiric treatment, as seen by a reduction in the size of the mass lesions.

Treatment
- **Sulfadiazine**, 25 mg/kg PO q6h, plus **pyrimethamine**, 200 mg PO on day 1, followed by 75 mg PO daily, is the therapy of choice.
- **Leucovorin**, 5–10 mg PO daily, should be added to prevent hematologic toxicity.
- For patients who are allergic to sulfonamides, clindamycin, 600 mg IV or PO q8h, can be used instead of sulfadiazine.
- Doses are reduced after 6 weeks of therapy.
- Secondary prophylaxis can be discontinued among patients with a sustained increase in CD4 count >200 cells/μL for more than 6 months as a result of response to ART and if the initial therapy is complete and there are no symptoms or signs attributable to toxoplasmosis.

Varicella-Zoster Virus

Diagnosis
- Varicella-zoster virus may cause typical dermatomal lesions or disseminated infection including retinal necrosis.
- May cause encephalitis, which is more common with ophthalmic distribution of facial nerve.

Treatment
Acyclovir, 10 mg/kg IV q8h for 7–14 days, is the recommended therapy. For milder cases, administration of acyclovir (800 mg PO five times a day), famciclovir (500 mg PO tid), or valacyclovir (1 g PO tid) for 1 week is usually effective.

JC Virus

Diagnosis
• Associated with progressive multifocal leukoencephalopathy. Symptoms include mental status changes, weakness, and disorders of gait.
• Characteristic periventricular and subcortical white matter lesions are seen on MRI.

Treatment
Potent ART has improved the survival of patients with progressive multifocal leukoencephalopathy.

CMV Retinitis

CMV retinitis accounts for 85% of CMV disease in patients with AIDS. It commonly develops in a setting of profound CD4 depletions (CD4 cell count <50 cells/μL).

Diagnosis
• CMV viremia can be detected by PCR and is usually present in end-organ disease but can also be seen in the absence of end-organ disease.
• The diagnosis of CMV retinitis is made based on characteristic findings during ophthalmoscopic exam.

Treatment
• Treatment of CMV retinitis can be local or systemic and is administered in two phases, induction and maintenance.
• **Ganciclovir** is given at an induction dosage of 5 mg/kg IV bid for 14–21 days and a maintenance dosage of 5 mg/kg IV daily indefinitely (unless immune reconstitution occurs). The most common side effect of ganciclovir is **myelotoxicity**, resulting in neutropenia. The neutropenia may respond to granulocyte colony-stimulating factor therapy. An intraocular ganciclovir implant is effective but does not provide systemic CMV therapy.
• **Valganciclovir**, a ganciclovir prodrug, has drug levels equivalent to those of IV ganciclovir. For induction, 900 mg PO bid for 14–21 days is given, followed by 900 mg once a day. **Treatment is indefinite unless immunologic recovery occurs.** Adverse effects are similar to those of ganciclovir.
• Alternatives include **IV foscarnet, IV cidofovir, and intraocular fomivirsen** (which does not provide systemic therapy). Both IV foscarnet and cidofovir administrations carry a significant risk of **nephrotoxicity**; therefore, adequate hydration and electrolyte monitoring (including calcium) are required.
• For other **invasive CMV disease**, the optimal therapy is with IV ganciclovir, PO valganciclovir, IV foscarnet, or a combination of two drugs (in persons with prior anti-CMV therapy), for at least 3–6 weeks. Foscarnet has the best CSF penetration and is the drug of choice for CMV encephalitis and myelopathy. Long-term maintenance therapy is indicated.

ESOPHAGITIS

Candida

General Principles
• The severity of infection depends on the degree of the patient's immunosuppression.
• Candidiasis is common in the HIV-infected host.
• Other causes of esophagitis include HSV, CMV, and *Histoplasma*.

Diagnosis
Location of infection can be oral, esophageal, or vaginal.

Treatment
• Oral and vaginal candidiasis usually responds to local therapy with troches or creams (**nystatin** or **clotrimazole**).
• For patients who do not respond or who have esophageal candidiasis, **fluconazole**, 100–200 mg PO daily, is the treatment of choice.

Special Considerations
Fluconazole-resistant candidiasis is increasing, especially in patients with advanced disease who have been receiving antifungal agents for prolonged periods.
• **Caspofungin or micafungin**, echinocandins, can be considered for refractory cases.
• **Itraconazole** oral suspension (200 mg bid) is occasionally effective, as is **posaconazole** oral solution, and posaconazole is generally better tolerated than itraconazole. **Voriconazole** may also be useful.

DIARRHEA

Cryptosporidium
Diagnosis
• *Cryptosporidium* causes chronic watery diarrhea with malabsorption in HIV-infected patients.
• Diagnosis is based on the visualization of the parasite in an acid-fast stain of stool.

Treatment
• No effective specific therapy has been developed as ART is essential.
• **Nitazoxanide**, 500 mg PO bid, may be effective.

Cyclospora, Isospora, Microsporidia, and *Campylobacter jejuni*
Diagnosis
These organisms cause chronic diarrhea. Microsporidia can also cause biliary tree disease in patients with advanced infection.

Treatment
• *Cyclospora* is treated with **TMP-SMX**, one double-strength (DS) tablet PO bid for 7–10 days. *Isospora* is treated with **TMP-SMX**, one DS tablet PO qid for 10 days, followed by chronic suppression with TMP-SMX, one DS tablet PO daily.
• Microsporidia are treated with **albendazole**, 400 mg PO bid, but this regimen has only modest success for *Enterocytozoon bieneusi* infections. Relapses are common when therapy is stopped.
• *C. jejuni* is treated with either azithromycin, 500 mg PO daily, or ciprofloxacin, 500–750 mg PO bid.

ASSOCIATED NEOPLASMS

Kaposi Sarcoma

GENERAL PRINCIPLES

Kaposi sarcoma is caused by co-infection with human herpesvirus-8 (HHV-8), also called Kaposi sarcoma–associated herpesvirus (KSHV).

DIAGNOSIS

In AIDS patients, it commonly presents as cutaneous lesions, but can be disseminated. The GI tract and lungs are the usual visceral organs involved.

TREATMENT

- Local therapy with **liquid nitrogen** or intralesional injection with alitretinoin or vinblastine has been used. Cryotherapy or radiation may be useful as well.
- Systemic therapy involves chemotherapy (e.g., liposomal doxorubicin, paclitaxel, liposomal daunorubicin, thalidomide, retinoids), radiation, and interferon-α.

Lymphoma

GENERAL PRINCIPLES

- Lymphomas commonly associated with AIDS are non-Hodgkin lymphoma, CNS and systemic lymphoma, and lymphomas of B-cell origin.
- **EBV** appears to be the associated pathogen.

DIAGNOSIS

- Primary CNS lymphomas are common and can be multicentric.
- Diagnosis is based on clinical symptoms, the presence of enhancing brain lesions, brain biopsy, and a positive EBV-PCR of the CSF.
- Other OIs need to be ruled out.
- Other potential extranodal sites of involvement including bone marrow, GI tract, and liver require tissue biopsy to confirm the diagnosis.

TREATMENT

Treatment involves **chemotherapy** and **radiation**.

Cervical and Perianal Neoplasias

GENERAL PRINCIPLES

- Both HIV-infected men and women are at high risk for HPV-related disease.
- Certain HPV subtypes such as 16 and 18 are oncogenic.
- Cancer can also arise from perianal condyloma acuminata.

DIAGNOSIS

- Screening for vaginal dysplasia with a Papanicolaou smear is indicated every 6 months during the first year and, if results are normal, annually thereafter.
- Screening for anal intraepithelial neoplasms is currently under evaluation and is recommended by some experts in populations such as MSM, any patient with a history of anogenital condylomas, and women with abnormal vulvar or cervical histology (*http:// hivguidelines.org/Content.aspx*).

TREATMENT

Refer to Chapter 22, Cancer, for specific treatments of these neoplasms.

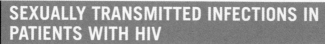

SEXUALLY TRANSMITTED INFECTIONS IN PATIENTS WITH HIV

For treatment, see Table 16-1.

Genital Herpes

HIV-infected individuals are more likely to have prolonged and severe disease as well as treatment failures due to the development of resistance. Treatment guidelines are slightly different for HIV-infected patients. See Table 16-1.

Genital Warts

GENERAL PRINCIPLES

Genital warts are caused by HPV. Different serotypes have been associated with the lesions, notably types 6 and 11. Other common HPV types (16, 18, 31, and 33) are associated with malignant transformation in different anatomic sites. Genital warts in HIV-infected persons are typically more resistant to treatment and have a higher chance of recurrence (*http://www.cdc.gov/STD/treatment/2006/genital-warts.htm*).

DIAGNOSIS

Diagnosis is made on the basis of physical exam and history. In some situations, biopsy of the lesions may be necessary.

TREATMENT

Local therapy is aimed at the removal of the warts. HPV vaccination is recommended in women and men under the age of 27 (see previous section on immunizations).

Syphilis

See the section on STIs for more complete information.

Additional Resources

- *www.aifsinfo.org*
- *www.aidsmeds.com*
- *www.thebody.com*
- *www.hivmedicine.com*
- *www.hivinsite.ucsf.edu*

17 Solid Organ Transplant Medicine

Rupinder Sodhi and Rowena Delos Santos

Solid Organ Transplant Basics

GENERAL PRINCIPLES

- Solid organ transplantation is a **treatment, not a cure**, for end-stage organ failure of the kidney, liver, pancreas, heart, and lung. Small intestine and vascularized composite allografts are performed in smaller numbers at specialized centers throughout the country. The benefits of organ replacement coexist with the risks of chronic immunosuppression. Thus, not all patients with organ failure are transplant candidates.
- Organs remain in short supply with increasing waiting times for potential recipients. **Living-donor transplants** are increasingly common in kidney transplantation and are being evaluated in liver and lung transplantation as a partial solution to this shortage. Xenotransplantation is **not** currently a viable option.
- **Immunologic considerations** prior to the transplant must be fully evaluated, including ABO compatibility with the donor, HLA typing, and some degree of immune response testing to the proposed donor. Newer protocols using desensitization techniques have had some success in overcoming these immunologic barriers.

DIAGNOSIS

- For indications and contraindications of heart, lung, kidney, and liver transplantations, see sections devoted to cardiology, pulmonology, nephrology, and hepatology.
- **Evaluation of the transplant patient.** The evaluation of the transplant recipient with general medical or surgical problems should encompass the details of the patient's organ transplant and treatment. Thus, the following should always be reviewed when taking a history from an organ transplant recipient:
  - Cause of organ failure
  - Treatment for organ failure prior to transplantation
  - Type and date of transplant
  - Cytomegalovirus (CMV) serology of donor and recipient
  - Induction immunosuppression, particularly use of antibody-based induction therapy
  - Initial allograft function (e.g., nadir creatinine, forced expiratory volume in 1 second [FEV_1], ejection fraction, synthetic function, and transaminases)
  - Current allograft function
  - Complications of transplantation (e.g., surgical problems, acute rejection, delayed graft function, infections, chronic organ dysfunction)
  - Current immunosuppression regimen and recent drug levels

TREATMENT

- **Immunosuppression.** Immunosuppressive medications are used to promote acceptance of a graft (induction therapy), to prevent rejection (maintenance therapy), and to reverse episodes of acute rejection (rejection therapy). These agents are associated with

527

immunosuppressive effects, immunodeficiency toxicities (e.g., infection and malignancy), and nonimmune toxicities (e.g., nephrotoxicity, diabetes mellitus, bone disease, gout, hyperlipidemia, cardiovascular disease, or neurotoxicity) (*N Engl J Med 2004;351:2715*). Immunosuppressive medications should only be prescribed and administered by physicians and nurses who have appropriate knowledge and expertise. Many variables factor into the choice and dose of drug, and the guidelines for each specific organ are different.

- **Glucocorticoids.** Glucocorticoids are immunosuppressive and anti-inflammatory. Their mechanisms of action include inhibition of cytokine transcription, induction of lymphocyte apoptosis, downregulation of adhesion molecule and major histocompatibility complex expression, and modification of leukocyte trafficking (*N Engl J Med 2005;353:1711*).
  - Side effects of chronic glucocorticoid therapy are well known.
  - As a result of the associated morbidity, steroids are tapered rapidly in the immediate posttransplant period to achieve maintenance doses of 0.1 mg/kg or less.
  - Further strategies are being developed to minimize side effects: steroid-free immunosuppression, rapid steroid tapering, and steroid withdrawal.
  - Although most long-term transplant recipients have abnormalities in the adrenal axis, increases in glucocorticoid therapy are not indicated for routine surgery or illness (*Arch Surg 2008;143:1222*).

- **Antiproliferative agents**
  - **Azathioprine** is a purine analog that is metabolized by the liver to 6-mercaptopurine (active drug), which in turn is catabolized by xanthine oxidase. Azathioprine inhibits DNA synthesis and thereby suppresses lymphocyte proliferation. The major dose-limiting toxicity of this agent is myelosuppression, which is usually reversible after dose reduction or discontinuation of the drug. The usual maintenance dose is 1.5–2.5 mg/kg/d in a single dose. Drug levels are generally not obtained. Azathioprine is generally considered safe in pregnancy.
  - **Mycophenolic acid (MPA)** is available in two forms: MPA or its precursor, mycophenolate mofetil (which is converted to the active metabolite, MPA). MPA inhibits the rate-limiting step in de novo purine synthesis. Because lymphocytes are dependent on the de novo pathway for purine synthesis, lymphocyte proliferation is selectively inhibited by MPA.
  - **Major adverse effects** of MPA are gastrointestinal disturbances (nausea, diarrhea, and abdominal pain) and hematologic disturbances (leukopenia and thrombocytopenia).
  - Antacids that contain magnesium and aluminum interfere with the absorption of MPA and should not be given concurrently.
  - Proton pump inhibitors can also interfere with the bioavailability of mycophenolate mofetil, but not enteric-coated MPA, which is absorbed in the small intestine.
  - MPA is not used in pregnancy due to its teratogenicity in animal models.
  - The usual dose is 1–2 g daily in divided doses, although lesser doses may be used with concomitant tacrolimus than cyclosporine (CsA), because of enterohepatic circulation affecting MPA levels. Additionally, the dosage of MPA should be reduced in chronic renal impairment. Drug levels can be obtained to verify absorption or compliance, but the clinical utility of MPA levels has not been determined.

- **Mammalian target of rapamycin (mTOR) inhibitors.** Sirolimus and everolimus inhibit the activation of a regulatory kinase, mTOR, and thus prohibit T-cell progression from the G_1 to the S phase of the cell cycle. Unlike the calcineurin inhibitors, mTOR inhibitors do not affect cytokine transcription but inhibit cytokine- and growth factor-induced cell proliferation.
  - The major adverse effects include hyperlipidemia (hypertriglyceridemia), anemia, proteinuria, difficulty with wound healing, cytopenias, peripheral edema, oral ulcers, and gastrointestinal symptoms, although other less common side effects are present.

- Although not directly nephrotoxic, mTOR inhibitors may compound the vasoconstriction of calcineurin inhibitors and potentiate their nephrotoxicity. Thus, mTOR inhibitors are best used alone or with steroids and/or other antiproliferative agents.
- Sirolimus interacts with CsA metabolism, making monitoring of both drugs difficult.
- The typical dose of sirolimus is 2–5 mg daily in a single dose. Everolimus is administered at 0.75–1.50 mg twice daily. Therapeutic drug monitoring is being perfected, with current trough levels between 5–15 ng/mL for sirolimus and 3–8 ng/mL for everolimus most commonly being used.
- Sirolimus should be avoided in moderate to advanced chronic kidney disease and immediately postoperatively because it is associated with poorer wound healing, delayed graft function (kidney transplant), anastomotic bronchial dehiscence (lung transplant), and hepatic artery thrombosis (liver transplant); limited data are available regarding use of everolimus in the immediate postoperative period.
- Sirolimus is not used in pregnant women due to teratogenicity in animal models.
- **Calcineurin inhibitors.** Calcineurin inhibitors inhibit T-lymphocyte activation and proliferation. **They remain the most commonly used immunosuppressant, despite their side effect of nephrotoxicity.** IV calcineurin inhibitors should be avoided because of their extreme toxicity and must never be given as a bolus under any circumstance.
  - **Cyclosporine (CsA)** is a cyclic 11-amino acid peptide derived from a fungus. Its major nonimmune side effect is nephrotoxicity due to glomerular afferent arteriolar vasoconstriction. This action leads to an immediate decline in glomerular filtration rate of up to 30% and a long-term vaso-occlusive fibrotic renal disease that often results in chronic kidney disease in recipients of all organ transplants. Angiotensin-converting enzyme inhibitors, mTOR inhibitors, volume depletion, and nephrotoxins may potentiate this effect. Acute nephrotoxicity is reversible with dose reduction; chronic nephrotoxicity is generally irreversible and nearly universally present in all patients after 8–10 years of therapy.
  - Other **adverse effects** include gingival hyperplasia, hirsutism, tremor, hypertension, glucose intolerance, hyperlipidemia, hyperkalemia, and rarely, thrombotic microangiopathy. CsA has a narrow therapeutic window, and doses are adjusted based on blood levels (recommended maintenance 12-hour trough levels of 100–300 ng/mL and 2-hour peak levels of 800–1200 ng/mL). Usual doses are 6–8 mg/kg/d in divided doses, with careful attention to levels and toxicities.
  - **Tacrolimus** is a macrolide and, like CsA, is nephrotoxic. Tacrolimus is more neurotoxic and diabetogenic than CsA, but it is associated with less hirsutism, hypertension, and gingival hyperplasia. Tacrolimus dosing is based on trough blood levels (recommended maintenance levels of 5–10 ng/mL). Usual starting dose is 0.15 mg/kg/d in divided doses.
- **Biologic agents**
  - **Polyclonal antibodies**
    - Antithymocyte globulin is produced by injecting human thymocytes into animals and collecting sera. This process generates antibodies against a wide variety of human immune system antigens. When subsequently infused into human patients, T lymphocytes are depleted as a result of complement-mediated lysis and clearance of antibody-coated cells by the reticuloendothelial system. Lymphocyte function is also disrupted by blocking and modulating the expression of cell surface molecules by the antibodies. Infusion is through a central vein over 4–6 hours. The most common side effects are fever, chills, and arthralgias.
    - Other important **adverse effects** include myelosuppression, serum sickness, and rarely, anaphylaxis. Two preparations are available: horse antithymocyte globulin (ATGAM) and rabbit antithymocyte globulin (Thymoglobulin). Current literature suggests that rabbit antithymocyte globulin is more efficacious. These drugs can be

used at the time of transplantation to promote engraftment ("induction") or as a subsequent treatment for acute rejection. The long-term risk of increased malignancy, particularly lymphoma, remains a concern with these agents.

○ **Monoclonal antibodies**

■ **Anti–interleukin-2 receptor monoclonal antibody.** Basiliximab (chimeric) is a monoclonal antibody that competitively inhibits the interleukin-2 receptor (CD25) and thereby inhibits activation of T cells. Chimerization results in antibodies with an extended half-life and minimizes the chance of developing antimurine antibodies. This drug is administered by a peripheral vein perioperatively at the time of transplantation and is associated with few side effects.

■ Belatacept, used in kidney transplants, is a fusion protein that blocks T-cell costimulation (CD80/86) and subsequent activation. It is contraindicated for use in nonrenal transplantation and additionally in patients seronegative for Epstein-Barr virus (EBV) due to increased posttransplant lymphoproliferative disease (PTLD) in EBV-seronegative recipients.

■ Other biologic agents used off-label in transplantation include **alemtuzumab**, a monoclonal antibody against CD52, a molecule present on B and T cells; **eculizumab**, a humanized monoclonal antibody blocking activation of complement protein C5; and **rituximab**, a chimeric monoclonal antibody against the B-cell protein CD20.

■ IV immunoglobulin **(IVIG)** has immunomodulatory effects. Due to these effects, IVIG is sometimes used in the treatment of antibody-mediated rejection. Side effects include flushing, myalgias, chills, headache, and rarely, anaphylaxis.

• **Infection prophylaxis**

○ **Immunization.** Pneumococcal and hepatitis B vaccination should be given at the time of pretransplant evaluation. Influenza A vaccination should be administered yearly. Live vaccines should be avoided after transplantation and if transplant is imminent (e.g., planned living donor kidney transplant) (*Am J Transplant 2004;4(suppl 10):160*). Varicella vaccination in seronegative patients and hepatitis A vaccination (particularly in liver transplant candidates) should be considered before transplant (*Clin Infect Dis 2009;49:1550*).

○ **Trimethoprim-sulfamethoxazole** prevents urinary tract infections, *Pneumocystis jirovecii* pneumonia, and *Nocardia* infections. The optimal dose and duration of prophylaxis have not been determined, although a minimum of 1 year is generally recommended. In sulfa-allergic patients, dapsone, aerosolized pentamidine, and atovaquone are alternatives.

○ **Acyclovir** prevents reactivation of herpes simplex virus (HSV) and varicella-zoster virus but is ineffective in CMV prophylaxis. HSV can be a serious infection in immunosuppressed individuals, and some form of prophylaxis should be used during the first year. Patients with recurrent HSV infections (oral or genital) should be considered candidates for long-term prophylaxis. Lifetime acyclovir should also be used in EBV-seronegative patients who receive an EBV-positive organ.

○ **Ganciclovir** or **valganciclovir** prevents reactivation of CMV infection when administered to patients who were previously CMV seropositive, received a CMV-positive organ, or both. Typically, they are administered for 3–12 months following transplantation. CMV hyperimmune globulin or IV ganciclovir can also be used for this purpose. Alternatively, patients can be monitored for the presence of CMV replication in the bloodstream by polymerase chain reaction before symptoms develop and can be treated preemptively.

○ **Fluconazole** or **ketoconazole** can be given to patients with a high risk of systemic fungal infections or recurrent localized fungal infections. Both medications increase CsA and tacrolimus levels (see Treatment under the Solid Organ Transplant Basics section).

○ **Nystatin suspension**, **clotrimazole** troches, or weekly **fluconazole** is used to prevent oropharyngeal candidiasis (thrush).

GRAFT REJECTION

Acute Rejection, Kidney

GENERAL PRINCIPLES

Most episodes of acute rejection occur in the first year after transplantation. The low incidence of acute rejection today usually entails a careful search for inadequate drug levels, noncompliance, or less common forms of rejection (such as antibody-mediated rejection or plasma cell rejection). Late acute rejection (>1 year after transplantation) usually results from inadequate immunosuppression or patient nonadherence.

Definition

An immunologically mediated, acute deterioration in renal function associated with specific pathologic changes on renal biopsy including lymphocytic interstitial infiltrates, tubulitis, and arteritis (cellular rejection) and/or glomerulitis, capillaritis, and positive staining of the peritubular capillaries for the complement component C4d (antibody-mediated rejection).

Epidemiology

Kidney allograft rejection currently occurs in only 10% of patients. Patients who do not receive induction therapy have a 20–30% incidence of acute rejection.

Associated Conditions

Diagnosis of acute renal allograft rejection is made by percutaneous renal biopsy after excluding prerenal azotemia via hydration and repeating laboratory tests. Further workup includes evaluation for calcineurin inhibitor nephrotoxicity (trough and/or peak levels and associated signs), infection (urinalysis and culture), obstruction (renal ultrasound), and surgical complications such as urine leak (renal scan). Newer techniques evaluating early markers of acute rejection in the blood and urine are being developed.

DIAGNOSIS

Clinical Presentation

Manifestations include an elevated serum creatinine, decreased urine output, increased edema, or worsening hypertension. Initial symptoms are often absent except for the rise in creatinine. Constitutional symptoms (fever, malaise, arthralgia, painful or swollen allograft) are uncommon in current practice.

Differential Diagnosis

Differential diagnosis varies with duration after transplantation (Table 17-1).

Acute Rejection, Lung

GENERAL PRINCIPLES

- Of the solid organ transplants, the lung is the most immunogenic organ. The majority of patients have at least one episode of acute rejection. Multiple episodes of acute rejection predispose to the development of chronic rejection (bronchiolitis obliterans syndrome).
- **Lung transplant rejection** occurs frequently and most commonly in the first few months after transplantation.

TABLE 17-1	Differential Diagnosis of Renal Allograft Dysfunction	
>1 Wk After Transplant	**<3 Mo After Transplant**	**>3 Mo After Transplant**
Acute tubular necrosis	Acute rejection	Prerenal azotemia
Hyperacute rejection	Calcineurin inhibitor toxicity	Calcineurin inhibitor toxicity
Accelerated rejection	Prerenal azotemia	Acute rejection (nonadherence, low levels)
Obstruction	Obstruction	Obstruction
Urine leak (ureteral necrosis)	Infection	Recurrent renal disease
Arterial or venous thrombosis	Interstitial nephritis	De novo renal disease
Atheroemboli	Recurrent renal disease BK virus nephropathy	Renal artery stenosis (anastomotic or atherosclerotic) BK virus nephropathy

DIAGNOSIS

Diagnosis is generally made by fiberoptic bronchoscopy with bronchoalveolar lavage and transbronchial biopsies.

Clinical Presentation

Manifestations are nonspecific and include fever, dyspnea, and a nonproductive cough. The chest radiograph is usually unchanged and is generally nondiagnostic even when abnormal (perihilar infiltrates, interstitial edema, pleural effusions). Change in pulmonary function testing is not specific for rejection, but a 10% or greater decline in forced vital capacity or FEV_1, or both, is usually clinically significant.

Differential Diagnosis

It is important to attempt to distinguish rejection from infection, because although the symptoms are similar, the treatments are markedly different.

Acute Rejection, Heart

GENERAL PRINCIPLES

Heart transplant recipients typically have two to three episodes of acute rejection in the first year after transplantation with a 50–80% chance of having at least one rejection episode, most commonly in the first 6 months.

DIAGNOSIS

• Diagnosis is established by endomyocardial biopsy performed during routine surveillance or as prompted by symptoms. None of the noninvasive techniques has demonstrated sufficient sensitivity and specificity to replace the endomyocardial biopsy. Repeated endomyocardial biopsies predispose to severe tricuspid regurgitation.

• **Manifestations** may include symptoms and signs of left ventricular dysfunction, such as dyspnea, paroxysmal nocturnal dyspnea, orthopnea, syncope, palpitations, new gallops, and elevated jugular venous pressure. Many patients are asymptomatic. Acute rejection may also be associated with a variety of tachyarrhythmias (atrial more often than ventricular).

Acute Rejection, Liver

GENERAL PRINCIPLES

• Many liver transplant recipients may be maintained on minimal immunosuppression. Acute rejection typically occurs within the first 3 months after transplant and often in the first 2 weeks after the operation. Acute rejection in the liver is generally reversible and does not portend a potentially serious adverse outcome as in other organs. Recurrent viral hepatitis is a much more frequent and morbid problem.
• **Liver transplant recipients** commonly experience acute allograft rejection, with at least 60% having one episode.

DIAGNOSIS

Diagnosis is made by liver biopsy after technical complications are excluded.

Clinical Presentation

Manifestations may be absent with only a slight elevation in transaminases, or patients may have signs and symptoms of liver failure including fever, malaise, anorexia, abdominal pain, ascites, decreased bile output, elevated bilirubin, and elevated transaminases.

Differential Diagnosis

Differential diagnosis of early liver allograft dysfunction includes primary graft nonfunction, preservation injury, vascular thrombosis, biliary anastomotic leak, or stenosis. These disorders should be excluded clinically or by Doppler ultrasonography. Late allograft dysfunction may be due to rejection, recurrent hepatitis B or C, CMV infection, EBV infection, cholestasis, or drug toxicity.

Acute Rejection, Pancreas

GENERAL PRINCIPLES

• The majority of rejection episodes occur within the first 6 months after transplant. Unlike other organs, clinical findings and biochemical markers correlate poorly with rejection; in particular, if hyperglycemia occurs due to rejection, it is often late, severe, and irreversible. Because 80% of pancreas transplants are performed with a simultaneous kidney transplant with the same immunologic status, renal allograft function and histopathology can be a valuable surrogate for diagnosis of pancreas allograft rejection.
• Most pancreas transplants are done with quadruple immunosuppression, consisting of an induction agent and triple maintenance immunosuppression, including corticosteroids. One-year posttransplant acute rejection rates range between 20–30%; this contributes significantly to early and late graft loss.

DIAGNOSIS

At time of surgery, the exocrine (digestive enzymes) secretions of the pancreas can be drained into the recipient's intestine (enteric drainage) or into the bladder (bladder drainage).

Serum amylase and lipase are used in both the enteric- and bladder-drained recipient to monitor for rejection but lack specificity. For the bladder-drained allograft, a fall in urinary amylase correlates with rejection. However, allograft biopsy remains the gold standard, demonstrating septal, ductal, and acinar inflammation and endotheliitis. If a recipient received a simultaneous kidney transplant from the same donor, the creatinine and renal biopsy may also be used to diagnose rejection, although isolated pancreas or kidney rejection may rarely occur.

Clinical Presentation

Manifestations may be absent with only a slight elevation in serum amylase and lipase or fall in urinary amylase (bladder drained). **Hyperglycemia is a late manifestation of rejection.**

Differential Diagnosis

Differential diagnosis of hyperglycemia includes thrombosis (affecting 7% of recipients), islet cell drug toxicity, steroid effect, infection, development of insulin resistance, or recurrent autoimmune disease. Differential diagnosis of elevated serum lipase includes graft pancreatitis, peripancreatic fluid/infection, obstruction, dehydration, and PTLD.

Chronic Allograft Dysfunction

GENERAL PRINCIPLES

- Chronic allograft dysfunction accounts for the vast majority of late graft losses and is the major obstacle to long-term graft survival.
- Chronic allograft dysfunction (formerly chronic rejection) is a slowly progressive, insidious decline in function of the allograft characterized by gradual vascular and ductal obliteration, parenchymal atrophy, and interstitial fibrosis.

DIAGNOSIS

- Diagnosis is often difficult and generally requires a biopsy. The process is mediated by immune and nonimmune factors.
- The manifestations of chronic rejection are unique to each organ system.

TREATMENT

To date, no effective therapy is available for established immune-mediated chronic allograft dysfunction. Some patients, particularly those with renal transplants, will require a second solid organ transplant. Current investigational strategies are aimed at prevention.

Complications

GENERAL PRINCIPLES

- **Infections**
  - **Posttransplant infections are a significant cause of morbidity and, in some cases, mortality for transplant recipients. Types of infections vary depending on the time since transplantation** (*N Engl J Med 1998;338:1741*) (Table 17-2).
  - **CMV infection** from reactivation of CMV in a seropositive recipient or new infection from a CMV-positive organ can lead to a wide range of presentations from a mild viral syndrome to allograft dysfunction, invasive disease in multiple organ systems, and

TABLE 17-2	Timing and Etiology of Posttransplant Infections	
Time Period	**Infectious Complication**	**Etiology**
<1 mo after transplant	Nosocomial pneumonia, wound infection, urinary tract infection, catheter-related sepsis, biliary, chest, or other drainage catheter infection	Bacterial or fungal infections
1–6 mo after transplant	Opportunistic infections	Cytomegalovirus *Pneumocystis jirovecii* *Aspergillus* spp. *Toxoplasma gondii* *Listeria monocytogenes* *Strongyloides stercoralis* West Nile virus Varicella-zoster virus (VZV)
	Reactivation of preexisting infections	*Mycobacteria* spp. Endemic mycoses Viral hepatitis
>6 mo after transplant	Community-acquired infections	Bacterial Tick-borne disease Influenza Metapneumovirus Norovirus
	Chronic progressive infection	Reactivated VZV (zoster) Hepatitis B Hepatitis C HIV Cytomegalovirus Epstein-Barr virus Papillomavirus Polyomavirus (BK)
	Opportunistic infections	*P. jirovecii* *L. monocytogenes* *Nocardia asteroides* *Cryptococcus neoformans* *Aspergillus* spp. West Nile virus

even death. CMV-seronegative patients who receive a CMV-seropositive organ are at substantial risk, particularly in the first year.

- Because of the potential progression and severity of untreated disease, treatment is usually indicated in viremic transplant patients without tissue diagnosis of invasive disease. Seroconversion with a positive IgM titer or a fourfold increase in IgM or IgG titer suggests acute infection; however, many centers now use polymerase chain reaction–based diagnostic techniques from blood samples, and treatment is usually administered in the patient with evidence of viremia (*J Am Soc Nephrol 2001;12:848*).
- Treatment is with oral valganciclovir, 450–900 mg PO bid, or IV ganciclovir, 2.5–5.0 mg/kg bid for 3–4 weeks or until clearance of the virus. Both drugs are adjusted

for renal function. Hyperimmune globulin is often used with ganciclovir for patients with organ involvement.

- Foscarnet and cidofovir are more toxic alternatives and should be reserved for ganciclovir-resistant cases.

○ **Hepatitis B and C.** Patients with active hepatitis or cirrhosis are not considered for nonhepatic transplantation. Immunosuppression increases viral replication in organ transplant recipients with either hepatitis B or C.

- **Hepatitis B** can recur as fulminant hepatic failure even in patients with no evidence of viral DNA replication before transplantation. In liver transplantation, the risk of recurrent hepatitis B virus infection can be reduced by the administration of hepatitis B immunoglobulin during and after transplantation. Lamivudine therapy initiated before transplantation to lower viral load has shown decreased likelihood of recurrent hepatitis B virus.

- **Hepatitis C** typically progresses slowly in nonhepatic transplants, and the effect of immunosuppression on mortality due to liver disease remains to be determined. Treatment protocols for hepatitis C in the nonhepatic transplant population are not yet established. Hepatitis C nearly always recurs in liver transplant recipients whose original disease was due to hepatitis C. Therapy for recurrent hepatitis C virus with ribavirin and interferon has been available, but treatment is evolving, with newer and effective therapies including protease inhibitors and polymerase inhibitors that achieve a sustained virologic response.

○ **EBV** plays a role in the development of PTLD. This life-threatening lymphoma is treated by withdrawal or reduction in immunosuppression and often aggressive chemotherapy. The role of newly discovered viral agents such as human herpesvirus (HHV)-6, HHV-7, HHV-8, and polyomavirus (BK and JC) after transplantation remains to be established. BK virus is known to cause interstitial nephritis, resulting in renal allograft loss, and occasionally ureteral stricture, resulting in obstruction. Because BK virus nephropathy results primarily from reactivation of latent BK in the transplanted organ, this is rarely seen in nonrenal transplant recipients.

○ **Fungal and parasitic infections**, such as *Cryptococcus*, *Mucor*, aspergillosis, and *Candida* spp., result in increased mortality after transplantation and should be aggressively diagnosed and treated. The role of prophylaxis with oral fluconazole has not been established.

• **Renal disease.** Chronic allograft dysfunction is the leading cause of allograft loss in renal transplant recipients. Chronic calcineurin inhibitor (CsA or tacrolimus) nephrotoxicity may also lead to chronic renal insufficiency and end-stage renal disease (ESRD), requiring dialysis or transplantation in recipients of lung, heart, liver, or pancreas transplants. The incidence of ESRD secondary to calcineurin inhibitor toxicity in recipients of solid organ transplants is at least 10%, and the incidence of significant chronic kidney disease approaches 50% (*N Engl J Med 2003;349:931*).

• **Malignancy** occurs in transplant patients with an overall incidence that is three- to four-fold higher than that seen in the general population (age matched). Cancers with an increased risk of fivefold or greater compared to the general population are Kaposi sarcoma, non-Hodgkin lymphoma, and skin, lip, vulvar, anal, and liver cancer, illustrating the oncogenic potential of associated viral infections (*JAMA 2011;306:1891*).

○ **Skin and lip cancers** are the most common de novo malignancies (40–50%) seen in transplant recipients, with an incidence 10–250 times that of the general population. Risk factors include immunosuppression, UV radiation, and human papillomavirus infection. These cancers develop at a younger age, and they are more aggressive in transplant patients. Protective clothing, sunscreens, and avoiding sun exposure are recommended. Examination of the skin is the principal screening test, and early diagnosis offers the best prognosis. The mTOR inhibitors may be better immunosuppressive choices in patients with recurrent skin cancer as long as no contraindications exist.

○ **PTLD** accounts for one-fifth of all malignancies after transplantation, with an incidence of approximately 1%. This is 30- to 50-fold higher than in the general population, and the risk increases with the use of antilymphocyte therapy for induction or rejection. The majority of these neoplasms are large-cell non-Hodgkin lymphomas of the B-cell type. PTLD results from EBV-induced B-cell proliferation in the setting of chronic immunosuppression. The EBV-seronegative recipient of a seropositive organ is at greatest risk. The presentation is often atypical and should always be considered in the patient with new symptoms. Diagnosis requires a high index of suspicion followed by a tissue biopsy. Treatment includes reduction or withdrawal of immunosuppression and chemotherapy.

SPECIAL CONSIDERATIONS

- **Important drug interactions** are always a concern given the polypharmacy associated with transplant patients. Before prescribing a new medication to a transplant recipient, always investigate drug interactions.
- The combination of **allopurinol and azathioprine** should be avoided due to the risk of profound myelosuppression.
- CsA and tacrolimus are metabolized by cytochrome P450 (3A4). Therefore, CsA and tacrolimus levels are decreased by drugs that induce cytochrome P450 activity, such as rifampin, isoniazid, barbiturates, phenytoin, and carbamazepine. Conversely, CsA and tacrolimus levels are increased by drugs that compete for cytochrome P450, such as verapamil, diltiazem, nicardipine, azole antifungals, erythromycin, and clarithromycin. Similar effects are seen with sirolimus and everolimus.
- **Tacrolimus and CsA** should not be taken together because of the increased risk of severe nephrotoxicity.
- Lower doses of MPA should be used when either tacrolimus or sirolimus is taken concurrently.
- Concomitant administration of CsA and sirolimus may result in a twofold increase in sirolimus levels; to avoid this drug interaction, CsA and sirolimus should be dosed 4 hours apart.

18 Gastrointestinal Diseases

C. Prakash Gyawali and Amit Patel

Gastrointestinal Bleeding

GENERAL PRINCIPLES

Acute gastrointestinal (GI) bleeding is a common clinical problem that results in substantial morbidity and health care costs, especially when it develops in hospitalized patients (*Gut 2011;60:1327*).

- **Overt GI bleeding** is the passage of fresh or altered blood in emesis or stool.
- **Occult GI bleeding** refers to a positive fecal occult blood test (stool guaiac or fecal immunochemical test) or iron deficiency anemia without visible blood in the stool.
- **Obscure GI bleeding** consists of GI blood loss of unknown origin that persists or recurs after negative initial endoscopic evaluation (*Gastroenterology 2007;133:1697*).

DIAGNOSIS

Clinical Presentation

History

- Hematemesis, coffee-ground emesis, and/or aspiration of blood or coffee-ground material from a nasogastric (NG) tube indicate an upper GI source of blood loss.
- **Melena**, black sticky stool with a characteristic odor, usually suggests an upper GI source, although small bowel and right-sided colonic bleeds can also result in melena.
- Various shades of **bloody stool (hematochezia)** are seen with distal small bowel or colonic bleeding, depending on the rate of blood loss and colonic transit. Rapid upper GI bleeding can present with hematochezia, typically associated with hemodynamic compromise or circulatory shock.
- **Anorectal bleeding** usually results in bright red blood coating the exterior of formed stool associated with distal colonic symptoms (e.g., rectal urgency, straining, or pain with defecation).
- **Anemia** from blood loss can cause fatigue, weakness, abdominal pain, pallor, or dyspnea.
- Estimation of the amount of blood loss is often inaccurate. If the baseline hematocrit is known, the drop in hematocrit provides a rough estimate of blood loss. In general, lower GI bleeding causes less hemodynamic compromise than upper GI bleeding.
- **Coagulation abnormalities** can propagate bleeding from a preexisting lesion in the GI tract. Disorders of coagulation (e.g., liver disease, von Willebrand disease, vitamin K deficiency, and disseminated intravascular coagulation) can influence the course of GI bleeding (see Chapter 20, Disorders of Hemostasis and Thrombosis).
- **Medications** known to affect the coagulation process or platelet function include warfarin, heparin, low–molecular-weight heparin, aspirin, NSAIDs, thienopyridines (clopidogrel [Plavix], prasugrel [Effient], ticlopidine [Ticlid]), thrombolytic agents, glycoprotein IIb/IIIa receptor antagonists (abciximab [ReoPro], eptifibatide [Integrilin], tirofiban [Aggrastat]), direct thrombin inhibitors (argatroban, bivalirudin, dabigatran etexilate), and direct factor Xa inhibitors (rivaroxaban [Xarelto], apixaban).
- **NSAIDs and aspirin** can result in mucosal damage anywhere in the GI tract. Therefore, dual antiplatelet therapy (e.g., clopidogrel plus aspirin) or concomitant aspirin and anticoagulation with warfarin can escalate the risk for GI bleeding by both initiating and propagating bleeding.

Physical Examination
- **Color of stool.** Direct examination of spontaneously passed stool or on **digital rectal examination (DRE)** can help localize the level of bleeding. Moreover, DRE may identify anorectal abnormalities including anal fissures, which induce extreme discomfort during the DRE.
- Fresh blood on an **NG aspirate** may indicate ongoing upper GI bleeding requiring urgent endoscopic attention (*Gastrointest Endosc 2004;59:172*). The aspirate should be considered positive only if blood or dark particulate matter ("coffee grounds") is seen; **hemoccult testing of NG aspirate has no clinical utility**. A bleeding source in the duodenum can result in a negative NG aspirate. Gastric lavage with water or saline may be useful in assessing the activity and severity of upper GI bleeding and in clearing the stomach of blood and clots before endoscopy. After a diagnosis of upper GI bleeding is made, the NG tube can be removed in a stable patient.
- Constant monitoring or frequent assessment of vital signs is necessary early in the evaluation, as a sudden increase in pulse rate or decrease in blood pressure (BP) may suggest recurrent or ongoing blood loss.
- If the baseline BP and pulse are within normal limits, sitting the patient up and/or having the patient stand may result in **orthostatic hemodynamic changes** (drop in systolic BP of >20 mm Hg, rise in pulse rate of >10 bpm). Orthostatic changes are seen with loss of 10–20% of the circulatory volume; supine hypotension suggests a >20% loss. Hypotension with a systolic BP of <100 mm Hg or baseline tachycardia >100 bpm suggests significant hemodynamic compromise that requires urgent volume resuscitation (*N Engl J Med 2008;359:928*).

Diagnostic Testing

Laboratories
- Complete blood cell (CBC) count
- Coagulation parameters (international normalized ratio [INR], partial thromboplastin time [PTT])
- Blood group, cross-matching of two to four units of blood
- Comprehensive metabolic profile (creatinine, blood urea nitrogen, liver function tests)

Diagnostic Procedures
- **Endoscopy**
  - **Esophagogastroduodenoscopy (EGD)**, with high diagnostic accuracy and therapeutic capability, is the preferred investigative test in upper GI bleeding. Volume resuscitation or blood transfusion should precede endoscopy in hemodynamically unstable patients. Patients with ongoing bleeding or at risk for an adverse outcome (Table 18-1) benefit most from urgent EGD, while stable patients can be endoscoped electively during the hospitalization. IV erythromycin (infusion of 125–250 mg completed 30 minutes before EGD) empties the stomach of blood and clots and improves visibility for EGD (*Gastrointest Endosc 2011;73:245*). Second-look EGD after hemostasis has no proven benefit in reducing surgical intervention or overall mortality (*J Gastroenterol Hepatol 2010;25:8*).
  - **Colonoscopy** can be performed after a rapid bowel purge in clinically stable patients; the purge solution can be infused through an NG tube when not tolerated orally. While diagnostic yield is highest with colonoscopy performed within 24 hours of presentation, (*Am J Gastroenterol 2005;100:2395*), patient outcome does not necessarily improve (*Am J Gastroenterol 2010;105:2636*). Therapeutic colonoscopy, however, may reduce transfusion requirements, need for surgery, and length of hospital stay. All patients with acute lower GI bleeding from an unknown source should eventually undergo colonoscopy during the initial hospitalization, regardless of the initial mode of investigation.
  - **Anoscopy** may be useful in the detection of internal hemorrhoids and anal fissures but does not replace the need for colonoscopy.

TABLE 18-1	Rockall Score for Risk Stratification of Acute Upper Gastrointestinal (GI) Bleeding	

		Variable	Points
Complete Rockall Score	**Clinical Rockall Score**	Age	
		<60 yr	0
		60–79 yr	1
		≥80 yr	2
		Shock	
		Heart rate >100 bpm	1
		Systolic blood pressure <100 mm Hg	2
		Coexisting illness	
		Coronary artery disease, congestive heart failure, other major illness	2
		Renal failure, hepatic failure, metastatic cancer	3
		Endoscopic diagnosis	
		No finding, Mallory-Weiss tear	0
		Peptic ulcer, erosive disease, esophagitis	1
		Cancer of the upper GI tract	2
		Endoscopic stigmata of recent bleeding	
		Clean based ulcer, flat pigmented spot	0
		Blood in upper GI tract, active bleeding, visible vessel, clot	2

A clinical score of 0 or a complete score of 2 or less indicate low risk for rebleeding or death. Adapted from Gralnek et al. *N Engl J Med* 2008;359:928, with permission.

- ○ **Push enteroscopy** allows evaluation of the proximal small bowel beyond reach of a standard EGD, especially if no source is found on careful colonoscopy.
- ○ **Capsule endoscopy** is most useful after the upper gut and the colon have been thoroughly examined and the bleeding source is suspected in the small bowel (*Gastroenterology 2007;133:1697*). In overt obscure GI bleeding, capsule endoscopy has higher diagnostic yield with similar long-term outcomes when compared with angiography (*Am J Gastroenterol 2012;107:1370*). However, images cannot be viewed in real time, exact localization within the small bowel cannot be pinpointed, and therapy cannot be administered; consequently, improvements in diagnostic yield may not translate into better outcomes (*Gastroenterology 2010;138:1673*).
- ○ **Single- and double-balloon enteroscopy** allows visualization of most of the small bowel through either an oral or anal approach. Balloons at the endoscope tip and overtube can be consecutively inflated and deflated to facilitate deep insertion into the small bowel.
- ○ **Intraoperative enteroscopy** may assist endoscopic therapy or surgical resection of an actively bleeding source in the small bowel.

- **CT enteroclysis** has value when both conventional endoscopy and capsule endoscopy are nondiagnostic in obscure-overt bleeding with prominent anemia (*Gastrointest Endosc 2011;73:1002*).
- **Tagged red blood cell (RBC) scanning** involves labeling RBCs with technetium-99m that may extravasate into the bowel lumen with active bleeding, detected as pooling of the radioactive tracer on gamma camera scanning, to identify the potential bleeding site. **CT angiography** may have similar benefit in localizing bleeding prior to catheter angiography (*J Vasc Interv Radiol 2010;21:848*). These tests are particularly useful in unstable active bleeding precluding urgent colonoscopy.
- **Arteriography** demonstrates extravasation of the dye into the intestine when bleeding rates exceed 0.5 mL/min, thereby localizing bleeding. Arteriography is often performed after bleeding is initially localized by other means. Selective cannulation and infusion of vasopressin vasoconstrict the bleeding vessel; moreover, the vessel can be embolized.

TREATMENT

- **Restoration of intravascular volume.** Two large-bore (16- to 18-gauge) IV lines or a central venous line should be urgently placed to provide IV fluid resuscitation. Circulatory shock may require volume administration using pressure infusion devices, guided by the patient's condition and degree of volume loss (*N Engl J Med 2008;359:928*). **Packed RBC transfusion** should be used for volume replacement whenever possible; O-negative blood or simultaneous multiple-unit transfusions may be indicated if bleeding is massive. Transfusion should be continued until hemodynamic stability is achieved and the hematocrit reaches ≥25–30%. Overcorrection of volume and blood counts does not necessarily improve outcome and may even be detrimental in variceal bleeding (*Aliment Pharmacol Ther 2010;32:215*).
- **Oxygen administration.** Supplemental oxygen enhances the oxygen-carrying capacity of blood and should be universally administered in acute GI bleeding.
- **Correction of coagulopathy.** Coagulopathy (INR ≥1.5) increases morbidity and mortality in acute GI bleeding (*Aliment Pharmacol Ther 2011;33:1010*) and should be corrected if possible. Platelet infusion may be indicated when the platelet count is <50,000/μL.
- **Endotracheal intubation** protects the airway and prevents aspiration in obtunded patients with massive hematemesis and in active variceal bleeding.
- **Risk stratification.** Validated risk stratification tools, such as the Rockall and Glasgow-Blatchford scores, are available to identify patients at highest risk for an adverse outcome (*Aliment Pharmacol Ther 2011;34:470*). The Rockall score (see Table 18-1) has a *clinical* component that is rapidly calculated at presentation and a *complete* final score that takes endoscopic findings into account (*Gut 1996;38:316*).

Medications

- **Nonvariceal upper GI bleeding.** Pre-endoscopic IV **proton pump inhibitors** (PPIs) (40 mg IV bolus bid or 80 mg IV bolus followed by 8 mg/h continuous infusion) impact the proportion of patients who have high-risk stigmata of hemorrhage and reduce need for endoscopic therapy in bleeding peptic ulcer disease (PUD) (*Am J Gastroenterol 2012;10:345*). However, meta-analysis does not show benefits in rebleeding, surgical intervention, or mortality between IV infusions and IV bolus therapy in unselected cases (*Arch Intern Med 2010;170:751*). PPI therapy, IV or oral (e.g., omeprazole 40 mg PO bid or equivalent), is more effective than IV histamine-2 receptor antagonist (H$_2$RA) therapy (*Am J Gastroenterol 2014;109:1005*).
- **Variceal bleeding. Octreotide** (an octapeptide that mimics endogenous somatostatin) infusion acutely reduces portal pressures and controls variceal bleeding, improving the

diagnostic yield and therapeutic success of subsequent endoscopy. Octreotide should be initiated immediately (50- to 100-μg bolus, followed by infusion at 25–50 μg/h) and continued for 3–5 days after EGD if variceal hemorrhage is confirmed (*Gastrointest Endosc 2014;80:221*). Both **terlipressin** and **octreotide** achieve similar hemostatic effects with comparable safety to octreotide as adjuvants to endoscopic therapy in variceal bleeding (*Hepatology 2014;60:954*; *Aliment Pharmacol Ther 2012;35:1267*). A 7-day course of antibiotic prophylaxis with an IV third-generation cephalosporin (ceftriaxone) is recommended (see Chapter 19, Liver Diseases) in any patient with cirrhosis and variceal bleeding; a fluoroquinolone is an alternative (*Hepatology 2009;49:2087*).

- **Thalidomide** may be an effective approach for refractory chronic bleeding from GI vascular malformations (*Gastroenterology 2011;141:1629*).

Other Nonpharmacologic Therapies

- **Endoscopic therapy**
  ○ **Therapeutic endoscopy** offers the advantage of endoscopic hemostasis. Therefore, EGD should be performed early in acute upper GI bleeding (within 12–24 hours).
  ○ **Variceal ligation** or **banding** is the endoscopic therapy of choice for esophageal varices, with endotracheal intubation for airway protection if bleeding is massive and the patient is obtunded (*Gastrointest Endosc 2014;80:221*). Variceal banding has value in both primary and secondary prophylaxis of variceal bleeding, with benefits similar to that from β-blocker therapy alone (*Gastroenterology 2010;139:1238*). Complications include superficial ulceration, dysphagia, and transient chest discomfort.
  ○ **Sclerotherapy** is also effective but is used mostly when variceal banding is not technically feasible.
  ○ Endoscopic injection of **cyanoacrylate (glue)** is more effective than β-blocker therapy in primary and secondary prophylaxis of gastric variceal bleeding, but not esophageal variceal bleeding (*Gut 2010;59:729*).
- **Transjugular intrahepatic portosystemic shunt (TIPS)** is a radiologic procedure wherein an expandable metal stent is deployed between the hepatic veins and the portal vein to reduce portal venous pressure in refractory esophageal and/or gastric variceal bleeding from portal hypertension (*Hepatology 2007;46:922*). Early TIPS may be of value in reducing treatment failure and mortality in acute variceal bleeding (*N Engl J Med 2010;362:2370*). Encephalopathy may occur in up to 25% of patients and is treated medically (see Chapter 19, Liver Diseases). Assessment with duplex Doppler ultrasound for TIPS stenosis is recommended if variceal bleeding recurs or if esophageal or gastric varices redevelop.
- **Balloon-occluded retrograde transvenous obliteration (BRTO)** is a newer treatment option for gastric variceal bleeding, where gastric varices are obliterated through a gastrorenal shunt (*J Gastroenterol Hepatol 2009;24:372*). BRTO appears to be equivalent to TIPS for short-term management of bleeding gastric varices (*J Vasc Interv Radiol 2014;25:355*).

Surgical Management

- **Emergent total colectomy** may rarely be required for massive, unlocalized, colonic bleeding; this should be preceded by EGD to rule out a rapidly bleeding upper source whenever possible. Certain lesions (e.g., neoplasia, Meckel diverticulum) require surgical resection for a cure.
- **Total or partial colectomy** may be required for ongoing or recurrent diverticular bleeding.
- **Splenectomy** is curative in bleeding gastric varices from splenic vein thrombosis.
- **Shunt surgery** (portacaval or distal splenorenal shunt) is now rarely performed; this can be considered in patients with good hepatic reserve.

SPECIAL CONSIDERATIONS

Cardiac Patients and Gastrointestinal Bleeding

- In acute coronary syndromes (ACS), GI bleeding increases 30-day all-cause mortality rates by a factor of almost 5 (*J Am Coll Cardiol 2009;29:1293*). Antiplatelet and anticoagulant therapy, especially dual antiplatelet therapy (e.g., aspirin plus clopidogrel), are significant risk factors. Among patients on low-dose aspirin with history of PUD bleeding, continuous aspirin therapy increases the risk for recurrent PUD bleeding (*Ann Intern Med 2010;152:1*).
- **PPI prophylaxis** decreases the risk of GI bleeding, without significant effects on the incidence of hospital-acquired pneumonia or 30-day mortality (*Aliment Pharmacol Ther 2011;34:519*).
- Despite concerns that PPIs competitively inhibit the cytochrome P450 enzyme that activates clopidogrel, randomized controlled trials have not substantiated higher vascular events with concurrent use of clopidogrel and PPI (*N Engl J Med 2010;11:363; Heart 2013;99:520*). Among PPIs, pantoprazole may have the least pharmacodynamic interaction with clopidogrel (*Eur J Gastroenterol Hepatol 2011;23:396*).
- **Left ventricular assist devices (LVADs),** used in end-stage heart failure, are associated with GI bleeding rates significantly higher than those seen with dual antiplatelet therapy or anticoagulation (*Clin Gastroenterol Hepatol 2014;12:1461*). Bleeding is predominantly overt and from upper GI sources, especially angiodysplastic lesions, making EGD or push enteroscopy the initial investigation of choice (*Gastrointest Endosc 2012;75:973*).

Dysphagia and Odynophagia

GENERAL PRINCIPLES

Definition

- **Oropharyngeal dysphagia** consists of difficulty in transferring food from the mouth to the esophagus, often associated with nasopharyngeal regurgitation and aspiration. Typical causes include neuromuscular or structural disorders involving the pharynx and proximal esophagus (*Gastroenterology 1999;116:452*).
- **Esophageal dysphagia** is the sensation of impairment in passage of food down the tubular esophagus. Potential etiologies include obstructive processes (such as webs, rings, neoplasia) or esophageal motor disorders (*Gastroenterology 1999;117:233*).
- **Odynophagia** is pain on swallowing food and fluids and may indicate the presence of esophagitis, particularly infectious esophagitis or pill esophagitis.

DIAGNOSIS

Oropharyngeal Dysphagia

- Assessment is initiated with a detailed neurologic exam. **Barium videofluoroscopy (modified barium swallow)** evaluates the oropharyngeal swallow mechanism and may identify laryngeal penetration.
- Ear, nose, and throat exam; flexible nasal endoscopy; and imaging studies may identify structural etiologies.
- Laboratory tests for polymyositis, myasthenia gravis, and other neuromuscular disorders should be considered in the absence of clear neurologic or structural etiologies.

Esophageal Dysphagia

- **EGD** is the initial test of choice, as it provides information on mucosal abnormalities, allows tissue sampling (to evaluate for esophageal eosinophilia, for instance), and offers the option of dilation, which should be performed for most esophageal strictures (*Gastrointest Endosc 2014;79:191*).

- **Barium swallow** has value in defining anatomy, especially subtle rings and strictures, which may only be seen with a barium pill or a solid barium bolus.
- Acute esophageal obstruction is best investigated with endoscopy. Barium studies should not be performed when esophageal obstruction is expected, as it may take several days for barium to clear, thereby delaying endoscopy. If a contrast study is needed, water-soluble contrast should be used in this setting.
- **Esophageal manometry,** preferably **high-resolution manometry (HRM)**, should be performed when other studies are normal or suggest an esophageal motility disorder. The image-based paradigm of Clouse plots on HRM provide several advantages over conventional manometry, including simplified testing procedures, easier analysis, and improved diagnostic utility (*Gastrointest Endosc Clin N Am 2014;24:527*).

TREATMENT

- Modification of diet and swallowing maneuvers may benefit patients with dysphagia, especially oropharyngeal dysphagia. Patients with dysphagia are typically advised to chew their food well and eat foods of soft consistencies.
- Enteral feeding through a gastrostomy tube is indicated in patients with frank tracheal aspiration on attempted swallowing.
- Endoscopic retrieval of an obstructing food bolus relieves acute dysphagia.
- Nutrition needs to be addressed in patients with prolonged dysphagia causing weight loss.

Medications

- Mucosal inflammation from reflux disease can be treated with acid suppression.
- Odynophagia generally responds to specific therapy when the cause is identified (e.g., PPIs for reflux disease, antimicrobial agents for infectious esophagitis). Viscous lidocaine swish-and-swallow solutions may afford symptomatic relief.
- Anticholinergic medication (e.g., transdermal scopolamine) helps drooling of saliva.
- **Glucagon** (2–4 mg IV bolus) or sublingual **nitroglycerin** can be attempted in acute food impaction, but meat tenderizer should not be administered.

Other Nonpharmacologic Therapies

- Esophageal dilation is performed for anatomic narrowings. Empiric bougie dilation performed when a defined narrowing is not identified may also provide symptomatic benefit.
- Pneumatic dilation of the lower esophageal sphincter (LES) is sometimes performed for achalasia (see Esophageal Motor Disorders section). Botulinum toxin injections into the LES provide temporary symptom relief in achalasia and in errors of LES relaxation (*Gastrointest Endosc 2014;79:191*).
- Esophageal stent placement can alleviate dysphagia in inoperable neoplasia.

Nausea and Vomiting

GENERAL PRINCIPLES

- Nausea and vomiting may result from side effects of medications, systemic illnesses, central nervous system (CNS) disorders, and primary GI disorders.
- Vomiting that occurs during or immediately after a meal can result from acute pyloric stenosis (e.g., pyloric channel ulcer) or from functional disorders, while vomiting within

30–60 minutes after a meal may suggest gastric or duodenal pathology. Delayed vomiting after a meal with undigested food from a previous meal can suggest gastric outlet obstruction or gastroparesis.
- Symptoms of gastroparesis may be indistinguishable from chronic functional nausea and vomiting with normal gastric emptying (*Clin Gastroenterol Hepatol 2011;9:567*).

DIAGNOSIS

- **Bowel obstruction and pregnancy should be ruled out.**
- **Medications** should be carefully scrutinized for potential offenders, and systemic illnesses (acute and chronic) should be evaluated as etiologies or contributing factors.
- Endoscopy and/or imaging should be considered in the setting of nonresolving or "red flag" symptoms, such as hematemesis or weight loss.

TREATMENT

- Correction of fluid and electrolyte imbalances is an important supportive measure.
- Oral intake should be limited to clear liquids, if tolerated. Many patients with self-limited illnesses require no further therapy.
- NG decompression may be required for patients with bowel obstruction or protracted nausea and vomiting of any etiology.
- Patients with protracted nausea and vomiting may require enteral feeding through jejunal tubes or, rarely, even total parenteral nutrition (TPN).

Medications

Empiric pharmacotherapy is often initiated while investigation is in progress or when the etiology is thought to be self-limited.
- **Phenothiazines and related agents.** Prochlorperazine (Compazine), 5–10 mg PO tid–qid, 10 mg IM or IV q6h, or 25 mg PR bid, and promethazine (Phenergan), 12.5–25.0 mg PO, IM, or PR q4–6h, may be effective. Drowsiness is a common side effect, and acute dystonic reactions or other extrapyramidal effects may occur.
- **Dopamine antagonists** include metoclopramide (10 mg PO 30 minutes before meals and at bedtime, or 10 mg IV PRN), a prokinetic agent that also has central antiemetic effects. Drowsiness and extrapyramidal reactions may occur, and a warning has been issued by the U.S. Food and Drug Administration (FDA) regarding the risk of permanent **tardive dyskinesia** with high-dose and/or long-term use (*Aliment Pharmacol Ther 2010;31:11*). Tachyphylaxis may limit long-term efficacy. Domperidone is an alternate agent that does not cross the blood–brain barrier and therefore has no CNS side effects; however, it is not uniformly available.
- **Antihistaminic agents** are most useful for nausea and vomiting related to motion sickness but may also be useful for other causes. Agents include diphenhydramine (Benadryl, 25–50 mg PO q6–8h or 10–50 mg IV q2–4h), dimenhydrinate (Dramamine, 50–100 mg PO or IV q4–6h), and meclizine (Antivert, 12.5–25.0 mg 1 hour before travel).
- **Serotonin 5-hydroxytryptamine-3 (5-HT$_3$) receptor antagonists. Ondansetron** (Zofran, 0.15 mg/kg IV q4h for three doses or 32 mg IV infused over 15 minutes beginning 30 minutes before chemotherapy) is effective in chemotherapy-associated emesis. It can also be used in emesis that is refractory to other medications (4–8 mg PO or IV up to q8h), especially the sublingual formulation.
- **Neurokinin-1 (NK-1) receptor antagonist. Aprepitant** (Emend, 125 mg PO day 1, 80 mg PO days 2 and 3) is an alternative agent intended for chemotherapy-induced nausea and vomiting.

Diarrhea

GENERAL PRINCIPLES

- **Acute diarrhea** consists of the abrupt onset of increased frequency and/or fluidity of bowel movements. Infectious agents, toxins, and drugs are the major causes of acute diarrhea. In hospitalized patients, pseudomembranous colitis, antibiotic- or drug-associated diarrhea, and fecal impaction should be considered (*Gastroenterology 2004; 127:287*).
- **Chronic diarrhea** consists of passage of loose stools with or without increased stool frequency for more than 4 weeks.

DIAGNOSIS

- Most acute infectious diarrheal illnesses last less than 24 hours and could be viral in etiology; therefore, stool studies are unnecessary in short episodes without fever, dehydration, or presence of blood or pus in the stool (*N Engl J Med 2004;350:38*).
- Stool cultures, *Clostridium difficile* toxin assay, ova and parasite examinations, and sigmoidoscopy may be warranted in patients with severe, prolonged, or atypical symptoms.
- The **fecal osmotic gap** can be calculated in patients with chronic diarrhea and voluminous watery stools as follows: $290 - 2(\text{stool } [Na^+] + \text{stool } [K^+])$. The osmotic gap is **<50 mOsm/kg in secretory diarrhea** but **>125 mOsm/kg in osmotic diarrhea**.
- A positive fecal occult blood test or fecal leukocyte test suggests inflammatory diarrhea.
- **Steatorrhea** is traditionally diagnosed by demonstration of fat excretion in stool of >7 g/d in a 72-hour stool collection while the patient is on a 100-g/d fat diet. Sudan staining of a stool specimen is an alternate test; >100 fat globules per high-power field (HPF) is abnormal.
- Laxative screening should be considered when chronic diarrhea remains undiagnosed.

Clinical Presentation

- **Acute diarrhea**
  - **Viral enteritis** and **bacterial infections** with *Escherichia coli* and *Shigella*, *Salmonella*, *Campylobacter*, and *Yersinia* spp. constitute the most common causes.
  - **Pseudomembranous colitis** is usually seen in the setting of antimicrobial therapy and is caused by toxins produced by *C. difficile* (*Am J Gastroenterol 2013;108:478*).
  - **Giardiasis** is confirmed by identification of *Giardia lamblia* trophozoites in the stool, in duodenal aspirate, or in small bowel biopsy specimens. A stool immunofluorescence assay is also available for rapid diagnosis.
  - **Amebiasis** may cause acute diarrhea, especially in travelers to areas with poor sanitation and in homosexual men. Stool examination for trophozoites or cysts of *Entamoeba histolytica* or a serum antibody test confirms the diagnosis.
  - **Medications** that can cause acute diarrhea include laxatives, antacids, cardiac medications (e.g., digitalis, quinidine), colchicine, and antimicrobial agents; symptoms typically respond to discontinuation.
  - **Graft-versus-host disease** should be considered when diarrhea develops after organ transplantation, especially bone marrow transplantation; **sigmoidoscopy with biopsies** should be pursued to confirm this diagnosis (*Aliment Pharmacol Ther 2013;38:955*).
- **Chronic diarrhea.** After a careful history, a thorough physical examination, and routine laboratory tests, chronic diarrhea can typically be classified into one of the following categories: watery diarrhea (secretory or osmotic), inflammatory diarrhea, or fatty diarrhea (steatorrhea) (*J Gastroenterol Hepatol 2014;29:6*).

TREATMENT

- Adequate hydration, including IV hydration in severe cases, represents an essential initial step in the therapy of diarrheal disease.
- Antibiotic-associated diarrhea and *C. difficile* infections can be prevented by restricting high-risk antibiotics and using antibiotics based on sensitivity analysis.
- Symptomatic therapy is useful in simple self-limiting GI infections where diarrhea is frequent or troublesome, while diagnostic workup is in progress, when specific management fails to improve symptoms, and/or when a specific etiology is not identified.
  ○ **Loperamide**, **opiates** (tincture of opium, belladonna, and opium capsules), and **anticholinergic agents** (diphenoxylate and atropine [Lomotil]) are the most effective non-specific antidiarrheal agents.
  ○ **Pectin** and **kaolin** preparations (bind toxins) and **bismuth subsalicylate** (antibacterial properties) are also useful in symptomatic therapy of acute diarrhea.
  ○ **Bile acid–binding resins** (e.g., cholestyramine) are beneficial in bile acid–induced diarrhea.
  ○ **Octreotide** is useful in hormone-mediated secretory diarrhea but can also be of benefit in refractory diarrhea.

Medications

- **Empiric antibiotic therapy** is only recommended in patients with moderate-to-severe disease and associated systemic symptoms while awaiting stool cultures. Antibiotics can increase the possibility of hemolytic-uremic syndrome associated with Shiga toxin–producing *E. coli* infections (*E. coli* O157:H7), especially in children and the elderly (*N Engl J Med 2000;342:1930*).
- Oral **metronidazole** is the treatment of choice for mild to moderate pseudomembranous colitis, whereas oral **vancomycin** can be used for resistant cases or intolerance to metronidazole (*Am J Gastroenterol 2013;108:478*). **Fidaxomicin** and **fecal microbiota transplant** represent newer treatment options (*Am J Gastroenterol 2014;109:1065*; see Chapter 14, Treatment of Infectious Diseases).
- Symptomatic amebiasis is treated with **metronidazole**, followed by **paromomycin** or **iodoquinol** to eliminate cysts.
- Therapy for giardiasis consists of metronidazole or tinidazole, with quinacrine representing an alternative agent.

SPECIAL CONSIDERATIONS

- **Opportunistic agents**, including *Cryptosporidium*, *Microsporidium*, cytomegalovirus (CMV), *Mycobacterium avium* complex (MAC), and *Mycobacterium tuberculosis*, may cause **diarrhea in patients with advanced HIV** (CD4 counts <50 cells/μL). However, *C. difficile* may be the most commonly identified bacterial pathogen (*Gut 2008;57:861*).
- Other causes of diarrhea in this population include venereal infections (syphilis, gonorrhea, chlamydia, herpes simplex virus [HSV]) as well as other nonvenereal infections (amebiasis, giardiasis, salmonellosis, shigellosis). Intestinal lymphoma and Kaposi sarcoma can also cause diarrhea.
- Stool studies (ova and parasites, culture), endoscopic biopsies, and serologic testing may assist in diagnosis. Management consists of specific therapy if pathogens are identified; symptomatic measures may be of benefit in idiopathic cases (*Gastroenterol Clin North Am 2012;41:677*).

Constipation

GENERAL PRINCIPLES

Definition

Constipation consists of infrequent (and frequently incomplete) bowel movements, sometimes associated with straining and passage of pellet-like stools.

Etiology

- Recent changes in bowel habits may suggest an organic cause, whereas long-standing constipation is more likely to be functional.
- **Medications** (e.g., calcium channel blockers, opiates, anticholinergics, iron supplements, barium sulfate) and systemic diseases (e.g., diabetes mellitus, hypothyroidism, systemic sclerosis, myotonic dystrophy) may contribute.
- Female gender, older age, lack of exercise, low caloric intake, low-fiber diet, and disorders that cause pain on defecation (e.g., anal fissures, thrombosed external hemorrhoids) are other risk factors (*Am Fam Physician 2011;84:299*).

DIAGNOSIS

- Colonoscopy and barium studies help rule out structural disease and may be particularly important in individuals >50 years without prior colorectal cancer screening or with alarm features such as anemia, blood in the stool, or new-onset symptoms (*Gastroenterology 2013;144:211*).
- Colonic transit studies, anorectal manometry, and defecography are reserved for resistant cases without a structural explanation after initial workup.

TREATMENT

- Regular exercise and adequate fluid intake are nonspecific measures.
- Increase in **dietary fiber** intake to 20–30 g/d may have value. However, fecal impactions should be resolved before fiber supplementation is initiated.

Medications

- **Laxatives**
  - **Emollient laxatives** such as docusate sodium, 50–200 mg PO daily, and docusate calcium, 240 mg PO daily, allow water and fat to penetrate the fecal mass. Mineral oil (15–45 mL PO q6–8h) can be given orally or by enema.
  - **Stimulant cathartics** such as castor oil, 15 mL PO, stimulate intestinal secretion and increase intestinal motility. Anthraquinones (cascara, 5 mL PO daily; senna, one tablet PO daily to qid) stimulate the colon by increasing fluid and water accumulation in the proximal colon. Bisacodyl (10–15 mg PO at bedtime, 10-mg rectal suppositories) stimulates colonic peristalsis, resulting in effective and well-tolerated treatment for chronic constipation (*Clin Gastroenterol Hepatol 2011;9:577*).
  - **Osmotic cathartics** include nonabsorbable salts or carbohydrates that cause water retention in the lumen of the colon. Magnesium salts include milk of magnesia (15–30 mL q8–12h) and magnesium citrate (200 mL PO), to be avoided in renal failure. Lactulose (15–30 mL PO bid–qid) can cause bloating as a side effect.
  - **Lubiprostone** (8–24 μg PO bid) is a selective intestinal chloride channel activator, causing movement of fluid into the bowel lumen and stimulating peristalsis, thus facilitating spontaneous bowel movements in chronic idiopathic constipation (*Clin Gastroenterol Hepatol 2015;13(2):29*).

- ○ **Linaclotide** (145–290 μg PO qday) is an agonist of the guanylate cyclase C receptor and also causes movement of fluid into the intestinal lumen, thereby improving symptoms of constipation (*N Engl J Med 2011;365:567*).
- **Enemas.** Sodium biphosphate (Fleet) enemas can be used for mild-to-moderate constipation and for bowel cleansing before sigmoidoscopy; these should be avoided in renal failure. Tap water enemas (1 L) are also useful. Oil-based enemas (cottonseed, Colace, hypaque) can be used in refractory constipation.
- **Polyethylene glycol** in powder form (MiraLax, 17 g PO daily to bid) can be used regularly or intermittently for the treatment of constipation.
- **Subcutaneous methylnaltrexone**, a selective peripherally acting μ-opioid receptor antagonist, is effective for rapid relief of opioid-induced constipation (*Am J Gastroenterol 2013;108:1566*; *N Engl J Med 2008;358:2332*). Prucalopride is approved in Europe for chronic constipation (*Aliment Pharmacol Ther 2010;32:1113*).
- **Bowel-cleansing agents.** Patients should be placed on a clear liquid diet the previous day and kept nothing by mouth (NPO) for 6 hours or overnight prior to colonoscopy. Patients may experience mild abdominal discomfort, nausea, and vomiting with the bowel preparation.
  - ○ An iso-osmotic **polyethylene glycol solution** (PEG, GoLYTELY, or NuLYTELY, 1 gallon, administered at a rate of 8 oz every 10 minutes) is commonly used as a bowel-cleansing agent before colonoscopy. Lower volume preparations, such as PEG (2 L or 0.5 gallon) with ascorbic acid or other laxatives, are alternatives (*Aliment Pharmacol Ther 2010;32:637*).

    Nonabsorbable phosphate (Fleet phosphosoda, 20–45 mL with 10–24 oz liquid, taken the day before and morning of the procedure), a hyperosmotic solution, draws fluid into the gut lumen and produces bowel movements in 0.5–6.0 hours. It is also available in pill form (Visicol or OsmoPrep, 32–40 tablets, taken at the rate of 3–4 tablets every 15 min with 8 oz fluid). Phosphosoda can result in severe dehydration, hyperphosphatemia, hypocalcemia, hypokalemia, hypernatremia, and acidosis. A dreaded rare complication is **acute phosphate nephropathy**, where calcium phosphate deposits cause irreversible dysfunction of renal tubules resulting in renal failure. Consequently, phosphosoda is only used in limited instances.
  - ○ **Split preparations.** Proximity of bowel preparation to procedure time improves effectiveness of cleansing and visualization during the procedure. Therefore, splitting bowel preparation into two doses may be useful, with one dose administered the evening prior and the second dose administered the morning of the procedure (*Am J Gastroenterol 2012;107:1036*; *Am J Gastroenterol 2010;105:1319*).
  - ○ **Two-day bowel preparation** is sometimes indicated in elderly or debilitated individuals when conventional bowel preparation is contraindicated, not tolerated, or ineffective. This consists of magnesium citrate (120–300 mL PO) administered on two consecutive days while the patient remains on a clear liquid diet; bisacodyl (30 mg PO or 10-mg suppository) is administered on both days.
  - ○ **Tap water enemas** (1-L volume) can cleanse the distal colon when colonoscopy is indicated in patients with proximal bowel obstruction.
- Other options: **Biofeedback therapy** and **sacral nerve stimulation** can be effective for idiopathic constipation resistant to medical treatment (*Gut 2010;59:333*).

LUMINAL GASTROINTESTINAL DISORDERS

Gastroesophageal Reflux Disease

GENERAL PRINCIPLES

Definition

Gastroesophageal reflux disease (GERD) is defined as symptoms and/or complications resulting from reflux of gastric contents into the esophagus and more proximal structures.

DIAGNOSIS

Clinical Presentation

* Typical esophageal symptoms of GERD include **heartburn** and **regurgitation**. GERD can also present as **chest pain**, where an important priority is to exclude a cardiac source before initiating a GI evaluation (*Am J Gastroenterol 2013;108:308*).
* **Extraesophageal manifestations** can include cough, laryngitis, asthma, and dental erosions.
* Symptom response to a therapeutic trial of PPIs can be diagnostic, but a negative response does not exclude GERD (*Gastroenterology 2008;135:1392*).

Differential Diagnosis

Other disorders that can result in esophagitis include:

* **Eosinophilic esophagitis (EoE)**, characterized by eosinophilic infiltration of esophageal mucosa, is increasingly recognized as an etiology for foregut symptoms.
  * Atopy (allergic rhinitis, eczema, asthma) is common, and food allergens may trigger the process. Transit symptoms (dysphagia) are prominent, but symptoms can also mimic GERD.
  * Common EGD findings include furrows, luminal narrowing, corrugations, and whitish plaques in the esophageal mucosa. The diagnosis of EoE is a clinicopathologic one, consisting of (a) symptoms related to esophageal dysfunction (such as dysphagia or food impaction), (b) ≥15 eosinophils per HPF on esophageal biopsies, and (c) exclusion of secondary causes of esophageal eosinophilia (such as GERD). Typically, a 2-month course of PPI bid should be given and followed by a repeat EGD with esophageal biopsies to rule out **PPI-responsive esophageal eosinophilia** and confirm the diagnosis of EoE (*Am J Gastroenterol 2013;108:679*).
  * First-line therapy for EoE includes **topical steroids** (swallowed fluticasone, 880–1760 μg/d in two to four divided doses, or swallowed budesonide, 2 mg/d in two to four divided doses); prednisone is an alternate option if topical steroids are ineffective (*Gastroenterology 2014;147:324*). Food allergen testing can be considered, but the yield is typically low. Regardless, elimination of dietary allergens is appropriate when identified. Concomitant GERD requires PPI therapy. Patients who do not respond to topical steroids may benefit from longer courses or higher doses of topical steroids, systemic steroids, elimination diet trials, or cautious esophageal dilation.
* **Infectious esophagitis** typically presents with dysphagia or odynophagia and is seen most often in immunocompromised states (AIDS, organ transplant recipients), esophageal stasis (abnormal motility [e.g., achalasia, scleroderma], mechanical obstruction [e.g., strictures]), malignancy, diabetes mellitus, and antibiotic use; however, it can rarely occur in the normal healthy host. The presence of typical oral lesions (thrush, herpetic vesicles) may suggest an etiologic agent. The usual presenting symptoms are dysphagia and odynophagia.
  * *Candida* **esophagitis** is the most common esophageal infection and typically occurs in the setting of esophageal stasis, impaired cell-mediated immunity from immunosuppressive therapy (e.g., with steroids or cytotoxic agents), malignancies, or AIDS. Endoscopic visualization of typical whitish plaques has near 100% sensitivity for diagnosis. Empiric antifungal agents are appropriate when concurrent oropharyngeal thrush is present, reserving endoscopy for nonresponse to therapy. **Fluconazole** 100–200 mg/d or **itraconazole** 200 mg/d for 14–21 days is recommended as initial therapy for *Candida* esophagitis; nystatin (100,000 units/mL, 5 mL tid for 3 weeks) and clotrimazole troches (10 mg four to five times a day for 2 weeks) are alternatives for oropharyngeal candidiasis. For infections refractory to azoles, a short course of parenteral **amphotericin B** (0.3–0.5 mg/kg/d) can be considered (*Best Pract Res Clin Gastroenterol 2008;22:639*).

- ○ **HSV esophagitis** is characterized by small vesicles and well-circumscribed ulcers on endoscopy and typical giant cells on histopathology. Viral antigen or DNA can be identified by immunofluorescent antibodies. Treatment consists of **acyclovir** 400–800 mg PO five times a day for 14–21 days or 5 mg/kg IV q8h for 7–14 days. **Famciclovir** and **valacyclovir** are alternate agents. The condition is usually self-limited in immunocompetent hosts (*Curr Opin Gastroenterol 2008;24:496*).
- ○ **CMV esophagitis**, which occurs almost exclusively in immunocompromised hosts, can cause erosions or frank ulcerations. **Ganciclovir** 5 mg/kg IV q12h or **foscarnet** 90 mg/kg IV q12h for 3–6 weeks can be used as initial therapy. Oral **valganciclovir** may also be effective.
- ○ Symptomatic relief can be achieved with 2% viscous **lidocaine** swish and swallow (15 mL PO q3–4h PRN) or **sucralfate** slurry (1 g PO qid).
- **Chemical esophagitis**
  - ○ Ingestion of caustic agents (alkalis, acids) or medications such as oral potassium, doxycycline, quinidine, iron, NSAIDs, aspirin, and bisphosphonates can result in mucosal irritation and damage.
  - ○ With caustic ingestions, cautious early EGD can evaluate the extent and degree of mucosal damage, and CT can rule out transmural esophageal necrosis in the setting of mucosal necrosis (*Best Pract Res Clin Gastroenterol 2013;27:679*).
  - ○ The offending medication should be discontinued if possible. Mucosal coating agents (sucralfate) and acid suppressive agents may help. A second caustic agent to neutralize the first is contraindicated.

Diagnostic Testing

- **Endoscopy** with biopsies is primarily indicated for avoiding misdiagnosis of alternate causes of esophageal symptoms (e.g., EoE), identification of complications, and evaluation of treatment failures. **Alarm symptoms** of dysphagia, odynophagia, early satiety, weight loss, or bleeding should prompt endoscopy (*N Engl J Med 2008;359:1700*).
- **Ambulatory pH or pH impedance monitoring** can be used to quantify esophageal acid exposure and reflux events and/or to assess symptom–reflux correlation in patients with ongoing symptoms despite acid suppression (especially if endoscopy is negative) or those with atypical symptoms. pH impedance testing detects all reflux events regardless of pH and is best performed off PPI therapy to increase yield; abnormal studies can predict symptomatic response to medical or surgical antireflux therapy (*Clin Gastroenterol Hepatol 2015;13(5):884*).
- **Esophageal manometry**, particularly HRM, may identify motor processes contributing to refractory symptoms.

TREATMENT

Medications

- Intermittent or prophylactic over-the-counter **antacids**, **H₂RAs**, and **PPIs** are effective with mild or intermittent symptoms.
- **PPIs** are more effective than standard-dose H₂RA and placebo in symptom relief and endoscopic healing of GERD. Modest gain is achieved by doubling the PPI dose in severe esophagitis or persistent symptoms. Continuous long-term PPI therapy is effective in maintaining remission of GERD symptoms, but the dose should be decreased after 8–12 weeks to the lowest dose that achieves symptom relief (*N Engl J Med 2008;359:1700*). Abdominal pain, headache, and diarrhea are common side effects. Long-term PPI use has been associated with bone demineralization, enteric infections, community-acquired pneumonia, and reduced circulating levels of vitamin B_{12} in observational studies, but benefits of PPI therapy continue to outweigh risks.

TABLE 18-2	Dosage of Acid-Suppressive Agents		
Medication Therapy	**Peptic Ulcer Disease**	**GERD**	**Parenteral**
Cimetidine[a]	300 mg qid 400 mg bid 800 mg at bedtime	400 mg qid 800 mg bid	300 mg q6h
Ranitidine[a]	150 mg bid 300 mg at bedtime	150–300 mg bid–qid	50 mg q8h
Famotidine[a]	20 mg bid 40 mg at bedtime	20–40 mg bid	20 mg q12h
Nizatidine[a]	150 mg bid 300 mg at bedtime	150 mg bid	
Omeprazole	20 mg daily	20–40 mg daily–bid	
Esomeprazole	40 mg daily	20–40 mg daily–bid	20–40 mg q24h
Lansoprazole	15–30 mg daily	15–30 mg daily–bid	30 mg q12–24h
Dexlansoprazole		30–60 mg daily	
Pantoprazole	20 mg daily	20–40 mg daily–bid	40 mg q12–24h or 80 mg IV, then 8 mg/h infusion

GERD, gastroesophageal reflux disease.
[a]Dosage adjustment required in renal insufficiency.

- Standard doses of **H₂RAs** (Table 18-2) can result in symptomatic benefit and endoscopic healing in up to half of patients. Dosage adjustments are required in renal insufficiency.
- Reflux inhibitors consist of γ-aminobutyric acid (GABA) type B receptor agonists that block transient LES relaxations. **Baclofen**, the prototype agent, reduces reflux events, but central side effects can be limiting (*Aliment Pharmacol Ther 2012;35:1036*).

Surgical Management

- Indications for **fundoplication** include the need for continuous PPIs, noncompliance or intolerance to medical therapy in patients who are good surgical candidates, ongoing nonacid reflux despite adequate medical therapy, and patient preference for surgery. When symptoms are controlled on PPI therapy, medical therapy and fundoplication are equally effective. Although fundoplication could provide better symptom control and quality of life in the short term, new postoperative symptoms and surgical failure can also occur (*Surg Endosc 2011;25:2547*).
- Elevated esophageal acid exposure and correlation of symptoms to reflux events on ambulatory pH monitoring predict a higher likelihood of a successful surgical outcome.
- Patients with medical treatment failures need careful evaluation to determine whether symptoms are indeed related to acid reflux before surgical options are considered; these patients often have other diagnoses including EoE, esophageal motor disorders, visceral hypersensitivity, and functional heartburn.
- Potential complications of surgery include dysphagia, inability to belch, gas-bloat syndrome, and bowel symptoms including flatulence, diarrhea, and abdominal pain.

Lifestyle/Risk Modification

- Patients with nocturnal GERD symptoms may benefit from elevating the head of the bed and avoiding meals within 2–3 hours before bedtime.
- Weight loss may benefit certain overweight patients with GERD.
- Lifestyle modifications alone are unlikely to resolve symptoms in the majority of GERD patients and should be recommended in conjunction with medications.

COMPLICATIONS

- **Esophageal erosion and ulceration** (esophagitis) can rarely lead to overt bleeding and iron deficiency anemia.
- **Strictures** can form when esophagitis heals, leading to dysphagia. Endoscopic dilation and maintenance PPI therapy typically resolve dysphagia from strictures.
- **Barrett esophagus (BE)** is a reflux-triggered change from normal squamous esophageal epithelium to specialized intestinal metaplasia and carries a 0.5% per year risk of progression to esophageal adenocarcinoma. Endoscopic screening for BE should be considered for patients with GERD who are at high risk (long duration of GERD symptoms, ≥50 years of age, male gender, Caucasian); patients who are found with BE should undergo periodic surveillance every 3 to 5 years in the absence of dysplasia (*Am J Gastroenterol 2013;108:308*). If high-grade dysplasia is found in the setting of BE, endoscopic therapy (usually radiofrequency ablation) is preferred to surveillance or surgery (*Gastroenterology 2012;143:336*).

Esophageal Motor Disorders

GENERAL PRINCIPLES

Definition

- **Achalasia** is the most easily recognized motor disorder of the esophagus, characterized by failure of the LES to relax completely with swallowing and aperistalsis of the esophageal body (*Am J Gastroenterol 2013;108:1238*).
- **Diffuse esophageal spasm** is a spastic disorder characterized by premature, nonperistaltic contractions in the esophageal body (*Gastroenterology 2011;141:469*).
- **Esophageal hypomotility disorders** are characterized by fragmented, ineffective, or absent esophageal peristalsis, sometimes with LES hypomotility, leading to reflux symptoms.

DIAGNOSIS

Clinical Presentation

- Presenting symptoms in achalasia can include dysphagia, regurgitation, chest pain, weight loss, and aspiration pneumonia.
- Diffuse esophageal spasm and other spastic disorders may have obstructive symptoms (dysphagia, regurgitation) but also perceptive symptoms (chest pain) from heightened esophageal sensitivity.
- LES hypomotility diminishes barrier function, and esophageal body hypomotility affects esophageal clearance of refluxed material, which can lead to prolonged reflux exposure and reflux complications.

Diagnostic Testing

- **Esophageal HRM** represents the gold standard for the diagnosis of esophageal motor disorders (*Neurogastroenterol Motil 2013;25:99*). HRM features categorize achalasia into

three subtypes that have symptomatic and therapeutic implications (*Neurogastroenterol Motil 2014;27:160*).
- **Barium radiographs** may demonstrate a typical appearance of a dilated intrathoracic esophagus with impaired emptying, an air-fluid level, absence of gastric air bubble, and tapering of the distal esophagus with a bird's beak appearance in achalasia. A beaded or cork-screw appearance may be seen with diffuse esophageal spasm. A dilated esophagus with an open LES and free gastroesophageal reflux may be seen with severe esophageal hypomotility.
- **Endoscopy** may help exclude a stricture or neoplasia of the distal esophagus in pre-sumed achalasia and spastic disorders. Hypomotility disorders may also manifest a dilated esophagus but with a gaping gastroesophageal junction and evidence of reflux disease.

TREATMENT

Medications
- **Smooth muscle relaxants** such as nitrates or calcium channel blockers administered im-mediately before meals may afford short-lived symptom relief in spastic disorders and achalasia, but symptom response is suboptimal. Phosphodiesterase inhibitors may pro-vide benefit in hypercontractile disorders but may be contraindicated in coronary disease.
- **Botulinum toxin** injection at endoscopy can improve dysphagia symptoms for several weeks to months in achalasia and spastic disorders with incomplete LES relaxation (*Am J Gastroenterol 2013;108:1238*). This approach may be useful in elderly and frail patients who are poor surgical risks or as a bridge to more definitive therapy.
- **Neuromodulators** (e.g., low-dose tricyclic antidepressants [TCAs]) may improve percep-tive symptoms (such as chest pain) associated with spastic motor disorders and achalasia.
- **Antisecretory therapy** with a PPI is recommended for reflux associated with esophageal hypomotility disorders. No specific promotility therapy exists. Antireflux surgery should be approached with caution in advanced hypomotility disorders.

Surgical Management
Disruption of the circular muscle of the LES using **pneumatic dilation** or surgical incision (**Heller myotomy**) can result in durable symptom relief in achalasia, with comparable symp-tom outcomes (*N Engl J Med 2011;364:1807*). Gastroesophageal reflux can result, treated with lifelong acid suppression or concurrent partial fundoplication during myotomy. Esoph-ageal perforation occurs in 3–5% of patients with pneumatic dilation, requiring prompt surgical repair. **Peroral endoscopic myotomy (POEM)** is a new technique with good short-term symptom improvement (*Gastroenterology 2013;145:309*; *Surgery 2013;154:885*).

COMPLICATIONS

- Complications of achalasia include aspiration pneumonia and weight loss.
- Achalasia is associated with a 0.15% risk of squamous cell cancer of the distal esophagus, a 33-fold higher risk relative to the nonachalasia population.

Peptic Ulcer Disease

GENERAL PRINCIPLES

Definition
PUD consists of mucosal breaks in the stomach and duodenum when corrosive effects of acid and pepsin overwhelm mucosal defense mechanisms. Other locations include esopha-gus, small bowel adjacent to gastroenteric anastomoses, and within a Meckel diverticulum.

Etiology

- *Helicobacter pylori*, a spiral, gram-negative, urease-producing bacillus, is responsible for at least half of all PUD and the majority of ulcers that are not due to NSAIDs.
- PUD can develop in 15–25% of **chronic NSAID and aspirin** users. Past history of PUD, age >60 years, concomitant corticosteroid or anticoagulant therapy, high-dose or multiple NSAID therapy, and presence of serious comorbid medical illnesses increase risk for PUD (*J Clin Gastroenterol 1997;24:2*).
- A gastrin-secreting tumor or **gastrinoma** accounts for <1% of all peptic ulcers.
- Gastric cancer or lymphoma may manifest as a gastric ulcer.
- When none of these etiologies are evident, PUD is designated idiopathic. Most idiopathic PUD could be due to undiagnosed *H. pylori* or undetected NSAID use.
- Cigarette smoking doubles the risk for PUD; it delays healing and promotes recurrence.

DIAGNOSIS

Clinical Presentation

- Epigastric pain or dyspepsia may be presenting symptoms; however, symptoms are not always predictive of the presence of ulcers. Epigastric tenderness may be elicited on abdominal palpation. Ten percent may present with a complication (see Complications).
- In the presence of **alarm symptoms** (weight loss, early satiety, bleeding, anemia, persistent vomiting, epigastric mass, and lack of response to PPI), EGD should be performed to assess for complications or alternate diagnoses.

Diagnostic Testing

- **Endoscopy** is the gold standard for diagnosis of peptic ulcers. **Barium studies** also have good sensitivity for diagnosis of ulcers, but smaller ulcers and erosions may be missed, and tissue sampling for *H. pylori* or cancer cannot be performed.
- **Serum *H. pylori* antibody testing** is the cheapest noninvasive test with a sensitivity of 85% and a specificity of 79% for the diagnosis of *H. pylori* infection. The antibody remains detectable as long as 18 months after successful eradication and cannot be used to document successful eradication of the organism.
- **Stool *H. pylori* antigen testing** has 91% sensitivity and 93% specificity for the diagnosis of *H. pylori* infection and can confirm eradication of *H. pylori* after triple therapy.
- **Rapid urease assay** (e.g., *Campylobacter*-like organism [CLO] test) and histopathologic examination of endoscopic biopsy specimens are commonly used for diagnosis in patients undergoing endoscopy but may be falsely negative in patients on PPI therapy.
- **Carbon-labeled urea breath testing** is the most accurate noninvasive test for diagnosis, with sensitivity and specificity of 95%; it is often used to document successful eradication after therapy of *H. pylori* infection (*BMJ 2008;337:a1400*).

TREATMENT

Medications

- Regardless of etiology, **acid suppression** forms the mainstay of therapy of PUD. Gastric ulcers are typically treated for 12 weeks and duodenal ulcers for 8 weeks.
- Oral PPI or H_2RA therapy will suffice in most instances (see Table 18-2). Dosage adjustment of H_2RAs is necessary in renal insufficiency. Cimetidine can impair metabolism of many drugs, including warfarin anticoagulants, theophylline, and phenytoin.
- Two antibiotics and a PPI (triple therapy) is the standard regimen for ***H. pylori* eradication**, which promotes healing and markedly reduces PUD recurrence. Several antimicrobial and antisecretory agent regimens are available (Table 18-3). Levofloxacin-based

TABLE 18-3	Regimens Used for Eradication of *Helicobacter pylori*
Medications and Doses	**Comments**
Clarithromycin (500 mg bid), amoxicillin (1 g bid), and PPI[a]	First-line therapy
Metronidazole (500 mg bid), amoxicillin (1 g bid), and PPI[a]	First-line therapy in setting of prior macrolide exposure
Clarithromycin (500 mg bid), metronidazole (500 mg bid), and PPI[a]	First-line therapy for penicillin-allergic patients
Amoxicillin (1 g bid) and PPI[a] for 5 days, followed by clarithromycin (500 mg bid), metronidazole (500 mg bid), and PPI[a] for another 5 days	Sequential therapy
Tetracycline (500 mg qid), metronidazole (250 mg qid), bismuth (525 mg qid), and PPI[a]	Bismuth-containing quadruple therapy; salvage regimen
Levofloxacin (250 mg bid), amoxicillin (1 g bid), and PPI[a]	Levofloxacin-based triple therapy; salvage regimen
Two antibiotics selected by sensitivity testing on culture, bismuth (525 mg qid), and PPI[a]	Culture-guided therapy (if failed multiple regimens)

PPI, proton pump inhibitor.
Duration of therapy: 10–14 days. When using salvage regimens after initial treatment failure, choose drugs that have not been used before.
[a]Standard doses for PPI: omeprazole 20 mg, lansoprazole 30 mg, pantoprazole 40 mg, rabeprazole 20 mg, all twice a day. Esomeprazole is used as a single 40-mg dose once a day.

sequential or triple therapy may be superior to standard triple therapy (clarithromycin, amoxicillin, PPI) (*Hepatogastroenterology 2011;58:1148*). Other regimens may include LOAD (levofloxacin, omeprazole, nitazoxanide, and doxycycline) for 7–10 days; ofloxacin, azithromycin, omeprazole, and bismuth for 14 days; and PPI, bismuth, tetracycline, and levofloxacin for 10 days (*Helicobacter 2014;19:74*; *Am J Gastroenterol 2011;106:1970*). Patients previously exposed to a macrolide antibiotic should be treated with a regimen that does not include clarithromycin.
- NSAIDs and aspirin should be avoided when possible; if continued, maintenance PPI therapy or a mucosal protective agent (misoprostol, 400–800 μg/d) is recommended (*Gut 2014;63:1061*).
- **Sucralfate** coats the eroded mucosal surface without blocking acid secretion and is often used in stress ulcer prophylaxis. Side effects include constipation and reduction of bioavailability of certain drugs (e.g., cimetidine, digoxin, fluoroquinolones, phenytoin, and tetracycline) when administered concomitantly.
- **Antacids** can be useful as supplemental therapy for pain relief in PUD.
- **Nonpharmacologic measures.** Cessation of cigarette smoking should be encouraged. Alcohol in high concentrations can damage the gastric mucosal barrier, but no evidence exists to link alcohol with ulcer recurrence.

Surgical Management
Surgery is still occasionally required for intractable symptoms, GI bleeding, Zollinger-Ellison syndrome, and complicated PUD. Surgical options vary depending on the location of the ulcer and the presence of complications.

SPECIAL CONSIDERATIONS

- **Zollinger-Ellison syndrome** is caused by a gastrin-secreting, non–β islet cell tumor of the pancreas or duodenum. Multiple endocrine neoplasia type I can be associated with this syndrome in one-quarter to one-third of patients (*Clin Gastroenterol Hepatol 2012;10:126*). The resultant hypersecretion of gastric acid can cause multiple PUD in unusual locations, ulcers that fail to respond to standard medical therapy, or recurrent PUD after surgical therapy. Diarrhea and GERD symptoms are common.
- Gastric acid output is typically >15 mEq/L, and gastric pH is <1.0. A fasting serum gastrin level while off acid suppression for at least 5 days serves as a screening test in patients who make gastric acid; a value >1000 pg/mL is seen in 90% of patients with Zollinger-Ellison syndrome. When serum gastrin is elevated but <1000 pg/mL, a secretin stimulation test may demonstrate a paradoxical 200-pg increment in serum gastrin level after IV secretin in patients with gastrinomas (*Aliment Pharmacol Ther 2009;29:1055*). High-dose PPIs are used for medical management. Specialized nuclear medicine scans (octreotide scans) can be useful in localizing the neoplastic lesion for curative resection. Long-term survival is principally related to underlying comorbidity rather than metastatic gastrinoma (*Dig Liver Dis 2011;43:439*).

COMPLICATIONS

- **GI bleeding** (see Gastrointestinal Bleeding section).
- **Gastric outlet obstruction** can occur with ulcers close to the pyloric channel and can manifest as nausea and vomiting, sometimes several hours after meals. Plain abdominal radiographs can show a dilated stomach with an air–fluid level. NG suction can decompress the stomach while fluids and electrolytes are repleted intravenously. Recurrence is common, and endoscopic balloon dilation or surgery is often necessary for definitive correction.
- **Perforation** occurs infrequently and usually necessitates emergent surgery. Perforation may occur in the absence of previous symptoms of PUD and may be asymptomatic in patients who are receiving glucocorticoids. A plain upright radiograph of the abdomen may demonstrate free air under the diaphragm.
- **Pancreatitis** can result from penetration into the pancreas from ulcers in the posterior wall of the stomach or duodenal bulb. The pain becomes severe and continuous, radiates to the back, and is no longer relieved by antisecretory therapy. Serum amylase may be elevated. CT scanning may be diagnostic. Surgery is often required for therapy.

MONITORING/FOLLOW-UP

- Repeat EGD or upper GI series should be performed 8–12 weeks after initial diagnosis of all gastric ulcers to document healing; repeat endoscopic biopsy should be considered for nonhealing ulcers to exclude the possibility of a malignant ulcer.
- Duodenal ulcers are almost never malignant; therefore, documentation of healing is unnecessary in the absence of symptoms.

Inflammatory Bowel Disease

GENERAL PRINCIPLES

- **Ulcerative colitis (UC)** is an idiopathic chronic inflammatory disease of the colon and rectum, characterized by mucosal inflammation and typically presenting with bloody diarrhea. Rectal involvement is almost universal.

- **Crohn disease (CD)** is characterized by transmural inflammation of the gut wall and can affect any part of the tubular GI tract.

DIAGNOSIS

Clinical Presentation

- Both disorders can present with diarrhea, weight loss, and abdominal pain. UC typically presents with bloody diarrhea. CD can also present with fistula formation, strictures, abscesses, or bowel obstruction.
- **Extracolonic manifestations** of inflammatory bowel disease (IBD) include arthritis, primary sclerosing cholangitis, and ocular and skin lesions.

Diagnostic Testing

- **Endoscopy** remains the preferred method for diagnosis, especially for UC, where contiguous inflammation is seen starting at the rectum and extending varying distances into the colon. Endoscopy may demonstrate colonic involvement in CD (erosions or ulcers with a patchy distribution and skip lesions); ileoscopy during colonoscopy may demonstrate terminal ileal involvement. **Histopathology** demonstrates chronic mucosal inflammation with crypt abscesses and cryptitis in UC and may demonstrate multinucleated giant cells and noncaseating granulomas in CD.
- Cross-sectional **imaging studies** (CT and MRI scans) have value in the evaluation of CD, especially when luminal narrowing (stricture) or extraluminal complications (abscess, fistula) are suspected. Although MRI and CT enterography both adequately assess disease activity and bowel involvement in CD, MRI may be superior to CT (*Gastroenterology 2014;146:374; Inflamm Bowel Dis 2011;17:1073*). Contrast radiography (small bowel follow-through series, barium enema) may also be useful, particularly in CD.
- **Serologic markers** play a limited role as adjuncts for diagnosis. Anti–*Saccharomyces cerevisiae* antibodies are typically seen in CD, and perinuclear antineutrophil cytoplasmic antibodies (p-ANCA) are seen in UC. C-reactive protein (CRP) and erythrocyte sedimentation rate (ESR) represent correlates for disease activity.
- ***C. difficile* colitis** is more frequent in IBD patients compared to non-IBD populations; therefore, **stool studies** are warranted to look for this organism with disease flares (*Clin Gastroenterol Hepatol 2007;5:339*). **CMV superinfection** can occur in patients on immunosuppressive agents and can be diagnosed by histopathology during endoscopy (*Am J Gastroenterol 2006;101:2857*).

TREATMENT

Medications

Treatment is based on the severity of disease, location, and associated complications (*Gastroenterology 2013;145:1459*). Management aims are to resolve the acute presentation and reduce future recurrences. Both UC and CD can be categorized into three categories of severity for management purposes:

- **Mild to moderate disease.** Patients have little to no weight loss and good functional capacity and are able to maintain adequate oral intake. UC patients have less than four bowel movements daily with no rectal bleeding or anemia, normal vital signs, and normal ESR, whereas CD patients have little or no abdominal pain. Treatment typically begins with aminosalicylates but can include antibiotics and glucocorticoids.
  - **5-Aminosalicylates (5-ASA).** Various formulations are available, each targeting different parts of the tubular gut, and are useful for both inducing and maintaining remission in mild to moderate disease. Infrequent hypersensitivity reactions include pneumonitis, pancreatitis, hepatitis, and nephritis.

Sulfasalazine reaches the colon intact, where it is metabolized to 5-ASA and a sulfapyridine moiety. Benefit is seen in UC or CD limited to the colon, either as initial therapy (0.5 g PO bid, increased as tolerated to 0.5–1.5 g PO qid) or to maintain remission (1 g PO bid–qid). The sulfapyridine moiety is responsible for side effects of headache, nausea, vomiting, and abdominal pain, which are treated with dose reduction. Skin rash, fever, agranulocytosis, hepatotoxicity, and paradoxical exacerbation of colitis are rare hypersensitivity reactions. Reversible reduction in sperm counts can be seen in males. Folic acid supplementation is recommended because sulfasalazine can impair folate absorption.

○ **Mesalamine.** Newer 5-ASA preparations lack the sulfa moiety of sulfasalazine and are associated with fewer side effects but can be expensive.

- **Asacol** is an oral formulation of 5-ASA released at a pH of 7 in the distal ileum. It is useful in UC and ileocecal/colonic CD at doses of 800–1600 mg PO tid.

- **Pentasa** has a time- and pH-dependent release mechanism that allows drug availability throughout the small bowel and colon. It is useful in diffuse small bowel involvement with CD but can also be used in UC in doses of 0.5–1.0 g PO qid.

- **Apriso** also has a pH-dependent release mechanism and distributes mesalamine throughout the colon when administered in doses of 1.5 g PO once daily.

- **Balsalazide** (**Colazal**) is cleaved by colonic bacteria to mesalamine and an inert molecule. Therefore, it is only useful for colonic disease, at doses of 2.25 g PO tid for active disease and 1.5 g PO bid for maintenance.

- **Multimatrix delivery system mesalamine** (**Lialda**) uses a novel delivery system that allows sustained 5-ASA release throughout the colon while decreasing frequency of administration. It is useful in colonic disease at doses of 1.2–2.4 g PO qday–bid.

○ **Olsalazine** (**Dipentum**) is a 5-ASA dimer cleaved by colonic bacteria and is useful in colonic disease. Significant diarrhea limits its use.

• **Antibiotics** are commonly used clinically in mild to moderate CD as well as perianal disease, but not in UC where the role of bacteria has not been established. Their role should be limited to colonic or ileocolonic CD, perianal disease, fistulas, and abscesses. Typical antibiotics used are **metronidazole** (250–500 mg PO tid) and **ciprofloxacin** (500 mg PO bid), usually concurrently, for 2–6 weeks.

○ **Budesonide** (Entocort; 6–9 mg PO qday) is a synthetic corticosteroid with first-pass liver metabolism that limits systemic toxicity while retaining local efficacy from high affinity to the glucocorticoid receptor, similar to oral corticosteroids. It is effective and safe for short-term use in mild to moderate ileocolonic CD and can replace mesalamine in inducing remission (*Gastroenterology 2013;145:1459*).

○ **Topical therapy** is useful in IBD limited to distal left colon. Topical mesalamine agents are superior to topical steroids or oral aminosalicylates for mild to moderate distal UC or ulcerative proctitis (*Am J Gastroenterol 2010;105:501*). Sitz baths, analgesics, hydrocortisone creams, and local heat may provide symptomatic benefit in perianal CD in conjunction with systemic therapy.

• **Moderate to severe disease** refers to CD patients who fail to respond to treatment for mild to moderate disease or those with significant weight loss, anemia, fever, abdominal pain or tenderness, and intermittent nausea and vomiting without bowel obstruction (*Am J Gastroenterol 2009;104:465*), or UC patients with more than six bloody bowel movements daily, fever, mild anemia, and elevated ESR. Predictive factors for moderate- to high-risk disease include age <30 years at initial diagnosis, extensive anatomic involvement, perianal and/or severe rectal disease, deep ulcers, prior surgical resection, and structuring or penetrating behavior (*Gastroenterology 2013;145:1459*). The goal of therapy is to induce remission rapidly with corticosteroids and to maintain remission with immunosuppressive agents and/or biologic agents as appropriate. Treatment is typically continued until the patient fails to respond to a particular agent or the agent is no longer tolerated.

- ○ **Glucocorticoids** are effective in inducing remission in moderate to severe disease, especially with flares of disease activity (*Gut 2011;60:571*).
  - ▪ **Prednisone** is started orally (typically 40–60 mg PO daily) and continued until symptom improvement. The dose can then be tapered on a weekly basis, because glucocorticoids are not recommended for maintenance therapy, and steroid-sparing alternatives should be sought for patients who appear dependent on these medications.
  - ▪ **Oral or parenteral glucocorticoids should not be prescribed before ruling out an infectious process and should not be initiated for the first time over the telephone.**
- ○ **Immunosuppressive agents**
  - ▪ **6-Mercaptopurine** (1.0–1.5 mg/kg/d PO), a purine analog, and **azathioprine** (1.5–2.5 mg/kg/d PO), its S-imidazole precursor, cause preferential suppression of T-cell activation and antigen recognition, and are useful in maintaining a glucocorticoid-induced remission in both UC and CD. Both azathioprine and 6-mercaptopurine are effective for inducing remission in active CD (*Cochrane Database Syst Rev 2010;16:CD000545*). Response may be delayed for up to 1–2 months, with optimal response occurring about 4 months after treatment initiation. Side effects include reversible bone marrow suppression, pancreatitis, and allergic reactions.
    - □ Determination of **thiopurine methyltransferase (TPMT)** enzyme activity prior to initiation of therapy will identify genetic polymorphisms that may predispose to toxicity with the use of these agents (*Gastroenterology 2006;130:935*).
    - □ Routine blood cell counts should be performed, initially every 1–2 weeks, to monitor for acute or delayed bone marrow suppression. On stable doses, testing can be performed every 3 months.
    - □ 6-Thioguanine (6-TG) metabolite levels assess adequacy of dosing, whereas high 6-methyl mercaptopurine (6-MMP) levels may predict hepatotoxicity. Addition of allopurinol to the regimen preferentially pushes metabolism toward the active metabolite (6-TG) rather than the toxic metabolite (6-MMP) (*Aliment Pharmacol Ther 2010;31:640*).
  - ▪ **Methotrexate** (15–25 mg IM or PO weekly) is effective as a steroid-sparing agent in CD but not UC. Side effects include hepatic fibrosis, bone marrow suppression, alopecia, pneumonitis, allergic reactions, and teratogenicity. In CD patients in remission, methotrexate is not as effective as azathioprine or infliximab for mucosal healing (*Aliment Pharmacol Ther 2011;33:714*), and methotrexate added to infliximab is no more effective than infliximab monotherapy (*Gastroenterology 2014;146:681*).
    - □ Baseline CXR and monitoring of CBC and liver function tests should be performed routinely.
    - □ Patients with abnormal transaminases may require a liver biopsy to assess for hepatic fibrosis prior to treatment, and subsequent biopsies are performed for significant elevations thereafter.
- ○ **Anti–tumor necrosis factor-α (anti–TNF-α) monoclonal antibodies** modify immune system function and are beneficial in moderate to severe CD refractory to other approaches, including immunosuppressives, and indicated both for induction and maintenance of remission. Benefit has also been demonstrated in moderate to severe UC (*Gut 2011;60:780*). **Infliximab (Remicade**; 5 mg/kg IV infusions at weeks 0, 2, and 6, followed by maintenance infusions every 8 weeks), **adalimumab (Humira**; 160 mg SC at week 0, then 80 mg SC at week 2, followed by 40 mg SC every 2 weeks), and **certolizumab pegol (Cimzia**; 400 mg SC at weeks 0, 2, and 4, followed by maintenance doses every 4 weeks) are the available anti–TNF-α agents. Combination therapy with infliximab and azathioprine is more effective than monotherapy with either agent in UC (*Gastroenterology 2014;146:392*). In addition to its role as an option for first-line therapy, adalimumab is also safe and effective for CD patients who have failed

infliximab therapy (*Aliment Pharmacol Ther 2010;32:1228*). However, because elective switching from IV infliximab to SC adalimumab is associated with loss of tolerance and efficacy, adherence to the first anti–TNF-α agent is encouraged (*Gut 2012;61:229*). In moderate to severe CD, infliximab plus azathioprine or infliximab monotherapy is more likely to attain steroid-free clinical remission than azathioprine monotherapy (*N Engl J Med 2010;362:1383*).

- Anti–TNF-α therapy has been associated with reactivation of latent TB; hence, placement of a purified protein derivative (PPD) skin test and CXR are essential prior to initiation of therapy (*Am J Gastroenterol 2010;105:501*). **Hepatitis B status** should also be assessed and vaccination provided prior to therapy. Opportunistic infections as well as infectious complications can develop, and congestive heart failure may worsen during therapy.
- Acute and delayed hypersensitivity reactions, or antibodies to infliximab and anti–double-stranded DNA antibodies, can develop with infliximab infusions. Local injection site reactions have been reported with adalimumab and certolizumab pegol therapy.
  ○ **Natalizumab** (**Tysabri**; 300-mg infusions at weeks 0, 4, and 8, followed by monthly infusions thereafter) is a humanized monoclonal antibody to α-4 integrin, a cellular adhesion molecule, used for moderate to severe CD refractory to all other approaches including anti–TNF-α antibodies. This agent may induce reactivation of human JC polyomavirus, causing progressive multifocal leukoencephalopathy (PML). Risk for PML can be minimized by avoiding concomitant immunosuppressive agents and close monitoring (*Am J Gastroenterol 2009;104:465*). Other infectious complications and acute hypersensitivity reactions are also possible.
  ○ **Vedolizumab** (**Entyvio**; 300-mg infusions at weeks 0 and 2, followed by infusions every 4–8 weeks), an α4β7 integrin antibody, has emerged as a new option for induction and maintenance of remission in both CD and UC (*N Engl J Med 2013;369:699*).
- **Severe or fulminant disease** describes patients typically hospitalized due to the severity of their symptoms. Fulminant CD patients have persistent symptoms despite conventional glucocorticoids or anti–TNF-α therapy or have high fevers, persistent vomiting, intestinal obstruction, intra-abdominal abscess, peritoneal signs, or cachexia (*Am J Gastroenterol 2009;104:465*). Fulminant colitis (both CD and UC) can present with profuse bloody bowel movements, significant anemia, systemic signs of toxicity (fever, sepsis, electrolyte disturbances, dehydration), and elevated laboratory markers of inflammation. **Toxic megacolon** occurs in 1–2% of UC patients, wherein the colon becomes atonic and modestly dilated, with significant systemic toxicity.
  ○ Supportive therapy consists of NPO status with NG suction if there is evidence of small bowel ileus. Dehydration and electrolyte disturbances are treated vigorously, and blood is transfused for severe anemia. Anticholinergic and opioid medication should be discontinued in toxic megacolon.
  ○ Initial investigation includes cross-sectional imaging to evaluate for intra-abdominal abscess. Blood cultures and stool studies to exclude *C. difficile* colitis are performed. Cautious flexible sigmoidoscopy may be done to determine severity of colonic inflammation and for biopsies to exclude CMV colitis.
  ○ Once infection is excluded, intensive medical therapy with IV **corticosteroids** (methylprednisolone 1 mg/kg body weight or equivalent to 40–60 mg of prednisone) and broad-spectrum antimicrobials should be initiated.
  ○ If response is not seen, **cyclosporine** infusion (2–4 mg/kg/d, to achieve blood levels of 200–400 ng/mL) and tacrolimus infusion represent options in fulminant UC colitis.
  ○ Nutritional support is administered as appropriate after 5–7 days; TPN is often indicated if enteral nutrition is not tolerated.
  ○ Clinical deterioration/lack of improvement despite 7–10 days of intensive medical management, evidence of bowel perforation, and peritoneal signs are indications for urgent total colectomy.

Surgical Management

- Surgery is generally reserved for fistulas, obstruction, abscess, perforation, or bleeding; medically refractory disease; and neoplastic transformation (*Gut 2011;60:571*). Stricturoplasty is an option for focal tight strictures; biopsies should be obtained to rule out cancer at stricture sites.
- In CD, recurrence close to the resected margins is common after bowel resection. Efforts should be made to avoid multiple resections in CD because of the risk of short bowel syndrome. Immunosuppressive agents should be discontinued before surgery and reinstituted if necessary during the postoperative period.
- **In UC, total colectomy is curative** and may be preferred over long-term immunosuppressive or biologic therapy.

Lifestyle/Risk Modification

- A low-roughage diet often can provide symptomatic relief in patients with mild to moderate disease or in patients with strictures.
- Patients with Crohn ileitis or ileocolonic resection may need vitamin B_{12} supplementation. Specific oral replacement of calcium, magnesium, folate, iron, vitamins A and D, and other micronutrients may be necessary in patients with small bowel CD.
- **TPN** can be administered in patients with food intolerance for greater than 4 or 5 days. Bowel rest has not been shown to reduce time to remission but can be used for nutritional maintenance and symptom relief while waiting for the effects of medical treatment or as a bridge to surgery.

SPECIAL CONSIDERATIONS

- In patients with both UC and Crohn colitis lasting longer than 8–10 years, annual or biennial **colonoscopic surveillance for neoplasia** with four-quadrant mucosal biopsies every 5–10 cm is recommended. Histopathologic evidence of any grade of dysplasia is an indication for total colectomy. Narrow-band imaging during colonoscopy may represent an alternative to chromoendoscopy for targeted biopsies in IBD (*Gastrointest Endosc 2011;74:840*).
- **Smoking cessation** is generally warranted for all patients with IBD. There is epidemiologic evidence of a protective effect on a limited number of patients with UC. However, nicotine has been shown to increase metabolism of many medications routinely used to treat IBD, decreasing their efficacy.
- **Venous thromboembolism.** Patients with IBD are at increased risk for both first and recurrent venous thromboembolism (*Gastroenterology 2011;139:779*).
- **Symptom control** is important as adjunct to therapy but must be used cautiously.
  - **Antidiarrheal agents** may be useful as an adjunctive therapy in selected patients with mild exacerbations or postresection diarrhea. They are contraindicated in severe exacerbations and toxic megacolon.
  - **Narcotics** should be used sparingly for pain control, because the chronicity of symptoms can lead to potential for dependence.

Functional Gastrointestinal Disorders

GENERAL PRINCIPLES

Definition

- Functional GI disorders are characterized by the presence of abdominal symptoms in the absence of a demonstrable organic disease process. Symptoms can arise from any part of the luminal gut.

- **Irritable bowel syndrome (IBS)**, primarily characterized by abdominal pain linked to altered bowel habits of at least 3 months in duration, is the best-recognized functional bowel disease.

DIAGNOSIS

- Clinical evaluation and investigation should be directed toward prudently excluding organic processes in the involved area of the gut while initiating therapeutic trials when functional symptoms are suspected.
- **Serologic tests for celiac sprue** are recommended in IBS patients. The prevalence of celiac sprue in diarrhea-predominant IBS patients is estimated at 3.6%, compared to 0.7% of the general population (*Am J Gastroenterol 2009;104:S1*).
- Patients >50 years old with new-onset bowel symptoms, patients with alarm symptoms (GI bleeding, anemia, weight loss, early satiety), and patients with symptoms not responding to empiric treatment need further workup with endoscopy. Routine cross-sectional imaging is not recommended with typical functional symptoms without alarm features.
- In young individuals with short-lived symptoms and no other explanation for dyspepsia, noninvasive testing for *H. pylori* can be considered (*BMJ 2008;337:a1400*).

TREATMENT

Patient education, reassurance, and help with diet and lifestyle modification are key to an effective physician–patient relationship. The psychosocial contribution to symptom exacerbation should be determined, and its management may be sufficient for many patients. Diets low in fermentable oligosaccharides, disaccharides, monosaccharides, and polyols (FODMAPs) appear to reduce functional GI symptoms in patients with IBS (*Gastroenterology 2014;146:67*).

Medications

- **Symptomatic management**
  - **Antiemetic agents** are useful in functional nausea and vomiting syndromes, in addition to neuromodulators.
  - When pain and bloating are the predominant symptoms, **antispasmodic** or **anticholinergic** medications (hyoscyamine, 0.125–0.25 mg PO/sublingual up to qid; dicyclomine, 10–20 mg PO qid) may provide short-term relief.
  - Stool frequency, but not abdominal pain, improves with increased dietary fiber (25 g/d) supplemented with PRN laxatives in constipation-predominant IBS.
  - **Loperamide** (2–4 mg, up to qid/PRN) can reduce stool frequency, urgency, and fecal incontinence.
  - Short-term nonabsorbable **antibiotic** therapy may improve bloating and diarrhea in IBS; long-term treatment has not been adequately studied. **Probiotics** (e.g., bifidobacteria) are sometimes beneficial (*Am J Gastroenterol 2009;104:S1*).
  - **Lubiprostone** (8 μg bid), a selective chloride channel activator, and **linaclotide** (290 μg daily), a guanylate cyclase C agonist, improve constipation-predominant IBS symptoms (*Gastroenterology 2014;147:1146; Clin Gastroenterol Hepatol 2014;12:616*). Moreover, polyethylene glycol 3350 plus electrolytes is suitable for use in constipation-predominant IBS (*Am J Gastroenterol 2013;108:1508*).
  - **Alosetron** (Lotronex, 1 mg daily to bid), a 5-HT$_3$ antagonist, is useful in women with diarrhea-predominant IBS (*Am J Gastroenterol 2009;104:1831*). However, its use is restricted to refractory diarrhea because of the rare potential for ischemic colitis.

- **Neuromodulators**
  - Low-dose **TCAs** (e.g., amitriptyline, nortriptyline, imipramine, doxepin: 25–100 mg at bedtime) have neuromodulatory and analgesic properties that are independent of their psychotropic effects. These can be beneficial, especially in pain-predominant functional GI disorders.
  - **Selective serotonin reuptake inhibitors (SSRIs)** (e.g., fluoxetine, 20 mg; paroxetine, 20 mg; sertraline, 50 mg; duloxetine, 20–60 mg) may also have efficacy, sometimes with better side effect profiles compared to TCAs.
  - **Cyclic vomiting syndrome (CVS)** is an increasingly recognized condition with stereotypic episodes of vigorous vomiting and asymptomatic intervals between episodes (*Aliment Pharmacol Ther 2011;34:263*). Treatment with low-dose TCAs or antiepileptic medications (zonisamide, levetiracetam) has prophylactic benefits (*Clin Gastroenterol Hepatol 2007;5:44*). Sumatriptan (25–50 mg PO, 5–10 mg transnasally, or 6 mg SC) or other triptans may abort an episode, especially if administered during a prodrome or early in the episode (*Cephalalgia 2011;31:504*). Established episodes may require IV hydration, scheduled IV antiemetics (ondansetron, prochlorperazine), benzodiazepines (lorazepam), and pain control with IV narcotics.

Acute Intestinal Pseudo-Obstruction (Ileus)

GENERAL PRINCIPLES

Definition

- **Acute intestinal pseudo-obstruction or ileus** consists of impaired transit of intestinal contents and obstructive symptoms (nausea, vomiting, abdominal distension, lack of bowel movements) without a mechanical explanation.
- **Acute colonic pseudo-obstruction** or **Ogilvie syndrome** describes massive colonic dilation without mechanical obstruction in the presence of a competent ileocecal valve, resulting from impaired colonic peristalsis (*Br J Surg 2009;96:229*).

Etiology

Ileus is frequently seen in the postoperative period. Narcotic analgesics administered for postoperative pain control may contribute, as can other medications that slow intestinal peristalsis (calcium channel blockers, anticholinergic medications, TCAs, antihistamines). Other predisposing causes include virtually any medical insult, particularly life-threatening systemic diseases, infection, vascular insufficiency, and electrolyte abnormalities. Etiology is similar for acute colonic pseudo-obstruction.

DIAGNOSIS

- A careful history and physical exam is essential in the initial evaluation.
- Conventional laboratory studies (CBC, complete metabolic profile, amylase, lipase) help in assessing for a primary intra-abdominal inflammatory process.
- **Obstructive series** (supine and upright abdominal radiograph with a CXR) determines the distribution of intestinal gas and assesses for the presence of free intraperitoneal air.
- **Additional imaging studies** assess for mechanical obstruction and inflammatory processes and include CT, contrast enema, and small bowel series.

TREATMENT

- Basic **supportive measures** consist of NPO, fluid replacement, and correction of electrolyte imbalances. Medications that slow GI motility (adrenergic agonists, TCAs, sedatives, narcotic analgesics) should be withdrawn or dose reduced. The ambulatory patient is encouraged to remain active and to undertake short walks.

- **Intermittent NG suction** prevents swallowed air from passing distally. In protracted cases, gastric decompression, either using an NG tube or a percutaneous endoscopic gastrostomy (PEG) tube, vents upper GI secretions and decreases vomiting and gastric distension.
- **Rectal tubes** help decompress the distal colon; more proximal colonic distension may necessitate **colonoscopic decompression**, especially when the cecal diameter approaches 9 cm. A flexible decompression tube can be left in the proximal colon during colonoscopy. Turning the patient from side to side may potentiate the benefit of colonoscopic decompression.

Medications

- **Neostigmine** (2 mg IV administered slowly over 3–5 minutes) is beneficial in selected patients with acute colonic distension. This can induce rapid reestablishment of colonic tone and is contraindicated if mechanical obstruction remains in the differential diagnosis. Side effects include abdominal pain, excessive salivation, symptomatic bradycardia, and syncope. A trial of neostigmine may be warranted before colonoscopic decompression in patients without contraindications (*N Engl J Med 1999;341:137*).
- **Methylnaltrexone** (**Relistor**; 8–12 mg SC per dose every other day) can be administered in settings where opioid medication use contributes to pseudo-obstruction.
- **Erythromycin** (200 mg IV) acts as a motilin agonist and stimulates upper gut motility; it has been used with some success in refractory postoperative ileus.
- **Alvimopan** is a peripherally acting μ-opioid receptor antagonist that enhances return of bowel function after abdominal surgery but has not been shown to shorten hospital stay (*Am Surg 2011;77:1460*).
- **Mosapride citrate** (15 mg PO tid), a 5-HT$_4$ receptor agonist, may reduce the duration of postoperative ileus when administered postoperatively (*J Gastrointest Surg 2011;15:1361*).
- **Prucalopride**, also a selective 5-HT$_4$ agonist, can relieve symptoms in patients with chronic intestinal pseudo-obstruction (*Aliment Pharmacol Ther 2012;35:48*).

Surgical Management

- **Surgical consultation** is required when the clinical picture is suggestive of mechanical obstruction or if peritoneal signs are present. Surgical exploration is reserved for acute cases with peritoneal signs, ischemic bowel, or other evidence for perforation.
- **Cecostomy** treats acute colonic distension when colonoscopic decompression fails.

PANCREATOBILIARY DISORDERS

Acute Pancreatitis

GENERAL PRINCIPLES

Definition

Acute pancreatitis consists of inflammation of the pancreas and peripancreatic tissue from activation of potent pancreatic enzymes within the pancreas, particularly trypsin.

Etiology

The most common causes are alcohol and gallstone disease, accounting for 75–80% of all cases. Less common causes include abdominal trauma, hypercalcemia, hypertriglyceridemia, and a variety of drugs. Post–endoscopic retrograde cholangiopancreatography

(ERCP) pancreatitis occurs in 5–10% of patients undergoing ERCP; prophylaxis with rectal NSAIDs or topical epinephrine and placement of prophylactic pancreatic duct stents can help prevent post-ERCP pancreatitis (*Aliment Pharmacol Ther 2013;38:1325*).

DIAGNOSIS

Clinical Presentation
Typical symptoms consist of acute onset of epigastric abdominal pain, nausea, and vomiting often exacerbated by food intake. Systemic manifestations can include fever, shortness of breath, altered mental status, anemia, and electrolyte imbalances, especially with severe episodes.

Diagnostic Testing
Laboratories
- Serum **lipase** is more specific and sensitive than serum **amylase**, although both are usually elevated beyond three times the upper limits of normal. These values do not correlate with severity or outcome of pancreatitis. Patients with renal insufficiency may have elevated enzymes at baseline from impaired clearance.
- Hepatic function testing may identify biliary obstruction as a possible etiology, and a lipid panel may suggest hypertriglyceridemia as the cause of acute pancreatitis.

Imaging
- **Dual-phase (pancreatic protocol) CT scan** is useful in the initial evaluation of severe acute pancreatitis but should be reserved for patients in whom the diagnosis is unclear, who fail to improve clinically within 48–72 hours, or in whom complications are suspected (*Am J Gastroenterol 2013;108:1400*). CT scan early in presentation may underestimate the severity of acute pancreatitis.
- **MRI with gadolinium** can also be used with at least similar efficacy, especially when CT is contraindicated. Magnetic resonance cholangiopancreatography (MRCP) is useful to detect a biliary source for pancreatitis before ERCP is performed (*Med Clin North Am 2008;92:889*).

TREATMENT

- **Aggressive volume repletion** with IV fluids must be undertaken, with careful monitoring of fluid balance, urine output, serum electrolytes (including calcium and glucose), and awareness of the potential for significant fluid sequestration within the abdomen. Intensive care unit monitoring may be necessary.
- Patients should receive **nothing PO** until they are free of pain and nausea. NG suction is reserved for patients with ileus or protracted emesis. TPN may be necessary when inflammation is slow to resolve (around 7 days) or if an ileus is present. However, early enteral feeding is preferred over TPN.
- Acid suppression may be necessary in severely ill patients with risk factors for stress ulcer bleeding, although it has not been shown to decrease symptom duration or severity (*Gastroenterology 2007;132:2022*).

Medications
- **Narcotic analgesics** are usually necessary for pain relief.
- Routine use of prophylactic antibiotics is not recommended in the absence of systemic infection (*Am J Gastroenterol 2013;108:1400*).

Other Nonoperative Therapies

Urgent **ERCP and biliary sphincterotomy** within 72 hours of presentation can improve the outcome of severe gallstone pancreatitis in the presence of biliary obstruction and is associated with fewer complications (*Ann Surg 2009;250:68*). This is thought to result from reduced biliary sepsis rather than true improvement of pancreatic inflammation.

Surgical Management

Cholecystectomy. A delay in cholecystectomy after gallstone pancreatitis carries a substantial risk of recurrent biliary events (*Br J Surg 2011;98:1446*).

COMPLICATIONS

- **Necrotizing pancreatitis** represents a severe form of acute pancreatitis, usually identified on dynamic dual-phase CT scanning with IV contrast. The presence of radiologically identified pancreatic necrosis increases the morbidity and mortality of acute pancreatitis. Increasing abdominal pain, fever, marked leukocytosis, and bacteremia suggest infected pancreatic necrosis that requires broad-spectrum antibiotics and often surgical debridement. CT-guided percutaneous aspiration for Gram stain and culture can confirm the diagnosis of infected necrosis. **Carbapenems** or a combination of a **fluoroquinolone** and **metronidazole** have good penetration into necrotic tissue.
- The presence of **pseudocysts** is suggested by persistent pain or high amylase levels. Complications include infection, hemorrhage, rupture (pancreatic ascites), and obstruction of adjacent structures. Asymptomatic nonenlarging pseudocysts can be followed clinically with serial imaging studies to resolution. Decompression of symptomatic or infected pseudocysts can be performed by percutaneous, endoscopic, or surgical techniques (*Gastrointest Endosc Clin N Am 2007;17:559*).
- **Infection.** Potential sources of fever include pancreatic necrosis, abscess, infected pseudocyst, cholangitis, and aspiration pneumonia. Cultures should be obtained, and broad-spectrum antimicrobials appropriate for bowel flora should be administered. In the absence of fever or other clinical evidence for infection, prophylactic antimicrobial therapy has no clear role in acute pancreatitis.
- **Pulmonary complications.** Atelectasis, pleural effusion, pneumonia, and acute respiratory distress syndrome can develop in severely ill patients (see Chapter 10, Pulmonary Diseases).
- **Renal failure** can result from intravascular volume depletion or acute tubular necrosis.
- **Other complications.** Metabolic complications include hypocalcemia, hypomagnesemia, and hyperglycemia. GI bleeding can result from stress gastritis, pseudoaneurysm rupture, or gastric varices from splenic vein thrombosis.

Chronic Pancreatitis

GENERAL PRINCIPLES

- Chronic pancreatitis represents inflammation, fibrosis, and atrophy of acinar cells resulting from recurrent acute or chronic inflammation of the pancreas.
- Most commonly seen with **chronic alcohol abuse**, it can also result from dyslipidemia, hypercalcemia, autoimmune disease, and exposure to various toxins. An inherited form (**hereditary pancreatitis**) is rarely seen; this can be associated with mutations in

genes encoding cationic trypsinogen (*PRSS1*) or pancreatic secretory trypsin inhibitor (*SPINK1*) (*Gastroenterology 2007;132:1557*).
• **Autoimmune pancreatitis (AIP)** represents an increasingly recognized subtype of chronic pancreatitis characterized by infiltration of IgG4-positive plasma cells in a classically sausage-shaped pancreas. AIP can be difficult to distinguish from pancreatic cancer on CT, but typically features diffuse narrowing of the main pancreatic duct without dilation. Initial treatment has traditionally been with high-dose steroids, although low-dose steroids may be similarly effective (*Pancreas 2014;43:261*). Relapses may occur in the pancreas or biliary tree, although retreatment with steroids is effective at inducing remission (*Gut 2013;62:1771*).

DIAGNOSIS

Clinical Presentation
Chronic abdominal pain, **exocrine insufficiency** from acinar cell injury and fibrosis (manifesting as weight loss and steatorrhea), and **endocrine insufficiency** from destruction of islet cells (manifesting as brittle diabetes) are the main clinical manifestations.

Diagnostic Testing
Laboratories
• Lipase and amylase may be elevated but are frequently normal and are nonspecific. Bilirubin, alkaline phosphatase, and transaminases may be elevated if there is concomitant biliary obstruction. A lipid panel and serum calcium should also be assessed.
• Indirect pancreatic function testing (such as secretin stimulation, fecal fat, and fecal elastase) can be performed but are not widely available and difficult to perform.

Imaging
• **Calcification** of the pancreas can be seen on imaging. Contrast-enhanced CT has a sensitivity of 75–90% and a specificity of 85% for the diagnosis of chronic pancreatitis, whereas MRCP is equivalent and a suitable alternative (*Gastroenterology 2007;132:1557*).
• **Endoscopic ultrasound (EUS)** has higher sensitivity for the diagnosis of chronic pancreatitis and is particularly useful for evaluating lesions concerning for neoplasia in the setting of chronic pancreatitis.

TREATMENT

Medications
• **Narcotic analgesics** are frequently required for control of pain, and narcotic dependence is common. **Neuromodulators** (TCAs, SSRIs) and **pregabalin** may improve symptoms and decrease reliance on narcotics (*Gastroenterology 2011;141:536*). In patients with mild to moderate exocrine insufficiency, the addition of oral pancreatic enzyme supplements may be beneficial for pain control.
• **Pancreatic enzyme supplements** are the mainstay of management of pancreatic exocrine insufficiency in conjunction with a low-fat diet (<50 g fat per day), facilitating weight gain and reduced stool frequency (*Aliment Pharmacol Ther 2011;33:1152*). Enteric-coated preparations (Pancrease or Creon, one to two capsules with meals) are stable at acid pH.
• **Fat-soluble vitamin** supplementation may be necessary.
• **Insulin** therapy is generally required for endocrine insufficiency, because the resultant diabetes mellitus is characteristically brittle and thus unresponsive to oral agents.
• When identified, treatment of the underlying disorder (e.g., hyperparathyroidism, dyslipidemia) is indicated. Alcohol cessation should be advised.

Other Nonoperative Therapies

- Patients with pancreatic duct obstruction from stones, strictures, or papillary stenosis may benefit from **ERCP and sphincterotomy**.
- Intractable pain may necessitate **celiac or splanchnic plexus block** (often EUS-guided) for short-term relief in selected patients or even surgery, such as a **Whipple procedure** or lateral pancreaticojejunostomy, in cases of a dilated pancreatic duct (*Aliment Pharmacol Ther 2009;29:979*).

Gallstone Disease

GENERAL PRINCIPLES

- **Asymptomatic gallstones (cholelithiasis)** are a common incidental finding for which no specific therapy is generally necessary (*J Gastroenterol Hepatol 2010;25:719*). Cholesterol stones are the most common type, but pigmented stones can be seen with hemolysis or infection. Risk factors include obesity, female gender, parity, rapid weight loss, ileal disease, and maternal family history.
- **Symptomatic cholelithiasis**, when upper abdominal symptoms are linked to gallstones, is typically treated surgically with cholecystectomy.
- **Acute cholecystitis** is caused most often by obstruction of the cystic duct by gallstones, but acalculous cholecystitis can occur in severely ill or hospitalized patients.

DIAGNOSIS

Clinical Presentation

- Cholelithiasis may present as **biliary colic**, a constant pain lasting for several hours, located in the right upper quadrant, radiating to the back or right shoulder, and sometimes associated with nausea or vomiting.
- Other presentations of gallstone disease include acute cholecystitis, acute pancreatitis, and cholangitis. Gallstone disease may rarely be associated with gallbladder cancer.
- Two-thirds of patients with **acute ascending cholangitis** present with right upper quadrant pain, fever with chills and/or rigors, and jaundice (**Charcot triad**), usually in the setting of biliary obstruction (choledocholithiasis, neoplasia, sclerosing cholangitis, biliary stent occlusion). The presence of hypotension and altered mentation defines the **Reynolds pentad**, which is seen less commonly.

Diagnostic Testing

- **Ultrasound scans** have a high degree of accuracy in diagnosis (sensitivity and specificity >95%) and are the preferred initial test.
- **Hydroxy iminodiacetic acid (HIDA)** scan can demonstrate nonfilling of the gallbladder in patients with acute cholecystitis, although false-negative results may be seen in acalculous cholecystitis.

TREATMENT

Medications

- **Supportive measures** include IV fluid resuscitation and broad-spectrum antimicrobial agents, especially in the event of complications such as acute cholecystitis with sepsis, perforation, peritonitis, abscess, or empyema formation.
- **Ursodeoxycholic acid** (8–10 mg/kg/d PO in two to three divided doses for prolonged periods) might be prudent in a select group of patients with small cholesterol stones in

normally functioning gallbladders who are at high risk for complications from surgical therapy. Side effects include diarrhea and reversible elevation in serum transaminases.

Other Nonpharmacologic Therapies

Percutaneous cholecystostomy can be performed under fluoroscopy in severely ill patients with acute cholecystitis who are not surgical candidates, especially for acalculous cholecystitis (*Am J Surg 2013;206:935*).

Surgical Management

Cholecystectomy is the therapy of choice for symptomatic gallstone disease and acute cholecystitis. Laparoscopic cholecystectomy compares favorably with the open procedure, with lower morbidity, lower cost, shorter hospital stay, and better cosmetic results (*Lancet 2006;368:230*).

COMPLICATIONS

- **Acute pancreatitis.** See Acute Pancreatitis section.
- **Choledocholithiasis.** Common bile duct obstruction, jaundice, biliary colic, cholangitis, or pancreatitis can result from stones retained in the common bile duct. The diagnosis can be made on ultrasonography, CT, or magnetic resonance cholangiography. ERCP with sphincterotomy and stone extraction is curative.
- **Acute ascending cholangitis** represents a medical emergency with high morbidity and mortality if biliary decompression is not performed urgently. The condition should be stabilized with IV fluids and broad-spectrum antibiotics. Drainage of the biliary tree can be performed through endoscopic (ERCP with sphincterotomy) or percutaneous approaches under fluoroscopic guidance.

OTHER GASTROINTESTINAL DISORDERS

Anorectal Disorders

- **Defecatory disorders** present with difficulty evacuating stool from the rectum or outlet constipation. The diagnosis is ideally made in the setting of compatible symptoms and abnormal testing, including DRE, balloon expulsion testing, barium defecography, MRI, anorectal manometry, and/or pelvic floor electromyography (*Am J Gastroenterol 2014;109:1141*). Management includes biofeedback therapy (*Gastroenterology 2014;146:37*).
- **Thrombosed external hemorrhoids** present as acutely painful, tense, bluish lumps covered with skin in the anal area. The thrombosed hemorrhoid can be surgically excised under local anesthesia for relief of severe pain. In less severe cases, oral analgesics, sitz baths (sitting in a tub of warm water), stool softeners, and topical ointments may provide symptomatic relief (*BMJ 2008;336:380*).
- **Internal hemorrhoids** commonly present with either bleeding or a prolapsing mass with straining. Bulk-forming agents such as fiber supplements are useful in preventing straining at defecation. Sitz baths and Tucks pads may provide symptomatic relief. Ointments and suppositories that contain topical analgesics, emollients, astringents, and hydrocortisone (e.g., Ansol-HC Suppositories, one per rectum bid for 7–10 days) may decrease edema but do not reduce bleeding. Hemorrhoidectomy or band ligation can be curative and is indicated in patients with recurrent or constant bleeding (*BMJ 2008;336:380*).
- **Anal fissures** present with acute onset of pain during defecation and are often caused by hard stool. Anoscopy reveals an elliptical tear in the skin of the anus, usually in

the posterior midline. Acute fissures heal in 2–3 weeks with the use of stool softeners, oral or topical analgesics, and sitz baths. The addition of oral or topical nifedipine to these conservative measures can improve pain relief and healing rates (*Am J Surg 2013;206:748*).

- **Perirectal abscess** commonly presents as a painful induration in the perianal area. Patients with IBD and immunocompromised states are particularly susceptible. Prompt drainage is essential to avoid the serious morbidity associated with delayed treatment. Antimicrobials directed against bowel flora (metronidazole, 500 mg PO tid, and ciprofloxacin, 500 mg PO bid) should be administered in patients with significant inflammation, systemic toxicity, or immunocompromised states.

Celiac Sprue

GENERAL PRINCIPLES

- Celiac sprue consists of chronic inflammation of proximal small bowel mucosa from an immunologic sensitivity to **gluten** (protein found in wheat, barley, and rye), resulting in malabsorption of dietary nutrients.
- Clinical presentation can vary greatly from asymptomatic iron deficiency anemia to significant diarrhea and weight loss. Other presenting features can include osteoporosis, dermatitis herpetiformis, abnormal liver enzymes, and abdominal pain; incidental recognition at endoscopy can also occur (*N Engl J Med 2007;357:1731*).
- More than 7% of patients with nonconstipated IBS have celiac-associated antibodies, suggesting that gluten sensitivity may trigger symptoms resembling IBS (*Gastroenterology 2011;141:1187*).

DIAGNOSIS

- Noninvasive serologic tests are highly sensitive and specific and should be checked while the patient is on a gluten-containing diet. Both **IgA anti–tissue transglutaminase (TTG) and antiendomysial antibodies** have accuracies close to 100%. Quantitative IgA levels should also be checked; IgG antibodies against TTG are checked if the patient is IgA deficient (*Am J Gastroenterol 2013;108:656*).
- EGD with small bowel biopsies is performed to confirm diagnosis with positive serologic testing or if suspicion remains high despite negative noninvasive testing. Classic biopsy findings include blunting or absence of villi and prominent intraepithelial lymphocytosis.
- Almost all patients with celiac sprue carry HLA-DQ2 and HLA-DQ8 molecules, so absence of these alleles has high negative predictive value when the diagnosis is in question or if patients are on a gluten-free diet.
- Nonceliac gluten sensitivity should only be considered after exclusion of celiac disease with appropriate testing; differentiation is important for risk identification for nutrient deficiency, complications, and family member risk.

TREATMENT

Medications

- Patients may require iron, folate, vitamin D, and vitamin B_{12} supplements.
- **Corticosteroids** (prednisone, 10–20 mg/d) may be required in refractory cases once inadvertent gluten ingestion has been excluded; immunosuppressive drugs have also been used (*N Engl J Med 2007;357:1731*).

Lifestyle/Risk Modification

- A **gluten-free diet** is first-line therapy and results in prompt improvement in symptoms. Dietary nonadherence is the most frequent cause for persistent symptoms.
- If symptoms persist despite a strict gluten-free diet, radiologic and endoscopic evaluation of the small bowel should be performed to rule out complications including collagenous colitis and **small bowel lymphoma**. However, the prognosis of adults with unrecognized celiac disease is good despite positive celiac antibodies; therefore, mass screening appears unnecessary (*Gut 2009;58:643*).

Diverticulosis and Diverticulitis

GENERAL PRINCIPLES

Definition

- **Diverticula** consist of outpouchings in the bowel, most commonly in the colon, but can also be seen elsewhere in the gut.
- **Diverticular bleeding** can occur from an artery at the mouth of the diverticulum.
- **Diverticulitis** results from microperforation of a diverticulum and resultant extracolonic or intramural inflammation.

DIAGNOSIS

Clinical Presentation

- Diverticulosis is most frequently asymptomatic. Although diverticulosis may be found in patients being investigated for symptoms of abdominal pain and altered bowel habits, a causal link is difficult to establish.
- Typical symptoms of diverticulitis include left lower quadrant abdominal pain, fevers and chills, and alteration of bowel habits. Localized left lower quadrant abdominal tenderness may be elicited on physical examination.

Diagnostic Testing

Laboratories

Diverticulitis may be associated with an elevated white blood cell (WBC) count with a left shift.

Imaging

- Diverticula are frequently seen on screening colonoscopy.
- Imaging studies, most commonly CT scans, can be useful in the diagnosis of diverticulitis.
- **Colonoscopy is contraindicated for 4–6 weeks after an episode of acute diverticulitis**, but should be performed after that interval to exclude a perforated neoplasm.

TREATMENT

- Increased dietary fiber is generally recommended in patients with diverticulosis, although no hard data exist to support its benefit (*Curr Opin Gastroenterol 2015;31:50*).
- A low-residue diet is recommended for mild diverticulitis, although no evidence exists to support this practice (*JAMA 2008;300:907*).

Medications

- Oral **antibiotics** (e.g., ciprofloxacin, 500 mg PO bid, and metronidazole, 500 mg PO tid for 10–14 days) may suffice for mild diverticulitis.

- Despite optimistic initial reports, mesalamine does not appear to be effective in preventing recurrence of diverticulitis in phase III controlled trials; no therapy has been proven to prevent recurrent diverticulitis (*Gastroenterology 2014;147:793*).
- Hospital admission, bowel rest, IV fluids, and broad-spectrum IV antimicrobial agents are typically required in moderate to severe cases.

Surgical Management

- Surgical consultation should be obtained early in moderate to severe diverticulitis, because operative intervention may be necessary should complications arise.
- Surgical resection may also be necessary in recurrent diverticulitis, typically after three or more recurrences at the same location.

Gastroparesis

GENERAL PRINCIPLES

Definition

Gastroparesis consists of abnormally delayed emptying of stomach contents into the small bowel in the absence of gastric outlet obstruction or ulceration, usually as a result of damage to the nerves or smooth muscle involved in gastric emptying.

Etiology

- **Mechanical obstruction should always be excluded.**
- In addition to evaluating for acute metabolic derangements and potential offending medications (narcotics, anticholinergic agents, chemotherapeutic agents, glucagon-like peptide-1 and amylin analogs), patients with gastroparesis should be screened for **diabetes mellitus**, thyroid dysfunction, neurologic disease, prior gastric or bariatric surgery, and autoimmune disorders (e.g., scleroderma).
- If no predisposing cause is identified, gastroparesis is designated **idiopathic**.

DIAGNOSIS

Clinical Presentation

Symptoms include nausea, bloating, and vomiting, usually hours after a meal.

Diagnostic Testing

- A **gastric-emptying study** (gamma camera scan after a radiolabeled meal) can confirm the diagnosis; medications that can delay gastric emptying should be stopped at least 48 hours prior to testing.
- Endoscopic evidence of retained food debris in the stomach after an overnight fast may be an indirect indicator of delayed gastric emptying.

TREATMENT

- First steps in management include fluid restoration, correction of electrolytes, nutritional support, and optimization of glucose control for diabetic patients. Indications for enteral feeding, preferably postpyloric, include unintentional loss of >10% of usual body weight and/or refractory symptoms requiring repeated hospitalizations (*Am J Gastroenterol 2013;108:18*).

- Nutritional consultation can help address nutritional deficiencies and optimize diet, especially to decrease dietary fat and insoluble fiber (*Gastroenterology 2011;141:486*). Small-particle-size diets reduce symptoms in patients with diabetic gastroparesis (*Am J Gastroenterol 2014;109:375*).

Medications

- **Metoclopramide** (10 mg PO qid half an hour before meals) often represents the first line of prokinetic therapy but has variable efficacy, and side effects (drowsiness, tardive dyskinesia, parkinsonism) may be limiting.
- **Domperidone** (20 mg PO qid before meals and at bedtime) does not cross the blood–brain barrier, but hyperprolactinemia can result. ECGs should be checked at baseline and on follow-up given the risk of QT prolongation.
- **Erythromycin** (125–250 mg PO tid or 200 mg IV) is a motilin receptor agonist and stimulates gastric motility, but tachyphylaxis limits long-term therapy.
- **Antiemetics** may improve associated nausea and vomiting but will not improve gastric emptying.

Surgical Management

- **Enteral feeding** through a jejunostomy feeding tube may be required for supplemental nutrition and is favored over TPN.
- **Gastric electrical stimulation** using a surgically implanted stimulator (Enterra) may reduce symptoms of nausea and vomiting in half of medically refractory patients, but gastric emptying is typically not enhanced by this approach (*Gastrointest Endosc 2011;74:496*).

Ischemic Intestinal Injury

GENERAL PRINCIPLES

- **Acute mesenteric ischemia** results from arterial (or rarely venous) compromise to the superior mesenteric circulation.
- Emboli and thrombus formation are the most common causes of acute mesenteric ischemia, although **nonocclusive mesenteric ischemia** from vasoconstriction can also give rise to the disorder.
- **Ischemic colitis** results from mucosal ischemia in the inferior mesenteric circulation during a low-flow state (hypotension, arrhythmias, sepsis, aortic vascular surgery) in patients with atherosclerotic disease. Vasculitis, sickle cell disease, vasospasm, and marathon running can also predispose to ischemic colitis.

DIAGNOSIS

Clinical Presentation

- Patients with acute mesenteric ischemia may present with abdominal pain, but physical examination and imaging studies can be unremarkable until infarction has occurred. As a result, diagnosis is late and mortality is high.
- Ischemic colitis may manifest as transient bleeding or diarrhea; severe insults can lead to stricture formation, gangrene, and perforation. The heterogeneity of clinical presentation of ischemic colitis helps explain why clinical suspicion is often low. Although recurrences of ischemic colitis are infrequent (<10% at 5 years), mortality is high (one-third at 5 years) and driven by unrelated causes (*World J Gastroenterol 2013;19:8042*).

Diagnostic Testing

- **Urgent angiography** is indicated if the suspicion for acute mesenteric ischemia is high.
- CT with contrast has high sensitivity and specificity for the diagnosis of primary acute mesenteric ischemia (*Radiology 2010;256:93*), whereas Doppler EUS may help exclude chronic mesenteric ischemia (*Dig Liver Dis 2011;43:470*).
- In patients with ischemic colitis, characteristic "**thumb-printing**" of the involved colon may be seen on plain radiographs of the abdomen.
- Colonoscopy may reveal mucosal erythema, edema, and ulceration, sometimes in a linear configuration; evidence of gangrene or necrosis is an indication for surgical intervention.

TREATMENT

- Treatment of acute mesenteric ischemia is essentially surgical and increasingly **endovascular**, whereas both arterial bypass and percutaneous angioplasty represent options for chronic mesenteric ischemia (*Br J Surg 2014;101:e100*).
- In patients with ischemic colitis, in the absence of peritoneal signs or evidence of gangrene or perforation, expectant management with fluid and electrolyte repletion, broad-spectrum antimicrobials, and maintenance of stable hemodynamics usually suffices.
- Evidence of gangrene or necrosis in the setting of ischemic colitis represents an indication for surgery.

19

Liver Diseases

Maria Samuel, Kristen Singer, and Mauricio Lisker-Melman

Evaluation of Liver Disease

GENERAL PRINCIPLES

- Liver disease can present as a spectrum of clinical conditions that ranges from asymptomatic disease to end-stage liver disease (ESLD).
- A comprehensive investigation combining thorough history and physical examination with diagnostic tests, liver histology, and imaging can often establish a precise diagnosis.

DIAGNOSIS

Clinical Presentation

History

History taking should be focused on the following:
- History of present illnesses
- Medicine usage and toxin exposure (including alcohol)
- Associated signs and symptoms—development of jaundice, ascites, edema, pruritus, encephalopathy, gastrointestinal (GI) bleeding
- Family history of liver disease
- Comorbid conditions: obesity, diabetes, hyperlipidemia, inflammatory bowel disease, systemic hypotension
- Risk factors for infection: IV/intranasal drug use, body piercings, tattooing, sexual history, travel to foreign countries, occupation

Physical Examination
- Detailed physical exam is necessary. Physical stigmata of acute and chronic liver disease may be subtle or absent.
  - Jaundice
  - Ascites, peripheral edema, pleural effusions
  - Hepatomegaly and splenomegaly
  - Gynecomastia, testicular hypotrophy
  - Muscle wasting
  - Telangiectasias, palmar erythema, pubic hair changes
- Specific liver disorders may be associated with distinctive physical abnormalities: arthritis, acne, skin color changes, Kayser-Fleischer rings, clubbing, platypnea, orthodeoxia, dyspnea, or S_3 gallop.

Diagnostic Testing

Laboratories
- **Serum enzymes.** Hepatic disorders associated predominantly with elevation in aminotransferases are referred to as hepatocellular; hepatic disorders with predominant elevation in alkaline phosphatase (ALP) are referred to as cholestatic.
  - Elevation of **aspartate aminotransferase (AST) and alanine aminotransferase (ALT)** indicates hepatocellular injury and necrosis.
  - **ALP** is an enzyme that is present in a variety of tissues (bone, intestine, kidney, leukocytes, liver, and placenta). The concomitant elevation of other hepatic enzymes

(e.g., γ-glutamyl transpeptidase [GGT] or 5′-nucleotidase) assists in establishing the hepatic origin of ALP. Serum ALP level is often elevated in biliary obstruction, space-occupying lesions or infiltrative disorders of the liver, and conditions that cause intrahepatic cholestasis (primary biliary cirrhosis [PBC], primary sclerosing cholangitis [PSC], drug-induced cholestasis).

- **Excretory products**
  - **Bilirubin** is a degradation product of hemoglobin and nonerythroid hemoproteins (e.g., cytochromes, myoglobin, catalases, and endothelial nitric oxide synthase). Total serum bilirubin is composed of conjugated (direct) and unconjugated (indirect) fractions. Unconjugated hyperbilirubinemia occurs as a result of excessive bilirubin production (hemolysis and hemolytic anemias, ineffective erythropoiesis, and resorption of hematomas), reduced hepatic bilirubin uptake (Gilbert syndrome and drugs such as rifampin and probenecid), or impaired bilirubin conjugation (Gilbert or Crigler-Najjar syndrome). Elevation of conjugated and unconjugated fractions occurs in Dubin-Johnson and Rotor syndromes and in conditions associated with intrahepatic (from hepatocellular, canalicular, or ductular damage) and extrahepatic (from mechanical obstruction) cholestasis.
  - **α-Fetoprotein (AFP)** is normally produced by fetal liver cells. Its production falls to normal adult levels of <10 ng/mL within 1 year of life. AFP is an insensitive and nonspecific biomarker for hepatocellular carcinoma (HCC), with a sensitivity and specificity of 61% and 81%, respectively, at a cutoff of 20 ng/mL, and 22% and 100%, respectively, at a cutoff of 200 ng/mL (*Gastroenterology 2010;138:493*). Levels of >400 ng/mL or a rapid doubling time are suggestive of HCC; mild to moderate elevations can also be seen in acute and chronic liver inflammation.

Imaging
- **Ultrasonography** is used to screen for dilation of the biliary tree and to detect gallstones and cholecystitis in patients with right-sided abdominal pain associated with abnormal liver blood tests. It can reveal and characterize liver masses, abscesses, and cysts. Color flow Doppler ultrasonography can assess patency and direction of blood flow in the portal and hepatic veins and is therefore used to monitor shunt patency following transjugular intrahepatic portosystemic shunt (TIPS). Ultrasonography is a frequently used modality for screening of HCC; however, this modality is less sensitive (tumors with diameters <2 cm) for the detection of HCC compared with CT or MRI. This technique is very operator dependent.
- **Helical CT scan** with IV contrast is useful in the evaluation of parenchymal liver disease. It has the added feature of contrast enhancement to define space-occupying lesions (e.g., abscess and tumor) and allows calculation of liver volume. Triple-phase CT (arterial, venous, and delayed phases) is indicated for liver mass evaluation. A delayed phase is useful when cholangiocarcinoma is suspected.
- **MRI** offers information similar to that provided by CT scan with the additional advantage of better characterization of liver lesions, fatty infiltration, and iron deposition. It is the modality of choice in patients with an allergy to iodinated contrast. This modality should not be used in patients with renal failure (glomerular filtration rate [GFR] <30 mL/min/1.73 m^2) due to the very low risk of gadolinium-associated nephrogenic systemic fibrosis. Of all the cross-sectional imaging techniques, MRI provides the highest tissue contrast. This, in conjunction with various contrast agents (especially hepatobiliary contrast agents), allows for definitive noninvasive characterization of liver lesions.
- **Magnetic resonance cholangiopancreatography (MRCP)** is a specialized version of MRI that provides an alternative noninvasive diagnostic modality for visualizing the intrahepatic and extrahepatic bile ducts. MRCP does not require contrast material to be administered into the ductal system.

Diagnostic Procedures

- **Percutaneous transhepatic cholangiography (PTC) and endoscopic retrograde cholangiopancreatography (ERCP)** involve the instillation of contrast into the biliary tree. They are most useful after the preliminary determination of abnormalities detected by ultrasonography, CT, or MRI/MRCP. These procedures allow for diagnostic and therapeutic maneuvers including biopsy, brushings, stenting, and placement of drains.
- **Percutaneous liver biopsy** is an invasive procedure that can be performed with or without radiographic (ultrasound or CT) guidance. Bleeding, pain, infection, injury to adjacent organs, and (rarely) death are potential complications. In the presence of coagulopathy, thrombocytopenia, and/or ascites, a biopsy can be obtained by the transjugular route. Suspicious liver lesions are usually biopsied with ultrasonographic or CT guidance. Laparoscopy is an alternative method for obtaining liver tissue.
- **Transjugular assessment of portal pressure** is an invasive procedure to measure the hepatic venous pressure gradient (HVPG), which is the difference between the wedged (representing the portal venous pressure) and the free hepatic venous pressures. The normal HVPG pressure is <6 mm Hg. HVPG >6 mm Hg is considered portal hypertension. Complications of portal hypertension such as ascites and esophageal varices usually manifest with HVPG >10 mm Hg.
- Noninvasive tests to assess fibrosis/cirrhosis, including AST-to-platelet ratio index (APRI), FibroScan, FibroTest/Fibrosure, transient elastography, and magnetic resonance spectroscopy, are being considered as alternative options to liver biopsy. Studies evaluating the combination of radiologic and serologic modalities to accurately detect the degree of fibrosis are under evaluation.

VIRAL HEPATITIS

The hepatotropic viruses include hepatitis A virus (HAV), hepatitis B virus (HBV), hepatitis C virus (HCV), hepatitis D virus (HDV), and hepatitis E virus (HEV) (Tables 19-1 and 19-2). Nonhepatotropic viruses (viruses that indirectly affect the liver) include Epstein-Barr virus, cytomegalovirus, herpesvirus, measles, Ebola, and others.

Acute viral hepatitis is defined by an array of symptoms that may vary from mild, nonspecific symptoms to acute or fulminant hepatic failure. This condition may resolve or progress to chronic hepatitis, in certain cases, or to liver failure as a consequence of diffuse necroinflammatory liver injury.

Acute or fulminant hepatic failure (FHF) is defined as the rapid development of severe liver injury with encephalopathy and coagulopathy in a patient without preexisting liver disease within <6 months from the onset of the acute illness.

Chronic viral hepatitis is defined as the presence of persistent (>6 months) virologic replication, as determined by serologic and molecular studies, with necroinflammatory and fibrotic injury. Symptoms and biochemical abnormalities may vary from none to moderate. Histopathologic classification of chronic viral hepatitis is based on etiology, grade, and stage. Grading and staging are measures of the severity of the inflammatory process and fibrosis, respectively. Chronic viral hepatitis may lead to cirrhosis and HCC.

Hepatitis A Virus

GENERAL PRINCIPLES

- HAV is an **RNA virus** that belongs to the **picornavirus family**. It is transmitted via the fecal–oral route and is the most common cause of acute viral hepatitis worldwide.
- Large-scale outbreaks due to contamination of food and drinking water can occur.
- The period of greatest infectivity is 2 weeks before the onset of clinical illness; virus shedding in infected patients' feces continues for 2–3 weeks after the onset of symptoms.

TABLE 19-1   **Clinical and Epidemiologic Features of Hepatotropic Viruses**

Organism	Hepatitis A	Hepatitis B	Hepatitis C	Hepatitis D	Hepatitis E
Incubation	15–45 d	30–180 d	15–150 d	30–150 d	30–60 d
Transmission	Fecal–oral	Blood Sexual Perinatal	Blood Sexual (rare) Perinatal (rare)	Blood Sexual (rare)	Fecal–oral Organ transplantation
Risk groups	Residents of and travelers to endemic regions Children and caregivers in daycare centers	Injection drug users Multiple sexual partners Men who have sex with men Infants born to infected mothers Health care workers	Injection drug users Transfusion recipients	Any person with hepatitis B virus Injection drug users	Residents of and travelers to endemic regions Zoonosis: workers in pig farms
Fatality rate	1.0%	1.0%	<0.1%	2–10%	1%
Carrier state	No	Yes	Yes	Yes	No
Chronic hepatitis	None	2–10% in adults; 90% in children <5 yr	70–85%	Variable	Rare
Cirrhosis	No	Yes	Yes	Yes	No

TABLE 19-2	Viral Hepatitis Serologies[a]			
Hepatitis	**Acute**	**Chronic**	**Recovered/Latent**	**Vaccinated**
HAV	IgM anti-HAV+	NA	IgG anti-HAV+	IgG anti-HAV+
HCV	All tests possibly negative HCV RNA+ Anti-HCV Ab+ in 8 wk after infection	Anti-HCV Ab+ HCV RNA+	Anti-HCV Ab+ HCV RNA−[b]	NA
HDV	IgM anti-HDV+[c] HDV Ag+[c]	IgG anti-HDV+[c]	IgG anti-HDV+[c]	Vaccination against HBV
HEV	IgM anti-HEV	NA	IgG anti-HEV	NA

Ab, antibody; HAV, hepatitis A virus; HCV, hepatitis C virus; HDV, hepatitis D virus; HEV, hepatitis E virus; NA, not applicable.
[a]For hepatitis B virus serologies, see Table 19-3.
[b]Negative HCV RNA results should be interpreted with caution. Differences are found in thresholds for detection among assays and among laboratories.
[c]Markers of HBV infection are also present because HDV cannot replicate in the absence of HBV.

DIAGNOSIS

- HAV can be silent (subclinical), especially in children and young adults. Symptoms vary from mild illness to FHF and commonly include malaise, fatigue, pruritus, headache, abdominal pain, myalgias, arthralgias, nausea, vomiting, anorexia, and fever.
- **Physical examination** may reveal jaundice, hepatomegaly, and in rare cases, lymphadenopathy, splenomegaly, or a vascular rash.
- **Aminotransferase** elevations range from 10–100 times the upper limit of normal.
- The diagnosis of acute HAV is made by the detection of **IgM anti-HAV antibodies**.
- The **recovery phase** and **immunity phase** are characterized by the presence of **IgG anti-HAV antibodies and the decline of IgM anti-HAV antibodies**.
- Liver biopsy is rarely needed.
- **FHF** is rare, but the risk increases with age: 0.1% in patients younger than 15 years to >1% in patients older than 40 years.

TREATMENT

- Supportive symptomatic treatment is recommended.
- Liver transplantation is an option for FHF.

OUTCOME/PROGNOSIS

- Almost all cases of acute HAV hepatitis will resolve in 4–8 weeks. HAV does not progress to chronicity.
- A prolonged cholestatic disease, characterized by persistent jaundice and waxing and waning of liver enzymes, is more frequently seen in adults.

Hepatitis B Virus

GENERAL PRINCIPLES

- **HBV** is a **DNA virus** that belongs to the **hepadnavirus family**. The United States is considered an area of low prevalence for the infection. Eight genotypes of HBV have been identified (A through H). The prevalence of HBV genotypes varies depending on the geographic location. Genotypes A, B, and C are the most prevalent in the United States.
- Modes of transmission include vertical (mother to infant) and horizontal (person to person) via the following routes: parenteral or percutaneous (e.g., injection drug use, needlestick injuries), direct contact with blood or open sores of an infected person, and sexual contact with an infected individual.
- The rate of progression from acute to chronic HBV is approximately 90% for a perinatal-acquired infection, 20–50% for infections acquired between the age of 1–5 years, and <5% for an adult-acquired infection.

DIAGNOSIS

Clinical Presentation

- According to the natural history of chronic HBV infection, three different **clinical phases** have been defined (Table 19-3):
  - Immune tolerant
  - Immune active (hepatitis B envelope antigen [HBeAg] positive and HBeAg negative)
  - Low replication
- **Extrahepatic manifestations** include polyarteritis nodosa, glomerulonephritis, cryoglobulinemia, serum sickness–like illness, membranous nephropathy, membranoproliferative glomerulonephritis, and papular acrodermatitis (predominantly in children).

Diagnostic Testing

- HBV antigens (hepatitis B surface antigen [HBsAg] and HBeAg) can be detected in the serum. In the liver tissue, **HBsAg** stains in the hepatocyte cytoplasm, and **hepatitis B core antigen (HBcAg)** stains in the hepatocyte nuclei.
- **HBV DNA** is the most accurate marker of viral replication. It is detected by polymerase chain reaction (PCR). Large population-based studies have demonstrated a correlation between HBV DNA levels and disease progression to cirrhosis, decompensation, and development of HCC (*Gastroenterology 2006;130:678*; *JAMA 2006;295:65*).
- For use of HBV markers in clinical practice, see Table 19-3.
- **Liver biopsy** is useful to assess the degree of inflammation (grade) and fibrosis (stage) as well as other potential histologic abnormalities in patients with chronic hepatitis. Liver histology is an important adjuvant diagnostic test in guiding treatment decisions.

TREATMENT

- The treatment goal is viral eradication or suppression to prevent progression to ESLD and HCC. End points of treatment include:
  - Maintained suppression of serum HBV DNA levels to undetectable levels
  - HBsAg clearance and seroconversion to antibody anti-HBs
  - HBeAg clearance and seroconversion to antibody anti-HBe
  - Normalization of serum ALT
  - Improvement in liver histology
- There are several treatment guidelines for patients with HBV. In general, all the guidelines (referred to in Table 19-4) recommend that patients with compensated cirrhosis

TABLE 19-3 Use of Hepatitis B Virus (HBV) Markers in Clinical Practice

Test	Acute HBV	Resolved Acute HBV	Immune-Tolerant Chronic HBV	Immune-Active Chronic HBV (wild-type)	Immune-Active Chronic HBV (pre-core or basal core promoter mutant)	Low-Replication Chronic HBV	Vaccine Immunity
HBsAg	+	−	+	+	+	+	−
HBeAg	+	−	+	+	−	−	−
Anti-HBs	−	+	−	−	−	−	+
Anti-HBe	−	+	−	−	+	+	−
IgM anti-HBc	+	−	−	−	−	−	−
IgG anti-HBc	−	+	−	+	+	+	−
HBV DNA	>10^6 IU/mL	Neg	>10$^{6-10}$ IU/mL	>10^6 IU/mL	>10$^{3-4}$ IU/mL	<10^2 IU/mL	Neg
ALT/AST	++++	Nor	Nor	+++	++	Nor	Nor

ALT, alanine aminotransferase; AST, aspartate aminotransferase; HBc, hepatitis B core antigen; HBeAg, hepatitis B e antigen; HBsAg, hepatitis B surface antigen; Neg, negative; Nor, normal.

TABLE 19-4 Treatment Guidelines for Chronic Hepatitis B

Guideline	HBeAg Positive			HBeAg Negative		
	HBV DNA	ALT	Liver Biopsy	HBV DNA	ALT	Liver Biopsy
AASLD (2009)	>20,000	>2× ULN	—	>20,000	>2× ULN	—
	>20,000	≤2× ULN	Biopsy[a]	2,000–20,000	<2× ULN	Biopsy[b]
EASL (2012)	>2,000	>ULN	Optional[c]	>2,000	>ULN	Optional[c]
	>20,000	>ULN	—	>20,000	>ULN	—
APASL (2012)	>20,000	>2× ULN	—	>2,000	>2× ULN	—
	>20,000	<2× ULN	Biopsy[a]	>2,000	<2× ULN	Optional[d]

AALSD, American Association for the Study of Liver Diseases; ALT, alanine aminotransferase; APASL, Asian Pacific Association for the Study of the Liver; EASL, European Association for the Study of the Liver; HBeAg, hepatitis B e antigen; HBV, hepatitis B virus; ULN, upper limit of normal (ULN for AALSD: 30 units/L for males, 19 units/L for females; ULN for EASL and APASL: 40 units/L).

[a]Biopsy indicated for >40 years of age, ALT persistently 1–2× ULN, and family history of hepatocellular carcinoma.

[b]Treat if abnormal.

[c]Biopsy may be substituted with noninvasive markers of fibrosis.

[d]Biopsy indicated for patients ≥40 years of age.

with HBV DNA levels >2000 IU/mL should be treated independently of the ALT level; those with HBV DNA levels <2000 IU/mL should be treated only if the ALT is elevated. Patients with decompensated cirrhosis should be treated regardless of HBV DNA level or serum ALT (*J Hepatol 2009;50:227*).
- Chronic hepatitis B immune-tolerant patients and chronic hepatitis B with low replication should not be treated.
- Indications for stopping treatment, as per the current guidelines, include the following. For HBeAg-positive patients, treatment can be discontinued after 6 months (American Association for the Study of Liver Diseases [AASLD]) or 12 months (European Association for the Study of the Liver [EASL] and Asian Pacific Association for the Study of the Liver [APASL]) after the induction of negative HBV DNA and seroconversion to anti-HBe. For HBeAg-negative patients, the treatment can be stopped after the loss of HBsAg (EASL and AASLD), whereas APASL recommends a minimum of 2 years of HBV DNA negativity at three testing points obtained 6 months apart.

Medications

Medications for the treatment of hepatitis B are divided into three main groups: nucleoside analogs (entecavir), nucleotide analogs (tenofovir), and the interferons (IFNs).
- **Entecavir** is a potent anti-HBV oral nucleoside (guanosine) analog and is well tolerated. Dose is 0.5–1.0 mg daily in naïve and lamivudine (LAM)-resistant patients. Entecavir has a high genetic barrier for resistance (1.2%) over several years. However, in patients resistant to LAM, the resistance to entecavir could be as high as 40%. In patients with renal impairment, dose adjustment is needed. Side effects include headache, upper respiratory tract infection, cough, nasopharyngitis, fatigue, and abdominal pain. Entecavir is pregnancy category C.
- **Tenofovir** is a potent anti-HBV oral nucleotide (acyclic) analog and is well tolerated. Dose is 300 mg daily. Tenofovir has a high genetic barrier for resistance; no clinical resistance has been identified thus far. It is rarely reported to induce renal failure and Fanconi syndrome and may also lead to decreased bone density. Tenofovir is pregnancy category B.
- **IFNs** (α2a and α2b, in their pegylated form) are antiviral, immunomodulatory, and antiproliferative glycoproteins that have been used in the treatment of chronic HBV for several years. IFNs are parenteral agents and associated with a poor tolerability profile, especially in patients with advanced liver disease. Long-term studies have shown a durable benefit in responders. Neither IFN nor pegylated IFN-α induces antiviral resistance. The IFNs are pregnancy category C.

PREVENTION

- **Preexposure prophylaxis**
  ○ **HBV vaccine** should be considered for everyone but particularly for individuals who belong to high-risk groups. HBV vaccines are safe.
  ○ HBV vaccination schedule includes three IM injections at 0, 1, and 6 months in infants or healthy adults. Protective antibody response (anti-HBs positive) is observed in >90% after the third dose.
- **Postexposure prophylaxis**
  ○ **Infants born to HBsAg-positive mothers should receive HBV vaccine and hepatitis B immunoglobulin (HBIg), 0.5 mL, within 12 hours of birth.** Immunized infants should be tested at approximately 12 months of age for HBsAg, anti-HBs, and anti-HBc.
  ○ Susceptible sexual partners of individuals with HBV and those with needlestick injury should receive HBIg (0.04–0.07 mL/kg) and the first dose of HBV vaccine at different sites as soon as possible (preferably within 48 hours but no more than 7 days after exposure). A second dose of HBIg should be administered 30 days after exposure, and the vaccination schedule should be completed.

○ Postexposure prophylaxis with HBIg plus a nucleotide or nucleoside analog should be used initially after liver transplantation to prevent HBV recurrence in certain patients.

OUTCOME/PROGNOSIS

Chronic hepatitis B
- Morbidity and mortality in chronic HBV are linked to level and persistence of viral replication. Spontaneous clearance of HBsAg occurs in 0.5% of patients annually.
- Once the diagnosis of chronic HBV is established, the 5-year cumulative incidence of developing cirrhosis ranges from 8–20%.
- Of patients with chronic HBV, 5–10% progress to HCC **with or without preceding cirrhosis**.

Hepatitis C

BASIC PRINCIPLES

- HCV is an RNA virus that belongs to the **flavivirus** family. There are six HCV genotypes with multiple subtypes. Genotype 1 accounts for about 75% and genotypes 2 and 3 account for about 20% of HCV infections in the United States.
- **HCV** is the most common chronic bloodborne infection and is a global health problem, with approximately **180 million carriers worldwide**.
- The most frequent mode of transmission is parenteral. Less common modes of transmission include high-risk sexual practices including men who have sex with men and perinatal transmission. Transmission by transfusion of blood products (and their derivatives) and organ transplantation has been reduced to near zero in developed countries due to sensitive screening methods.

DIAGNOSIS

Clinical Presentation
- The incubation period varies from 15–150 days.
- **Acute HCV hepatitis** is defined as presenting within 6 months of the exposure to HCV. During this time, there is a 20–50% chance of spontaneous resolution of infection (*Am J Gastroenterol 2008;103:1283*). Symptoms may vary from mild illness to FHF. Malaise, fatigue, pruritus, headache, abdominal pain, myalgias, arthralgias, nausea, vomiting, anorexia, and fever are nonspecific symptoms.
- **Chronic HCV hepatitis** runs an indolent course, sometimes for decades. Fatigue is a common symptom. The disease may only become clinically apparent late in the natural course, when symptoms are associated with advanced liver disease.
- **Extrahepatic manifestations** include mixed cryoglobulinemia (10–25% of patients with HCV), glomerular diseases (mixed cryoglobulinemia syndrome, membranous nephropathy, polyarteritis nodosa), porphyria cutanea tarda, cutaneous necrotizing vasculitis, lichen planus, lymphoma, diabetes mellitus, and other autoimmune disorders.

Diagnostic Testing
- **Antibodies against HCV (anti-HCV)** may be undetectable for the first 8 weeks after infection. These antibodies are detected by enzyme immunoassay (EIA). **Antibodies do not confer immunity.** The test has a sensitivity of 95–99% and a lower specificity. A false-positive test (anti-HCV positive with HCV RNA negative) may be detected in

the setting of autoimmune hepatitis (AIH) or hypergammaglobulinemia. A false-negative test (anti-HCV negative with HCV RNA positive) may be seen in immunosuppressed individuals and in patients on hemodialysis.

- **HCV RNA** can be detected by **PCR** in serum as early as **1–2 weeks after infection** (qualitative and quantitative assays). It is expressed in IU/mL, with lower limits of detection approaching 10 IU/mL. HCV RNA determination is useful for both diagnosis and treatment purposes.
- **HCV genotypes and subtypes** can be detected by commercially available serologic and molecular assays. HCV genotype influences the response to treatment.
- **Liver biopsy** is useful to score the degree of inflammation (grade) and fibrosis (stage) in the liver of chronically infected patients. It is useful to grade the amount of liver steatosis and guide treatment decisions.
- Noninvasive markers of fibrosis are increasingly being used as an alternative to liver biopsy.

TREATMENT

- Acute infection: Monitor for spontaneous clearance, which is rare after 4 months. Although pegylated IFN monotherapy induces a sustained virologic response (SVR) in 80–94% of patients without ribavirin for a 24-week period independent of the genotype, current AASLD guidelines recommend to treat as described for chronic HCV infection.
- Treatment should be considered for patients with chronic HCV. Patients with limited life expectancy due to non–liver-related comorbid conditions do not require treatment.
- The highest priority for treatment should be given to patients with advanced liver disease, co-infected (HIV and HBV) patients, patients with extrahepatic manifestations, and those with recurrent HCV after liver transplantation.
- The **goal of treatment** of HCV-infected persons is eradication of HCV, as determined by an SVR. SVR is defined as absence of detectable HCV RNA 12 weeks after completion of therapy. SVR reduces morbidity and end-stage complications of HCV infection including cirrhosis, HCC, and mortality (*Ann Intern Med 2013;158:3297*).

Medications

- Current regimens for the treatment of chronic HCV are IFN-free regimens. Medications for HCV treatment include the following:
  - **Ribavirin** is a guanosine analog antiviral agent (nucleoside inhibitor). It is generally not effective when used alone but plays an important role in combination treatment.
  - **Direct-acting antivirals (DAAs)** target specific nonstructural proteins of the virus, resulting in disruption of viral replication. Current treatment regimens for HCV include the combination of more than one DAA with or without ribavirin.
    - **Nonstructural proteins 3/4A (NS3/4A) protease inhibitors (PIs)** include the first-generation PIs telaprevir and boceprevir, which are no longer in use. Currently approved NS3/4A PIs include simeprevir and paritaprevir. Paritaprevir is boosted with ritonavir in for HCV treatment.
    - **NS5A inhibitors** include ledipasvir and ombitasvir.
    - **NS5B nucleos(t)ide polymerase inhibitors (NPIs)** include sofosbuvir and dasabuvir.
- The selection of a particular treatment regimen is dependent on several factors that are determined by a combination of clinical, biochemical, serologic, molecular, and imaging modalities and fibrosis score:
  - Treatment naïve (those who have never received any treatment for HCV) or treatment experienced (those who have failed an HCV treatment regimen)
  - HCV genotype and subtype
  - Stage or degree of liver fibrosis
  - Potential drug interactions
  - Comorbid conditions

TABLE 19-5		Treatment for Genotype 1 Chronic Hepatitis C Virus Infection		
Drug Regimen	**Dose**	**Duration of Treatment**	**Efficacy (%) Sustained Virological Response**	
Sofosbuvir + Ledipasvir	1 tab/d	12 wk	**Naïve** Cirrhotic 94 Noncirrhotic[a] 99	**Experienced** Cirrhotic[b] 100 Noncirrhotic 95
Sofosbuvir (SOF) Simeprevir (SMV)	1 tab/d (SOF) 1 tab/d (SMV)	12 wk	**Naïve** 93[c]	**Experienced** F0–F1 97 F2 96 F3–F4[d] 93
Paritaprevir + Ritonavir + Ombitasvir (3D) Dasabuvir (DSV)	2 tab/d (3D) 1 tab BID (DSV) +/− Ribavirin	12 wk	**Genotype 1b** Noncirrhotic *Experienced* 100 *Naïve* 100 Cirrhotic *Experienced* 86–100 *Naïve* 100	**Genotype 1a**[e] Noncirrhotic *Experienced* 94–100 *Naïve* 96 Cirrhotic *Experienced* 80–100 *Naïve* 92

SVR, sustained virologic response.
[a]Naïve, noncirrhotic, viral load <6 million → treat for 8 weeks; SVR 95%.
[b]24 weeks of treatment, SVR 98%.
[c]24 weeks of treatment, SVR 100%.
[d]Treatment for 12 and 24 weeks resulted in similar efficacy for regimen containing ribavirin. For nonribavirin regimen, treatment for 24 weekly yielded SVR of 100%.
[e]For cirrhosis, genotype 1a, 24 weeks of treatment resulted in an SVR of 96% for naïve and experienced patients.

- **Chronic infection:** Treatment options vary depending on genotype and subtype, all with similar efficacy.
- **Genotypes 1–3** are the most commonly encountered genotypes in North America and Europe. Refer to Tables 19-5, 19-6, and 19-7 for specific treatment recommendations for genotypes 1a, 1b, 2, and 3. **Current treatments are all oral and IFN free.**
- **Genotypes 4–6** are rarely encountered in North America, and data on treatment are limited, particularly for genotypes 5 and 6. Current recommendations suggest the following treatments for **treatment-naïve** individuals:
  - **Genotype 4:** similar for genotype 1 (see Table 19-5)
  - Genotype 5: sofosbuvir plus peginterferon and weight-based ribavirin for 12 weeks
  - Genotype 6: ledipasvir-sofosbuvir for 12 weeks or sofosbuvir plus peginterferon and weight-based ribavirin for 12 weeks

PREVENTION

No preexposure prophylaxis or vaccine exists. Prevention of high-risk behaviors and lifestyle modifications should be encouraged.

OUTCOME/PROGNOSIS

HCC develops in approximately **1–2% of patients per year** and rarely occurs in the absence of cirrhosis.

TABLE 19-6	Treatment for Genotype 2 Chronic Hepatitis C Virus Infection		
	Dose	**Length of Treatment**	**Efficacy (SVR in %)**
Sofosbuvir (SOF) + RBV			
Naïve	1 tab SOF + RBV	12 wk	97 (noncirrhotic) 83–100 (cirrhotic)
Experienced	1 tab SOF + RBV	12 wk	92–96 (noncirrhotic) 88–94 (cirrhotic)
SOF + daclatasvir (DAC)	1 tab SOF + 1 tab DAC	24 wk	92

RBV, ribavirin; SVR, sustained virologic response.

OTHER HEPATITIS VIRUSES

Hepatitis D

HDV is a circular RNA virus and is the only member of the genus *Delta virus*. It is found throughout the world and is endemic to the Mediterranean basin, the Middle East, and portions of South America (Amazon basin). Outside these areas, infections occur primarily in individuals who have received transfusions or in injection drug users. In countries such as the United States where HDV infection is rare, testing for HDV infection is not necessary in all patients with HBV infection. **HDV requires the presence of HBV for infection and replication.** In patients with coinfection (acute hepatitis B and D), the course is transient and self-limited. The rate of progression to chronicity is similar to the one reported for acute HBV. **IFN-α** is the **treatment of choice** for chronic hepatitis D.

TABLE 19-7	Treatment for Genotype 3 Chronic Hepatitis C Virus Infection		
	Dose	**Length of Treatment**	**Efficacy (SVR in %)**
Sofosbuvir (SOF) + RBV +/− interferon (IFN)			
Naïve	1 tab SOF + RBV	24 wk	94 (noncirrhotic) 92 (cirrhotic)
Naïve, noncirrhotic	1 tab SOF + RBV + IFN	12 wk	97
Experienced	1 tab SOF + RBV	24 wk	87 (noncirrhotic) 60 (cirrhotic)
SOF + daclatasvir (DAC)			
Naïve	1 tab SOF + 1 tab DAC	12 wk	97 (noncirrhotic) 58 (cirrhotic)
Experienced	1 tab SOF + 1 tab DAC	12 wk	94 (noncirrhotic) 69 (cirrhotic)

RBV, ribavirin; SVR, sustained virologic response.

Hepatitis E

HEV is an **RNA virus** that belongs to the Hepeviridae family. Hepatitis E is considered a zoonotic disease, and reservoirs include pigs, wild boar, deer, and potentially other species. Transmission closely resembles that of HAV (i.e., **fecal–oral route**). Acute hepatitis E is clinically indistinguishable from other acute viral hepatitis and is usually a self-limited illness. Hepatitis E can cause chronic infection (HEV RNA for >6 months). Most cases have occurred in solid organ transplant recipients or immunosuppressed individuals (e.g., HIV). In a recent retrospective, multicenter study of 59 transplant recipients with chronic hepatitis E, the use of ribavirin monotherapy for 3 months achieved an SVR of 78% (*N Engl J Med 2014;370(12):1111*).

DRUG-INDUCED LIVER INJURY

GENERAL PRINCIPLES

- The National Institutes of Health (NIH) maintains a searchable database of drugs, herbal medications, and dietary supplements that have been associated with drug-induced liver injury (DILI) at *http://livertox.nih.gov/*. Over 1000 drugs and herbals have been associated with DILI.
- There are three major classifications of DILI that occur as a result of both intrinsic and idiosyncratic hepatotoxicity:
  - Hepatocellular injury refers to injury to the liver cell.
  - Cholestatic injury refers to injury to the biliary system or to hepatocytes with resulting intrahepatic cholestasis
  - Mixed hepatocellular and cholestatic injury refers to injury to both the liver cell and the biliary system.
- DILI is associated with approximately 50% of all the cases of FHF in the United States, with acetaminophen being the most common causative agent. Acute DILI can progress to chronic injury in 5–10% of cases. Patients with chronic DILI may go on to develop significant fibrosis or cirrhosis and have signs and symptoms associated with cirrhosis or hepatic decompensation.
- Other less common types of DILI include chronic hepatitis, chronic cholestasis, granulomatous hepatitis, fibrosis or cirrhosis, and carcinogenesis.

DIAGNOSIS

Clinical Presentation

- The acute presentation can be clinically silent. When symptoms are present, they are nonspecific and include nausea/vomiting, general malaise, fatigue, jaundice, pruritus, and abdominal pain. In the acute setting, the majority of patients will recover after cessation of the offending drug.
- Fever and rash may also be seen in association with hypersensitivity reactions.

Diagnostic Criteria

- Clinical suspicion
- Temporal relation of liver injury to drug usage
- Resolution of liver injury after the suspected agent has been discontinued (except in cases of chronic DILI)

Diagnostic Testing

Biochemical abnormalities
- **Hepatocellular injury:** AST and ALT elevation more than two times the upper limit of normal.

- **Cholestatic injury:** ALP and conjugated bilirubin elevation more than two times the upper limit of normal.
- **Mixed injury** includes increases in all of the mentioned biochemical abnormalities to more than two times the upper limit of normal.

Diagnostic Procedures
Liver biopsy is sometimes needed.

TREATMENT

Nonpharmacologic Therapies
- Treatment includes cessation of offending drug and institution of supportive measures.
- An attempt to remove the agent from the GI tract should be made in most cases of acute toxic ingestion using lavage or cathartics (see Chapter 28, Toxicology).
- Management of acetaminophen overdose is a medical emergency (see Chapter 28, Toxicology).

Surgical Management
Liver transplantation may be an option for patients with drug-induced FHF.

OUTCOME/PROGNOSIS

Prognosis of DILI is often unique to the offending medication.

ALCOHOLIC LIVER DISEASE

GENERAL PRINCIPLES

- Alcoholism is a significant medical and socioeconomic problem.
- In 2012, 3.3 million deaths, or 5.9% of all global deaths, were attributable to alcohol consumption. Approximately 17 million US adults age 18 and older (7.2% of this age group) had an alcohol use disorder in 2012.
- The spectrum of alcoholic liver disease includes fatty liver, alcoholic hepatitis, and alcoholic cirrhosis.
- Fatty liver is the most commonly observed abnormality and occurs in up to 90% of alcoholics.
- In all of the excessive alcohol users, between 10–20% develop cirrhosis and 35% develop alcoholic hepatitis. More than half of the latter will progress to cirrhosis.
- Alcoholic cirrhosis is a common cause of ESLD and HCC.

DIAGNOSIS

Clinical Presentation
- **Fatty liver**
  - Patients are usually asymptomatic.
  - Clinical findings include hepatomegaly and mild liver enzyme abnormalities.
- **Alcoholic hepatitis**
  - Alcoholic hepatitis may be clinically silent or severe enough to lead to rapid development of hepatic failure and death.
  - Clinical features include fever, abdominal pain, anorexia, nausea, vomiting, weight loss, and jaundice.
  - In severe cases, patients may develop transient portal hypertension.

- **Alcoholic cirrhosis**
  - The presentation is variable, from clinically silent disease to decompensated cirrhosis.
  - Patients frequently give a history of drinking until the onset of symptoms.
  - Alcoholics may underestimate or minimize their reported alcohol abuse.

Diagnostic Testing

Laboratories
- In alcoholic fatty liver, laboratory tests may be normal or demonstrate **mild elevation in serum aminotransferases** (AST greater than ALT) and ALP.
- In alcoholic hepatitis, laboratory tests typically demonstrate elevation in serum aminotransferases (AST greater than ALT with a 2:1 ratio) and ALP. Hyperbilirubinemia (conjugated) and elevated prothrombin time (PT)/international normalized ratio (INR) may also be observed.
  - Laboratory abnormalities associated with a poor prognosis include renal failure, leukocytosis, a markedly elevated total bilirubin, and elevation of PT/INR that does not normalize with subcutaneous or IV vitamin K. Administration of oral vitamin K is not recommended due to poor gut absorption in patients with jaundice (*Clin Liver Dis 2012;16:371*).
- A number of classification systems have been developed to risk stratify patients with alcoholic hepatitis and assess response to treatment:
  - **Discriminant function (DF)** = $4.6 \times (PT_{patient} - PT_{control})$ + serum bilirubin. Scores <32 and >32 have 93% and 68% 1-month survival, respectively.
  - **The Glasgow Alcoholic Hepatitis Score (GAHS)** incorporates patient age, white blood cell count, blood urea, PT/INR, and serum bilirubin (Table 19-8). A score <9 has no difference in survival between untreated and steroid-treated patients. A score >9 has a difference in 1-month survival between untreated (52% 1-month survival) and steroid-treated (78% 1-month survival) patients (*Gut 2007;56:1743*).
  - The **Lille model** incorporates age, renal insufficiency, albumin, PT, bilirubin, and the evolution of bilirubin at day 7 (bilirubin on day 7 – bilirubin on day 0) to predict 6-month mortality in patients with severe alcoholic hepatitis who have received corticosteroid therapy. In a prospective study, a score of ≥0.45 was associated with a lower 6-month survival compared to a score <0.45 (25% vs. 85%). A score >0.45 suggests that a patient is not responding to glucocorticoid therapy (*Hepatology 2007;45:1348*).

Diagnostic Procedures
- The typical histopathologic findings in alcoholic liver disease include hepatocyte ballooning with and without Mallory-Denk bodies, lobular inflammation, necrosis of hepatocytes, periportal fibrosis, perivenular and pericellular fibrosis, ductal proliferation, and fatty changes.

TABLE 19-8	The Glasgow Alcoholic Hepatitis Score		
	Points Given		
Variable	**1**	**2**	**3**
Age	<50	≥50	—
WBC ($\times 10^9$/L)	<15	≥15	—
Urea (mmol/L)	<5	≥5	—
INR	<1.5	1.5–2.0	>2.0
Bilirubin (μmol/L)	<125	125–250	>250

INR, international normalized ratio; WBC, white blood cell.

- The indication of liver biopsy depends on the clinical assessment of the patient. It may be helpful if alternate diagnoses are being considered.

TREATMENT

- The cornerstone of treatment is abstinence from alcohol.
- Nutritional status should be evaluated and corrected accordingly. Nutrition should be oral or by a small-bore feeding tube. Peripheral parenteral nutrition (PPN) and total parenteral nutrition (TPN) are alternative options. Good nutrition improves nitrogen balance, may improve liver tests, and may decrease hepatic fat accumulation, but generally does not enhance survival.

Medications

Treatment of acute alcoholic hepatitis with corticosteroids is controversial. However, there is evidence that patients with a DF >32 and GAHS >9 may have a short-term benefit from steroid therapy. An early decrease in bilirubin levels after 1 week of treatment portends a better prognosis (Lille score).

- **Oral prednisolone** (40 mg/d PO for 4 weeks, followed by a taper over 2–4 weeks) is a steroid treatment for patients with severe alcoholic hepatitis. Prednisolone is preferred (but not demonstrated to be better) over prednisone as the latter requires conversion to its active form, prednisolone, within the liver. In a recent trial, prednisolone demonstrated a beneficial effect on short-term mortality (28 days), but not on the medium- or long-term mortality (90 days and 1 year, respectively) (*N Engl J Med 2015;372:1619*).
- **Pentoxifylline** (400 mg PO tid for 4 weeks) is a nonselective phosphodiesterase inhibitor that, in a recent trial, did not show improved outcomes in this patient group (*N Engl J Med 2015;372:1619*).

Surgical Management

Patients with cirrhosis and ESLD can be evaluated for liver transplantation but are required to abstain from alcohol for 6 months prior to evaluation, maintain abstinence, and be part of a rehabilitation program.

OUTCOME/PROGNOSIS

- Fatty liver may be reversible with abstinence.
- In alcoholic hepatitis, prognosis depends on the severity of presentation and alcohol abstinence. The in-hospital mortality for severe cases is approximately 50% due to complications including sepsis and renal failure.
- In alcoholic cirrhosis, prognosis is variable and depends on the degree of liver decompensation. Abstinence from alcohol may promote significant liver chemistry improvement.

IMMUNE-MEDIATED LIVER DISEASES

Autoimmune Hepatitis

GENERAL PRINCIPLES

AIH is a chronic unresolving inflammation of the liver of unknown cause, associated with circulating autoantibodies and hyperglobulinemia.

- Women are affected more than men (gender ratio, 3.6:1).
- Extrahepatic manifestations may be found in 30–50% of patients and include synovitis, celiac disease, Coombs-positive hemolytic anemia, autoimmune thyroiditis, Graves disease, rheumatoid arthritis, ulcerative colitis, and other immune-mediated processes.

Two types of AIH have been proposed based on differences in their immunologic markers. They have a good response to corticosteroid therapy.
- **Type I AIH** is the most common form of the disease and constitutes 80% of AIH cases. It is associated with antinuclear antibodies (ANAs) and anti–smooth muscle antibodies (SMAs).
- **Type 2 AIH** is characterized by antibodies to liver/kidney microsome type 1 (anti-LKM1) and/or liver cytosol type 1 (anti-LC1). This type is predominately seen in children and young adults (*J Hepatol 2015;62:S100*).

DIAGNOSIS

Clinical Presentation

- Aminotransferase elevations are generally more prominent than those of bilirubin and ALP, although a cholestatic picture marked by high levels of conjugated bilirubin and ALP can be seen.
- Elevation of serum globulins, particularly γ-globulins (IgG), is characteristic of AIH. Hyperglobulinemia is generally associated with circulating autoantibodies, which are helpful in identifying AIH.
- In approximately 30–40% of cases, the clinical presentation is similar to acute viral hepatitis. A smaller percentage of patients may present in FHF or with asymptomatic elevation of serum ALT. It presents with cirrhosis in at least 25% of patients.
- The most common symptoms at presentation include fatigue, jaundice, myalgias, anorexia, diarrhea, acne, abnormal menses, and right upper quadrant abdominal discomfort.
- Patients with AIH may overlap with clinical and histologic findings consistent with other liver diseases (e.g., PBC, PSC, Wilson disease, and autoimmune cholangitis).
- Diagnostic criteria have been codified by an international panel (*Hepatology 2002;36(2):479*). This same panel has since put forth simplified diagnostic criteria based on autoantibodies, IgG, histology, and the exclusion of viral hepatitis (*Hepatology 2010;51(6):7*).

Diagnostic Testing

Liver biopsy is recommended for definitive diagnosis.
- **"Piecemeal necrosis" or interface hepatitis** with lobular or panacinar inflammation (lymphocytic and plasmacytic infiltration) are the histologic hallmarks of the disease.
- Histologic changes, such as ductopenia or destructive cholangitis, may indicate overlap syndromes combining characteristics of AIH, PSC, PBC, or autoimmune cholangitis.

TREATMENT

Treatment should be started in patients with elevated serum aminotransferase levels (>5 times upper limit of normal), hyperglobulinemia, and histologic features of interface hepatitis, bridging, or multiacinar necrosis.

Medications

- Therapy consists of prednisone (50–60 mg/d PO) as monotherapy or at a lower dose (30 mg/d PO) in conjunction with azathioprine (50 mg or up to 1–2 mg/kg). The dose of prednisone is tapered down every 10–15 days, whereas the dose of azathioprine remains unchanged. As the AIH biochemical abnormalities subside, the maintenance regimen with combination therapy is continued for 1 year. The prednisone is then gradually stopped, and during the second year, treatment is with azathioprine monotherapy. At the end of the second year, a liver biopsy is obtained to reassess histologic regression. If the histology has normalized, in association with biochemical remission, options include discontinuation of the immuno-suppression with close follow-up to assess new flares or continuing the maintenance therapy.

- The combination of prednisone and azathioprine decreases corticosteroid-associated side effects; however, azathioprine should be used with caution in patients with pretreatment cytopenias or thiopurine methyltransferase deficiency.
- **Budesonide** (6–9 mg/d PO), in combination with azathioprine (1–2 mg/kg/d PO), may also result in normalization of AST and ALT, with fewer steroid-specific side effects, in **noncirrhotic** adults with AIH (*Gastroenterology 2010;139(4):1198*).
- Other treatment alternatives for suboptimal response or treatment failures include mycophenolate mofetil, tacrolimus, cyclosporine, and budesonide.

Surgical Management
- Liver transplantation should be considered in patients with ESLD and those with AIH-mediated FHF.
- After transplantation, recurrent AIH is seen in approximately 15% of patients. De novo AIH or immunologically mediated hepatitis, defined as hepatitis with histologic features similar to AIH in patients transplanted for nonautoimmune diseases, has been described in about 5% of transplant recipients.

MONITORING/FOLLOW-UP

- About 90% of adults have improvements in the serum aminotransferase, bilirubin, and γ-globulin levels within the first 2 weeks of treatment.
- Histologic improvement lags behind clinical and laboratory improvement by 3–8 months.

OUTCOME/PROGNOSIS

- The overall goal of treatment is normalization of aminotransferases, hyperglobulinemia (IgG), and liver histology.
- Remission is achieved in 65% and 80% of patients within 1.5 and 3.0 years of treatment, respectively.
- Relapses occur in at least 20–50% of patients after cessation of therapy and require retreatment.

Primary Biliary Cirrhosis

GENERAL PRINCIPLES

Primary biliary cirrhosis or primary biliary cholangitis (PBC) is a cholestatic hepatic disorder of unknown etiology with autoimmune features.
- It most often affects middle-aged women (>90%) and is more commonly described in Caucasians. It is caused by granulomatous destruction of the interlobular bile ducts, which leads to progressive ductopenia and cholestasis.
- Cholestasis is generally slowly progressive and can lead to cirrhosis and eventually liver failure.
- Extrahepatic manifestations include keratoconjunctivitis sicca (Sjögren), renal tubular acidosis, gallstones, thyroid disease, scleroderma, Raynaud phenomenon, CREST syndrome (calcinosis, Raynaud phenomenon, esophageal dysmotility, sclerodactyly, and telangiectasia), and celiac disease.

DIAGNOSIS

Clinical Presentation
- Fatigue, jaundice, and pruritus are often the most troublesome symptoms.
- Patients may present de novo with manifestations of ESLD.

- Although there are no exam findings that are specific for PBC, xanthomata and xanthelasma can be a clue to underlying cholestasis.

Diagnostic Testing

- Antimitochondrial antibodies are present in >90% of patients.
- Typical features include elevated levels of ALP, total bilirubin, cholesterol, and IgM.

Diagnostic Procedures
Liver biopsy is helpful for both diagnosis and staging.

TREATMENT

Medications

- No curative therapy is available; treatment aims to slow progression of disease.
- **Ursodeoxycholic acid (UDCA)** (13–15 mg/kg/d PO) is a bile acid derivative with hepatocyte cytoprotective properties that stimulates hepatocellular and ductular secretions. Traditionally, UDCA has been suggested to reduce mortality when given long term. However, recent meta-analyses have suggested an advantage of using a combination of UDCA plus steroids or UDCA plus bezafibrates over UDCA monotherapy (outcomes measured were all-cause mortality and liver transplantation). UDCA plus bezafibrates had a greater side effect profile compared to the other treatment options (*Medicine 2015;94(11):1*).
- **Obeticholic acid** (OCA; 10–50 mg/d PO) is a derivative of the primary bile acid chenodeoxycholic acid and affects bile acid homeostasis. This agent is expected to be approved by the US Food and Drug Administration (FDA) soon. In a trial of patients with PBC who had an inadequate response to UDCA, a 3-month treatment with OCA plus UDCA significantly reduced levels of ALP, GGT, and ALT when compared to UDCA plus placebo (*Gastroenterology 2015;148:751*).

Surgical Management

- Liver transplantation is an option in advanced disease.
- Recurrent PBC after transplantation has been documented at a rate of 20% over 10 years.

OUTCOME/PROGNOSIS

- PBC progresses along a path of increasingly severe histologic damage (florid bile duct lesions, ductular proliferation, fibrosis, and cirrhosis).
- Progression to cirrhosis and liver failure may occur years from diagnosis.

Primary Sclerosing Cholangitis

GENERAL PRINCIPLES

PSC is a cholestatic liver disorder characterized by inflammation, fibrosis, and obliteration of the extrahepatic and/or intrahepatic bile ducts.

- Patients with PSC can be subdivided into those with **small duct** and **large duct involvement**. Small duct disease is defined as typical histologic features of PSC with a normal cholangiogram. In classic PSC, characteristic strictures of the biliary tree can be detected by cholangiography. Patients with small duct disease have a more favorable prognosis (*Hepatology 2002;35:1494*).
- The peak incidence is at about age 40 years. Most patients are middle-aged men, and the male-to-female ratio is 2:1.
- PSC is frequently associated with inflammatory bowel disease (70% of patients have concomitant ulcerative colitis). The clinical course of these conditions is not correlated.

DIAGNOSIS

Clinical Presentation

- Clinical manifestations include intermittent episodes of jaundice, hepatomegaly, pruritus, weight loss, and fatigue. Patients slowly progress to cirrhosis.
- Acute cholangitis is defined as an infection of the biliary ductal system usually caused by bacteria ascending from its junction with the duodenum and is a frequent complication in patients with strictures of the biliary ducts. Symptoms of acute cholangitis include fever, chills, rigors, jaundice, and right upper quadrant pain.
- Cholangiocarcinoma is the most frequent neoplasm associated with PSC. Patients with PSC have a 15% lifetime risk of developing cholangiocarcinoma (*Curr Gastroenterol Rep 2015;17:17*).

Diagnostic Testing

- The diagnosis of PSC should be considered in individuals with inflammatory bowel disease who have increased levels of ALP even in the absence of symptoms of hepatobiliary disease.
- **ANA** is positive in up to 50% of cases, and perinuclear antineutrophil cytoplasmic antibody (p-ANCA) is positive in 80% of cases.
- MRCP is the preferred diagnostic study of choice.

Diagnostic Procedures

- ERCP can confirm the diagnosis of PSC by demonstrating strictures or irregularities of the intrahepatic or extrahepatic bile ducts. It also allows duct brushings and biopsies to be obtained to evaluate for associated malignancy. Intraductal endoscopy provides direct visualization of the biliary ducts with the advantage of direct tissue sampling.
- Liver biopsy is helpful in the diagnosis of small-duct PSC, in the exclusion of other diseases, and in staging. Characteristic histologic findings include concentric periductal fibrosis ("onion skinning"), degeneration of bile duct epithelium, ductular proliferation, ductopenia, and cholestasis.
- Fluorescent in situ hybridization (FISH) allows for molecular assessment of malignancy from tissue obtained by brushing or biopsy.

TREATMENT

Medications

- At this time, there is no established medical treatment for PSC. Clinical trials for the utilization of nuclear receptor ligands (fibrates, OCA, and TGR5 receptor ligand), novel bile acid therapies, and simtuzumab are under investigation.
- Several randomized, placebo-controlled trials comparing the use of UDCA (13–23 mg/kg/d) showed improvement of liver tests in the UDCA group compared to placebo. However, there was no difference in long-term survival or time to liver transplantation between both groups. UDCA (>28 mg/kg/d) was associated with a higher risk of serious adverse events including death and transplantation and is **not** currently recommended for **PSC therapy** (*Gastroenterology 2013;145:521*).
- Episodes of cholangitis should be managed with IV antibiotics and endoscopic therapy.

Other Nonpharmacologic Therapies

- ERCP can be useful to dilate and stent dominant strictures.
- Surgical management
  - Colectomy for ulcerative colitis does not affect the course of PSC.
  - Patients with decompensated cirrhosis or recurrent cholangitis should be referred for liver transplantation.
  - Selected hilar cholangiocarcinomas may be considered for liver transplantation
  - Recurrent PSC after liver transplantation has been documented.

COMPLICATIONS OF CHOLESTASIS

Nutritional Deficiencies

GENERAL PRINCIPLES

Any condition that blocks bile excretion (at the level of the liver cell level or the biliary ducts) is defined as cholestasis. Laboratory manifestations of cholestasis include elevated levels of ALP and bilirubin.

- **Nutritional deficiencies** result from fat malabsorption.
- **Fat-soluble vitamin deficiency** (vitamins A, D, E, and K) is often present in advanced cholestasis and is particularly common in patients with steatorrhea.

DIAGNOSIS

Clinical Presentation

- Characteristic manifestations of vitamin deficiencies are discussed in Chapter 2, Nutrition Support.
- Patients with steatorrhea may give a history of oily, foul-smelling diarrhea that may stick to the toilet bowl or be difficult to flush.

Diagnostic Testing

- 25-Hydroxyvitamin D serum concentrations reflect the total body stores of vitamin D. Vitamin D deficiency in the setting of malabsorption and steatorrhea is a good surrogate clinical marker for total body concentrations of other fat-soluble vitamins.
- Stool can be tested for fecal fat. Both spot tests and 24-hour collections can be done.

TREATMENT

Medications

Vitamin supplements are available to correct deficiencies.

Osteoporosis

GENERAL PRINCIPLES

- Osteoporosis is defined as a decrease in the amount of bone (mainly trabecular bone), leading to a decrease in its structural integrity and increase in the risk of fractures.
- The relative risk of osteopenia in cholestasis is 4.4 times greater than the general population, matched for age and gender. Osteoporosis is more commonly seen in clinical cholestasis due to PBC.

DIAGNOSIS

Bone mineral density should be measured by dual-energy X-ray absorptiometry (DEXA) in all patients at the time of diagnosis and during follow-up (every 1–2 years).

TREATMENT

Treatment of bone disease includes weight-bearing exercise, oral calcium supplementation (1.0–1.5 g/d), bisphosphonate therapy, and vitamin D supplementation.

Pruritus

GENERAL PRINCIPLES

The pathophysiology is debated and may be due to the accumulation of bile acid compounds or endogenous opioid agonists.

DIAGNOSIS

Patients with cholestasis may present with itching in the setting of a normal or elevated bilirubin level.

TREATMENT

Medications

First Line
- Pruritus is best treated with cholestyramine, a basic anion exchange resin. It binds bile acids and other anionic compounds in the intestine and inhibits their absorption. The dose is 4 g mixed with water before and after the morning meal, with additional doses before lunch and dinner. The maximum recommended dose is 16 g/d. Cholestyramine should be administered apart from other vitamins or medications to prevent impaired absorption.
- Colestipol, another similar resin, is also available.

Second Line
- Antihistamines (hydroxyzine, diphenhydramine, or doxepin, 25 mg PO at bedtime) and petrolatum may provide symptomatic relief.
- Rifampin (150–600 mg/d) and naltrexone (25–50 mg/d) are reserved for intractable pruritus. Long-term therapy with rifampin is associated with minor, transient elevations in serum aminotransferase levels in 10–20% of patients—abnormalities that usually do not require dose adjustment or discontinuation. In rare instances, it can induce severe forms of DILI.

METABOLIC LIVER DISEASES

GENERAL PRINCIPLES

Wilson disease (WD) is an autosomal recessive disorder (*ATP7B* gene on chromosome 13) that results in progressive copper overload.
- Female-to-male ratio is 2:1.
- Absent or reduced function of ATP7B protein leads to decreased hepatocellular excretion of copper into bile. This results in hepatic copper accumulation and injury. Eventually, copper is released into the bloodstream and deposited in other organs, notably the brain, kidneys, and cornea.
- Extrahepatic manifestations include Kayser-Fleischer rings in the Descemet membrane in the periphery of the cornea due to copper deposition (diagnosed on slit-lamp examination), Coombs-negative hemolytic anemia, renal tubular acidosis, arthritis, and osteopenia.

DIAGNOSIS

Clinical Presentation
- The average age at presentation of liver dysfunction is 6–20 years, but it can manifest later in life. Liver disease can be highly variable, ranging from asymptomatic with only mild biochemical abnormalities to FHF.

- Most patients with the FHF presentation of WD have a characteristic pattern of clinical findings including Coombs-negative hemolytic anemia with features of acute intravascular hemolysis, rapid progression to renal failure, a rise in serum aminotransferases from the beginning of clinical illness (typically <2000 IU/L), and normal or markedly subnormal serum ALP (typically <40 IU/L) (*Hepatology 2008;47:2090*).
- The diagnosis of WD should be considered in patients with unexplained liver disease with or without neuropsychiatric symptoms, first-degree relatives with WD, or individuals with FHF (with or without hemolysis).
- Neuropsychiatric disorders usually occur later, most of the time in association with cirrhosis. The manifestations include asymmetric tremor, dysarthria, ataxia, and psychiatric features.

Diagnostic Testing

- Low serum ceruloplasmin level (<20 mg/dL), elevated serum free copper level (>25 μg/dL), and elevated 24-hour urinary copper level (>100 μg) are seen in patients with WD.
- The liver histology (massive necrosis, steatosis, glycogenated nuclei, chronic hepatitis, fibrosis, cirrhosis) findings are nonspecific and depend on the presentation and stage of the disease. Elevated hepatic copper levels of >250 μg/g dry weight (normal <40 μg/g) on biopsy are highly suggestive of WD.
- Mutation analysis by whole-gene sequencing is possible and should be performed on individuals in whom the diagnosis is difficult to establish by clinical and biochemical testing. Many patients are compound heterozygotes for mutations in the *ATP7B* gene, making identification of mutations difficult.

TREATMENT

Medications

Treatment is with the copper-chelating agents penicillamine and trientine. Zinc salts that block the intestinal absorption of copper are also used.

- **Penicillamine** 1–2 g/d (in divided doses bid or qid) and pyridoxine 25 mg/d (to avoid vitamin B_6 deficiency during treatment) are indicated in patients with hepatic failure. Use may be limited by side effects (e.g., hypersensitivity, bone marrow suppression, proteinuria, systemic lupus erythematosus, Goodpasture syndrome). Penicillamine should never be given as initial treatment to patients with neurologic symptoms.
- **Trientine** 1–2 g/d (in divided doses bid or qid) may also be used in hepatic failure. This has similar side effects as penicillamine but at a lower frequency. The risk of neurologic worsening with trientine is less than with penicillamine.
- **Zinc salts** 50 mg tid are indicated in patients with chronic hepatitis and cirrhosis in the absence of hepatic failure. Other than gastric irritation, zinc has an excellent safety profile.

Surgical Management

Liver transplantation is the only therapeutic option in FHF or in patients with progressive dysfunction despite chelation therapy.

MONITORING/FOLLOW-UP

- For monitoring, serum copper and ceruloplasmin, liver biochemistries, INR, complete blood cell count, urinalysis (especially for those on chelation therapy), and physical examination should be performed regularly, at least twice annually.
- The 24-hour urinary excretion of copper should be measured annually while on medication. More frequent monitoring may be needed if there is suspicion of noncompliance or if dose adjustment is required. The estimated serum free copper may be elevated or low in situations of nonadherence and overtreatment, respectively.
- First-degree relatives of any newly diagnosed patient with WD should be screened for WD.

OUTCOME/PROGNOSIS

After liver transplantation, in the absence of neurologic symptoms, patients require no further medical treatment.

Hereditary Hemochromatosis

GENERAL PRINCIPLES

Hereditary hemochromatosis (HH) is an autosomal recessive disorder of iron overload.
- This is the most common inherited form of iron overload affecting Caucasian populations. One in 200–400 Caucasian individuals are homozygous for hemochromatosis (*HFE*) gene mutations. It rarely manifests clinically before middle age (40–60 years).
- HH is most frequently caused by a missense mutation (C282Y) in the *HFE* gene located on chromosome 6. **Approximately 90% of patients with HH are homozygote for the C282Y mutation.** Less frequent mutations that lead to HH include H63D and S65C and the compound heterozygous C282Y/H63D and C282Y/S65C mutations.
- Secondary iron overload states include thalassemia major, sideroblastic anemia, chronic hemolytic anemias, iatrogenic parenteral iron overload, chronic hepatitis B and C, alcohol-induced liver disease, porphyria cutanea tarda, and aceruloplasminemia.

DIAGNOSIS

Clinical Presentation
- Presentation varies from **asymptomatic disease** to **cirrhosis** and HCC.
- Clinical findings include slate-colored skin, diabetes, cardiomyopathy, arthritis, hypogonadism, and hepatic dysfunction.

Diagnostic Testing
Diagnosis is based on laboratory testing, imaging, and liver biopsy.
- The diagnosis is suggested by **high fasting transferrin saturation (>45%) (serum iron divided by the total iron binding capacity)**. Other nonspecific laboratory tests include elevated serum iron and ferritin levels. **Ferritin level >1000 ng/mL is an accurate predictor of the degree of fibrosis in patients with HH.**
- If transferrin saturation is >45% and ferritin is elevated, then check for C282Y homozygosity. If patient is a C282Y homozygote, then:
  ○ If ferritin <1000 ng/mL and liver enzymes are normal, proceed to therapeutic phlebotomy.
  ○ If ferritin >1000 ng/mL or liver enzymes are elevated, proceed to liver biopsy for histology and hepatic iron concentration (HIC).
- The normal content of iron in the liver ranges from 250–1500 μg/g dry weight. In patients with HH, HIC ranges from 2000–30,000 μg/g dry weight.
- In patients with elevated transferrin saturation and heterozygosity of the C282Y mutation, exclude other liver or hematologic diseases and consider liver biopsy.
- **MRI** is the modality of choice for noninvasive quantification of iron storage in the liver and for noninvasive surveillance of HCC. It allows for repeated measures and minimizes sampling error.

TREATMENT

Therapy consists of **phlebotomy** every 7–15 days (500 mL blood) until iron depletion is confirmed by a ferritin level of 50–100 ng/mL and a transferrin saturation of <40%. Maintenance phlebotomy of one or two units of blood three to four times a year is continued for life, unless there are contraindications for rapid mobilization of iron stores (i.e., heart failure).

Medications

- **Iron chelation with deferoxamine** is an alternative to phlebotomy, but it is often more expensive and has side effects such as GI distress, visual and auditory impairments, and muscle cramps. Deferoxamine binds free iron, facilitates urinary excretion, and is recommended only when phlebotomy is contraindicated. Deferoxamine is only given IV, IM, or SC.
- Deferasirox is an oral iron chelator that selectively binds iron, forming a complex that is excreted through the feces.

Surgical Management

Liver transplantation may be considered in cases of HH with cirrhosis.

OUTCOME/PROGNOSIS

- The survival rate in appropriately treated noncirrhotic patients is identical to that of the general population.
- Patients who undergo liver transplantation for hemochromatosis have better survival rates if they are iron depleted via phlebotomy prior to transplantation compared to patients who are iron overloaded prior to transplantation (*Gastroenterology 2010;139:393*).
- The relative risk for HCC is approximately 20, with an annual incidence of 3–4%. Patients with HH and advanced fibrosis or cirrhosis should be screened annually for HCC (*Hepatology 2011;54(1):328*).

α_1-Antitrypsin Deficiency

GENERAL PRINCIPLES

- α_1-Antitrypsin (α_1AT) deficiency is an autosomal recessive disease associated with accumulation of misfolded α_1AT in the endoplasmic reticulum of hepatocytes. The most common allele is protease inhibitor M (PiM—normal), followed by PiS and PiZ (deficient variants). African Americans have a lower frequency of these alleles.
- The most prevalent deficiency alleles Z and S are derived from European ancestry (*Am J Gastroenterol 2008;103:2136*).
- α_1AT deficiency can also be associated with emphysema in early adulthood, as well as other extrahepatic manifestations including panniculitis, pancreatic fibrosis, and membranoproliferative glomerulonephritis.

DIAGNOSIS

Clinical Presentation

- The disease may present as neonatal cholestasis or, later in life, as chronic hepatitis, cirrhosis, or HCC.
- The presence of significant pulmonary and hepatic disease in the same patient is rare (1–2%).

Diagnostic Testing

- Low serum α_1AT level (10–15% of normal) will flatten the α_1-globulin curve on serum electrophoresis.
- Deficient α_1AT phenotype (PiSS, PiSZ, and PiZZ).
- Elevated AST and ALT.

Diagnostic Procedures

Liver biopsy shows characteristic periodic acid–Schiff–positive diastase-resistant globules in the periportal hepatocytes.

TREATMENT

Currently, there is no specific medical treatment for liver disease associated with α_1AT deficiency. Gene therapy for α_1AT deficiency is a potential future alternative.

Surgical Management

Liver transplantation is an option for those with cirrhosis and is curative, with survival rates of 90% at 1 year and 80% at 5 years.

OUTCOME/PROGNOSIS

- Chronic hepatitis, cirrhosis, or HCC may develop in 10–15% of patients with the PiZZ phenotype during the first 20 years of life.
- Controversy exists as to whether liver disease develops in heterozygotes (PiMZ, PiSZ, PiFZ).

MISCELLANEOUS LIVER DISORDERS

Nonalcoholic Fatty Liver Disease

GENERAL PRINCIPLES

- Nonalcoholic fatty liver disease (NAFLD) is a clinicopathologic syndrome that encompasses several clinical entities that range from simple steatosis to steatohepatitis, fibrosis, ESLD, and HCC in the absence of significant alcohol consumption (*Gastroenterology 2002;123:1705*).
- Nonalcoholic steatohepatitis (NASH) is part of the spectrum of NAFLD and is defined as the presence of hepatic steatosis and inflammation with hepatocyte injury (ballooning) with or without fibrosis.
- NAFLD is associated with an increasing prevalence of type 2 diabetes, obesity, and the metabolic syndrome in the US population.

DIAGNOSIS

Clinical Presentation

The disease may vary from asymptomatic liver fatty infiltration to advanced fibrosis, cirrhosis, and HCC.

Diagnostic Testing

- When patients with hepatic steatosis detected on imaging have symptoms or signs attributable to liver disease or have abnormal liver biochemistries, they should be evaluated for NAFLD and worked up accordingly.
- In patients with hepatic steatosis detected on imaging who lack any liver-related symptoms or signs and have normal liver biochemistries, it is reasonable to assess for metabolic risk factors (e.g., obesity, glucose intolerance, dyslipidemia) and alternate causes for hepatic steatosis such as significant alcohol consumption or medications.

- The distinction between NAFLD and NASH is determined by liver biopsy. Liver biopsy remains the diagnostic gold standard. However, the decision to perform a liver biopsy should take into account the specific clinical questions that are relevant to each case.
- Noninvasive predictive models, serum biomarkers, and imaging studies are increasingly used as surrogate measures of liver fibrosis, inflammation, and steatosis, without replacing liver biopsy.
- Normal liver enzymes are observed in up to 80% of patients. When present, these elevations are mild. Aminotransferases greater than two times normal may be predictive of fibrosis across different populations.
- Imaging studies such as ultrasonography, CT scan, and MRI may detect moderate to severe steatosis.

TREATMENT

Nonpharmacologic Therapies

Therapies to correct or control associated conditions are warranted (weight loss through diet and exercise, tight control of diabetes and insulin resistance, appropriate treatment of hyperlipidemia, and discontinuation of possible offending agents).

Medications

Despite inconclusive data on a long-term therapy safety profile, guidelines support the use of pioglitazone (45 mg/d) and vitamin E (800 IU/d) in nondiabetics with biopsy-proven NASH (*Hepatology 2012;55(6):2005*).

Surgical Management

Liver transplantation should be considered in patients with cirrhosis.

OUTCOME/PROGNOSIS

- Approximately 25% of patients with simple steatosis will progress to NASH.
- Progression to NASH cirrhosis has been reported at a rate of 11% over a 15-year period (*Clin Liver Dis 2012;16:397*).

Ischemic Hepatitis

GENERAL PRINCIPLES

Ischemic hepatitis results from acute liver hypoperfusion. Clinical circumstances associated with acute hypotension or hemodynamic instability include severe blood loss, substantial burns, cardiac failure, heat stroke, sepsis, sickle cell crisis, and others.

DIAGNOSIS

Clinical Presentation

Ischemic hepatitis presents with an acute and frequently transient and severe rise of aminotransferases during or following an episode of liver hypoperfusion.

Diagnostic Testing

- Laboratory studies show a rapid rise in levels of serum AST, ALT (>1000 mg/dL), and lactate dehydrogenase (LDH) within 1–3 days of the insult.
- Total bilirubin, ALP, and INR may initially be normal but subsequently rise as a result of reperfusion injury.

Diagnostic Procedures

Liver biopsy is not routinely needed, because the diagnosis can usually be made with clinical history. Classic histologic features include variable degrees of zone 3 (centrilobular) necrosis with collapse around the central vein. Coexistent features may include passive congestion, sinusoidal distortion, fatty change, and cholestasis. Inflammatory infiltrates are rare.

TREATMENT

Treatment consists of supportive care and correction of the underlying condition that caused the circulatory collapse.

OUTCOME/PROGNOSIS

Prognosis is dependent on rapid and effective treatment of the underlying condition.

Hepatic Vein Thrombosis

GENERAL PRINCIPLES

Hepatic vein thrombosis (HVT), also known as Budd-Chiari syndrome, causes hepatic venous outflow obstruction. It has multiple etiologies and a variety of clinical consequences.
- Thrombosis is the main factor leading to obstruction of the hepatic venous system, frequently in association with myeloproliferative disorders, antiphospholipid antibody syndrome, paroxysmal nocturnal hemoglobinuria, factor V Leiden, protein C and S deficiency, Jak-2 mutation, and contraceptive use (*Dig Liver Dis 2011;43:503*).
- Membranous obstruction of the inferior vena cava (IVC) and stenosis of the IVC anastomosis after liver transplantation are conditions that present clinically similar to HVT.
- Less than 20% of cases are idiopathic.

DIAGNOSIS

Clinical Presentation

Patients may present with acute, subacute, or chronic illness characterized by ascites, hepatomegaly, and right upper quadrant abdominal pain. Other symptoms may include jaundice, encephalopathy, GI bleeding, and lower extremity edema.

Diagnostic Testing

- Serum-to-ascites albumin gradient (SAAG) is >1.1 g/dL. Serum albumin, bilirubin, AST, ALT, and PT/INR are usually abnormal.
- Laboratory evaluation to identify a hypercoagulable state should be performed (see Chapter 20, Disorders of Hemostasis and Thrombosis).
- Doppler ultrasound can be used as a screening test. Definitive diagnosis is made with magnetic resonance venography, hepatic venography, or cavography.

TREATMENT

Medications

Nonsurgical treatment includes anticoagulation, thrombolytics, diuretics, angioplasty, stents, and TIPS.

Surgical Management

Liver transplantation is an option in selected patients.

Portal Vein Thrombosis

GENERAL PRINCIPLES

Portal vein thrombosis (PVT) is seen in a variety of clinical settings, including abdominal trauma, cirrhosis, malignancy, hypercoagulable states, intra-abdominal infections, pancreatitis, and after portocaval shunt surgery and splenectomy.

DIAGNOSIS

Clinical Presentation
- PVT can present as an acute or chronic condition.
- The acute phase may go unrecognized. Symptoms include abdominal pain/distension, nausea, anorexia, weight loss, diarrhea, or features of the underlying disorder.
- Chronic PVT may present with variceal hemorrhage or other manifestations of portal hypertension.

Diagnostic Testing
- In patients with no obvious etiology, a hypercoagulable workup should be performed.
- **Ultrasonographic Doppler** examination is sensitive and specific for establishing the diagnosis. Portal venography, CT, or magnetic resonance venography can also be used.

TREATMENT

Medications
- In patients with acute PVT with or without cirrhosis, anticoagulation is recommended in the absence of any obvious contraindications. Treatment is aimed to prevent further thrombosis and recanalization, to treat complications and concurrent disease, and to identify underlying risk factors (*Neth J Med 2009;67:46*).
- In patients with chronic PVT, anticoagulation is not recommended.

Other Nonpharmacologic Therapies
In the setting of chronic PVT, treatment should focus on the complications of portal hypertension and include nonselective β-blockers, endoscopic banding for varices, and diuretics for ascites.

Surgical Management
Portosystemic derivative surgery carries a high morbidity and mortality, especially in patients with cirrhosis. In some instances where surgery is precluded or the thrombus expands despite adequate anticoagulation, interventional radiology may be able to deploy a TIPS. This may then theoretically resolve symptomatic portal hypertension and prevent the thrombus recurrence or extension by the creation of a portosystemic shunt (*Nat Rev Gastroenterol Hepatol 2014;11:435*).

FULMINANT HEPATIC FAILURE

GENERAL PRINCIPLES

- FHF is a condition that includes evidence of a combination of coagulation abnormalities and any degree of mental alteration (encephalopathy) in a patient without preexisting liver disease and with an illness of <26 weeks in duration.

- Terms signifying length of illness in FHF such as hyperacute (<7 days), acute (7–21 days), and subacute (>21 days to <26 weeks) are not frequently used because they do not have prognostic significance (*Gastroenterol Clin North Am 2011;40:523*).
- In 20% of cases, no clear cause is identified. Acetaminophen hepatotoxicity and viral hepatitis are the most common causes of FHF. Other causes include AIH, drug and toxin exposure, ischemia, acute fatty liver of pregnancy, WD, and Reye syndrome.
- Acute inflammation with varying degrees of necrosis and collapse of the liver's architectural framework are the typical histologic changes seen in FHF.

DIAGNOSIS

Clinical Presentation

- Patients may present with mild to severe mental status changes in the setting of moderate to severe acute hepatitis and coagulopathy.
- Patients may develop cardiovascular collapse, acute renal failure, cerebral edema, and sepsis.

Diagnostic Testing

- Aminotransferases are typically elevated and, in many cases, are >1000 IU/L.
- INR >1.5 that does not correct with the administration of vitamin K is characteristic.
- Workup to determine the etiology of FHF should include acute viral hepatitis panel, serum drug screen (including acetaminophen level), ceruloplasmin, AIH serologies, and pregnancy test.
- Right upper quadrant ultrasound with Doppler may be obtained to evaluate obstruction of hepatic venous inflow or outflow.
- CT of the head may be obtained to evaluate and track progression of cerebral edema; however, the radiologic findings may lag behind its development and do not substitute for serial bedside assessments of neurologic status.
- Liver biopsy is seldom used to establish etiology or prognosis. Given the presence of coagulopathy, a transjugular approach to liver biopsy may be attempted if necessary.

TREATMENT

- Supportive therapy (quiet dark room, avoid patient stimulation, maintain head of bed elevation to 30 degrees) in the intensive care unit (ICU) setting with liver transplant capabilities is essential.
- Precipitating factors, such as infection, should be identified and treated. Blood glucose, electrolytes, acid–base balance, coagulation parameters, and fluid status should be serially monitored.
- Sedatives should be avoided to appropriately gauge the patient's mental status.
- *N*-acetylcysteine (NAC) may be used in cases of FHF in which acetaminophen ingestion is suspected or when circumstances surrounding admission is inadequate. NAC also appears to improve spontaneous survival when given during early hepatic encephalopathy stages (grades I and II) even in the setting of nonacetaminophen FHF.
- Fresh frozen plasma and the use of recombinant activated factor VIIa should be considered in the setting of active bleeding or when invasive procedures are required.
- Cerebral edema and intracranial hypertension are related to the severity of encephalopathy. In patients with grade III or IV encephalopathy, intracranial pressure monitoring should be considered (intracranial pressure should be maintained below 20 mm Hg and cerebral perfusion pressure should be maintained above 50 mm Hg). Management of cerebral edema, when identified by CT imaging, includes intubation with sedation to avoid overstimulation, elevation of the head of the bed,

use of mannitol (0.5–1.25 g/kg of 20% solution), and/or use of hypertonic saline (30% hypertonic saline at a rate of 5–20 mL/h to maintain a serum sodium of 145–155 mmol/L) (*Hepatology 2004;39(2):464*). Lactulose is not indicated for encephalopathy in this setting. Its use may result in increased bowel gas that can interfere with the surgical approach for liver transplantation.
- Therapeutic hypothermia (chilled to 32°C) is an adjunct therapy in patients with grade III or IV hepatic encephalopathy or uncontrolled intracranial hypertension; it may be used as a bridge to liver transplantation in some patients.
- Liver transplantation should be urgently considered in cases of severe FHF. Poor prognostic indicators in acetaminophen-induced FHF include arterial pH <7.3, INR >6.5, creatinine >2.3 mg/dL, and encephalopathy grades III through IV (King's College Criteria).

OUTCOME/PROGNOSIS

- In the United States, 45% of adults with FHF have a spontaneous recovery, 25% undergo liver transplantation, and 30% die without liver transplantation (*Curr Opin Organ Transplant 2011;16:289*).
- Death often results from progressive liver failure, GI bleeding, cerebral edema, sepsis, or arrhythmia.
- A rapid decline in aminotransferases correlates poorly with prognosis and does not always indicate an improved response to therapy.

CIRRHOSIS

- Cirrhosis is a chronic condition characterized by diffuse replacement of liver cells by fibrotic tissue, which creates a nodular-appearing distortion of the normal liver architecture. Advanced fibrosis represents the end result of many etiologies of liver injury.
- Cirrhosis affects nearly 5.5 million Americans, and in 2009, it was the 12th leading cause of death in the United States.
- The most common etiologies are alcohol-related liver disease, chronic viral infection, and NASH (diagnosis and treatment discussed earlier in respective sections).
- Main complications of cirrhosis include portal hypertension with various clinical manifestations (ascites, esophageal and gastric varices, portal hypertensive gastropathy and colopathy, hypersplenism, gastric antral vascular ectasia, spontaneous bacterial peritonitis [SBP], hepatorenal syndrome [HRS], hepatic encephalopathy, and HCC). Frequent laboratory abnormalities encountered in a patient with cirrhosis include anemia, leukopenia, thrombocytopenia, hypoalbuminemia, coagulopathy, and hyperbilirubinemia.

Portal Hypertension

GENERAL PRINCIPLES

- Portal hypertension is the main complication of cirrhosis and is characterized by increased resistance to portal flow and increased portal venous inflow. Portal hypertension is established by measuring the pressure gradient between the hepatic vein and the portal vein (normal portosystemic pressure gradient is approximately 3 mm Hg).
- Direct and indirect clinical consequences of portal hypertension appear when the portosystemic pressure gradient exceeds 10 mm Hg (*Dig Liver Dis 2011;43:762*).

- Causes of portal hypertension in patients without cirrhosis include idiopathic portal hypertension, schistosomiasis, congenital hepatic fibrosis, sarcoidosis, cystic fibrosis, arteriovenous fistulas, splenic and portal vein thrombosis, HVT (Budd-Chiari syndrome), myeloproliferative diseases, nodular regenerative hyperplasia, and focal nodular hyperplasia.

DIAGNOSIS

Portal hypertension frequently complicates cirrhosis and presents with ascites, splenomegaly, and GI bleeding from varices (esophageal or gastric), portal hypertensive gastropathy (PHG), gastric antrum vascular ectasia (GAVE), or portal hypertensive colopathy.
- Ultrasonography, CT, and MRI showing cirrhosis, splenomegaly, collateral venous circulation, and ascites are suggestive of portal hypertension.
- Upper endoscopy may show varices (esophageal or gastric), PHG, or GAVE.
- Transjugular portal pressure measurements may be performed to calculate the portosystemic pressure gradient.

TREATMENT

Treatment of GI bleeding due to portal hypertension is covered in Chapter 18, Gastrointestinal Diseases.

Ascites

GENERAL PRINCIPLES

Ascites is the abnormal (>25 mL) accumulation of fluid within the peritoneal cavity. Other causes of ascites, unrelated to portal hypertension, include cancer (peritoneal carcinomatosis), heart failure, tuberculosis, myxedema, pancreatic disease, nephrotic syndrome, surgery or trauma to the lymphatic system or ureters, and serositis.

DIAGNOSIS

- Presentation ranges from ascites detected only by imaging methods to a distended, bulging, and sometimes tender abdomen. Percussion of the abdomen may reveal shifting dullness.
- **SAAG** is calculated as serum albumin minus the ascites albumin; a gradient ≥1.1 indicates portal hypertension–related ascites (97% specificity). A SAAG of <1.1 is found in nephrotic syndrome, peritoneal carcinomatosis, serositis, TB, and biliary or pancreatic ascites.
- Ultrasonography, CT, and MRI are sensitive methods to detect ascites.
- **Diagnostic paracentesis** (60 mL) should be performed in the setting of new-onset ascites, suspicion of malignant ascites, or to rule out SBP. **Therapeutic paracentesis** (large volume) should be performed when tense ascites causes significant discomfort or respiratory compromise or when suspecting abdominal compartment syndrome.
- Routine diagnostic testing should include SAAG calculation, red and white blood cell counts and differential, total protein, and culture. Amylase and triglyceride measurement, cytology, and mycobacterial smear/culture can be performed to confirm specific diagnoses.
- Bleeding, infection, persistent ascites leak, and intestinal perforation are possible complications.

• Large-volume paracentesis (>7 L) may lead to circulatory collapse, encephalopathy, and renal failure. Concomitant administration of IV albumin (5–8 g/L ascites removed) can be used to minimize these complications, especially in the setting of renal insufficiency or the absence of peripheral edema.

TREATMENT

Medications

• **Diuretic therapy** is initiated along with **salt restriction** (<2 g sodium or 88 mmol Na^+/d). Diuretics should be used with caution, or their use should be discontinued in patients with an increasing serum creatinine level.
• **Spironolactone** 100 mg PO daily is indicated. The daily dose can be increased by 50–100 mg every 7–10 days to a maximum dose of 400 mg until satisfactory weight loss or side effects occur. Hyperkalemia and gynecomastia are common side effects. Other potassium-sparing diuretics such as amiloride, triamterene, or eplerenone are substitutes that can be used in patients in whom painful gynecomastia develops.
• **Loop diuretics**, such as furosemide (20–40 mg, increasing to a maximum dose of 160 mg PO daily) or bumetanide (0.5–2.0 mg PO daily), can be added to spironolactone.
• Patients should be observed closely for signs of dehydration, electrolyte disturbances, encephalopathy, muscle cramps, and renal insufficiency. Nonsteroidal anti-inflammatory agents may blunt the effect of diuretics and increase the risk of renal dysfunction.

Other Alternative Therapies

• TIPS is effective in the management of refractory or hard-to-treat ascites.
• Complications of TIPS include shunt occlusion, bleeding, infection, cardiopulmonary compromise, hepatic encephalopathy, hepatic failure, and death.

Spontaneous Bacterial Peritonitis

GENERAL PRINCIPLES

• SBP is an infectious complication of portal hypertension–related ascites defined as >250 neutrophils/μL in the ascites fluid.
• Bacterascites is defined as culture-positive ascites in the presence of normal neutrophil counts (<250 neutrophils/μL) in the ascites fluid. This condition may be spontaneously reversible or the first step in the development of SBP. In the presence of signs or symptoms of infection, bacterascites should be treated like SBP.
• Risk factors for SBP include ascites fluid protein concentration <1 mg/dL, acute GI bleeding, and a prior episode of SBP.

DIAGNOSIS

Clinical Presentation

SBP may be asymptomatic. Clinical manifestations include abdominal pain and distention, fever, decreased bowel sounds, and worsening hepatic encephalopathy. Cirrhotic patients with ascites and evidence of any clinical deterioration should undergo diagnostic paracentesis to exclude SBP.

Diagnostic Testing

The diagnosis is confirmed when >250 neutrophils/μL are found in the ascites fluid. Gram stain reveals the organism in only 10–20% of samples.

- Ascites cultures are more likely to be positive when 10 mL of the fluid is inoculated into two blood culture bottles at the bedside.
- The most common organisms are *Escherichia coli*, *Klebsiella*, and *Streptococcus pneumoniae*. Polymicrobial infection is uncommon and should lead to the suspicion of secondary bacterial peritonitis. Checking total protein, LDH, and glucose on ascites fluid is helpful in distinguishing secondary bacterial peritonitis from SBP.

TREATMENT

Medications

- Patients with SBP should receive empiric antibiotic therapy with IV third-generation cephalosporins (ceftriaxone, 1 g IV daily, or cefotaxime, 1–2 g IV q6–8h, depending on renal function). Therapy should be tailored based on culture results and antibiotic susceptibility. Paracentesis should be repeated if no clinical improvement occurs in 48–72 hours, especially if the initial fluid culture was negative (*Hepatology 2009;49:2087*).
- Oral quinolones can be considered a substitute for IV third-generation cephalosporins in the absence of vomiting, shock, grade II (or higher) hepatic encephalopathy, or serum creatinine >3 mg/dL (*Hepatology 2009;49:2087*).
- Patients with <250 neutrophils/μL in the ascites fluid and signs or symptoms of infection (fever or abdominal pain or tenderness) should also receive empiric antibiotic therapy (*Hepatology 2009;49:2087*).
- Concomitant use of albumin 1.5 g/kg body weight at time of diagnosis and 1.0 g/kg body weight on day 3 improves survival and prevents renal failure in SBP (*Am J Gastroenterol 2009;104:1802*).

Primary Prophylaxis (No Prior History of SBP)
Patients with severe liver disease with ascitic fluid protein <1.5 mg/dL along with impaired renal function (creatinine ≥1.2, blood urea nitrogen ≥25, or serum Na ≤130) or liver failure (Child score ≥9 and bilirubin ≥3) should be treated with long-term norfloxacin 400 mg PO daily.

Secondary Prophylaxis (After the First Episode of SBP)
Norfloxacin 400 mg PO daily is the treatment of choice for prevention of recurrent SBP (*Hepatology 1990;12:716*). Alternative treatments include Bactrim double strength, levofloxacin, or ciprofloxacin.

Acute Kidney Injury in Patients with Cirrhosis and Hepatorenal Syndrome

GENERAL PRINCIPLES

Acute kidney injury (AKI) in decompensated cirrhosis is a common complication. Revised consensus recommendations define AKI as an increase in serum creatinine ≥0.3 mg/dL within 48 hours or a percentage increase of serum creatinine ≥50% from a known or presumed baseline within the prior 7 days (*J Hepatol 2015;62:968*). HRS results from severe peripheral vasodilatation, which leads to renal vasoconstriction. The definition of HRS-AKI (type I HRS) is provided in Table 19-9. Common precipitating factors include systemic bacterial infections, SBP, GI hemorrhage, and large-volume paracentesis without volume expansion. HRS is a diagnosis of exclusion.

TABLE 19-9	Diagnostic Criteria of HRS-AKI

- Diagnosis of cirrhosis and ascites
- Diagnosis of AKI (an increase in serum creatinine ≥0.3 mg/dL within 48 hours or a percentage increase of serum creatinine ≥50% from a known or presumed baseline within the prior 7 days)
  - Stage 1: increase in serum creatinine ≥0.3 mg/dL or an increase ≥1.5- to 2-fold from baseline
  - Stage 2: increase in serum creatinine >2- to 3-fold from baseline
  - Stage 3: increase in serum creatinine >3-fold from baseline, >4 mg/dL with an acute increase ≥0.3 mg/dL, or initiation of renal replacement therapy
- No response after 2 consecutive days of diuretic withdrawal and plasma volume expansion with albumin 1 g/kg
- Absence of shock
- No current or recent use of nephrotoxic drugs (NSAIDs, aminoglycosides, iodinated contrast media, etc.)
- No macroscopic signs of structural kidney injury, defined as:
  - Absence of proteinuria (>500 mg/d)
  - Absence of microhematuria (>50 RBCs per high-power field)
  - Normal findings on renal ultrasonography

AKI, acute kidney injury; HRS, hepatorenal syndrome; RBC, red blood cell.
Adapted from Angeli P, Gines P, Wong F, et al. Diagnosis and management of acute kidney injury in patients with cirrhosis: revised consensus recommendations of the International Club of Ascites. *J Hepatol* 2015;62:968–74.

DIAGNOSIS

HRS is observed in cirrhotic patients with ascites, with and without hyponatremia. HRS has been divided into two types.
- **Type I** HRS is characterized by the acute onset of rapidly progressive renal failure (<2 weeks) unresponsive to volume expansion.
- **Type II** HRS progresses more slowly but relentlessly and often clinically manifests as diuretic-resistant ascites.

TREATMENT

Medication
Specific medical therapy is only recommended for type I HRS.
- Terlipressin (vasopressin analog) is not FDA approved for use in the United States. In a placebo-controlled trial, 34% of patients who received terlipressin had a reversal of their HRS in comparison to 13% who received placebo (*Gastroenterology 2008;134:1360*).
- SC somatostatin analogs (octreotide) and oral α-adrenergic agonist (midodrine) with IV albumin is a commonly used regimen for the management of HRS in the United States.

Other Nonpharmacologic Therapies
Hemodialysis may be indicated in patients listed for liver transplantation.

Surgical Management
Liver transplantation may be curative. Patients receiving hemodialysis for more than 12 weeks should be considered for liver and kidney transplantation.

OUTCOME/PROGNOSIS

Without treatment, patients with type I HRS have a poor prognosis, with death occurring within 1 to 3 months of onset. Patients with type II HRS have a longer median survival.

Hepatic Encephalopathy

GENERAL PRINCIPLES

- Hepatic encephalopathy is the syndrome of disordered consciousness and altered neuromuscular activity that is seen in patients with acute or chronic hepatocellular failure or portosystemic shunting.
- The grades of hepatic encephalopathy are dynamic and can rapidly change.
  - Grade I: Sleep reversal pattern, mild confusion, irritability, tremor, asterixis
  - Grade II: Lethargy, disorientation, inappropriate behavior, asterixis
  - Grade III: Somnolence, severe confusion, aggressive behavior, asterixis
  - Grade IV: Coma
- **Precipitating factors** include medication noncompliance to lactulose, azotemia, FHF, opioids or sedative-hypnotic medications, acute GI bleeding, hypokalemia and alkalosis (diuretics and diarrhea), constipation, infection, high-protein diet, progressive hepatocellular dysfunction, and portosystemic shunts (surgical or TIPS).

DIAGNOSIS

- Asterixis (flapping tremor) is present in stage I through III encephalopathy. This motor disturbance is not specific to hepatic encephalopathy.
- The electroencephalogram shows slow, high-amplitude, and triphasic waves.
- Determination of blood ammonia level is not a sensitive or specific test for hepatic encephalopathy.

TREATMENT

Medications include nonabsorbable disaccharides (lactulose, lactitol, and lactose in lactase-deficient patients) and antibiotics (neomycin, metronidazole, and rifaximin).
- **Lactulose**, 15–45 mL PO (or via nasogastric tube) bid–qid, is the first choice for treatment of hepatic encephalopathy. Lactulose dosing should be adjusted to produce three to five soft stools per day. Oral lactulose should not be given to patients with ileus or possible bowel obstruction. In the acute phase, a starting dose of 30 mL every 2 hours is recommended. This can then be transitioned to every 4 hours, 6 hours, and then 8 hours once the patient starts having bowel movements.
- **Lactulose enemas** (prepared by the addition of 300 mL lactulose to 700 mL distilled water) may also be administered in patients who cannot tolerate oral intake.
- **Rifaximin** is an oral nonsystemic broad-spectrum antibiotic that is used at a dose of 550 mg PO bid with no serious adverse events. In a placebo-controlled trial, rifaximin reduced the risk of hepatic encephalopathy and the time to first hospitalization over a 6-month period.
- **Neomycin** can be given by mouth (500–1000 mg q6h) or as a retention enema (1% solution in 100–200 mL isotonic saline). Approximately 1–3% of the administered dose of neomycin is absorbed with the attendant risk of ototoxicity and nephrotoxicity.
- In a randomized controlled trial, combination therapy with lactulose and rifaximin was more effective than lactulose alone for management of hepatic encephalopathy (*Am J Gastroenterol 2013;108(9):1458*).

Hepatocellular Carcinoma

GENERAL PRINCIPLES

HCC frequently occurs in patients with cirrhosis, especially when associated with viral hepatitis (HBV or HCV), alcoholic cirrhosis, α_1AT deficiency, and hemochromatosis.

DIAGNOSIS

Clinical Presentation

• Clinical presentation is directly proportional to the stage of disease. HCC may present with right upper quadrant abdominal pain, weight loss, and hepatomegaly.
• Suspect HCC in a cirrhotic patient who develops manifestations of liver decompensation.
• Surveillance for HCC should be performed every 6 months with a sensitive imaging study. The combination of imaging with AFP is not recommended because it is unlikely to provide a gain in the detection rate. In patients with hepatitis B, surveillance should begin after age 40 years even in the absence of cirrhosis.

Diagnostic Testing

• AFP (see earlier section Evaluation of Liver Disease).
• Investigational serum markers for HCC include lens culinaris agglutinin-reactive AFP, des-γ-carboxyprothrombin (DCP), α-L-fucosidase, and glypican-3 (GPC3).
• Liver ultrasound, triple-phase CT, and MRI with contrast are sensitive and often used for detection of HCC (see Table 19-10 for Organ Procurement and Transplantation

TABLE 19-10	Organ Procurement and Transplantation Network (OPTN) Imaging Criteria for the Diagnosis of Hepatocellular Carcinoma (HCC)
OPTN Class 5	Meets all diagnostic criteria for HCC and may qualify for automatic MELD exception points.
Class 5A: ≥1 cm and <2 cm measured on late arterial or portal venous phase	Increased contrast enhancement in late hepatic arterial phase *and* washout during later phases *and* peripheral rim enhancement (capsule or pseudocapsule). A single solitary OPTN class 5A does not earn MELD exception points, but the combination of two or three OPTN class 5A nodules constitutes eligibility for transplantation.
Class 5A-g: same size as OPTN class 5A HCC	Increased contrast enhancement in late hepatic arterial phase *and* growth by ≥50% or more on serial CT or MRI obtained ≤6 months apart.
Class 5B: maximum diameter ≥2 cm and ≤5 cm	Increased contrast enhancement in late hepatic arterial phase *and* either washout *or* peripheral rim enhancement (capsule or pseudocapsule) *or* growth by ≥50% or more on serial CT or MRI obtained ≤6 months apart.
Class 5T	Prior regional treatment for HCC.
Class 5X: maximum diameter ≥5 cm	Increased contrast enhancement in late hepatic arterial phase *and* either washout *or* peripheral rim enhancement (capsule or pseudocapsule).

MELD, Model for End-Stage Liver Disease.
Adapted from *Radiology* 2013;266(2):376–82.

Network criteria for diagnosis of HCC). Liver biopsy should be considered for patients at risk for HCC with suspicious liver lesions >1 cm with noncharacteristic imaging features (absence of arterial hypervascularity and venous or delayed phase washout).

TREATMENT

Surgical Management

- Hepatic resection is the treatment of choice in noncirrhotic patients.
- Liver transplantation is the treatment of choice for select cirrhotic patients who fall into Milan criteria (single HCC <5 cm or up to three nodules <3 cm).
- Milan criteria are used by the United Network for Organ Sharing (UNOS) for priority status (exception points) for liver transplantation candidacy in patients with HCC.

Nonpharmacologic Therapies

- Transarterial chemoembolization (TACE) improves survival in selected patients. It is recommended as first-line palliative therapy for nonsurgical patients with large or multifocal HCC who do not have vascular invasion or metastatic disease (*Hepatology 2011;53:1020*).
- Selected patients with tumors beyond Milan criteria HCC can be downstaged to meet Milan criteria with TACE, radiofrequency ablation (RFA), and transarterial radioembolization (TARE) prior to liver transplantation

Medications

- **Sorafenib** is a small molecule that inhibits tumor cell proliferation and angiogenesis. In patients with advanced HCC, median survival and radiologic progression were 3 months longer for patients treated with sorafenib compared to placebo (*N Engl J Med 2008;359:378*). Currently, there are several new medications being investigated for the treatment of HCC that inhibit angiogenesis, epidermal growth factor receptor, and mammalian target of rapamycin (mTOR).
- **Chemotherapy.** There are no consistently effective combination cytotoxic agents for the management of HCC.

OUTCOME/PROGNOSIS

Early diagnosis is essential because surgical resection and liver transplantation can improve long-term survival (*Hepatology 2011;53:1020*). Liver transplantation has demonstrated, in patients meeting Milan criteria, a recurrence-free survival of 80–90% at 3–4 years. Advanced HCC that is beyond Milan criteria has a dismal prognosis, with a 5-year survival of 0–10%.

LIVER TRANSPLANTATION

GENERAL PRINCIPLES

- Liver transplantation is an effective therapeutic option for irreversible acute liver disease and ESLD for which available therapies have failed. Whole cadaveric livers and partial livers (split-liver, reduced-size, and living-related) are used in the United States as sources for liver transplantation. There continues to be a disparity between supply and demand of suitable livers for transplantation.
- The Model for End-Stage Liver Disease (MELD) score allows for prioritization for liver transplantation. It is calculated by a formula that takes into account serum bilirubin, serum creatinine, and INR. Patients are regularly evaluated for a liver transplantation

when they achieve a MELD of 15. Patients are considered for "exception MELD points" for conditions such as HCC within Milan criteria, hepatopulmonary syndrome, portopulmonary hypertension, polycystic liver disease, familial amyloidosis, and unusual tumors.

- Patients with cirrhosis should be considered for transplant evaluation when they have a decline in hepatic synthetic or excretory functions, ascites, hepatic encephalopathy, or complications such as HRS, HCC, recurrent SBP, or variceal bleeding.
- Candidates for liver transplantation are evaluated by a multidisciplinary team that includes hepatologists, transplant surgeons, transplant nurse coordinators, social workers, psychologists, and financial coordinators.
- General **contraindications** to liver transplant include severe and uncontrolled extrahepatic infection, advanced cardiac or pulmonary disease, extrahepatic malignancy, multiorgan failure, unresolved psychosocial issues, medical noncompliance issues, and ongoing substance abuse (e.g., alcohol and illegal drugs).

TREATMENT

Immunosuppressive, infectious, and long-term complications are discussed in Chapter 17, Solid Organ Transplant Medicine.

20

Disorders of Hemostasis and Thrombosis

Kristen M. Sanfilippo, Brian F. Gage, Tzu-Fei Wang, and Roger D. Yusen

Hemostatic Disorders

GENERAL PRINCIPLES

Normal hemostasis involves a sequence of interrelated reactions that lead to platelet aggregation (primary hemostasis) and activation of coagulation factors (secondary hemostasis) to produce a durable vascular seal.

- **Primary hemostasis** consists of an immediate but temporary response to vessel injury, where platelets and von Willebrand factor (**vWF**) interact to form a primary hemostatic plug.
- **Secondary hemostasis** results in formation of a fibrin clot (Figure 20-1). Injury exposes extravascular tissue factor to blood, which initiates activation of factors VII and X and prothrombin. Subsequent activation of factors XI, VIII, and V leads to generation of thrombin, conversion of fibrinogen to fibrin, and formation of a durable clot (*Semin Thromb Hemost 2009;35:9*).

DIAGNOSIS

Clinical Presentation

History

A detailed history can assess bleeding risk or severity, determine congenital or acquired etiology, and evaluate for primary or secondary hemostatic defects.

- Prolonged bleeding after dental extractions, circumcision, menstruation, labor and delivery, trauma, or surgery may suggest an underlying bleeding disorder.
- Family history may suggest an inherited bleeding disorder.

Physical Examination

- Primary hemostasis defects often cause mucosal bleeding and excessive bruising.
  - Petechiae: <2 mm subcutaneous bleeding, do not blanch with pressure, typically present in areas subject to increased hydrostatic force (the lower legs and periorbital area)
  - Ecchymoses: >3 mm black-and-blue patches due to rupture of small vessels from trauma
- Secondary hemostasis defects can result in **hematomas**, hemarthroses, or delayed bleeding after trauma or surgery.

Diagnostic Testing

Laboratories

The history and physical exam guide test selection. Initial studies should include platelet count, prothrombin time (**PT**), activated partial thromboplastin time (**aPTT**), and a blood smear.

- **Primary hemostasis tests**
  - A low **platelet count** requires review of blood smear to rule out platelet clumping artifact or giant platelets.

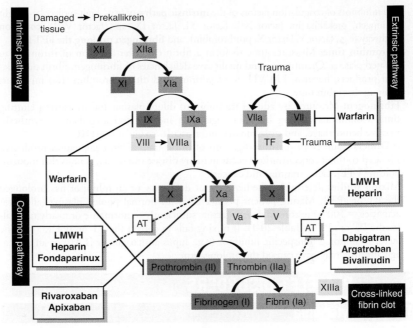

Figure 20-1. Coagulation cascade. *Solid arrows* indicate activation. *Solid* or *dashed lines* that run into a vertical line are associated with drugs represent a point of inhibition. Extrinsic pathway includes the right upper portion of cascade above factor X. Intrinsic pathway includes the left upper portion of the cascade above factor X. Common pathway includes the lower portion of the cascade from factor X and below. AT, antithrombin; LMWH, low-molecular-weight heparin; TF, tissue factor.

- ○ The **platelet function assay-100 (PFA-100)** instrument assesses vWF-dependent platelet activation in flowing citrated whole blood. Patients with von Willebrand disease (**vWD**) and qualitative platelet disorders can have prolonged PFA-100 closure times. Anemia (hematocrit <30%) and thrombocytopenia (platelet <100 × 10⁹/L) can cause prolonged closure times.
- ○ **In vitro platelet aggregation** studies measure platelet secretion and aggregation in response to platelet agonists (see Qualitative Platelet Disorders section).
- ○ Laboratory evaluation of vWD includes measurement of vWF antigen (**vWF:Ag**) and **vWF activity** and **vWF multimer analysis**.
- **Secondary hemostasis** (Figure 20-1)
  - ○ **PT:** Measures time to form a fibrin clot after adding thromboplastin (tissue factor and phospholipid) and calcium to citrated plasma. Sensitive (i.e., elevated PT) to deficiencies of **extrinsic pathway** (factor VII), **common pathway** (factors X and V and prothrombin), and **fibrinogen** and to use of vitamin K antagonists and direct factor Xa and thrombin (IIa) inhibitors. Reporting a PT ratio as an international normalized ratio (**INR**) reduces interlaboratory variation (*Thromb Haemost 1983;49:238*) in monitoring warfarin use.
  - ○ **aPTT:** Measures the time to form a fibrin clot after activation of citrated plasma by calcium, phospholipid, and negatively charged particles. Besides heparin, low-molecular-weight heparin (**LMWH**), fondaparinux, and direct anti-Xa and thrombin (IIa) inhibitors, deficiencies

and inhibitors of coagulation factors of the **intrinsic pathway** (e.g., high-molecular-weight kininogen, prekallikrein, factor XII, factor XI, factor IX, and factor VIII), **common pathway** (e.g., factor V, factor X, prothrombin), and **fibrinogen prolong the aPTT**.

○ **Thrombin time:** Measures time to form a fibrin clot after addition of thrombin to citrated plasma. Quantitative and qualitative deficiencies of fibrinogen, fibrin degradation products, heparin, LMWH, fondaparinux, and direct thrombin (IIa) inhibitors prolong thrombin time.

○ **Fibrinogen:** Measured by adding thrombin to dilute plasma and measuring clotting time. Conditions causing hypofibrinogenemia include decreased hepatic synthesis, massive hemorrhage, and disseminated intravascular coagulation (**DIC**).

○ **D-Dimers** result from plasmin digestion of fibrin (i.e., fibrin degradation products). Elevated D-dimer concentrations occur in many disease states (i.e., venous thromboembolism [**VTE**], DIC, trauma, and cancer).

○ **Mixing studies** determine whether a factor deficiency or an inhibitor has prolonged the PT or aPTT. Mixing patient plasma 1:1 with normal pooled plasma (all factor activities = 100%) restores deficient factors sufficiently to normalize or nearly normalize the PT or aPTT (Table 20-1). If mixing fails to correct the PT or aPTT, a specific factor inhibitor, a nonspecific inhibitor (e.g., lupus anticoagulant [**LA**]), or an anticoagulant drug may have caused the prolongation.

PLATELET DISORDERS

Thrombocytopenia

• **Thrombocytopenia** is defined as a platelet count of $<140 \times 10^9/L$.
• Thrombocytopenia occurs from decreased production, increased destruction, or sequestration of platelets (Table 20-2).

Immune Thrombocytopenia

GENERAL PRINCIPLES

Immune thrombocytopenia (ITP) is an acquired immune disorder in which antiplatelet antibodies cause shortened platelet survival and suppress megakaryopoiesis leading to thrombocytopenia and increased bleeding risk (*Blood 2009;113:6511*). Etiologies of ITP include idiopathic (primary), associated with coexisting conditions (secondary), or drug induced.

TABLE 20-1	Factor Deficiencies That Cause Prolonged Prothrombin Time and/or Activated Partial Thromboplastin Time and Correct with 50:50 Mix
Assay Result	**Suspected Factor Deficiencies**
↑ aPTT; normal PT	XII, XI, IX, VIII, HMWK, PK
↑ PT; normal aPTT	VII
↑ PT and ↑ aPTT	II, V, X, or fibrinogen

aPTT, activated partial thromboplastin time; HMWK, high-molecular-weight kininogen; PK, prekallikrein; PT, prothrombin time.

TABLE 20-2	Classification of Thrombocytopenia

Decreased Platelet Production	Increased Platelet Clearance

Marrow failure syndromes
 Congenital
 Acquired: Aplastic anemia, paroxysmal
   nocturnal hemoglobinuria
 Hematologic malignancies
 Marrow infiltration: Cancer, granuloma
 Myelofibrosis: Primary or secondary
 Nutritional: Vitamin B_{12} and folate
   deficiencies
 Physical damage to the bone marrow:
   Radiation, alcohol, chemotherapy
	Immune-mediated mechanisms
	 Immune thrombocytopenic
	 Thrombotic thrombocytopenic pur-
	   pura/hemolytic-uremic syndrome
	 Posttransfusion purpura
	 Heparin-induced thrombocytopenia
	 Non–immune-mediated mechanisms
	 DIC
	 Local consumption (aortic aneurysm)
	 Acute hemorrhage

Increased Splenic Sequestration	**Infections Associated with Thrombocytopenia**
Portal hypertension Felty syndrome Lysosomal storage disorders Infiltrative hematologic malignancies Extramedullary hematopoiesis	HIV, HHV-6, ehrlichiosis, rickettsia, malaria, hepatitis C, CMV, Epstein- Barr, *Helicobacter pylori, Escherichia coli* O157

CMV, cytomegalovirus; DIC, disseminated intravascular coagulation; HHV-6, human herpesvirus 6.

Epidemiology

Adult primary **ITP** has an incidence of 3.3 cases per 10^5 persons (*Am J Hematol 2010;85:174*).

Etiology

- In **primary ITP**, autoantibodies bind to platelet surface antigens and cause premature clearance by the reticuloendothelial system in addition to immune-mediated suppression of platelet production.
- **Secondary ITP** occurs in the setting of systemic lupus erythematosus (**SLE**), antiphospholipid antibody syndrome (**APS**), HIV, hepatitis C virus (**HCV**), *Helicobacter pylori*, and lymphoproliferative disorders (*Blood 2009;113:6511*).
- **Drug-dependent ITP** results from drug–platelet interactions prompting antibody binding (*N Engl J Med 2007;357:580*). Medications linked to thrombocytopenia include quinidine and quinine; platelet inhibitors abciximab, eptifibatide, tirofiban, and ticlopidine; antibiotics linezolid, rifampin, sulfonamides, and vancomycin; the anticonvulsants phenytoin, valproic acid, and carbamazepine; analgesics acetaminophen, naproxen, and diclofenac; cimetidine; and chlorothiazide (*Ann Intern Med 2005;142:474*).

DIAGNOSIS

Clinical Presentation

- **ITP** typically presents as mild mucocutaneous bleeding and petechiae or incidental thrombocytopenia. Occasionally, ITP can present as major bleeding.
- Risk of bleeding is highest with platelet counts $<30 \times 10^9$/L (*Blood 2011;117:1490*).

Diagnostic Testing

Normalization of platelet counts with discontinuation of suspected drug and confirmation if thrombocytopenia recurs when rechallenged support the diagnosis of **drug-induced ITP**.

Laboratories
- Review a peripheral blood smear to confirm automated platelet count and assess for platelet clumping and to determine platelet, red cell, and white cell morphologies.
- Laboratory tests do not confirm the diagnosis of primary ITP, although they help to exclude secondary causes. Primary **ITP** often has the scenario of isolated thrombocytopenia in the absence of a likely underlying causative disease or medication.
- Test for infection-associated causes (e.g., HIV, HCV) (*Blood 2011;117:4190*).
- Serologic tests for antiplatelet antibodies generally do not help diagnose **ITP** because of poor sensitivity and low negative predictive value (**NPV**) (*Am J Hematol 2005;78:193*).

Diagnostic Procedures
Diagnosis of ITP does not typically require bone marrow examination, although it can help to exclude other causes in select patients with additional complete blood cell (**CBC**) abnormalities, unresponsiveness to immune suppression therapy, or atypical signs or symptoms (*Blood 2011;117:4190*).

TREATMENT

- The decision to treat **primary ITP** depends on the severity of thrombocytopenia and bleeding risk. The therapeutic goal is a safe platelet count to prevent major bleeding (typically $\geq 30 \times 10^9$/L) and minimization of treatment-related toxicities.
- Initial therapy, when indicated, consists of **glucocorticoids** (typically prednisone 1 mg/kg/d orally, followed by a slow taper over weeks to months). Nonresponders to glucocorticoids or patients with active bleeding may also receive IV immunoglobulin (**IVIG**; 1 g/kg for one to two doses). Rh-positive patients may also receive anti-D immunoglobulin (**WinRho**) (ineffective postsplenectomy). WinRho works by forming anti–D-coated red blood cell (**RBC**) complexes, which bind to splenic macrophages, saturate the reticuloendothelial system, and prevent platelet destruction. WinRho may cause severe hemolysis and requires postinfusion monitoring. Reduce WinRho dose if hemoglobin (**Hgb**) <10 g/dL and avoid when the Hgb is <8 g/dL. Most primary ITP cases respond to therapy within 1–3 weeks.
- 30–40% of patients will relapse during a steroid taper (**relapsed/refractory ITP**).
- Two-thirds of patients with refractory ITP will obtain a durable complete response following **splenectomy**. Administer pneumococcal, meningococcal, and *Haemophilus influenzae* type B vaccines before (preferred) or after splenectomy.
- Treatment options for those who fail splenectomy include single or combined therapies with prednisone, IVIG, androgen therapy with danazol, other immunosuppressive agents, **rituximab** (anti-CD20 monoclonal antibody) (*Blood 2011;117:4190*), and/or thrombopoietin receptor (**TPO-R**) agonists.
- There are two TPO-R agonists for treatment of refractory primary ITP patients with increased bleeding risk: **romiplostim** (Nplate), dosed SC weekly, and **eltrombopag** (Promacta), taken orally once a day. TPO-R agonists produce durable platelet count improvements in a majority of refractory ITP patients beginning 5–7 days after initiation. Potential complications include thromboembolic events and bone marrow fibrosis (*Lancet 2011;377:393; Lancet 2008;371:395*).
- Management of **secondary ITP** may include a combination of treatment for the underlying disease and therapies similar to those used for management of primary ITP.
- Platelet transfusion for severe drug-induced thrombocytopenia may decrease risk of bleeding. IVIG, steroids, and plasmapheresis have uncertain benefit.

Thrombotic Thrombocytopenic Purpura and Hemolytic-Uremic Syndrome

GENERAL PRINCIPLES

Definition

Thrombotic thrombocytopenic purpura (TTP) and **hemolytic-uremic syndrome (HUS)** are thrombotic microangiopathies (**TMAs**) caused by platelet–vWF aggregates and platelet–fibrin aggregates, respectively, resulting in thrombocytopenia, microangiopathic hemolytic anemia (**MAHA**), and organ ischemia. Usually, clinical and laboratory features permit differentiation of TTP from HUS. TMA may occur in association with DIC, HIV infection, malignant hypertension, vasculitis, organ and stem cell transplant–related toxicity, adverse drug reactions, and pregnancy-related complications of preeclampsia/eclampsia and **HELLP** (**h**emolysis, **e**levated **l**iver enzymes, **l**ow **p**latelets) syndrome.

Epidemiology

Sporadic TTP has an incidence of approximately 11.3 cases per 10^6 persons, occurring more frequently in women and African Americans (*J Thromb Haemost 2005;3:1432*). **Typical HUS** usually occurs in gastroenteritis outbreaks affecting children. Adults may present with both **typical** and **atypical** (non–gastroenteritis-associated) variants of **HUS**.

Etiology

- Autoantibody-mediated removal of plasma vWF-cleaving protease: A disintegrin and metalloproteinase with a thrombospondin type 1 motif, member 13 (ADAMTS13), leading to elevated levels of abnormally large vWF multimers, typically causes **sporadic TTP** (*N Engl J Med 1998;339:1578*). The abnormal vWF multimers spontaneously adhere to platelets and may produce occlusive vWF–platelet aggregates in the microcirculation and subsequent microangiopathy. Second-hit events may involve endothelial dysfunction or injury.
- Severe ADAMTS13 deficiency does not cause HUS and other types of TMA, with the exception of some cases associated with HIV and pregnancy.
- **Typical or enteropathic HUS** has an association with *Escherichia coli* (O157:H7) production of Shiga-like toxins in Shiga toxigenic *E. coli* HUS (**STEC-HUS**).
- **HUS** can also be associated with transplantation, endothelial-damaging drugs, and pregnancy (*Kidney Int Suppl 2009;112:S8*).
- Inherited or acquired defects in regulation of the alternative complement pathway are present in 30–50% of atypical HUS cases (*Annu Rev Path Mech Dis 2008;3:249*).

DIAGNOSIS

Clinical Presentation

- The complete clinical pentad of **TTP**, present in <30% of cases, includes **consumptive thrombocytopenia, MAHA, fever, renal dysfunction, and fluctuating neurologic deficits**.
- The findings of thrombocytopenia and MAHA should raise suspicion for **TTP-HUS** in the absence of other identifiable causes.
- Patients with autosomal recessive inherited ADAMTS13 deficiencies have relapsing TTP (Upshaw-Schulman syndrome).
- Diarrhea, usually bloody, and abdominal pain often precede STEC-HUS.
- Marked renal dysfunction usually occurs in HUS.

Diagnostic Testing

- TMAs produce schistocytes (fragmented red cells) and thrombocytopenia on blood smears. The findings of anemia, elevated reticulocyte count, low or undetectable haptoglobin, and elevated lactate dehydrogenase (**LDH**) support the presence of hemolysis.
- Sporadic TTP has TMA findings, normal PT and aPTT, mild to moderate azotemia, very low or undetectable ADAMTS13 enzyme activity, and often detectable ADAMTS13 inhibitory antibody.
- Typical HUS has TMA and acute renal failure. *E. coli* O157 stool culture has a higher sensitivity than Shiga toxin assays. However, stool samples obtained after diarrhea has resolved reduce the sensitivity of both tests (*Kidney Int 2009;75:S29*).
- In the absence of precipitating risk factors, testing for **atypical HUS** should include molecular and serologic tests for complement regulator factor H and I mutations or autoantibodies through reference laboratories.

TREATMENT

- The mainstay of therapy for **TTP** consists of rapid treatment with plasma exchange (**PEX**) of 1.0–1.5 plasma volumes daily. PEX is continued for several days after normalization of platelet count and LDH.
  - If PEX is not available or will be delayed, infuse **fresh frozen plasma (FFP)** immediately to replace ADAMTS13.
  - Common practice includes the administration of **glucocorticoids**: prednisone 1 mg/kg PO per day. Consider a brief course of high-dose corticosteroids (methylprednisolone 0.5–1.0 g/d IV) in critically ill or PEX nonresponding patients (*Blood 2010;116:4060*).
  - Platelet transfusion in the absence of severe bleeding is relatively contraindicated due to potential risk of additional microvascular occlusions.
  - 90% of treated patients have a remission; however, relapses may occur days to years later.
  - Therapy with **rituximab** can achieve durable remissions following TTP relapses (*Ann Intern Med 2003;138:105*; *Thromb Haemost 2009;101:233*).
  - **Immunosuppression** with cyclophosphamide, azathioprine, or vincristine and splenectomy may have success in the treatment of refractory or relapsing TTP (*Ann Hematol 2002;81:7*; *Blood 2000;96:1223*).
- **STEC-HUS** does not usually improve with PEX, and treatment remains supportive. Antibiotic therapy does not hasten recovery or minimize toxicity for STEC-HUS.
- **TMA associated with calcineurin inhibitors** (cyclosporine, tacrolimus), typically given in the transplant setting, usually responds to drug dose reduction or discontinuation of the offending agent.
- **Atypical HUS** often leads to chronic renal failure necessitating dialysis.
- In 2011, the US Food and Drug Administration (**FDA**) approved eculizumab for treatment of **atypical HUS**. Eculizumab is a humanized monoclonal antibody that binds to complement protein C5, blocking its cleavage into C5a and the cytotoxic membrane attack complex C5b-9, thus inhibiting complement activation (*Blood 2011;118:3303*).
- *Neisseria meningitides* vaccination is recommended 2 weeks prior to starting eculizumab; however, in **atypical** HUS, this grace period is typically not possible.

Heparin-Induced Thrombocytopenia

GENERAL PRINCIPLES

Definition

Heparin-induced thrombocytopenia (HIT) is an acquired hypercoagulable disorder associated with use of heparin or heparin-like products and due to autoantibodies targeting the anticoagulant and platelet factor 4 (**PF4**) complexes. HIT typically presents with thrombocytopenia or a decrease in platelet count by at least 50% from preexposure baseline. Major complications of HIT consist of arterial and venous thromboembolic events.

Epidemiology

The incidence of **HIT** ranges from 0.1–1.0% in medical and obstetric patients receiving prophylactic and therapeutic unfractionated heparin (**UFH**), to >1–5% in patients receiving prophylactic UFH after cardiothoracic surgery (*Chest 2012;141:e495s*). Patients exposed only to LMWH have a low incidence of HIT (*Thromb Res 2009;124:189*). HIT rarely occurs in association with the synthetic pentasaccharide fondaparinux (*N Engl J Med 2007;356:2653*).

Etiology

Immune-responsive patients produce autoantibodies that bind to PF4/heparin complexes, which can activate platelets, cause thrombocytopenia, and lead to clot formation through increased thrombin generation (*Blood 2003;101:31*).

DIAGNOSIS

Clinical Presentation

- **HIT** usually develops within 5–14 days of heparin exposure (**typical-onset HIT**). Exceptions include **delayed-onset HIT**, which occurs after stopping heparin, and **early-onset HIT**, which starts within the first 24 hours of heparin administration in patients with recent exposure to heparin (*Chest 2012;141:e495s*).
- Suspect HIT when thrombocytopenia occurs during heparin exposure by any route in the absence of other causes of thrombocytopenia.
- The **4T scoring system** (Table 20-3) determines HIT pretest probability and has an NPV of >95% (*J Thromb Haemost 2006;4:759*).

TABLE 20-3	4T Scoring System for Pretest Probability of Heparin-Induced Thrombocytopenia		
T Category	**0 Points**	**1 Point**	**2 Points**
Thrombocytopenia	PLT fall <30% or nadir <10 × 10^9/L	PLT fall 30–50% or nadir 10–19 × 10^9/L	PLT fall >50% and nadir ≥20 × 10^9/L
Timing of thrombocytopenia	≤4 d without prior exposure	Likely within 5–10 d, not clear; >10 d; ≤1 d (with exposure 31–100 d)	Within 5–10 d of exposure or ≤1 d (with exposure in last 30 d)
Thrombotic event	No thrombus	Thrombus recurrence or progression; erythematous skin lesion; suspected thrombus	Confirmed thrombus; skin necrosis; acute reaction after UFH bolus
Other causes for thrombocytopenia	Definite	Possible	None apparent

PLT, platelets; UFH, unfractionated heparin.
Sum the points for each of the four categories to determine the clinical probability: high (6–8 points), intermediate (4–5 points), low (0–3 points).
Data from *J Thromb Haemost 2006;4:759–65* and *J Thromb Haemost 2010;8:1483–5*.

- HIT rarely causes severe thrombocytopenia (platelet count <20 × 10⁹/L) and bleeding.
- **Thromboembolic complications** occur in 30–75% of HIT patients (i.e., heparin-induced thrombocytopenia and thrombosis [**HITT**]). Thrombosis can precede, be concurrent with, or follow thrombocytopenia.
- HIT causing venous thrombi at heparin injection sites produces full-thickness skin infarctions, sometimes in the absence of thrombocytopenia.
- HIT can cause systemic allergic responses following an IV bolus of heparin characterized by fever, hypotension, dyspnea, and cardiac arrest.

Diagnostic Testing

- Obtain surveillance platelet counts every 2–3 days during heparin exposure in patients with >1% risk of HIT (*Chest 2012;141:e495s*).
- For suspected HIT, laboratory tests for PF4 antibodies improve diagnostic accuracy.
  ○ PF4 antibodies in patients' serum is a sensitive screening test but lacks specificity.
  ○ Specificity improves when a positive enzyme-linked immunosorbent assay (**ELISA**) is quantified in optical density (**OD**) units. The higher the OD, the more likely it is that the patient has HIT.
- There are two functional assays for HIT: serotonin release assay (**SRA**) and heparin-induced platelet activation (**HIPA**; more common in Europe).
  ○ Both tests detect PF4 antibodies in patients' serum capable of activating control platelets in the presence of heparin.
  ○ Both tests have high specificity for HIT but lower sensitivity than ELISA.
  ○ Testing in reference laboratories typically delays results for days.
- For a low clinical probability of HIT, testing for HIT antibodies is *not* indicated.
  ○ For a moderate to high clinical probability of HIT, PF4 ELISA testing is indicated. A negative PF4 ELISA effectively rules out HIT.
  ○ A functional test (SRA or HIPA) should confirm a positive PF4 ELISA to improve testing specificity.

TREATMENT

- Because HIT test results are not often immediately available, clinical assessment should determine initial management.
- When HIT is strongly suspected or confirmed, **eliminate all heparin exposure**.
- Patients with HIT are at high risk for VTE and require alternative anticoagulation (*Blood 2012;119:2209*) with a parenteral direct thrombin inhibitor (**DTI**) (i.e., **argatroban or bivalirudin**), although fondaparinux also has been used (*J Thromb Haemost 2011;9:2389*). Do not use LMWH in patients with HIT.
- Assess for symptomatic VTE, and screen (e.g., lower extremity venous compression ultrasound) to assess for asymptomatic VTE, because VTE warrants a full course of anticoagulation (*Blood 2003;101:31*).
- Start warfarin only after the platelet count normalizes, at an initial dose no greater than 5 mg daily, overlapping with a DTI for 5 days, to reduce the risk of limb gangrene due to ongoing hypercoagulable conditions and depletion of proteins C and S.
- DTIs prolong the INR and require careful monitoring when transitioning from DTI to warfarin (see Medications under Approach to Venous Thromboembolism).
- Avoid using oral DTI and anti-Xa inhibitors because they have not been adequately evaluated for safety and efficacy in HIT patients with or without thrombosis.
- The recommended duration of anticoagulation therapy for HIT depends on the clinical scenario: 4 weeks for **isolated HIT** (without thrombosis) and 3 months for **HIT-associated thrombosis** (*Chest 2012;141:e495s*) (see treatment duration in Approach to Venous Thromboembolism section).

Posttransfusion Purpura

GENERAL PRINCIPLES

Definition

Posttransfusion purpura (PTP), a rare syndrome characterized by the formation of alloantibodies against platelet antigens, most commonly HPA-1a, follows blood component transfusion and causes severe thrombocytopenia.

Epidemiology

PTP has an incidence of 1 in 50,000 to 100,000 blood transfusions, although approximately 2% of the population has a potential risk for PTP based on the frequency of HPA-1b/1b.

Etiology

Glycoprotein (GP) IIIa has a polymorphic epitope called HPA-1a/b, the antigen most commonly involved in PTP. **PTP** typically occurs in HPA-1a/1b–negative multiparous women or previously transfused patients when reexposed to HPA-1a by transfusion. An amnestic response produces alloantibodies to the HPA-1a, which appear to also recognize the patient's HPA-1a–negative platelets and cause thrombocytopenia via platelet destruction.

DIAGNOSIS

- In **PTP**, severe thrombocytopenia ($<15 \times 10^9$/L) usually occurs within 7–10 days of transfusion.
- Confirmation of suspected **PTP** requires detection of platelet alloantibodies.

TREATMENT

Although spontaneous platelet recovery eventually occurs, bleeding may require treatment. Effective therapies include IVIG and plasmapheresis. Transfusion with platelets from a donor who lacks the causative epitope (typically HPA-1a) does not clearly have higher efficacy than random platelet transfusion. Reserve transfusion for patients with PTP and severe bleeding (*Am J Hematol 2004;76:258*).

Gestational Thrombocytopenia

GENERAL PRINCIPLES

Definition

Gestational thrombocytopenia (platelet counts $\geq 70 \times 10^9$/L) is a benign, mild thrombocytopenia associated with pregnancy.

Epidemiology

Gestational thrombocytopenia spontaneously occurs in approximately 5–7% of otherwise uncomplicated pregnancies (*Clin Obstet Gynecol 1999;42:327*).

Etiology

The mechanism of gestational thrombocytopenia remains unknown.

DIAGNOSIS

Clinical Presentation

Gestational thrombocytopenia occurs in the third trimester of pregnancy. The mother has no symptoms, and the fetus remains unaffected.

Differential Diagnosis

Other causes of thrombocytopenia during pregnancy include **ITP, preeclampsia, eclampsia, HELLP syndrome, TTP, and DIC.**

Diagnostic Testing

To distinguish between gestational thrombocytopenia and other syndromes, diagnostic testing includes an evaluation for infection and hypertension and laboratory testing for hemolysis and liver dysfunction.

OUTCOME/PROGNOSIS

Gestational thrombocytopenia and thrombocytopenia associated with preeclampsia and eclampsia usually resolve promptly after delivery.

Thrombocytosis

GENERAL PRINCIPLES

Definition

Thrombocytosis is defined as a platelet count of $>450 \times 10^9/L$ by the World Health Organization (WHO).

Etiology

Thrombocytosis has reactive and clonal etiologies that may coexist.
- **Reactive thrombocytosis** may occur during recovery from thrombocytopenia; after splenectomy; or in response to iron deficiency, acute infectious or chronic inflammatory states, trauma, and malignancies.
  - ○ Low risks of thrombosis or bleeding.
  - ○ Platelets normalize after improvement of the underlying disorder.
  - ○ If accompanied by thrombotic complications, evaluate for an underlying myeloproliferative disorder.
- **Essential thrombocytosis (ET)** is a chronic myeloproliferative disorder. Eventual progression to myelofibrosis, acute myeloid leukemia, or myelodysplastic syndrome occurs in a minority of ET patients (*Br J Haematol 2005;130:153*).

DIAGNOSIS

Clinical Presentation

History
ET may present as an incidental discovery or present with thrombotic or hemorrhagic symptoms. The risk of thrombosis increases with age, prior thrombosis, duration of disease, and other comorbidities (*Blood 1999;93:417*). Erythromelalgia, due to microvascular occlusive platelet thrombi, presents as intense burning or throbbing of the extremities, typically involving the feet. Cold exposure usually relieves symptoms. Hemorrhage typically occurs with platelet counts $>1000 \times 10^9/L$, and acquired deficiencies of large vWF multimers often accompany hemorrhage patients with ET (*Blood 1993;82:1749*).

Physical Examination

Approximately 50% of ET patients develop mild splenomegaly. Typical signs of erythromelalgia include erythema and warmth of affected digits.

Diagnostic Criteria

In 2008, the **WHO** revised criteria (requires all four) included (*Curr Hematol Malig Rep 2007;4:33*):
- Sustained platelet count >450 × 10⁹/L
- Bone marrow biopsy showing increased mature megakaryocytes and no increase in erythropoiesis or granulopoiesis
- Exclusion of chronic myelogenous leukemia (**CML**), polycythemia vera, and primary myelofibrosis according to WHO criteria
- Presence of *JAK2V617F* mutation or other clonal marker (*Lancet 2005;365:1054*), **or**, if clonal marker not present, no evidence for reactive thrombocytosis (*Leukemia 2008;22:14*)

TREATMENT

Patients requiring cytoreduction include those with high risk of thrombosis (age >60 years or a history of thrombosis). The majority of thrombotic complications occur at modest platelet count elevations. Treatment typically aims for a platelet count of ≤400 × 10⁹/L. Platelet-lowering drugs include **hydroxyurea** and **anagrelide** or **interferon-α** in pregnant patients or females in their childbearing years (*Blood 2001;97:863*).
- Hydroxyurea and anagrelide provide equivalent platelet count control, but anagrelide causes more complications (*N Engl J Med 2005;353:33*).
- Anagrelide side effects include palpitations, atrial fibrillation, fluid retention, and headache.
- Plateletpheresis rapidly lowers platelet counts, although it is reserved for patients who have acute arterial thrombosis.

Qualitative Platelet Disorders

GENERAL PRINCIPLES

Qualitative platelet disorders present with mucocutaneous bleeding and excessive bruising with an adequate platelet count, PT, and aPTT and normal screening tests for vWD. Most potent platelet defects produce prolonged PFA-100 closure times. However, a normal PFA-100 does not exclude qualitative platelet disorders, and high clinical suspicion of a disorder should lead to further testing.

Classification

- **Inherited disorders** of platelet function include receptor, signal transduction, cyclooxygenase, secretory (e.g., storage pool disease), adhesion, or aggregation defects. In vitro platelet aggregation studies can identify patterns of agonist responses consistent with a particular defect, such as the rare autosomal recessive disorders of adhesion in **Bernard-Soulier syndrome** (lack of GP Ib/IX [vWF receptor]) and aggregation in **Glanzmann thrombasthenia** (lack of GP IIb/IIIa [fibrinogen receptor]).
- **Acquired** platelet defects are more common than hereditary platelet qualitative disorders.
  - Conditions associated with acquired qualitative defects include metabolic disorders (uremia, liver failure), myeloproliferative diseases, myelodysplasia, acute leukemia, monoclonal gammopathy, and cardiopulmonary bypass platelet trauma.
  - **Drug-induced** platelet dysfunction is a side effect of many drugs, including high-dose penicillin, aspirin (ASA) and other **NSAIDs**, and ethanol. Other drug classes, such

as β-lactam antibiotics, β-blockers, calcium channel blockers, nitrates, antihistamines, psychotropic drugs, tricyclic antidepressants, and selective serotonin reuptake inhibitors, cause platelet dysfunction in vitro, but they rarely cause bleeding.
- Certain **foods and herbal products** may affect platelet function including omega-3 fatty acids, garlic and onion extracts, ginger, gingko, ginseng, and black tree fungus. Patients should stop using herbal medications and dietary supplements ≥1 week before major surgery (*Thromb Res 2005;117:49*; *Anaesthesia 2002;57:889*).

TREATMENT

- Reserve platelet transfusions for major bleeding episodes. Anecdotal reports have described successful control of severe bleeding with recombinant factor VIIa (**rFVIIa**).
- Treatment of **uremic platelet dysfunction** can include dialysis to improve uremia; desmopressin (**DDAVP**) 0.3 μg/kg IV to stimulate release of vWF from endothelial cells; or conjugated estrogens (0.6 mg/kg IV daily for 5 days) (*Nat Clin Pract Nephrol 2007;3:138*) and platelet transfusions in actively bleeding patients, although transfused platelets rapidly acquire the uremic defect. Transfusion or erythropoietin (**EPO**) to increase a hematocrit toward 30% might assist in hemostasis (*Am J Kidney Dis 1991;18:44*; *Br J Haematol 1985;59:139*).
- **Reversal of drug-induced platelet dysfunction**
  - **NSAIDs** other than ASA reversibly inhibit cyclooxygenase (**COX**). Their effects only last several days. **COX-2 inhibitors** have antiplatelet activity in large doses, but they have a minimal effect on platelets at therapeutic doses.
  - **Aspirin** irreversibly inhibits COX-1 and COX-2. Its effects diminish over 7–10 days due to new platelet production.
  - **Thienopyridines** inhibit platelet aggregation by irreversibly (clopidogrel and prasugrel) or reversibly (ticagrelor) blocking platelet adenosine diphosphate (ADP) receptor P2Y12.
  - **Dipyridamole**, alone or in combination with ASA (Aggrenox), inhibits platelet function by increasing intracellular cyclic adenosine monophosphate (**cAMP**).
  - **Abciximab, eptifibatide, and tirofiban** block platelet IIb/IIIa–dependent aggregation (see Chapter 4, Ischemic Heart Disease).
  - Platelet transfusion compensates for drug-induced platelet dysfunction, except immediately following tirofiban and eptifibatide therapy.
  - Hold antiplatelet agents for 7 days before elective invasive procedures.

INHERITED BLEEDING DISORDERS

Hemophilia A

GENERAL PRINCIPLES

Definition
Hemophilia A is an X-linked recessive coagulation disorder due to mutations in the gene encoding factor VIII.

Epidemiology
Hemophilia A affects approximately 1 in 5000 live male births. Approximately 40% of cases occur in families with no prior history of hemophilia, reflecting the high rate of spontaneous germline mutations in the factor VIII gene (*N Engl J Med 2001;344:1773*).

DIAGNOSIS

Clinical Presentation

- Patients with severe hemophilia experience frequent spontaneous hemarthroses and hematomas, hematuria, and delayed posttraumatic and postoperative bleeding. Repeated bleeding into a "target" joint causes chronic synovitis and hemophilic arthropathy.
- Moderate hemophiliacs have fewer spontaneous bleeding episodes, and mild hemophiliacs may only bleed excessively after trauma or surgery.

Diagnostic Testing

Factor VIII activity: Severe (<1%), moderate (1–5%), and mild (>5–<40%).
Mild hemophiliacs with factor VIII ≥30% may not have a prolonged aPTT.

TREATMENT

Medications

First Line

- Mild to moderate hemophilia A with minor bleeding:
  - **DDAVP** (0.3 μg/kg IV infused over 30 minutes, or 150 μg intranasally [Stimate, 1.5 mg/mL] each nostril) increases factor VIII activity three- to fivefold. Because all patients do not have an expected response to DDAVP, they should undergo a DDAVP challenge to assess responsiveness. To avoid tachyphylaxis, no more than three consecutive doses should be given per week (*Blood 1997;90:2515*).
- Mild to moderate hemophilia A with major bleeding *or* severe hemophilia A with any bleeding:
  - **Factor VIII replacement** is the mainstay of therapy with many hemophiliac patients able to do home infusion.
  - **Factor VIII concentrate** increases factor VIII activity by 2% for every 1 IU/kg infused; thus a 50 IU/kg IV bolus raises factor VIII activity by 100% over baseline. Extended treatment should follow with 25 IU/kg IV bolus q12h to maintain sufficient levels.
  - One to three doses of **factor VIII** concentrates targeting peak plasma activities of 30–50% typically stop mild hemorrhages.
  - Major traumas and surgery require maintenance of levels >80%.
  - Adjust doses based on peak and trough factor VIII levels to achieve individualized targets based on bleeding risk.
  - Continuous infusion of factor VIII provides a safe and effective alternative to intermittent infusion (*Haemophilia 2006;12:212*; *Haemophilia 2012;18:753*).

Second Line

Second-line factor VIII sources include **cryoprecipitate** and **FFP**.

Hemophilia B

GENERAL PRINCIPLES

Definition

Hemophilia B is an X-linked recessive coagulation disorder secondary to mutations in the gene encoding factor IX.

Epidemiology

Hemophilia B affects approximately 1 in 30,000 male births.

Diagnostic Testing

Factor IX activity. Hemophilia A (factor VIII) and B (factor IX) use the same severity scale based on degree of decreased factor activity.

Clinical Presentation

Hemophilia B remains clinically indistinguishable from hemophilia A.

TREATMENT

Therapy of hemophilia B consists of **factor IX replacement** with either **plasma-derived factor IX** or **recombinant factor IX** (BeneFIX).
- DDAVP lacks efficacy because it does **not** increase factor IX levels.
- Postinfusion peak targets, duration of therapy, and laboratory monitoring for treatment of hemophilia B–related bleeding are similar to those for hemophilia A.
- Every 1 IU/kg of factor IX replacement typically raises plasma factor IX activity by 1%. Factor IX has a half-life of 18–24 hours.

COMPLICATIONS OF HEMOPHILIA A AND B THERAPY

- Alloantibodies to factors VIII and IX in response to replacement therapy develop in approximately 20% and 12% of severe hemophilia A and B patients, respectively. These alloantibodies neutralize infused factor VIII or IX.
- Determining the titer of a factor VIII or IX inhibitor, using a laboratory assay that reports inhibitor strength in Bethesda units (**BUs**), predicts inhibitor behavior and guides therapy.
- Treatment options for factor VIII or IX inhibitors include the following (*Lancet 2012;379:1447*):
  ○ Large doses of factor VIII or IX concentrates overcome inhibitors for patients with weak inhibitors (BU <5).
  ○ Because factor VIII or IX concentrates will not overcome inhibitors in patients with high titers (BU >5), bypassing agents, such as recombinant factor VII or activated prothrombin complex concentrate (aPCC), need to be used (*Blood 2007;109:546*).
    ■ **rFVIIa** (NovoSeven) is dosed at 90 µg/kg every 2 hours until hemostasis occurs.
    ■ **aPCC** (most commonly used is Factor Eight Inhibitor Bypassing Activity [FEIBA]) is dosed at 75–100 IU/kg q12h. FEIBA contains activated factors VII, VIII, XI, and X and thrombin, and it can cause thrombosis or DIC.

von Willebrand Disease

GENERAL PRINCIPLES

Classification

vWD has three main types (*J Thromb Haemost 2006;4:2103*).
- **Type 1 vWD** is due to a quantitative deficiency of vWF (70–80% of cases).
- **Type 2 vWD**, due to a qualitative defect of vWF, includes four subtypes (2A, 2B, 2M, 2N).
  ○ Type 2A: reduced vWF high-molecular-weight multimer
  ○ Type 2B: pathologically enhanced platelet affinity to vWF
  ○ Type 2M: reduced platelet affinity to vWF
  ○ Type 2N: defective factor VIII binding to vWF
- **Type 3 vWD** has a virtual complete lack of vWF (*Blood 2001;97:1915*).

Epidemiology

vWD, the most common inherited bleeding disorder, affects around 0.1–1% of the population.

Etiology

Most forms of **vWD** have an autosomal dominant inheritance with variable penetrance, although autosomal recessive forms (types 2N and 3) exist. vWF circulates as multimers of variable size and facilitates adherence of platelets to injured vessel walls and stabilizes factor VIII in plasma.

DIAGNOSIS

Clinical Presentation

Clinical findings consist of mucocutaneous bleeding (epistaxis, menorrhagia, gastrointestinal bleeding), easy bruising, and bleeding from trauma or surgery.

Diagnostic Testing

Testing for suspected vWD should include vWF:Ag, vWF ristocetin cofactor (vWF:RCo), and factor VIII activity. See the American Society of Hematology pocket guide on vWD.

TREATMENT

Goal of therapy is to raise vWF:RCo and factor VIII activity to ensure adequate hemostasis. vWF:RCo activities >50% control most hemorrhages.
- **DDAVP** 0.3 µg/kg IV can be used to treat type 1 vWD. Because only two-thirds of patients will respond, a test dose should assess for a response. For responders undergoing **minor invasive procedures**, infuse 1 hour before, followed by q12–24h for three more doses postoperatively, with or without oral antifibrinolytic drugs (i.e., aminocaproic acid or tranexamic acid).
  ○ DDAVP does not effectively treat most type 2 or type 3 vWD patients.
  ○ DDAVP is contraindicated in type 2B vWD because of the risk of thrombocytopenia.
  ○ Common side effects of DDAVP include hyponatremia, nausea, and flushing. Patients should limit fluid intake to 1200 mL/d within 24 hours of any dose.
- **vWF plasma-derived concentrate transfusions** (Alphanate, Humate-P, and Wilate) should aim to raise vWF:RCo activity to approximately 100% and maintain it between 50–100% until sufficient hemostasis occurs (typically 5–10 days). Cryoprecipitate is a second-line vWF source. Indications for concentrate transfusions:
  ○ Type 1 vWD-DDAVP nonresponders
  ○ Type 1 vWD with major bleeding or surgery
  ○ All other vWD types requiring hemostasis treatment

ACQUIRED COAGULATION DISORDERS

Vitamin K Deficiency

GENERAL PRINCIPLES

Vitamin K deficiency is usually caused by malabsorption states or poor dietary intake combined with antibiotic-associated loss of intestinal bacterial colonization. Hepatocytes require vitamin K to complete the synthesis (γ-carboxylation) of clotting factors (X, IX, VII, prothrombin) and the natural anticoagulant proteins C and S.

DIAGNOSIS

Vitamin K deficiency is suspected when an at-risk patient has a prolonged PT that corrects after a 1:1 mix with normal pooled plasma.

TREATMENT

Vitamin K replacement can be given by mouth (e.g., phytonadione 5 mg PO daily) in patients who have had poor dietary intake. When malabsorption is present, vitamin K can be repleted parenterally. IV administration of vitamin K has more reliable absorption than SC and is the preferred parenteral route.

Liver Disease

GENERAL PRINCIPLES

Liver disease can impair hemostasis (see Figure 20-1) because hepatocytes produce coagulation factors, with the exception of vWF and factor VIII. Coagulopathy is typically mild with stable liver disease until patients decompensate. Other hemostatic complications include thrombocytopenia due to splenic sequestration, DIC, hyperfibrinolysis, and cholestasis (which impairs vitamin K absorption). Although PT/INR and aPTT prolongations imply an increased risk of bleeding, they do not reflect concurrent reductions in protein C and protein S. Liver disease has a fragile balance of procoagulant and anticoagulant activities, which can easily be disrupted by infection, renal insufficiency, and vasomotor dysfunction (*Blood 2010;116:878*).

TREATMENT

- **Vitamin K** replacement may shorten a prolonged PT/INR due to a vitamin K antagonist, dietary deficiency, or cholestasis.
- **FFP** may be indicated for patients who are bleeding or require an invasive procedure and have abnormal coagulation parameters but may cause volume overload. A common threshold is PT >1.5 control despite limited supportive evidence.
- **Cryoprecipitate**, 1.5 units/10 kg body weight, corrects hypofibrinogenemia (<100 mg/dL).
- **Prothrombin complex concentrate (PCC)**, but safety and efficacy are unproven.
- Randomized controlled trials failed to show a hemostasis benefit for **recombinant factor VIIa** in GI bleeding (*Hepatology 2008;47:1604*).
- Reserve **platelet transfusions** for active bleeding or prior to invasive procedures, such as liver biopsy, in patients with thrombocytopenia (<50 × 10^9/L).

Disseminated Intravascular Coagulation

GENERAL PRINCIPLES

Etiology

DIC occurs in a variety of systemic illnesses that include sepsis, trauma, burns, shock, obstetric complications, and malignancies (notably, acute promyelocytic leukemia).

Pathophysiology

Exposure of tissue factor to the circulation generates excess thrombin, leading to platelet activation, consumption of coagulation factors (including fibrinogen) and regulators (antithrombin [**AT**] and proteins C and S), fibrin generation, generalized microthrombi, and reactive fibrinolysis.

DIAGNOSIS

Clinical Presentation

Consequences of **DIC** include bleeding, organ dysfunction secondary to microvascular thrombi and ischemia, and less often, large arterial and venous thrombosis (*Br J Haematol 2009;145:24*).

Diagnostic Testing

No one test confirms diagnosis of DIC. The International Society on Thrombosis and Haemostasis (**ISTH**) devised a clinical scoring system for objective detection of DIC (Table 20-4). Serial "DIC panels" help assess clinical management and prognosis.

TREATMENT

Treatment consists of supportive care and correction of the underlying disorder if possible. **FFP**, **cryoprecipitate**, and **platelets** can be administered when needed clinically (e.g., bleeding or surgery), rather than strictly based on a laboratory threshold. Administer adjusted-dose IV **heparin** to patients with large-vessel venous or arterial thrombi. Nonbleeding patients who have DIC should receive thromboprophylaxis with heparin.

Acquired Inhibitors of Coagulation Factors

GENERAL PRINCIPLES

Acquired inhibitors of coagulation factors may occur de novo (autoantibodies) or may develop in hemophiliacs (alloantibodies) following factor VIII or IX infusions. The most common acquired inhibitor is directed against factor VIII. De novo cases often arise in patients with underlying lymphoproliferative or autoimmune disorders.

DIAGNOSIS

Patients with factor VIII inhibitors present with an abrupt onset of bleeding or bruising, prolonged aPTT that does not correct after 1:1 mixing with normal plasma, markedly decreased factor VIII activity, and a normal PT. Patients rarely develop autoantibodies that

TABLE 20-4	International Society on Thrombosis and Haemostasis Disseminated Intravascular Coagulation Scoring System		
Use only in patients with an underlying condition known to be associated with DIC.			
	0 Points	**1 Point**	**2 Points**
Thrombocytopenia	$>100 \times 10^9/L$	$\leq100 \times 10^9/L$	$\leq50 \times 10^9/L$
D-Dimer	Normal	$<10 \times$ upper limit of normal	$\geq10 \times$ upper limit of normal
PT Prolongation	<3 s	3–6 s	>6 s
Fibrinogen	>100 mg/dL	≤100 mg/dL	

DIC, disseminated intravascular coagulation.
Sum the points for each of the four categories to determine the clinical probability of having DIC: compatible with overt DIC ≥5 points, and suggestive of nonovert DIC <5 points.
Data from *Thromb Haemost 2001;86:132* and *Crit Care Med 2004;32:24167*.

inhibit other factors (II, V, X) and subsequently prolong aPTT and PT, which do not correct after mixing studies.

TREATMENT

Bleeding complications in patients with factor VIII inhibitors (autoantibodies) are managed in the same manner as for hemophiliacs with alloantibodies to factor VIII (see Inherited Bleeding Disorders section). Long-term therapy consists of immunosuppression with prednisone or prednisolone ± cyclophosphamide to reduce production of the autoantibody (*Blood 2012;120:47*). The use of rituximab has become increasingly more common (*Br J Haematol 2014;165:600*).

VENOUS THROMBOEMBOLIC DISORDERS

Approach to Venous Thromboembolism

GENERAL PRINCIPLES

Definition
- **Thromboses** or blood clots may occur in veins, arteries, or chambers of the heart.
- **VTE** refers to **deep vein thrombosis (DVT)** or **pulmonary embolism (PE)**.
- **Thrombophlebitis** consists of inflammation in a vein due to a blood clot.
- **Superficial thrombophlebitis** may occur in any superficial vein.

Classification
The anatomic location of DVT/PE, clot burden, and sequelae may affect prognosis and treatment recommendations.
- Thromboses can be classified as **deep** or **superficial** and as **proximal** or **distal**.
  - Avoid using the term **superficial femoral vein** because it really refers to part of the **femoral vein (a deep vein)**.
  - **Proximal** lower extremity DVTs occur in or superior to the popliteal vein (or the confluence of tibial and peroneal veins), whereas **distal** DVTs occur inferiorly.
- Location in the pulmonary arterial system characterizes **PEs** as **central/proximal** (main pulmonary artery, lobar, or segmental) or **distal** (subsegmental).

Epidemiology
- Without treatment, half of patients with proximal lower extremity DVT develop PE.
- DVTs in the upper extremities are often related to an indwelling catheter and can cause PE.
- DVT may occur concomitantly with superficial thrombophlebitis.

Etiology
- Venous thromboemboli arise under conditions of **blood stasis**, **hypercoagulability** (changes in the soluble and formed elements of the blood), or venous **endothelial dysfunction/injury**.
- Hypercoagulable states may have an inherited or acquired etiology (see Risk Factors section).
- **Superficial thrombophlebitis** occurs in association with varicose veins, trauma, infection, and hypercoagulable disorders.
- Other causes of pulmonary arterial occlusion *include in situ* thrombi (e.g., sickle cell disease), marrow fat embolism, amniotic fluid embolism, pulmonary artery sarcoma, and fibrosing mediastinitis.

Risk Factors

- Risk factors for VTE can be categorized as inherited, acquired, or unknown (idiopathic).
- **Inherited thrombophilic disorders** are suggested by spontaneous VTE at a young age (<50 years), recurrent VTE, VTE in first-degree relatives, thrombosis in unusual anatomic locations (i.e., abdominal), and recurrent fetal loss.
- The most common inherited risk factors for VTE include gene mutations **(factor V Leiden and prothrombin gene G20210A)** and deficiencies of the natural anticoagulants **protein C, protein S, and AT.**
- **Homocystinuria,** a rare autosomal recessive disorder caused by deficiency of cystathionine-β-synthase, leads to extremely high plasma homocysteine and causes early onset arterial and venous thromboembolic events. Mild elevation of homocysteine may be caused by a mutation in methylenetetrahydrofolate reductase (*MTHFR*), but does not cause VTE (*Arch Intern Med 2007;167:497*; *Br J Haematol 2008;141:529*). Therefore, *MTHFR* mutation should not be included in the thrombophilia testing.
- Spontaneous VTE in unusual locations, such as cavernous sinus, mesenteric vein, or portal vein, may be the initial presentation of paroxysmal nocturnal hemoglobinuria **(PNH)** or myeloproliferative disorders.
- **Spontaneous (idiopathic) VTEs** have a high risk of recurrence (8–10% per year) regardless of the presence of an inherited thrombophilia (*N Engl J Med 2001;344:1222*).
- **Acquired hypercoagulable** states may arise secondary to malignancy, immobilization, infection, trauma, surgery, collagen vascular diseases, nephrotic syndrome, HIT, DIC, medications (e.g., estrogen), and pregnancy.
- Acquired **autoantibodies** associated with HIT and APS can cause arterial or venous thrombi.
- **APS** is a hypercoagulable disorder that requires the presence of at least one clinical **and** one laboratory criterion (*J Thromb Haemost 2006;4:295*).
  - **APS clinical criteria:**
    - Unprovoked arterial or venous thrombosis in any tissue or organ *or*
    - Pregnancy morbidities (unexplained late fetal death; premature birth complicated by eclampsia, preeclampsia, placental insufficiency; or ≥ three unexplained consecutive spontaneous abortions at <10 weeks of gestation or one at ≥10 weeks).
  - **APS laboratory criteria:**
    Presence of autoantibodies
    - **LA,** anticardiolipin, or β_2-glycoprotein-1 antibodies
    - Confirmation of positive autoantibody tests (must be done at least 12 weeks apart)
    - Approximately 10% of patients with SLE have an LA; however, most patients with an LA do not have SLE.
  - APS may include **other features,** such as thrombocytopenia, valvular heart disease, livedo reticularis, neurologic manifestations, and nephropathy.

Prevention

Identifying patients at high risk for VTE and instituting prophylactic measures should remain a high priority (see Chapter 1, Inpatient Care in Internal Medicine).

DIAGNOSIS

Clinical Presentation

- **Pain, edema, redness, and warmth** in an affected extremity **are the most common symptoms of a DVT**. Pretest assessment of the probability of a DVT provides useful information when combined with the results of compression ultrasound, D-dimer test, or both, in determining whether to exclude or accept the diagnosis of DVT or perform additional imaging studies (*Lancet 1997;350:1795*).
- **Superficial thrombophlebitis** presents as a tender, warm, erythematous, and often palpable thrombosed vein. Accompanying DVT may produce additional symptoms and signs.

- **PE** may produce shortness of breath, chest pain (pleuritic), hypoxemia, hemoptysis, pleural rub, new right-sided heart failure, and tachycardia (*Ann Intern Med 1998;129:997*). Validated clinical risk factors for a PE in outpatients who present to an emergency department include signs and symptoms of DVT, high clinical suspicion of PE, tachycardia, immobility in the past 4 weeks, history of VTE, active cancer, and hemoptysis (*Ann Intern Med 2001;135:98*).

Differential Diagnosis

- The **differential diagnoses of DVT** include cellulitis, Baker cyst, hematoma, venous insufficiency, postphlebitic syndrome, lymphedema, sarcoma, arterial aneurysm, myositis, rupture of the gastrocnemius, and abscess.
- **Symmetric, bilateral lower extremity edema** suggests heart, renal, or liver failure as the cause of the signs and symptoms.
- The **differential diagnosis of PE** includes dissecting aortic aneurysm, pneumonia, acute bronchitis, pericardial or pleural disease, heart failure, costochondritis, rib fracture, and myocardial ischemia.

Diagnostic Testing

Clinical Probability Assessment

Clinical decision rules help to exclude VTE when used in combination with other diagnostic tests (such as normal D-dimer).

- Clinical predictors of PE include prior VTE, heart rate ≥100 bpm, recent surgery/immobilization, hemoptysis, cancer, signs of a DVT (e.g., unilateral edema), and an alternative diagnosis less likely than PE. Patients who have one or fewer of these predictors (i.e., a low simplified Wells score) are unlikely to have a PE. The combination of a low Wells score and a normal D-dimer essentially rules out a PE (*Ann Intern Med 2011;154:709*).
- Clinical predictors of DVT from Wells criteria include heart rate ≥100 bpm, recent lower limb trauma/surgery/immobilization, bedridden state, cancer, lower extremity vein proximal tenderness, swelling of entire lower extremity, significant calf size asymmetry, pitting edema, dilated collateral lower extremity superficial veins, and alternative diagnoses less likely than DVT. Patients who have one or fewer of these predictors (i.e., low Wells score) are unlikely to have a DVT (*Lancet 1997;350:1795*).

Laboratories

- D-**Dimer** and fibrin degradation products may increase during VTE but are nonspecific.
  - D-Dimer testing for VTE has a low positive predictive value (**PPV**) and specificity; **patients with a positive test require further evaluation**.
  - A sensitive quantitative D-dimer assay has a high enough NPV to exclude a **DVT** when the objectively defined clinical probability is low and/or a noninvasive test is negative (*Ann Intern Med 2004;140:589; JAMA 2006;295:199*).
  - In the setting of a moderate to high clinical pretest probability (e.g., patients with cancer), a negative D-dimer does not have sufficient NPV for excluding the presence of DVT or PE (*Ann Intern Med 1999;131:417; Arch Intern Med 2001;161:567*).
  - Compared to a fixed D-dimer cutoff of 500 μg/L, upward age adjustment of the cutoff (age × 10 in patients at least age 50 years) will increase the number of patients who can have PE excluded based on the combination of D-dimer testing and objective clinical probability assessment (*JAMA 2014;311:1117*).
- Signs and symptoms of the **APS** should lead to laboratory evaluation.
  - Serologic tests (e.g., IgG and IgM β_2-glycoprotein-1 antibodies, and IgG and IgM cardiolipin antibodies) or clotting assays (e.g., LA) detect APS, and performing both improves sensitivity.
  - LAs may prolong the aPTT or PT/INR, although they do not predispose to bleeding.
- In the setting of spontaneous VTE at unusual sites, use flow cytometry to assess for missing antigens on red cells and leukocytes and detect **PNH**.

Imaging
- **DVT-specific testing** (*Chest 2012;141:e351S*)

  Initial diagnostic imaging for suspected acute DVT typically consists of **compression ultrasound,** called **duplex examination** when performed with Doppler testing, of the veins (*Am J Respir Crit Care Med 1999;160:1043*), although some other diagnostic options include magnetic resonance venography, **CT** venography, and venography.
  - In addition to assessing for DVT, imaging may detect other pathology (see Differential Diagnosis section).
  - Compression ultrasound has a high sensitivity in **symptomatic** patients and a low sensitivity in **asymptomatic** patients.
  - Compression ultrasound has a low sensitivity for detecting **calf** DVT and may fail to visualize parts of the deep femoral vein, upper extremity venous system, and pelvic veins.
  - Compression ultrasound may have difficulty distinguishing between acute and **chronic** DVT.
  - **Lower extremity venous compression ultrasound** may help diagnose or exclude VTE in patients who have suspected PE and a nondiagnostic ventilation/perfusion (**V/Q**) scan, nondiagnostic or negative chest CT with high suspicion of PE, or contraindications to or difficulty completing imaging for PE (see PE-specific testing section).
  - **Serial testing** can improve the diagnostic yield of compression ultrasound. If a patient with a clinically suspected lower extremity DVT has a negative initial noninvasive test and no satisfactory alternative explanation, one can withhold anticoagulant therapy and repeat testing at least once 3–14 days later.
  - **Ultrasound is recommended to exclude DVT in the setting of superficial venous thrombosis** (*Ann Intern Med 2010;152:218*).
- **PE-specific testing**
  - **Contrast-enhanced spiral (helical) chest CT**
    - PE protocol chest CT requires IV administration of iodinated contrast.
    - Contraindications to spiral CT include renal dysfunction and dye allergy.
    - Used according to standardized protocols in conjunction with expert interpretation, spiral CT has good accuracy for detection of large (proximal) PEs, but it has lower sensitivity for detecting small (distal) emboli (*N Engl J Med 2006;354:2317*).
    - The sensitivity of CT for PE improves by combining the CT pulmonary angiography results with objective grading of clinical suspicion.
    - **Clinical suspicion discordant with the objective test finding** (e.g., high suspicion with a negative CT scan or low suspicion with a positive CT scan) **should lead to further testing**.
    - Advantages of CT scan over V/Q scan includes more diagnostic information (positive or negative) with fewer indeterminate or inadequate studies and the detection of alternative or concomitant diagnoses, such as dissecting aortic aneurysm, pneumonia, and malignancy (*JAMA 2007;298:2743*).
  - **V/Q scan**
    - V/Q scans require administration of radioactive material (via inhaled and IV routes).
    - V/Q scans may be classified as normal, nondiagnostic (i.e., very low probability, low probability, intermediate probability), or high probability for PE.
    - V/Q scans are most useful in a patient with a normal CXR, because nondiagnostic V/Q scans commonly occur in the setting of an abnormal CXR.
    - Use of clinical suspicion improves the accuracy of V/Q scanning. In patients with normal or high-probability V/Q scans and matching pretest clinical suspicion, the testing has a PPV of 96% (*JAMA 1990;263:2753*).
  - **Pulmonary angiography**
    - Angiography requires placement of a pulmonary artery catheter, infusion of IV contrast, and exposure to radiation.
    - Contraindications to angiography include renal dysfunction and dye allergy.
    - Less invasive tests (i.e., CT angiography) have mostly replaced pulmonary angiography.

○ **Electrocardiogram, troponin and brain natriuretic peptide (BNP) levels, arterial blood gas, CXR, and echocardiogram** may to help assess clinical probability of PE, cardiopulmonary reserve, and potential benefit of thrombolysis (see thrombolytic therapy in Medications section).

○ **Studies do not support extensive screening for an associated occult malignancy** in patients with a first, unprovoked VTE (*N Engl J Med 2015;373:697-704*). However, such patients should undergo a comprehensive history and physical examination, routine blood work, age- and gender-appropriate cancer screening (e.g., colonoscopy, mammography, Papanicolaou smear, prostate-specific antigen), and specific cancer screening tests indicated for distinct populations (e.g., chest CT to search for lung cancer in smokers of advanced age).

TREATMENT

• **VTE therapy** should aim to prevent recurrent VTE, consequences of VTE (i.e., postphlebitic syndrome [i.e., pain, edema, and ulceration], pulmonary arterial hypertension, and death), and complications of therapy (e.g., bleeding and HIT/HITT).

• Clinicians should perform standard laboratory tests (i.e., CBC, PT/INR, and aPTT) and assess bleeding risk before starting anticoagulants.

• Unless contraindications exist, **initial treatment of VTE should consist of anticoagulation** with IV or SC UFH, SC LMWH, SC pentasaccharide (fondaparinux), or a rapid-onset targeted oral anticoagulant (see Medications).

Medications

• **Anticoagulants, oral**

○ **Warfarin, an oral anticoagulant**, inhibits reduction of vitamin K to its active form and leads to depletion of the vitamin K–dependent clotting factors II, VII, IX, and X, and proteins C, S, and Z.

▪ The initial INR rise primarily reflects warfarin-related depletion of factor VII; the depletion of factor II takes several days due to its relatively long half-life.

▪ Because of the rapid depletion of the anticoagulant protein C and a slower depletion of factor II, patients might develop increased hypercoagulability during the first few days of warfarin therapy if warfarin is not combined with a parenteral anticoagulant (*Thromb Haemost 1997;78:785*).

▪ The **starting dose** of warfarin depends on many factors and ranges from 2–4 mg in older or petite patients to 10 mg in young, robust patients (*www.warfarindosing .org*). Patients with polymorphisms in genes for cytochrome P450 2C9 or vitamin K epoxide reductase (*VKORC1*) may benefit from lower dose warfarin initiation. Use the INR to adjust dosing.

▪ **Treatment of DVT/PE with warfarin requires overlap therapy with a parenteral anticoagulant** (UFH, LMWH, or pentasaccharide) for at least 4–5 days and until the INR reaches at least 2.0.

□ For most indications, **target INR** is 2.5 with a therapeutic range of 2–3.

□ Patients with **mechanical mitral valves** require a higher level of anticoagulation (INR target range 2.5–3.5) and typically benefit from concomitant low-dose ASA.

▪ **INR monitoring should occur frequently during the first month of warfarin therapy (e.g., twice weekly for 1–2 weeks, then weekly for 2 weeks, then less frequently).**

□ Patients receiving a stable warfarin dose should have INR monitoring performed approximately monthly, although patients with labile INRs should have more frequent monitoring (e.g., weekly). Typical dose adjustments after the first couple of weeks of therapy change the weekly dose by 10–25%.

- □ The addition or discontinuation of medications, especially amiodarone, certain antibiotics (e.g., rifampin, sulfamethoxazole), or antifungal drugs (e.g., fluconazole), should trigger more frequent INR monitoring and may require dose adjustments >25%.
- □ In eligible patients, home INR monitoring may improve INR control and patient satisfaction (*N Engl J Med 2010;363:1608*).
- □ Compliant patients who have unacceptable INR lability likely benefit from a target-specific oral anticoagulant other than warfarin.
  - ○ **Target-specific oral anticoagulants** (Table 20-5): These currently include two categories, **DTI** (dabigatran) and **direct Xa inhibitors** (rivaroxaban, apixaban, and edoxaban)
    - As compared to warfarin, these oral anticoagulants have a more rapid onset, shorter half-life, wider therapeutic window, and more predictable pharmacokinetics. These features allow for sole oral therapy without the need for an overlapping parenteral agent (with the exception of edoxaban for VTE), no need for titration or dose adjustments in patients with normal renal function, and no need for routine monitoring.
    - Compared to warfarin, the target-specific anticoagulants have a lower risk of intracranial hemorrhage (*J Thromb Haemost 2014;12:320*).
    - Issues of concern include the lack of antidotes, risk of thrombosis due to missed doses, and drug level effects based on renal function.
    - In the United States, currently available oral direct Xa inhibitors include rivaroxaban, apixaban, and edoxaban.
- • **Anticoagulants, parenteral**
  - ○ **UFH** inactivates thrombin and factor Xa via AT.
    - At usual doses, UFH prolongs aPTT and thrombin time, although it has variable effect on the PT.
    - Because the anticoagulant effects of UFH normalize within hours of discontinuation and **protamine sulfate** reverses it even faster, UFH is the anticoagulant of choice during initial therapy for patients with a high risk of bleeding.
    - Abnormal renal function does not typically affect UFH dosing.
    - For **DVT prophylaxis**, the typical dosage is 5000 units SC q8–12h, and aPTT monitoring is not necessary.
    - For **therapeutic anticoagulation**, UFH is usually administered IV with a bolus (e.g., 80 units/kg) followed by continuous infusion (e.g., 18 units/kg/h) that has a dose titration based on standard protocols (i.e., heparin nomogram), usually to a goal aPTT of 2- to 2.5-fold of normal range (see Table 20-5).
  - ○ **LMWHs**, produced by chemical or enzymatic cleavage of UFH, indirectly inactivate thrombin and factor Xa via AT.
    - Because LMWH inactivates factor Xa to a greater extent than it does thrombin (IIa), LMWH minimally prolongs the aPTT.
    - Factor Xa monitoring is not needed, except in special circumstances: renal dysfunction, morbid obesity, or pregnancy. For therapeutic anticoagulation, peak factor Xa levels, measured 4 hours after an SC dose, should be 0.6–1.0 IU/mL for q12h dosing and 1–2 IU/mL for q24h dosing (*Blood 2002;99:3102*).
    - Different LMWH preparations have different dosing recommendations (see Table 20-5).
    - Given the renal clearance of LMWHs, they are generally contraindicated in patients with creatinine clearance (**CrCl**) <10 mL/min, and patients with a CrCl of 10–30 mL/min require dose adjustments (e.g., enoxaparin 1 mg/kg daily).
    - **LMWH** is the first choice in **pregnant** women (without artificial heart valves) with thrombosis. Warfarin is teratogenic, at least during the first trimester.
  - ○ **Fondaparinux**, a synthetic pentasaccharide structurally similar to the region of the heparin molecule that binds AT, functions as a selective indirect factor Xa inhibitor.
    - Because fondaparinux inhibits factor Xa and does not inhibit thrombin, it does not prolong the aPTT.

TABLE 20-5   Anticoagulant Dosing for Treatment of Venous Thromboembolism

Anticoagulant	Mechanism of Action	Initial Treatment Dose(s)	Subsequent Dose	Contraindications[a]
Warfarin	Vitamin K antagonist	2–10 mg; overlapped for 4–5 d with a faster-acting anticoagulant; goal INR 2–3 (see www.warfarindosing.org)	Adjusted per INR	Pregnancy
Apixaban	Direct FXa inhibitor	10 mg PO bid × 7 d	5 mg PO bid	
Edoxaban	Direct FXa inhibitor	Initially treat with parenteral anticoagulant for 5–10 d	60 mg PO daily, or 30 mg PO daily (if CrCl 30–50 mL/min, body weight ≤60 kg, or using strong P-gp inhibitor)	
Rivaroxaban	Direct FXa inhibitor	15 mg PO bid × 21 d	20 mg PO daily	CrCl <30 mL/min
Dabigatran	Direct thrombin (FIIa) inhibitor	Initially treat with parenteral anticoagulant for 5–10 d	150 mg bid (CrCl >30 mL/min)	CrCl <15 mL/min
Dalteparin	FXa > FIIa inhibition	200 IU/kg SC daily	Transition to oral agent or, for cancer patients, after 30 d of initial therapy, reduce dose to 150 IU/kg SC daily	HIT; hypersensitivity to pork
Enoxaparin	FXa > FIIa inhibition	1 mg/kg SC q12h or 1.5 mg/kg SC q24h; lower dose if CrCl <30 mL/min	Transition to long-term oral agent[b]	HIT; hypersensitivity to pork

Fondaparinux	Binds to antithrombin, primarily inhibiting FXa	Weight <50 kg: 5 mg SC daily Weight 50–100 kg: 7.5 mg SC daily Weight >100 kg: 10 mg SC daily	Transition to long-term oral agent[b]	CrCl <30 mL/min
Tinzaparin	FXa > FIIa inhibition	175 IU/kg SC daily	Transition to long-term oral agent[b]	HIT
Unfractionated heparin	Binds to antithrombin	Continuous IV: Goal aPTT 2.0–2.5× normal range	Transition to long-term oral agent[b]	HIT; hypersensitivity to pork

aPTT, activated partial thromboplastin time; CrCl, creatinine clearance; FIIa, factor IIa; FXa, factor Xa; HIT, heparin-induced thrombocytopenia; INR, international normalized ratio; P-gp, P-glycoprotein.

aInvasive procedures (e.g., neuraxial anesthesia), bleeding, and bleeding diathesis (e.g., liver disease, thrombocytopenia) are contraindications to all anticoagulants.

bFor venous thromboembolism (VTE) treatment, overlap therapy of warfarin and parenteral agent should be at least 5 days, until the INR is at least 2. Low-molecular-weight heparin can be prescribed long term for VTE (e.g., in setting of cancer).

- Dosing of fondaparinux is weight based (see Table 20-5; *Ann Intern Med 2004; 140:867*).
- Similar to the LMWHs, factor Xa monitoring is not routinely used.
- Fondaparinux is not recommended for patients with CrCl <30 mL/min.
  ◦ **Argatroban** is a synthetic DTI used for **HIT** therapy.
  - Argatroban has a half-life of <1 hour, and a reversal agent is not available.
  - Argatroban is infused IV at an initial rate of ≤2 μg/kg/min. Special patient populations require lower initial infusion rates: patients with recent cardiac surgery, heart failure, hepatic dysfunction, or anasarca (*Chest 2012;141:e495S*).
  - aPTT monitoring should occur 2 hours after beginning the infusion, and the infusion rate should undergo adjustment to achieve a therapeutic aPTT (1.5–3.0 times the patient's baseline aPTT).
  - Overlap argatroban therapy with warfarin therapy for at least 5 days and until warfarin leads to a therapeutic INR. During warfarin coadministration, argatroban should be discontinued for an INR >4, and the INR should be measured again within 4–6 hours.
  ◦ **Bivalirudin** is a DTI with an indication for treatment of **HIT** in the setting of percutaneous coronary intervention in patients receiving ASA.
  - Bivalirudin has a half-life of 25 minutes in patients with normal renal function.
  - Because of its renal clearance, bivalirudin requires dose adjustment of the infusion rate in patients with renal insufficiency.
  - Bivalirudin dosing for HIT should start at a rate of 0.15–0.20 mg/kg/h IV with titration to a target aPTT 1.5–2.5 times baseline. An initial bolus dose is not recommended (*Chest 2012;141:e495s; Pharmacotherapy 2008;28:1115*). Lower rates should be initiated for patients with renal insufficiency (*Ann Pharmacother 2011;45:1185*).
  - aPTT monitoring during bivalirudin therapy should occur 2 hours after a dose change.
  - The interpretation of the INRs in patients receiving warfarin must take into account the increased PT/INR caused by bivalirudin.
- **Thrombolytic therapy**
  ◦ Thrombolytic therapy (e.g., alteplase or recombinant tissue plasminogen activator as a 100-mg IV infusion over 2 hours) is indicated for patients with **PE** and systemic hypotension who do not have a high risk of bleeding (*Chest 2012;141:e419S*).
  ◦ Thrombolytic therapy also should be considered in normotensive patients who have PE associated with right ventricular dysfunction and elevated troponin (*Eur Heart J 2014;35:3033*). Despite the prevention of hemodynamic decompensation and a possible mortality benefit, use of thrombolysis in this situation remains controversial because of an increased risk of major bleeding (especially hemorrhagic stroke in the elderly) in comparison to heparin therapy alone (*N Engl J Med 2014;370:1402; JAMA 2014;311:2414*).
  ◦ Thrombolytic therapy has been used in selected cases of DVT. The main indication is DVT leading to venous congestion that compromises the arterial supply to the limb. The **CaVenT trial** showed that thrombolysis in patients with massive iliofemoral DVT reduced postthrombotic syndrome but increased bleeding (*Lancet 2012;379:31*).
- **Duration of anticoagulation for DVT or PE**
  ◦ **Duration of anticoagulation** should be individualized and based on risk of recurrent VTE, risk of hemorrhage, and patient preference (*Chest 2012;141:e419S*).
  ◦ Patients with a **first episode of VTE due to reversible risk factors** (e.g., surgery, major trauma, estrogen therapy) have a low risk of recurrence (≤2% per year), and 3 months of anticoagulation are recommended (*Blood 2014;123:1794; Chest 2012;141:e419S*). Provoked distal DVTs can be treated with 6 weeks (*BMJ 2011;342:d3036*) to 3 months of anticoagulation.
  ◦ Guidelines recommend at least 3 months of anticoagulant therapy for patients with a **first episode of VTE** associated with less compelling and transient risk factors, such as prolonged travel, oral contraceptive pills/hormone replacement therapy, or minor injury (*Chest 2012;141:e419S*).

- ○ For **unprovoked PE**, many experts anticoagulate for >3 months in patients with low to moderate risk of bleeding. Some experts recommend long-term anticoagulation for men with low to moderate risk of bleeding and an unprovoked PE (*Ann Intern Med 2015;162:27*).
- ○ Patients with **cancer and VTE** should continue anticoagulation until cancer resolution or development of a contraindication. LMWH is the treatment of choice in cancer-associated VTE due to superior efficacy over warfarin (*Lancet Oncol 2008;9:577*).
- ○ For patients with a **first VTE and one inherited hypercoagulable risk factor**, consider an extended anticoagulation duration, depending on the type of thrombophilia.
  - ▪ Heterozygous factor V Leiden or heterozygous prothrombin 20210A modestly increases the odds of recurrence (relative risk, 1.6 and 1.4, respectively); prolonged anticoagulation is not recommended. Deficiency of protein S, protein C, or AT carries a significant risk of recurrence (*JAMA 2009;301:2472*); long-term anticoagulation is recommended.
  - ▪ For patients with a **first VTE and APS or two inherited risk factors**, indefinite anticoagulation should be considered.
- ○ Patients with **recurrent idiopathic VTE** should receive extended-duration anticoagulation, unless a contraindication develops or patient preferences or high bleeding risk dictate otherwise (*Chest 2012;141:e419S*).
- ○ Patients with a history of VTE, especially those with risk factors, should possibly receive prophylactic anticoagulation (e.g., low-dose LMWH SC) during **periods of increased VTE risk**.

Other Nonpharmacologic Therapies

- **Leg elevation** is useful for the treatment of edema associated with DVT.
- **Ambulation** is encouraged for patients with DVT, especially after improvement of pain and edema, although strenuous lower extremity activity should initially be avoided.
- **Fitted below-the-knee graduated compression stockings** can reduce swelling after DVT, but does not prevent DVT recurrence, and the reduction of postthrombotic syndrome is controversial (*Lancet 2013;383:880*).
- In patients with **congenital AT deficiency**, infusion of **AT concentrate** can be used for an acute thrombosis (*Br J Haematol 1982;50:531*).
- **Inferior vena cava (IVC) filters** are mainly indicated for acute DVTs when there are **absolute contraindications to anticoagulation** (e.g., bleeding). They may also be used when a recurrent VTE has occurred despite therapeutic anticoagulation.
  - ○ Prophylactic IVC filters in patients with acute DVT/PE halve the risk of recurrent PE; however, they do not decrease mortality, and they increase DVT recurrence (*Circulation 2005;112:416*).
  - ○ Several types of **temporary/retrievable IVC filters** exist and provide a physical barrier against emboli from the lower extremities. To reduce the risks from retrievable IVC filters, they should be removed when they are no longer indicated. However, if an IVC filter placed for VTE is left in place after a bleeding contraindication has resolved, guidelines recommend a full course of anticoagulation (*Chest 2012;141:e419S*).
- **Catheter embolectomy, often combined with local thrombolytic therapy,** can treat large, proximal, acute PE and DVT. This approach is primarily considered for patients with PE and hypotension who have failed systemic thrombolytic therapy or who have contraindications to it (*Chest 2012;141:e419S*).

Surgical Management

Surgical embolectomy should be considered in patients with life-threatening massive PE who have contraindications to or have failed thrombolytic therapy (*Chest 2012;141:e419S*). Predictors of life-threatening massive PE include signs of cardiovascular dysfunction (e.g., elevated plasma BNP, tachycardia, hypotension, right ventricular strain on echocardiogram, and right ventricular enlargement on chest CT) (*Circulation 2004;110:3276*).

SPECIAL CONSIDERATIONS

Anticoagulant Bridging

- **Perioperative management of anticoagulation** requires close coordination with the surgical service (see Perioperative Medicine in Chapter 1) to address timing of interventions and therapeutic changes with the aim of VTE prevention and avoidance of bleeding.
- **Invasive procedures** usually require discontinuation of anticoagulation.
  - For patients receiving warfarin, to achieve a preoperative INR ≤1.4, stop the warfarin therapy 4–5 days before the invasive procedure.
  - If an INR around 1.7 is acceptable for the procedure, the warfarin dose can be halved for 4 days preoperatively (*Clin Lab Haematol 2003;25:127*).
  - In situations where a clinician aims to minimize the patient's time off therapeutic anticoagulation, parenteral anticoagulation should be initiated when the INR becomes subtherapeutic (approximately 3 days after the last warfarin dose) but should be stopped 6–48 hours prior to the procedure (depending on the half-life of the parenteral drug).
  - In some instances, IV UFH is the preferred bridging therapy (e.g., pregnant woman with a mechanical heart valve).
  - After the procedure, resume warfarin and/or parenteral anticoagulation as soon as hemostasis and bleeding risk reach an acceptable level, typically within 24 hours (*J Thromb Haemost 2014;12:1254*).
- Studies are needed to address the risks and benefits of anticoagulation for **isolated subsegmental PE.**
- **Upper extremity acute DVT** (*N Engl J Med 2011;364:861*) that involves axillary or more proximal vein(s) should receive standard-duration (e.g., 3 months) anticoagulation. If the DVT is associated with a functioning central venous catheter, it does not need to be removed, but anticoagulation should be continued as long as the catheter is in place (*Chest 2012;141:e419S*).
- **Isolated calf acute DVT** without severe symptoms or risk factors for extension may undergo serial imaging in 1–2 weeks instead of anticoagulation. Clot extension should lead to full-dose anticoagulation. Alternatively, treat with 6–12 weeks of anticoagulation in patients at low risk of bleeding.
- **Superficial vein thrombophlebitis (SVT)**
  - **Small SVTs (<5 cm in length)** and SVT associated with IV infusion therapy do not require anticoagulation; treatment consists of oral NSAIDs and warm compresses.
  - Treatment of **extensive SVT (e.g., >5 cm in length)** with a short course of prophylactic doses of fondaparinux (2.5 mg SC daily for 6 weeks) (*N Engl J Med 2010;363:1222*) or LMWH (e.g., enoxaparin 40 mg SC daily for 10 days) (*Arch Intern Med 2003;163:1657*) decreases the incidence of SVT recurrence, SVT extension, and VTE (*Chest 2012;141:e419S*) but increases the risk of bleeding.
  - **Recurrent SVT** may be treated with anticoagulation or vein stripping (*Br J Haematol 1982;50:531*).
- **Chronic PE** occurs in 2–4% of patients with PE (*N Engl J Med 2011;364:351*), and patients with this disorder should undergo evaluation for chronic thromboembolic pulmonary hypertension (CTPH). Those with CTPH should undergo extended-duration anticoagulation, consideration of IVC filter placement, consideration of riociguat therapy (*N Engl J Med 2013;369:330*), and evaluation by an experienced team for possible pulmonary thromboendarterectomy.

COMPLICATIONS

- **Bleeding** is the major complication of anticoagulation.
  - Up to 2% of patients who receive short-term anticoagulation for VTE therapy experience major bleeding.

- For patients receiving chronic oral therapy, the annual incidence of major bleeding is approximately 1–3% per year.
- Concomitant use of **antiplatelet agents** increases the risk of bleeding.
- Major bleeding in a patient with an acute VTE should lead to the discontinuation of anticoagulation and consideration of a temporary IVC filter. Reinitiation of anticoagulation should occur after the bleeding events have resolved, and the IVC filter can be removed at that time.

- **INR elevation** on warfarin
  - Asymptomatic minor INR elevations <5 should be managed by holding or reducing warfarin dose until the INR returns to the appropriate range and then resuming warfarin at a lower dose.
  - Moderate elevation (INR ≥5 but <9) of the INR in asymptomatic patients should be treated by holding one or more warfarin doses. Treatment with oral vitamin K_1 1–5 mg does not reduce the risk of hemorrhage in this setting as compared to warfarin cessation alone and is not routinely recommended (*Ann Intern Med 2009;150:293*).
  - Severe elevation (INR ≥9) should be treated with vitamin K (e.g., oral vitamin K_1 2–10 mg) (*Thromb Res 2004;113:205*) unless the INR is likely to be spurious.

- **Bleeding with warfarin**
  - **Vitamin K replacement** should be given PO or IV. Vitamin K has variable absorption when administered SC, especially in edematous patients. IV vitamin K carries the risk of anaphylactoid reactions. With adequate replacement therapy, the INR should begin to normalize within 12 hours and normalize completely in 24–48 hours (*Ann Intern Med 2002;137:251*). Serious hemorrhages should be treated with vitamin K (10 mg) by slow IV infusion and four-factor PCC. When four-factor PCC is not available, three-factor PCC and/or FFP (two or three units) can be used. Because of the long half-life of warfarin (approximately 36 hours), vitamin K should be repeated every 8–12 hours to prevent INR rebound.
  - Although expensive and potentially thrombogenic (*N Engl J Med 2010;363:1791*), **rFVIIa** may stop life-threatening bleeding (*Br J Haematol 2002;116:178*).

- **Bleeding with UFH, LMWH, and pentasaccharide**
  - Discontinuation usually sufficiently restores normal hemostasis.
  - With moderate to severe bleeding, FFP may reduce bleeding.
  - For patients receiving **UFH** who develop major bleeding, heparin can be completely reversed by infusion of **protamine sulfate** in situations where the potential benefits outweigh the risks (e.g., intracranial bleed, epidural hematoma, retinal bleed).
  - Approximately 1 mg of protamine sulfate IV neutralizes 100 units of heparin, up to a maximum dose of 250 mg. The dose can be given as a loading dose of 25–50 mg by slow IV injection over 10 minutes, with the rest of the dose over 12 hours.
  - Heparin serum concentrations decline rapidly due to a short half-life after IV administration, and the amount of protamine required decreases based on time since heparin treatment.
  - For major bleeding associated with **LMWH**, protamine sulfate neutralizes only approximately 60% of LMWH (*Reg Anesth Pain Med 2003;28:172*). Protamine does not reverse **pentasaccharide** (e.g., **fondaparinux**).
  - For patients with serious bleeding on fondaparinux, concentrated factor VIIa may be used.

- **Bleeding with target-specific oral anticoagulants**
  - No antidotes are FDA approved at this time. FFP rarely adequately addresses bleeding associated with direct oral anticoagulants.
  - **Bleeding with apixaban, edoxaban, rivaroxaban:** Four-factor PCC can reverse direct factor Xa inhibitors, but evidence is limited to animal studies or case reports (*Circulation 2011;124(14):1573*). aPCC or factor VII concentrate may decrease bleeding. The high degree of albumin binding in plasma does not allow dialysis to significantly lower these drug concentrations.

- ○ **Bleeding with dabigatran:** Neither factor VII concentrate nor PCC adequately reverse dabigatran (*Circulation 2011;124(14):1573*), although they have been used in the clinical setting. Because the majority of dabigatran remains unbound to plasma proteins, **hemodialysis** will decrease the drug concentration and lower the thrombin clotting time. In a prospective cohort study, idarucizumab (5 g IV), a monoclonal antibody that binds to free and thrombin-bound dabigatran and neutralizes its activity, completely reversed the anticoagulation effect of dabigatran in minutes (*N Engl J Med 2015;373:511*). Idarucizumab currently does not have FDA approval.
- **Occult gastrointestinal or genitourinary bleeding** is a relative and not absolute contraindication to anticoagulation, although its presence prior to or during anticoagulation warrants an investigation for underlying disease.
- **Warfarin-induced skin necrosis**, associated with rapid depletion of protein C, may occur during initiation of warfarin therapy.
  - ○ Necrosis occurs most often in areas with a high percentage of adipose tissue, such as breast tissue, and it can be life threatening.
  - ○ Therapeutic anticoagulation with an immediate-acting anticoagulant (e.g., UFH, LMWH) and/or avoiding "loading doses" of warfarin prevents warfarin-induced skin necrosis.
- **Warfarin is absolutely contraindicated in early** (i.e., first-trimester) **pregnancy** because of the **risk of teratogenicity**, and it is often avoided during the entire **pregnancy** because of the **risk of fetal bleeding**, although it is safe for infants of nursing mothers.
- **Osteoporosis** may occur with long-term heparin or warfarin use (*Arch Intern Med 2006;166:241*).

MONITORING/FOLLOW-UP

- For a suspicious clinical presentation, **testing for intrinsic hypercoagulable risk factors** ideally should wait until the patient is in stable health and off anticoagulation therapy for at least 2 weeks (e.g., at the end of a standard course of treatment) **to avoid false-positive results** for nongenetic testing.
  - ○ Although uncommon, if reasons exist to screen for hypercoagulable risk factors around the time of diagnosis, collect blood for **factor V Leiden and prothrombin gene mutations and LA**.
  - ○ If done, blood collection for **protein C, protein S, and AT activity and antigen level** testing should occur while patients are not on anticoagulation and should be avoided in the setting of acute thrombosis. If testing occurs near the time of the acute VTE, normal protein C, protein S, and AT tests rule out congenital deficiencies, and abnormally low results require confirmation through repeat testing (or screening first-degree relatives) to rule out a temporary deficiency related to the acute thrombosis.
- Although **testing for PE in patients with DVT and testing for DVT in patients with PE** will produce many positive findings, such testing rarely affects therapy.
- **Outpatient therapy** is appropriate for most DVTs and for selected (low-risk) PEs (*Lancet 2011;378:41*).
- Decisions regarding the **prolongation of anticoagulation duration** remain controversial in patients with residual thrombosis on compression ultrasonography at the end of standard-duration anticoagulation for proximal DVT (*Ann Intern Med 2009;150:577*) or in those with a positive D-dimer weeks after completing a standard duration of therapy for VTE (*N Engl J Med 2006;355:1780*). Prolonged-duration anticoagulation reduces VTE recurrence but increases bleeding.
- After completion of anticoagulation for an unprovoked VTE, **low-dose ASA** reduces the risk of arterial and venous thrombosis (*N Engl J Med 2012;366:1959; N Engl J Med 2012;367:1979*).

21

Hematologic Disorders and Transfusion Therapy

Amy Zhou, Tom Regenbogen, Ronald Jackups, and Morey Blinder

ANEMIA

Anemia Introduction

GENERAL PRINCIPLES

Definition

Anemia is defined as a decrease in circulating red blood cell (RBC) mass; the usual criteria in adults being hemoglobin (Hgb) <12 g/dL or hematocrit (Hct) <36% for nonpregnant women and Hgb <13 g/dL or Hct <39% in men.

Classification

Anemia can be broadly classified into three etiologic groups: **blood loss (acute or chronic), decreased RBC production, and increased RBC destruction (hemolysis).** It is also described morphologically as microcytic, normocytic, or macrocytic.

DIAGNOSIS

Anemia is always caused by an underlying disorder; thus, a careful evaluation to determine the etiology is required in each case.

Clinical Presentation

Based on the history, one can often discern timeline (acute, subacute, or chronic), severity, and the underlying etiology.
- Acute anemia: Patients with abrupt onset of anemia tolerate diminished red cell mass poorly. Patients may have symptoms of fatigue, malaise, dizziness, syncope, or angina.
- Chronic anemia: In contrast to acute anemia, patients with stable chronic anemia are occasionally asymptomatic or minimally symptomatic. However, patients usually have symptoms when Hgb <7 g/dL.
- The following history will aid in the evaluation and management of anemia:
  ○ Gastrointestinal (GI) hemorrhage
  ○ Obstetric and menstrual history
  ○ Comorbidities associated with anemia such as GI resection or malabsorption, renal disease, rheumatologic disease, or other chronic inflammatory conditions
  ○ Comorbid conditions that may be exacerbated by anemia, such as cardiovascular disease
  ○ Family history of anemia
  ○ Prescribed and over-the-counter medicines including herbal supplements, alcohol consumption, diet, ethnic background, and religious beliefs pertaining to blood transfusions
  ○ Symptoms suggestive of other cytopenias (such as bruising thrombocytopenia) or infections (neutropenia)

Physical Examination

Common signs and symptoms of anemia include pallor, tachycardia, hypotension, dizziness, tinnitus, headaches, loss of concentration, fatigue, and weakness. Atrophic glossitis, angular cheilosis, koilonychias (spoon nails), and brittle nails are more common in severe long-standing anemia. Patients may also experience reduced exercise tolerance, dyspnea on exertion, and heart failure. High-output heart failure and shock may be seen in the most severe cases.

Diagnostic Testing

Laboratories

- The complete blood count (CBC) and reticulocyte count will guide further laboratory testing because they provide a morphologic classification and assessment of RBC production.
- The Hgb level is a measure of the concentration of Hgb in blood as expressed in grams per deciliter (g/dL), whereas the Hct is the percentage of RBC in blood. Hgb and Hct are unreliable indicators of red cell mass in the setting of rapid shifts of intravascular volume (i.e., an acute bleed).
- The most useful red cell indices are:
  - Mean corpuscular volume (MCV): mean volume of the red cells. Normal range: 80–100 fL.
    - **Microcytic: MCV <80 fL**
    - **Normocytic: MCV of 80–100 fL**
    - **Macrocytic: MCV >100 fL**
  - Red cell distribution width (RDW): A reflection of the variability in the size of the red cells and is proportional to the standard deviation of the MCV. **An elevated RDW indicates an increased variability in RBC size.**
  - Mean cellular hemoglobin (MCH): Describes the concentration of Hgb in each cell, and an elevated level is often indicative of spherocytes or a hemoglobinopathy.
- **The relative reticulocyte count** measures the percentage of immature red cells in the blood and reflects production of RBCs in the bone marrow (BM).
  - A normal RBC has a life span of approximately 120 days, and the reticulocytes circulate for about 1 day; therefore, the normal reticulocyte count is 1–2%.
  - In the setting of anemia from blood loss, the BM should increase its production of RBCs in proportion to loss of RBCs, and thus a 1% reticulocyte count in the setting of anemia is inappropriate.
  - **The reticulocyte index** (RI) is a determination of the BM's ability to respond to anemia and is calculated by % reticulocytes/maturation correction × actual Hct/normal Hct (normally 45). The maturation correction factor is 1.0 for Hct >30%, 1.5 for 24–30%, 2.0 for 20–24%, and 2.5 for <20%.
  - **RI <2 with anemia indicates decreased production of RBCs (hypoproliferative anemia). RI >2 with anemia may indicate hemolysis or bleeding,** leading to increased compensatory production of reticulocytes (hyperproliferative anemia).
- The **peripheral smear** is reviewed to assess the morphologic characteristics of RBC including the shape, size, presence of inclusions, and orientation of cells in relation to each other. RBCs can appear in many abnormal forms, such as acanthocytes, schistocytes, spherocytes, or teardrop cells, and abnormal orientation such as agglutination or Rouleaux formation. Each is associated with several specific disease processes.

Diagnostic Procedures

A **BM biopsy** may be indicated in cases of unexplained normocytic anemias with a low reticulocyte count or with anemias associated with other cytopenias. The biopsy may confirm a myelophthisic process (i.e., presence of teardrop or fragmented cells, nucleated RBCs, or immature white blood cells [WBCs] on peripheral blood smear) in the setting of pancytopenia.

ANEMIAS ASSOCIATED WITH DECREASED RED BLOOD CELL PRODUCTION

Iron Deficiency Anemia

GENERAL PRINCIPLES

- **Iron deficiency** is the most common cause of anemia in the ambulatory setting and is usually microcytic.
- The most common causes of iron deficiency are blood loss (e.g., menses, GI blood loss), decreased absorption (e.g., achlorhydria, celiac disease, bariatric surgery, *Helicobacter pylori* infection), and increased iron requirement (e.g., pregnancy).
- It is important to determine the cause of iron deficiency, and in the absence of menstrual bleeding, evaluation of the GI tract should be performed to identify a source and exclude occult malignancy.

DIAGNOSIS

Clinical Presentation

- Patients often present with fatigue or malaise that is typically worsened with activity, as well as pica (consumption of substances such as ice, starch, or clay). Iron deficiency is also associated with restless leg syndrome.
- Pallor is a common physical finding in patients with anemia. Rarely, splenomegaly, koilonychia ("spoon nail"), and glossitis (i.e., Plummer-Vinson syndrome) can be seen with severe iron deficiency.

Diagnostic Testing

Peripheral blood smear may show hypochromia (increased central pallor of RBCs), microcytosis, and pencil-shaped cells.

Laboratories
- **Ferritin** is the primary storage form for iron in the liver and BM and is the best surrogate marker of iron stores.
  - A ferritin level of <10 ng/mL in women or <20 ng/mL in men is a specific marker of low iron stores.
  - Ferritin is an acute-phase reactant, so normal levels may be seen in inflammatory states despite low iron stores. **A serum ferritin level of >200 ng/mL generally excludes an iron deficiency**; however, in renal dialysis patients, a functional iron deficiency may be seen with a ferritin up to 500 ng/mL.
- **Iron, total iron binding capacity (TIBC), and transferrin saturation** are often used in combination with ferritin to diagnose iron deficiency anemia. Serum iron level alone is often unreliable given its significant fluctuation based on patients' diets.
- **Reticulocyte count is often normal or decreased in iron deficiency anemia.**

TABLE 21-1	Oral Iron Preparations	
Preparation	**Common Dosing Regimen**	**Elemental Iron (mg per dose)**
Ferrous sulfate	325 mg tid	65
Ferrous gluconate	300 mg tid	36
Ferrous fumarate	100 mg tid	33
Iron polysaccharide complex	150 mg bid	150
Carbonyl iron	50 mg bid–tid	50

Diagnostic Procedures

A **BM biopsy** that shows absent staining for iron is the definitive test to diagnose iron deficiency anemia and is helpful when the serum tests do not clearly demonstrate the diagnosis.

TREATMENT

- **Oral iron therapy.** Given in stable patients with mild symptoms. Several different preparations are available (Table 21-1).
  - Iron is best absorbed on an empty stomach, and 3–10 mg of elemental iron can be absorbed daily.
  - Oral iron ingestion may induce a number of GI side effects, including epigastric distress, bloating, and constipation. As a result, nonadherence is a common problem. These side effects can be decreased by initially administering the drug with meals or once per day and increasing the dosage as tolerated. Concomitant treatment with a stool softener can also alleviate these symptoms.
  - Ferrous sulfate is the most commonly prescribed formulation. If there are unacceptable side effects, consider using a lower dose or an alternative formulation such as ferrous gluconate or ferrous fumarate, which contain lower amounts of elemental iron and may be better tolerated.
  - Administration of vitamin C along with iron improves absorption by maintaining the iron in the reduced state. Certain medications (e.g., H_2 blockers, proton pump inhibitors) and foods (e.g., coffee, tea, phosphate-containing carbonated beverages) may decrease iron absorption, and patients should be made aware of these effects when prescribed oral iron therapy.
  - The total iron deficit may be calculated using the patient's baseline Hgb and body weight (*http://www.globalrph.com/irondeficit.htm*).
  - In general, patients responding to oral iron therapy should see an increase in reticulocyte count within 1 week of therapy followed by an increase in Hgb in 2–4 weeks. Treatment should be continued until the total iron deficit is replete.
- **Parenteral iron therapy** (Table 21-2). There are several formulations of IV iron, and indications for parenteral iron over oral iron include:
  - Poor absorption (e.g., inflammatory bowel disease, malabsorption).
  - Very high iron requirements that cannot be met with oral supplementation (e.g., ongoing bleeding)
  - Intolerance to oral preparations
  - Relative iron deficiency in chronic kidney disease (CKD)

Specific Considerations

- IV iron infusion **should not be given** in patients with an active infection (i.e., fever) due to concern for increased adverse reactions.

TABLE 21-2	IV Iron Preparations	
Preparation	**IV Administration**	**Caution**
Iron dextran (INFeD, Dexferrum)	The entire dose may be diluted and infused in one setting; 1000 mg can be given over 1 h.	A 0.5-mL test dose should be given; observe patient for at least 1 h prior to full dose.
Iron sucrose (Venofer)	Administered undiluted as slow IV injection or infusion in diluted solution: Injection: 100 mg over 2–5 min 200 mg over 2–5 min Infusion: 100 mg/100 mL over 15 min 300 mg/250 mL over 1.5 h 400 mg/250 mL over 2.5 h >500 mg/250 mL over 3.5 h	
Ferric gluconate (Ferrlecit)	Injection: 125 mg over 10 min Infusion: 125 mg/100 mL over 1 h	
Ferumoxytol (Feraheme)	510 mg over 20 min; given as 2 doses 7 d apart	Observe patient for at least 30 min after administration. Serious hypersensitivity reactions have been observed with rapid IV injection (<1 min).
Ferric carboxymaltose (Injectafer)	750 mg over 15–30 min; given as 2 doses 7 d apart	

- **Iron dextran** (INFeD, Dexferrum) **may be the least expensive and allows for high-dose repletion in a single dose**; however, infusion can be complicated by serious side effects including **anaphylaxis**.
  - An IV **test dose** of 0.5 mL should be administered over 5–10 minutes at 30–60 minutes prior to the full dose. Methylprednisolone, diphenhydramine, and 1:1000 epinephrine 1-mg ampule (for SC administration) should be immediately available at all times during the infusion.
  - A dose of 1000 mg can be administered over 1 hour (*Am J Hematol 2011;86(10):860*).
  - Delayed reactions to IV iron, such as arthralgia, myalgia, fever, pruritus, and lymphadenopathy, may be seen within 3 days of therapy and usually resolve spontaneously or with NSAIDs.
- **Second-generation irons** include **ferric gluconate** (Ferrlecit) and **iron sucrose** (Venofer) and can be given at a faster infusion rate than iron dextran. Anaphylaxis is rare, and a test dose is often not needed; however, a single infusion cannot be used to replenish the entire iron deficit. Higher doses of iron sucrose (i.e., >400 mg/250 mL doses) are associated with a higher adverse event rate.
- **Third-generation irons** include **ferumoxytol** (Feraheme) and **ferric carboxymaltose** (Injectafer) and allow for administration of a high dose with a rapid infusion. A rare complication is severe hypotension, which can be related to the rapidity of the injection. Of note, ferumoxytol is also available as an MRI contrast agent, and radiology should be made aware if a patient received ferumoxytol within 3 months of a scheduled MRI study.

Thalassemia

GENERAL PRINCIPLES

Definition

The **thalassemia syndromes** are inherited disorders characterized by reduced Hgb synthesis associated with mutations in either the α- or β-gene of the molecule (Table 21-3).

Etiology

- **β-Thalassemia** results in a decreased production of β-globin and a resultant excess of α-globin, forming insoluble α-tetramers and leading to ineffective erythropoiesis.
  - **β-Thalassemia minor (trait)** occurs with one gene abnormality with underproduction of β-chain globin. Patients are asymptomatic and present with microcytic, hypochromic RBCs and Hgb levels >10 g/dL.
  - **β-Thalassemia intermedia** occurs with dysfunction in both β-globin genes so that anemia is more severe (Hgb, 7–10 g/dL).
  - **β-Thalassemia major** (Cooley anemia) is caused by severe abnormalities of both genes that produce no β-globin and generally requires lifelong transfusion support.
- **α-Thalassemia** occurs with a deletion of one or more of the four α-globin genes, leading to a β-globin excess.
  - Mild microcytosis and mild hypochromic anemia (Hgb >10 g/dL) are seen with the loss of one or two α-globin genes (silent carrier and α-thal trait), whereas Hgb H disease (deletion of three α-globin genes) results in splenomegaly and hemolytic anemia.
  - In patients with Hgb H disease, transfusion or splenectomy is often not necessary until after the second or third decades of life. In addition, oxidant drugs similar to those that

TABLE 21-3	Thalassemias			
	Genotype	Hemoglobin (g/dL)	Mean Corpuscular Volume (fL)	Transfusion Dependent
α-Thalassemia				
Silent carrier	$\alpha\alpha/\alpha-$	Normal	None	No
Trait	$\alpha-/\alpha-$ or $\alpha\alpha/--$	>10	<80	No
Hemoglobin H	$\alpha-/--$	7–10	<70	+/−
Hydrops fetalis	$--/--$	Incompatible with life		
β-Thalassemia (Thal)				
Silent carrier	β/β^1	>10	<80	No
β-Thal minor (trait)	β/β^0	>10	<80	No
β-Thal intermedia	β^1/β^1	7–10	65–75	+/−
β-Thal major	β^1/β^0 or β^0/β^0	<7	<70	Yes

β^+, β-thalassemia genes produce some β-globin chains but with impaired synthesis; β^0, β-thalassemia genes produce no β-globin chains.

exacerbate glucose-6-phosphate dehydrogenase (G6PD) deficiency should be avoided because increased hemolysis may occur.
- ○ Hydrops fetalis occurs with the loss of all four α-globin genes and is incompatible with life.

DIAGNOSIS

Diagnostic Testing

- Peripheral smear may show microcytic hypochromic RBCs, along with poikilocytosis and nucleated RBCs.
- Hgb electrophoresis is diagnostic for β-thalassemia showing an increased percentage of Hgb A2 (α2δ2) and Hgb F (α2γ2).
- Silent carriers with a single α-chain loss have an essentially normal electrophoresis. Those with Hgb H disease have increased Hgb H (β-tetramers). The diagnosis of α-thalassemia is made by α-globin gene analysis.

TREATMENT

- Patients with thalassemia trait require no specific treatment.
- In patients with more severe forms of the disease, RBC transfusions to maintain an Hgb level of 9–10 g/dL are needed to prevent the skeletal deformities that result from accelerated erythropoiesis.
- In severe forms of thalassemia, repeated transfusions result in tissue iron overload, which may cause congestive heart failure (CHF), hepatic dysfunction, glucose intolerance, and secondary hypogonadism. **Iron chelation therapy** delays or prevents these complications. Once clinical organ deterioration has begun, it may not be reversible.
- **Chelation therapy** is indicated for transfusion-associated iron overload from any cause. It is indicated in patients with iron infusion burden of >20 units of packed RBCs and ferritin consistently >1000 ng/mL.
  - ○ Deferoxamine, 40 mg/kg SC or IV over 8–12 hours continuous infusion (*N Engl J Med 2011;364(2):146*).
  - ○ Deferasirox 20–40 mg/kg/d (as Exjade) is an effective oral agent. Side effects of deferasirox include moderate to severe GI disturbances and skin rash. A recently available formulation of deferasirox (Jadenu) is dosed at 70% of Exjade and seems to be better tolerated. Dose can be titrated every 3–6 months based on ferritin level. Efficacy is similar to that of deferoxamine.
  - ○ Chelation therapy should be continued until ferritin levels of <1000 mg/L are maintained.
- Hydroxyurea (15–35 mg/kg/d) to increase Hgb F may reduce transfusion requirements in some patients with β-thalassemia.
- Stem cell transplantation (SCT) is the only curative therapy and should be considered in young patients with thalassemia major who have HLA-identical donors. Gene therapy is the subject of ongoing research and holds promise (*Blood 2011;118(13):3479*).

Surgical Management

Splenectomy should be considered in patients with accelerated (more than two units/month) transfusion requirements. To decrease the risk of postsplenectomy sepsis, immunization against *Pneumococcus*, *Haemophilus influenzae*, and *Neisseria meningitidis* should be administered at least 2 weeks before surgery if not previously vaccinated (see Appendix A, Immunizations and Postexposure Therapies). Splenectomy is not recommended if the patient is younger than 5–6 years because of the risk of sepsis.

Sideroblastic Anemias

GENERAL PRINCIPLES

Definition
Sideroblastic anemias are hereditary or acquired RBC disorders characterized by abnormal iron metabolism associated with the presence of ring sideroblasts in the BM aspirate and normal cytogenetics.

Etiology
- Acquired
  - Primary sideroblastic anemia (myelodysplastic syndrome [MDS])
  - Sideroblastic anemia secondary to drugs (i.e., chloramphenicol, cycloserine, ethanol, isoniazid, pyrazinamide), lead or zinc toxicity, chronic ethanol use, or copper deficiency
- Hereditary
  - X-linked
  - Autosomal
  - Mitochondrial

DIAGNOSIS

A BM examination including cytogenetics is needed to evaluate for the presence of ring sideroblasts or other abnormal marrow forms.

TREATMENT

- Remove any possible offending agent.
- Pyridoxine 50–200 mg daily may be used to treat hereditary sideroblastic anemias.

Macrocytic/Megaloblastic Anemia

GENERAL PRINCIPLES

Definition
Megaloblastic anemia is a term used to describe disorders of impaired DNA synthesis in hematopoietic cells but that affect all proliferating cells.

Etiology
- Almost all cases are due to folic acid or vitamin B_{12} deficiency.
- **Folate deficiency** results from a negative folate balance arising from malnutrition, malabsorption, or increased requirement (pregnancy, hemolytic anemia).
  - Patients on slimming diets, alcoholics, the elderly, and psychiatric patients are particularly at risk for nutritional folate deficiency.
  - **Pregnancy and lactation** require three- to fourfold increased daily folate needs and are commonly associated with megaloblastic changes in maternal hematopoietic cells, leading to a dimorphic (combined folate and iron deficiency) anemia.
  - Folate malabsorption can also be seen in celiac disease.
  - Drugs that can interfere with folate absorption include ethanol, trimethoprim, pyrimethamine, diphenylhydantoin, barbiturates, and sulfasalazine.
  - Dialysis-dependent patients require more folate intake because of increased folate losses.

- ○ Patients with hemolytic anemia, such as sickle cell anemia, require increased folate for accelerated erythropoiesis and can present with aplastic crisis (rapidly falling RBC counts) with folate deficiency.
- **Vitamin B_{12} deficiency** occurs insidiously over 3 or more years because daily vitamin B_{12} requirements are low (6–9 μg/d), whereas total body stores are 2–5 mg.
  - ○ Because multivitamins, bread, and cereals are enriched in folic acid, the hematologic manifestations of vitamin B_{12} deficiency may be obscured, and neurologic symptoms may be the sole presenting features.
  - ○ Vitamin B_{12} deficiency occurs in up to 20% of untreated patients within 8 years of partial gastrectomy and in almost all patients with total gastrectomy or pernicious anemia (PA). Older patients with gastric atrophy may develop a food-bound vitamin B_{12} deficiency in which vitamin B_{12} absorption is impaired. In nonvegan adults, vitamin B_{12} deficiency is almost always due to malabsorption.
  - ○ PA usually occurs in individuals who are older than 40 years (mean age of onset, 60 years). Up to 30% of patients have a positive family history. PA is associated with other autoimmune disorders (Graves disease 30%, Hashimoto thyroiditis 11%, and Addison disease 5–10%). Of patients with PA, 90% have antiparietal cell immunoglobulin (IgG) antibodies, and 60% have anti-intrinsic factor antibodies.
  - ○ Other etiologies include pancreatic insufficiency, bacterial overgrowth, and intestinal parasites (*Diphyllobothrium latum*).

DIAGNOSIS

Clinical Presentation

- Folate-deficient patients may present with sleep deprivation, fatigue, and manifestations of depression, irritability, or forgetfulness.
- In addition to symptoms of anemia, vitamin B_{12} deficiency may demonstrate neurologic symptoms, such as peripheral neuropathy, paresthesias, lethargy, hypotonia, and seizures.
- Important physical findings include signs of poor nutrition, pigmentation of skin creases and nail beds, or glossitis. Jaundice or splenomegaly may indicate ineffective and extramedullary hematopoiesis. Vitamin B_{12} deficiency may cause decreased vibratory and positional sense, ataxia, paresthesias, confusion, and dementia. Neurologic complications may occur even in the absence of anemia and may not fully resolve despite adequate treatment. **Folic acid deficiency does not result in neurologic disease.**

Diagnostic Testing

Laboratories

- Macrocytic anemia is usually present unless there is also a coincident cause of microcytic anemia present, and leukopenia and thrombocytopenia may occur.
- The peripheral smear may show anisocytosis, poikilocytosis, and macro-ovalocytes; hypersegmented neutrophils (containing more than six nuclear lobes) are common.
- Lactate dehydrogenase (LDH) and indirect bilirubin are typically elevated, reflecting ineffective erythropoiesis and premature destruction of RBCs (intramedullary hemolysis).
- Serum vitamin B_{12} and folate levels should be measured.
- RBC folate is a more accurate indicator of body folate stores than serum folate, particularly if measured after folate therapy or improved nutrition has been initiated.
- **Serum methylmalonic acid (MMA) and homocysteine (HC)** may be useful when the vitamin B_{12} is between 100–400 pg/mL (or borderline low per the laboratory reference range). MMA and HC are elevated in vitamin B_{12} deficiency; only HC is elevated in folate deficiency.
- Detecting **antibodies to intrinsic factor** is specific for the diagnosis of PA.

Diagnostic Procedures

BM biopsy may be necessary to rule out MDS or acute leukemia because these disorders may present with findings similar to those of megaloblastic anemia.

TREATMENT

- Potassium supplementation may be necessary when treatment is initiated to avoid potentially serious arrhythmias due to transient hypokalemia induced by enhanced hematopoiesis.
- Reticulocytosis should begin within 1 week of therapy, followed by a rising of Hgb over 6–8 weeks.
- Coexisting iron deficiency is present in one-third of patients and is a common cause for an incomplete response to therapy.
- Folic acid 1 mg daily is given until the deficiency is corrected. High doses of folic acid (5 mg daily) may be needed in patients with malabsorption syndromes.
- Vitamin B_{12} deficiency is corrected by administering cyanocobalamin. Initial treatment (1 mg/d intramuscular cyanocobalamin) is typically administered in the setting of severe anemia, neurologic dysfunction, or chronic malabsorption. After 1 week of daily therapy, a commonly employed regimen is 1 mg/wk given for 4 weeks and then 1 mg/month for life.
- High-dose enteral therapy (1000–2000 μg/d PO) may be considered in those without neurologic involvement who refuse parenteral therapy (*Blood 2008;112:2214*).
- After the initial repletion, patients who decline or cannot take parenteral therapy may be prescribed oral cyanocobalamin tablets or syrup 1000 μg/d as maintenance.

Anemia of Chronic Renal Insufficiency

GENERAL PRINCIPLES

Anemia of chronic renal insufficiency is attributed primarily to decreased endogenous erythropoietin (EPO) production and may occur as the creatinine clearance declines to below 50 mL/min. Other causes including iron deficiency may contribute to the etiology (see the previous description).

DIAGNOSIS

- Laboratory evaluation typically reveals a normal MCV.
- Peripheral smear: The RBCs are often hypochromic, with the occasional presence of echinocytes (burr cells).
- If the patient's creatinine level is >1.8 mg/dL, the primary cause of the anemia can be assumed to be EPO deficiency and/or iron deficiency, and an EPO level is unnecessary.
- Iron status should be evaluated in patients who are undergoing dialysis by obtaining levels of ferritin and transferrin saturation. Oral iron supplementation is not effective in CKD; therefore, parenteral iron to maintain a ferritin level of >500 ng/mL is recommended (*Kidney Int 2005;68:2846*).

TREATMENT

- Treatment has been revolutionized by erythropoiesis-stimulating agents (ESAs) including epoetin alfa and darbepoetin alfa (Table 21-4).
- Therapy is initiated in predialysis patients who are symptomatic.
- Objective benefits of reversing anemia include enhanced exercise capacity, improved cognitive function, elimination of RBC transfusions, and reduction of iron overload.

TABLE 21-4	Erythropoietin Dosing	

	Agent and Initial Dose (SC or IV)	
Indication	**Erythropoietin**[a]	**Darbepoetin**[b]
Chemotherapy-induced anemia from nonmyeloid malignancy, multiple myeloma, lymphoma; anemia secondary to malignancy or myelodysplastic syndrome	40,000 units/wk or 150 units/kg 3 times a week	2.25 μg/kg/wk or 100 μg/wk or 200 μg/2 wk or 500 μg/3 wk
Anemia associated with renal failure	50–150 units/kg 3 times a week	0.45 μg/kg/wk
Anemia associated with HIV infection	100–200 units/kg 3 times a week	Not approved
Anemia of chronic disease	150–300 units/kg 3 times a week	Not approved
Anemia in patients unwilling or unable to receive RBCs; anemic patients undergoing major surgery	600 units/kg/wk × 3 300 units/kg/d × 1–2 wk	Not recommended

RBC, red blood cell.
[a]Dose increase after 48 weeks up to 900 units/kg/wk or 60,000 units/wk; discontinue if hematocrit (Hct) is >40%; resume when Hct is <36% at 75% of previous dose.
[b]Dose increase after 6 weeks up to 4.5 mg/kg/wk or 150 mg/wk or 300 mg/2 wk; hold dose if Hct is >36%, then resume when Hct is <36% at 75% of previous dose.

Subjective benefits include increased energy, enhanced appetite, better sleep patterns, and improved sexual activity.
- Administration of ESAs can be IV (hemodialysis patients) or SC (predialysis or peritoneal dialysis patients). In dialysis and predialysis patients with CKD, **the target Hgb should be between 11–12 g/dL and should not exceed 12 g/dL**. Hgb and Hct should be measured at least monthly while receiving an ESA. Dose adjustments should be made to maintain the target Hgb. The US Food and Drug Administration (FDA) requires ESA prescribers to be certified by a risk evaluation and mitigation strategy (REMS).
- Side effects of ESAs: Targeting higher Hgb levels and/or exposure to high doses of ESAs is associated with a greater risk of cardiovascular complications and mortality. In addition, a higher Hct level from ESAs increases the risk of stroke, heart failure, hypertension, and deep vein thrombosis (*N Engl J Med 2006;355:2085*).
- **Suboptimal responses to ESA therapy** are most often due to iron deficiency, inflammation, bleeding, infection, malignancy, malnutrition, and aluminum toxicity.
  ○ Because anemia is a powerful determinant of life expectancy in patients on chronic dialysis, IV iron administration has become first-line therapy for individuals with transferrin saturation <20% and/or ferritin <500 ng/mL. It has also been shown to reduce the ESA dosage required to correct anemia.
  ○ A ferritin level and transferrin saturation should be tested at least monthly during the initiation of ESA therapy with a goal ferritin level of >200 ng/mL and a transferrin saturation of >20% in dialysis-dependent patients and a ferritin level of >100 ng/mL and a transferrin saturation of >20% in predialysis or peritoneal dialysis patients.
  ○ Iron therapy is unlikely to be useful if the ferritin level is >500 ng/mL.
  ○ Secondary hyperparathyroidism that causes BM fibrosis and relative ESA resistance may also occur.

Anemia of Chronic Disease

GENERAL PRINCIPLES

- Anemia of chronic disease (ACD) often develops in patients with long-standing inflammatory diseases, malignancy, autoimmune disorders, and chronic infection.
- Etiology is multifactorial, including defective iron mobilization during erythropoiesis, inflammatory cytokine-mediated suppression of erythropoiesis, and impaired EPO response to anemia. Hepcidin is a critical regulator of iron homeostasis and is normally low when iron is deficient, allowing for increased iron absorption and utilization. Chronic inflammation increases hepcidin levels and causes a functional iron deficiency due to impaired iron recycling and utilization. Hepcidin is renally cleared, suggesting a role in anemia of chronic renal disease (*Biochim Biophys Acta 2012; 1823(9):1434*).

DIAGNOSIS

- Anemia is normocytic in 75% of cases and microcytic in the remainder of cases.
- The soluble transferrin receptor level is helpful in differentiating ACD (normal) and iron deficiency (elevated) when the ferritin is indeterminate. Measurement of serum hepcidin may become part of the standard evaluation of anemia when the assay becomes widely available.
- Iron studies may show low serum iron and TIBC.
- Ferritin level below 30 ng/mL suggests coexisting iron deficiency and should be treated with supplemental iron. Clinical responses to IV iron therapy may occur in patients with ferritin levels up to 100 ng/mL.

TREATMENT

- Therapy for ACD is directed toward the underlying disease and eliminating exacerbating factors such as nutritional deficiencies and marrow-suppressive drugs.
- Note that IV iron should not be administered in the setting of active infection. Enteral iron is typically ineffective in ACD due to reduced intestinal absorption of iron.
- ESA therapy should be considered if the patient is transfusion dependent or has symptomatic anemia. ESA therapy is discontinued when the Hgb is >11 g/dL to reduce risk of cardiovascular adverse events. Suboptimal (<1 g/dL) increase in Hgb 2 weeks after ESA dose prompts a reevaluation of iron stores.
  - Effective doses of ESA are higher than those reported in anemia from renal insufficiency.
  - If no responses have been observed at 900 units/kg/wk, further dose escalation is unlikely to be effective.

Anemia in Cancer Patients

Although ESA therapy has been shown to reduce transfusion requirements in chemotherapy-related anemia, their use remains controversial due to evidence of increased mortality risk in cancer patients (*Cochrane Database Syst Rev 2012;12:CD003407*). In addition, ESAs are ineffective in patients who are not receiving chemotherapy and have not been shown to increase quality of life (*J Clin Oncol 2005;23:5960*). They confer an elevated risk of thrombosis likely regardless of baseline Hgb level. Current guidelines recommend ESA therapy should only be considered in transfusion-dependent patients with Hgb level <10 g/dL who are receiving chemotherapy with palliative intent and do not have high risks for thromboembolism. As of 2010, the FDA requires prescribers to enroll in a REMS program termed APPRISE (Assisting Providers and Cancer Patients with Risk Information for the Safe Use of ESAs), which provides written documentation that adequate patient counseling of the risks has been performed.

Anemia Associated with HIV Disease

- Anemia is the most common cytopenia in patients with HIV; the prevalence increases as the disease progresses and the CD4 count drops (*Am J Med 2004;116(suppl 7A):27S*).
- *Mycobacterium avium* complex infections are frequently associated with severe anemia. Diagnosis is established on BM examination or culture. Treatment of *M. avium* complex is described in Chapter 16, Sexually Transmitted Infections, Human Immunodeficiency Virus, and Acquired Immunodeficiency Syndrome.
- Parvovirus B19 should be considered in HIV-infected patients with transfusion-dependent anemia and a low reticulocyte count.
  ○ Laboratory studies: Parvovirus by polymerase chain reaction from serum or BM.
  ○ Treatment with IV immunoglobulin (IVIG) 0.4 g/kg daily for 5–10 days results in erythropoietic recovery. Relapses have occurred between 2–6 months and can be successfully managed with maintenance IVIG at a dose of 0.4 g/kg IV every 4 weeks (*Ann Intern Med 1990;113(12):926*).

Aplastic Anemia

GENERAL PRINCIPLES

- Aplastic anemia (AA) is a disorder of hematopoietic stem cells that usually presents with pancytopenia.
- Most cases are acquired and idiopathic, but AA can also arise from an inherited BM failure syndrome such as Fanconi anemia. Approximately 20% of cases may be associated with drug or chemical exposure (Table 21-5).
- 10% of cases are associated with viral illnesses (e.g., viral hepatitis, Epstein-Barr virus, cytomegalovirus [CMV]).

DIAGNOSIS

Diagnostic Criteria

AA is a diagnosis of exclusion, and other causes of pancytopenia should be ruled out. Prognosis in AA is dependent on disease severity and patient age (*Br J Haematol 2009; 147(1):43*):

- Moderate or nonsevere AA
  ○ BM cellularity <30%
  ○ Absence of criteria for severe AA
  ○ At least two of three blood lines are lower than normal
- Severe AA
  ○ BM cellularity <25% with normal cytogenetics, OR
  ○ BM cellularity <50% with normal cytogenetics, and <30% residual hematopoietic cells, AND two of three peripheral blood criteria:
    ■ Absolute neutrophil count (ANC) <500/μL
    ■ Platelet count <20,000/μL
    ■ Absolute reticulocyte count <20,000/μL
  ○ No other hematologic disease

TABLE 21-5	Commonly Used Drugs That Can Induce Red Blood Cell Disorders		
Sideroblastic Anemia	**Aplastic Anemia**[a]	**G6PD Deficiency**	**Immune Hemolytic Anemia**
Chloramphenicol	Acetazolamide	Dapsone	Cephalosporins (cefo-
Cycloserine	Antineoplastic	Doxorubicin	tetan, ceftriaxone)
Ethanol	drugs	Methylene blue	Penicillins (piperacillin)
Isoniazid	Carbamazepine	Nalidixic acid	Purine nucleoside ana-
Pyrazinamide	Chloramphenicol	Nitrofurantoin	logues (fludarabine,
	Gold salts	Phenazopyridine	cladribine)
	Hydantoins	Primaquine	NSAIDs (diclofenac,
	Penicillamine	Sulfacetamide	ibuprofen)
	Sulfonamides	Sulfamethoxazole	Quinidine
	Phenylbutazone	Sulfanilamide	Quinine
	Quinacrine	Sulfapyridine	Rifampin
			Sulfonamides
			(trimethoprim/
			sulfamethoxazole)

G6PD, glucose-6-phosphate dehydrogenase.
[a]Drugs with .30 cases reported; many other drugs rarely are associated with aplastic anemia and are considered low risk.
Data compiled from multiple sources. Agents listed are available in the United States.

- Very severe AA
  - The criteria of severe AA are met, AND
  - ANC <200/µL

Diagnostic Testing

BM biopsy is required for diagnosis. Morphology of BM may be difficult to distinguish from hypocellular MDS and paroxysmal nocturnal hemoglobinuria (PNH). Evidence of dysplasia or abnormal cytogenetics is suggestive of MDS. PNH clones can be detected by flow cytometry of the blood or BM.

TREATMENT

- Suspected offending drugs should be discontinued and exacerbating factors corrected. Rarely, spontaneous recovery of normal hematopoiesis can occur, usually within 1–2 months of discontinuing the offending drug.
- Once the diagnosis is established, care should be provided in a center experienced with AA.
- Therapy is optional in moderate AA unless there is transfusion dependence; however, severe or very severe AA requires urgent treatment given the high risk of infectious and hemorrhagic complications.
- AA typically does not respond to EPO. Granulocyte colony-stimulating factor may be effective in some patients and can be used while awaiting definitive therapy; however, there is no clear evidence of survival benefit with the use of these agents.
- Immunosuppressive treatment with cyclosporine and antithymocyte globulin (ATG) should be considered in patients with severe AA who do not undergo an SCT (*Blood 2012;120(6):1185-96*). Overall response rate at 3 months is between 60–80%, and most responses occur by 6 months.

- Corticosteroids have not been shown to be effective and can increase the risk of infections and **should not** be used in the treatment of AA.
- **SCT.** Early referral to a center that is experienced in managing AA is recommended. When feasible, SCT from an HLA-identical sibling is generally recommended and has achieved a long-term survival rate of 60–70%.
- **Transfusions in AA.** Transfusions with RBCs should be kept to a minimum. Prophylactic platelet transfusions are generally recommended if the platelet count is <10,000/μL. Transfusion of irradiated, leukocyte-depleted blood products is preferred to decrease the risk of alloimmunization.
- **Eltrombopag,** 50–150 mg/d, a thrombopoietin agonist, has been shown to be effective in some patients who do not respond to cyclosporine and ATG and may be an option for patients with refractory severe AA (*Blood 2014;123(12):1818–25*).

ANEMIAS ASSOCIATED WITH INCREASED RED BLOOD CELL DESTRUCTION

Anemias Associated with Increased Erythropoiesis

GENERAL PRINCIPLES

Definition

Anemias associated with increased erythropoiesis (i.e., an elevated reticulocyte count) are caused by bleeding or destruction of RBCs (hemolysis) and may exceed the capacity of normal BM to correct the Hgb. Bleeding is much more common than hemolysis.

Etiology

- **Blood loss.** If no obvious source, suspect occult loss into GI tract, retroperitoneum, thorax, or deep compartments of thigh depending on history (recent instrumentation, trauma, hip fracture, coagulopathy).
- **Hemolysis** can be categorized into two broad groups based on the cause of destruction: intrinsic (caused by deficits inherit to the RBC) and extrinsic (caused by factors external to the RBC).
  - In general, intrinsic causes are inherited, whereas extrinsic causes tend to be acquired. Intrinsic disorders are a result of defects of the red cell membrane (i.e., hereditary spherocytosis), Hgb composition (i.e., sickle cell disease), or enzyme deficiency (i.e., G6PD deficiency).
  - Extrinsic disorders can result from antibodies (i.e., cold or warm reactive immunoglobulin), infectious agents (i.e., malaria), trauma, chemical agents (i.e., venom), or liver disease.
  - Hemolytic disorders are also commonly categorized by the location of RBC destruction: intravascular (within the circulation) or extravascular (within the macrophage-monocyte system typically in the liver or spleen).

DIAGNOSIS

Laboratory assessment of patients with suspected hemolysis should include:
- **Decreased Hgb** and **Hct.**
- **Elevated reticulocyte count** (occurs within 3–5 days of onset).
- **Elevated LDH** and **indirect hyperbilirubinemia** reflect increased RBC turnover.
- **Decreased haptoglobin** due to binding of intravascular Hgb.
- The **direct Coombs test** (direct antiglobulin testing [DAT]) is an indicator of the presence of antibodies or complement bound to RBC.

- The **indirect Coombs test** indicates the presence of antibody in the plasma.
- A peripheral blood smear is essential and can aid in determining the etiology of hemolysis. Intravascular hemolysis may reveal red cell fragmentation (i.e., schistocytes, helmet cells), whereas spherocytes indicate extravascular hemolysis. Polychromasia and nucleated RBCs are indicators of increased erythropoiesis.

Sickle Cell Disease

GENERAL PRINCIPLES

- Sickle cell disease (SCD) is a group of hereditary Hgb disorders in which Hgb undergoes a sickle shape transformation under conditions of deoxygenation.
- The most common are homozygous sickle cell anemia (Hgb SS) or other double-heterozygous conditions (Hgb SC, Hgb S–β°, or Hgb S–β+ thalassemia).
- Newborn screening programs for hemoglobinopathies identify most patients in infancy.
- In the United States, the incidence of SCD is approximately 1 in 625 births.
- **Sickle cell trait** is present in 8–10% of African Americans (*N Engl J Med 1973;288:31*). It is generally considered to be a benign hereditary condition, but high-altitude hypoxia is associated with splenic infarction, whereas intense physical exertion has been associated with sudden death.
- Sickle cell trait has been associated with an increased risk of CKD; thus, minimizing other risk factors for kidney disease is likely to benefit these patients (*JAMA 2014;312(20):2115–25*).

DIAGNOSIS

Diagnostic Testing
- Hgb analysis by high-pressure liquid chromatography is most commonly used in the diagnosis of hemoglobinopathies.
- Laboratory abnormalities include anemia (mean Hgb in SCD, 8 g/dL), reticulocytosis (3–15%), indirect hyperbilirubinemia, elevated LDH, and decreased or absent haptoglobin. Leukocytosis (10,000–20,000/μL) and thrombocytosis (>450,000/μL) are common, due to enhanced stimulation of the marrow compartment and autosplenectomy.
- Peripheral smear shows sickle-shaped RBCs, target cells (particularly in Hgb SC and Hgb S−β thalassemia), and Howell-Jolly bodies, indicative of functional asplenism.

Clinical Presentation
- Clinical presentation of SCD is heterogeneous and is dependent on type and degree of hemoglobinopathy. The most common clinical manifestations of SCD result from hemolysis and/or vascular occlusions.
- Vascular occlusions include pain crises, avascular necrosis, priapism, and acute chest syndrome, whereas hemolytic complications include pulmonary hypertension, cholelithiasis, and leg ulcers. Strokes and renal medullary infarctions are complications of both.
- **Vaso-occlusive complications (VOCs)** result from polymerization of deoxygenated Hgb S. These polymerized RBCs assume the classic sickle shape and develop a marked loss of deformability, leading to vaso-occlusion.
  - **Acute painful episodes ("sickle cell pain crisis")**
    - Sickle cell pain crisis is the most common VOC and manifestation of SCD.
    - Pain is typically in the long bones, back, chest, and abdomen.
    - Precipitating factors can include stress, infection, dehydration, alcohol, and weather. However, a majority of cases have no identifiable trigger.

- Typical duration of the episode is 2–6 days.
- Higher levels of fetal Hgb (Hgb F) seem to be protective against VOC.
  - **Acute chest syndrome** is a life-threatening emergency that occurs when decreased oxygen saturation (<90%) leads to increased intravascular sickling and irreversible occlusion of the microvasculature in the pulmonary circulation. It is diagnosed based on a pulmonary infiltrate involving at least one complete segment and one of the following: fever, hypoxemia, tachypnea, respiratory failure, chest pain, or wheezing. ACS precipitated by infection tends to be less severe than pulmonary embolism or fat emboli as the inciting events.
  - **Priapism** often presents in adolescence and may result in impotence.
  - **Retinopathy** is caused by chronic vaso-occlusion of the retina, which causes proliferative retinopathy and may lead to complications including vitreous hemorrhage and retinal detachment.
  - **Functional asplenia** results from recurrent splenic infarcts due to sickling and eventually results in the loss of splenic function. The majority of cases occur before the age of 1 year. Functional asplenia places patients at higher risk of infection, especially with encapsulated organisms.
  - **Avascular necrosis (AVN)** is the result of infarction of bone trabeculae and occurs most commonly in the femoral and humeral heads. Up to 50% of adults affected by SCD can manifest AVN, which is a leading cause of pain and disability.
- **Hemolytic complications**
  - **Cholelithiasis** is present in >80% of patients and is primarily due to bilirubin stones. It may lead to acute cholecystitis or biliary colic.
  - **Leg ulceration** occurring at the ankle is often chronic and recurring.
  - **Pulmonary hypertension** has been linked to several hemolytic disorders and can occur in up to 60% of patients with SCD (*N Engl J Med 2004;350:857*). The pathophysiology is unclear but may be the result of nitric oxide depletion.
- **Renal medulla infarction** is the result of repeated occlusion of renal medullary capillaries, resulting in CKD in many patients. This can lead to isosthenuria (inability to concentrate urine) and hematuria, predisposing patients to dehydration and thus increasing the risk of VOC.
- **Neurologic complications** occur in up to 25% of patients with SCD by the age of 45 years (*Am J Med 1978;65:461*) and include cerebrovascular accidents (transient ischemic attacks, infarction, cerebral hemorrhage), seizure, and sensory hearing loss. Ischemic stroke is felt to result from recurrent endothelial injury from hemolysis and vaso-occlusion, resulting in intimal hyperplasia with large-artery vasculopathy (*Stroke 2011;42:227*). High cerebral flow rate (>200 cm/s) detected by transcranial Doppler has been associated with increased risk of stroke in children. This risk is greatly reduced by routine transfusion or exchange therapy (*N Engl J Med 1998;339:5*). Current recommendations for adults include evaluation for known additional stroke risk factors with management accordingly (*Circulation 2006;113:e873*).
- **Infections** typically occur in tissues susceptible to vaso-occlusive infarcts (i.e., lungs, bone, kidney). The most common infectious organisms include *Streptococcus pneumoniae*, *Staphylococcus aureus*, *Salmonella* spp., *Mycoplasma pneumoniae*, or *H. influenzae*. Vaccinations are a key mechanism in prevention.
- **Aplastic "crisis"** occurs when there is a transient halt of erythropoiesis due to an inciting event causing a sudden decrease in Hgb. The most common etiology in children with SCD is parvovirus B19 infection. Folate deficiency should also be suspected because of the chronic increased requirements for erythropoiesis.
- **Pregnancy** in a patient with sickle cell anemia should be considered high risk and is associated with increased spontaneous abortions or premature delivery, along with increased occurrence of vaso-occlusive crises.

TREATMENT

- Evidence-based management of SCD has been recently updated and is available online at *http://www.nhlbi.nih.gov/health-pro/guidelines/sickle-cell-disease-guidelines*.
- **Acute painful episodes.** Management of **acute painful episodes** consists of rehydration (3–4 L/d), evaluation for and management of infections, analgesia, and if needed, antipyretic and empiric antibiotic therapy.
  - ○ **Opioids** (see Chapter 1, Inpatient Care in Internal Medicine, see the section on opioids in the Medication section, under Pain) are typically used and are effectively administered by a **patient-controlled analgesia pump,** allowing the patient to self-administer medication within a set limit of infusions (lockout interval) and basal rate. Morphine (2 mg/h basal rate with boluses of 2–10 mg every 6–10 minutes) is the drug of choice for moderate or severe pain. If patient-controlled analgesia is not used, morphine (0.1–0.2 mg/kg IV q2–3h) or hydromorphone (0.02–0.04 mg/kg IV q2–3h) is recommended.
  - ○ Transfusion therapy has no role in the treatment of uncomplicated vaso-occlusive crises.
  - ○ Supplemental oxygen does not benefit acute pain crisis unless hypoxia is present.
- **Acute chest syndrome.** Multimodal treatment includes adequate analgesia, volume resuscitation, supplemental oxygen and incentive spirometry, and blood transfusion. It is unclear whether exchange transfusion is superior to simple RBC transfusion; however, it is standard practice to perform exchange transfusion for moderate to severe cases, whereas simple transfusion to >10 g/dL for mild cases may be sufficient. The presentation of acute chest syndrome is clinically indistinguishable from pneumonia; thus, empiric broad-spectrum antibiotics should also be administered.
- **Priapism** is initially treated with hydration and analgesia. Persistent erections for more than 24 hours may require transfusion therapy or surgical drainage.
- **AVN** management consists of local heat, analgesics, and avoidance of weight bearing. Hip and shoulder arthroplasty are often effective at decreasing symptoms and improving function.
- **Cholelithiasis.** Induced acute cholecystitis should be treated medically with antibiotics followed by cholecystectomy when the attack subsides. Elective cholecystectomy for asymptomatic gallstones is controversial.
- **Leg ulcers** should be treated with rest, leg elevation, and intensive local care. Wet to dry dressings should be applied three to four times per day. A zinc oxide–impregnated bandage (Unna boot), changed weekly for 3–4 weeks, can be used for nonhealing or more extensive ulcers.
- There is no standard therapy for treatment of **pulmonary hypertension** in SCD, with clinical trials of sildenafil showing conflicting results (*Br J Haematol 2005;130:445*; *Blood 2001;118:855*); thus, patients should be referred to a clinical specialist.
- **Acute cerebrovascular accident** should be managed based on current standards. Long-term transfusions to maintain the Hgb S concentration to <50% for at least 5 years significantly reduce the incidence of recurrence.
- Patients with suspected **aplastic crisis** require hospitalization. Therapy includes folic acid, 5 mg/d, as well as supportive RBC transfusions.
- **Iron chelation therapy** can be used to prevent or treat iron overload in patients with high transfusion requirements.

Risk Modification

- **Dehydration and hypoxia** should be avoided because they may precipitate or exacerbate irreversible sickling.
- **Folic acid** (1 mg PO daily) is administered to patients with SCD because of chronic hemolysis.
- **Hydroxyurea** (15–35 mg/kg PO daily) has been shown to increase levels of Hgb F and significantly decreases the frequency of VOC and acute chest syndrome in adults with

SCD (*N Engl J Med 1995;332:1317*). In practice, the dose is increased until the ANCs are between 2000–4000/µL.

- **Antimicrobial prophylaxis** with penicillin VK, 125 mg PO bid to age 3 years and then 250 mg PO bid until age 5 years, is effective at reducing risk of infection (*N Engl J Med 1986;314:1593*). Patients who are allergic to penicillin should receive erythromycin 10 mg/kg PO bid. Prophylaxis should be stopped at age 5 years to avoid development of resistant organisms (*J Pediatr 1995;127:685*).
- **Immunizations** against the usual childhood illnesses should be given to children with SCD, including hepatitis B vaccine. After 2 years of age, a polyvalent pneumococcal vaccine should be administered. Yearly influenza vaccine is recommended.
- **Ophthalmologic examinations** are recommended yearly in adults because of the high incidence of proliferative retinopathy.
- Local and regional anesthesia can be used without special precautions. Care should be taken to avoid volume depletion, hypoxia, and hypernatremia. For surgery with general anesthesia, RBC transfusions to increase the Hgb to 10 g/dL is as effective as more aggressive thresholds to decrease postoperative complications (*N Engl J Med 1995;333:206*).

Glucose-6-Phosphate Dehydrogenase Deficiency

GENERAL PRINCIPLES

G6PD deficiency represents the most common disorder of RBC metabolism worldwide. Deficiency of G6PD renders RBCs more susceptible to oxidative damage through decreased glutathione reduction, leading to chronic or acute episodic hemolysis in the presence of oxidative stress.

Classification

More than 400 variants of G6PD are recognized. The severity of hemolysis depends on the degree of deficiency present (*Blood Rev 2007;21:267*).
- Milder forms, such as those seen in men of African heritage in the United States, result in self-limiting acute hemolytic episodes (G6PD A⁻).
- More severe forms, such as the Mediterranean variant, can result in severe hemolysis.
- The most severe type causes a chronic, hereditary, nonspherocytic hemolytic anemia in the absence of an inciting cause.

Epidemiology

- X-linked inheritance; thus degree of involvement in females is dependent on lyonization.
- In the United States, 10% of African American males are affected by a mild form.
- G6PD is felt to be protective against malaria, thus accounting for its prevalence in malaria-stricken areas.
- Hemolysis is triggered by exposure to mediators of oxidative stress (i.e., drugs [see Table 21-5]), infections, and fava beans.

DIAGNOSIS

- Examination of a peripheral blood smear reveals presence of "bite cells" and **Heinz bodies** (represents precipitated Hgb within RBCs).
- Diagnosis is determined by showing deficient amounts of reduced nicotinamide adenine dinucleotide phosphate (NADPH) generated from NADP using quantitative spectrophotometric analysis or rapid fluorescent screening test.
- False-negative results may occur in patients with high levels of reticulocytes or in patients recently transfused because these cells have innately higher levels of G6PD.

TREATMENT

• Hemolytic episodes tend to be self-limiting; the mainstay of treatment is supportive.
• The underlying cause of oxidative stress should be addressed (i.e., treatment of infection, removal of drug).

Autoimmune Hemolytic Anemia

GENERAL PRINCIPLES

Definition

Autoimmune hemolytic anemia (AIHA) results from autoantibodies targeted to antigens on the patient's own RBCs, resulting in extravascular hemolysis (removal of RBC by tissue macrophages in the liver or spleen).

Classification

There are two main causes of AIHA: warm and cold AIHA. Warm AIHA antibodies interact best with RBCs at 37°C, whereas cold AIHA antibodies are most active at temperatures below 37°C and almost always fix complement.

Etiology

• Warm antibody AIHA is usually caused by an IgG autoantibody. It may be idiopathic or secondary to an additional process (i.e., lymphoma, chronic lymphocytic leukemia [CLL], collagen vascular disorder, or drugs [see Table 21-5]).
• Cold antibody AIHA is typically caused by an IgM autoantibody (in cold agglutinin disease).
  ○ The acute form is often secondary to an infection (*Mycoplasma*, Epstein-Barr virus).
  ○ The chronic form is usually due to a paraprotein associated with lymphoma, CLL, or Waldenström macroglobulinemia (WM) in approximately one-half of cases and is usually idiopathic in the others.

DIAGNOSIS

Diagnostic Testing

• Laboratory data usually identify hemolysis with anemia, reticulocytosis, elevated LDH, decreased haptoglobin, and indirect hyperbilirubinemia.
• Peripheral blood smear may show spherocytes, occasional fragmented RBCs, polychromasia, and nucleated RBCs.
• The hallmark of diagnosis is by a positive **DAT (also known as a direct Coombs test)**. The DAT detects the presence of IgG or complement bound to the RBC surface and may be falsely negative in cases of IgM-mediated hemolysis.
  ○ Warm AIHA: IgG+ and/or C3+
  ○ Cold AIHA: IgG− and C3+
• The indirect antiglobulin test (indirect Coombs) detects the presence of autoantibodies in the serum but also detects alloantibodies in the serum from alternate causes including from transfusion or maternal–fetal incompatibility.
• An elevated cold agglutinin titer is seen with cold AIHA.
• If secondary AIHA is suspected, a workup for the underlying cause should be performed.

TREATMENT

• Initial therapy should be aimed at correcting complications from the hemolytic anemia. Definitive therapy should include identification and treatment of any underlying cause.

- **RBC transfusions may exacerbate hemolysis** with hemolysis of transfused cells. Autoantibodies may confound plasma antibody screens and conventional cross-matches, and therefore, alloantibodies may go undetected. **In life-threatening circumstances, transfusion of universal donor (O negative) blood is appropriate.**
- **Warm AIHA**
  - First-line treatment involves **glucocorticoids**, such as prednisone 1 mg/kg/d, which is effective in 70–80% of patients. They decrease macrophage clearance of antibody-coated RBCs. Response is typically seen in 7–10 days. When hemolysis has abated, glucocorticoids can be tapered over 2–3 months. Rapid steroid taper can result in relapse.
  - Second-line treatments include **splenectomy**, which should be considered for steroid-resistant AIHA, and **rituximab**, a monoclonal antibody directed against CD20 antigen expressed on B cells. Rituximab 375 mg/m^2 weekly for four doses has been shown to be effective in 80–90% of cases, and responses to treatment are observed with monotherapy or in combination with corticosteroids (*Haematologica 2014;99(10):1547*). Low-dose rituximab, 100 mg weekly for four doses, has also demonstrated efficacy in AIHA (*Haematologica 2007;92:1695*).
  - Additional immunosuppressive therapies have also been used such as azathioprine, cyclophosphamide, cyclosporine, and mycophenolate mofetil.
  - Treatment for relapsed/refractory cases includes IVIG, danazol, plasma exchange, alemtuzumab, and high-dose cyclophosphamide.
- **Idiopathic cold AIHA**
  - Avoidance of cold exposure can minimize exacerbations. RBC transfusions at 37°C and keeping the room warm can prevent exacerbation of hemolysis.
  - Glucocorticoids and splenectomy have low efficacy in treatment.
  - Plasma exchange removes approximately 80% of IgM, thus offering effective control of the disease.
  - Rituximab has shown to be effective in some cases (*Blood 2004;103(8):2925*).

Drug-Induced Hemolytic Anemia

GENERAL PRINCIPLES

- **Drug-induced hemolytic anemia** is anemia resulting from exposure to a medication. Table 21-5 lists common offending medications.
- Hemolysis occurs by several mechanisms such as drug-induced antibodies, hapten formation, and immune complexes. The most commonly implicated agents are cephalosporins, penicillins, NSAIDs, and quinine or quinidines.

TREATMENT

The initial treatment may be similar to treatment of warm AIHA with corticosteroids if the etiology is unclear, but if drug-induced hemolytic anemia is suspected, the most important treatment is discontinuation of the offending agent.

Microangiopathic Hemolytic Anemia

GENERAL PRINCIPLES

Definition

Microangiopathic hemolytic anemia (MAHA) is a syndrome of traumatic intravascular hemolysis causing fragmentation of the RBCs that are seen on peripheral blood smear (schistocytes). It is not a specific diagnosis but suggests a limited differential diagnosis.

Etiology

Possible causes of MAHA include **mechanical heart valve**, **malignant hypertension**, **vasculitis**, **adenocarcinoma**, **preeclampsia/eclampsia**, **disseminated intravascular coagulation (DIC)**, **thrombotic thrombocytopenic purpura (TTP)**, and **hemolytic-uremic syndrome (HUS)/atypical HUS** (see Chapter 20, Disorders of Hemostasis and Thrombosis, for a discussion of DIC, TTP, and HUS/atypical HUS).

DIAGNOSIS

MAHA is established by confirming the presence of hemolysis with laboratory data and identifying RBC fragments (schistocytes) on peripheral blood smear.

TREATMENT

The treatment depends on the underlying etiology of microangiopathy.

WHITE BLOOD CELL DISORDERS

Leukocytosis and Leukopenia

GENERAL PRINCIPLES

Definition

- Leukocytosis is an elevation in the absolute WBC count (>10,000 cells/µL).
- Leukopenia is a reduction in the WBC count (<3500 cells/µL).

Etiology

- **Leukocytosis**
  - An elevated WBC can be the normal response of BM to an infectious or inflammatory process, steroid, β-agonist or lithium therapy, splenectomy, or stress, and is usually associated with an **absolute neutrophilia**.
  - Occasionally, leukocytosis is due to a primary BM disorder in WBC production, maturation, or death (apoptosis). This may occur in the setting of leukemia or myeloproliferative disorders and can affect any cell in the leukocyte lineage.
  - A **"leukemoid reaction"** is defined as an excessive WBC response usually reserved for neutrophilia (>50,000/µL) due to a reactive cause.
  - Lymphocytosis is less commonly encountered and is typically associated with atypical infections (i.e., viral), medication use, or leukemia/lymphoma.
- **Leukopenia**
  - Leukopenia can occur in response to infection (i.e., HIV), inflammation, primary BM disorders (i.e., malignancy), medications, environmental exposure (i.e., heavy metals or radiation), and vitamin deficiencies.
  - Many cases are medication induced (i.e., chemotherapeutic or immunosuppressive drugs).
  - Idiopathic chronic benign neutropenia is often caused by an antineutrophil antibody or an inherited disorder.

DIAGNOSIS

Diagnostic Testing

Laboratories
- Review of the peripheral smear is very helpful in the evaluation of WBC disorders. The presence of blasts is concerning for acute leukemia and warrants emergent evaluation.

- Flow cytometry of the blood may help determine if there is an underlying clonal process in lymphocytosis (i.e., CLL).
- A BCR-ABL molecular study may be warranted in cases of unexplained neutrophilia to diagnose chronic myeloid leukemia (CML), especially if there is associated eosinophilia or basophilia.
- Additional laboratory abnormalities are related to the underlying disorder and may include elevation in LDH and uric acid from high cell turnover in acute leukemia.
- An infectious workup should be performed as indicated, including assessment for HIV.
- Prothrombin time, international normalized ratio, partial thromboplastin time, and fibrinogen should also be considered, especially if acute promyelocytic leukemia is suspected because this can be associated with DIC.

Diagnostic Procedures
A BM biopsy with ancillary studies such as cytogenetics, special stains, and flow cytometry may be required to establish the diagnosis.

TREATMENT

- The primary goal of therapy is treatment of the underlying cause.
- See Chapter 22, Cancer, for the treatment of acute and chronic leukemia.
- If symptoms of **leukostasis** are present (neurologic symptoms, dyspnea, hypoxia, or fever), emergent leukopheresis should be done to decrease WBC burden and relieve symptoms.
- Growth factor support should be considered in patients with chronic neutropenia and ongoing infections until the neutropenia resolves (see Oncologic Emergencies in Chapter 22, Cancer).

PLATELET DISORDERS

Discussed in Chapter 20, Disorders of Hemostasis and Thrombosis.

BONE MARROW DISORDERS

Myelodysplastic Syndrome

Discussed in Chapter 22, Cancer.

Myeloproliferative Disorders

GENERAL PRINCIPLES

Myeloproliferative disorders (MPDs) are a group of disorders characterized by clonal expansion of a hematopoietic stem cell resulting in overproduction of mature, largely functional cells. The 2008 World Health Organization (WHO) designated seven conditions as MPDs, including polycythemia vera (PV), essential thrombocytosis (ET) (discussed in Chapter 22, Cancer), CML (discussed in Chapter 22, Cancer), primary myelofibrosis (PMF), chronic neutrophilic leukemia, chronic eosinophilic leukemia, and mast cell disease (*Cancer 2009;17:3842*). The most common MPDs include PV, ET, CML, and PMF. This section will focus on PV and PMF.

TABLE 21-6	Diagnostic Criteria for Polycythemia Vera	

Presence of *JAK2* Mutation	Absence of *JAK2* Mutation	
	Four Major **or** Three Major + Two Minor	
	Major Criteria	**Minor Criteria**
Hct >52% in males	Hct >60% in males	Platelets >450,000/μL
Hct >48% in females	Hct >56% in females	Neutrophils >10,000/μL
	Palpable splenomegaly No secondary erythrocytosis Presence of genetic mutations (excludes *JAK2*)	Radiographic splenomegaly Low serum erythropoietin

Hct, hematocrit.

DIAGNOSIS

Diagnostic Criteria

• **PV**

Criteria for the diagnosis of PV have been updated and include Hct >52% in males or >48% in females in addition to presence of *JAK2* mutation. In the absence of *JAK2* mutation, four major criteria or three major and two minor criteria need to be met for diagnosis (*N Engl J Med 2006;355:2452*) (Table 21-6).

• **PMF**

The WHO diagnostic criteria for PMF are listed in Table 21-7 (*Blood 2007;110:1092*). All three major criteria and at least two minor criteria need to be met for the diagnosis.

TABLE 21-7	Diagnostic Criteria for Primary Myelofibrosis

Major Criteria

Presence of megakaryocyte proliferation and atypia, usually accompanied by either reticulin and/or collagen fibrosis
Not meeting WHO criteria for PV, CML, MDS, or other myeloid neoplasm
Presence of *JAK2* or other clonal marker, or no evidence of bone marrow fibrosis due to underlying inflammatory or neoplastic diseases in the absence of a clonal marker

Minor Criteria

Leukoerythroblastosis
Increase in serum LDH level
Anemia
Palpable splenomegaly

CML, chronic myelogenous leukemia; LDH, lactate dehydrogenase; MDS, myelodysplastic syndrome; PV, polycythemia vera; WHO, World Health Organization.

Diagnostic Testing

Laboratories
- Patients with PV typically present with an elevated Hct and platelet count (>400,000/µL), the presence of *JAK2* mutation (>95%), and decreased EPO level.
- Patients with PMF may present with leukocytosis or cytopenias and may have mutations in *JAK2* (50%), *MPL* (10%), or calreticulin (*CALR*) (40%).

Diagnostic Procedures
A BM biopsy should be included in the diagnostic workup of PMF, but not necessarily in PV. Cytogenetic studies should be performed for PMF because they have a significant impact on prognosis (*J Clin Oncol 2011;29(4):392*).

TREATMENT

- **PV:** The main goal of treatment is to decrease the risk of thrombotic complications. Treatment includes serial phlebotomy along with aspirin 81 mg/d. Hydroxyurea may be added depending on the risk for thrombosis.
  - In patients with low risk for thrombosis (age <60 years, no history of thrombosis): serial phlebotomy to keep goal Hct <45% in men and <42% in women.
  - Patients with high risk for thrombosis (age >60 years, prior thrombosis) should be treated with serial phlebotomy and hydroxyurea.
  - Ruxolitinib 10 mg twice a day, a JAK inhibitor first approved for treatment of myelofibrosis, was recently approved by the FDA for the treatment of PV in patients who fail hydroxyurea therapy. It improves the Hct and improves pruritus (*N Engl J Med 2015;372(5):426*).
- **PMF:** Patients are risk stratified based on several prognostic scoring systems and treatment depends on risk category. Treatment may not be needed for low-risk patients.
  - Low-dose aspirin should be started to decrease the risk of thrombosis in the absence of significant thrombocytopenia.
  - Cytoreductive agents such as hydroxyurea have been used historically to improve leukocytosis but do not significantly improve constitutional symptoms or splenomegaly and can cause myelosuppression.
  - Allogeneic hematopoietic SCT is the only curative therapy and should be considered for high-risk patients.
  - Ruxolitinib is useful for the treatment of patients with intermediate-1 and -2 risk myelofibrosis. It is effective in improving constitutional symptoms and splenomegaly. The main side effect is myelosuppression, and initial dosing is dependent on the platelet count.
  - Splenectomy may be considered for painful splenomegaly in patients intolerant to or not responsive to the JAK inhibitor.
  - Involved-field radiotherapy may also offer symptomatic relief for drug-refractory splenomegaly or sites of extramedullary hematopoiesis; however, the effects are usually transient.

MONOCLONAL GAMMOPATHIES

Monoclonal Gammopathy of Unknown Significance

GENERAL PRINCIPLES

Definition
Monoclonal gammopathy of unknown significance (MGUS) is a commonly occurring premalignant condition characterized by the presence of a small (<10%) population of

neoplastic, clonal plasma cells in the BM that occurs in the absence of any end-organ damage. Progression to a more serious disorder including multiple myeloma, WM, or primary amyloidosis occurs at a rate of approximately 1% per year.

DIAGNOSIS

- Patients with MGUS are asymptomatic and diagnosed when a monoclonal protein is detected on serum protein electrophoresis (SPEP) during workup of an elevated protein or other unrelated clinical finding. Most of the gammopathies are identified as IgG, but gammopathies in all immunoglobulin classes occur.
- Serum free light chain assay is used in both prognosis of MGUS and in the diagnosis of multiple myeloma.
- The Multiple Myeloma International Working Group identified diagnostic criteria for MGUS in 2003. All three criteria are required:
  ○ Presence of a serum monoclonal protein (M protein) IgG, IgA, or IgM <3 g/dL
  ○ Presence of clonal BM plasma cells comprising <10% of the marrow
  ○ Absence of end-organ damage attributed to the underlying plasma cell disorder, such as hypercalcemia, renal insufficiency, anemia, or lytic bone lesions

TREATMENT

There is currently no treatment recommended for MGUS. The vast majority of patients will not progress to a malignant disease. Generally, it is accepted practice to follow these patients annually with an evaluation that includes SPEP, urine protein electrophoresis (UPEP), CBC, serum creatinine, and calcium. If patients develop symptoms concerning for a malignant plasma cell disease, they should undergo an extensive evaluation.

PROGNOSIS

MGUS can evolve into a malignant lymphoproliferative disorder. Factors for higher risk of progression include an M protein >1.5 g/dL, non-IgG monoclonal gammopathy, and abnormal serum free light chain ratio (<0.26 or >1.65).

Multiple Myeloma

Discussed in Chapter 22, Cancer.

Waldenström Macroglobulinemia

WM is an uncommon IgM monoclonal disorder also known as lymphoplasmacytic lymphoma, characterized by mild hematologic abnormalities, and accompanied by tissue infiltration including lymphadenopathy, splenomegaly, or hepatomegaly. Because of its high molecular weight and concentration, IgM gammopathy can lead to hyperviscosity (central nervous system, visual, cardiac) manifestations. In these cases, emergent plasmapheresis to decrease IgM concentration is indicated. Asymptomatic patients may be observed initially, whereas durable responses have been observed in those requiring chemotherapy (*Blood 2014;124(9):1404–11*). The Bruton tyrosine kinase inhibitor ibrutinib received FDA approval in January 2015 based on an overall response rate of 62% in a study of 63 patients with WM (*N Engl J Med 2015;372:1430*).

Amyloidosis

GENERAL PRINCIPLES

Primary (AL) amyloidosis is an infiltrative disorder due to monoclonal, light chain deposition in various tissues most often involving the kidney (renal failure, nephrotic syndrome), heart (nonischemic cardiomyopathy), peripheral nervous system (neuropathy), and GI tract/liver (macroglossia, diarrhea, nausea, vomiting). Unexplained findings in any of these organ systems should prompt evaluation for amyloidosis.

DIAGNOSIS

- SPEP, UPEP, and serum free light chains may detect an M protein that is found in >90% of patients with AL amyloidosis. Congo red staining for amyloid in tissue or marrow establishes the diagnosis, and additional staining may identify the subtype of amyloid.
- Secondary (AA) amyloidosis is caused by chronic inflammation but occasionally may be idiopathic. In the absence of a measurable M protein, consider secondary amyloidosis or transthyretin-related hereditary amyloidosis because these are nonclonal disorders.
- Several effective chemotherapy regimens have been developed during the last decade (*Oncology 2012;26(2):152*). However, treatment of amyloidosis is difficult, and progressive organ failure is frequent. Cardiac involvement generally portends the worst prognosis. Transthyretin-related hereditary amyloidosis may be cured by liver transplantation.

Transfusion Medicine

GENERAL PRINCIPLES

Transfusion is a commonly used therapy for a variety of hematologic and hemostatic disturbances. The benefits and risks must be carefully weighed in each situation because blood products are a limited resource with potentially life-threatening side effects.

TREATMENT

- **Packed RBCs (pRBCs)**. RBC transfusion is indicated to increase the oxygen-carrying capacity of blood in anemic or bleeding patients.
  - Hgb threshold for transfusion (*Ann Intern Med 2012;157:49*):
    - Stable patient, no cardiac risk: 7 g/dL (*N Engl J Med 1999;340:409*).
    - Cardiac risk factors: 8 g/dL (*N Engl J Med 2011;365:2453*).
    - Active acute coronary syndrome: Thresholds have not been established; higher thresholds (8–10 g/dL) may be considered.
  - One unit of pRBCs increases the Hgb level by approximately 1 g/dL or Hct by 3% in the average adult.
  - If the cause of anemia is easily treatable (e.g., iron or folic acid deficiency) and no cerebrovascular or cardiopulmonary compromise is present, it is preferable to avoid transfusion.
- **Fresh frozen plasma (FFP):** Plasma transfusion is used to replace certain plasma proteins, usually coagulation factors, to treat bleeding or as bleeding prophylaxis for patients undergoing invasive procedures.
  - Common indications include:
    - Acquired coagulopathy in a patient with serious or massive bleeding
    - Warfarin overdose with life-threatening bleeding: consider using four-factor (II, VII, IX, X) prothrombin complex concentrates instead
    - Factor deficiencies for which specific factor concentrates are unavailable

- ○ The usual dose is 10 to 20 mL/kg. One unit of FFP contains approximately 250 mL of plasma and 250 units of factor activity for each factor.
- ○ Plasma should not be used as a volume expander and is usually not indicated in patients who are not currently bleeding, even those with an abnormal PT or activated PTT. In the case of warfarin overdose with a very prolonged PT but no bleeding, vitamin K should be used instead.
- **Platelets:** Platelet transfusion is indicated to prevent or treat bleeding in a thrombocytopenic patient or patients with dysfunctional platelets (e.g., due to aspirin).
  - ○ Platelet count threshold for transfusion (*Ann Intern Med 2015;162:205*):
    - Nonbleeding, stable inpatients: 10×10^9/L (*N Engl J Med 2013;368:1771*).
    - Nonbleeding, stable outpatients: 20×10^9/L.
    - Central line placement in a stable patient: 20×10^9/L.
    - Major invasive procedures or bleeding: 50×10^9/L.
    - High-risk surgery (e.g., neurosurgery) or life-threatening bleeding may require higher thresholds.
  - ○ Most platelet infusions are from a single donor collected by platelet pheresis rather than pooled platelets from a number of individuals
  - ○ One unit of single donor platelets increases the platelet count by 30–50×10^9/L.
  - ○ Platelets have a short shelf life (<5 days) and are stored at room temperature; they must never be placed on ice or refrigerated, which can cause platelet activation.
  - ○ **Platelet refractoriness** (poor platelet recovery after transfusion) may be due to immunologic causes (anti-ABO, anti-HLA, or antiplatelet antibodies) or nonimmunologic causes (e.g., sepsis, DIC, fever, active bleeding, splenic sequestration, certain drugs). Immunologic causes are likely if a 10- to 60-minute posttransfusion platelet count shows little increment and may be prevented in future transfusions by the use of ABO- and/or HLA-compatible platelets (*Br J Haematol 2008;142:348*).
- **Cryoprecipitate**
  - ○ Cryoprecipitate contains the cold-precipitated portion of plasma and is enriched in the following factors:
    - Fibrinogen
    - von Willebrand factor (vWF)
    - Factor VIII
    - Factor XIII
  - ○ It is most commonly indicated to replace **fibrinogen** in patients with hypofibrinogenemia or DIC, and should not be used to replace vWF or factor VIII, for which specific products exist.
  - ○ One unit increases fibrinogen concentration by approximately 7–8 mg/dL. Doses are frequently ordered in pools of 5 or 10 units.

SPECIAL CONSIDERATIONS

- **Pretransfusion testing**
  - ○ The **type and screen** procedure tests the recipient's RBCs for the A, B, and D (Rh) antigens and also screens the recipient's serum for antibodies against other RBC antigens.
  - ○ The **cross-match** tests the recipient's serum for antibodies against antigens on a specific donor's RBCs and is performed for each unit of blood that is dispensed for a patient.
- **Modifications of blood products**
  - ○ **Leukoreduction** is performed by the use of filters to eliminate WBC contamination before storage or at the bedside. Indicated for all patients to reduce the risk of the following transfusion complications:
    - Nonhemolytic febrile transfusion reactions
    - Transfusion-transmitted CMV infection
    - Formation of HLA alloantibodies

- ○ **CMV-seronegative** blood products may be indicated for immunocompromised patients who are CMV seronegative to reduce the risk of CMV transmission. However, prestorage leuko-reduced products are considered equivalently "CMV reduced risk" and can be used in place of CMV-seronegative products.
- ○ **Irradiation** eliminates immunologically competent lymphocytes in order to prevent transfusion-associated graft-versus-host disease and is indicated for certain immunocompromised patients, BM transplant recipients, or patients who receive directed donations from HLA-matched donors or relatives.
- ○ **Washing** of blood products is rarely indicated but should be considered for patients in whom plasma proteins may cause a serious reaction (e.g., recipients with IgA deficiency or a history of anaphylactic reactions).
- **Blood administration**
  - ○ Patient and blood product identification procedures must be carefully followed to avoid any transfusion-related errors including ABO-incompatible transfusion.
  - ○ The IV catheter should be at least 18 gauge to allow adequate flow.
  - ○ All blood products should be administered through a 170- to 260-μm "standard" filter to prevent infusion of macroaggregates, fibrin, and debris.
  - ○ Patients should be observed with vital signs for the first 10–15 minutes of each transfusion for adverse effects and at regular intervals thereafter.
  - ○ RBC infusion is typically administered over 1–2 hours, with a maximum of 4 hours.
- **Emergency transfusion** may be considered in situations in which massive blood loss has resulted in cardiovascular compromise.
  - ○ Before the patient's ABO type can be confirmed, "emergency release" blood may be used, consisting of uncross-matched group O pRBCs and group AB or A plasma.
  - ○ If **massive transfusion** (replacement of ≥10 units of pRBCs in <24 hours) is indicated, hemostatic components (plasma, platelets, and cryoprecipitate) should be included to correct the loss and dilution of hemostatic factors. In addition, care must be taken to manage the potential iatrogenic complications of massive transfusion, such as hypothermia, hypocalcemia (due to the citrated preservative solution), and hyperkalemia.

COMPLICATIONS

- **Transfusion-transmitted infections**
  - ○ Donors and blood products are screened for HIV-1/2, human T-lymphotropic virus 1/2 (HTLV-1/2), hepatitis B, hepatitis C, West Nile virus, syphilis, *Trypanosoma cruzi* (Chagas), and bacteremia (platelets only).
  - ○ Viral transmission may occur when donors are in the "window period" (i.e., undetectable to testing).
    - ▪ The risk of hepatitis B transmission is approximately 1 in 1,000,000; other tested viruses have a transmission risk of <1 in 1,000,000.
    - ▪ CMV transmission risk may be reduced in immunocompromised patients by the use of CMV-seronegative or prestorage leuko-reduced products.
  - ○ Bacterial transmission may occur from either a donor infection or a contaminant at the time of collection or processing.
    - ▪ Platelet transfusions are more likely than RBCs to have bacterial contamination because they are stored at room temperature.
    - ▪ The most common organisms identified are *Yersinia enterocolitica* in RBCs and *Staphylococcus* spp. in platelets.
- **Noninfectious hazards of transfusion**
  - ○ **Acute hemolytic transfusion reactions** are usually caused by **preformed antibodies** in the recipient and are characterized by intravascular hemolysis of the transfused RBCs soon after the administration of ABO-incompatible blood.

- **Fever, chills, back pain, chest pain, nausea, vomiting, anxiety, and hypotension** may develop. Acute renal failure with hemoglobinuria may occur. In the unconscious patient, hypotension or hemoglobinuria may be the only manifestation.
- If a hemolytic transfusion reaction is suspected, **the transfusion should be stopped immediately and all IV tubing should be replaced**. Samples of the patient's blood should be delivered to the blood bank along with the remainder of the suspected unit for repeat of the cross-match. Direct and indirect Coombs tests should be performed, and the plasma and freshly voided urine should be examined for free Hgb.
- Management includes preservation of intravascular volume and protection of renal function. Urine output should be maintained at ≥100 mL/h with the use of IV fluids and diuretics or mannitol, if necessary. The excretion of free Hgb can be aided by alkalinization of the urine. Sodium bicarbonate can be added to IV fluids to increase the urinary pH to ≥7.5.
  ○ **Delayed hemolytic transfusion reactions** typically occur 3–10 days after transfusion and are caused by either a primary or an anamnestic antibody response to specific RBC antigens on donor RBCs.
- Hgb and Hct levels may fall.
- The DAT is usually positive, depending on when follow-up testing is conducted.
- Reactions may at times be severe; these cases should be treated similarly to acute hemolytic reactions.
  ○ **Nonhemolytic febrile transfusion reactions** are characterized by fevers and chills.
- Cytokines released from white cells are thought to be the cause.
- Treatment and future prophylaxis may include acetaminophen and prestorage leuko-reduced blood products.
  ○ **Allergic reactions** are characterized by urticaria and, in severe cases, bronchospasm and hypotension.
- The reactions are due to plasma proteins that elicit an IgE-mediated response. The reaction may be specific to the plasma proteins of a particular donor and therefore may occur infrequently or never again.
- Treatment and future prophylaxis may include antihistamines such as diphenhydramine or corticosteroids.
- **Anaphylactic reactions** may require the addition of corticosteroids and washed or plasma-reduced products. Additionally, check serum immunoglobulins, because patients with IgA deficiency who receive IgA-containing blood products may experience anaphylaxis with small exposure to donor plasma.
  ○ **Transfusion-associated circulatory overload** (TACO) is a relatively common yet under-recognized complication of blood transfusion. Volume overload with pulmonary edema and signs of CHF may be seen when patients with cardiovascular compromise are transfused. The clinical and radiographic features may be difficult to distinguish from that of transfusion-related acute lung injury (TRALI) (*Crit Care Med 2006;34(5 suppl):S109*). Slowing the rate of transfusion and judicious use of diuretics help prevent this complication, as well as avoidance of unnecessary transfusion.
  ○ **TRALI** is indistinguishable from acute respiratory distress syndrome and occurs within 6 hours of a transfusion.
- Symptoms include dyspnea, hypoxemia, and possibly fever.
- New or worsening pulmonary edema is typically seen on CXR, as with TACO.
- Anti-HLA or antineutrophil antibodies in the donor's serum directed against the recipient's WBCs are thought to cause the disorder.
- On recognition, transfusions must be stopped and the blood bank notified so that other products from the donor(s) in question may be quarantined.
- Hypoxemia resolves rapidly, typically in about 24 hours, but ventilatory assistance may be required during that time.

- Despite clinical or radiographic findings that suggest pulmonary edema, data indicate that diuretics have no role and may be detrimental (*Blood 2005;105(6):2266*).
  - **Transfusion-associated graft-versus-host disease** is a rare but serious complication usually seen in immunocompromised patients (and immunocompetent patients receiving blood from a relative) and is thought to result from the infusion of immunocompetent donor T lymphocytes.
    - Symptoms include rash, elevated liver function tests, and severe pancytopenia.
    - Mortality is >80%.
    - **Irradiation** of blood products for at-risk patients prevents this disease.
  - **Posttransfusion purpura** is a rare syndrome of severe thrombocytopenia and purpura or bleeding that starts 7–10 days after exposure to blood products. This disorder is described in Chapter 20, Disorders of Hemostasis and Thrombosis, in the Platelet Disorders section.

22

Cancer

Siddhartha Devarakonda, Daniel Morgensztern,
and Ramaswamy Govindan

Cancer is the leading cause of mortality in developed countries and the second leading cause of death in developing countries. It is estimated that nearly 589,430 people will die from cancer in the United States in 2015 (*CA Cancer J Clin 2015;65:5*). The most common malignancies in the United States are lung cancer, prostate cancer, breast cancer, and colon cancer (Table 22-1). However, cancer death rates have declined over the past decade due to advances in drug development and availability of better supportive care. Improved understanding of the molecular pathways operative in cancer cells has led to the development of targeted agents and personalized treatment approaches that continue to demonstrate meaningful clinical benefit. This chapter provides an overview of cancer therapy.

Approach to the Cancer Patient

GENERAL PRINCIPLES

- The median age at diagnosis for all cancers in the United States is 67 years (*CA Cancer J Clin 2008;58:71*).
- The lifetime probability of being diagnosed with cancer is 43% in males and 38% in females.
- Tobacco use is the most common cause of cancer death and is associated with lung, head and neck, esophageal, gastric, pancreatic, kidney, and bladder cancers.
- Diet, obesity, inactivity, and height have also been shown to be associated with increased risk of developing selected cancers.
- Chronic inflammatory states such as ulcerative colitis and infections such as HIV, hepatitis, Epstein-Barr virus (EBV), human papillomavirus (HPV), and *Helicobacter pylori* are also associated with increased cancer risk.
- Several familial cancer syndromes have been described to date, which have important implications for cancer screening (Table 22-2).
- Prior exposure to cytotoxic chemotherapy or radiation therapy is associated with an increased risk of developing secondary cancers. For instance, exposure to alkylating agents or topoisomerase II inhibitors increases the risk of developing treatment-related leukemia, and exposure to radiation therapy increases risk for developing cancers such as breast cancer, angiosarcoma, and osteosarcoma.

DIAGNOSIS

- Obtaining tissue is crucial for facilitating a definitive tissue diagnosis, examining molecular features, and treatment planning.
- **Cytology** specimens often consist of only a few malignant cells that are obtained either invasively through biopsy (fine-needle or core biopsies), brushings (Pap smear or endoscopic), or aspiration of body fluids (blood, cerebrospinal fluid [CSF], pleural, pericardial, or peritoneal) or noninvasively though collection of fluids such as sputum and urine. Although these approaches are relatively less invasive compared to surgical approaches and easier to pursue, cytologic samples are often inadequate for molecular testing. Furthermore, the loss of tissue architecture also makes it challenging to diagnose certain malignancies such as lymphomas.

TABLE 22-1	Most Common Cancer Diagnoses and Rates of Death in the United States for 2015			
Sites	New Cases			Deaths
	Both Sexes	Male	Female	Total
Lung	221,200	115,610	105,590	158,040
Prostate	220,800	220,800		27,540
Breast	234,190	2,350	231,840	40,730
Colon	93,090	45,890	47,200	49,700

- **Histology** specimens are obtained through large-core needle biopsies, excisional biopsies, or surgical resection. These specimens are ideal for diagnosing most malignancies and provide enough tissue for molecular testing. However, these procedures are more invasive and not feasible in all patients.

STAGING

- Once a tissue diagnosis is obtained, most cancer patients will require additional imaging, procedures, and laboratory testing for determining the disease burden and stage. This workup is cancer and patient specific, and also varies by local and institutional patterns of practice. Organizations such as the American Society of Clinical Oncology (ASCO), National Comprehensive Cancer Network (NCCN), and European Society of Medical Oncology (ESMO) review available evidence and issue periodic recommendations to guide appropriate staging workup and management.
- Cancer stage provides an assessment of the extent of tumor dissemination, which is crucial for treatment.
  - Most malignancies are staged according to the tumor, lymph node, and metastasis (TNM) system from stages I to IV. The T classification is based on the size and extent of local invasion. The N classification describes the extent of lymph node involvement, and the M classification is based on the presence or absence of distant metastasis.
  - Performance status provides a quantitative measure of a patient's generalized well-being and quality of life. It has important implications for treatment planning (Table 22-3).

TREATMENT

Surgical Management

- Surgical resection is often performed with curative intent, although selected patients may benefit from palliative surgery that is performed for debulking large tumor masses (e.g., ovarian cancer), increasing the efficacy of immunotherapy (e.g., renal cell carcinoma), or relieving symptoms (e.g., mastectomy for local control in a patient with metastatic disease).
- Surgery can facilitate staging and guide subsequent therapeutic decisions (adjuvant treatment), including chemotherapy or radiation therapy.
- Surgical resection of isolated metastatic sites in selected patients can improve survival. Examples include solitary brain metastases, pulmonary metastases from sarcomas, and liver metastases from colorectal cancer.

TABLE 22-2	List of Selected Familial Cancer Syndromes with High Penetrance	
Syndrome	**Defect**	**Associated Cancer Type**
Ataxia-telangiectasia	*ATM*	Multiple; predominantly leukemia and lymphoma
Birt-Hogg-Dube	*BHD*	Chromophobe RCC
Bloom syndrome	*BLM*	Multiple
Cowden syndrome	*PTEN*	Multiple; predominantly breast, thyroid, RCC, endometrial
Familial adenomatous polyposis	*APC*	Colorectal, desmoid
Fanconi anemia	*DNA* repair complex	Multiple; predominantly MDS and AML
Hereditary breast–ovarian cancer	*BRCA1* and *BRCA2*	Multiple; predominantly breast, ovarian
Hereditary diffuse gastric cancer	*CDH1*	Gastric, lobular breast cancer
Hereditary leiomyomatosis and RCC	*FH*	Papillary RCC
Lynch syndrome (HNPCC)	Mismatch repair	Multiple; predominantly colorectal
Hereditary papillary RCC	*MET*	Papillary RCC
Juvenile polyposis syndrome	*MADH4 (SMAD4), BMPR1A*	Digestive tract and pancreas
Li-Fraumeni syndrome	*TP53*	Multiple
MEN type 1	*MEN1*	Islet cell tumors
MEN type 2	*RET*	Medullary thyroid cancer
Neurofibromatosis type 1	*NF1*	MPNST, glioma
Neurofibromatosis type 2	*NF2*	Meningioma, glioma, schwannoma
Nijmegen breakage syndrome	*NBS1*	Predominantly lymphoma
Peutz-Jeghers syndrome	*LKB1 (STK11)*	Multiple; predominantly breast, GI, pancreas
Retinoblastoma, hereditary	*RB*	Retinoblastoma, primitive neuroectodermal tumor
Rothmund-Thomson syndrome	*RECQL4*	Osteosarcoma
Tuberous sclerosis (TS)	*TSC1, TSC2*	RCC, giant cell astrocytoma
von Hippel-Lindau	*VHL*	Clear cell RCC
Xeroderma pigmentosum	Nucleotide excision repair	Multiple, cutaneous

AML, acute myeloid leukemia; GI, gastrointestinal; HNPCC, hereditary nonpolyposis colorectal cancer; MDS, myelodysplastic syndrome; MEN, multiple endocrine neoplasia; MPNST, malignant peripheral nerve sheath tumor; RCC, renal cell carcinoma.

TABLE 22-3	Eastern Cooperative Oncology Group (ECOG) and Karnofsky Score	
ECOG	**Karnofsky Score Correlate**	**Description**
0	100	Fully active, able to carry on all predisease performance without restriction.
1	80–90	Restricted in physically strenuous activity but ambulatory and able to carry out work of a light or sedentary nature (e.g., light housework, office work).
2	60–70	Ambulatory and capable of all self-care but unable to carry out any work activities. Up and about >50% of waking hours.
3	40–50	Capable of only limited self-care, confined to bed or chair >50% of waking hours.
4	20–30	Completely disabled. Cannot carry on any self-care. Totally confined to bed or chair.
5	0	Dead.

From Oken MM, Creech RH, Tormey DC, et al. Toxicity and response criteria of the Eastern Cooperative Oncology Group. *Am J Clin Oncol* 1982;5:649.

Principles of Radiation

- Radiation is used for treatment of benign and malignant diseases. Commonly used forms of radiation include external-beam photons and electrons. Photons are usually x-rays or γ-rays. With the exception of stereotactic radiation to the brain, γ-rays are rarely used today. Protons and neutrons are other forms of external-beam radiation. Electrons are mostly useful for treating skin and superficial tumors.
- Brachytherapy is an alternative method of radiation therapy, where radioactive sources are placed close to or in contact with their target tissue. This ensures a higher dose delivery to the targeted tissue over a short duration of time. Brachytherapy sources can be temporary (e.g., iridium-192 in cervical cancer) or permanent (e.g., iodine-125 in prostate cancer).
- Radioactive substances can also be administered systemically. For instance, iodine-131 is administered orally for treating thyroid cancer, yttrium-90 microspheres are injected into the liver vasculature in hepatocellular cancer, and radium-223 is dosed intravenously in patients with prostate cancer and skeletal metastases.
- Radiation planning is designed to deliver a precise dose of radiation to a tumor while sparing surrounding tissues.
- **Curative** intent radiotherapy is used in several settings.
  - **Neoadjuvant:** Preoperative therapy intended to reduce both the extent of surgery and the risk of local relapse. Radiation in this setting is almost always administered in combination with chemotherapy.
  - **Adjuvant:** Postoperative therapy intended to reduce the risk of local relapse.
  - **Definitive:** High dose with curative intent.
  - **Concurrent chemoradiation:** Chemotherapy with definitive radiation is associated with increased efficacy but at a cost of increased toxicity compared to either chemotherapy or radiation alone.
- **Palliative** radiotherapy is used in lower dosing to reduce symptoms, including bone pain, obstruction, bleeding, and neurologic symptoms.

- The total dose of radiation administered is usually spread out over time (fractionated). This allows time for normal tissue repair and increases the probability of delivering radiation to tumor cells in a radiosensitive phase of cell cycle. Radiation treatments are usually delivered either through conventional fractionation, hypofractionation, hyperfractionation, or accelerated fractionation schedules.
  - **Conventional fractionation** consists of daily fractions typically of 1.8–2.0 Gy, usually delivered 5 days per week.
  - **Hypofractionation** refers to delivery of larger fraction sizes once daily and a lower total dose.
  - **Hyperfractionation** refers to the delivery of smaller doses per fraction and a higher total dose.
  - **Accelerated fractionation** refers to the delivery of smaller fraction sizes, more frequently, and over a shorter duration of time, while keeping the total dose administered the same or slightly lower.

Principles of Chemotherapy

- Cytotoxic chemotherapy targets all dividing cells and has broad toxicities.
- In patients with resectable disease, chemotherapy may be used prior to the surgery (neoadjuvant) or following complete resection (adjuvant).
- Chemotherapy is typically given in 2-, 3-, or 4-week cycles. In most regimens, IV treatment is given on the first few days of the cycle, with no further treatment until the next cycle. In other regimens, treatments are administered weekly for 2–3 weeks, with 1 week off between cycles.
- **Curative** intent chemotherapy includes neoadjuvant, adjuvant, and chemoradiation protocols in solid tumors. Chemotherapy alone is curative in many lymphomas, leukemias, and germ cell tumors.
- **Palliative** chemotherapy is used in advanced solid tumors and relapsed hematologic malignancies, with a focus on prolonging survival and improving the quality of life.
- Most agents have a very narrow therapeutic index, and dosing is based on body surface area (mg/m^2). Chemotherapy toxicities are widely variable and can be life threatening.

Principles of Targeted Therapy

- The advent of molecularly targeted agents has led to marked advances in the treatment of selected malignancies.
- The most common classes of drugs are monoclonal antibodies and receptor tyrosine kinase inhibitors (TKIs). Monoclonal antibodies are administered IV and by standard nomenclature have names that end with the stem -mab. Substems indicate the source and target of the antibody. The most common source substems in oncology include -xi- indicating a chimeric antibody (e.g., cetuximab), -zu- indicating humanized antibody (e.g., bevacizumab), and -u- indicating fully human antibodies (e.g., ipilimumab). The most common target substems include -ci- indicating circulatory system (e.g., bevacizumab), -tu- indicating tumor (e.g., cetuximab), and -li- indicating immune system (e.g., ipilimumab).
- TKIs are administered orally and have names that end with -ib. The most common substems include -ti- indicating tyrosine kinase inhibition (e.g., imatinib) and -zom- indicating proteasome inhibition (e.g., bortezomib).
- Most antibodies are used in combination with chemotherapy or radiation, whereas most TKIs are used as single agents.
- Toxicities of targeted therapies are unique to each agent, although specific classes of drugs can be associated with characteristic side effects.
  - Inhibitors of the epidermal growth factor receptor (EGFR) frequently cause an acne-like rash on the face and upper chest, which can be severe. Treatment is typically with topical corticosteroids or oral minocycline.

TABLE 22-4	Summary of Selected Response Evaluation Criteria in Solid Tumors (RECIST) 1.1 Criteria
Measurable lesions	Tumor: >10 mm in longest diameter (LD) on axial CT or MRI
	Lymph node: >15 mm in short axis on CT
Method	Sum of longest diameter (SLD) of the lesions in axial plane. Up to five target lesions (two per organ).
Response	
Complete response (CR)	Disappearance of all nonnodal target lesions. All target lymph nodes must be <10 mm in short axis.
Partial response (PR)	At least 30% decrease in the SLD of target lesions, with baseline sum of diameters as reference.
Progressive disease (PD)	New lesions or SLD increased by ≥20%.
Stable disease (SD)	Neither PR nor PD.

- Inhibitors of human epidermal growth factor receptor 2 (HER2) are associated with a reversible decline in cardiac systolic function, which should be monitored in these patients periodically.
- Inhibitors of angiogenesis are associated with endothelial toxicity, leading to hypertension, proteinuria, delayed wound healing, mild cardiac toxicity, increased risk of bleeding, thromboembolism, and gastrointestinal (GI) perforation/fistula. All antiangiogenics should be held in the perioperative period.

Assessing Response to Therapy

Objective assessment of changes in tumor burden, i.e., tumor shrinkage or progression, is crucial for planning cancer treatment and evaluating the efficacy of experimental interventions. Criteria such as the Response Evaluation Criteria in Solid Tumors (RECIST) are commonly used for this purpose (Table 22-4).

Lung Cancer

GENERAL PRINCIPLES

Epidemiology and Etiology

Lung cancer is the most common cause of cancer death in the United States, with an estimated 158,040 deaths in 2015. Smoking is the greatest risk factor for lung cancer, with over 90% of cases being tobacco related. The risk of smoking-related lung cancer persists for 20–30 years after quitting smoking. Other environmental risks include exposure to asbestos and radon.

Pathology

Non–small-cell lung cancer (NSCLC) accounts for over 85% of cases. The most common histologic subtypes are adenocarcinoma and squamous cell carcinoma. Small-cell lung cancer (SCLC) is associated with a rapid tumor growth and early development of metastases compared to NSCLC.

Screening

- In 2011, the National Lung Screening Trial (NLST) research team showed a 20% relative reduction in lung cancer mortality and a 6.7% relative reduction in all-cause mortality (*N Engl J Med 2011;365:395*). The NLST included more than 50,000 asymptomatic current and former smokers at high risk for developing lung cancer. Participants were randomly assigned to screening with baseline low-dose chest CT (LDCT) or CXR, followed by annual scans at years 1 and 2.
- The number needed to screen to prevent one lung cancer death was 320 in the NLST.
- Based on these data, the US Preventive Services Task Force (USPSTF) currently recommends annual screening for lung cancer with LDCT in current smokers or former smokers who quit within the past 15 years, are between 55–80 years old, and have a 30-pack-year smoking history.

DIAGNOSIS

Clinical Presentation

- Symptoms in patients with lung cancer can be related to local disease (cough, dyspnea, wheezing, hemoptysis), intrathoracic extension (hoarseness from recurrent laryngeal nerve involvement, dysphagia, chest wall pain, Horner syndrome, symptoms related to brachial plexus involvement, superior vena cava syndrome), systemic metastases (fever, jaundice, bone pain, headaches, back pain), or paraneoplastic syndromes.
- Paraneoplastic syndromes in lung cancer typically include hypercalcemia,, hyponatremia from syndrome of inappropriate antidiuretic hormone secretion, and hypertrophic pulmonary osteoarthropathy.

Diagnostic Testing

- Any patient with a smoking history and concerning pulmonary symptoms should undergo a chest CT scan. A normal CXR does not exclude lung cancer. Diagnosis can be made from pleural fluid cytology, bronchoscopy with biopsy, brushings or washings, or ultrasound/CT-guided needle biopsy. Core needle biopsy is preferable to fine-needle aspiration (FNA).
- Staging evaluation in all patients should include a CT scan of the chest and abdomen. Additional imaging depends on the initial findings. In potentially curable patients, evaluation may also include brain MRI, positron emission tomography (PET)/CT scan, and mediastinoscopy.

TREATMENT

- **NSCLC**
  - Stages I and II: Surgery is the preferred therapy. Radiation therapy is an option for those who are not candidates for surgical resection. Postoperative platinum doublet chemotherapy improves overall survival in patients with surgically resected stage II and III NSCLC.
  - Stage III: The standard therapy is concurrent radiation and chemotherapy. Surgery is indicated for selected patients.
  - Stage IV: The standard treatment is with chemotherapy.
    - Frontline platinum-based doublet chemotherapy provides modest improvement in survival compared to best supportive care, and there is no difference in outcomes among the multiple regimens (*N Engl J Med 2002;346:92*).
    - EGFR TKIs, such as erlotinib or afatinib, should be considered as frontline therapy in patients whose tumors harbor activating mutations in *EGFR* (*J Thorac Oncol 2015;10:S1*).

- Crizotinib and ceritinib are TKIs effective in patients with tumors harboring the *EML4-ALK* fusion gene (*J Clin Oncol 2013;31:1105*). Crizotinib is also associated with marked clinical activity in tumors harboring *ROS1* rearrangements (*N Engl J Med 2014;371:1963*).
- Nivolumab, which targets the programmed death-1 (PD-1) receptor, has been approved for patients with previously treated metastatic squamous cell lung cancer.
- **SCLC**
  - Limited stage (stages I to III): The standard therapy is concurrent radiation therapy and chemotherapy with a platinum agent (carboplatin or cisplatin) plus etoposide.
  - Extensive stage (stage IV): The treatment of choice is with chemotherapy, usually with a platinum agent (cisplatin or carboplatin) plus etoposide.
  - Prophylactic cranial irradiation is recommended for all patients with limited stage and selected patients with extensive stage after completion of initial therapy.

Breast Cancer

GENERAL PRINCIPLES

Epidemiology and Etiology

Breast cancer is the most common cancer in women in developed countries and is expected to account for 29% of new cancers in women in 2015. Nearly 231,840 patients develop breast cancer per year in the United States, and less than 1% of cases are reported in men. *BRCA1* and *BRCA2* mutations are associated with a 57% and 49% cumulative risk of breast cancer by age 70, respectively (*J Clin Oncol 2007;25:1329*). However, less than 10% of all breast cancers are attributable to mutations involving susceptibility genes. Alcohol consumption, early menarche, late menopause, nulliparity, postmenopausal obesity, hormone replacement therapy, and delayed first pregnancy are all risk factors for breast cancer. Women receiving mantle field radiation for Hodgkin disease also carry a higher lifetime risk.

Pathology

- Noninvasive: Ductal carcinoma in situ (DCIS) and lobular carcinoma in situ (LCIS).
- Invasive: Ductal carcinoma is more common than lobular carcinoma.
- Estrogen receptor (ER) is expressed in nearly 75% of all cases. ER positivity (ER+) is associated with good prognosis and responsiveness to endocrine therapies.
- Progesterone receptor expression (PR+) usually correlates with ER expression.
- Approximately 20% of tumors are HER2 positive (HER2+) by immunohistochemistry (IHC) or fluorescent in situ hybridization (FISH). HER2 positivity is associated with higher grade cancers, but HER2+ breast cancers have a very good outcome when treated with HER2-directed targeted therapies (e.g., trastuzumab).

Screening and Prevention

- The American Cancer Society (ACS) recommends a clinical breast exam every 3 years between 20–39 years of age and annually thereafter. The role of self-breast examination is controversial and should only be performed as an adjunct to clinical exam and mammography.
- The ideal age to begin screening mammography and optimal screening intervals are unknown, and recommendations vary among organizations and clinicians.
- The ACS recommends annual mammography from age 40, for as long as the person does not have serious illnesses that shorten life expectancy. MRI along with mammography is indicated in select individuals with a strong family history of breast cancer.

- Prophylactic mastectomy and oophorectomy are recommended for carriers of *BRCA1* or *BRCA2* mutations.
- Chemoprevention with tamoxifen and raloxifene is an option in women who are at high risk for developing breast cancer (family history and LCIS).

DIAGNOSIS

Clinical Presentation

Most breast cancers are identified by screening tests, but patients can present with a painless, palpable mass in the breast or axilla. Some patients may have nipple discharge, pain, and skin changes associated with the mass and nipple retraction. Patients with inflammatory breast cancer can complain of a "warm" breast and erythema. Inflammatory breast cancer is rare, but patients with these symptoms should be promptly evaluated by a clinician experienced with this diagnosis.

Diagnostic Testing

- Patients with palpable breast masses require diagnostic mammograms and ultrasonography. Patients with axillary mass and no detectable breast mass by routine imaging and examination should receive an MRI to identify occult cancer. Any clinically concerning mass needs to be biopsied irrespective of its radiographic appearance.
- CXR is routinely obtained. Bone scan and CT imaging are indicated in patients with stage III or higher disease, localizing symptoms, and abnormal laboratory values that suggest liver or skeletal involvement. CT scans can be considered in patients with stage II disease with node involvement.

TREATMENT

Surgery

- Lumpectomy (breast conservation therapy) with adjuvant radiation is equivalent to mastectomy (*N Engl J Med 1995;332:907*).
- Sentinel lymph node biopsy is the most common procedure for evaluation of regional lymph nodes.
- Whole-breast radiation therapy with radiotherapy boost to the tumor bed is recommended for patients following breast conservation surgery (BCS). Postmastectomy radiation is recommended in selected patients.

Endocrine Therapies

- Tamoxifen is an estrogen antagonist used in ER+ breast cancer. Fulvestrant is an ER antagonist that is approved for use in postmenopausal women.
- Luteinizing hormone–releasing hormone (LHRH) agonists (goserelin, leuprolide) can be used for ovarian suppression in premenopausal women, as an alternative to oophorectomy.
- Aromatase inhibitors (AIs) are the most commonly used endocrine drugs in postmenopausal patients and work by blocking androgen to estrogen conversion in peripheral tissues. These agents (letrozole, anastrozole, exemestane) can be used in conjunction with ovarian suppression in premenopausal women.

Treatment by Stage

- **DCIS and LCIS (stage 0)**

  Mastectomy or lumpectomy with negative margins followed by adjuvant radiation. Repeat resections for positive margins may be necessary. Tamoxifen is typically used if the tumor is ER+.

- **Resectable breast cancer (stages I–III)**
  - Surgical approach depends on the size of the tumor, patient preference, and the presence or absence of contraindications to BCS. Contraindications for BCS include multicentric disease, extensive microcalcifications, and previous irradiation. Neoadjuvant (preoperative) chemotherapy or hormonal therapy can be used to shrink larger tumors to facilitate BCS.
  - For ER+ and/or PR+ cancers, adjuvant endocrine therapy with tamoxifen or a combination of AI and ovarian suppression is recommended in premenopausal women (*N Engl J Med 2014;371:107*). For postmenopausal women, an AI is standard of care. Treatment duration is 5–10 years.
  - Adjuvant chemotherapy is generally recommended based on node involvement, tumor size, and ER, PR, and HER2 status.
  - Adjuvant treatment with the HER2 inhibitor trastuzumab dramatically reduces rate of relapse and improves survival in HER2+ breast cancer (*N Engl J Med 2005; 353:1673*).
  - Pertuzumab is another HER2 inhibitor that has recently been approved for the treatment of HER2+ cancer in the neoadjuvant and metastatic settings (*N Engl J Med 2012;366:109*).
- **Treatment of metastatic breast cancer**
  - Radiation therapy is urgently needed for brain metastases and can be used for symptomatic bone metastases.
  - Endocrine therapy is usually preferred in ER+/PR+ patients. Upfront use of chemotherapy can be considered in ER+/PR+ patients with visceral metastases. ER–/PR– metastatic breast cancer requires chemotherapy.
  - HER2+ metastatic breast cancer requires HER2-directed targeted drugs, such as trastuzumab, pertuzumab, T-DM1, or lapatinib, and these are typically combined with chemotherapy.
  - Bone-strengthening agents, such as bisphosphonates or denosumab (an anti-RANKL antibody), are recommended for patients with bone metastases to reduce risks of fracture or other bone complications.

Head and Neck Cancer

GENERAL PRINCIPLES

Head and neck squamous cell cancer (HNSCC) includes carcinoma of the lip, oral cavity, pharynx, nasopharynx, and larynx. It is estimated that nearly 59,000 patients will be diagnosed with HNSCC in the year 2015. Tobacco use and alcohol consumption are associated with increased risk of developing HNSCC. HPV infection is implicated in oropharyngeal squamous cell carcinomas, and the incidence of HPV-associated HNSCC has quadrupled since the 1980s. EBV infection is associated with nasopharyngeal cancers.
- **Field cancerization** is an important concept in HNSCC. Given the diffuse nature of mucosal exposure to tobacco smoke, the primary cancer site is often surrounded by areas of premalignant lesions (carcinoma in situ and dysplasia). For this reason, patients with tobacco-associated HNSCC are at increased risk for developing secondary cancers.
- **Leukoplakia and erythroleukoplakia** are premalignant lesions of the oral mucosa. Leukoplakia refers to a white mucosal patch that cannot be scraped off, whereas erythroleukoplakia appears red and velvety. Erythroleukoplakias are associated with a higher risk of malignant transformation.

DIAGNOSIS

Clinical Presentation

Patients with HNSCC can present with a variety of symptoms depending on the primary tumor site: oral mass, nonhealing ulcers, trismus from invasion of pterygoid muscles, dysphagia, odynophagia, otitis media from eustachian tube blockage, hoarseness, neck mass, weight loss, and cranial nerve palsies. Nasopharyngeal tumors can invade the cavernous sinus and frequently affect the abducens and trigeminal nerves. Salivary gland tumors, which can have nonsquamous pathology, can invade the facial nerve and cause facial nerve–related symptoms.

Diagnostic Testing

- Comprehensive ear, nose, and throat (ENT) evaluation with fiberoptic endoscopy or mirror exam is required. Particular attention should be paid to assess dentition. Functional evaluation that includes assessment of swallowing, biting, chewing, and speech should be performed.
- Examination under anesthesia is a critical component of staging. Imaging should include a panorex to evaluate dentition and mandibular bony involvement. A CT of the neck and chest should be obtained to evaluate lymph node involvement and rule out pulmonary metastases, respectively. Whole-body PET can be considered in select patients.
- p16 positivity on IHC is used as a surrogate for HPV infection and is an independent favorable prognostic factor for survival (*N Engl J Med 2010;363:24*).
- **Stage classification:** Stage I to II disease does not show lymph node involvement. Stage III tumors are larger (defined as >4 cm for most sites) or have isolated lymph node involvement. Stage IVA/B tumors are locally advanced tumors or show bilateral or bulky cervical lymph node involvement. Stage IVC tumors are associated with distant metastasis.

TREATMENT

- Early stage (I–II): Either surgery or definitive radiation.
- Locally advanced (stage III–IVA/B): Treatment approaches include:
  - Definitive surgical resection followed by adjuvant radiation with or without chemotherapy
  - Concurrent chemotherapy with radiation
  - Induction chemotherapy followed by concurrent chemotherapy with radiation or radiation alone
- Metastatic (stage IVC): Palliative chemotherapy.
- **Chemotherapy:** Cisplatin is the chemotherapy agent commonly used in combination with radiation for definitive treatment. Induction regimens usually involve a platinum combination with drugs such as 5-fluorouracil (5FU) and a taxane (paclitaxel or docetaxel).
- **Targeted therapy:** Cetuximab, a monoclonal antibody against EGFR, can be used in combination with definitive radiation in patients who cannot tolerate traditional chemotherapeutic regimens or in combination with cisplatin and 5FU for the treatment of metastatic disease (*N Engl J Med 2008;359:1116*).
- **Surgery:** Nodal neck dissection is an important part of surgical management. Radical neck dissection refers to surgical removal of lymph nodes from all five neck stations unilaterally, along with excision of the internal jugular vein, spinal accessory nerve, and sternocleidomastoid. Modified neck dissections spare some of these structures.
- **Organ sparing:** Chemoradiation or induction chemotherapy followed by radiation can potentially spare patients from undergoing a total laryngectomy and improve quality of life.

- **Supportive care:** Dental evaluation is indicated prior to radiation. Patients undergoing definitive radiation or adjuvant radiation may develop severe mucositis requiring the placement of gastric feeding tube for nutrition. Surgery may lead to loss of speech, swallowing dysfunction, permanent tracheostomy, and disfigurement. Swallowing impairment can lead to aspiration. Radiation can result in severe xerostomia.

Sarcoma

GENERAL PRINCIPLES

Epidemiology and Etiology

In the United States, approximately 14,000 patients will be diagnosed with sarcomas in the year 2015. Risk increases with age. Predisposing factors include prior radiation, chemical and chemotherapy exposure, genetic syndromes, Paget disease of the bone, HIV/human herpesvirus 8 (HHV8) infection (Kaposi sarcoma), and chronic lymphedema (lymphangiosarcoma, also known as Stewart-Treves syndrome).

Pathology

Soft tissue sarcomas consist of at least 50 different types of histologies. Review by a pathologist who has expertise in the diagnosis of sarcoma is recommended.

DIAGNOSIS

Clinical Presentation

Symptoms depend on the site of disease. Sarcomas arising in extremities can present as a painless soft tissue mass. Visceral sarcomas can be associated with GI bleeding, early satiety, dysphagia, dyspepsia, or vaginal bleeding. Retroperitoneal tumors can result in early satiety, nausea, paresthesias, or abdominal mass and pain.

Diagnostic Testing

Initial imaging studies include MRI for sarcomas involving the extremities or pelvis and CT for retroperitoneal and visceral sarcomas. PET/CT maybe helpful in high-grade sarcomas. Chest imaging with radiography and CT is important because the majority of sarcomas first metastasize to the lungs.

Treatment

Early stage (stages I–III)
- Surgical excision is the mainstay of therapy. Adjuvant radiotherapy is often indicated in patients with large (>5 cm) tumors and positive or equivocal margins when re-excision is not feasible.
- Although the role of neoadjuvant and adjuvant chemotherapy is controversial, patients should be seen in conjunction with a center that has extensive experience in the treatment of sarcoma.

Metastatic disease
- Palliative chemotherapy is the primary mode of treatment. Doxorubicin, ifosfamide, gemcitabine, docetaxel, dacarbazine, and pazopanib are commonly used.
- Metastasectomy can be considered in patients with oligometastatic disease to the lungs.
- **GI stromal tumor (GIST):** The most common site is stomach, followed by small bowel. Surgery should be performed if feasible. Most GISTs overexpress KIT and are highly responsive to imatinib. Adjuvant and/or neoadjuvant imatinib can be considered in select patients.

- **Ewing sarcoma:** This tumor is usually responsive to chemotherapy. Metastatic disease can be potentially cured with chemotherapy in a few cases.

GASTROINTESTINAL MALIGNANCIES

Esophageal Cancer

GENERAL PRINCIPLES

Epidemiology and Etiology

Esophageal cancer is estimated to account for nearly 15,590 deaths in the United States in 2015. Esophageal cancer is three to four times more common in men than in women. Risk factors include tobacco, alcohol, obesity, gastroesophageal reflux disease, Barrett esophagus, achalasia, and caustic injury.

Pathology

Adenocarcinomas are most common in the lower third of the esophagus and at the gastro-esophageal junction and have had a sharp increase in incidence over the last few decades in the United States. Squamous cell carcinomas are more common in the upper and middle esophagus.

DIAGNOSIS

Clinical Presentation

Patients usually present with progressive dysphagia and weight loss. Other symptoms include odynophagia, cough, regurgitation, and hoarseness.

Diagnostic Testing

- The diagnosis is usually established through upper endoscopy with biopsy.
- Staging workup includes CT of the chest and abdomen (with or without PET) to determine the presence of distant metastases. For patients without distant metastases, endoscopic ultrasonography (EUS) is required for the definition of tumor depth and lymph node status.
- Tumors located above the carina increase the risk of tracheoesophageal (TE) fistula formation and should be evaluated with bronchoscopy. Patients with TE fistulas often present with postprandial cough and aspiration pneumonias.

TREATMENT

- **Resectable disease:** Patients with resectable disease are candidates for esophagectomy with or without preoperative chemotherapy and radiation (*N Engl J Med 2012;366:2074*), depending on the extent of disease.
- **Unresectable primary disease:** Patients diagnosed with locally advanced disease are usually managed by concurrent chemoradiation.
- **Metastatic disease** is treated with palliative chemotherapy, usually with regimens including 5FU, platinum, and a taxane or anthracycline agent. Ramucirumab, an antibody against vascular endothelial growth factor receptor-2 (VEGFR-2), is approved for use in the second-line setting in combination with paclitaxel or as a single agent (*Lancet 2014;383:31*).
- **Trastuzumab** can be used in combination with chemotherapy in patients with *HER2*-amplified esophageal or gastroesophageal junction metastatic adenocarcinomas.

Gastric Cancer

GENERAL PRINCIPLES

Epidemiology and Etiology

The highest incidence rates for gastric cancer are in eastern Asia, eastern Europe, and South America, whereas the lowest incidence is in North America and Africa. Gastric cancer will account for an estimated 10,720 deaths in 2015 in the United States. Risk factors include *H. pylori* infection, previous partial gastrectomy for benign ulcer, achlorhydria associated with pernicious anemia, cigarette smoking, and blood group A. Hereditary diffuse gastric cancer is an inherited type of gastric cancer in families with germline *CDH1* (E-cadherin) mutations.

Pathology

More than 90% are adenocarcinomas. Tumors may be subdivided according to the Lauren classification into intestinal or diffuse types. Intestinal type is more common in older patients and has a better prognosis. Diffuse type, the most common subtype in the United States, is more prevalent in younger patients and is associated with a worse prognosis. Linitis plastica (leather bottle stomach) refers to a diffusely infiltrating type of gastric adenocarcinoma. Nearly 15–20% of patients with gastric cancer have *HER2* amplification or overexpression.

DIAGNOSIS

Clinical Presentation

The most common symptoms are weight loss, decreased appetite, and abdominal discomfort. Dysphagia may occur with gastroesophageal junction tumors, and persistent vomiting may occur if there is pyloric obstruction. Physical exam may show metastases to the left supraclavicular node (Virchow node) or periumbilical node (Sister Mary Joseph node).

Diagnostic Testing

Diagnosis is established by upper endoscopy. CT of the chest and abdomen should be obtained in all patients, and CT of the pelvis should be performed in women to exclude ovarian involvement (Krukenberg tumor). Other tests include *H. pylori* testing, EUS, and PET scan. Staging laparoscopy may be indicated prior to surgery in select patients for assessing peritoneal involvement.

TREATMENT

- Medically fit patients with resectable disease should undergo surgery. Chemotherapy or chemoradiation is commonly used, either before or after the resection, except in patients with very early stage disease.
- Patients with unresectable disease are treated with palliative chemotherapy. Trastuzumab can be used in combination with chemotherapy in patients with HER2-positive gastric cancers. Trastuzumab and anthracyclines should not be administered concurrently due to increased cardiotoxicity.
- Prophylactic total gastrectomy is recommended in carriers of *CDH1* germline mutations.

Colorectal Cancer

GENERAL PRINCIPLES

Epidemiology and Etiology

Colorectal cancer is the third most common malignancy worldwide. The incidence is higher in Western industrialized countries, with 93,090 cases estimated to be diagnosed in the United States in 2015. Although the incidence of colorectal cancer in adults age 50 years or older is declining, largely due to screening colonoscopy, the incidence among young adults (age 20–49 years) has increased over the last few decades. Risk factors include age >50 years, physical inactivity, obesity, diet with increased red meat and decreased fiber, personal history of polyps or colorectal cancer, inflammatory bowel disease, and hereditary syndromes such as Lynch syndrome and familial adenomatous polyposis (FAP).

DIAGNOSIS

Clinical Presentation

The most common symptoms include lower GI bleeding, abdominal pain, change in bowel habits, and obstruction. Patients can also rarely present with perforation, peritonitis, and fever. Any unexplained iron deficiency anemia should be evaluated with upper and lower endoscopy to evaluate for a GI malignancy. Colorectal carcinomas are also identified through screening colonoscopies.

Diagnostic Testing

- A thorough family history must be obtained to rule out a hereditary cancer syndrome, especially in younger (<50 years) patients.
- Diagnosis is typically made through colonoscopy with biopsy.
- Imaging studies include CT scan of the chest, abdomen, and pelvis. PET scan is not routinely indicated but is useful in patients being considered for definitive resection of oligometastatic disease.
- Additional studies include serum carcinoembryonic antigen (CEA) levels.

TREATMENT

- **Localized disease** should be treated with surgical resection. Adjuvant chemotherapy is indicated in patients with stage III disease and may also be beneficial in selected patients with stage II disease. The preferred regimen in the adjuvant setting includes 5FU (or capecitabine), leucovorin, and oxaliplatin (FOLFOX).
- **Unresectable metastatic disease** is treated with combination palliative chemotherapy, usually including 5FU plus leucovorin, capecitabine, and oxaliplatin (FOLFOX or XELOX), or irinotecan (FOLFIRI). The combination of bevacizumab, a vascular endothelial growth factor (VEGF) monoclonal antibody, and chemotherapy improves survival compared with chemotherapy alone. EGFR antibodies, cetuximab and panitumumab, are associated with improved outcomes when combined with chemotherapy in tumors lacking *KRAS* and *NRAS* gene mutations (*N Engl J Med 2013;369:1023*).
- **Surgical resection of metastatic disease**, with a curative intent, can be attempted in patients with a limited number of liver or lung metastases. Aggressive chemotherapy can be employed in selected patients initially presenting with unresectable liver metastases to achieve maximal response and make them eligible for resection.

Treatment of Rectal Cancer

Patients without metastatic disease should undergo endorectal ultrasound or pelvic MRI for the evaluation of tumor depth and lymph node status.
- **Early stage disease:** The treatment of choice is resection. Low anterior resection (LAR) is suitable for tumors located in the middle and upper third of the rectum, whereas abdominoperineal resection (APR) might be warranted in low-lying cancers. Preoperative radiation can be considered in low-lying cancers with an attempt to convert APR to a sphincter-preserving LAR.

- **Locally advanced disease:** These patients are usually treated with 5FU (or capecitabine)-based neoadjuvant chemoradiation followed by surgery and adjuvant chemotherapy (FOLFOX).
- **Metastatic disease:** The standard of care is palliative chemotherapy with the same drugs used in colon cancer.

Pancreatic Cancer

GENERAL PRINCIPLES

Epidemiology and Etiology

Pancreatic cancer is the fourth most common cause of cancer-related death in the United States, estimated to result in 40,560 deaths in 2015. Incidence increases with age, with median age at diagnosis between 60 and 80 years. Risk factors include cigarette smoking, obesity, inactivity, diabetes, chronic nonhereditary and hereditary pancreatitis, and inherited syndromes such as ataxia telangiectasia and hereditary intestinal polyposis syndrome (Peutz-Jeghers).

Pathology

Pancreatic adenocarcinoma is the most common subtype. Pancreatic neuroendocrine tumors are less common, associated with a better prognosis, and managed differently.

DIAGNOSIS

Clinical Presentation

Common symptoms include painless jaundice, anorexia, weight loss, and abdominal pain. Pancreatic cancer should be suspected when diabetes mellitus develops suddenly in patients older than 50 years.

Diagnostic Testing

Diagnosis is usually suspected by the presence of a pancreatic mass or dilated biliary duct on CT scan or ultrasound. Those without metastatic disease will require endoscopic retrograde cholangiopancreatography or EUS-guided FNA. Pancreatic protocol CT (triple-phase, contrast-enhanced, helical CT) with thin slices is often recommended to evaluate tumor resectability.

- Resectability is defined based on the extent of vascular involvement and often involves the absence of distant metastases, superior mesenteric artery encasement (more than half of vessel circumference), and direct involvement of celiac artery, hepatic arteries, and inferior vena cava.
- In case of metastatic disease, biopsy of the metastatic lesion is preferred.
- CA19-9 is not a reliable diagnostic marker because it can be elevated in patients with benign biliary obstruction and falsely low in 10% of patients who are Lewis-negative phenotypes.

STAGING

Based on imaging, pancreatic cancer is classified as resectable, borderline resectable, locally advanced, or metastatic disease. The definition of borderline resectability can be variable but usually involves focal abutment of vasculature by the pancreatic tumor.

TREATMENT

- **Resectable disease:** Surgical resection is the only potentially curative therapy, which is typically a pancreaticoduodenectomy (Whipple procedure). At presentation, only 15%

of patients present with resectable disease. Patients who have adequately recovered from surgery may benefit from adjuvant chemotherapy (usually including gemcitabine) and radiation because nearly 70% of patients will experience a distant relapse.

- **Borderline resectable and locally advanced disease:** For borderline resectable disease, induction chemotherapy and chemoradiotherapy are often used to induce response, which may increase the probability of resection with negative margins. For unresectable locally advanced disease, palliative chemotherapy with or without radiation is used for disease control.
- **Metastatic disease** is treated with palliative chemotherapy.
- FOLFIRINOX, a combination chemotherapy regimen consisting of oxaliplatin, irinotecan, 5FU, and leucovorin, is an option for use in patients with good performance status (*N Engl J Med 2011;364:1817*). The combination of gemcitabine with albumin-bound paclitaxel (nab-paclitaxel) can also be used in patients with good performance status. Patients who are unable to tolerate these regimens can be treated with single-agent gemcitabine.

Hepatocellular Carcinoma

GENERAL PRINCIPLES

Epidemiology and Etiology

An estimated 35,660 patients are estimated to be diagnosed with liver and intrahepatic bile duct tumors in 2015 in the United States. Risk factors include chronic viral hepatitis B or C, autoimmune hepatitis, nonalcoholic steatohepatitis (NASH), hemochromatosis, and cirrhosis (primary biliary or from other causes such as aflatoxin, alcohol, etc.). Most patients with hepatocellular carcinoma (HCC) have cirrhosis.

SCREENING

Patients with chronic hepatitis B (Asian males >40 years, Asian females >50 years, African or African American ethnicity, or family history of HCC) and all patients with cirrhosis irrespective of etiology are candidates for screening. Ultrasonography every 6–12 months is the preferred screening modality.

DIAGNOSIS

Clinical Presentation

Common symptoms include abdominal pain, anorexia with weight loss, jaundice, and vomiting. Invasion of the hepatic veins may cause Budd-Chiari syndrome, characterized by tender hepatomegaly and tense ascites. HCC should be suspected in patients with stable cirrhosis who decompensate rapidly. Most common paraneoplastic syndromes include hypoglycemia, hypercalcemia, dysfibrinogenemia, and erythrocytosis.

Diagnostic Testing

- The classic feature of HCC in CT is rapid enhancement during the arterial phase of contrast administration, followed by "washout" during the later venous phases. Lesions <1 cm have low probability of being HCC and should be followed with repeated imaging to detect growth suspicious of malignancy.
- Tumors that do not show the radiologic hallmarks for HCC may need biopsy for diagnosis.
- It is important to assess liver function in patients with HCC through scoring systems such as the Child-Pugh classification.

Treatment

- **Surgery** is the only curative option. Liver transplant should be considered in patients ineligible for surgery. To be deemed eligible for transplantation, patients are required to fulfill the Milan criteria, which include single tumor ≤5 cm or up to three tumors <3 cm, absence of macrovascular invasion, and absence of extrahepatic disease.
- **Other local therapies** such as percutaneous ethanol injection, radiofrequency ablation, cryoablation, transarterial chemoembolization, and radiation can be considered in select patients for palliation or to control tumor growth.
- **Chemotherapy** has minimal efficacy in HCC. Sorafenib is well tolerated and improves survival modestly compared to best supportive care (*N Engl J Med 2008;359:378*).

GENITOURINARY MALIGNANCIES

Renal Cancer

GENERAL PRINCIPLES

Epidemiology and Etiology

Renal cell carcinoma (RCC) is estimated to result in approximately 14,080 deaths in the United States in 2015. It is more commonly diagnosed in men, and the risk increases with age. Other risk factors include tobacco smoking, obesity, and hypertension.

Pathology

RCC is a malignancy of the renal parenchyma. Clear cell RCC is the most common subtype (80–85%), followed by papillary (15%) and chromophobe (5%) RCCs. Transitional cell (urothelial) carcinoma of the renal pelvis is treated as bladder cancer.

DIAGNOSIS

Clinical Presentation

Most patients in the United States are diagnosed by incidental findings on CT scan. The most common symptoms are anemia, hematuria, cachexia, and fever. The classic triad of flank pain, hematuria, and a palpable mass is uncommonly seen. Hypercalcemia is the most common paraneoplastic manifestation of RCC. Although erythrocytosis from erythropoietin production can be seen in RCC, anemia is more common. Stauffer syndrome refers to a paraneoplastic syndrome characterized by nonmetastatic hepatic dysfunction seen in RCC.

Diagnostic Testing

CT is usually sufficient for staging. MRI and magnetic resonance angiography (MRA) may be useful for further evaluation of the collecting system and inferior vena cava for involvement. The role of PET imaging is limited because normal renal tissue excretes fluorodeoxyglucose in the urine and has a high background activity. RCC often spreads to brain and bone, and thus, symptomatic patients should undergo additional imaging with CT, MRI, or bone scan to look for sites of metastasis. In patients without metastatic disease, resection can be both diagnostic and therapeutic.

TREATMENT

- **Localized disease:** The treatment of choice is surgery. A nephron-sparing approach (partial nephrectomy) can be considered if feasible.

- **Locally advanced disease:** The treatment of choice is radical nephrectomy, which involves removal of the Gerots fascia, perirenal fat, regional lymph nodes, and ipsilateral adrenal gland. There is no role for adjuvant therapy
- **Metastatic disease**
  - Surgery is an option in patients with oligometastatic disease. Cytoreductive nephrectomy followed by immunotherapy with interferon-α (IFN-α) can be considered in patients with resectable primary tumors and good performance status. Emerging data also suggest a benefit of cytoreductive surgery in patients treated with VEGF-targeted therapies, and randomized trials addressing this are ongoing.
  - Targeted agents approved for metastatic RCC include the VEGF inhibitors sunitinib, sorafenib, pazopanib, and axitinib, and the mammalian target of rapamycin (mTOR) inhibitors temsirolimus and everolimus. The choice of therapy depends on the histology, patient risk category, and adverse effect profile of targeted therapies.
  - **Immunotherapy** with high-dose interleukin (IL)-2 and IFN-α were predominantly used before the advent of targeted therapies. However, high-dose IL-2 should be considered in select patients with good performance status given the potential for durable cures in a small subset (approximately 5–15%) of patients. The role of newer immunotherapies targeting PD-1 and PD-L1 is actively being investigated (*N Engl J Med 2012;366:2443*).

Bladder Cancer

GENERAL PRINCIPLES

Bladder cancer is one of the more commonly diagnosed malignancies in the United States, with 74,000 estimated cases in 2015. Transitional cell or urothelial carcinoma is the most common histology. Tobacco smoking, chronic cystitis from long-term indwelling catheters, previous pelvic radiation or prolonged cyclophosphamide use, and exposure to benzene and other industrial chemicals are all risk factors. Bladder cancer is three times more common in men than in women, with a median age at diagnosis of 65. *Schistosoma haematobium* infection is linked to squamous cell bladder cancer.

DIAGNOSIS

Clinical Presentation

Most patients present with hematuria (microscopic or macroscopic). Lower urinary tract symptoms such as increased frequency, urgency, and dysuria can be seen in patients with bladder neck tumors.

Diagnostic Testing

The presence of >3 red blood cells per high-power field (HPF) is considered significant hematuria. Hematuria should be evaluated with urine cytology, upper tract imaging (IV pyelogram or CT), and cystoscopy with transurethral resection of bladder tumor (TURBT).

STAGING

Bladder cancers are broadly divided into non–muscle-invasive, muscle-invasive, and metastatic cancers. Cystoscopy with biopsies or TURBT determines the depth of invasion; imaging is not reliable to distinguish noninvasive from muscle-invasive disease in the majority of cases.

TREATMENT

The following describes treatment options by stage.

- **Superficial tumors** (no muscle invasion, stages 0–I) are treated with TURBT. Intravesicular bacille Calmette-Guérin (BCG) vaccine instillation reduces recurrence, and both induction and maintenance courses can be used. Intravesicular chemotherapy (typically mitomycin C) can be used in cases of BCG failure.
- **Muscle-invasive disease** is defined by the invasion of muscle or adjacent tissue (stages II and III). The treatment of choice is radical cystectomy with urinary diversion by creating an ileal conduit. Neoadjuvant chemotherapy has been shown to provide a survival benefit and should be considered in appropriate patients. For patients who cannot get neoadjuvant treatment, adjuvant chemotherapy can help reduce recurrences. Radiation, often with concurrent chemotherapy, is an alternative to surgery if resection cannot be performed.
- **Metastatic disease**, including node-positive or distant disease, is managed with chemotherapy, most commonly the combination of gemcitabine and cisplatin or methotrexate, vinblastine, doxorubicin, and cisplatin (MVAC).

Prostate Cancer

GENERAL PRINCIPLES

Epidemiology and Etiology

Prostate cancer is the most common cancer in men in the United States, with an estimated 220,800 new cases and 27,540 deaths in 2015. African American ethnicity, family history, and a high-fat/low-vegetable diet are a few predisposing risk factors.

Screening

The absolute risk reduction in mortality from annual prostate-specific antigen (PSA) is modest and should be discussed with patients older than 50 years of age with known risk factors. The USPSTF currently does not recommend annual PSA-based screening, although there are conflicting data from American and European trials looking at the benefit of prostate cancer screening.

DIAGNOSIS

Clinical Presentation

The most common presentation in the United States is asymptomatic elevation in PSA. Digital rectal examination (DRE) findings of asymmetric induration or nodules are suggestive, and any palpable nodule should be biopsied. Less common symptoms are obstructive symptoms, new-onset erectile dysfunction, hematuria, or hematospermia. Bone is the most common site of metastatic involvement, and patients with skeletal metastases can present with pain, fractures, and nerve root compression.

Diagnostic Testing

DRE supplemented by transrectal ultrasound helps in assessing T stage. PSA testing and Gleason scoring in the initial biopsy are important in staging and risk category assessment. Although patients with high-risk disease are likely to benefit from routine imaging (CT, MRI, or bone scan) for detection of metastatic disease, symptom-directed imaging is appropriate in patients with low-risk disease.

- Gleason grades range from 1 to 5. Grade 1 is assigned to well-differentiated and grade 5 to poorly differentiated gland pattern. **Gleason score** is the sum of the grades for the primary and secondary patterns seen on the biopsy.

- Risk categorization: Based on these characteristics, tumors are classified as low (PSA ≤10 ng/mL, Gleason score <7, and stage up to T2a), intermediate (PSA >10 to ≤20 ng/mL, Gleason score 7, and stage T2b), or high (PSA >20 ng/mL, Gleason score >7, and stage T2c) risk.

Staging

Early stage disease (T1–T2) is confined to the prostate, and locally advanced disease (T3–T4) is defined by local invasion. Stage IV disease is defined by nodal involvement and metastatic disease.

TREATMENT

The most important predictors of outcome are pretreatment PSA levels, Gleason score, and clinical TNM stage.

- **Early stage disease:** Outcomes are equivalent with radical prostatectomy, external-beam radiation, or brachytherapy. Late toxicities are variable but usually include incontinence and erectile dysfunction. Active surveillance is a suitable option for men with low-risk disease.
- **Locally advanced disease** is often treated with different combinations of surgical, radiation, and hormonal therapy. Surgery (if previous radiation), radiation (if previous prostatectomy), brachytherapy, and sometimes systemic hormonal therapy can be considered in patients who show an asymptomatic increase in PSA levels after surgery or radiation. Adjuvant or "salvage" radiation should be offered to patients with adverse pathologic features after prostatectomy even in the absence of a PSA recurrence.
- **Metastatic disease** is incurable and is initially treated with surgical or medical castration with an LHRH agonist or antagonist, termed androgen deprivation therapy (ADT), because testosterone/androgens play a major role in tumor growth. The antiandrogens flutamide or bicalutamide may be added for combined androgen blockade (CAB), which has shown marginal improvements in overall survival compared with LHRH monotherapy in meta-analyses. **Castration-resistant disease** is diagnosed in patients who experience disease progression on hormonal therapy. The term "castration resistance" does not necessarily imply complete resistance to therapies that block androgen stimulation. Chemotherapy with docetaxel, cabazitaxel, abiraterone, enzalutamide, radium-223, and sipuleucel-T are treatment options for these patients. Sipuleucel-T is an autologous cell-based vaccine targeting prostatic acid phosphatase.

Testicular Cancer and Germ Cell Tumors

GENERAL PRINCIPLES

Epidemiology

Testicular cancers are relatively rare tumors with about 8000 cases annually in the United States. However, they are the most common tumors diagnosed in men age 15–35 years. Nonseminomatous tumors are more common in younger men, whereas seminomas are more common after age 30 years. Incidence is higher in Caucasians than in patients of other ethnicities. Other risk factors include cryptorchidism and Klinefelter syndrome.

Pathology

Fifty percent of testicular cancers are seminomas, and the remainder are nonseminomas or of mixed histology. Nonseminomas include embryonal carcinoma, teratoma, chorio carcinoma, and yolk sac tumors. Pure seminomas carry a better prognosis compared to nonseminomas or mixed histology tumors.

DIAGNOSIS

Clinical Presentation

The most common presentation is that of a painless testicular mass, but patients can also present with testicular pain, hydrocele, or gynecomastia. Advanced testicular cancer can present with back or flank pain, fevers, night sweats, and weight loss.

Diagnostic Testing

Tumor markers, including α-fetoprotein (AFP), β-human chorionic gonadotropin (β-hCG), and lactate dehydrogenase (LDH), should be ordered. In patients with pure seminomas, AFP is not elevated; thus, elevated AFP suggests a focus of undetected nonseminoma. Preoperative CT of the abdomen and pelvis and CXR should be performed.

STAGING

Staging is based on TNM status and serum markers (S). In general, stage I represents disease confined to the scrotum, stage II indicates lymph node involvement, and stage III is defined by the presence of visceral metastases.

TREATMENT

- Stage I: The treatment of choice is orchiectomy. Adjuvant radiation to retroperitoneal nodes, retroperitoneal nodal dissection, chemotherapy with carboplatin, and active surveillance are possible adjuvant management approaches based on histology and other risk features such as lymphatic or vascular involvement.
- Stages II–III: Chemotherapy with BEP (bleomycin, etoposide, and cisplatin) results in high rates of cure, particularly in seminomas, and a minimum of three cycles is administered. Second-line chemotherapy regimens include VeIP (vinblastine, ifosfamide, cisplatin) and TIP (paclitaxel, ifosfamide, cisplatin). High-dose chemotherapy with stem cell therapy may be used in more advanced cases refractory to initial treatment.
- Sperm banking should be discussed with all patients prior to beginning treatment.

GYNECOLOGIC MALIGNANCIES

Cervical Cancer

GENERAL PRINCIPLES

Epidemiology and Etiology

Cervical cancer death rates have declined by almost 80% between 1930 and 2010 because of the widespread implementation of screening programs. In countries that lack a cervical cancer screening and prevention program, cervical cancer is the second most common cancer seen in women. The most important risk factor is persistent HPV infection, detected in >99% of tumors, usually HPV-16 and -18. Other risk factors include early onset of sexual activity, multiple sexual partners, high-risk partner, history of sexually transmitted disease, and chronic immunosuppression (HIV infection).

Pathology

The most common histology seen is squamous cell carcinoma followed by adenocarcinoma.

Prevention

The prophylactic quadrivalent HPV vaccine protects against types 6, 11, 16, and 18 (Gardasil), whereas the bivalent vaccine protects against HPV-16 and -18. Vaccinated women should continue routine Pap smears because the vaccine is not effective against all HPV subtypes. Cervical cancer screening should begin at age 21 years.

DIAGNOSIS

Clinical Presentation

Patients with early stage lesions are commonly asymptomatic and diagnosed incidentally on Pap smear, which underscores the importance of screening. Symptoms observed at presentation include irregular or heavy vaginal bleeding or postcoital bleeding. Patients with advanced disease may present with back pain, hematochezia from bowel involvement, or vaginal passage of urine or stool.

Diagnostic Testing

Diagnosis is obtained through cervical cytology and biopsy. A large cone biopsy is recommended in women without gross cervical lesions or with microinvasive disease to define depth of lesion. Clinical exam, CXR, IV pyelogram, proctosigmoidoscopy, and cystoscopy are required to assess International Federation of Gynecology and Obstetrics (FIGO) stage. CT, MRI, and PET imaging are used to guide treatment.

TREATMENT

Patients with early stage disease are treated with hysterectomy and/or pelvic radiation. Chemoradiation can be used in locally advanced tumors and as adjuvant therapy in high-risk patients following hysterectomy. Metastatic disease is treated with chemotherapy.

Endometrial Cancer

GENERAL PRINCIPLES

Epidemiology

Endometrial cancer is the most common gynecologic cancer in the United States, estimated to account for 54,870 new cases in 2015. Risk factors include obesity, unopposed estrogen, early menarche, late menopause, nulliparity, chronic anovulation, and tamoxifen use. Patients with hereditary cancer syndromes, such as Lynch syndrome, have increased incidence of endometrial cancer.

Pathology

There are two molecularly and morphologically distinct histologic subtypes:
• Type I: These are associated with exposure to unopposed estrogen (exogenous use, chronic anovulation, obesity, diabetes, nulliparity, and late menopause).
• Type II: These are more sporadic and not associated with the same risk factors as type I. These tumors show nonendometrioid histologies (serous, clear cell) and are associated with an aggressive behavior.

DIAGNOSIS

Clinical Presentation

The most common presentation is abnormal vaginal bleeding. Any vaginal bleeding in a postmenopausal woman, including spotting and staining, should be evaluated.

Diagnostic Testing

Tissue diagnosis is obtained through endometrial biopsy or through dilation and curettage. Cystoscopy, proctoscopy, and radiologic imaging might be necessary following clinical evaluation. Surgical exploration and staging are indicated in medically fit patients.

TREATMENT

- Surgery is indicated for staging and treatment.
- Patients with cervical extension (stage II) may benefit from adjuvant radiotherapy.
- Patients with extrauterine disease extension and those with distant metastases are treated with chemotherapy. Surgical cytoreduction prior to chemotherapy is a treatment option in a few women with metastatic disease.
- Chemotherapy, radiation, and hormone therapy are considered for patients in whom surgical staging and debulking is not feasible.

Ovarian Cancer

GENERAL PRINCIPLES

Epidemiology

Ovarian cancer is the leading cause of gynecologic mortality in the United States, with 14,180 deaths estimated in 2015. Risk factors include early menarche, late menopause, nulligravidity, family history, and familial syndromes including patients with *BRCA1* and *BRCA2* mutations and Lynch syndrome. Oral contraception use and pregnancy are associated with a low risk of ovarian cancer, suggesting a role for ovulation in malignant transformation.

Pathology

Most tumors are seen in patients between the ages of 40 and 65 years, and the majority of tumors are epithelial. Nonepithelial ovarian malignancies (germ cell, sex cord-stromal, and mixed) are seen in younger patients.

DIAGNOSIS

Clinical Presentation

Patients with early stage disease have nonspecific symptoms including bloating and abdominal discomfort. Patients usually have advanced disease at presentation and may have increasing abdominal girth, ascites, and abdominal pain.

Diagnostic Testing

- Cancer antigen 125 (CA-125) is elevated in most patients but is not specific.
- Surgical staging is an important aspect of management and is usually performed without prior histologic diagnosis for tumor debulking.

TREATMENT

- Stage I (without pelvic extension): Surgery is the preferred treatment.
- Stage II (extension to uterus, fallopian tubes, or other pelvic tissues): Treatment includes surgery and adjuvant chemotherapy.
- Stage III (peritoneal or lymph node involvement) and IV (distant metastasis): The treatment of choice is cytoreductive surgery and systemic chemotherapy with platinum and taxane agents administered intravenously (with or without intraperitoneal chemotherapy).

- Poly-ADP-ribose phosphorylase (PARP) inhibitors are associated with activity in patients with ovarian cancer carrying *BRCA* mutations. Olaparib is the first PARP inhibitor to be approved for use in ovarian cancer.
- **Germ cell ovarian cancers** are rare, typically occur in younger women, and are curable with chemotherapy.
- **Stromal tumors** usually present in early stages and are commonly cured with resection alone.

Cancer of Unknown Primary

GENERAL PRINCIPLES

Definition

Cancer of unknown primary site is defined as biopsy-proven malignancy for which the primary site of origin cannot be identified after a thorough history and physical examination, blood tests, and routine imaging studies.

Pathology

These malignancies are classified using light microscopy into adenocarcinoma (60%), poorly differentiated carcinoma/poorly differentiated adenocarcinoma (29%), squamous cell carcinoma (5%), poorly differentiated malignant neoplasm (5%), and neuroendocrine carcinoma (1%). Further identification usually requires specialized tests including IHC staining, electron microscopy, and genetic analysis.

DIAGNOSIS

In most cases, it is required to perform several studies to facilitate a diagnosis. Routine tests include pelvic and rectal examination, urinalysis, stool occult blood testing, and tumor marker testing in select patients (e.g., PSA in older men and β-hCG and AFP in younger men). CT of the chest, abdomen, and pelvis and symptom-oriented endoscopy are often warranted. PET scans are particularly useful in identifying the primary site in squamous cell carcinomas involving the cervical lymph nodes. IHC, electron microscopy, cytogenetic analysis for identifying characteristic abnormalities, and molecular profiling can yield important diagnostic clues and guide treatment.

TREATMENT

Treatment for favorable subgroups of patients with cancer of unknown primary is tailored to the likely primary site of origin (Table 22-5). Most patients who have unfavorable disease are treated with an empiric combination chemotherapy regimen, such as carboplatin and paclitaxel.

Melanoma

GENERAL PRINCIPLES

Epidemiology and Etiology

It is estimated that nearly 73,870 new cases of cutaneous melanoma will be diagnosed in 2015 in the United States. Lifetime risk of melanoma is higher among Caucasians (1 in 50) compared to African Americans (1 in 1000). Exposure to UV radiation, increased number of nevi (>50), history of >5 atypical nevi, large congenital nevi, immune suppression, and

TABLE 22-5	Treatment Recommendations for Selected Favorable Subgroups of Cancer of Unknown Primary
Subgroup	**Treat for**
Women with adenocarcinoma involving the axillary nodes	Stage II or III breast cancer
Women with papillary serous adenocarcinoma in the peritoneal cavity	Stage III ovarian carcinoma
Men with blastic bone metastases and elevated prostate-specific antigen	Prostate cancer
Men with poorly differentiated midline carcinoma	Extragonadal germ cell tumor
Squamous cell carcinoma of the cervical lymph nodes	Locally advanced head and neck cancer
Single metastasis	Local treatment with surgery or radiation therapy

familial risk (*CDKN2A* mutations) are known risk factors. Uveal (5%) and mucosal (1%) melanomas are rare.

Pathology

The most common types are superficial spreading (most common), nodular, lentigo maligna, acral lentiginous, and rare variants such as nevoid and desmoplastic. In most instances, histologic subtype does not influence staging or management (with the exception of desmoplastic melanoma, in which sentinel node biopsy may not be required). Breslow thickness, mitotic rate, ulceration, and presence or absence of disease at resection margins are important elements of histology that influence management and prognosis.

DIAGNOSIS

Clinical Presentation

Melanoma should be suspected in persons with pigmented skin lesions with **a**symmetry, **b**order irregularity, **c**olor variegation, **d**iameter >6 mm, or **e**volution (change in characteristics) (ABCDEs of melanoma). Patients can present with pigmented lesions that itch, bleed, or show ulceration at diagnosis. Desmoplastic melanoma can present as a firm cutaneous mass.

Diagnostic Testing

The workup often involves adequate sampling of the lesion, IHC for markers of melanocytic origin (e.g., S100, MART1, HMB45), and genotype testing for detection of mutations in the *BRAF* gene (the V600E variant in particular). Primary lesions >0.75 mm in Breslow thickness, with ulceration, ≥ 1 mitoses/mm^2, or lymphovascular invasion, require a sentinel lymph node biopsy. CT imaging of chest, abdomen, and pelvis with or without PET can be considered in patients with node-positive disease. Patients with metastatic disease require brain MRI.

TREATMENT

- **Localized disease:** The treatment of choice is resection with wide margins (0.5–2 cm depending on Breslow thickness). Patients with stage IIB–III benefit from adjuvant treatment with IFN-α2b. The role of newer therapies in the adjuvant setting is being investigated.
- **Metastatic disease:** There has been substantial progress in the management of metastatic melanoma.
  - *BRAF* **mutant:** About 50% of patients harbor the V600E mutation. These patients benefit from therapy with the BRAF inhibitors vemurafenib or dabrafenib, either alone or in combination with MEK inhibitors such as trametinib (*N Engl J Med 2015;372:30*).
  - **Immunotherapy:** Ipilimumab, an antibody against cytotoxic T-lymphocyte–associated protein 4 (CTLA4); nivolumab, a PD-1–directed antibody; and pembrolizumab, a PD-L1–directed antibody, are immunotherapies currently approved for use in patients with metastatic melanoma. Preliminary data support a role for concurrent therapy with nivolumab and ipilimumab (*N Engl J Med 2013;369:122*). Autoimmune endocrinopathies, pneumonitis, and colitis have been reported in patients treated with these drugs and may warrant treatment discontinuation if severe.

Central Nervous System Tumors

GENERAL PRINCIPLES

Epidemiology and Etiology

Brain and other central nervous system (CNS) tumors are estimated to be diagnosed in 22,850 patients in 2015. Ionizing radiation and familial cancer syndromes such as neurofibromatosis types 1 and 2, Li Fraumeni syndrome, and Von Hippel-Lindau syndrome are known risk factors.

Pathology

Meningiomas, gliomas, pituitary tumors, and embryonal tumors are the predominantly encountered primary CNS tumors in adults. The World Health Organization (WHO) classification further classifies gliomas based on their histology (e.g., astrocytoma, oligodendroglioma) and grade (I–IV).

DIAGNOSIS

Clinical Presentation

Patients with brain tumors typically present with a variety of symptoms ranging from headache, nausea, vomiting, seizures, and focal deficits to global neurologic dysfunction, based on the extent of mass effect and location of the tumor.

Diagnostic Testing

Workup includes MRI of the brain and molecular testing of the surgical biopsy or resected tumor specimen for *MGMT* methylation, 1p/19q co-deletion, and *IDH1* mutation, which may help guide therapy.

TREATMENT

- Gross total resection should be attempted in all patients, when possible. If resection is not feasible, a biopsy should be obtained for diagnosis and molecular testing.

- **Grade I tumors:** The treatment of choice is surgical excision.
- **Grade II tumors:** The treatment of choice is surgical excision. Recent data seem to favor treatment with adjuvant PCV (procarbazine, lomustine, and vincristine) and radiation in selected patients undergoing subtotal resection.
- **Grade III tumors:** The standard treatment is surgical excision followed by radiation and chemotherapy with either temozolomide or PCV.
- **Grade IV tumors/glioblastoma multiforme (GBM):** The treatment of choice is surgical excision or maximal debulking followed by concurrent chemoradiation with temozolomide and adjuvant temozolomide upon completion of chemoradiation. Bevacizumab is approved for recurrent GBM. Treatment is often individualized for elderly patients.
- **Meningioma:** Can be observed in asymptomatic patients for lesions that do not seem to be expanding. Surgical excision can be curative. Radiation is an option for inoperable tumors and in the adjuvant setting.

HEMATOLOGIC MALIGNANCIES

Myelodysplastic Syndrome

GENERAL PRINCIPLES

Epidemiology and Etiology

- Myelodysplastic syndromes (MDSs) comprise a heterogeneous group of myeloid neoplasms that are broadly characterized by cytopenias associated with a dysmorphic and usually cellular bone marrow and an increased risk of leukemic transformation. The median age at diagnosis is $\geq$65 years for de novo MDS. Cytopenias in MDS are due to clonal abnormalities of marrow cells affecting one or more cell lines. Therapy-related myeloid neoplasms, including acute myeloid leukemia (AML) and MDS, account for 10–20% of all myeloid neoplasms.
- Environmental factors such as exposure to chemicals, radiation, and chemotherapy, as well as genetic syndromes and benign hematologic disorders (such as paroxysmal nocturnal hemoglobinuria), have been associated with an increased risk of MDS.
- Chromosome abnormalities occur in up to 80% of cases, leading to accumulation of multiple genetic lesions, loss of tumor suppressor genes, and/or activating oncogene mutations.

Pathology

The current WHO classification system includes the following subclasses of MDS: refractory cytopenia with unilineage dysplasia (anemia, neutropenia, or thrombocytopenia); refractory cytopenia with multilineage dysplasia; refractory anemia with ring sideroblasts; refractory anemia with excess blasts (RAEB; 5–20%), which may be subdivided into RAEB-1 (5–9% blasts) and RAEB-2 (10–19% blasts); MDS with isolated deletion of 5q; and MDS unclassified.

DIAGNOSIS

Clinical Presentation

Symptoms can be related to bone marrow failure including fatigue, fever, bruising, or bleeding. Some cases are discovered incidentally through routine blood work. Leukopenia can be related to frequent infections. Sweet syndrome (acute febrile neutrophilic dermatosis) during the course of MDS may herald leukemic transformation.

Diagnostic Testing

Complete blood counts usually show anemia alone or as part of bicytopenia or pancytopenia. Macrocytosis is common. Platelet count can be normal or low. Peripheral blood smear can show dimorphic erythrocytes and large platelets. Neutrophils can be hypogranulated and have abnormally segmented nuclei (pseudo–Pelger-Huet cells). Obtaining a bone marrow aspirate and biopsy is important. The bone marrow is usually hypercellular. Cytogenetic analyses and FISH are required to identify chromosomal abnormalities, which aid in prognostication and planning therapy.

TREATMENT

- Therapy for MDS is generally unsatisfactory, and stem cell transplantation is the only curative option. A prognostic scoring system such as the Revised International Prognostic Scoring System (IPSS-R) (Table 22-6) is often used to determine patient risk category and influences treatment.
- Asymptomatic patients with low risk can be followed without specific therapy.
- Patients with very-low-risk or low-risk MDS and symptomatic anemia and a low erythropoietin level (<500 mU/mL) can be treated with erythropoiesis-stimulating agents. Treatment with immunosuppressive agents such as antithymocyte globulin and cyclosporine can be considered in patients with high erythropoietin levels. Patients who are young (age <60 years), have hypocellular MDS, express HLA-DR15, and demonstrate a paroxysmal nocturnal hemoglobinuria clone are more likely to respond to immunosuppression.
- Treatment with hypomethylating agents such as 5-azacytidine or decitabine can be considered in patients not suitable for immunosuppression. Treatment with 5-azacytidine has been associated with improved blood counts and a modest survival benefit compared to best supportive care.
- 5q-deleted MDS is associated with a good prognosis and higher probability of response to treatment with lenalidomide.
- Patients with high- and very-high-risk MDS are candidates for stem cell transplantation if eligible. Therapy with hypomethylating agents can be considered in those not eligible for transplant.

Acute Myeloid Leukemia

GENERAL PRINCIPLES

Epidemiology and Etiology

AML is the most common type of acute leukemia in adults. Median age at presentation is around 65 years. Risk factors are similar to those of MDS. Antecedent MDS increases the risk of AML.

Pathology

The current WHO classification (Table 22-7) includes the following categories: AML with recurrent genetic abnormalities; AML with MDS-related changes; therapy-related AML; AML, not otherwise specified (NOS); myeloid sarcoma; myeloid proliferations related to Down syndrome; and blastic plasmacytoid dendritic neoplasms.

The AML NOS category includes the French-American-British (FAB) subtypes M0 (AML minimally differentiated), M1 (AML without maturation), M2 (AML with maturation), M4 (acute myelomonocytic leukemia), M5 (acute monocytic leukemia), M6 (acute erythroleukemia), and M7 (acute megakaryoblastic leukemia). FAB subtype M3 (acute promyelocytic leukemia [APL]) is classified as AML with recurrent genetic abnormalities due to the presence of t(15;17).

TABLE 22-6 Revised International Prognostic Scoring System (IPSS-R) for Myelodysplastic Syndromes

Score	Cytogenetics	Marrow Blasts (%)	Hemoglobin (g/dL)	Neutrophils (× 10⁹/L)	Platelets (× 10⁹/L)
0	Very good: −Y, del(11q)	≤2	≥10	≥0.8	≥100
0.5				<0.8	50–99
1	Good: normal, del(5q), del(12p), del(20q), double including del(5q)	2.1–4.9	8–9.9		<50
1.5			<8		
2	Intermediate: del(7q), +8, +19, i(17q), any other single or double independent clones	5–10			
3	Poor: −7, inv(3)/t(3q)/del(3q), double including −7/del(7q), complex with 3 abnormalities	>10			
4	Very poor: complex with >3 abnormalities				

Total Score	Risk Category	Median Overall Survival (years)	Median Time to 25% Acute Myeloid Leukemia Risk (years)
≤1.5	Very low	8.8	NR
2.0–3.0	Low	5.3	10.8
3.5–4.5	Intermediate	3	3.2
5.0–6.0	High	1.6	1.4
>6.0	Very high	0.8	0.73

TABLE 22-7	Acute Leukemias with Recurrent Genetic Abnormalities
Acute Myeloid Leukemia	**Acute Lymphoblastic Leukemia (ALL)**
Recurrent genetic abnormalities	**Recurrent genetic abnormalities**
t(8;21); *RUNX1-RUNX1T1*	t(9;22); *BCR1-ABL*
inv(16) or t(16;16); *CEFB-MYH11*	t(V;11); *V/MLL* (*MLL* rearranged)
t(15;17); *PML-RARA*	t(12;21); *TEL/AML1* (*ETV6-RUNX1*)
t(9;11); *MLLT3-MLL*	t(1;19); *E2A-PBX1*
t(6;9); *DEK-NUP214*	t(5;14); *IL3-IGH*
inv(3) or t(3;3); *RPN1-EVI1*	ALL with hyperdiploidy
t(1;22); *RBM15-MKL1*	Hypodiploid ALL
Provisional entities at molecular level	
NPM1 mutated	
CEBPA mutated	

DIAGNOSIS

Clinical Presentation

Symptoms are usually related to bone marrow failure, including fatigue, fever, bruising, or bleeding. Most patients present with pancytopenia and circulating blast forms. Patients with a high blast percentage are at risk for leukostasis, manifested by dyspnea, chest pain, headaches, confusion, and cranial nerve palsies. Extramedullary tissue invasion by leukemic cells (most commonly with AML-M5) can result in hepatomegaly, splenomegaly, lymphadenopathy, rashes (leukemia cutis), gingival hypertrophy, CNS dysfunction, cranial neuropathies, or infiltrative masses (granulocytic sarcomas or chloromas).

Diagnostic Testing

In the WHO system, AML is defined by the presence of ≥20% blasts in the bone marrow and/or in the peripheral blood. AML with t(8;21), inv(16), and t(15;17) can be diagnosed irrespective of the blast percentage. Bone marrow specimens should be submitted for flow cytometry, molecular testing, and cytogenetics. This information is used to classify AML into prognostic groups and guide treatment (*Blood 2010;115:453*).

TREATMENT

- **Remission induction:** Induction chemotherapy consists of a 7 + 3 regimen that includes administration of cytarabine over 7 days in combination with an anthracycline (daunorubicin or idarubicin) on the first 3 days. Approximately 60–80% of AML patients achieve remission with induction chemotherapy. However, patients achieving remission eventually relapse without additional consolidation therapy.
- **Consolidation:** Options include high-dose cytarabine with or without subsequent stem cell transplantation. Optimal consolidation strategy is dependent on disease risk category (Table 22-8).
- Acute promyelocytic leukemia (AML-M3) is characterized by increased cure rates. Treatment includes the use of all-*trans*-retinoic acid (ATRA) and arsenic trioxide.

TABLE 22-8	Cytogenetic Abnormalities in Acute Myeloid Leukemia and Associated Prognosis	
Risk Group	**Cytogenetic and Molecular Features**	**Preferred Consolidation Strategy**
Favorable	t(15;17), t(8;21), inv(16). Mutated *NPM1* without mutated *FLT3*-ITD, or mutated *CEBPA*	Chemotherapy
Intermediate	Normal cytogenetics. Mutated *FLT3*-ITD, t(9;22)	Allogeneic transplant
Unfavorable	Complex karyotype (defined as ≥3 abnormalities, excluding the favorable-risk cytogenetics), monosomal karyotype, inv(3), t(6;9), *MLL* rearranged, del(5q), −5, −7, +8	Allogeneic transplant

Acute Lymphoblastic Leukemia

GENERAL PRINCIPLES

Epidemiology and Etiology

Acute lymphoblastic leukemia (ALL) is the most common childhood leukemia. The median age at presentation is 35 years with a bimodal distribution including one peak at 4–5 years and a second gradual increase after the age of 50 years. Advanced age is a poor prognostic factor.

Pathology

ALL can arise from B- or T-lymphocyte progenitors. The WHO classifies ALL into three categories: B cell with recurrent genetic abnormalities, T cell, and B cell, not otherwise specified (see Table 22-7).

DIAGNOSIS

Clinical Presentation

Symptoms include fatigue, fever, and bleeding. Leukostasis is uncommon, even with high white blood cell counts. Lymphadenopathy and splenomegaly are present in approximately 20% of cases. CNS may be involved at presentation, manifesting as headache or cranial nerve palsies.

Diagnostic Testing

Basic workup is similar to that required in AML. Immunophenotyping is often necessary to distinguish ALL from AML.

TREATMENT

• Several complex regimens such as the Berlin-Frankfurt-Munster (BFM); hyperfractionated cyclophosphamide, vincristine, doxorubicin, and dexamethasone (Hyper-CVAD); Cancer and Leukemia Group B (CALGB) 8811; and the German Multicenter ALL (GMALL) regimen have been described in ALL. Treatment is usually subdivided into induction, consolidation, and maintenance (usually administered over a course of 2 years) phases.

- Because of the high risk of CNS relapse, prophylactic intrathecal therapy is administered during the induction and consolidation phases.
- Allogeneic stem cell transplantation is an option in relapsed ALL and in patients with high-risk disease.

Chronic Myeloid Leukemia

GENERAL PRINCIPLES

Epidemiology and Etiology

Chronic myeloid leukemia (CML) accounts for nearly 14% of leukemias diagnosed in the United States, with a median age at diagnosis of 65 years.

Pathology

- CML is associated with the fusion of two genes, *BCR* on chromosome 22 and *ABL1* on chromosome 9, resulting in the *BCR-ABL1* fusion gene (Philadelphia chromosome). The fusion protein is associated with deregulated kinase activity.
- The natural history of CML is a triphasic process with a chronic phase, an accelerated phase, and a blast phase. Chronic phase is associated with an asymptomatic accumulation of differentiated myeloid cells in the marrow, spleen, and circulation. CML patients will invariably progress to accelerated and blast phases without treatment.

DIAGNOSIS

Clinical Presentation

Patients can present in any of three phases, although the majority present in the chronic phase of their illness. Symptoms are usually related to splenomegaly (pain, left abdominal mass, early satiety) or anemia. Peripheral blood counts show increased white blood cells with all levels of granulocytic differentiation, from myeloblasts to segmented neutrophils. Transformation from chronic phase to blast phase can be insidious through the accelerated phase or abrupt.

Diagnostic Testing

The presence of the *BCR-ABL1* rearrangement by cytogenetics, FISH, or polymerase chain reaction (PCR) in the peripheral blood or bone marrow confirms the diagnosis of CML. Quantitative PCR (qPCR) is performed prior to treatment initiation to establish a baseline and then every 3 months to monitor response to treatment.

TREATMENT

- Most patients are initially treated with oral TKIs such as imatinib, dasatinib, and nilotinib. The choice of agent typically depends on treatment-related adverse effects and patient preference. Phase III trials comparing second-generation TKIs (dasatinib or nilotinib) to imatinib as initial therapy for CML in chronic phase have demonstrated faster and deeper responses with the former.
- Complete hematologic remission (CHR) is defined as normalization of peripheral blood counts and absence of splenomegaly, whereas complete cytogenetic response (CCyR) is defined by the absence of Philadelphia chromosome metaphases on bone marrow cytogenetic analysis; major molecular remission (MMR) is defined by qPCR when *BCR-ABL1* transcripts in the peripheral blood are ≤0.1% on the International Scale (IS). Complete molecular remission (CMR) defined by the absence of *BCR-ABL1* transcripts by qPCR is a misleading term because a very low burden of malignant clone may still be present in

these patients, and therefore, it has been proposed to not use this term any more. CHR and/or *BCR-ABL1* transcripts in the marrow ≤10% (IS) by 3 months, CCyR and/or *BCR-ABL1* transcripts in the marrow ≤1% (IS) by 6 months, and *BCR-ABL1* transcripts in the marrow ≤0.1% (IS) by 12 months after starting a TKI constitute an optimal response to therapy (*Blood 2013;122:872*).

• Failure to achieve treatment milestones often requires switching therapies. Many patients who respond initially to first-line TKIs may eventually develop acquired resistance. For patients with resistance, ponatinib and omacetaxine are available, although they do not provide long-term disease control.

• Stem cell transplantation can be considered in patients who relapse after initial response to TKIs and/or who develop resistance to TKIs.

• Blast crises are more challenging to manage, and treatment often involves TKIs, chemotherapy, and stem cell transplantation.

Chronic Lymphocytic Leukemia

GENERAL PRINCIPLES

Epidemiology and Etiology

Chronic lymphocytic leukemia (CLL) is the most common form of leukemia in Western countries. CLL carries the highest familial risk of all hematologic malignancies, highlighting the importance of inheritable risk factors. Monoclonal B lymphocytosis (MBL) precedes the development of CLL with a rate of 1.1% per year. MBL is characterized by the presence of less than 5000 monoclonal B cells/μL with no other features of a lymphoproliferative disorder (*N Engl J Med 2008;359:575*).

Pathology

The diagnosis of CLL requires the presence of more than 5000 lymphocytes/μL and characteristic cell surface markers including the B-cell antigens CD19, CD20, and CD23. Of note, CD5, a T-cell antigen, is found in virtually all cases of CLL.

STAGING

The classification of CLL, based on the extent of systemic infiltration of lymphocytes, is used to determine the prognosis and initiation of treatment (Table 22-9). Molecular and cytogenetic markers have become increasingly useful for prognostication.

TABLE 22-9	Chronic Lymphocytic Leukemia Clinical Staging
Rai	**Binet**
Stage 0: Lymphocytosis	Stage A: Lymphocytosis
Stage 1: Lymphadenopathy	Stage B: Lymphadenopathy in ≥3 areas
Stage 2: Splenomegaly	Stage C: Hgb <10 g/dL or platelets <100,000/μL
Stage 3: Hgb <11 g/dL	
Stage 4: Platelets <100,000/μL	

Hgb, hemoglobin.

DIAGNOSIS

Clinical Presentation

Most patients are diagnosed while asymptomatic. When present, symptoms include fatigue, weight loss, lymphadenopathy, anemia, thrombocytopenia, and infections. Patients can also present with a hemolytic anemia, immune thrombocytopenia, or Richter syndrome, which is a malignant transformation of CLL to diffuse large B-cell lymphoma.

Diagnostic Testing

Flow cytometry aids in the identification of CLL surface markers on B cells. FISH of the peripheral blood for evaluating 17p, 11q, and 13q deletion, and trisomy 12, mutation status of Ig heavy chain variable region (IGHV), and assessing the expression of ZAP70 and CD38 are of prognostic importance.

TREATMENT

- Many patients do not require treatment at the time of initial diagnosis.
- **Active disease** as defined by the International Workshop on CLL is an indication for treatment. Active disease is characterized by progressive marrow failure, massive or symptomatic splenomegaly (>6 cm below costal margin) or lymphadenopathy (>10 cm in longest diameter), progressive lymphocytosis (>50% increase in 2 months or doubling time of <6 months), autoimmune anemia and/or thrombocytopenia that is poorly responsive to standard therapy, and the presence of constitutional symptoms (*Blood 2008;111:5446*).
- Treatment options include oral alkylating agents (chlorambucil, cyclophosphamide, bendamustine), purine analogues (fludarabine, cladribine), and monoclonal antibodies such as rituximab (anti-CD20), ofatumumab (anti-CD20), and alemtuzumab (anti-CD52), either as single agents or in combination. Idelalisib, a PI3K inhibitor, has been associated with improved survival and response rates in patients with relapsed CLL (*N Engl J Med 2014;370:997*).

Hairy Cell Leukemia

GENERAL PRINCIPLES

Epidemiology

Hairy cell leukemia is a rare disorder, most commonly seen in elderly men.

Diagnostic Testing

Peripheral blood leukocytes have the characteristic "hairy" appearance and are tartrate-resistant acid phosphatase (TRAP) positive. Flow cytometry is positive for CD20, CD11c, CD103, CD123, cyclin D1, and annexin A1. The majority of patients with hairy cell leukemia harbor the *BRAF* V600E mutation.

DIAGNOSIS

Clinical Presentation

Most patients present with malaise and fatigue. Splenomegaly and hepatomegaly may be evident on exam. With more advanced disease, pancytopenia develops, and patients may present with bleeding or recurrent infections.

TREATMENT

- The decision to treat is based on the development of cytopenias, symptomatic splenomegaly, constitutional symptoms, and recurrent infections.
- Cladribine and pentostatin are typically used for treatment. However, both of these agents induce significant and prolonged immunosuppression.

Hodgkin Lymphoma

GENERAL PRINCIPLES

Epidemiology and Etiology

The incidence of Hodgkin lymphoma (HL) follows a bimodal distribution with the first peak at age 25 years and second peak after the age of 50 years. EBV and HIV infections, autoimmune conditions, and immunosuppressant use have been described as risk factors for HL.

Pathology

- HL is subdivided into nodular lymphocyte predominant (NLPHL) and classical HL (nodular sclerosis, lymphocyte-rich, mixed-cellularity, lymphocyte-depleted) subtypes.
- The Reed-Sternberg (RS) cells consistently express the CD30 and CD15 antigens. CD30 is a marker of lymphocyte activation that is expressed by reactive and malignant lymphoid cells. CD15 is a marker of late granulocytes, monocytes, and activated T cells that is not normally expressed by cells of B lineage. In contrast to the other histologic subtypes, RS cells are infrequent in NLPHL. Instead, "popcorn cells" are seen within a background of inflammatory cells in NLPHL.

DIAGNOSIS

Clinical Presentation

Most patients present with painless lymphadenopathy. B symptoms are more common in advanced stages.

Diagnostic Testing

FNA is often inadequate to make a diagnosis, and an excisional biopsy may be required. Workup includes history and physical, complete blood cell counts, chemistry, LDH, erythrocyte sedimentation rate (ESR), CT, PET, and bone marrow exam.

STAGING

The Ann Arbor staging system classifies lymphomas into four stages (Table 22-10). Patients with early stage disease (stages I–II) are further stratified into favorable and unfavorable risk categories. Favorable risk is defined by the presence of not more than two sites of disease, mediastinal width less than one-third of maximal thoracic diameter, ESR <50 mm/h (30 mm with B symptoms), and absence of extranodal extension (*N Engl J Med 2010;363:640*).

TREATMENT

The treatment of choice for HL is chemotherapy with ABVD (doxorubicin, bleomycin, vinblastine, dacarbazine), with or without radiation, depending on the stage and risk category. Relapsed disease is treated with salvage chemotherapy with or without stem cell transplantation. Brentuximab vedotin, a CD30-directed antibody-drug conjugate, has been recently approved for treatment of refractory and relapsed HL.

TABLE 22-10	Ann Arbor Staging of Lymphomas[a]

Stage	Description
I	Involvement of a single lymph node region (I) or single extralymphatic organ (IE).
II	Involvement of ≥2 lymph node regions in the same side of the diaphragm.
III	Involvement of lymph node regions in both sides of the diaphragm.
IV	Diffuse or disseminated involvement of one or more extralymphatic organs.

[a]**Modifying features:** A, absence of B features; B, presence of B features; E, involvement of a single extranodal site contiguous or proximal to the involved nodal site; S, spleen involvement; X, bulky disease defined as lymph node ≥10 cm than one-third of mediastinum.

Non-Hodgkin Lymphoma

GENERAL PRINCIPLES

Epidemiology and Etiology

Non-Hodgkin lymphoma (NHL) is the fifth most common malignancy in the United States with an estimated 71,850 new cases in 2015. Risk factors include immunodeficiency, autoimmune disorders, bacterial infections (*H. pylori*, *Borrelia burgdorferi*, and *Chlamydia psittaci*), viral infections (HIV, EBV, HHV8, and human T-lymphotropic virus-1), and immunosuppression in the setting of previous transplantation.

Pathology

NHL may be broadly divided into indolent (e.g., follicular, marginal, small lymphocytic), aggressive (e.g., diffuse large B cell, mantle cell, peripheral T cell, anaplastic T cell), and very aggressive (Burkitt lymphoma, lymphoblastic) tumors. Several recurrent chromosomal abnormalities have been described in patients with NHL (Table 22-11).

DIAGNOSIS

Clinical Presentation

Clinical manifestations depend on the histologic subtype and can be characteristic in some rare subtypes of NHL. For instance, pruritic plaques can be seen in mycosis fungoides (a primary cutaneous T-cell NHL), marked hepatosplenomegaly in mantle cell lymphoma, and isolated splenomegaly in splenic marginal zone lymphomas.

Diagnostic Testing

Essential workup often includes history, physical exam, complete blood cell count, chemistry, PET/CT, and bone marrow biopsy. The CSF evaluation is indicated in patients with high-grade lymphomas, HIV-related lymphomas, and involvement of the epidural space, nasopharynx, and paranasal sinuses. Patients suspected to have primary CNS lymphomas require an ophthalmologic exam. Occasionally, patients with aggressive lymphomas can present with a spontaneous tumor lysis syndrome (TLS) (Table 22-12).

STAGING

Patients are staged by the Ann Arbor classification. Patients with aggressive lymphoma are usually stratified according to the International Prognostic Index, which uses five adverse

TABLE 22-11	Selected Chromosomal Abnormalities in B-Cell Non-Hodgkin Lymphomas	
Cytogenetic Abnormality	**Histology**	**Oncogene**
t(14;18)	Follicular, DLBCL	*BCL2*
t(11;14)	Mantle cell	Cyclin D1
t(1;14)	MALT lymphoma	*BCL10*
t(11;18)	Marginal zone/extranodal marginal zone	
t(2;5)	ALK-positive anaplastic large-cell lymphoma	*ALK*
t(9;14)	Lymphoplasmacytic lymphoma	
8q24 translocations t(8;14) t(2;8) t(8;22)	Burkitt lymphoma	*MYC*

DLBCL, diffuse large B-cell lymphoma; MALT, mucosa-associated lymphoid tissue.

prognostic factors: age >60 years, Ann Arbor stage III or IV, abnormal serum LDH, two or more extranodal sites involved, and Eastern Cooperative Oncology Group performance status of ≥2. Five-year survival rates for patients with 0–1, 2, 3, or 4–5 risk factors are 73%, 51%, 43%, and 26%, respectively (*N Engl J Med 1993;329:987*).

TREATMENT

Indolent Lymphomas
Stage I–II
- Observation, involved-field radiotherapy (IFRT), single-agent rituximab, rituximab with chemotherapy, and combined-modality therapy with rituximab, chemotherapy, and IFRT are all options.
- Gastric mucosa-associated lymphoid tissue (MALT) lymphomas are related to *H. pylori* infection and respond well to *H. pylori*–directed therapy (*Gut 2012;61:507*).

TABLE 22-12	Defining Features of Tumor Lysis Syndrome
Manifestation	**Features**
Laboratory	1. Uric acid ≥8 mg/dL or 25% increase from baseline 2. Potassium ≥6 mEq/dL or 25% increase from baseline 3. Phosphorus ≥6.5 mg/dL or 25% increase from baseline 4. Calcium ≤7 mg/dL or 25% decrease from baseline
Clinical	1. Creatinine ≥1.5× upper normal limit 2. Cardiac arrhythmia or sudden death 3. Seizure

Gastric MALT lymphomas that do not respond to or relapse after *H. pylori* therapy, and other isolated extranodal lymphomas (salivary gland, breast, conjunctiva) may be treated with IFRT.

Stage III–IV

There is no convincing evidence to support early intervention versus "watchful waiting" in asymptomatic patients (*Lancet Oncol 2014;15:424*). Older patients with low-volume disease and no symptoms can be observed. A combination of rituximab and chemotherapy or single-agent rituximab can be used for treatment.

Relapsed disease

First-line therapy can be repeated in patients who were in first remission for >1–2 years. Radioimmunotherapy (RIT) with ibritumomab (anti-CD20 antibody conjugated with yttrium-90), idelalisib, lenalidomide, and stem cell transplant are all effective options.

Aggressive Lymphomas

Diffuse Large B-Cell Lymphoma

Stage I–II

Limited-stage disease is managed with chemotherapy (rituximab, cyclophosphamide, doxorubicin, vincristine, and prednisone [R-CHOP]) with or without IFRT.

Stage III–IV

- Patients beginning therapy for aggressive lymphomas should be monitored closely for signs of TLS and should receive adequate IV hydration and appropriate prophylaxis with allopurinol and/or rasburicase.
- Chemotherapy with R-CHOP is the standard. Patients with *MYC* translocations, especially those with "double-hit" lymphomas (combined translocations of *MYC* and either *BCL2* or *BCL6*), have significantly worse outcomes.
- **CNS prophylaxis** with intrathecal chemotherapy or high-dose methotrexate should be considered for patients with testicular, orbital, epidural, paranasal sinus, or extensive bone marrow involvement with elevated LDH.
- Primary CNS lymphoma is treated with complex regimens that usually incorporate high-dose methotrexate, cytarabine, and rituximab with consideration for consolidation with stem cell transplantation (*J Clin Oncol 2013;31:3061*). Whole-brain radiation alone is reserved for elderly patients who are ineligible for aggressive chemotherapy.

Burkitt Lymphoma

Burkitt lymphomas are usually treated with complex multidrug protocols and CNS prophylaxis.

Mantle Cell Lymphoma

Chemotherapy regimens such as rituximab plus Hyper-CVAD alternating with high-dose methotrexate and cytarabine, or brentuximab and rituximab are often used. Consolidation with stem cell transplantation can be considered in first remission. Maintenance rituximab is considered in select patients.

Relapsed disease

- Younger patients without significant comorbidities are candidates for stem cell transplantation at relapse. Several effective salvage regimens such as ICE (ifosfamide, carboplatin, etoposide), DHAP (dexamethasone, cisplatin, cytarabine), and ESHAP (etoposide, methylprednisone, cytarabine, cisplatin) are available. Rituximab can be added to patients with B-cell lymphomas.
- Allogeneic transplantation should be considered in patients with relapsed Burkitt or lymphoblastic lymphoma, refractory disease at relapse, or a duration of remission of <1 year after initial therapy.

Multiple Myeloma

GENERAL PRINCIPLES

Multiple myeloma (MM) is the second most frequent hematologic malignancy after NHL. The median age at diagnosis is 66 years. A small percentage of cases are familial.

DIAGNOSIS

Clinical Presentation

The most common presentation is anemia. Patients can also have bone pain, renal failure, fatigue, elevated creatinine, weight loss, and hypercalcemia. Patients with extramedullary plasmacytomas can present with radiculopathy, cord compression, or CNS involvement.

Diagnostic Testing

Initial evaluation includes routine blood work, β_2-microglobulin (B2M), serum and urine protein electrophoresis, serum free light chain estimation, skeletal survey, and bone marrow exam. The diagnosis is confirmed by the presence of 10% or more clonal plasma cells in the bone marrow or a biopsy-proven plasmacytoma, with evidence of end-organ damage (hypercalcemia, renal dysfunction, anemia, or bone lesions). A clonal marrow plasma cell percentage of ≥60%, κ or λ free light chain ratio of ≥100, and the presence of one or more focal lesions on MRI are also criteria for diagnosis of myeloma because they are associated with a high risk of progression to end-organ damage (*Lancet Oncol 2014;15:e538*).

STAGING

- The International Staging System for MM uses B2M and albumin to stratify patients into: stage I (B2M <3.5 mg/dL and albumin >3.5 g/dL), stage II (albumin <3.5 g/dL or B2M 3.5–5.5 mg/dL), and stage III (B2M >5.5 mg/dL).
- Cytogenetic features (Table 22-13) can be used for risk stratification and guiding treatment (*Am J Hematol 2014;89:999*).

TREATMENT

- Transplant-eligible patients are offered autologous stem cell transplantation following approximately 4 months of treatment with one of the previously mentioned regimens,

TABLE 22-13	Risk Stratification in Myeloma Based on mSMART (Mayo Stratification for Myeloma and Risk-Adapted Therapy) Model	
Standard Risk	**Intermediate Risk**	**High Risk**
Trisomies, t(11;14), and t(6;14)	t(4;14), 1q gain, deletion 13, hypodiploidy, complex karyotype	17p del, t(14;16), and t(14;20) High-risk gene expression profile signature

Adapted from Mikhael JR1, Dingli D, Roy V, et al. Management of newly diagnosed symptomatic multiple myeloma: updated Mayo Stratification of Myeloma and Risk-Adapted Therapy (mSMART) consensus guidelines 2013. *Mayo Clin Proc.* 2013;88(4):360–76.

whereas initial therapy is continued for 12–18 months in transplant-ineligible patients.
* Maintenance therapy with either lenalidomide or bortezomib is considered following initial therapy based on the patient's risk category.

Principles of Stem Cell Transplantation

GENERAL PRINCIPLES

Background
* Hematopoietic stem cell transplantation (HSCT) involves the infusion of either allogeneic (different donor) or autologous (patient's own) stem cells following administration of intense chemotherapy and/or radiation.
* Autologous transplantation involves collection, cryopreservation, and reinfusion of a patient's own stem cells. This allows administration of myelosuppressive doses of chemotherapy with the intent of maximizing the efficacy of therapy.
* Allogeneic transplantation refers to the infusion of stem cells collected from either HLA-matched or -mismatched donors. In addition to facilitating the administration of high doses of chemotherapy, allogeneic transplantation also allows for an immunologic effect mediated by donor T and natural killer (NK) cells (graft-versus-tumor effect).

Indications
* Stem cell transplantation can be considered for patients with progressive or residual disease that is thought to be chemoresponsive or susceptible to graft-versus-tumor effect. MM and lymphoma are the most common indications for autotransplantation, whereas MDS and leukemia are the most common indications for allotransplantation.
* Allogeneic transplantations are also considered in other nonmalignant disorders, such as congenital immune deficiencies, sickle cell anemia, thalassemia, and inborn errors of metabolism.

Donor Selection
Appropriate donor selection is crucial and is based on the following factors:
* HLA typing: Major histocompatibility class I and II alleles code for HLA proteins that are expressed on the cell surface and play a major role in immune recognition. High-resolution typing of 10 HLA alleles (e.g., HLA-A, HLA-B, HLA-C, HLA-DRB1, and HLA-DQB1) is the current standard.
* The chance of any given sibling being a full HLA match is only 25%. Patients who lack HLA-identical siblings should have a search for HLA-matched donors through the National Marrow Donation Program (NMDP), although chances of finding an HLA-matched unrelated donor is significantly influenced by the patient's ethnicity.
* Partial HLA-mismatched transplantations, umbilical cord blood, and haploidentical transplantations (3/6 match) are alternate sources of marrow for patients without matched sibling or unrelated donors
* Cytomegalovirus (CMV)-negative donors are preferred for CMV-negative patients.

Source of Stem Cells
* Bone marrow can be obtained under anesthesia through repeated aspirations from the iliac crest.
* Stem cells can be collected from peripheral blood by leukopheresis after mobilization with granulocyte colony-stimulating factor (G-CSF) and plerixafor (CXCR4 antagonist).

Complications

- Hematopoietic transplantation is often preceded by the use of intense chemotherapy and sometimes total-body radiation to clear residual disease and immunosuppress the host. Depending on the extent of myelosuppression achieved as a result of this conditioning, regimens are classified as myeloablative, reduced intensity, or nonmyeloablative.
- **Graft-versus-host disease (GVHD):** Occurs when the donor T cells react with recipient tissues, leading to acute and/or chronic inflammation. The most common tissues affected are the skin, liver, gut, cornea, and lungs. Acute and chronic GVHD are associated with significant morbidity and mortality in allogeneic transplantation patients. Chronic GVHD can result in diarrhea and sclerodermatous-type skin changes. The prophylaxis and treatment of GVHD include the use of corticosteroids and a myriad of immunosuppressants including cyclosporine, methotrexate, sirolimus, mycophenolate, and tacrolimus.
- **Infections:** Due to the intense conditioning and heavy immunosuppression, transplant patients are susceptible to a variety of infections in the peritransplant setting. The postengraftment period is complicated by susceptibility to CMV, *Pneumocystis jirovecii* pneumonia, and *Aspergillus* infections.

ONCOLOGIC EMERGENCIES

The most common oncology emergencies are febrile neutropenia, TLS, malignant hypercalcemia, spinal cord compression, superior vena cava syndrome, and brain metastases with increased intracranial pressure (Table 22-14).

Febrile Neutropenia

GENERAL PRINCIPLES

- Febrile neutropenia (FN) is defined as an absolute neutrophil count (ANC) of $<500/\mu L$, with a single core temperature of $>38.3°C$ or a persistent temperature (>1 hour) of $>38.0°C$.
- Risk of FN is proportional to the duration of neutropenia.
- Although most solid tumor chemotherapy regimens are associated with a brief (<5 day) duration of neutropenia, neutropenia with leukemia and transplantation regimens can be more persistent.
- Risk is also increased with regimens that cause mucositis (inflammation and ulceration of the oral and GI mucosa).

DIAGNOSIS

- Evaluation should include a complete physical exam including assessment of catheter sites, perianal region, and mucosal surfaces. DRE should not be performed, considering the potential risk for bacterial translocation.
- Cultures of blood and urine and CXR in all patients, along with stool and sputum cultures in symptomatic patients, should be obtained.

TREATMENT

- Emergent IV antibiotic therapy is critical to prevent life-threatening sepsis.
  - Antibiotics with coverage of gram-negative bacilli (including *Pseudomonas aeruginosa*) must be used.
  - Empiric coverage of methicillin-resistant *Staphylococcus aureus* (MRSA) with vancomycin or linezolid is not recommended unless patients are unstable or have active oral mucositis, evidence of a catheter-related infection, or a recent infection with MRSA.

TABLE 22-14	Oncologic Emergencies		
Emergency	**Etiology**	**Presentation**	**Management**
Neutropenic fever	Infectious	Temperature >38.3°C or >38°C two times 1 h apart	1. Antibiotic coverage: gram-negative with pseudomonal activity, and gram-positive if risk factors (catheters, pneumonia, mucositis, *Staphylococcus* colonization, sepsis), and also fungal if unstable 2. IV hydration and supportive care as appropriate
Tumor lysis syndrome (TLS)	Massive lysis of cancer cells (mostly with chemotherapy)	Hyperuricemia, hyperkalemia, hyperphosphatemia, hypocalcemia, AKI, cardiac arrhythmias, and/or seizures	1. Prevention with IV fluids and prophylactic allopurinol or rasburicase based on estimated risk of TLS 2. Treatment: Aggressive hydration, rasburicase, dialysis
Hypercalcemia	Humoral, PTHrP, bone metastasis, calcitriol mediated (lymphomas)	Dehydration, CNS symptoms, constipation, ileus, weakness, cardiac (bradycardia, short QT, prolonged PR, etc.)	1. IV hydration 2. Bisphosphonates or denosumab (if low creatinine clearance) 3. Calcitonin (if symptomatic, rapid onset) 4. Steroids can be useful
Spinal cord compression (SCC)	Metastatic or involvement of spine in SCC	SCC: pain, weakness, sensory loss, incontinence, ataxia	1. Steroids 2. Neurosurgery consultation 3. RT 4. Chemotherapy can be considered in few cases of SCC

Superior vena cava (SVC) syndrome	Obstruction of SVC by primary or metastatic cancer (mostly intrathoracic)	Dyspnea, stridor (laryngeal edema), facial and upper extremity swelling, risk of cerebral edema and herniation	1. Histologic diagnosis is important 2. Consider upfront endovascular stent and RT if comatose or respiratory compromise 3. Treatment depends on tumor type: SCLC, lymphoma, germ cell: chemotherapy; NSCLC: RT; thymic tumors: surgery
Hyperleukocytosis with leukostasis	Intravascular accumulation of blasts, with or without DIC	Chest pain, respiratory distress, stupor, TLS, DIC	1. Leukapheresis: symptomatic patients (count threshold AML $>50 \times 10^3/\mu L$, ALL and CML $>150 \times 10^3/\mu L$, CLL $>500 \times 10^3/\mu L$); asymptomatic patients (AML $>100 \times 10^3/\mu L$, ALL $>200 \times 10^3/\mu L$) 2. Hydroxyurea for cytoreduction

AKI, acute kidney injury; ALL, acute lymphoblastic leukemia; AML, acute myeloid leukemia; CLL, chronic lymphocytic leukemia; CML, chronic myeloid leukemia; CNS, central nervous system; DIC, disseminated intravascular coagulation; NSCLC, non–small-cell lung cancer; PTHrP, parathyroid hormone–related protein; RT, radiotherapy; SCLC, small-cell lung cancer.

- Antimicrobial regimen should be tailored to treat the source of infection, if one is identified.
- Empiric antifungal therapy should be considered if fever persists for >72 hours.
- Gram-negative coverage should continue until ANC is >500/µL.
- Low-risk patients (afebrile for 24 hours after antibiotics, negative culture results, and expected duration of myelosuppression for <1 week) can be treated as outpatients with oral, broad-spectrum antibiotics such as fluoroquinolone, amoxicillin/clavulanic acid, or trimethoprim-sulfamethoxazole.
- Consuming raw fruits and vegetables is not associated with excessive risk for infection in neutropenic patients.
- White cell growth factors
  - G-CSF is the most commonly used growth factor and is given SC in doses of 5 µg/kg/d.
  - Although growth factors can reduce the duration of hospitalization for FN, they have not been shown to improve survival.
  - Growth factors should not be given within 24 hours after chemotherapy or during radiation because of the potential for increased myelosuppression.
  - Prophylactic growth factors are used when the predicted risk of FN is high and the neutropenia is predicted to result in chemotherapy delays.

Tumor Lysis Syndrome

GENERAL PRINCIPLES

- TLS is a group of metabolic disturbances resulting from significant tumor breakdown with release of intracellular products into the circulation.
- TLS occurs in tumors that grow rapidly and are sensitive to cytotoxic chemotherapy. The risk of TLS is high in patients with acute leukemias and high-grade lymphomas, bulky tumors, elevated pretreatment LDH and uric acid levels, and renal dysfunction.
- TLS can also be spontaneous (not treatment related).

DIAGNOSIS

TLS is characterized by the presence of certain laboratory and clinical criteria (see Table 22-14).

TREATMENT

- The most important intervention to prevent TLS is aggressive hydration to maintain a urine output of at least 100 mL/m^2/h.
- Prophylactic strategies include the use of the xanthine oxidase inhibitor allopurinol prior to treatment initiation.
- Rasburicase is a recombinant enzyme that degrades uric acid that can be used for the prophylaxis and treatment of hyperuricemia. It is indicated in patients with an elevated uric acid level prior to treatment initiation and those at a high risk for developing hyperuricemia (predicted based on tumor type, tumor burden, and pretreatment LDH level).
- Hyperkalemia is an immediate threat and should be treated aggressively.
- Calcium administration should be restricted in symptomatic patients with hypocalcemia or hyperkalemia to prevent risk of metastatic calcification in the setting of hyperphosphatemia.
- Hyperphosphatemia should be treated with phosphate binders.
- Patients with persistent electrolyte abnormalities (hyperkalemia, hyperphosphatemia, and high calcium-phosphate products) and a pronounced decrease in urine output require renal replacement therapy.

Malignant Hypercalcemia

GENERAL PRINCIPLES

- Malignant hypercalcemia is a common paraneoplastic syndrome and occurs in nearly 10–20% of cancer patients.
- A serum total calcium level of >10.5 g/dL is generally considered elevated. Measuring ionized calcium can be necessary and helpful in patients with abnormal serum albumin levels.
- Osteolysis and humoral hypercalcemia through tumor production of parathyroid hormone (PTH), PTH-related protein (PTHrP), or vitamin D analogs are the predominant mechanisms of hypercalcemia.

DIAGNOSIS

Classic symptoms usually develop with total calcium levels above 12 mg/dL and include polyuria, polydipsia, anorexia, constipation, nausea, vomiting, and confusion. Patients are usually severely hypovolemic due to excessive fluid losses and limited intake.

TREATMENT

- Aggressive hydration with normal saline is important. Diuretics should not be used unless volume overload is present.
- IV bisphosphonates, pamidronate 90 mg or zoledronic acid 4 mg, inhibit bone resorption and are used in the management of severe or symptomatic hypercalcemia. Zoledronic acid is contraindicated in patients with severe renal dysfunction.
- Calcitonin can be used in patients with severe symptomatic hypercalcemia for short-term and immediate control of calcium levels.
- Hypercalcemia caused by tumor production of vitamin D analogs may respond to corticosteroids.

Malignant Spinal Cord Compression

GENERAL PRINCIPLES

Malignant spinal cord compression (MSCC) affects approximately 5–10% of patients with cancer and is commonly seen in patients with lung, breast, prostate, and lymphoid malignancies.

DIAGNOSIS

- The study of choice for MSCC is MRI of the entire spine.
- Most patients present with back pain and local tenderness in the involved region. Pain is worse in a recumbent position and aggravated by sneezing, coughing, or bearing down (Valsalva maneuver). Other symptoms include weakness, sensory loss, and bladder or bowel incontinence.
- Timely diagnosis and intervention are crucial to prevent permanent neurologic damage.

TREATMENT

- Patients suspected of having MSCC should be started on glucocorticoids. Treatment should not be delayed for imaging. The most commonly used corticosteroid regimen is a 10-mg dexamethasone loading dose, followed by 4 mg every 4–6 hours.

- Consultation from surgical and radiation oncology services should be obtained in a timely fashion. Outcomes are better with surgery compared to radiation therapy in patients who are surgical candidates.
- Systemic chemotherapy can be used to treat patients with chemosensitive tumors.

Superior Vena Cava Syndrome

GENERAL PRINCIPLES

- Cancer-related superior vena cava (SVC) syndrome results from obstruction of blood flow through the SVC through invasion, external compression, or thrombosis in the setting of a malignancy.
- The severity and rapidity of symptom onset depends on the rate at which the SVC is occluded and if there has been enough time for collateral venous drainage to develop.
- Lung cancer, lymphomas, thymic neoplasms, germ cell tumors, mesothelioma, and other solid tumors that cause mediastinal involvement are the cancers that are commonly associated with SVC syndrome.

DIAGNOSIS

- Symptoms can range from asymptomatic interstitial edema of the head and neck to life-threatening complications, such as airway narrowing from upper airway or laryngeal edema and cerebral herniation and ischemia secondary to cerebral edema, as a consequence of venous outflow obstruction.
- Facial plethora, cyanosis, and arm edema are often observed. Physical exam can show presence of venous collaterals on the chest and neck. Close attention should be paid to detect stridor, headaches, or confusion.
- Contrast-enhanced CT scan of the chest allows identification of the underlying cause and level of obstruction.

TREATMENT

- Management of SVC depends on the presentation and underlying malignancy. Patients presenting with stridor from laryngeal edema and stupor from cerebral edema need emergent management with stent placement and/or radiation. Upfront radiation prior to obtaining a histologic diagnosis in patients who are stable can obscure a pathologic diagnosis and should not be pursued.
- Steroids have a role in the management of patients with steroid-responsive tumors such as lymphomas and thymomas. Their role in the management of other cancers is unclear and not recommended. Although steroids have anecdotally been used to control edema in patients with airway obstruction, they have not been systematically studied for use in this setting.
- Every effort should be made to obtain a pathologic diagnosis in a timely fashion because this information is crucial to plan management. Chemotherapy is the treatment of choice for patients with cancers such as SCLC, lymphomas, and germ cell tumors that tend to be chemosensitive.
- Stent placement and radiotherapy may be required for management and symptom relief of SVC syndrome in patients with less chemoresponsive tumors such as NSCLC. Anticoagulation is indicated in patients with SVC thrombosis.

Hyperleukocytosis with Leukostasis

Hyperleukocytosis refers to an elevated white blood cell count (often $>100 \times 10^9/L$) as a result of leukemic proliferation. Leukostasis is a medical emergency as a result of hypoperfusion due to the elevated blast count. The clinical features and emergent management of leukostasis have been summarized in Table 22-14.

Brain Metastases with Increased Intracranial Pressure

GENERAL PRINCIPLES

* Brain metastases are common in patients with malignancies. Patients with lung cancer, breast cancer, and melanoma have the highest incidence of brain metastases.
* Most lesions are supratentorial and located at the junction of gray and white matter.

DIAGNOSIS

* Headache, confusion, and focal neurologic deficits are the most common symptoms. However, nearly a third of these patients can be asymptomatic.
* CT scan of the head with IV contrast or a brain MRI is required for diagnosis.

TREATMENT

* Increased intracranial pressure from peritumoral edema or hemorrhage can lead to cerebral herniation and death in untreated patients.
* Symptomatic treatment with dexamethasone at an initial dose of 10 mg, followed by 4 mg every 6 hours, usually relieves symptoms.
* Treatment approach depends on several factors including the type of malignancy, its treatment responsiveness, location, number, and size.
* Neurosurgery, stereotactic radiosurgery or whole-brain radiation, and occasionally treatment with chemotherapy or targeted therapies are the commonly employed modalities of treatment.
* Anticonvulsants are indicated only in patients with seizures.

MANAGEMENT OF TREATMENT TOXICITIES

Nausea

GENERAL PRINCIPLES

* Historically, nausea was one of the most debilitating side effects of chemotherapy. The advent and use of effective antiemetic therapies have made chemotherapy much more tolerable for cancer patients.
* Incidence of chemotherapy-induced nausea and vomiting (CINV) is widely variable and depends on both drug and dose used.
* CINV can be categorized as acute (<24 hours) or delayed (>24 hours). Acute CINV is an important predictor of delayed CINV.
* **Prevention** of CINV is more effective than treatment. Commonly used prophylactic agents include:
  ○ Dexamethasone, which has active antiemetic properties. It is frequently administered via IV prior to chemotherapy (premedication) and continued orally for 2–3 days with certain chemotherapy regimens.
  ○ 5-Hydroxytryptamine-3 (5-HT^3) receptor antagonists (ondansetron, granisetron, dolasetron, palonosetron), which are highly effective and widely used as premedications.
  ○ Aprepitant, which is used with highly emetogenic regimens.

TREATMENT

- Posttreatment nausea should not be immediately assumed to be secondary to chemotherapy. Secondary causes, including bowel obstruction, brain metastasis with cerebral edema, constipation, narcotics, and gastroenteritis, should all be considered.
- Initial treatment with prochlorperazine is often effective. Lorazepam and other anxiolytics also have antiemetic properties. 5-HT$_3$ antagonists are less effective in treatment than in prevention but are frequently used. Olanzapine has also been studied and found to be active in treating CINV.

Diarrhea

GENERAL PRINCIPLES

- Diarrhea is a common side effect of many chemotherapies (irinotecan, 5FU, capecitabine), targeted agents (erlotinib, cetuximab, sunitinib, lapatinib), and newer immunotherapies (ipilimumab, nivolumab, pembrolizumab).
- Diarrhea can also be a symptomatic manifestation of the underlying cancer (such as carcinoid syndrome in neuroendocrine tumors).

DIAGNOSIS

- Obtaining a good history and accurately assessing the type of cancer a patient has, treatments received and their timing, history of bone marrow transplantation (GVHD), immunosuppressant regimen and recent dose adjustments, and recent antibiotic use are all very crucial.
- Imaging of the abdomen, *Clostridium difficile* testing, and even obtaining a colonoscopy might be required in selected patients (e.g., ipilimumab-related colitis).
- Special attention should be paid to transplant patients because testing serum levels of immunosuppressants and testing for opportunistic infections constitute an important part of workup.

TREATMENT

- Hydration to avoid volume depletion is critical.
- Patients who test positive for *C. difficile* should be appropriately managed with suitable antibiotics such as metronidazole and/or oral vancomycin.
- Empiric and aggressive treatment with loperamide can be considered in patients with chemotherapy-related diarrhea. When loperamide is ineffective, diphenoxylate, atropine, or other similar agents can be used.
- Timely initiation of steroid therapy is important in immunotherapy and GVHD-related diarrhea.

SUPPORTIVE CARE: COMPLICATIONS OF CANCER

Cancer Pain

GENERAL PRINCIPLES

- The two main mechanisms for pain are nociceptive (somatic or visceral) and neuropathic.
  - Nociceptive pain is caused by stimulation of pain receptors and neuropathic pain by direct injury to the peripheral nervous system or CNS.

- ○ Somatic pain typically occurs with bone metastases, musculoskeletal inflammation, or after surgery and is characterized by a well-localized, dull, or aching pain.
- ○ Visceral pain results from tumor infiltration and compression or distention of viscera and is described as diffuse, deep, squeezing, and pressure-like sensation.
- ○ Neuropathic pain occurs due to tumor infiltration of peripheral nerves, roots, or spinal cord, as well as chemical injury caused by chemotherapy, radiotherapy, or surgery. This pain is described as a sharp or burning sensation.
- These three types of pain may occur alone or in combination in the same patient.
- Cancer pain in adults may be classified into three levels on the basis of a 0 to 10 numerical scale: mild pain (1–3), moderate pain (4–6), and severe pain (7–10).

TREATMENT

- Cancer pain is usually managed through a stepwise approach (the "WHO ladder"), according to the level of pain.
  - ○ Step 1: Patients with mild pain and not taking opioids may be treated with nonopioid analgesics including NSAIDs or acetaminophen.
  - ○ Step 2: Patients with no response to nonopioids or moderate pain are treated with weak opioids such as codeine, hydrocodone, and oxycodone, either alone or in combination with acetaminophen.
  - ○ Step 3: Severe pain is treated with opioids such as morphine, hydromorphone, methadone, or transdermal fentanyl.
- Tramadol, which has weak affinity to μ-opioid receptors and is considered a nonopioid drug, can be used in patients with mild to moderate pain not responding to NSAIDs and those who wish to defer opioid treatment.
- Co-analgesics should be considered in specific cases.
  - ○ Systemic corticosteroids may be useful in pain caused by bone metastases, increased cranial pressure, spinal cord compression, and nerve compression or infiltration.
  - ○ Tricyclic antidepressants, such as nortriptyline, and anticonvulsants, such as gabapentin, are commonly indicated in neuropathic pain.
  - ○ Bisphosphonates (zoledronic acid and pamidronate) and radiolabeled agents (strontium-89 and samarium-153) may help in treating bone metastases–related pain.
- Common side effects of opioid therapy include constipation, nausea, respiratory depression, and sedation. Constipation should be prevented with the prophylactic use of combined stimulant laxative and stool softener. If symptoms persist, patients may benefit from the addition of a third agent, including lactulose, magnesium citrate, polyethylene glycol, or enema.
- Patients who experience inadequate pain control despite aggressive opioid therapy or who cannot tolerate opioid titration due to side effects may benefit from interventional therapies, such as regional infusion of analgesics and neuroablative or neurostimulatory procedures.
- Uncontrolled pain should be treated as a medical emergency. Patients in acute pain may often require opioids dosed through a patient-controlled analgesia delivery system. These patients require close monitoring.

Bone Metastasis

GENERAL PRINCIPLES

Commonly seen in patients with prostate, breast, lung, kidney, and bladder cancers and myeloma.

DIAGNOSIS

Bone scan (nuclear imaging with technetium-99m) is sensitive for blastic lesions but not lytic lesions). Concerning lesions on bone scan should be evaluated with plain radiograph films or CT to identify lesions at risk for pathologic fracture.

TREATMENT

- Pain should be managed aggressively with opioids. NSAIDs may offer additional relief.
- Lesions at risk for fracture should be treated surgically or with radiation therapy.
- Bisphosphonates and RANK ligand inhibitors may reduce the risk of fracture and reduce pain.

Pleural Effusion

GENERAL PRINCIPLES

Pleural effusions are common in patients with primary lung cancer, mesothelioma, advanced breast cancer, and lymphoma.

DIAGNOSIS

Routine thoracentesis with cytologic evaluation is typically adequate. Effusions with negative cytology can be further evaluated with pleuroscopy or open pleural biopsy (see Chapter 10, Pulmonary Diseases).

TREATMENT

- Prompt and complete drainage by therapeutic thoracentesis is necessary to avoid chronic fibrosis and trapped lung. Observation for rate of reaccumulation after initial drainage is appropriate for most patients. Rapidly reaccumulating effusions (<1 month) should be treated aggressively.
- Pleurodesis (obliteration of the pleural space by fibrosis) by complete drainage and instillation of a sclerosant (usually talc) can prevent recurrence of most malignant effusions.
- Placement of an indwelling pleural catheter for intermittent outpatient drainage is another alternative. Pleural fibrosis and resolution of the effusion occurs over several weeks in most patients.
- Medical therapy may be sufficient for managing effusions in breast cancer and lymphoma.

Fatigue

GENERAL PRINCIPLES

- Common symptom in cancer, occurring in an estimated 80% of patients with advanced disease.
- Close attention should be paid to any signs of underlying depression, which should be managed appropriately.

TREATMENT

- First step in the treatment is the identification of treatable contributing factors such as pain, poor nutrition, emotional distress, sleep disturbance, and comorbidities (anemia,

infection, organ dysfunction). Appropriate pain management, nutrition support, sleep therapy, exercise, and necessary supportive care can help address some of these issues.
• Transfusion support and erythropoietin may be helpful in selective patients with anemia.
• Psychostimulants such as methylphenidate or modafinil can prove helpful in some patients with severe symptoms.

Anorexia and Cachexia

GENERAL PRINCIPLES

• Anorexia is defined as loss of appetite with associated weight loss.
• Cachexia is a metabolic syndrome characterized by profound involuntary weight loss.

TREATMENT

• In addition to caloric supplementation, patients may benefit from pharmacologic therapy.
• Megestrol acetate is active, with symptomatic improvement in <1 week. Despite the quick increase in the appetite, it may take several weeks to achieve weight gain. Megestrol is also associated with an increased risk of thromboembolism.
• Dexamethasone provides a short-lived improvement, usually without significant weight gain.
• Dronabinol has limited benefits in anorexia and is associated with sedation.

23 Diabetes Mellitus and Related Disorders

Cynthia J. Herrick and Janet B. McGill

Diabetes Mellitus

GENERAL PRINCIPLES

- **Diabetes mellitus (DM)** is a group of metabolic diseases characterized by hyperglycemia resulting from defects in insulin secretion, insulin action, or both. In 2012, DM was present in 12.3% of persons over the age of 20 years in the United States and 25.9% of those over the age of 65 years. A substantial percentage of affected persons are not diagnosed. Type 2 diabetes (T2DM) represents 90–95% of all cases of diabetes, with type 1 diabetes (T1DM) and other causes representing the remaining 5–10% (*National Diabetes Statistics Report, 2014 http://www.cdc.gov/diabetes/pdfs/data/2014-report-estimates-of-diabetes-and-its-burden-in-the-united-states.pdf*).
- Persons with diabetes are at risk for microvascular complications, including retinopathy, nephropathy, and neuropathy, and are at increased risk for macrovascular disease.
- T2DM is accompanied by hypertension (approximately 75%) and hyperlipidemia (>50%) in adult patients and is considered a "cardiac risk equivalent" because of the excess risk for macrovascular disease, cardiovascular disease (CVD) events, and mortality (*Diabetes Care 2012;35(suppl 1):S11*).

Classification

DM is classified into four clinical classes (*Diabetes Care 2015;38(suppl 1):S8*).

- T1DM accounts for <10% of all cases of DM and results from a cellular-mediated autoimmune destruction of the beta (β) cells of the pancreas.
- T2DM accounts for >90% of all cases of diabetes. T2DM is characterized by insulin resistance followed by reduced insulin secretion from β cells that are unable to compensate for the increased insulin requirements.
- **Other specific types of DM** include those that result from genetic defects in insulin secretion or action (monogenic diabetes such as neonatal diabetes and maturity-onset diabetes of the young), pancreatic surgery or disease of the exocrine pancreas (cystic fibrosis), endocrinopathies (e.g., Cushing syndrome, acromegaly), or drugs (corticosteroids, antiretroviral, atypical antipsychotics), and diabetes associated with other syndromes.
- **Gestational DM** (GDM) is glucose intolerance with onset or diagnosis during pregnancy. The prevalence of GDM depends on the criteria used for diagnosis and varies by age and ethnic group (generally from 5–6% of pregnancies to 15–20% of pregnancies). Diagnostic criteria for GDM vary based on practice location with a two-step method (50-g, 1-hour screen followed by 100-g, 3-h oral glucose tolerance test [OGTT]) used in the United States and a one-step method (75-g, 2-hour OGTT) more common internationally (*Diabetes Care 2015;38(suppl 1):S13*). About 60% of women with GDM will develop T2DM in the ensuing 5–10 years, and all remain at an increased risk for the development of T2DM later in life (*http://www.cdc.gov/diabetes/pubs*).
  - All patients with GDM should undergo diagnostic testing 6–12 weeks postpartum with a 2-h OGTT or fasting plasma glucose and every 1–3 years thereafter to determine whether abnormal carbohydrate metabolism has persisted or is recurrent (*Diabetes Care 2015;38(suppl 1):S79*).

○ Weight loss and exercise are encouraged to decrease the risk of persistent prediabetes or T2DM after delivery.

DIAGNOSIS

- Progression from impaired fasting glucose or impaired glucose tolerance to T2DM occurs at the rate of 2–22% (average, about 12%) per year depending on the population studied.
- Lifestyle modification, including a balanced hypocaloric diet to achieve 7% weight loss in overweight patients and regular exercise of ≥150 minutes per week, is recommended for persons with prediabetes to prevent progression to T2DM (*Diabetes Care 2015;38(suppl 1):S31*).
- Metformin may be considered in patients with prior GDM, those with body mass index ≥35, or those with progressive hyperglycemia (*Diabetes Care 2015;38(suppl 1):S32*).
- See Table 23-1.

TREATMENT

- **Goals of therapy** are alleviation of symptoms; achievement of glycemic, blood pressure, and lipid targets; and prevention of acute and chronic complications of diabetes.
- Glycemic control recommendations are the same for T1DM and T2DM: Fasting and preprandial capillary blood glucose (BG) 80–130 mg/dL (3.9 to 7.2 mmol/L), postprandial capillary BG <180 mg/dL (<10 mmol/L), and A1C <7% or as close to normal as possible while avoiding significant hypoglycemia (*Diabetes Care 2015;38(suppl 1):S37*). The American Association of Clinical Endocrinologists (AACE) and European Association for the Study of Diabetes (EASD) recommend an A1C target of <6.5% (*Endocr Pract 2011;17(suppl 2):1*). This degree of glycemic control has been associated with the lowest risk for microvascular complications in patients with T1DM (*N Engl J Med 1993;329:978*) as well as T2DM (*BMJ 2000;321:405; Lancet 1998;352:837*).

TABLE 23-1	Diagnosis of Diabetes
Prediabetes Diagnosis (increased risk for developing diabetes)	**Diabetes Diagnosis**
A1C 5.7–6.4%	A1C ≥6.5%[a]
Fasting plasma glucose (FPG) 100–125 mg/dL (5.6–6.9 mmol/L) (impaired fasting glucose)	FPG ≥126 mg/dL (7.0 mmol/L)[a]
Oral glucose tolerance test (OGTT): glucose 140–199 mg/dL (7.8–11.0 mmol/L) 2 h after 75-g glucose load (impaired glucose tolerance)	OGTT: glucose ≥200 mg/dL (11.1 mmol/L) 2 h after 75-g glucose load[a]
	Symptoms of diabetes (polyuria, polydipsia, fatigue, weight loss) and random plasma glucose level ≥200 mg/dL (11.1 mmol/L)

[a]Should be repeated unless unequivocal hyperglycemia is present.

- Intensive diabetes therapy leading to tight glycemic control in patients with risk factors for CVD has been associated with increased mortality (*N Engl J Med 2011;364:818*; *N Engl J Med 2008;359:1577*). Hypoglycemia was implicated as the cause of higher mortality in one, but not all, of the studies (*N Engl J Med 2008;359:1577*). Less tight glycemic goals may be appropriate for patients with a history of cardiovascular (CV) events or those at high risk for CV events.
- The blood pressure target for patients with diabetes is <140/90 mm Hg, but a lower goal of <130/80 mm Hg may be considered for younger patients. The use of either an angiotensin-converting enzyme (ACE) inhibitor or an angiotensin receptor blocker (ARB) is recommended as first-line therapy. For patients not at goal, a thiazide diuretic should be added if the glomerular filtration rate (GFR) is >30 mL/min/1.73 m^2 and a loop diuretic added if the GFR is <30 mL/min/1.73 m^2 (*Diabetes Care 2015;38(suppl 1):s49*; *JAMA 2014;311:511*).
- High-intensity statin therapy (atorvastatin 40–80 mg daily or rosuvastatin 20–40 mg daily) is recommended in all patients with diabetes and overt CVD as well as patients age 40–75 with CVD risk factors (10-year atherosclerotic CVD risk score ≥7.5%). Moderate-intensity statin therapy can be considered in patients age 40–75 with no other CVD risk factors and in patients <40 or >75 with CVD risk factors (*Circulation 2014;129(suppl 2):S11*).
- Aspirin therapy should be advised in patients with diabetes who are older than 40 years or who have other risk factors. Low doses (75–162 mg) are appropriate for primary prevention (*Diabetes Care 2015;38(suppl 1):S54*).
- **Assessment of glycemic control** consists of the following:
  ○ **Self-monitoring of blood glucose (SMBG)** is recommended for all patients who take insulin and provides useful information for those on noninsulin therapies. Patients using multiple daily injections or insulin pumps should test themselves three or more times daily. Less frequent testing may be appropriate for those on noninsulin therapies. Although most SMBG is done before meals and at bedtime, periodic testing 1–2 hours after eating may be necessary to achieve postprandial glucose targets (*Diabetes Care 2015;38(suppl 1):S33*).
  ○ **Continuous glucose monitoring (CGM)** has been shown to reduce A1C in adults older than 25 years on intensive insulin therapy. CGM measures interstitial glucose, which provides a close approximation of BG values. Hypoglycemia and hyperglycemia alarms may help patients with widely fluctuating BG levels or hypoglycemia unawareness. CGM is supplemental to SMBG (*N Engl J Med 2008;359:1464*).
  ○ **A1C** provides an integrated measure of BG values over the preceding 2–3 months. A1C should be obtained every 3 months in patients not at goal or when either diabetes therapy or clinical condition changes and twice yearly in well-controlled patients. A1C should confirm results of SMBG, and discordant values should be investigated. An A1C level that is higher than expected should be evaluated by a diabetes educator to ensure meter accuracy, appropriate technique, and frequency of testing. When the A1C is lower than expected, blood loss, transfusion, hemolysis, and hemoglobin variants should be considered. The correlation between A1C and mean plasma glucose is sufficiently strong that laboratory reports may include both the A1C result and the estimated average glucose (*Diabetes Care 2015;38(suppl 1):S34*).
  ○ **Ketones** can be detected in a fingerstick blood sample by measuring β-hydroxybutyrate with the handheld glucose/ketone meter, Precision Xtra. Urine ketones can be qualitatively identified, using Ketostix or Acetest tablets. Patients with T1DM should test for ketones during febrile illness, for persistent elevation of glucose (>300 mg/dL), or if signs of impending diabetic ketoacidosis (e.g., nausea, vomiting, abdominal pain) develop. Testing for β-hydroxybutyrate is useful in emergency departments to determine whether a patient with hyperglycemia has ketonemia (*Acad Emerg Med 2006;13(6):683*). Hospital laboratories measure serum ketones including acetone, acetoacetate, and β-hydroxybutyrate.

MANAGEMENT

Comprehensive diabetes management includes coordinated diet, exercise, and medication plans. **Patient education** in medical nutrition therapy, exercise, SMBG, medication use, and insulin dosing and administration is integral to the successful management of diabetes.

Medical Nutrition Therapy

- Medical nutrition therapy includes dietary recommendations for a healthy, balanced diet to achieve adequate nutrition and maintain an ideal body weight (*Diabetes Care 2015;38(suppl 1):S21*).
- Caloric restriction is recommended for overweight individuals, with individualized targets that may be as low as 1000–1500 kcal/d for women and 1200–1800 kcal/d for men depending on activity level and starting body weight.
- Caloric intake is usually distributed as follows: 45–65% of total calories as carbohydrates, 10–30% as protein, and <30% as total fat (<7% saturated fat) with <300 mg/d of cholesterol.
- In patients with low-density lipoprotein cholesterol >100 mg/dL (2.6 mmol/L), total fat should be restricted to <25% of total calories, saturated fat to <7% of calories, and cholesterol to <200 mg/d.
- Patients with progressive kidney disease may benefit from restriction of protein intake to 0.8 g/kg/d. Patients with severe chronic kidney disease (CKD) will need additional restrictions of potassium- and phosphorus-containing foods.
- "Carbohydrate counting" is a useful skill for patients on intensified insulin therapy who adjust insulin doses based on the carbohydrate content of meals and snacks.

Exercise

Exercise improves insulin sensitivity, reduces fasting and postprandial BG levels, and offers numerous metabolic, CV, and psychological benefits in diabetic patients.
- In general, 150 minutes per week is recommended as part of a healthy lifestyle and has been shown to assist with the prevention and management of T2DM.
- Patients may need individualized guidance regarding exercise, and they are more likely to exercise when counseled by their physician to do so.

Diabetes Mellitus in Hospitalized Patients

GENERAL PRINCIPLES

Diabetes-specific indications for hospitalization

- **Diabetic ketoacidosis (DKA)** is characterized by a plasma glucose level of >250 mg/dL (14 mmol/L) in association with an arterial pH <7.30 or serum bicarbonate level of <15 mEq/L and moderate ketonemia or ketonuria (*Diabetes Care 2009;32:1336*).
- **Hyperosmolar hyperglycemic state (HHS)** includes marked hyperglycemia (≥600 mg/dL) and elevated serum osmolality (>320 mOsm/kg), often accompanied by impaired mental status (*Diabetes Care 2009;32:1336*).
- **Hypoglycemia** is an indication for hospitalization if it is induced by a sulfonylurea (SFU) medication, is due to a deliberate drug overdose, or results in coma, seizure, injury, or persistent neurologic change.
- **Newly diagnosed T1DM** or newly recognized GDM can be indications for hospitalization, even in the absence of ketoacidosis.
- **Patients with T2DM** are rarely admitted to the hospital for initiation or change in insulin therapy unless hyperglycemia is severe and associated with mental status change or other organ dysfunction.

Management of diabetes in hospitalized patients
- Hyperglycemia (BG ≥140 mg/dL [7.8 mmol/L]) is a common finding in hospitalized patients and may be due to previously diagnosed diabetes, undiagnosed diabetes, medications, or stress-induced hyperglycemia. Up to 40% of general medical and surgical patients exhibit hyperglycemia, and approximately 80% of intensive care unit (ICU) patients will demonstrate transient or persistent hyperglycemia. Patients with T1DM should be clearly identified as such at the time of admission.
- A1C can help identify previously undiagnosed diabetes in hospitalized patients and may assist with the evaluation of prior glucose control. A1C is not accurate in patients who are severely anemic, bleeding, or hemolyzing or who have been transfused.
- Data are limited regarding use of noninsulin therapies in inpatients.
- Medication reconciliation on admission should include a careful assessment of home diabetes medications, level of glucose control, kidney function, expected diagnostic studies and treatments, and the possible need for insulin treatment.
- Patients who are required to fast for diagnostic testing or treatments should have all non-insulin therapies stopped.
- **Patients hospitalized for reasons other than diabetes and are eating normally** may continue or restart outpatient diabetes treatments, unless specifically contraindicated.
- Use of noninsulin therapies may be appropriate in psychiatric units, rehabilitation settings, or stable patients preparing for discharge.
- **Glucose targets for inpatients** aim to reduce morbidity and mortality, while minimizing hypoglycemia.
  ○ In critical care settings, the glucose target is 140–180 mg/dL (7.8–10.0 mmol/L) with frequent monitoring recommended to avoid hypoglycemia (*N Engl J Med 2009;360:1283*).
  ○ In noncritical care settings, the glucose target is <140 mg/dL (7.8 mmol/L) fasting and premeal and <180 mg/dL (10.0 mmol/L) postmeal or on a random glucose check with reassessment of the insulin regimen if glucose falls below 100 mg/dL (5.6 mmol/L) (*Endocr Pract 2009;15:353*; *J Clin Endocrinol Metab 2012;97:16*; *Diabetes Care 2015;38(suppl 1):S80*).

Management of hyperglycemia in critical care settings
- Variable IV insulin infusion is recommended for critical illness, emergency surgery, or major surgery. Numerous algorithms have been published that direct insulin dose adjustments based on capillary BG values performed hourly at the bedside.
- An IV infusion of a dextrose-containing solution or other caloric source should be provided to prevent hypoglycemia and ketosis. For fluid-restricted patients, 10% dextrose in water (D10W) can be infused at a rate of 10–25 mL/h to provide a steady, consistent source of calories.
- An intermediate- or long-acting insulin should be given 2 hours prior to insulin infusion discontinuation.

Management of hyperglycemia in non–critical care hospital settings
- BG should be checked on admission in all patients and monitored four times per day in hyperglycemic patients, especially in patients treated with insulin.
- Scheduled insulin with basal, nutritional, and correction components provides superior glycemic control compared with correction or "sliding scale" insulin alone (*Diabetes Care 2007;30:2181*; *Diabetes Care 2011;34:256*).
- For patients who are naïve to insulin, the starting dose of basal insulin should equal 0.2 units/kg or 0.1 units/lb. Scheduled premeal insulin should be 0.2 units/kg divided by three meals.
  Example: Your patient weighs 80 kg. The starting insulin dose should be 16 units of long-acting insulin plus 5 units of rapid-acting insulin before each meal. A correction dose of 1–2 units per 50 mg/dL of BG, beginning at 140 mg/dL, can be added to the premeal doses.

- Patients with T1DM should continue their home insulin doses and may continue the use of an insulin pump if there is a hospital policy in place to do so. Insulin doses in patients with T2DM should be reduced by 20% on admission. If their home insulin dose is excessive compared to a weight-based dose of 0.4–0.5 units/kg or distribution between basal and premeal insulin is uneven, further reductions and adjustments may be necessary.
- Meal-time insulin doses should be given shortly before or immediately after meals, and the correction factor or sliding scale dose should be added to the premeal dose.
- The glucose threshold for sliding scale (corrective) insulin should be higher at bedtime, or corrective insulin should not be given at bedtime. Adjustments in the next-day basal or premeal insulin doses are indicated if correction doses of insulin are frequently required or if clinical status or medications change.
- Extreme hyperglycemia (≥300 mg/dL [16.7 mmol/L]) on more than one consecutive test should prompt testing for ketoacidosis with electrolytes and ketone measurements.
- Hypoglycemia should be treated promptly with oral or IV glucose, and the capillary BG should be repeated every 10 minutes until >100 mg/dL (5.5 mmol/L) and stable. Reevaluation of scheduled doses and assessment of risk factors for hypoglycemia (declining renal function, hepatic impairment, poor intake) should be undertaken for any BG <70 mg/dL (3.9 mmol/L) (*Endocr Pract 2006;12:458*).
- **Enteral nutrition** (*Mayo Clin Proc 1996;71:587*). Intermittent tube feeds should be matched by either short-acting (human regular) insulin or intermediate-acting (human NPH [Neutral Protamine Hagedorn]) insulin. Patients with baseline hyperglycemia may need a basal insulin dose in addition to the doses given to cover tube feeds. For example, nighttime enteral feeding lasting 6–8 hours should be managed with NPH, with or without a basal insulin dose. NPH can be given three to four times daily for continuous tube feeds, allowing a change in insulin dose if the feeding is interrupted.
- **Total parenteral nutrition (TPN).** Patients supported with TPN are likely to develop hyperglycemia, and some require large amounts of insulin. See Chapter 2, Nutrition Support, for insulin management of patients on TPN.

Diabetic Ketoacidosis

GENERAL PRINCIPLES

Epidemiology

DKA, a potentially fatal complication of diabetes, occurs in up to 5% of patients with T1DM annually and can occur in insulin-deficient patients with T2DM.

Pathophysiology

DKA is a catabolic condition that results from severe insulin deficiency, often in association with stress and activation of counter-regulatory hormones (e.g., catecholamines, glucagon).

Risk Factors

Precipitating factors for DKA include inadvertent or deliberate interruption of insulin therapy, sepsis, trauma, myocardial infarction (MI), and pregnancy. DKA may be the first presentation of T1DM and, rarely, T2DM.

Prevention

DKA can be prevented in many cases, and its occurrence suggests a breakdown in education, communication, and problem solving. Therefore, diabetes education should be reinforced at every opportunity, with special emphasis on (a) self-management skills during sick days; (b) the body's need for more, rather than less, insulin during such illnesses; (c) testing of blood or urine for ketones; and (d) procedures for obtaining timely and preventive medical advice.

DIAGNOSIS

History

- Patients may describe a variety of symptoms including polyuria, polydipsia, weight loss, nausea, vomiting, and vaguely localized abdominal pain generally in the setting of persistent hyperglycemia. A high index of suspicion is warranted because clinical presentation may be nonspecific.
- Tachycardia; decrease of capillary filling; rapid, deep, and labored breathing (Kussmaul respiration); and fruity breath odor are common physical findings.
- Prominent gastrointestinal (GI) symptoms and abdominal tenderness on exam may give rise to suspicion for intra-abdominal pathology.
- Dehydration is invariable, and respiratory distress, shock, and coma can occur.

Diagnostic Testing

- Anion gap metabolic acidosis.
- Positive serum β-hydroxybutyrate or ketones (a semiquantitative measurement of acetone, acetoacetate, and β-hydroxybutyrate) and positive urine ketones.
- Plasma glucose ≥250 mg/dL. Euglycemic DKA (plasma glucose <200 mg/dL) has been described in pregnancy, alcohol ingestion, fasting or starvation, during hospitalization, and in patients with both T1DM and T2DM treated with sodium-glucose cotransport (SGLT-2) inhibitors (*http://www.fda.gov/Safety/MedWatch/SafetyInformation/SafetyAlertsforHumanMedicalProducts/ucm446994.htm*).
- Hyponatremia, hyperkalemia, azotemia, and hyperosmolality are other possible findings.
- A focused search for a precipitating infection is recommended if clinically indicated.
- An ECG should be obtained to evaluate electrolyte abnormalities and for unsuspected myocardial ischemia.

TREATMENT

Management of DKA should preferably be conducted in an ICU (Table 23-2). **If treatment is conducted in a non-ICU setting, close monitoring is mandatory until ketoacidosis resolves and the patient's condition is stabilized.** The therapeutic priorities are fluid replacement, adequate insulin administration, and potassium repletion. Administration of bicarbonate, phosphate, magnesium, or other therapies may be advantageous in selected patients.

- **Monitoring of therapy**
  - BG levels should be monitored hourly, serum electrolyte levels every 2–4 hours, and arterial blood gas values as often as necessary for a severely acidotic or hypoxic patient.
  - Serum sodium tends to rise as hyperglycemia is corrected; failure to observe this trend suggests that the patient is being overhydrated with free water.
  - Serial serum ketone measurements are not necessary because ketonemia may persist after clinical recovery and because the most commonly used assays measure all ketones, not just β-hydroxybutyrate. Restoration of renal buffering capacity by normalization of the serum bicarbonate level and closure of the anion gap are more reliable indices of metabolic recovery.
  - Use of a flowchart is an efficient method of tracking clinical data (e.g., weight, fluid balance, mental status) and laboratory results during the management of DKA.
  - Telemetry is recommended given the propensity to electrolyte abnormalities.
- **IV antimicrobial therapy** should be started promptly for documented or suspected bacterial, fungal, and other treatable infections. Empiric broad-spectrum antibiotics can be started in septic patients pending results of blood cultures. Note that DKA

TABLE 23-2 Treatment of Diabetic Ketoacidosis

IV Fluids
Goals: First, replete circulating volume and then replenish total-body water deficit
Estimate fluid deficit by subtracting current weight from recent dry weight
Usually 7–9% of body weight
Hypotension → >10% loss of body fluids
(*Diabetes Care 2004;27:S94*)

Replete circulating volume
0.9% saline: 1 L bolus then 500–1000 mL/h if cardiac and renal function normal
Replenish total-body water deficit
0.45% saline (0.9% saline if hyponatremic): 150–500 mL/h
Adjust repletion according to BP, UOP, exam; no faster than 3 mOsm/kg/h; aim for positive fluid balance over 12–24 h

Insulin
Goals: Turn off ketogenesis; correct hyperglycemia

Do not start until K >3.5 mmol/L
Bolus: 0.1 units/kg
Infusion: 0.1 units/kg/h
(Regular insulin 100 units in 100 mL 0.9% saline at 10 mL/h = 10 units/h)
Goal decrease in BG = 50–75 mg/dL/h
Avoid correcting >100 mg/dL/h to reduce risk of osmotic encephalopathy
Continue at 1–2 units per hour until HCO$_3$ >15 mEq/L, clinical improvement, AND anion gap closed
Administer SC basal insulin 2 h prior to stopping insulin infusion

Dextrose (5%)
Goal: Prevent hypoglycemia

Add when BG <250 mg/dL
Consider giving glucose as a separate infusion of 50–100 mL/h (2-bag approach). Concurrently reduce insulin infusion to 0.05 units/kg/h

Potassium as KCl
Goal: Prevent hypokalemia as insulin shifts potassium into the cell

Add to fluids at 10–20 mEq/h

Bicarbonate

NOT routinely recommended
May consider if (a) shock/coma; (b) pH <6.9; (c) HCO$_3$ <5 mEq/L; (d) cardiac/respiratory dysfunction; or (e) severe hyperkalemia
50–100 mEq in 1 L 0.45% saline over 30–60 min; follow arterial pH
Avoid hypokalemia by adding 10 mEq KCl

Phosphate and magnesium

NOT routinely recommended
May give KPhos IV fluids if not eating
May give 10–20 mEq of magnesium Sulfate IV with ventricular arrhythmias

BG, blood glucose; BP, blood pressure; HCO$_3$, bicarbonate; K, potassium; KCl, potassium chloride; KPhos, potassium phosphate; UOP, urine output.

is not typically accompanied by fever, so infection must be considered in a febrile patient.

COMPLICATIONS

Complications of DKA include life-threatening conditions that must be recognized and treated promptly.

- **Lactic acidosis** may result from prolonged dehydration, shock, infection, and tissue hypoxia in DKA patients. Lactic acidosis should be suspected in patients with refractory metabolic acidosis and a persistent anion gap despite optimal therapy for DKA. Management includes adequate volume replacement, control of sepsis, and judicious use of bicarbonate.
- **Arterial thrombosis** manifesting as stroke, MI, or an ischemic limb occurs with increased frequency in DKA. However, routine anticoagulation is not indicated except as part of the specific therapy for a thrombotic event.
- **Cerebral edema** is observed more frequently in children than in adults.
  ○ Symptoms of increased intracranial pressure (e.g., headache, altered mental status, papilledema) or a sudden deterioration in mental status after initial improvement in a patient with DKA should raise suspicion for cerebral edema.
  ○ Overhydration with free water and excessively rapid correction of hyperglycemia are known risk factors. Watch for a decrease in serum sodium level or failure to rise during therapy.
  ○ Neuroimaging with a CT scan can establish the diagnosis. Prompt recognition and treatment with IV mannitol is essential and may prevent neurologic sequelae in patients who survive cerebral edema.
- **Rebound ketoacidosis** can occur due to premature cessation of IV insulin infusion or inadequate doses of SC insulin after the insulin infusion has been discontinued. All patients with T1DM and patients with T2DM who develop DKA (indicating severe insulin deficiency) require both basal and premeal insulin in adequate doses to avoid recurrence of metabolic decompensation.

Hyperosmolar Hyperglycemic State

GENERAL PRINCIPLES

HHS is one of the most serious life-threatening complications of T2DM (*J Clin Endocrinol Metab 2008;93:1541*).

Epidemiology

- HHS occurs primarily in patients with T2DM, and in 30–40% of cases, it is the initial presentation of a patient's diabetes (*Emerg Med Clin North Am 2005;23:629*).
- HHS is significantly less common than DKA, with an incidence of <1 case per 1000 person-years.

Pathophysiology

- Ketoacidosis is absent because the ambient insulin level may effectively prevent lipolysis and subsequent ketogenesis yet is inadequate to facilitate peripheral glucose uptake and to prevent hepatic residual gluconeogenesis and glucose output.
- Precipitating factors include dehydration, stress, infection, stroke, noncompliance with medications, dietary indiscretion, and alcohol and cocaine abuse. Impaired glucose excretion is a contributory factor in patients with renal insufficiency or prerenal azotemia.

DIAGNOSIS

Clinical Presentation

In contrast to DKA, the onset of HHS is usually insidious. Several days of deteriorating glycemic control are followed by increasing lethargy. Clinical evidence of severe dehydration is the rule. Some alterations in consciousness and focal neurologic deficits may be found at presentation or may develop during therapy. Therefore, repeated neurologic assessment is recommended.

Differential Diagnosis

The differential diagnosis of HHS includes any cause of altered level of consciousness, including hypoglycemia, hyponatremia, severe dehydration, uremia, hyperammonemia, drug overdose, and sepsis. Seizures and acute stroke-like syndromes are common presentations.

Diagnostic Testing

Clinical findings include (a) hyperglycemia, often >600 mg/dL; (b) plasma osmolality >320 mOsm/L; (c) absence of ketonemia; and (d) pH >7.3 and serum bicarbonate level of >20 mEq/L. Prerenal azotemia and lactic acidosis can develop. Although some patients will have detectable urine ketones, most patients do not have a metabolic acidosis. Lactic acidosis may develop from an underlying ischemia, infection, or other cause.

TREATMENT

- See Table 23-3 for detailed treatment recommendations.
- **Underlying illness.** Detection and treatment of any underlying predisposing illness are critical in the treatment of HHS. Antibiotics should be administered early, after appropriate cultures, in patients in whom infection is known or suspected as a precipitant to HHS. A high index of suspicion should be maintained for underlying pancreatitis, GI bleeding, renal failure, and thromboembolic events, especially acute MI.

COMPLICATIONS

Complications of HHS include thromboembolic events (cerebral and MI, mesenteric thrombosis, pulmonary embolism, and disseminated intravascular coagulation), cerebral edema, adult respiratory distress syndrome, and rhabdomyolysis.

MONITORING/FOLLOW-UP

- **Monitoring of therapy.** Use of a flowchart is helpful for tracking clinical data and laboratory results.
- Initially, BG levels should be monitored every 30–60 minutes and serum electrolyte levels every 2–4 hours; frequency of monitoring can be decreased during recovery.
- Neurologic status must be reassessed frequently; persistent lethargy or altered mentation indicates inadequate therapy. On the other hand, relapse after initial improvement in mental status suggests too rapid correction of serum osmolarity.

Type 1 Diabetes

GENERAL PRINCIPLES

A comprehensive approach is necessary for successful management of T1DM. A team approach that includes the expertise of physicians, diabetes educators, dietitians, and other members of the diabetes care team offers the best chance of success.

TABLE 23-3	Treatment of Hyperosmolar Hyperglycemic State
IV Fluids Goals: Restore hemodynamic stability and intravascular volume by fluid replacement; this is the primary treatment and supersedes insulin; patients often require much more fluid than with diabetic ketoacidosis	**Replete circulating volume** 0.9% saline **Replenish total-body water deficit** 0.45% saline Aim for positive fluid balance over 24–72 h; may require 10–12 L
Potassium as KCl Goal: Prevent hypokalemia as insulin shifts potassium into the cell	Add to fluids at 10–20 mEq/h; begin as soon as urine output confirmed
Insulin Goals: Plays a secondary role; slowly corrects hyperglycemia	**Do not start until K >3.5 mmol/L** **Bolus: 5–10 units (if BG >600 mg/dL); smaller bolus if BG <600 mg/dL** **Infusion: 0.10–0.15 units/kg/h** Avoid correcting >100 mg/dL/h to reduce risk of osmotic encephalopathy **Administer SC basal insulin 2 h prior to stopping insulin infusion**
Dextrose (5%) Goal: Prevent hypoglycemia	Add when BG 250–300 mg/dL Can give as a separate infusion of 50–100 mL/h (two-bag approach) Concurrently reduce insulin infusion to 1–2 units/h
Bicarbonate	NOT routinely recommended May be required if concurrent lactic acidosis

BG, blood glucose; K, potassium; KCl, potassium chloride.

DIAGNOSIS

T1DM can present at any age, and because of the variable prodrome of hyperglycemia, the diagnosis can be challenging in adults.

- The rate of destruction of β cells is rapid in infants and children and slower in adults. Therefore, ketoacidosis as an initial presentation is more common in young patients.
- T1DM is characterized by severe insulin deficiency. Exogenous insulin is required to control BGs, prevent DKA, and preserve life. Ketosis develops in 8–16 hours and ketoacidosis in 12–24 hours without insulin.
- Early in the course of T1DM, some insulin secretory capacity remains, and the insulin requirement may be lower than expected (0.3–0.4 units/kg). Tight control of BG level from the onset has been shown to preserve the residual β-cell function and prevent or delay later complications.
- Latent autoimmune diabetes in adults (LADA) is characterized by mild to moderate hyperglycemia at presentation that often responds to noninsulin therapies initially. Adults with LADA will have one or more β cell–specific autoantibodies and tend to require insulin therapy sooner than patients with classic T2DM (months to years).
- T1DM should be suspected when there is a family history of T1DM, thyroid disease, or other autoimmune disease. Presentation with ketoacidosis suggests T1DM, but confirmatory tests may be useful to guide therapy.

- Autoantibodies include islet cell autoantibodies (ICA), antibodies to insulin, antibodies to glutamic acid decarboxylase (anti-GAD), antibodies to zinc transporter 8 (ZnT8), and antibodies to tyrosine phosphatases IA-2 and IA-2β. Measuring one or more of these autoantibodies along with a C-peptide can help to confirm the diagnosis of T1DM; however, 20% of insulin-deficient adults are antibody negative (*Diabetes Care 2015;38(suppl 1):S10*).

TREATMENT

Treatment of T1DM requires lifelong insulin replacement and careful coordination of insulin doses with food intake and activity.

- **Insulin preparations.** After SC injection, there is individual variability in the duration and peak activity of insulin preparations and day-to-day variability in the same subject (Table 23-4).
- **SC insulin administration.** The abdomen, thighs, buttocks, and upper arms are the preferred sites for SC insulin injection. Absorption is fastest from the abdomen, followed by the arm, buttocks, and thigh, probably as a result of differences in blood flow. Injection sites should be rotated within the regions, rather than randomly across separate regions, to minimize erratic absorption. Exercise or massage over the injection site may accelerate insulin absorption.

TABLE 23-4	**Approximate Kinetics of Insulin Preparations**		
Insulin Type	**Onset of Action (h)**	**Peak Effect (h)**	**Duration of Activity (h)**
Rapid acting			
Lispro, aspart, glulisine	0.25–0.50	0.50–1.50	3–5
Regular	0.50–1.00	2–4	6–8
Technosphere insulin	0.25–0.5	1.0–1.5	2–3
Intermediate acting			
NPH	1–2	6–12	18–24
Lente[a]	1–2	6–12	18–24
Long acting[b]			
Detemir	3–4	8–12	18–24
Glargine	4–6	Possible[c]	20–24
Ultralente[a]	3–4	Variable	18–24
PZI[a]	3–4	Unclear	18–24

PZI, protamine zinc insulin.
[a]Not available in the United States; possibly generic manufacturers.
[b]Some patients with type 1 diabetes have improved control when the long-acting basal insulin is given twice a day rather than once daily.
[c]Insulin dosage and individual variability in absorption and clearance rates affect pharmacokinetic data. Duration of insulin activity is prolonged in renal failure. After a lag time of approximately 5 hours, insulin glargine generally has a flat peakless effect over a 22- to 24-hour period; however, broad peaks can occur.

- **Regular human insulin is now available in an inhaled form as technosphere insulin (Afrezza).** This comes in four- and eight-unit cartridges for rapid-acting insulin administration. Onset occurs at 0.2–0.25 hour with peak effect within the first hour and a duration of action of 3 hours. It is contraindicated in patients with asthma or chronic obstructive pulmonary disease because of risk of bronchospasm. Pulmonary function tests are required prior to starting and at regular intervals during therapy.
- A regimen of **multiple daily insulin injections** that include basal, premeal, and correction doses is preferred to obtain optimal control in both hospitalized patients and outpatients. This regimen implies that capillary glucose monitoring will occur four times daily, 10–30 minutes before meals and at bedtime.
  - The **insulin requirement** for optimal glycemic control is approximately 0.5–0.8 units/kg/d for the average nonobese patient. A conservative total daily dose (TDD) of 0.4 units/kg/d is given initially to a newly diagnosed patient; the dose is then adjusted, using SMBG values. Higher doses may be required in obese or insulin-resistant patients, in adolescents, and in the latter part of pregnancy.
  - Basal insulin (administered as NPH twice daily, detemir once or twice daily, or glargine once daily) should provide 40–50% of the TDD of insulin and should be adjusted by 5–10% daily until the fasting glucose is consistently <130 mg/dL. In general, basal insulin is given regardless of nothing by mouth (NPO) or dietary status and should not be held without a direct order.
  - Premeal or bolus doses of insulin (given only if eating) are adjusted according to the BG, the anticipated carbohydrate intake, and anticipated activity level. The total premeal complement should roughly equal the total basal dose, with one-third given before or after each meal. Rapid-acting insulins (lispro, aspart, or glulisine) are preferred, but regular human insulin can be used.
  - The third component of a comprehensive insulin regimen is "correction factor" insulin, which is similar to sliding scale, adjusted according to the premeal fingerstick glucose testing and the patient's estimated insulin sensitivity. In general, thinner patients should use a less aggressive scale than heavier or more insulin-resistant patients. Correction factor and premeal doses should use the same insulin and be given together in the same syringe.
- **Continuous SC insulin infusion** using an insulin pump is widely used for insulin delivery in patients with T1DM and increasingly in T2DM. It is a useful tool but does not automatically improve glucose control without patient self-management.
  - A typical regimen provides 50% of total daily insulin as basal insulin and the remainder as multiple preprandial boluses of insulin, using a programmable insulin pump. A rapid-acting insulin (aspart, lispro, or glulisine) is used to fill the pump and is infused continuously to provide basal insulin.
  - Insulin pumps have advanced features that allow patients to fine-tune their basal and bolus doses but require diabetes education to use the pump to its full potential. Patients must check their blood sugars regularly because DKA can occur rapidly if the insulin infusion is disrupted (i.e., faulty infusion set).

Type 2 Diabetes

GENERAL PRINCIPLES

- T2DM results from defective insulin secretion followed by loss of β-cell mass in response to increased demand as a result of insulin resistance (*Diabetes 1988;37:667*).
- T2DM is usually diagnosed in adults, with both incidence and prevalence increasing with age; however, T2DM now accounts for up to one-third of new cases of diabetes diagnosed between the ages of 5 and 15 years.

- T2DM is associated with obesity, family history of diabetes, history of GDM or prediabetes, hypertension, physical inactivity, and race/ethnicity. African Americans, Latinos, Asian Indians, Native Americans, Pacific Islanders, and some groups of Asians have a greater risk of developing T2DM than Caucasians.
- T2DM may be asymptomatic and, therefore, can remain undiagnosed for months to years.
- The loss of pancreatic β cells is progressive. Insulin secretion is usually sufficient to prevent ketosis, but DKA or HHS can develop during severe stress. T2DM in patients who present with or later develop ketosis or DKA, but who do not require insulin between episodes, is termed ketosis-prone T2DM.
- The mechanisms underlying the β-cell loss in T2DM are unknown, but programmed cell death in response to genetic and environmental factors has been demonstrated in animal models (*Diabetes 2003;52:2304*).

TREATMENT

Medications

- The achievement of glycemic control requires individualized therapy and a comprehensive approach that incorporates lifestyle and pharmacologic interventions. Guidelines have been published by several professional organizations regarding the choice and sequence of antidiabetic therapy (*Endocr Pract 2015;15:e6*; *Diabetes Care 2015:38 (supplement 1)*).
- Considerations for selecting noninsulin therapy (Table 23-5) in patients with T2DM include the following:
  - Oral therapy should be initiated early in conjunction with diet and exercise.
  - Metformin is the recommended first-line therapy if tolerated.
  - Monotherapy with maximum doses of insulin secretagogues, metformin, or thiazolidinediones (TZDs) yields comparable glucose-lowering effects.
  - The glucose-lowering effects of metformin, insulin secretagogues, and DPP-4 inhibitors and glucagon-like peptide-1 (GLP-1) analogs are observed within days to weeks, whereas the maximum effect of TZDs may not be observed for several weeks to months.
  - Combination therapy with two or more oral or injectable agents may be needed at the time of diagnosis to achieve A1C and glucose targets in patients presenting with significant hyperglycemia and will likely be needed as β-cell function deteriorates over time. The AACE recommends dual therapy for initial A1C ≥7.5% and triple therapy or insulin for initial A1C >9%. A preference for medications with lower risk of hypoglycemia (GLP-1 receptor agonists, DPP-4 inhibitors, SGLT-2 inhibitors) is indicated (*Endocr Pract 2015;15:e6*). The American Diabetes Association (ADA) recommends proceeding to two-drug, three-drug, and injectable combinations if the A1C goal is not achieved in 3-month increments. Dual therapy is recommended at the time of diagnosis if the A1C is >9%. A particular order of therapy after metformin is not specified and will depend on patient comorbidities and preferences (*Diabetes Care 2015;38:145*).
  - About 60% of patients on monotherapy may have worsening of metabolic control during the first 5 years of therapy, and concurrent use of two or more medications with different mechanisms of action may be necessary (*Am J Med 2010;123(suppl 3):S38*).
  - Insulin therapy should be considered for patients presenting in DKA or with very high glucose levels (A1C >10%). Insulin therapy can sometimes be stopped after glucose toxicity is corrected but may need to be continued in patients with persistent insulin deficiency.
  - Because pancreatic β-cell function is required for the glucose-lowering effects of all noninsulin therapies, many patients will require insulin replacement therapy at some point. Insulin therapy can be initiated with basal insulin in addition to other therapies. Nonsecretagogue therapies can be continued with premixed insulin or with a basal/bolus regimen.

TABLE 23-5	Noninsulin Medications for Diabetes	
Oral therapies	Renal Dosing Necessary?	Main Adverse Effects
Biguanide: inhibits hepatic glucose output and stimulates glucose uptake by peripheral tissues. Weight neutral. Hold for 48 h after radiographic contrast procedure. Avoid in patients with cardiogenic or septic shock, CHF, severe liver disease, hypoxemia, and tissue hypoperfusion.		
Metformin (available in liquid and long-acting formulations)	Avoid if serum Cr ≥1.4 mg/dL in women or ≥1.5 mg/dL in men	GI symptoms (20–30%); lactic acidosis (3/100,000 patient-years)
Sulfonylureas (SFU): increase insulin secretion by binding specific β-cell receptors. Give 30–60 min before food. NEVER give if fasting. Start with lowest dose and increase over days to weeks to optimal dose (usually half the maximum approved dose).		
Glyburide (glibenclamide)	Avoid if CrCl <50 mL/min	Hypoglycemia, weight gain; avoid with renal insufficiency; caution in elderly
Glipizide	Yes; if CrCl <50 mL/min	Same; fewer problems in kidney disease
Glimepiride	Start lowest dose and titrate slowly	Same; fewer problems in kidney disease
Gliclazide[a]		Same; fewer problems in kidney disease
Meglitinides: increase insulin secretion; much shorter onset and half-life than SFUs. Dose before each meal. NEVER give if fasting.		
Nateglinide • Give 10 minutes before meal • Metabolized by cytochrome P450	No	Hypoglycemia, weight gain; not as severe as SFUs
Repaglinide	Yes; if CrCl ≤40 mL/min	Same
Mitiglinide[a] • Give 30 minutes before meal		Same

α-Glucosidase inhibitors: block polysaccharide and disaccharide breakdown and decrease postprandial hyperglycemia. Give with food. Start with low dose and increase weekly. Do not use in patients with intestinal disease.

Acarbose	Avoid if serum Cr >2.0 mg/dL	Gas, bloating, diarrhea, abdominal pain (25–50%); transaminase elevations
Miglitol	Avoid if serum Cr >2.0 mg/dL	Gas, bloating, diarrhea, abdominal pain (25–50%)
Voglibose[a]	No; Not renally excreted; not studied in CKD	Same

Thiazolidinediones: increase insulin sensitivity in muscle, adipose tissue, and liver. Start with low dose and increase after several weeks. Avoid in patients with New York Heart Association class III/IV heart failure. Caution in patients with coronary artery disease, hypertension, long-standing diabetes, left ventricular hypertrophy, preexisting edema or edema on therapy, insulin use, advanced age, renal failure, and aortic or mitral valve disease (*Diabetes Care 2004;27:256*).

Pioglitazone • Alters levels of medicines metabolized by CYP3A4	No	Edema, heart failure, fractures in women, increased risk of bladder cancer?—not seen in recent analysis of >1 million patients (*Diabetologia 2015;58(3):49*); rare hepatotoxicity; mild pancytopenia

DPP-4 inhibitors: inhibit enzyme that breaks down endogenous GLP (incretin secreted from intestinal L cells). Increased GLP reduces blood glucose by inhibiting glucagon release and stimulating insulin secretion. Avoid in patients with a history of pancreatitis.

Alogliptin	Yes; if CrCl <60 mL/min	Anaphylaxis, angioedema, skin reactions, liver injury, URI
Linagliptin	No	Anaphylaxis, angioedema, exfoliative skin reactions, URI
Saxagliptin	Yes; if CrCl ≤50 mL/min	Urticaria, facial edema, URI
Sitagliptin	Yes; if CrCl <50 mL/min	AKI, ESRD, anaphylaxis, angioedema, exfoliative skin reactions, URI
Vildagliptin[a] (not indicated in severe hepatic impairment, LFT >3× upper limit of normal)	Yes; if CrCl <50 mL/min; not indicated in severe renal impairment	Blistering skin lesions in animals, increased LFTs

(continued)

TABLE 23-5	Noninsulin Medications for Diabetes *(Continued)*	
	Renal Dosing Necessary?	**Main Adverse Effects**
SGLT-2 inhibitors: inhibit sodium glucose cotransporter 2 in the proximal renal tubule, decreasing glucose reabsorption by the kidney.		
Canagliflozin	Yes; if eGFR 45 to <60 mL/min/1.73 m^2	Female genital mycotic infections, urinary tract infections, polyuria; hypotension, volume depletion, renal failure; increased LDL-C
Dapagliflozin	Not indicated for eGFR <60 mL/min/1.73 m^2	Same; possible increased risk for bladder cancer
Empagliflozin	Not indicated for eGFR <45 mL/min/1.73 m^2	Same
Bile acid sequestrants		
Colesevelam hydrochloride (contraindicated in bowel obstruction or GI motility disorders; pregnancy class B; can be used in renal and hepatic disease; take on an empty stomach)	No	Constipation, reduced absorption of some medications; raises triglycerides
Dopamine agonists		
Bromocriptine mesylate (do not use with other dopamine agonists or antagonists)	No	Nausea, asthenia, dizziness, headache, constipation, diarrhea

SC injectable therapies

GLP-1 analogs: structurally similar to endogenous GLP-1 but resist breakdown by DPP-4. They have a longer half-life and reach higher levels in blood and tissues. They are given by injection and can improve satiety and result in weight loss. Avoid in patients with history of pancreatitis. Avoid in patients with history of medullary thyroid cancer or MEN2 given increased C-cell tumors in rodents (all except immediate-release exenatide).

Albiglutide (dosed weekly)	No; monitor for GI side effects in patients with renal impairment	URI, diarrhea, nausea, injection site reaction
Dulaglutide (dosed weekly)	No; monitor for GI side effects in patients with renal impairment	Diarrhea, nausea, vomiting, abdominal pain, decreased appetite
Exenatide (dosed twice daily)	Do not use in severe renal impairment or ESRD; caution with moderate renal impairment or history of renal transplant	Nausea, vomiting, GI distress, reported cases of pancreatitis
Exenatide extended release (dosed weekly)	Do not use in severe renal impairment or ESRD; caution with moderate renal impairment or history of renal transplant	Nausea, vomiting, injection site reaction, headache, diarrhea, dyspepsia
Liraglutide (dosed once daily)	Caution when initiating or escalating dose in patients with renal impairment	Headache, nausea, diarrhea, urticaria

Amylin analogs: blunt postprandial blood glucose response

Pramlintide acetate (given as a separate injection with meals; insulin dose reduction is required when starting)	Not defined with CrCl <20 mL/min	Nausea, vomiting, diarrhea, headache, hypoglycemia

AKI, acute kidney injury; CKD, chronic kidney disease; CHF, congestive heart failure; Cr, creatinine; CrCl, creatinine clearance; DPP-4, dipeptidyl peptidase-4; eGFR, estimated glomerular filtration rate; ESRD, end-stage renal disease; GI, gastrointestinal; GLP, glucagon-like peptide; LDL-C, low-density lipoprotein cholesterol; LFT, liver function test; MEN2, multiple endocrine neoplasia type 2; URI, upper respiratory infection.
Please refer to country-specific prescribing information before using any of the antidiabetes therapies.
[a]Not available in the United States.

○ The toxicity profile of some oral and injectable antidiabetic agents may preclude their use in patients with preexisting illnesses.

• **Insulin therapy** in T2DM is indicated in the following:
  ○ Patients in whom oral or injectable agents have failed to achieve or sustain glycemic control
  ○ Metabolic decompensation: DKA, HHS
  ○ Newly diagnosed patients with severe hyperglycemia
  ○ Pregnancy and other situations in which oral agents are contraindicated

• **The success of insulin therapy** depends on both the adequacy of the insulin TDD (0.6 to >1.0 units/kg of body weight per day) and the appropriateness of the insulin regimen for a given patient to achieve target glucose and A1C values.
  ○ A once-daily injection of intermediate- or long-acting insulin at bedtime or before breakfast (basal insulin) added to oral or injectable agents may achieve the target A1C goal.
  ○ Premeal insulin may be required if basal insulin plus other agents is not adequate. Short- or rapid-acting insulin administered before meals can be added to a basal insulin. Alternatively, a premixed insulin can be given twice daily before breakfast and dinner. In general, the secretagogues are discontinued when premeal insulin is added, but sensitizing and other agents are continued on the basis of the individual patient needs.
  ○ The TDD of insulin required to achieve glycemic targets varies widely in patients with T2DM and is based on body mass index, the continuation of oral agents, and the presence of comorbid conditions. Large doses of insulin (>100 units/d) may be required for optimal glycemic control. Weight gain with insulin use is a concern.
  ○ Insulin-induced hypoglycemia, the most dangerous side effect, may increase CV event rates and death. Avoidance of hypoglycemia while achieving an A1C as low as can be safely achieved requires close collaboration between physician, patient, and diabetes educators. The frequency of hypoglycemia increases as patients approach normal A1C levels or when deterioration of kidney function occurs.

• **Concentration.** The standard insulin concentration is 100 units/mL (U-100), with vials containing 1000 units in 10 mL. A highly concentrated form of regular insulin containing 500 units/mL (Humulin U-500) is available for the rare patient with severe insulin resistance (usually T2DM). The vial size for U-500 insulin is 20 mL. A newly approved insulin glargine formulation that is 300 units/mL (U-300) is being marketed as Toujeo. It should be noted that Toujeo has less glucose-lowering effect when compared unit by unit to Lantus (i.e., the Toujeo dose required to achieve the same blood sugars will be more than the Lantus dose divided by 3).

• **Mixed insulin therapy.** Short- and rapid-acting insulins (regular, lispro, aspart, and glulisine) can be mixed with NPH insulin in the same syringe for convenience. The rapid-acting insulin should be drawn first, cross-contamination should be avoided, and the mixed insulin should be injected immediately. Commercial premixed insulin preparations do not allow dose adjustment of individual components but are convenient for patients who are unable or unwilling to do the mixing themselves. Premixed insulins are an option for patients with T2DM who have a regular eating and activity schedule and, in general, should not be used in T1DM.

CHRONIC COMPLICATIONS OF DIABETES MELLITUS

• Prevention of long-term complications is one of the main goals of diabetes management. Appropriate treatment of established complications may delay their progression and improve quality of life.

- **Microvascular complications** include diabetic retinopathy, nephropathy, and neuropathy. These complications are directly related to hyperglycemia. Tight glycemic control has been shown to reduce the development and progression of these complications.

Diabetic Retinopathy

GENERAL PRINCIPLES

Classification

- Diabetic retinopathy (DR) is classified as background retinopathy (microaneurysms, retinal infarcts, lipid exudates, cotton wool spots, and/or microhemorrhages) with or without macular edema and proliferative retinopathy. Background DR is also known as preproliferative retinopathy.
- Other ocular abnormalities associated with diabetes include cataract formation, dyskinetic pupils, glaucoma, optic neuropathy, extraocular muscle paresis, floaters, and fluctuating visual acuity. The latter may be related to changes in BG levels.
- The presence of floaters may be indicative of preretinal or vitreous hemorrhage; immediate referral for ophthalmologic evaluation is warranted.

Epidemiology

The incidence of DR and vision impairment has dropped significantly with improved management of glycemia, blood pressure, and lipids in patients with both T1DM and T2DM. Early identification and treatment of DR have further reduced vision impairment once it is diagnosed. DR is less frequent in T2DM, but maculopathy may be more severe. DR is still the leading cause of vision loss in adults younger than age 65 years (*N Engl J Med 2012;366:1227*).

DIAGNOSIS

Annual examination by an ophthalmologist is recommended at the time of diagnosis of all T2DM patients and at the beginning of puberty or 3–5 years after diagnosis for patients with T1DM. Dilated eye examination should be repeated annually by an optometrist or ophthalmologist because progressive DR can be completely asymptomatic until sudden loss of vision occurs. Early detection of DR is critical because therapy is more effective before severe maculopathy or proliferation develops. Any diabetic patient with visual symptoms should be referred for ophthalmologic evaluation (*Diabetes Care 2012;35(suppl 1):S64*).

TREATMENT

The first line of treatment is glycemic control, which has been shown to reduce the incidence and progression of DR in patients with T1DM or T2DM. Blood pressure control was also shown to be effective in the United Kingdom Prospective Diabetes Study (UKPDS), and treatment with either an ACE inhibitor (ACE-I) or ARB has demonstrated additional utility in preventing DR. Fenofibrate, used with simvastatin, reduced the risk of progression of DR in the ACCORD and FIELD clinical trials (*N Engl J Med 2012;366:1227*). Background retinopathy is not usually associated with loss of vision unless macular edema is present (25% of cases). The development of macular edema or proliferative retinopathy (particularly new vessels near the optic disk) requires elective laser photocoagulation therapy to preserve vision. Intraocular injections of vascular endothelial growth factor (VEGF)-neutralizing antibodies or glucocorticoids improve vision outcomes in macular edema but have side effects. Vitrectomy is indicated for patients with vitreous hemorrhage or retinal detachment.

Diabetic Nephropathy

GENERAL PRINCIPLES

Epidemiology

Approximately 25–45% of patients with either type of diabetes develop clinically evident diabetic nephropathy during their lifetime. Diabetic nephropathy is the leading cause of end-stage renal disease (ESRD) in the United States and a major cause of morbidity and mortality in patients with diabetes (*Med Clin North Am 2004;88:1001*).

Risk Factors

The newest ADA guidelines no longer distinguish between microalbuminuria and macroalbuminuria, defining albuminuria as urinary albumin-to-creatinine ratio ≥30 mg/g (*Diabetes Care 2015;38(suppl 1):S58*). The mean duration from diagnosis of T1DM to the development of overt proteinuria has increased significantly and is now >25 years. The time from the occurrence of proteinuria to ESRD has also increased and is now >5 years. In T2DM, albuminuria can be present at the time of diagnosis. Poor glycemic control is the major risk factor for diabetic nephropathy, but hypertension and smoking are contributors. Obesity may contribute to kidney damage in T2DM. Due to the widespread use of ACE inhibitor and ARB agents for the treatment of hypertension, impaired kidney function may occur in the absence of albuminuria (*Diabetes Care 2015;38(suppl 1):S60*).

Prevention

Prevention of diabetic nephropathy starts at the time of diagnosis with achievement of glycemic, blood pressure, and lipid targets. Smoking cessation is also important. Annual screening for albuminuria and measurement of serum creatinine identify those with early damage who are at risk of progression. Annual screening should be performed in T1DM patients who have had diabetes for >5 years and all T2DM patients starting at diagnosis.

Associated Conditions

- Patients with proteinuria (albumin/creatinine >300 mg/g) are at higher risk for anemia due to loss of transferrin and poor production of erythropoietin and should be screened at any stage of CKD and treated.
- **Patients with CKD are at higher risk for CVD and mortality**, so management of other CV risk factors is particularly important in this group of patients.
- Hypovitaminosis D should be corrected, and secondary hyperparathyroidism should be prevented or treated as early as possible.
- Diabetic patients with CKD may be at risk for hyperkalemia and metabolic acidosis, which should be identified and managed accordingly.

DIAGNOSIS

Diagnostic Testing

- Measurement of the albumin-to-creatinine ratio (normal, <30 mg of albumin/g of creatinine) in a random urine sample is recommended for screening. At least two to three measurements within a 6-month period should be performed to establish the diagnosis of diabetic nephropathy (*Diabetes Care 2003;26:S94*).
- Measurement of serum creatinine and serum urea nitrogen should be performed annually, along with calculation of the estimated GFR. Patients with diabetes may have reduced kidney function without manifesting albumin in their urine. Testing and treatment of

associated disorders such as anemia, secondary hyperparathyroidism, hyperkalemia, and acid–base disturbances should begin when the estimated GFR is $<$60 mL/min/1.73 m^2, or during stage 3 CKD (see Chapter 13, Renal Diseases).

TREATMENT

Intensive control of both diabetes and hypertension is important to reduce the rate of progression of CKD due to diabetes. The current guideline by the Eighth Joint National Committee suggests treating to a target blood pressure of $<$140/90 mm Hg in patients with diabetes, including those with evidence of CKD (*JAMA 2014;311:511*).

Medications
- Antihypertensive treatment with ACE inhibitor or ARB drugs is recommended as first-line therapy for all patients with diabetes and hypertension. These agents have been shown to reduce progression of both retinopathy and nephropathy and may be considered in patients with normal blood pressure or prehypertension.
- Diuretics are considered second line, followed by calcium channel blockers, β-blockers, or centrally acting agents (*JAMA 2014;311:511*).

Lifestyle/Risk Modification
- Dietary protein intake of 0.8 g/kg/d (based on ideal body weight) is recommended. Further reduction does not alter glycemic control, CVD risk, or kidney function decline (*Diabetes Care 2015;38(suppl 1):S58*).
- Avoidance of renal toxins is important for preservation of kidney function.

Diabetic Neuropathy

GENERAL PRINCIPLES

Classification
Diabetic neuropathy can be classified as (a) subclinical neuropathy, determined by abnormalities in electrodiagnostic and quantitative sensory testing; (b) diffuse symmetrical polyneuropathy with distal symmetric sensorimotor losses $\pm$ autonomic syndromes; and (c) focal syndromes.

Epidemiology
Distal symmetric polyneuropathy (DPN) is the most common neuropathy in developed countries and accounts for more hospitalizations than all the other diabetic complications combined. Sensorimotor DPN is a major risk factor for foot trauma, ulceration, and Charcot arthropathy, and is responsible for 50–75% of nontraumatic amputations (*Med Clin N Am 2004;88:947*).

Prevention
- Sensation in the lower extremities should be documented at least annually, using a combination of modalities such as a light-touch monofilament, tuning fork (frequency of 128 Hz), pinprick, or temperature.
- Foot examination should be conducted at least annually to evaluate the presence of musculoskeletal deformities, skin changes, and pulses, in addition to the sensory examination.

TREATMENT

- **Painful peripheral neuropathy** responds variably to treatment with tricyclic antidepressants (e.g., amitriptyline 10–150 mg PO at bedtime), topical capsaicin (0.075% cream), or anticonvulsants (e.g., carbamazepine 100–400 mg PO bid, gabapentin 900–3600 mg/d, or pregabalin 150–300 mg/d). Patients should be warned about adverse effects, including sedation and anticholinergic symptoms (tricyclics), burning sensation (capsaicin), and blood dyscrasias (carbamazepine). α-Lipoic acid (600 mg bid) and high-dose thiamine (50–100 mg tid) have been tested in early DPN. Vitamin B_{12} should be checked and replaced if low.

- **Orthostatic hypotension** is a manifestation of autonomic neuropathy, but other etiologies (e.g., dehydration, anemia, medications) should be excluded. Treatment is symptomatic and includes postural maneuvers, use of compressive garments (e.g., Jobst stockings), and intravascular expansion using sodium chloride 1–4 g PO qid and fludrocortisone 0.1–0.3 mg PO daily. Hypokalemia, supine hypertension, and congestive heart failure (CHF) are some adverse effects of fludrocortisone.
- **Intractable nausea and vomiting** may be manifestations of impaired GI motility from autonomic neuropathy. **DKA** should be ruled out when nausea and vomiting are acute. Other causes of nausea and vomiting, including adrenal insufficiency, should be excluded.
  ○ **Management of diabetic gastroenteropathy** can be challenging. Frequent, small meals (six to eight per day) of soft consistency that are low in fat and fiber provide intermittent relief. Parenteral nutrition may become necessary in refractory cases.
  ○ **Pharmacologic therapy** includes the prokinetic agent metoclopramide, 10–20 mg PO (or as a suppository) before meals and at bedtime, and erythromycin, 125–500 mg PO qid. Extrapyramidal side effects (tremor and tardive dyskinesia) from the antidopaminergic actions of metoclopramide may limit therapy.
  ○ **Cyclical vomiting** that is unrelated to a GI motility disorder or other clear etiology may also occur in diabetic patients and appears to respond to amitriptyline 25–50 mg PO at bedtime.
- **Diabetic cystopathy**, or bladder dysfunction, results from impaired autonomic control of detrusor muscle and sphincteric function. Manifestations include urgency, dribbling, incomplete emptying, overflow incontinence, and urinary retention. Recurrent urinary tract infections are common in patients with residual urine. Treatment with bethanechol 10 mg tid or intermittent self-catheterization may be required to relieve retention.
- **Chronic, persistent diarrhea** in patients with diabetes is probably multifactorial. Celiac disease and inflammatory bowel diseases should be ruled out, particularly in patients with T1DM. Pancreatic mass is reduced with long-standing diabetes, so the possibility of exocrine pancreatic dysfunction should be considered. Bacterial overgrowth has been considered as an etiology but is difficult to diagnose. Empiric treatment with broad-spectrum antibiotics (e.g., azithromycin, tetracycline, cephalosporins) along with metronidazole may be beneficial. Antifungal agents and probiotic replacement can be tried. If diarrhea persists, loperamide or octreotide 50–75 mg SC bid can be effective in patients with intractable diarrhea.

MACROVASCULAR COMPLICATIONS OF DIABETES MELLITUS

Coronary Heart Disease

GENERAL PRINCIPLES

- Coronary heart disease (CHD), stroke, and peripheral vascular disease (PVD) are responsible for 80% of deaths in persons with diabetes (*Lancet 1997;350(suppl 1):S123*) (see Chapter 4, Ischemic Heart Disease).

- **Coronary artery disease (CAD)** occurs at a younger age and may have atypical clinical presentations in patients with diabetes (*Lancet 1997;350(suppl 1):SI23*).
  - MI carries a worse prognosis, and angioplasty gives less satisfactory results in diabetic patients.
  - Persons with diabetes have an increased risk of ischemic and nonischemic heart failure and sudden death.

Risk Factors

Risk factors for macrovascular disease that are common in persons with diabetes include insulin resistance, hyperglycemia, albuminuria, hypertension, hyperlipidemia, cigarette smoking, and obesity.

Prevention

- CV risk factors should be assessed at least annually and treated aggressively (see treatment goals in the following text). ECG should be obtained yearly. Stress tests, with or without imaging, should be reserved for those with typical or atypical chest pain or those with abnormalities on ECG (*Diabetes Care 2012;35(suppl 1):S64*).
- Screening asymptomatic persons with cardiac stress test has not been shown to reduce mortality or events in asymptomatic patients with T2DM (*JAMA 2009;301:1547*).
- Aspirin 81–325 mg/d has proven beneficial in secondary prevention of MI or stroke in diabetic patients and may be considered for persons over age 40 years with diabetes.

TREATMENT

- Aggressive risk factor reduction lowers the risk of both microvascular and macrovascular complications in patients with diabetes.
  - Glycemic control should be optimized to A1C <7% and as close to normal as possible in the first few years after diagnosis. Patients with long-standing T2DM may have increased risk of mortality with very tight glycemic control (A1C <6.5%), particularly if multiple agents are required and the risk of hypoglycemia increases.
  - Hypertension should be controlled to a target blood pressure of <140/90 mm Hg (or <130/80 mm Hg if this can be achieved without adverse effects).
  - Hyperlipidemia should be treated appropriately, with a high-intensity statin in patients with known CHD. High-density lipoprotein cholesterol levels of >50 mg/dL and triglyceride levels of <150 mg/dL should be achieved.
  - Cigarette smoking should be actively discouraged, and weight loss should be promoted in obese patients.
- **Management of diabetes after acute MI**
  Hyperglycemia (glucose >110 mg/dL), with or without a history of diabetes, is an independent predictor of in-hospital mortality and CHF in patients admitted for acute MI (*Lancet 2000;355:773*). However, the results of the studies that investigated tight glucose control with insulin in the setting of acute MI in T2DM patients are inconclusive (*BMJ 1997;314:1512; J Am Coll Cardiol 1995;26:57; Eur Heart J 2005;26:650*). Nevertheless, given the consistent epidemiologic association, it is reasonable to expect that glucose-lowering effects in acute conditions could lead to clinical benefit.

Peripheral Vascular Disease

GENERAL PRINCIPLES

Diabetes and smoking are the strongest risk factors for PVD. In diabetic patients, the risk of PVD is increased by age, duration of diabetes, and presence of peripheral neuropathy.

PVD is a marker for systemic vascular disease involving coronary, cerebral, and renal vessels. Diabetic patients with PVD have increased risk for subsequent MI or stroke regardless of the PVD symptoms.

DIAGNOSIS

Clinical Presentation

Symptoms of PVD include intermittent claudication, rest pain, tissue loss, and gangrene, but patients with diabetes may have fewer symptoms due to concomitant neuropathy.

Physical Examination

Physical examination findings include diminished pulses, dependent rubor, pallor on elevation, absence of hair growth, dystrophic toenails, and cool, dry, fissured skin.

Diagnostic Testing

- The ankle-to-brachial index (ABI), defined as the ratio of the systolic blood pressure in the ankle divided by the systolic blood pressure at the arm, is the best initial diagnostic test. An ABI <0.9 by a handheld, 5- to 10-MHz Doppler probe has a 95% sensitivity for detecting angiogram-positive PVD (*Int J Epidemiol 1988;17:248*).
- ABI should be performed in diabetic patients with signs or symptoms of PVD.

TREATMENT

- Risk factors should be controlled, with similar goals described for CAD (see the previous text).
- Antiplatelet agents such as clopidogrel (75 mg/d) have additional benefits when compared with aspirin in diabetic patients with PVD (*Diabetes Care 2003;26:3333*).
- Patients with intermittent claudication could also benefit from exercise rehabilitation and cilostazol (100 mg bid). This medication is contraindicated in patients with CHF.

MISCELLANEOUS COMPLICATIONS

Erectile Dysfunction

GENERAL PRINCIPLES

Epidemiology

It is estimated that 40–60% of men with diabetes have erectile dysfunction (ED), and the prevalence varies depending on the age of the patient and duration of diabetes. In addition to increasing age, ED is associated with smoking, poor glycemic control, low high-density lipoprotein, neuropathy, and retinopathy.

Etiology

ED in diabetic patients is multifactorial. It can result from nerve damage, impaired blood flow (vascular insufficiency), adverse drug effects, low testosterone, psychological factors, or a combination of these etiologies.

DIAGNOSIS

Evaluation should include a measurement of total or bioavailable testosterone. If the total testosterone is <300 mg/dL, the test should be repeated in the morning (does not have to be fasting, but a blood draw before 9:00 a.m. is appropriate) along with a prolactin and prostate-specific antigen (PSA).

TREATMENT

- If testosterone is low, and both PSA and prostate examination are normal, then testosterone replacement can be tried with either testosterone enanthate, 200 mg every 2–3 weeks, or a topical gel (AndroGel or Testim).
- A trial of phosphodiesterase type 5 inhibitors (sildenafil, tadalafil, vardenafil) is often warranted in addition to hormonal correction (if indicated). Typical doses include sildenafil 50-100 mg, vardenafil 10 mg, or tadalafil 10 mg 1 hour prior to sexual activity. Tadalafil can also be administered as a daily medication at lower doses (2.5 to 5 mg/d). Referral to a urology specialist should be considered if the problem persists. CV status should be considered before starting these agents. **This drug class should not be used concurrently with nitrates** to prevent severe and potentially fatal hypotensive reactions. Macular edema should also be ruled out before starting these agents.

Hypoglycemia

GENERAL PRINCIPLES

Classification

Hypoglycemia is uncommon in patients not treated for diabetes. Iatrogenic factors usually account for hypoglycemia in the setting of diabetes, whereas hypoglycemia in the nondiabetic population could be classified as fasting or postprandial hypoglycemia. **Iatrogenic hypoglycemia** complicates therapy with insulin or SFUs and is a limiting factor to achieving glycemic control during intensive therapy in patients with DM (*Diabetes Care 2003;26:1902*).

Risk Factors

Hypoglycemia resulting from too intensive diabetes management may increase the risk of mortality in older patients with a long duration of diabetes and should be avoided.
- Risk factors for iatrogenic hypoglycemia include skipped or insufficient meals, unaccustomed physical exertion, misguided therapy, alcohol ingestion, and drug overdose.
- Recurrent episodes of hypoglycemia impair recognition of hypoglycemic symptoms, thereby increasing the risk for severe hypoglycemia (hypoglycemia unawareness).
- Hypoglycemia unawareness results from defective glucose counterregulation with blunting of autonomic symptoms and counterregulatory hormone secretion during hypoglycemia. Seizures or coma may develop in such patients without the usual warning symptoms of hypoglycemia.
- Hypoglycemia unrelated to diabetes therapy is an infrequent problem in general medical practice.

DIAGNOSIS

Clinical Presentation

- Hypoglycemia is a clinical syndrome in which low serum (or plasma) glucose levels lead to symptoms of sympathetic–adrenal activation (sweating, anxiety, tremor, nausea, palpitations, and tachycardia) from increased secretion of counterregulatory hormones (e.g., epinephrine).
- Neuroglycopenia occurs as the glucose levels decrease further (fatigue, dizziness, headache, visual disturbances, drowsiness, difficulty speaking, inability to concentrate, abnormal behavior, confusion, and ultimately loss of consciousness or seizures).

Differential Diagnosis

Plasma or capillary BG values should be obtained, whenever feasible, to confirm hypoglycemia.

- Any patient with a serum glucose concentration of <60 mg/dL should be suspected of having a hypoglycemic disorder, and further evaluation is required if the value is <50 mg/dL.
- Absence of symptoms with these levels of glucose suggests the possibility of artifactual hypoglycemia. These levels are usually accompanied by symptoms of hypoglycemia. Detailed evaluation is usually required in a healthy-appearing patient, whereas hypoglycemia may be readily recognized as part of the underlying illness in a sick patient (*N Engl J Med 1986;315:1245*). Major categories include fasting and postprandial hypoglycemia.
- **Fasting hypoglycemia** can be caused by inappropriate insulin secretion (e.g., insulinoma), alcohol abuse, severe hepatic or renal insufficiency, hypopituitarism, glucocorticoid deficiency, or surreptitious injection of insulin or ingestion of an SFU.
  - These patients present with neuroglycopenic symptoms, but episodic autonomic symptoms may be present. Occasionally, patients with recurrent seizures, dementia, and bizarre behavior are referred for neuropsychiatric evaluation, which may delay timely diagnosis of hypoglycemia.
  - **Definitive diagnosis** of fasting hypoglycemia requires hourly BG monitoring during a supervised fast lasting up to 72 hours and measurement of plasma insulin, C-peptide, and SFU metabolites if hypoglycemia (<50 mg/dL) is documented. Patients who develop hypoglycemia and have measurable plasma insulin and C-peptide levels without SFU metabolites require further evaluation for an insulinoma.
- **Postprandial hypoglycemia** often is suspected, but seldom proven, in patients with vague symptoms that occur 1 or more hours after meals.
  - **Alimentary hypoglycemia** should be considered in patients with a history of partial gastrectomy or intestinal resection in whom recurrent symptoms develop 1–2 hours after eating. The mechanism is thought to be related to too rapid glucose absorption, resulting in a robust insulin response. These symptoms should be distinguished from dumping syndrome, which is not associated with hypoglycemia and occurs in the first hour after food intake. Frequent small meals with reduced carbohydrate content may ameliorate symptoms.
  - **Functional hypoglycemia.** Symptoms that are possibly suggestive of hypoglycemia, which may or may not be confirmed by plasma glucose measurement, occur in some patients who have not undergone GI surgery. This condition is referred to as "functional hypoglycemia." The symptoms tend to develop 3–5 hours after meals. Current evaluation and management of functional hypoglycemia are imprecise; some patients show evidence of impaired glucose tolerance and may respond to dietary therapy.

TREATMENT

Isolated episodes of mild hypoglycemia may not require specific intervention. Recurrent episodes require a review of lifestyle factors; adjustments may be indicated in the content, timing, and distribution of meals, as well as medication dosage and timing. Severe hypoglycemia is an indication for supervised treatment.

- **Readily absorbable carbohydrates** (e.g., glucose and sugar-containing beverages) can be administered orally to conscious patients for rapid effect. Alternatively, milk, candy bars, fruit, cheese, and crackers may be used in some patients with mild hypoglycemia. Hypoglycemia associated with acarbose or miglitol therapy should preferentially be treated with glucose. Glucose tablets and carbohydrate supplies should be readily available to patients with DM at all times.
- **IV dextrose** is indicated for severe hypoglycemia, in patients with altered consciousness, and during restriction of oral intake. An initial bolus, 20–50 mL of 50% dextrose, should

be given immediately, followed by infusion of 5% dextrose in water (D5W) (or D10W) to maintain BG levels above 100 mg/dL. Prolonged IV dextrose infusion and close observation are warranted in SFU overdose, in the elderly, and in patients with defective counterregulation.

- **Glucagon**, 1 mg IM (or SC), is an effective initial therapy for severe hypoglycemia in patients unable to receive oral intake or in whom an IV access cannot be secured immediately. Vomiting is a frequent side effect, and therefore, care should be taken to prevent the risk of aspiration. A glucagon kit should be available to patients with a history of severe hypoglycemia; family members and roommates should be instructed in its proper use.

PATIENT EDUCATION

- **Education** regarding etiologies of hypoglycemia, preventive measures, and appropriate adjustments to medication, diet, and exercise regimens is an essential task to be addressed during hospitalization for severe hypoglycemia.
- **Hypoglycemia unawareness** can develop in patients who are undergoing intensive diabetes therapy. These patients should be encouraged to monitor their BG levels frequently and take timely measures to correct low values (<60 mg/dL). In patients with very tightly controlled diabetes, slight relaxation in glycemic control and scrupulous avoidance of hypoglycemia may restore the lost warning symptoms.

Endocrine Diseases

William E. Clutter

DISORDERS OF THE THYROID GLAND

Evaluation of Thyroid Function

GENERAL PRINCIPLES

The major hormone secreted by the thyroid is **thyroxine (T_4)**, which is converted by deiodinases in many tissues to the more potent **triiodothyronine (T_3)**. Both are bound reversibly to plasma proteins, primarily **thyroxine-binding globulin (TBG)**. Only the free (unbound) fraction enters cells and produces biologic effects. T_4 secretion is stimulated by **thyroid-stimulating hormone (TSH)**. In turn, TSH secretion is inhibited by T_4, forming a negative feedback loop that keeps free T_4 levels within a narrow normal range. Diagnosis of thyroid disease is based on clinical findings, palpation of the thyroid, and measurement of plasma TSH and thyroid hormones.

DIAGNOSIS

Clinical Presentation
Thyroid palpation determines the size and consistency of the thyroid and the presence of nodules, tenderness, or a thrill.

Diagnostic Testing
- **Plasma TSH is the best initial test in most patients with suspected thyroid disease.** TSH levels are elevated in very mild primary hypothyroidism and are suppressed in very mild hyperthyroidism. Thus, **a normal plasma TSH level excludes hyperthyroidism and primary hypothyroidism.** Because even slight changes in thyroid hormone levels affect TSH secretion, **abnormal TSH levels are not specific for clinically important thyroid disease.** Changes in plasma TSH lag behind changes in plasma T_4, and TSH levels may be misleading when plasma T_4 levels are changing rapidly, as during treatment of hyperthyroidism.
  - TSH levels may be suppressed in severe nonthyroidal illness, in mild (or subclinical) hyperthyroidism, and during treatment with dopamine or high doses of glucocorticoids. Also, TSH levels remain suppressed for some time after hyperthyroidism is corrected.
  - Plasma TSH is mildly elevated (up to 20 microunits/mL) in some euthyroid patients recovering from nonthyroidal illnesses and in mild (or subclinical) hypothyroidism.
  - TSH levels are usually within the reference range in secondary hypothyroidism and cannot diagnose this rare form of hypothyroidism.
- **Plasma free T_4** confirms the diagnosis and assesses the severity of hyperthyroidism when plasma TSH is <0.1 microunits/mL. It is also used to diagnose secondary hypothyroidism and adjust thyroxine therapy in patients with pituitary disease. Most laboratories measure free T_4 by immunoassay.
- **Free T_4 measured by equilibrium dialysis** is the most reliable measure of unbound T_4, but results are seldom rapidly available. It is needed only in rare cases in which the diagnosis is not clear from measurement of plasma TSH and free T_4 by immunoassay.

- **Effect of nonthyroidal illness on thyroid function tests.** Many illnesses alter thyroid tests without causing true thyroid dysfunction (the nonthyroidal illness or euthyroid sick syndrome). These changes must be recognized to avoid mistaken diagnosis.
  - **The low T_3 syndrome** occurs in many illnesses, during starvation, and after trauma or surgery. Conversion of T_4 to T_3 is decreased, and plasma T_3 levels are low. Plasma free T_4 and TSH levels are normal. This may be an adaptive response to illness, and thyroid hormone therapy is not beneficial.
  - **The low T_4 syndrome** occurs in severe illness. TSH levels decrease early in severe illness, sometimes to <0.1 microunits/mL. In prolonged illness, free T_4 may also fall below normal. During recovery, TSH rises, sometimes to levels slightly above the normal range (rarely >20 microunits/mL).
  - Some drugs affect thyroid function tests (see Table 24-1). Iodine-containing drugs (**amiodarone** and radiographic contrast media) may cause hyperthyroidism or hypothyroidism in susceptible patients. In general, plasma TSH levels are a reliable guide to whether true hyperthyroidism or hypothyroidism is present.

TABLE 24-1	**Effects of Drugs on Thyroid Function Tests**
Effect	**Drug**
Decreased free and total T_4	
True hypothyroidism (TSH elevated)	Iodine (amiodarone, radiographic contrast)
	Lithium
	Some tyrosine kinase inhibitors
	Some immune modulators (e.g., interferon-α)
Inhibition of TSH secretion	Glucocorticoids
	Dopamine
Multiple mechanisms (TSH normal)	Phenytoin
Decreased total T_4 only	
Decreased TBG (TSH normal)	Androgens
Inhibition of T_4 binding to TBG (TSH normal)	Furosemide (high doses)
	Salicylates
Increased free and total T_4	
True hyperthyroidism (TSH <0.1 microunits/mL)	Iodine (amiodarone, radiographic contrast)
	Some immune modulators (e.g., interferon-α)
Inhibited T_4 to T_3 conversion (TSH normal)	Amiodarone
Increased free T_4 only	
Displacement of T_4 from TBG in vitro (TSH normal)	Heparin, low-molecular-weight heparin
Increased total T_4 only	
Increased TBG (TSH normal)	Estrogens, tamoxifen, raloxifene

T_3, triiodothyronine; T_4, thyroxine; TBG, thyroxine-binding globulin; TSH, thyroid-stimulating hormone.

Hypothyroidism

GENERAL PRINCIPLES

Etiology

- **Primary hypothyroidism** (due to disease of the thyroid itself) accounts for >90% of cases.
- **Chronic lymphocytic thyroiditis (Hashimoto disease)** is the most common cause and may be associated with Addison disease and other endocrine deficits. Its prevalence is greater in women and increases with age.
- **Iatrogenic hypothyroidism** due to thyroidectomy or radioactive iodine (RAI; iodine-131) therapy is also common.
- Transient hypothyroidism occurs in postpartum thyroiditis and subacute thyroiditis, usually after a period of hyperthyroidism.
- **Drugs that may cause hypothyroidism** include iodine-containing drugs, lithium, interferon (IFN)-α, IFN-β, interleukin-2, thalidomide, bexarotene, and sunitinib.
- Secondary hypothyroidism due to TSH deficiency is uncommon but may occur in any disorder of the pituitary or hypothalamus. However, it rarely occurs without other evidence of pituitary disease.

DIAGNOSIS

Clinical Presentation

History

Most symptoms of hypothyroidism are nonspecific and develop gradually. They include cold intolerance, fatigue, somnolence, poor memory, constipation, menorrhagia, myalgias, and hoarseness. Hypothyroidism is readily treatable and should be suspected in any patient with compatible symptoms.

Physical Examination

Signs include slow tendon reflex relaxation, bradycardia, facial and periorbital edema, dry skin, and nonpitting edema (myxedema). Mild weight gain may occur, but hypothyroidism does not cause marked obesity. Rare manifestations include hypoventilation, pericardial or pleural effusions, deafness, and carpal tunnel syndrome.

Diagnostic Testing

- Laboratory findings may include hyponatremia and elevated plasma levels of cholesterol, triglycerides, and creatine kinase.
- In suspected primary hypothyroidism, plasma TSH is the best initial test.
  - A normal value excludes primary hypothyroidism, and a markedly elevated value (>20 microunits/mL) confirms the diagnosis.
  - Mild elevation of plasma TSH (<20 microunits/mL) may be due to recovery from nonthyroidal illness, but usually indicates mild (or subclinical) primary hypothyroidism, in which thyroid function is impaired but increased secretion of TSH maintains normal plasma free T$_4$ levels. These patients may have nonspecific symptoms that are compatible with hypothyroidism and a mild increase in serum cholesterol and low-density lipoprotein cholesterol. They develop clinical hypothyroidism at a rate of 2.5% per year.
- If secondary hypothyroidism is suspected because of evidence of pituitary disease, plasma free T$_4$ should be measured. Plasma TSH levels are usually within the reference range in secondary hypothyroidism and cannot be used alone to make this diagnosis. Patients with secondary hypothyroidism should be evaluated for other pituitary hormone deficits and for a mass lesion of the pituitary or hypothalamus (see Disorders of Anterior Pituitary Function section).

- **In severe nonthyroidal illness**, the diagnosis of hypothyroidism may be difficult. Plasma free T_4 measured by routine assays may be low.
  - **Plasma TSH is the best initial diagnostic test.** A normal TSH value is strong evidence that the patient is euthyroid, except when there is evidence of pituitary or hypothalamic disease or in patients treated with dopamine or high doses of glucocorticoids. Marked elevation of plasma TSH (>20 microunits/mL) establishes the diagnosis of primary hypothyroidism.
  - Moderate elevations of plasma TSH (<20 microunits/mL) may occur in euthyroid patients recovering from nonthyroidal illness and are not specific for hypothyroidism. Plasma free T_4 should be measured if TSH is moderately elevated or if secondary hypothyroidism is suspected, and patients should be treated for hypothyroidism if plasma free T_4 is low. Thyroid function in these patients should be reevaluated after recovery from illness.

TREATMENT

Thyroxine is the drug of choice. The average replacement dose is 1.6 μg/kg PO daily, and most patients require doses between 75–150 μg/d. In elderly patients, the average replacement dose is lower. The need for lifelong treatment should be emphasized. Thyroxine should be taken 30 minutes before a meal, because some foods interfere with its absorption, and should not be taken with medications that affect its absorption (see the following text).

- **Initiation of therapy.** Young and middle-aged adults should be started on 1.6 μg/kg/d. This regimen gradually corrects hypothyroidism, because several weeks are required to reach steady-state plasma levels of T_4. In otherwise healthy elderly patients, the initial dose should be 50 μg/d. Patients with cardiac disease should be started on 25 μg/d and monitored carefully for exacerbation of cardiac symptoms.
- **Dose adjustment and follow-up**
  - **In primary hypothyroidism, the goal of therapy is to maintain plasma TSH within the normal range.** Plasma TSH should be measured 6–8 weeks after initiation of therapy. The dose of thyroxine should then be adjusted in 12- to 25-μg increments at intervals of 6–8 weeks until plasma TSH is normal. Thereafter, annual TSH measurement is adequate to monitor therapy. TSH should also be measured in the first trimester of pregnancy, because the thyroxine dose requirement often increases at this time (see the following text). Overtreatment, indicated by a subnormal TSH, should be avoided because it increases the risk of osteoporosis and atrial fibrillation.
  - **In secondary hypothyroidism, plasma TSH cannot be used to adjust therapy.** The goal of therapy is to maintain the **plasma free T_4** near the middle of the reference range. The dose of thyroxine should be adjusted at 6- to 8-week intervals until this goal is achieved. Thereafter, annual measurement of plasma free T_4 is adequate to monitor therapy.

COMPLICATIONS

- **Situations in which thyroxine dose requirements change.** Difficulty in controlling hypothyroidism is most often due to **poor compliance** with therapy. Other causes of increasing thyroxine requirement include:
  - Malabsorption due to intestinal disease or drugs that interfere with thyroxine absorption (e.g., calcium carbonate, ferrous sulfate, cholestyramine, sucralfate, aluminum hydroxide)
  - Drug interactions that increase thyroxine clearance (e.g., estrogen, rifampin, carbamazepine, phenytoin) or block conversion of T_4 to T_3 (amiodarone)
  - Pregnancy, in which thyroxine requirements often increase in the first trimester (see the following text)
  - Gradual failure of remaining endogenous thyroid function after RAI treatment of hyperthyroidism

- **Pregnancy.** Thyroxine dose increases by an average of 50% in the first half of pregnancy (*J Clin Endocrinol Metab 2012;97:2543*). In women with primary hypothyroidism, plasma TSH should be measured as soon as pregnancy is confirmed and monthly thereafter through the second trimester. The thyroxine dose should be increased as needed to maintain plasma TSH within the lower half of the normal range to avoid fetal hypothyroidism.
- **Subclinical hypothyroidism** should be treated if any of the following are present: (a) symptoms compatible with hypothyroidism, (b) goiter, (c) hypercholesterolemia that warrants treatment, or (d) plasma TSH >10 microunits/mL (*Thyroid 2014;24:1670*). Untreated patients should be monitored annually, and thyroxine should be started if symptoms develop or serum TSH increases to >10 microunits/mL.
- **Urgent therapy** for hypothyroidism is rarely necessary. Most patients with hypothyroidism and concomitant illness can be treated in the usual manner. However, hypothyroidism may impair survival in critical illness by contributing to hypoventilation, hypotension, hypothermia, bradycardia, or hyponatremia.
  - Hypoventilation and hypotension should be treated intensively, along with any concomitant diseases. Confirmatory tests (plasma TSH and free T_4) should be obtained before thyroid hormone therapy is started.
  - **Thyroxine, 50–100 μg IV, can be given q6–8h for 24 hours**, followed by 75–100 μg IV daily until oral intake is possible. No clinical trials have determined the optimum method of thyroid hormone replacement, but this method rapidly alleviates hypothyroidism while minimizing the risk of exacerbating underlying coronary disease or heart failure. **Rapid correction is warranted only in extremely ill patients. Vital signs and cardiac rhythm should be monitored carefully to detect early signs of exacerbation of heart disease. Hydrocortisone**, 50 mg IV q8h, is recommended during rapid replacement of thyroid hormone, because this therapy may precipitate adrenal crisis in patients with adrenal failure.

Hyperthyroidism

GENERAL PRINCIPLES

- Evidence-based recommendations have been developed to guide the treatment of patients with hyperthyroidism and thyrotoxicosis (*Thyroid 2011:21:593*).
- **Graves disease** causes most cases of hyperthyroidism, especially in young patients. This **autoimmune** disorder may also cause **proptosis** (exophthalmos) and pretibial myxedema, neither of which is found in other causes of hyperthyroidism.
- **Toxic multinodular goiter (MNG)** may cause hyperthyroidism in older patients.
- Unusual causes include **iodine-induced hyperthyroidism** (precipitated by drugs such as **amiodarone** or radiographic contrast media), thyroid adenomas, subacute thyroiditis (painful tender goiter with transient hyperthyroidism), painless thyroiditis (nontender goiter with transient hyperthyroidism, most often seen in the postpartum period), and surreptitious ingestion of thyroid hormone. TSH-induced hyperthyroidism is extremely rare.

DIAGNOSIS

Clinical Presentation

History
- Symptoms include heat intolerance, weight loss, weakness, palpitations, oligomenorrhea, and anxiety.

TABLE 24-2	Differential Diagnosis of Hyperthyroidism
Type of Goiter	**Diagnosis**
Diffuse, nontender goiter	Graves disease or painless thyroiditis
Multiple thyroid nodules	Toxic multinodular goiter
Single thyroid nodule	Thyroid adenoma
Tender painful goiter	Subacute thyroiditis
Normal thyroid gland	Graves disease, painless thyroiditis, or factitious hyperthyroidism

- **In the elderly**, hyperthyroidism may present with only atrial fibrillation, heart failure, weakness, or weight loss, and a high index of suspicion is needed to make the diagnosis.

Physical Examination
- Signs include brisk tendon reflexes, fine tremor, proximal weakness, stare, and eyelid lag. Cardiac abnormalities may be prominent, including sinus tachycardia, atrial fibrillation, and exacerbation of coronary artery disease or heart failure.
- Key differentiating physical exam findings (Table 24-2) include the following:
  - The presence of proptosis or pretibial myxedema, seen only in Graves disease (although many patients with Graves disease lack these signs)
  - A diffuse nontender goiter, consistent with Graves disease or painless thyroiditis
  - Recent pregnancy, neck pain, or recent iodine administration, suggesting causes other than Graves disease

Diagnostic Testing
- In rare cases, **24-hour radioactive iodine uptake (RAIU)** is needed to distinguish Graves disease or toxic MNG (in which RAIU is elevated) from postpartum thyroiditis, iodine-induced hyperthyroidism, or factitious hyperthyroidism (in which RAIU is very low).
- In suspected hyperthyroidism, plasma TSH is the best initial diagnostic test.
  - A TSH level >0.1 microunits/mL excludes clinical hyperthyroidism. If plasma TSH is <0.1 microunits/mL, **plasma free T_4** should be measured to determine the severity of hyperthyroidism and as a baseline for therapy. If plasma free T_4 is elevated, the diagnosis of clinical hyperthyroidism is established.
  - **If plasma TSH is <0.1 microunits/mL but free T_4 is normal**, the patient may have clinical hyperthyroidism due to elevation of plasma T_3 alone; and plasma T_3 should be measured in this case.
  - Very **mild (or subclinical) hyperthyroidism** may suppress TSH to <0.1 microunits/mL, and thus suppression of TSH alone does not confirm that symptoms are due to hyperthyroidism.
  - TSH may also be suppressed by **severe nonthyroidal illness** (see Evaluation of Thyroid Function section).

TREATMENT
- Some forms of hyperthyroidism (subacute or postpartum thyroiditis) are transient and require only **symptomatic therapy**. A β-adrenergic antagonist (such as **atenolol** 25–100 mg daily) relieves symptoms of hyperthyroidism, such as palpitations, tremor, and anxiety, until hyperthyroidism is controlled by definitive therapy or until transient

forms of hyperthyroidism subside. The dose is adjusted to alleviate symptoms and tachycardia, then reduced gradually as hyperthyroidism is controlled.

- Three methods are available for definitive therapy (none of which controls hyperthyroidism rapidly): RAI, thionamides, and subtotal thyroidectomy (*Thyroid 2011;21:593*).
  - During treatment, patients are followed by clinical evaluation and measurement of plasma free T_4. Plasma TSH is useless in assessing the initial response to therapy, because it remains suppressed until after the patient becomes euthyroid.
  - Regardless of the therapy used, all patients with Graves disease require lifelong follow-up for recurrent hyperthyroidism or development of hypothyroidism.
- **Choice of definitive therapy**
  - **In Graves disease, RAI therapy is the treatment of choice for almost all patients.** It is simple and highly effective but **cannot be used in pregnancy. Propylthiouracil (PTU) should be used to treat hyperthyroidism in pregnancy.** Thionamides achieve long-term control in fewer than half of patients with Graves disease, and they carry a small risk of life-threatening side effects. Thyroidectomy should be used in patients who refuse RAI therapy and who relapse or develop side effects with thionamide therapy.
  - **Other causes of hyperthyroidism.** Toxic MNG and toxic adenoma should be treated with RAI (except in pregnancy). Transient forms of hyperthyroidism due to thyroiditis should be treated symptomatically with atenolol. Iodine-induced hyperthyroidism is treated with thionamides and atenolol until the patient is euthyroid. Although treatment of some patients with amiodarone-induced hyperthyroidism with glucocorticoids has been advocated, **nearly all patients with amiodarone-induced hyperthyroidism respond well to thionamide therapy** (*Circulation 2002;105:1275*).
- **RAI therapy**
  - A single dose permanently controls hyperthyroidism in 90% of patients, and further doses can be given if necessary.
  - A **pregnancy test** is done immediately before therapy in potentially fertile women.
  - A 24-hour RAIU is usually measured and used to calculate the dose.
  - Thionamides interfere with RAI therapy and should be stopped at least 3 days before treatment. If iodine treatment has been given, it should be stopped at least 2 weeks before RAI therapy.
  - **Follow-up.** Usually, several months are needed to restore euthyroidism. Patients are evaluated at 4- to 6-week intervals, with assessment of clinical findings and plasma free T_4.
    - If thyroid function stabilizes within the normal range, the interval between follow-up visits is gradually increased to annual intervals.
    - If symptomatic hypothyroidism develops, thyroxine therapy is started (see Hypothyroidism section).
    - If symptomatic hyperthyroidism **persists after 6 months, RAI treatment is repeated**.
  - **Side effects**
    - **Hypothyroidism** occurs in most patients within the first year and continues to develop at a rate of approximately 3% per year thereafter.
    - Because of the release of stored hormone, a slight rise in plasma T_4 may occur in the first 2 weeks after therapy. This development is important only in **patients with severe cardiac disease**, which may worsen as a result. Such patients should be treated with thionamides to restore euthyroidism and to deplete stored hormone before treatment with RAI.
    - There is no convincing evidence that RAI has a clinically important effect on the course of Graves eye disease.
    - It does not increase the risk of malignancy or cause congenital abnormalities in the offspring of women who conceive after RAI therapy.

- **Thionamides.** Methimazole and PTU inhibit thyroid hormone synthesis. PTU also inhibits extrathyroidal deiodination of T_4 to T_3. Once thyroid hormone stores are depleted (after several weeks to months), T_4 levels decrease. These drugs have no permanent effect on thyroid function. **In the majority of patients with Graves disease, hyperthyroidism recurs within 6 months after therapy is stopped.** Spontaneous remission of Graves disease occurs in approximately one-third of patients during thionamide therapy, and in this minority, no other treatment may be needed. Remission is more likely in mild, recent-onset hyperthyroidism and if the goiter is small. Because of a better safety profile, **methimazole should be used instead of PTU** except in specific situations (see the following text).
  - **Initiation of therapy.** Before starting therapy, patients must be warned of side effects and precautions. Usual starting doses are methimazole, 10–40 mg PO daily, or PTU, 100–200 mg PO tid; higher initial doses can be used in severe hyperthyroidism.
  - **Follow-up.** Restoration of euthyroidism takes up to several months.
    - Patients are evaluated at 4-week intervals with assessment of clinical findings and plasma free T_4. If plasma free T_4 levels do not fall after 4–8 weeks, the dose should be increased. Doses as high as methimazole, 60 mg PO daily, or PTU, 300 mg PO qid, may be required.
    - Once the plasma free T_4 level falls to normal, the dose is adjusted to maintain plasma free T_4 within the normal range.
    - No consensus exists on the optimal duration of therapy, but periods of 6 months to 2 years are usually used. Patients must be monitored carefully for recurrence of hyperthyroidism after the drug is stopped.
- **Side effects** are most likely to occur within the first few months of therapy.
  - Minor side effects include rash, urticaria, fever, arthralgias, and transient leukopenia.
  - **Agranulocytosis** occurs in 0.3% of patients treated with thionamides. Other life-threatening side effects include **hepatitis**, vasculitis, and drug-induced lupus erythematosus. These complications usually resolve if the drug is stopped promptly.
  - **Patients must be warned to stop the drug immediately if jaundice or symptoms suggestive of agranulocytosis develop (e.g., fever, chills, sore throat)** and to contact their physician promptly for evaluation. Routine monitoring of the white blood cell count (WBC) is not useful for detecting agranulocytosis, which develops suddenly.
- **Subtotal thyroidectomy.** This procedure provides long-term control of hyperthyroidism in most patients.
  - Surgery may trigger a perioperative exacerbation of hyperthyroidism, and patients should be prepared for surgery by one of two methods.
    - **A thionamide** is given until the patient is nearly euthyroid. **Supersaturated potassium iodide (SSKI)**, 40–80 mg (one to two drops) PO bid, is then added 1–2 weeks before surgery. Both drugs are stopped postoperatively.
    - **Atenolol** (50–100 mg daily) is started 1–2 weeks before surgery. The dose of atenolol is increased, if necessary, to reduce the resting heart rate below 90 bpm and is continued for 5–7 days postoperatively. SSKI is given as mentioned earlier.
  - **Follow-up.** Clinical findings and plasma free T_4 and TSH should be assessed 4–6 weeks after surgery.
    - If thyroid function is normal, the patient is seen at 3 and 6 months and then annually.
    - If symptomatic hypothyroidism develops, thyroxine therapy is started.
    - Hyperthyroidism persists or recurs in 3–7% of patients.
  - **Complications** of thyroidectomy include **hypothyroidism** and **hypoparathyroidism**. Rare complications include permanent vocal cord paralysis, due to recurrent laryngeal nerve injury, and perioperative death. The complication rate appears to depend on the experience of the surgeon.

SPECIAL CONSIDERATIONS

- **Subclinical hyperthyroidism** (*J Clin Endocrinol Metab 2011;96:59*) is present when the plasma TSH is suppressed to <0.1 microunits/mL but the patient has no symptoms that are definitely caused by hyperthyroidism and plasma levels of free T_4 and T_3 are normal.
  - Subclinical hyperthyroidism increases the risk of **atrial fibrillation** in patients older than 60 years and those with heart disease and predisposes to **osteoporosis** in postmenopausal women; it should be treated in these patients.
  - Asymptomatic young patients with mild Graves disease can be observed for spontaneous resolution of hyperthyroidism or the development of symptoms or increasing free T_4 levels that warrant treatment.
- **Urgent therapy** is warranted when hyperthyroidism exacerbates heart failure or acute coronary syndromes and in rare patients with severe hyperthyroidism complicated by fever and delirium (sometimes called thyroid storm). Concomitant diseases should be treated intensively, and confirmatory tests (serum TSH and free T_4) should be obtained before therapy is started.
  - **PTU 300 mg PO q6h or methimazole 60 mg/d PO should be started immediately.**
  - **Iodide** (**SSKI**, two drops PO q12h) should be started to inhibit thyroid hormone secretion rapidly.
  - **Propranolol**, 40 mg PO q6h (or an equivalent dose IV), should be given to patients with angina or myocardial infarction, and the dose should be adjusted to prevent tachycardia. β-Adrenergic antagonists may benefit some patients with heart failure and marked tachycardia but can further impair left ventricular systolic function. In patients with clinical heart failure, it should be given only with careful monitoring of left ventricular function.
  - Plasma free T_4 is measured every 4–6 days. When free T_4 approaches the normal range, the doses of methimazole and iodine are gradually decreased. RAI therapy should be scheduled 2–4 weeks after iodine is stopped.
- **Hyperthyroidism in pregnancy.** If hyperthyroidism is suspected, plasma TSH should be measured. Plasma TSH declines in early pregnancy but rarely to <0.1 microunits/mL (*Endocrinol Metab Clin North Am 2011;40:739*).
  - If TSH is <0.1 microunits/mL, the diagnosis should be confirmed by measurement of plasma free T_4.
  - RAI is contraindicated in pregnancy, and therefore, patients should be treated with PTU. Methimazole is not used in the first trimester because it is associated with certain congenital defects. The dose should be adjusted at 4-week intervals to maintain the plasma free T_4 near the upper limit of the normal range to avoid fetal hypothyroidism. The dose required often decreases in the later stages of pregnancy.
  - Atenolol, 25–50 mg PO daily, can be used to relieve symptoms while awaiting the effects of PTU.
  - The fetus and neonate should be monitored for hyperthyroidism. The maternal plasma level of thyroid-stimulating immunoglobulin should be measured in the third trimester to assess this risk.

Euthyroid Goiter and Thyroid Nodules

GENERAL PRINCIPLES

- The diagnosis of euthyroid goiter is based on palpation of the thyroid and evaluation of thyroid function. If the thyroid is enlarged, the examiner should determine whether the enlargement is **diffuse or multinodular or whether a single palpable nodule is present**. All three forms of euthyroid goiter are common, especially in women.

- Thyroid scans and ultrasonography (US) provide no useful additional information about goiters that are diffuse by palpation and should not be performed in these patients.
- Between 30–50% of people have nonpalpable thyroid nodules that are detectable by ultrasound. These nodules rarely have any clinical importance, but their incidental discovery may lead to unnecessary diagnostic testing and treatment.
- **Diffuse goiter**
  - Almost all euthyroid diffuse goiters in the United States are due to **chronic lymphocytic thyroiditis (Hashimoto thyroiditis)**. Because Hashimoto thyroiditis may also cause hypothyroidism, plasma TSH should be measured.
  - Diffuse goiters are usually asymptomatic, and therapy is seldom required. Patients should be monitored regularly for the development of hypothyroidism.
- **MNG**
  - MNG is common in older patients, especially women. Most patients are asymptomatic and require no treatment.
  - In a few patients, **hyperthyroidism** (toxic MNG) develops (see Hyperthyroidism section).
  - In rare patients, the gland compresses the trachea or esophagus, causing dyspnea or dysphagia, and treatment is required. Thyroxine treatment has little, if any, effect on the size of MNGs. RAI therapy reduces gland size and relieves symptoms in most patients. Subtotal thyroidectomy can also be used to relieve compressive symptoms.
  - Evaluation for thyroid carcinoma with needle biopsy is warranted if there is a dominant nodule (a nodule that is disproportionately larger than the rest). Some centers have adopted a policy of performing thyroid US in all patients with MNG and evaluating all nodules larger than 1 cm by needle biopsy. This policy dramatically increases the number of thyroid biopsies and the cost of managing this common condition. There is no evidence that routine thyroid US improves clinical outcomes in patients with MNG.
- **Single thyroid nodules**
  - **Single palpable thyroid nodules** are usually benign, but about 5% are thyroid carcinomas.
  - Clinical findings that increase the risk of carcinoma include the presence of cervical lymphadenopathy, a history of radiation to the head or neck, and a family history of medullary thyroid carcinoma or multiple endocrine neoplasia syndromes type 2A or 2B. A hard, fixed nodule, recent nodule growth, or hoarseness due to vocal cord paralysis also suggests malignancy.
  - Most patients with thyroid carcinomas have none of these risk factors, and all **palpable single thyroid nodules should be evaluated with needle aspiration biopsy**. Patients with thyroid carcinoma should be managed in consultation with an endocrinologist.
  - Nodules with benign cytology should be reevaluated periodically by palpation. Thyroxine therapy has little or no effect on the size of single thyroid nodules and is not indicated.
  - Some centers routinely use US for thyroids that contain a palpable thyroid nodule and biopsy all nodules that meet size and imaging criteria.

DISORDERS OF ADRENAL FUNCTION

Adrenal Failure

GENERAL PRINCIPLES

- Adrenal failure may be due to disease of the adrenal glands (**primary adrenal failure, Addison disease**), with deficiency of both cortisol and aldosterone and elevated plasma adrenocorticotropic hormone (ACTH), or due to ACTH deficiency caused by disorders of the pituitary or hypothalamus (**secondary adrenal failure**), with deficiency of cortisol alone.
- **Primary adrenal failure** is most often due to **autoimmune adrenalitis**, which may be associated with other endocrine deficits (e.g., hypothyroidism).

- Infections of the adrenal gland such as tuberculosis and histoplasmosis may cause adrenal failure.
- **Hemorrhagic adrenal infarction** may occur in the postoperative period, in coagulation disorders and hypercoagulable states, and in sepsis. Adrenal hemorrhage often causes abdominal or flank pain and fever; CT scan of the abdomen reveals high-density bilateral adrenal masses.
- Adrenal failure may develop in patients with AIDS, caused by adrenal lymphoma, disseminated cytomegalovirus, mycobacterial infection, or fungal infection.
- Less common etiologies include adrenoleukodystrophy that causes adrenal failure in young men and drugs such as ketoconazole and etomidate that inhibit steroid hormone synthesis.
- **Secondary adrenal failure** is most often due to **glucocorticoid therapy**; ACTH suppression may persist for a year after therapy is stopped. Any disorder of the pituitary or hypothalamus can cause ACTH deficiency, but other evidence of these disorders is usually obvious.

DIAGNOSIS

Clinical Presentation
- Adrenal failure should be suspected in patients with hypotension, weight loss, persistent nausea, hyponatremia, or hyperkalemia.
- **Clinical findings** in adrenal failure are nonspecific, and without a high index of suspicion, the diagnosis of this potentially lethal but readily treatable disease is easily missed.
  - ○ Symptoms include anorexia, nausea, vomiting, weight loss, weakness, and fatigue. Orthostatic hypotension and hyponatremia are common.
  - ○ Symptoms are usually chronic, but **shock** may develop suddenly and is fatal unless promptly treated. Often, this adrenal crisis is triggered by illness, injury, or surgery. All these symptoms are due to cortisol deficiency and occur in both primary and secondary adrenal failure.
- Hyperpigmentation (due to marked ACTH excess) and hyperkalemia and volume depletion (due to aldosterone deficiency) occur only in primary adrenal failure.

Diagnostic Testing
- **The cosyntropin (Cortrosyn) stimulation test** is used for diagnosis. Cosyntropin, 250 μg, is given IV or IM, and **plasma cortisol is measured 30 minutes later**. The normal response is a stimulated plasma cortisol >18 μg/dL. This test detects primary and secondary adrenal failure, except within a few weeks of onset of pituitary dysfunction (e.g., shortly after pituitary surgery; see Disorders of Anterior Pituitary Function section).
- The distinction between primary and secondary adrenal failure is usually clear.
- Hyperkalemia, hyperpigmentation, or other autoimmune endocrine deficits indicate primary adrenal failure, whereas deficits of other pituitary hormones, symptoms of a pituitary mass (e.g., headache, visual field loss), or known pituitary or hypothalamic disease indicate secondary adrenal failure.
- If the cause is unclear, the **plasma ACTH** level distinguishes primary adrenal failure (in which it is markedly elevated) from secondary adrenal failure.
- Most cases of primary adrenal failure are due to autoimmune adrenalitis, but other causes should be considered. Radiographic evidence of adrenal enlargement or calcification indicates that the cause is infection or hemorrhage.
- Patients with secondary adrenal failure should be tested for other pituitary hormone deficiencies and should be evaluated for a pituitary or hypothalamic tumor (see Disorders of Anterior Pituitary Function section).

TREATMENT

- **Adrenal crisis** with hypotension must be treated immediately. Patients should be evaluated for an underlying illness that precipitated the crisis.
- **If the diagnosis of adrenal failure is known, hydrocortisone, 100 mg IV q8h**, should be given, and **0.9% saline with 5% dextrose** should be infused rapidly until hypotension is corrected. The dose of hydrocortisone is decreased gradually over several days as symptoms and any precipitating illness resolve, then changed to oral maintenance therapy. Mineralocorticoid replacement is not needed until the dose of hydrocortisone is <100 mg/d.
- **If the diagnosis of adrenal failure has not been established**, a single dose of **dexamethasone**, 10 mg IV, should be given, and a rapid infusion of 0.9% saline with 5% dextrose should be started. A **Cortrosyn stimulation test** should be performed, regardless of the time of day. Dexamethasone is used because it does not interfere with measurement of plasma cortisol. After the 30-minute plasma cortisol measurement, hydrocortisone, 100 mg IV q8h, should be given until the test result is known.
- **Maintenance therapy** in all patients requires cortisol replacement with prednisone. Most patients with primary adrenal failure also require replacement of aldosterone with fludrocortisone.
  - **Prednisone**, 5 mg PO every morning, should be started. The dose is then adjusted with the goal being the lowest dose that relieves the patient's symptoms, to prevent osteoporosis and other signs of Cushing syndrome. Most patients require doses between 4.0–7.5 mg PO daily. Concomitant therapy with rifampin, phenytoin, or phenobarbital accelerates glucocorticoid metabolism and increases the dose requirement.
  - **During illness, injury, or the perioperative period, the dose of glucocorticoid must be increased.**
  - For minor illnesses, the patient should double the dose of prednisone for 2–3 days. If the illness resolves, the maintenance dose is resumed.
  - **Vomiting requires immediate medical attention**, with IV glucocorticoid therapy and IV fluid. Patients can be given a 4-mg vial of dexamethasone to be self-administered IM for vomiting or severe illness if medical care is not immediately available.
  - **For severe illness or injury**, hydrocortisone, 50 mg IV q8h, should be given, with the dose tapered as severity of illness wanes. The same regimen is used in **patients undergoing surgery**, with the first dose of hydrocortisone given preoperatively. The dose can be tapered to maintenance therapy by 2–3 days after uncomplicated surgery.
- **In primary adrenal failure, fludrocortisone, 0.1 mg PO daily**, should be given. The dose is adjusted to maintain blood pressure (supine and standing) and serum potassium within the normal range; the usual dosage is 0.05–0.20 mg PO daily.
- **Patients should be educated in management of their disease**, including adjustment of prednisone dose during illness. They should wear a medical identification tag or bracelet.

Cushing Syndrome

GENERAL PRINCIPLES

- Cushing syndrome (*J Clin Endocrinol Metab 2008;93:1526*) is most often **iatrogenic**, due to therapy with glucocorticoid drugs.
- **ACTH-secreting pituitary microadenomas (Cushing disease)** account for 80% of cases of endogenous Cushing syndrome.
- Adrenal tumors and ectopic ACTH secretion account for the remainder.

DIAGNOSIS

Clinical Presentation

- Findings include truncal obesity, rounded face, fat deposits in the supraclavicular fossae and over the posterior neck, hypertension, hirsutism, amenorrhea, and depression. More specific findings include thin skin, easy bruising, reddish striae, proximal muscle weakness, and osteoporosis.
- Hyperpigmentation or hypokalemic alkalosis suggests Cushing syndrome due to ectopic ACTH secretion.
- Diabetes mellitus develops in some patients.

Diagnostic Testing

- **Diagnosis** is based on increased cortisol excretion, lack of normal feedback inhibition of ACTH and cortisol secretion, or loss of the normal diurnal rhythm of cortisol secretion. Three initial tests are available:
  - The best initial test is the **24-hour urine cortisol** measurement;
  - Alternatively, an **overnight dexamethasone suppression test** may be performed (1 mg dexamethasone given PO at 11:00 p.m.; plasma cortisol measured at 8:00 a.m. the next day; normal range: plasma cortisol <2 μg/dL); or
  - Salivary cortisol may be measured at home during the nadir of normal plasma cortisol at 11:00 p.m.
- All these tests are very sensitive, and a normal value virtually excludes the diagnosis. If the overnight dexamethasone suppression test or 11:00 p.m. salivary cortisol is abnormal, 24-hour urine cortisol should be measured.
  - If the 24-hour urine cortisol excretion is more than 3–4 times the upper limit of the reference range in a patient with compatible clinical findings, the diagnosis of Cushing syndrome is established.
  - In patients with milder elevations of urine cortisol, a **low-dose dexamethasone suppression test** should be performed. Dexamethasone, 0.5 mg PO q6h, is given for 48 hours, starting at 8:00 a.m. Urine cortisol is measured during the last 24 hours, and plasma cortisol is measured 6 hours after the last dose of dexamethasone. Failure to suppress plasma cortisol to <2 μg/dL and urine cortisol to less than the normal reference range is diagnostic of Cushing syndrome.
  - Testing should not be done during severe illness or depression, which may cause false-positive results. Phenytoin therapy also causes a false-positive test by accelerating metabolism of dexamethasone.
- After the diagnosis of Cushing syndrome is made, tests to determine the cause are best done in consultation with an endocrinologist.

Incidental Adrenal Nodules

GENERAL PRINCIPLES

- Adrenal nodules are a common incidental finding on abdominal imaging studies.
- Most incidentally discovered nodules are benign adrenocortical tumors that do not secrete excess hormone.

DIAGNOSIS

In patients without a known malignancy elsewhere, the diagnostic issues are whether a syndrome of hormone excess or an adrenocortical carcinoma is present.

Clinical Presentation

Patients should be evaluated for hypertension, symptoms suggestive of pheochromocytoma (episodic headache, palpitations, and sweating), and signs of Cushing syndrome (see Cushing Syndrome section).

Differential Diagnosis

- The differential diagnosis includes adrenal adenomas causing Cushing syndrome or primary hyperaldosteronism, pheochromocytoma, adrenocortical carcinoma, and metastatic cancer.
- The imaging characteristics of the nodule may suggest a diagnosis but are not specific enough to obviate further evaluation.

Diagnostic Testing

- **Plasma potassium, metanephrines, and dehydroepiandrosterone sulfate** should be measured, and an **overnight dexamethasone suppression** test should be performed.
- **Patients who have potentially resectable cancer elsewhere** and in whom an adrenal metastasis must be excluded may require positron emission tomography.
- Patients with hypertension (especially if they have hypokalemia) should be evaluated for primary hyperaldosteronism by measuring the ratio of plasma aldosterone (in nanograms per deciliter [ng/dL]) to plasma renin activity (in ng/mL/h). If the ratio is <20, the diagnosis of primary hyperaldosteronism is excluded, whereas a ratio >50 makes the diagnosis very likely. Patients with an intermediate ratio should be further evaluated in consultation with an endocrinologist.
- An abnormal overnight dexamethasone suppression test should be evaluated further (see Cushing Syndrome section).
- Elevation of plasma dehydroepiandrosterone sulfate or a large nodule suggests adrenocortical carcinoma.

TREATMENT

- Most incidental nodules are <4 cm in diameter, do not produce excess hormone, and do not require therapy. One **repeat imaging procedure** 3–6 months later is recommended to ensure that the nodule is not enlarging rapidly (which would suggest an adrenal carcinoma).
- A policy of resecting all nodules >4 cm in diameter appropriately treats the great majority of adrenal carcinomas while minimizing the number of benign nodules that are removed unnecessarily.
- If clinical or biochemical evidence of a pheochromocytoma is found, the nodule should be resected after appropriate α-adrenergic blockade with phenoxybenzamine.

DISORDERS OF ANTERIOR PITUITARY FUNCTION

GENERAL PRINCIPLES

- The anterior pituitary gland secretes **prolactin**, **growth hormone**, and four **trophic hormones**, including corticotropin (ACTH), thyrotropin (TSH), and the gonadotropins, luteinizing hormone and follicle-stimulating hormone. Each trophic hormone stimulates a specific target gland.
- Anterior pituitary function is regulated by hypothalamic hormones that reach the pituitary via portal veins in the pituitary stalk. The predominant effect of hypothalamic

regulation is to stimulate secretion of pituitary hormones, except for prolactin, which is inhibited by hypothalamic dopamine secretion.
- Secretion of trophic hormones is also regulated by negative feedback by their target gland hormone, and the normal pituitary response to target hormone deficiency is increased secretion of the appropriate trophic hormone.
- **Anterior pituitary dysfunction** can be caused by disorders of either the pituitary or hypothalamus.

Etiology

- **Pituitary adenomas** are the most common pituitary disorder. They are classified by size and function.
  - **Microadenomas** are <10 mm in diameter and cause clinical manifestations only if they produce excess hormone. They are too small to produce hypopituitarism or mass effects.
  - **Macroadenomas** are >10 mm in diameter and may produce any combination of pituitary hormone excess, hypopituitarism, and mass effects (headache, visual field loss).
  - **Secretory adenomas** produce prolactin, growth hormone, or ACTH.
  - **Nonsecretory macroadenomas** may cause hypopituitarism or mass effects.
  - **Nonsecretory microadenomas** are common incidental radiographic findings, seen in approximately 10% of the normal population, and do not require therapy.
- **Other pituitary or hypothalamic disorders**, such as head trauma, pituitary surgery or radiation, and postpartum pituitary infarction (Sheehan syndrome) may cause hypopituitarism. Other tumors of the pituitary or hypothalamus (e.g., craniopharyngioma, metastases) and inflammatory disorders (e.g., sarcoidosis, Langerhans cell histiocytosis) may cause hypopituitarism or mass effects.

DIAGNOSIS

Clinical Presentation

- In **hypopituitarism** (deficiency of one or more pituitary hormones), gonadotropin deficiency is most common, causing amenorrhea in women and androgen deficiency in men. Secondary hypothyroidism or adrenal failure rarely occurs alone. Secondary adrenal failure causes deficiency of cortisol but not of aldosterone; hyperkalemia and hyperpigmentation do not occur, although life-threatening adrenal crisis may develop.
- **Hormone excess** most commonly results in **hyperprolactinemia**, which can be due to a secretory adenoma or due to nonsecretory lesions that damage the hypothalamus or pituitary stalk. Growth hormone excess **(acromegaly)** and ACTH and cortisol excess **(Cushing disease)** are caused by secretory adenomas.
- **Mass effects** due to pressure on adjacent structures, such as the optic chiasm, include headaches and loss of visual fields or acuity. Hyperprolactinemia may also be due to mass effect. **Pituitary apoplexy** is sudden enlargement of a pituitary tumor due to hemorrhagic necrosis.
- **Asymptomatic pituitary adenomas incidentally discovered on imaging.**

Diagnostic Testing

- If an incidental microadenoma is found on imaging done for another purpose, the patient should be evaluated for clinical evidence of hyperprolactinemia, Cushing disease, or acromegaly (*J Clin Endocrinol Metab 2011;96:894*).
- Plasma prolactin and **insulin-like growth factor 1** (IGF-1) should be measured, and tests for Cushing syndrome should be performed if symptoms or signs of this disorder are evident.
- If no pituitary hormone excess exists, therapy is not required. Whether such patients need repeat imaging is not established, but the risk of enlargement is clearly small.

- Incidental discovery of a macroadenoma is unusual. Patients should be evaluated for hormone excess and hypopituitarism. Most macroadenomas should be treated because they are likely to grow further.

Hypopituitarism

DIAGNOSIS

Clinical Presentation

Hypopituitarism may be suspected in the presence of clinical signs of target hormone deficiency (e.g., hypothyroidism) or pituitary mass effects.

Diagnostic Testing

Laboratories

- **Laboratory evaluation** for hypopituitarism begins with evaluation of **target hormone function**, including **plasma free T$_4$** and a **Cortrosyn stimulation test** (see Adrenal Failure section).
  - If recent onset of secondary adrenal failure is suspected (within a few weeks of evaluation), the patient should be treated empirically with glucocorticoids and should be tested 4–8 weeks later because the Cortrosyn stimulation test cannot detect secondary adrenal failure of recent onset.
  - In men, plasma testosterone should be measured. The best evaluation of gonadal function in women is the menstrual history.
- **If a target hormone is deficient**, its trophic hormone is measured to determine whether target gland dysfunction is secondary to hypopituitarism. An elevated trophic hormone level indicates primary target gland dysfunction. In hypopituitarism, trophic hormone levels are not elevated and are usually within (not below) the reference range. Thus, **pituitary trophic hormone levels can be interpreted only with knowledge of target hormone levels**, and **measurement of trophic hormone levels alone is useless in the diagnosis of hypopituitarism**. If pituitary disease is obvious, target hormone deficiencies may be assumed to be secondary, and trophic hormones need not be measured.

Imaging

Anatomic evaluation of the pituitary gland and hypothalamus is best done by MRI. However, hyperprolactinemia and Cushing disease may be caused by microadenomas too small to be seen. The prevalence of incidental microadenomas should be kept in mind when interpreting MRIs. Visual acuity and **visual fields** should be tested when imaging suggests compression of the optic chiasm.

TREATMENT

- Secondary adrenal failure should be treated immediately, especially if patients are to undergo surgery (see Adrenal Failure section).
- Treatment of secondary hypothyroidism should be monitored by measurement of **plasma free T$_4$** (see Hypothyroidism section).
- Infertility due to gonadotropin deficiency may be correctable, and patients who wish to conceive should be referred to an endocrinologist.
- Treatment of hypogonadism in premenopausal women requires replacement of estrogen and progesterone. This can be conveniently done with combination oral contraceptives.
- Treatment of hypogonadism in men requires testosterone replacement, with either topical testosterone gel, 40–50 mg applied daily, or by injection of testosterone enanthate or testosterone cypionate, 100–200 mg IM every 2 weeks.

- Treatment of growth hormone deficiency in adults has been advocated by some, but the long-term benefits, risks, and cost-effectiveness of this therapy are not established.
- Treatment of pituitary macroadenomas generally requires transsphenoidal surgical resection, except for prolactin-secreting tumors.

Hyperprolactinemia

GENERAL PRINCIPLES

- In women, the most common causes of pathologic hyperprolactinemia are prolactin-secreting pituitary **microadenomas** and **idiopathic hyperprolactinemia** (Table 24-3).
- In men, the most common cause is a prolactin-secreting **macroadenoma**.
- Hypothalamic or pituitary lesions that cause deficiency of other pituitary hormones often cause hyperprolactinemia.
- **Medications** are an important cause in both men and women (*Pituitary 2008;11:209*).

DIAGNOSIS

Clinical Presentation

- In women, hyperprolactinemia causes amenorrhea or irregular menses and infertility. Only approximately half of these women have galactorrhea. Prolonged estrogen deficiency increases the risk of osteoporosis. Plasma prolactin should be measured in women with amenorrhea, whether or not galactorrhea is present. Mild elevations should be confirmed by repeat measurements.
- In men, hyperprolactinemia causes androgen deficiency and infertility but not gynecomastia; mass effects and hypopituitarism are common.
- The history should include medications and symptoms of pituitary mass effects or hypothyroidism.

Diagnostic Testing

Testing for hypopituitarism is needed only in patients with a macroadenoma or hypothalamic lesion. **Pituitary imaging** should be performed in most cases, because large nonfunctional pituitary or hypothalamic tumors may present with hyperprolactinemia.

TABLE 24-3	Major Causes of Hyperprolactinemia
Pregnancy and lactation	
Prolactin-secreting pituitary adenoma (prolactinoma)	
Idiopathic hyperprolactinemia	
Drugs (e.g., phenothiazines, metoclopramide, risperidone, verapamil)	
Interference with synthesis or transport of hypothalamic dopamine	
Hypothalamic lesions	
Nonsecretory pituitary macroadenomas	
Primary hypothyroidism	
Chronic renal failure	

TREATMENT

- For **microadenomas and idiopathic hyperprolactinemia** (*J Clin Endocrinol Metab 2011;96:273*), most patients are treated because of infertility or to prevent estrogen deficiency and osteoporosis.
- Some women may be observed without therapy by periodic follow-up of prolactin levels and symptoms. In most patients, hyperprolactinemia does not worsen, and prolactin levels sometimes return to normal. Enlargement of microadenomas is rare.
- **The dopamine agonists bromocriptine** and **cabergoline** suppress plasma prolactin and restore normal menses and fertility in most women.
  - ○ Initial dosages are bromocriptine, 1.25–2.50 mg PO at bedtime with a snack, or cabergoline, 0.25 mg twice a week.
  - ○ Plasma prolactin levels are initially obtained at 2- to 4-week intervals, and doses are adjusted to the lowest dose required to maintain prolactin in the normal range. In general, the maximally effective doses are bromocriptine 2.5 mg tid and cabergoline 1.5 mg twice a week.
  - ○ **Side effects** include nausea and orthostatic hypotension, which can be minimized by increasing the dose gradually and usually resolve with continued therapy. Side effects are less severe with cabergoline.
  - ○ Initially, women should use barrier contraception, because fertility may be restored quickly.
  - ○ **Women who want to become pregnant** should be managed in consultation with an endocrinologist.
  - ○ **Women who do not want to become pregnant** should be followed with clinical evaluation and plasma prolactin levels every 6–12 months. Every few years, plasma prolactin may be measured after the dopamine agonist has been withdrawn for several weeks, to determine whether the drug is still needed. Follow-up imaging studies are not warranted unless prolactin levels increase substantially.
- **Prolactin-secreting macroadenomas** should be treated with a dopamine agonist, which usually suppresses prolactin levels to normal, reduces tumor size, and improves or corrects abnormal visual fields in 90% of cases.
  - ○ If mass effects are present, the dose should be increased to maximally effective levels over a period of several weeks. Visual field tests, if initially abnormal, should be repeated 4–6 weeks after therapy is started.
  - ○ Pituitary imaging should be repeated 3–6 months after initiation of therapy. If tumor shrinkage and correction of visual abnormalities are satisfactory, therapy can be continued indefinitely, with periodic monitoring of plasma prolactin levels.
  - ○ The full effect on tumor size may take more than 6 months. Further pituitary imaging is probably not warranted unless prolactin levels rise despite therapy.
  - ○ **Transsphenoidal surgery** is indicated to relieve mass effects if the tumor does not shrink or if visual field abnormalities persist during dopamine agonist therapy. However, the likelihood of surgical cure of a prolactin-secreting macroadenoma is low, and most patients require further therapy with a dopamine agonist.
  - ○ **Women with prolactin-secreting macroadenomas should not become pregnant** unless the tumor has been resected surgically or has decreased markedly in size with dopamine agonist therapy, because the risk of symptomatic enlargement during pregnancy is 15–35%. Contraception is essential during dopamine agonist treatment.

Acromegaly

GENERAL PRINCIPLES

Acromegaly is the syndrome caused by growth hormone excess in adults and is due to a growth hormone–secreting pituitary adenoma in the vast majority of cases (*J Clin Endocrinol Metab 2014;99:3933*).

DIAGNOSIS

Clinical Presentation

Clinical findings include thickened skin and enlargement of hands, feet, jaw, and forehead. Arthritis or carpal tunnel syndrome may develop, and the pituitary adenoma may cause headaches and vision loss. Mortality from cardiovascular disease is increased.

Diagnostic Testing

- **Plasma IGF-1**, which mediates most effects of growth hormone, is the best diagnostic test. Marked elevations establish the diagnosis.
- If IGF-1 levels are only moderately elevated, the diagnosis can be confirmed by giving 75 mg glucose orally and measuring serum growth hormone every 30 minutes for 2 hours. Failure to suppress growth hormone to <1 ng/mL confirms the diagnosis of acromegaly. Once the diagnosis is made, the pituitary should be imaged.

TREATMENT

The treatment of choice is transsphenoidal resection of the pituitary adenoma. Most patients have macroadenomas, and complete tumor resection with cure of acromegaly is often impossible. If IGF-1 levels remain elevated after surgery, radiotherapy is used to prevent regrowth of the tumor and to control acromegaly.

Medications

- The somatostatin analog **octreotide** in depot form can be used to suppress growth hormone secretion while awaiting the effect of radiation. A dose of 10–40 mg IM monthly suppresses IGF-1 to normal in about 60% of patients. Side effects include cholelithiasis, diarrhea, and mild abdominal discomfort.
- **Pegvisomant** is a growth hormone antagonist that lowers IGF-1 to normal in almost all patients. The dose is 10–30 mg SC daily. Few side effects have been reported, but patients should be monitored for pituitary adenoma enlargement and transaminase elevation.

METABOLIC BONE DISEASE

Osteomalacia

GENERAL PRINCIPLES

- Osteomalacia is characterized by defective mineralization of osteoid. Bone biopsy reveals increased thickness of osteoid seams and decreased mineralization rate, assessed by tetracycline labeling.
- Suboptimal vitamin D nutrition, indicated by plasma 25-hydroxy vitamin D (25[OH]D) levels <30 ng/mL, is very common and contributes to the development of osteoporosis (*J Clin Endocrinol Metab 2011;96:1911*).

Etiology

- Dietary vitamin D deficiency
- Malabsorption of vitamin D and calcium due to intestinal, hepatic, or biliary disease
- Disorders of vitamin D metabolism (e.g., renal disease, vitamin D–dependent rickets)
- Vitamin D resistance
- Chronic hypophosphatemia
- Renal tubular acidosis
- Hypophosphatasia

DIAGNOSIS

Clinical Presentation
- Clinical findings include diffuse skeletal pain, proximal muscle weakness, waddling gait, and propensity to fractures.
- Osteomalacia should be suspected in a patient with osteopenia, elevated serum alkaline phosphatase, and either hypophosphatemia or hypocalcemia.

Diagnostic Testing
Laboratories
- Serum alkaline phosphatase is elevated. Serum phosphorus, calcium, or both may be low.
- **Serum 25(OH)D** levels may be low, establishing the diagnosis of vitamin D deficiency or malabsorption.

Imaging
Radiographic findings include osteopenia and radiolucent bands perpendicular to bone surfaces (pseudofractures or Looser zones). Bone density is decreased.

TREATMENT

- **Dietary vitamin D deficiency** can initially be treated with ergocalciferol 50,000 international units (IU) PO weekly for 8 weeks to replete body stores, followed by long-term therapy with 2000 IU/d.
- **Malabsorption of vitamin D** may require continued therapy with high doses such as 50,000 IU PO per week. The dose should be adjusted to maintain serum 25(OH)D levels above 30 ng/mL. Calcium supplements, 1 g PO daily–tid, may also be required. Serum 25(OH)D and serum calcium should be monitored every 6–12 months to avoid hypercalcemia.

Paget Disease

GENERAL PRINCIPLES

Paget disease of bone is a focal skeletal disorder characterized by rapid, disorganized bone remodeling. It usually occurs after the age of 40 years and most often affects the pelvis, femur, spine, and skull (*J Clin Endocrinol Metab 2014;99:4408*).

DIAGNOSIS

Clinical Presentation
- Clinical manifestations include bone pain and deformity, degenerative arthritis, pathologic fractures, neurologic deficits due to nerve root or cranial nerve compression (including deafness), and rarely, high-output heart failure and osteogenic sarcoma.
- Most patients are asymptomatic, with disease discovered incidentally because of elevated serum alkaline phosphatase or a radiograph taken for other reasons.

Diagnostic Testing
Laboratories
Serum alkaline phosphatase is elevated, reflecting the activity and extent of disease. Serum and urine calcium are usually normal but may increase with immobilization, as after a fracture.

Imaging
The radiographic appearance is usually diagnostic. A bone scan will reveal areas of skeletal involvement, which can be confirmed by radiography.

TREATMENT

Indications for therapy include (a) bone pain due to Paget disease, (b) nerve compression syndromes, (c) pathologic fracture, (d) elective skeletal surgery, (e) progressive skeletal deformity, (f) immobilization hypercalcemia, and (g) asymptomatic involvement of weight-bearing bones or the skull.

Medications

Bisphosphonates inhibit excessive bone resorption, relieve symptoms, and restore serum alkaline phosphatase to normal in most patients. **Zoledronic acid**, 5 mg IV by a single infusion, is the drug of choice. The effectiveness of therapy is monitored by measuring serum alkaline phosphatase annually. Therapy can be repeated if serum alkaline phosphatase rises above normal. Bisphosphonates are not recommended in patients with renal insufficiency.

25 Arthritis and Rheumatologic Diseases

Zarmeena Ali, María González-Mayda, and Tiphanie Vogel

Basic Approach to the Rheumatic Diseases

Arthritis is any medical process affecting a joint or joints, causing pain, swelling, and stiffness. Pain from a true articular process is usually present throughout the complete range of motion of a particular joint, whereas pain from a **periarticular process** is usually evident at a single point in the range of motion, and it is elicited by palpation in a specific area corresponding to a tendon, ligament, or bursa.

Arthritis can be categorized as an inflammatory or noninflammatory process and by the number and type of joints involved.

DIAGNOSIS

Evidence of an inflammatory process includes the presence of morning stiffness lasting more than an hour, worsening of symptoms with inactivity, or constitutional symptoms. Skin rashes, uveitis, scleritis, mouth ulcers, and serositis among others may give clues to an underlying arthropathy or connective tissue disease. Physical exam may reveal swelling, warmth, or erythema. Synovial fluid analysis should be sent for cell count, microscopic examination for crystals, Gram stain, and cultures. Ancillary lab test and imaging are helpful in supporting a diagnosis if their use is directed by the specific findings on the history and physical exam.

TREATMENT

The etiology of most rheumatologic disorders is unknown. Therapeutic approaches involve either local or systemic administration of analgesic, anti-inflammatory, immunomodulatory, or immunosuppressive drugs.

Medications

- **NSAIDs** exert their effects by inhibiting the constitutive (COX-1) and inducible (COX-2) isoforms of cyclooxygenase, producing a mild to moderate anti-inflammatory and analgesic effect. Individual responses to these agents are variable. If one drug is not effective during a 2- to 3-week trial, another should be tried.
  - **Side effects**
    - **Gastrointestinal (GI) toxicity** manifests clinically as dyspepsia, nausea, vomiting, or GI bleeding. Nausea and dyspepsia often respond to the addition of a histamine-2 (H_2)-blocking agent or proton pump inhibitor or to a change in NSAID. Direct GI irritation can be minimized by administration after food, by the use of enteric-coated preparations, and by use of the lowest effective dose. All NSAIDs, however, have a systemic effect on the GI mucosa, resulting in increased permeability to gastric acid. Most serious GI bleeds during NSAID use occur without prior GI symptoms.

Risk factors for GI bleed include a history of duodenal–gastric ulceration, age >60, smoking, ethanol use, high dose of NSAIDs, and concomitant use of corticosteroids, anticoagulants (i.e., aspirin, warfarin, clopidogrel), or selective serotonin reuptake inhibitors. The use of proton pump inhibitors such as **omeprazole** 20 mg PO daily decreases the risk of NSAID-induced gastric or duodenal ulceration. **Misoprostol**, a synthetic prostaglandin E analog, is another alternative but may cause diarrhea and is an abortifacient. Consider *Helicobacter pylori* testing prior to beginning NSAIDs, especially in patients with high risk of duodenal–gastric ulceration. If the test is positive, treat accordingly (see Chapter 18, Gastrointestinal Diseases).

- **Acute renal failure** due to reversible renal ischemia is the most common form of renal toxicity; however, nephrotic syndrome and acute interstitial nephritis may also occur. **Risk factors** for acute renal failure include preexisting renal dysfunction, congestive heart failure (CHF), cirrhosis with ascites, and a concomitant angiotensin-converting enzyme (ACE) inhibitor or angiotensin receptor blocker (ARB). Periodic monitoring of renal function is recommended, particularly in elderly patients.

- **Platelet dysfunction** can be caused by all NSAIDs, particularly aspirin, which is a covalent inhibitor of COX. NSAIDs should be used cautiously or avoided in patients with a bleeding diathesis and those taking warfarin. NSAIDs should be discontinued 5–7 days before surgical procedures.

- **Hypersensitivity reactions** are often seen in patients with a history of asthma, nasal polyps, or atopy. NSAIDs may cause a variety of type I hypersensitivity-like reactions, including urticaria, asthma, and anaphylactoid shock, presumably by increasing leukotriene synthesis. Patients with a hypersensitivity reaction to one NSAID should avoid all NSAIDs and selective COX-2 inhibitors.

  ○ **Other side effects: Central nervous system** (CNS) toxicity (headaches, dizziness, dysphoria, confusion, aseptic meningitis) is uncommon. Tinnitus and deafness can complicate NSAID use, particularly with high-dose salicylates. **Blood dyscrasias**, including aplastic anemia, have been observed as isolated case reports with ibuprofen, piroxicam, indomethacin, and phenylbutazone. **Dermatologic reactions** and **elevations in transaminases** have also been described. **A metabolic acidosis and respiratory alkalosis** can be seen with high doses of salicylates. Nonacetylated salicylates have been reported to have less toxicity but also may be less effective. The use of NSAIDs in general may be associated with an increased risk for **cardiovascular thrombotic events** and might diminish the cardioprotective effect of aspirin.

- **Selective COX-2 inhibitors** exhibit selective inhibition of COX-2, thereby reducing inflammation while preserving the homeostatic functions of constitutive COX-1–derived prostaglandins. The anti-inflammatory and analgesic efficacy is similar to that of traditional NSAIDs. Celecoxib is the only selective COX-2 inhibitor approved in the United States.

  ○ **Side effects**

    - Some data demonstrate that **GI symptoms** and **GI ulcerations are reduced** with these agents in comparison to NSAIDs. The potential gastroduodenal-sparing effect of selective COX-2 inhibitors may be eliminated by concurrent warfarin therapy or the use of low-dose aspirin therapy for primary or secondary prevention of cardiovascular or cerebrovascular disease (*JAMA 2000;284:1247*).

    - Acute kidney injury might be precipitated in patients taking selective COX-2 inhibitors, similar to COX-1 inhibitors.

  ○ **Platelet function** is not impaired, making selective COX-2 inhibitors a good anti-inflammatory option for patients with thrombocytopenia, hemostatic defects, or chronic anticoagulation. In patients who are taking warfarin, however, the international normalized ratio (INR) should be monitored after the addition of a COX-2 inhibitor (as with any medication change). In addition, there has been controversy as to whether the inhibition of prostacyclin but not thromboxane by these agents may promote clotting.

- ○ Patients with hypersensitivity reactions to NSAIDs should not use a COX-2 inhibitor. Celecoxib should be used with caution in patients with sulfonamide allergy.
- ○ An increase in blood pressure and a dose-related **increase in cardiovascular events** (i.e., CHF exacerbation) have been associated with the use of this medication.
- **Glucocorticoids** exert a pluripotent anti-inflammatory effect via the inhibition of inflammatory mediator gene transcription.
  - ○ **Preparations, dosages, and routes of administration:** The goal of therapy **is to suppress** disease activity with the minimum effective dosage. **Prednisone** (PO) and **methylprednisolone** (IV) are generally the preferred drugs because of cost and half-life considerations. IM absorption is variable and therefore is not advised. The following are **relative anti-inflammatory potencies** of common glucocorticoid preparations: cortisone, 0.8; hydrocortisone, 1.0; prednisone, 4.0; methylprednisolone, 5.0; dexamethasone, 25.0.
  - ○ **Side effects:** Adverse effects are related to dosage and duration of administration and, except for cataracts and osteoporosis, can be minimized by alternate-day administration once the disease is controlled.
    - ▪ **Adrenal suppression:** Glucocorticoids suppress the hypothalamic–pituitary–adrenal axis. Assume functional suppression in patients receiving more than 20 mg of prednisone (or the equivalent) daily for more than 3 weeks, patients receiving an evening dose for more than a few weeks, or patients with cushingoid appearance. Adrenal suppression is unlikely if the patient has received any dose of steroids for less than 3 weeks or if using alternate-day therapy. Adrenal suppression is minimized by dosing in the morning and using a single daily low dose of a short-acting preparation, such as prednisone, for a short period. In patients who are receiving chronic glucocorticoid therapy, hypoadrenalism (anorexia, weight loss, lethargy, fever, and postural hypotension) may occur at times of severe stress (e.g., infection, major surgery) and should be treated with stress doses of glucocorticoids.
    - ▪ **Immunosuppression:** Glucocorticoid therapy reduces resistance to infections. **Bacterial infections** in particular are related to the dosage of glucocorticoids and are a major cause of morbidity and mortality. Minor infections may become systemic, quiescent infections may be activated, and organisms that usually are nonpathogenic may cause disease. Local and systemic signs of infection may be partially masked, although fever associated with infection generally is not suppressed. A skin test for TB should be performed before glucocorticoid therapy is instituted, and if it is positive, TB should be treated appropriately. For patients on prolonged high-dose therapy, consider prophylaxis with trimethoprim-sulfamethoxazole (TMP-SMX) and acyclovir to prevent *Pneumocystis jirovecii* and varicella-zoster viral infections.
    - ▪ **Endocrine abnormalities:** Endocrine abnormalities include a **cushingoid habitus**, hirsutism, and induced or aggravated hyperglycemia, rarely associated with ketoacidosis. Hyperglycemia is not a contraindication to therapy and may require treatment with insulin therapy. Fluid and electrolyte abnormalities include hypokalemia and sodium retention, which may induce or aggravate hypertension.
    - ▪ **Osteoporosis** with vertebral compression fractures is common among patients who are receiving long-term glucocorticoid therapy. **Supplemental calcium**, 1.0–1.5 g/d PO, should be given along with **vitamin D**, 1000 units daily PO, as soon as steroid therapy is begun. Bisphosphonates or teriparatide (recombinant human parathyroid hormone [1-34]) is indicated in postmenopausal women and in premenopausal women or men who are at high risk for osteoporosis (*Nat Rev Rheumatol. 2015;11(2):98–109*). Determination of baseline bone density is appropriate in these patients. A weight-bearing exercise program and avoidance of alcohol and tobacco are recommended.
    - ▪ **Steroid myopathy** generally involves the hip and shoulder girdle musculature. Muscles are weak but not tender, and in contrast to inflammatory myositis, serum creatine

kinase, aldolase, and electromyography are normal. The myopathy usually improves with a reduction in glucocorticoid dosage and resolves slowly with discontinuation.

■ **Ischemic bone necrosis** (aseptic necrosis, avascular necrosis) caused by glucocorticoid use often is multifocal, most commonly affecting the femoral head, humeral head, and tibial plateau. Early changes can be demonstrated by bone scan or MRI.

○ **Other adverse effects:** Changes in **mental status** ranging from mild nervousness, euphoria, and insomnia to severe depression or psychosis may occur. **Ocular effects** include increased intraocular pressure (sometimes precipitating glaucoma) and the formation of posterior subcapsular cataracts. **Hyperlipidemia**, **menstrual irregularities**, increased perspiration with **night sweats**, and **pseudotumor cerebri** also may occur.

• **Immunomodulatory and immunosuppressive drugs**, also known as **disease-modifying antirheumatic drugs (DMARDs)**, include a number of pharmacologically diverse agents that exert anti-inflammatory or immunosuppressive effects. They are characterized by a delayed onset of action and the potential for serious toxicity. Consequently, they should be prescribed with the guidance of a rheumatologist and in cooperative patients who are willing to comply with meticulous follow-up. The specific agents will be discussed in relation to the diseases for which they are indicated. Examples of these agents include methotrexate, azathioprine, hydroxychloroquine, sulfasalazine, cyclosporine, rituximab, and etanercept.

Nonpharmacologic Therapies

• **Joint aspiration should be performed in one of three instances: effusion of unclear etiology**, symptomatic relief in a patient with known arthritis diagnosis, and monitoring treatment response in **infectious arthritis**. Intra-articular glucocorticoid therapy can be used to suppress inflammation when only one or a few peripheral joints are inflamed and infection has been excluded. Intra-articular hyaluronic acid derivatives are used for the treatment of knee osteoarthritis (OA). The joint should be aspirated to remove as much fluid as possible before injection. **Glucocorticoid preparations** include methylprednisolone acetate, triamcinolone acetonide, and triamcinolone hexacetonide. The dose used is arbitrary, but the following guidelines based on volume are useful: large joints (knee, ankle, shoulder), 1–2 mL; medium joints (wrists, elbows), 0.5–1.0 mL; and small joints of the hands and feet, 0.25–0.50 mL. **Lidocaine** (or its equivalent), up to 1 mL of a 1% solution, can be mixed in a single syringe with the glucocorticoid to promote immediate relief but is not generally used in the digits.

• **Contraindications:** Cellulitis overlying the site to be injected is an absolute contraindication. Significant hemostatic defects and bacteremia are relative contraindications to joint aspiration and injection.

• **Complications**
  ○ **Postinjection synovitis** may develop rarely as a result of phagocytosis of glucocorticoid ester crystals. Reactions usually resolve within 48–72 hours. More persistent symptoms suggest the possibility of iatrogenic infection, which occurs rarely (<0.1% of patients).
  ○ Localized skin depigmentation and atrophy along with accelerated deterioration of bone and cartilage may occur when frequent injections are administered over an extended period. Therefore, any single joint should be injected no more frequently than every 3–6 months.

Infectious Arthritis and Bursitis

GENERAL PRINCIPLES

• **Infectious arthritis** is generally categorized into gonococcal and nongonococcal disease.
• **Nongonococcal infectious arthritis** in adults tends to occur in patients with previous joint damage or compromised host defenses. It is caused most often by *Staphylococcus*

aureus (60%) and *Streptococcus* spp. Gram-negative organisms are less common and typically seen with IV drug abuse, neutropenia, concomitant urinary tract infection, or postoperative status.
- **Gonococcal arthritis** causes one-half of all septic arthritis in otherwise healthy, sexually active young adults.

DIAGNOSIS

Clinical Presentation
- **Nongonococcal infectious arthritis** usually presents with fever and an acute monoarticular arthritis, although multiple joints may be affected by hematogenous spread of pathogens.
- **Gonococcal arthritis** often includes migratory or additive polyarthralgias, followed by tenosynovitis or arthritis of the wrist, ankle, or knee, and vesicopustular skin lesions on the extremities or trunk (disseminated gonococcal infection).

Diagnostic Testing
- **Joint aspiration should be performed and synovial fluid sent for** Gram stain, cell count with differential, and cultures. Cultures of blood and other possible extra-articular sites of infection also should be obtained.
- Synovial fluid Gram stain may be positive in 50–70% of nongonococcal infectious arthritis cases.
- Gram staining of synovial fluid is positive in **less than 25% of cases** of gonococcal arthritis. Cultures of synovial fluid are positive in 20–50% of cases. Bacteriologic assessment of the throat, cervix, urethra, and rectum may aid in establishing the diagnosis.

TREATMENT

- **Empiric antimicrobial therapy** should be started immediately based on the clinical situation.
  - With a positive Gram stain and culture, antibiotic coverage can be tailored accordingly.
  - With a nondiagnostic Gram stain, antibiotics should be chosen to cover *S. aureus, Streptococcus* spp., and *Neisseria gonorrhoeae*. Vancomycin 15 mg/kg IV every 12 hours and ceftriaxone 1 g IV every 24 hours are good initial treatment choices. Cefepime instead of ceftriaxone is preferred if *Pseudomonas* infection is suspected.
  - IV antimicrobials are given for at least 2 weeks, followed by 1–2 weeks of oral antimicrobials, with the course of therapy tailored to the patient's response.
  - Treatment of gonococcal arthritis is with an IV antibiotic, generally ceftriaxone, 1–2 g IV daily. After clinical improvement is noted, usually 48 hours after IV antibiotics, therapy is continued with an oral antibiotic to complete 7–14 days of treatment. Cefixime, 400 mg PO bid, or amoxicillin, 500–850 mg PO bid, may be used. **Treatment of coexisting *Chlamydia* infection** with azithromycin or doxycycline should also be considered.
  - Oral and intra-articular antimicrobials are not appropriate as initial therapy.
- **Drainage** of the affected joint is needed to decrease the possibility of permanent joint damage. **Surgical drainage** or arthroscopic lavage and drainage are indicated for (a) a septic hip; (b) joints in which the anatomy, large amounts of tissue debris, or loculation of pus prevent adequate needle drainage; (c) septic arthritis with coexistent osteomyelitis; (d) joints that do not respond in 3–5 days to appropriate therapy; and (e) prosthetic joint infection.

• **General supportive measures** include splinting of the joint, which may help to relieve pain. However, prolonged immobilization can result in joint stiffness. An **NSAID** is useful to reduce pain and increase joint mobility but should not be used until response to antimicrobial therapy has been demonstrated by symptomatic and laboratory improvement.

SPECIAL CONSIDERATIONS

Nonbacterial infectious arthritis is common with many viral infections, especially hepatitis B, rubella, mumps, infectious mononucleosis, parvovirus, enterovirus, and adenovirus.
• It is generally self-limiting, lasting for <6 weeks, and responds well to a conservative regimen of rest and NSAIDs.
• Arthralgias (often severe) or a reactive arthritis can also be a manifestation of HIV infection.
• Fungi and mycobacterium can cause septic arthritis and should be considered in patients with chronic monoarticular arthritis.

Septic Bursitis

GENERAL PRINCIPLES

• Usually involves the olecranon or prepatellar bursa and can be differentiated from septic arthritis by localized, fluctuant superficial swelling and by **relatively painless joint motion** (particularly extension).
• Most patients have a history of previous trauma to the area or an occupational predisposition (e.g., "housemaid's knee," "writer's elbow").
• *S. aureus* is the most common pathogen of septic bursitis.

DIAGNOSIS AND TREATMENT

• Aspiration of the joint is performed, with antibiotic therapy guided by Gram stain and culture of bursa fluid. Aspiration can be repeated if fluid reaccumulates. Surgical drainage is indicated only if adequate needle drainage is not possible.
• Oral antibiotics (guided by Gram stain and culture of bursa fluid) and outpatient management are usually appropriate. Preventive measures (e.g., knee pads) should be used in patients with occupational predispositions to septic bursitis.

Lyme Disease

GENERAL PRINCIPLES

Lyme disease is caused by the tick-borne spirochete *Borrelia burgdorferi*.

DIAGNOSIS

• Typical manifestations begin with an erythematous annular rash **(erythema migrans)** and flu-like symptoms.
• Arthralgias, myalgias, meningitis, neuropathy, and cardiac conduction defects may follow in weeks to a few months. Months later, in untreated patients, an intermittent or chronic oligoarticular arthritis, characteristically including the knee, may develop.
• The diagnosis is based on the clinical picture and exposure in an endemic area and **supported by serology**. A two-tiered serologic assay with enzyme-linked immunosorbent assay (ELISA) and IgG western blot for *B. burgdorferi* is uniformly positive by the time frank

arthritis develops. False positives occur, however, and may signify prior infection. *B. burgdorferi* DNA can be detected by polymerase chain reaction in synovial fluid in 85% of cases.

TREATMENT

Antibiotic therapy is required, generally with doxycycline 100 mg PO bid or amoxicillin 500 mg PO tid for 28 days. NSAIDs are a useful adjunct for arthritis.

Crystal-Induced Synovitis

GENERAL PRINCIPLES

Definition

Deposition of microcrystals in joints and periarticular tissues results in **gout**, **pseudogout**, and **apatite disease**.

Classification

- Clinical phases of gout can be divided into asymptomatic hyperuricemia, acute gouty arthritis, and chronic arthritis.
- **Asymptomatic hyperuricemia** is defined as serum uric acid levels >7 mg/dL without arthritis.
- Men are much more commonly affected by gouty arthritis than women. Most premenopausal women with gout have a family history of the disease.

Etiology

- **Primary gouty arthritis** is characterized by hyperuricemia that is usually because of underexcretion of uric acid (90% of cases) rather than its overproduction. Urate crystals may be deposited in the joints, subcutaneous tissues (tophi), and kidneys.
- **Secondary gout**, like primary gout, can be caused by either defective renal excretion or overproduction of uric acid. Intrinsic renal disease, diuretic therapy, low-dose aspirin, cyclosporine, and ethanol all interfere with renal excretion of uric acid. Starvation, lactic acidosis, dehydration, preeclampsia, and diabetic ketoacidosis also can induce hyperuricemia. Overproduction of uric acid occurs in myeloproliferative and lymphoproliferative disorders, hemolytic anemia, polycythemia, and cyanotic heart disease.
- **Pseudogout** results when calcium pyrophosphate dihydrate crystals deposited in bone and cartilage are released into synovial fluid and induce acute inflammation. **Risk factors** include older age, advanced OA, neuropathic joint, gout, hyperparathyroidism, hemochromatosis, diabetes mellitus, hypothyroidism, and hypomagnesemia.

DIAGNOSIS

Clinical Presentation

- **Acute gouty arthritis** presents as an excruciating attack of pain, usually in a single joint of the foot or ankle. Occasionally, a polyarticular onset can mimic rheumatoid arthritis (RA). Acute gouty arthritis attacks can be precipitated by surgery, dehydration, fasting, binge eating, or heavy ingestion of alcohol.
- **Chronic gouty arthritis:** With time, acute gouty attacks occur more frequently, asymptomatic periods are shorter, and chronic joint deformity may appear.
- **Pseudogout** may present as an **acute monoarthritis or oligoarthritis**, mimicking gout, or as a **chronic polyarthritis** resembling RA or OA. Usually the knee or wrist is affected, although any synovial joint can be involved.

• **Apatite/basic calcium phosphate crystals** may cause periarthritis, tendonitis, or a destructive arthritis.

Diagnostic Testing

Laboratories
• A definitive diagnosis of gout or pseudogout is made by finding **intracellular crystals** in synovial fluid examined with a compensated polarized light microscope. **Urate crystals** are needle shaped and strongly negatively birefringent. **Calcium pyrophosphate dihydrate crystals** are pleomorphic and weakly positively birefringent. Hydroxyapatite complexes and basic calcium phosphate complexes can be identified only by electron microscopy and mass spectroscopy.
• Serum uric acid level is normal in 30% of patients with acute gout.
• **Apatite disease** should be suspected when no crystals are present in the **synovial fluid**.

Imaging
• Erosions with overhanging borders may be seen on imaging with gout.
• If pseudogout is suspected, films of the wrists, knees, and pubic symphysis may be ordered. These are the most common sites for chondrocalcinosis, a finding that is supportive of (but not diagnostic for) pseudogout.
• Hydroxyapatite disease may be suspected by finding poorly defined cloud-like calcific deposits in the periarticular area on imaging.

TREATMENT

• **Asymptomatic hyperuricemia** is not routinely treated. However, patients should be monitored closely for the development of complications if the serum uric acid level is at least 12 mg/dL in men or 10 mg/dL in women. Urate-lowering therapy should then be considered.
• **Management of secondary gout** includes treatment of the underlying disorder and urate-lowering therapy.
• Treatment of **apatite disease** is similar to that for pseudogout.
• **Acute gout**
  ○ Although the acute gouty attack will subside spontaneously over several days, prompt treatment can abort the attack within hours.
  ○ **NSAIDs** are the treatment of choice due to ease of administration and low toxicity. Clinical response may require 12–24 hours, and initial doses should be high, followed by rapid tapering over 2–8 days. One approach is to use indomethacin, 50 mg PO q8h for 2 days, followed by 25 mg PO q8h for 3–7 days. Long-acting NSAIDs are generally not recommended for acute gout.
  ○ **Glucocorticoids** are useful when NSAIDs are contraindicated. An intra-articular injection of glucocorticoids produces rapid dramatic relief. Alternatively, prednisone, 40–60 mg PO daily, can be given until a response is obtained and then should be tapered rapidly.
  ○ **Colchicine is most effective if given in the first 12–24 hours** of an acute attack and usually brings relief in 6–12 hours. A dose of 1.2 mg is given at onset of symptoms, and 0.6 mg is taken 1 hour after the initial dose (1.8 mg over 1 hour). This regimen decreases the GI side effects noted with previous higher dose therapies.
  ○ **Urate-lowering drugs should not be started during an acute gouty attack even if the uric acid is elevated.**
• **Chronic gouty arthritis**
  ○ **Colchicine**, 0.6 mg PO daily or bid, can be used prophylactically for acute attacks. The dosage needs to be adjusted in patients with renal insufficiency. Colchicine 0.6 mg every other day or every 3 days should be considered in patients with a creatinine

clearance between 10 and 34 mL/min. Aspirin (uricoretentive), diuretics, high alcohol intake, and foods high in purines (sweetbreads, anchovies, shellfish, sardines, liver, and kidney) should be avoided. Weight loss should be encouraged. Frequent gout attacks, tophi, joint damage, and urate nephropathy are indications for urate-lowering therapy. **Maintenance colchicine, 0.6 mg PO daily or bid, should be given for a few days before manipulation of the uric acid level to prevent precipitation of an acute attack.** In patients without tophi, prophylactic colchicine can be discontinued after 6 months once serum urate levels are <6 mg/dL and no acute attacks have been documented by the patient (*Arthritis Rheum 2004;51(3):321*). In patients with tophi, duration of prophylaxis is uncertain but consider discontinuation 6 months after resolution of tophi.

- **Allopurinol**, a xanthine oxidase inhibitor, is effective therapy for hyperuricemia in most patients.
  - **Dosage and administration:** Initial dosage varies and should be adjusted for renal and hepatic dysfunction. Daily doses can be increased by 100 mg every 2–4 weeks to achieve the minimum maintenance dosage that will keep the uric acid level below 6 mg/dL, which is below the limit of solubility of monosodium urate in serum. The concomitant use of a uricosuric agent may hasten the mobilization of tophi. **Allopurinol should be continued during an acute gout flare if already started, and use of NSAIDs, colchicine, or steroids to abort the attack be considered.**
  - **Side effects: Hypersensitivity reactions** from a minor skin rash to a diffuse exfoliative dermatitis associated with fever, eosinophilia, and a combination of renal and hepatic injury occur in up to 5% of patients. Patients who have mild renal insufficiency and are receiving diuretics are at greatest risk. Severe cases are potentially fatal and usually require glucocorticoid therapy. Allopurinol may potentiate the effect of oral anticoagulants and blocks metabolism of azathioprine and 6-mercaptopurine, necessitating a 60–75% reduction in dosage of these cytotoxic drugs.
- **Febuxostat** is a nonpurine selective inhibitor of the xanthine oxidase. It is significantly more expensive than allopurinol. The starting dose is 40 mg/d, with titration to 80 mg/d if needed.
- **Uricase** catabolizes uric acid to the more soluble compound allantoin. It is available in the United States for the treatment of tumor lysis syndrome in a recombinant form **(rasburicase).** IV **pegloticase** is a recombinant polyethylene glycol–conjugated form of uricase given every 2 weeks that has been shown to provide sustained reductions in plasma uric acid levels to less than the therapeutic target of 6 mg/dL in a substantial proportion of patients with chronic gout who are refractory to, or intolerant of, conventional urate-lowering therapy. The drug is discontinued if serum uric acid levels fail to reach target or are noted to rise above 6 mg/dL on two consecutive times. There is a high risk of anaphylaxis and infusion reactions with this medication, and thus, it is administered in a controlled setting with health care professionals who are familiar with the medication.
- **Uricosuric drugs** lower serum uric acid levels by blocking renal tubular reabsorption of uric acid. A 24-hour measurement of creatinine clearance and urine uric acid should be obtained before therapy is started, because these drugs are **ineffective with glomerular filtration rates of <50 mL/min.** They are also not recommended for patients who already have high levels of urine uric acid (800 mg/24 h) because of the risk of urate stone formation. Risk of urate stone formation can be minimized by maintaining a high fluid intake and by alkalinizing the urine. If these drugs are being used when an acute gouty attack begins, they should be continued while other drugs are used to treat the acute attack.
  - **Probenecid**
    - Initial dosage is 500 mg PO daily, which can be raised in 500-mg increments every week until serum uric acid levels normalize or urine uric acid levels exceed 800 mg/24 h. The maximum dose is 3000 mg/d. Most patients require a total of 1.0–1.5 g/d in two to three divided doses.

□ Salicylates and probenecid are antagonistic and should not be used together.

□ Probenecid decreases renal excretion of penicillin, indomethacin, and sulfonylureas.

□ Side effects are minimal.

- **Sulfinpyrazone** has uricosuric efficacy similar to that of probenecid; however, it also inhibits platelet function. The initial dosage of 50 mg PO bid can be increased in 100-mg increments weekly until serum uric acid levels normalize, to a maximum dose of 800 mg/d. Most patients require 300–400 mg/d in three to four divided doses.

- **Pseudogout**
  ○ As in gout, the therapy of choice for most patients is a brief high-dose course of an **NSAID. Oral corticosteroids, intra-articular corticosteroids**, and **colchicine** may also relieve symptoms promptly.
  ○ **Maintenance therapy** with colchicine may diminish the number of recurrent attacks. Allopurinol or uricosuric agents have no role in treating pseudogout.
  ○ Treatment of underlying disease (hyperparathyroidism, hypothyroidism, hemochromatosis) will also help in disease management.

Rheumatoid Arthritis

GENERAL PRINCIPLES

RA is a systemic disease of unknown etiology that is characterized by a symmetric inflammatory polyarthritis, extra-articular manifestations (rheumatoid nodules, pulmonary fibrosis, serositis, scleritis, vasculitis), and serum rheumatoid factor (RF) in up to 80% of patients. The course of RA is variable but tends to be chronic and progressive.

DIAGNOSIS

Clinical Presentation

- Most patients describe the insidious onset of pain, swelling, and morning stiffness in the hands and/or wrists or feet.
- Synovitis may be evident upon exam of the metacarpophalangeal, proximal interphalangeal, wrist, or other joints. Rheumatoid nodules may be palpated most commonly on extensor surfaces.
- Clinical criteria for the diagnosis of RA are available (*Arthritis Rheum 2010;62:2569*). Suspect the diagnosis in patients presenting with symmetric arthritis in three or more joints especially involving small joints and associated with morning stiffness lasting more than 30 minutes.

Diagnostic Testing

RF may be positive in 80% of patients. Cyclic citrullinated peptide (CCP) antibodies may be detected in 50–60% of patients with early RA.

- CCP antibodies are more specific (>90%) for RA than is the RF, which can also be elevated in the setting of hepatitis C and other chronic infections.
- Hand and wrist radiographs may show early changes of erosions or periarticular osteopenia.
- Musculoskeletal MRI and ultrasonography are more sensitive than plain radiographs and may be used in equivocal cases to demonstrate clinically inapparent synovitis or erosions.

TREATMENT

Most patients can benefit from an early aggressive treatment program that combines medical, rehabilitative, and surgical services designed with three distinct goals: (a) early suppression of inflammation in the joints and other tissues, (b) maintenance of joint and muscle function and prevention of deformities, and (c) repair of joint damage to relieve pain or improve function.

- **DMARDs** appear to alter the natural history of RA by retarding the progression of bony erosions and cartilage loss. Because RA may lead to substantial long-term disability (and is associated with increased mortality), the standard of care is to initiate therapy with such agents early in the course of RA. Once a clinical response has been achieved, the chosen drug usually is continued indefinitely at the lowest effective dosage to prevent relapse.
  - **An established diagnosis of RA along with any evidence of disease activity is an indication to initiate disease-modifying therapy.** Initial monotherapy with NSAIDs or steroids is no longer considered appropriate under usual circumstances.
  - **Methotrexate** typically is the initial choice for moderate to severe RA. **Leflunomide** is also an alternative. **Hydroxychloroquine** or **sulfasalazine** can be used as the initial choice in very mild RA. If response to the initial agent is unsatisfactory after an adequate trial (or if limiting toxicity supervenes), other DMARDs or a biologic agent can be added or substituted.
- **Methotrexate**, a purine inhibitor and folic acid antagonist, is useful in treating synovitis, regardless of the underlying disease process. RA is its most common indication. It is also useful for myositis and may improve the leukopenia of Felty syndrome.
  - **Dosage and administration:** Typically, methotrexate is administered as a single PO dose once a week starting with 7.5–10.0 mg. Clinical response is usually noted in 4–8 weeks. The dosage can be increased by 2.5- to 5.0-mg increments every 2–4 weeks to a maximum of 25 mg/wk or until improvement is observed. Dosages above 20 mg/wk are generally given by SC injection to promote absorption.
  - **Contraindications and side effects:** Methotrexate is **teratogenic** and should not be used during pregnancy. It should also be avoided in patients with significant hepatic or renal impairment. **Folic acid supplementation** at a dosage of 1–2 mg daily may reduce toxicity without attenuating efficacy. Concomitant use of TMP-SMX should be avoided. Serologic testing for hepatitis B and C should be included before initiation of therapy.
    - **Minor side effects** include GI intolerance, stomatitis, rash, headache, and alopecia.
    - **Bone marrow suppression** may occur, particularly at higher doses. Blood and platelet counts should be obtained before initiation, every 4 weeks during the first 3–4 months or if the dose is changed, and every 8 weeks thereafter. **Macrocytosis** may herald serious hematologic toxicity and is an indication for folate supplementation, dose reduction, or both.
    - **Cirrhosis** occurs rarely with long-term use. Aspartate transaminase (AST), alanine transaminase (ALT), and serum albumin should be obtained initially at 4- to 8-week intervals during the first 3–4 months of therapy or if the dose is changed. Patients on a stable dose should be monitored every 8–12 weeks after 3 months of therapy and every 12 weeks after 6 months of therapy. Liver biopsy should be considered if the liver function tests are persistently abnormal or if the liver function tests are abnormal in 6 of 12 monthly determinations (five of nine determinations if measured every 6 weeks). Alcohol consumption increases the risk of methotrexate hepatotoxicity.
    - **Hypersensitivity pneumonitis** may occur but usually is reversible. Distinction from the interstitial lung disease (ILD) associated with RA may be difficult. Patients with preexisting pulmonary parenchymal disease may be at increased risk. **New or worsening symptoms of dyspnea or cough in a patient on methotrexate should prompt evaluation for pneumonitis.**
    - **Rheumatoid nodules** may develop or worsen, paradoxically, in some patients on methotrexate.

- **Sulfasalazine** is useful for treating synovitis in the setting of RA and seronegative spondyloarthropathies.
  - **Dosage:** Initial dosage is 500 mg PO daily, with increases in 500-mg increments weekly until a total daily dose of 2000–3000 mg (given in evenly divided doses) is reached. Clinical response usually occurs in 6–10 weeks.
  - **Contraindications and side effects: Sulfasalazine should be used with extreme caution in patients with glucose-6-phosphate dehydrogenase deficiency. Sulfasalazine should not be used in patients with sulfa allergy.** Nausea is the principal adverse effect and can be minimized by the use of the enteric-coated preparation of the drug. Hematologic toxicity, including a reduction in any cell line and aplastic anemia, rarely occurs. Periodic monitoring of blood and platelet counts is recommended.
- **Hydroxychloroquine** is an antimalarial agent that is used to treat dermatitis, alopecia, and synovitis in systemic lupus erythematosus (SLE) and mild synovitis in RA.
  - **Dosage:** Hydroxychloroquine typically is given at a dosage of 4–6 mg/kg PO daily (200–400 mg) after meals to minimize dyspepsia and nausea.
  - **Contraindications and side effects: Hydroxychloroquine should be used with caution in patients with porphyria, glucose-6-phosphate dehydrogenase deficiency, or significant hepatic or renal impairment.** It is safe during pregnancy. The most common side effects are allergic skin eruptions and nausea. Serious ocular toxicity (corneal deposits and retinopathy) occurs, but is rare with currently recommended dosages. Ophthalmologic evaluation should be performed on an annual basis.
- **Leflunomide** is a pyrimidine inhibitor that has been approved for the treatment of RA.
  - **Dosage and administration:** Treatment is begun with 10 or 20 mg PO daily. Clinical response is generally seen within 4–8 weeks.
  - **Contraindications and side effects:** Leflunomide is **teratogenic** and has a very long half-life. Women who plan to become pregnant must discontinue the drug and complete a course of elimination therapy with cholestyramine, 8 g PO tid for 11 days. Plasma levels should then be verified to be <0.02 mg/L on two separate tests at least 14 days apart before pregnancy is considered. Leflunomide is **contraindicated in patients with significant hepatic dysfunction** or in those who are receiving rifampin. **GI side effects** are the most common. **Diarrhea** occurs in up to 20% of patients and may require discontinuation of the drug. Dosage reduction to 10 mg/d may provide relief while maintaining efficacy, and loperamide can be used for symptomatic relief. **Elevations in serum transaminase levels** may occur and should be measured at baseline and then monitored periodically. The dosage should be reduced for confirmed twofold elevations, and greater elevations should be treated with cholestyramine and discontinuation of leflunomide. **Rash** and **alopecia** may occur during therapy.
- **Anticytokine therapies** directed at specific cytokines have been developed. These agents are considered **biologic DMARDs**.
  - **Tumor necrosis factor (TNF) inhibitors** have been approved for treatment of RA and seronegative spondyloarthropathies. These agents are used in patients with moderate to severe RA who have failed a trial of one or more DMARDs. The effect of these agents on synovitis can be dramatic, with responsive patients reporting the onset of symptomatic benefits within 1–2 weeks. In addition to their symptomatic benefits, these agents appear to retard joint damage significantly.
    - **Etanercept is a fusion protein** that consists of the ligand-binding portion of the human TNF receptor linked to the Fc portion of human IgG. It binds to TNF, blocking its interaction with cell surface receptors, thus inhibiting the inflammatory and immunoregulatory properties of TNF. It is given in a dosage of 25 mg SC twice a week or 50 mg SC weekly.
    - **Infliximab** is a chimeric monoclonal antibody that binds specifically to human TNF-α, blocking its proinflammatory and immunomodulatory effects. It is given by IV infusion in conjunction with methotrexate to reduce production of neutralizing

antibodies against infliximab. The recommended treatment regimen includes infliximab infusions of 3 mg/kg at initiation, at 2 and 6 weeks, and every 8 weeks thereafter, along with methotrexate at a dose of at least 7.5 mg/wk.

- **Adalimumab** is a recombinant human IgG-1 monoclonal antibody that is specific to human TNF-α. It is given in a dosage of 40 mg SC every other week.
- **Golimumab** is a human monoclonal antibody that binds to human TNF-α. It can be given as a monthly injection or an infusion every 8 weeks after an initial loading dose.
- **Certolizumab pegol** is a pegylated humanized Fab′ fragment of an anti–TNF-α monoclonal antibody. It is given monthly after an initial loading dose.
  ○ **Contraindications and side effects**
    - **Serious infections and sepsis**, including fatalities, have been reported during the use of TNF-blocking agents. These drugs are contraindicated in patients with acute or chronic infections, and if serious infection or sepsis occurs, the drug should be stopped. Those with a history of recurrent infections and those with underlying conditions that may predispose to infection should be treated with caution and counseled to be vigilant for signs and symptoms of infection. Upper respiratory and sinus infections are most common. TB has also been noted, and **a tuberculin skin test and CXR should be obtained before beginning therapy**. These agents are also contraindicated in patients with CHF (usually with a left ventricular ejection fraction <30%). Patients undergoing elective surgical procedures can omit the dose that is scheduled to be given before surgery and the next dose scheduled to follow the surgery as long as their wound has completely healed.
    - **Local injection site reactions** are common with SC administration, particularly during the first month of therapy. Reactions are generally self-limited and do not require discontinuation of therapy. Serious systemic allergic reactions are rare but may occur with infliximab infusions.
    - **Other adverse effects** may include induction of antinuclear antibodies and, rarely, a lupus-like illness. A demyelinating disorder has been described as well as exacerbations of preexisting multiple sclerosis. The risk of nonmelanoma skin cancer is increased in patients who receive TNF blockers. It is unclear whether the frequency of occurrence of lymphoma is increased in patients who receive these agents. A black box warning, however, has been placed on the package insert of these agents.
- **Interleukin inhibitors**
  ○ **Anakinra** is a recombinant interleukin (IL)-1 receptor antagonist that is approved for use in RA. It blocks binding of IL-1 to its receptor, thus inhibiting the proinflammatory and immunomodulatory actions of IL-1.
    - It is given in a dosage of 100 mg SC daily. Similar to TNF blockers, it should not be prescribed to patients with ongoing or recurrent infections.
    - **Adverse effects** include an increased frequency of bacterial infections and injection site reactions.
  ○ **Tocilizumab** is an antagonist of soluble and membrane-bound IL-6 receptors. It is given as an IV infusion or as an SC injection at a dose of 162 mg either weekly or every other week depending on the patient's weight. Side effects include increased infections, neutropenia, and elevations in cholesterol.
- **B-cell–directed therapy: Rituximab** is a monoclonal antibody directed against CD20, a cell surface receptor found on B cells. CD20-positive B cells in peripheral blood are rapidly depleted after two infusions of 1 g of rituximab 2 weeks apart. Methotrexate is generally used as background therapy. The infusion can be repeated in 6- to 12-month intervals, based on patient symptoms.
  ○ **Contraindications and side effects:** Rituximab has rarely been reported to cause reactivation of JC virus, leading to the clinical syndrome of progressive multifocal leukoencephalopathy (PML), which is uniformly fatal.

- ○ **Infusion reactions** are more common with the first dose and rarely fatal. Antihistamines, IV steroids, and acetaminophen are routinely given prior to infusion.
- ○ **Infectious complications** are a concern, as with all biologics, but appear to be less frequent than in anti-TNF–treated patients.
- **Abatacept** is a fusion protein comprising the CTLA-4 molecule and the Fc portion of IgG-1. It blocks selective co-stimulation of T cells. It is given as an IV infusion of 500–1000 mg every 4 weeks. It is also available as a SC formulation that can be given 125 mg SC weekly with or without an initial loading dose. It is approved in patients with an inadequate response to biologic or nonbiologic DMARDs.
  - ○ **Infections** occur slightly more often than in placebo-treated patients. Opportunistic infections have not been observed. **Infusion reactions** are much less common than with rituximab or infliximab.
  - ○ **Chronic obstructive pulmonary disease exacerbations and respiratory infections** are more common in patients with moderate to severe obstructive lung disease when treated with abatacept.
- **Combinations of DMARDs** can be used if the patient has a partial response to the initial agent.
  - ○ Common combination therapies include methotrexate with hydroxychloroquine, sulfasalazine, or both. Methotrexate is commonly combined with TNF antagonists because there is evidence for additive efficacy and for a decrease in the formation of human antichimeric antibodies against the TNF blocker. Methotrexate is often used in combination with rituximab or abatacept. Methotrexate and leflunomide may have additive hepatotoxicity, and this combination should be used cautiously.
  - ○ **Combination therapy with two biologic agents is contraindicated because of increased infectious complications.**
  - ○ **NSAIDs or selective COX-2 inhibitors** may be used as an adjunct to DMARD therapy. **Glucocorticoids are not curative** but may delay the formation of erosions with other **DMARDs** and are among the most potent anti-inflammatory drugs available.
    - ▪ **Indications for glucocorticoids** include (a) symptomatic relief while waiting for a response to a slow-acting immunosuppressive or immunomodulatory agent, (b) persistent synovitis despite adequate trials of DMARDs and NSAIDs, and (c) severe constitutional symptoms (e.g., fever and weight loss) or extra-articular disease (vasculitis, episcleritis, or pleurisy).
    - ▪ **Oral administration** of prednisone 5–20 mg daily usually is sufficient for the treatment of synovitis, whereas severe constitutional symptoms or extra-articular disease may require up to 1 mg/kg PO daily. Although alternate-day glucocorticoid therapy reduces the incidence of undesirable side effects, some patients do not tolerate the increase in symptoms that may occur on the off day.
    - ▪ **Intra-articular administration** may provide temporary symptomatic relief when only a few joints are inflamed. The beneficial effects of intra-articular steroids may persist for days to months and may delay or negate the need for systemic glucocorticoid therapy.

Nonpharmacologic Therapies

- **Acute care** of inflammatory arthritides involves joint protection and pain relief. Proper joint positioning and splints are important elements in joint protection. Heat is a useful analgesic.
- **Subacute disease** therapy should include a gradual increase in passive and active joint movement.
- **Chronic care** encompasses instruction in joint protection, work simplification, and performance of activities of daily living. Adaptive equipment, splints, orthotics, and mobility

aids may be useful, and specific exercises designed to promote normal joint mechanics and to strengthen affected muscle groups are useful.

Surgical Management

- **Corrective surgical procedures** including synovectomy, total joint replacement, and joint fusion may be indicated in patients with RA to reduce pain and to improve function.
- **Carpal tunnel syndrome** is common, and surgical repair may be curative if local injection therapy is unsuccessful.
- **Synovectomy** may be helpful if major involvement is limited to one or two joints and if a 6-month trial of medical therapy has failed, but usually it is only of temporary benefit.
- **Surgical fusion of joints** usually results in freedom from pain but also in total loss of motion; this is tolerated well in the wrist and thumb.
- **Cervical spine fusion** of C1 and C2 is indicated for significant cervical subluxation (>5 mm) with associated neurologic deficits. Patients with long-standing RA undergoing elective surgical procedures should have a lateral cervical spine radiograph in flexion and extension performed to screen for subluxation.

Immunizations

- Immune response to influenza and pneumococcal vaccinations in patients receiving methotrexate and biologic therapies may be attenuated, although usually adequate. **Influenza** vaccinations should be given to patients prior to starting therapy with all nonbiologic DMARDs, and **pneumococcal** vaccinations should be given to patients starting leflunomide, methotrexate, or sulfasalazine if the patients' vaccinations were not current. In addition, periodic pneumococcal vaccinations and annual influenza vaccinations should be considered for all patients receiving biologic agents, in accordance with the Centers for Disease Control and Prevention (CDC) recommendations for appropriate use and timing of these vaccinations.
- Hepatitis B vaccination is recommended if risk factors for this disease exist and if hepatitis B vaccination has not previously been administered.
- Live vaccines (e.g., varicella-zoster vaccine, oral polio, rabies) are contraindicated during biologic therapy but should be considered before initiation of biologic therapy or high-dose steroids.

COMPLICATIONS

- **Patients with RA and a single joint inflamed out of proportion to the rest of the joints must be evaluated for coexistent septic arthritis.** This complication occurs with increased frequency in RA and carries 20–30% mortality.
- **Sjögren syndrome**, characterized by failure of exocrine glands, occurs in a subset of patients with RA, producing sicca symptoms (dry eyes and mouth), parotid gland enlargement, dental caries, and recurrent tracheobronchitis. **Treatment** is symptomatic with artificial tears and saliva or with pilocarpine up to 5 mg PO qid. Cevimeline, 30 mg tid, can also be considered. Assiduous dental and ophthalmologic care is recommended, and drugs that suppress lacrimal–salivary secretion further should be avoided.
- **Felty syndrome:** The triad of RA, splenomegaly, and granulocytopenia also occurs in a small subset of patients, and these patients are at risk for recurrent bacterial infections and nonhealing leg ulcers.
- Approximately 70% of patients show irreversible joint damage on radiography within the first 3 years of disease. Work disability is common, and life span may be shortened.

Osteoarthritis

GENERAL PRINCIPLES

OA, or **degenerative joint disease**, is characterized by deterioration of articular cartilage with subsequent formation of reactive new bone at the articular surface. The joints most commonly affected are the distal and proximal interphalangeal joints of the hands and joints of the hips, knees, and cervical and lumbar spine.

Epidemiology

The disease is more common in the elderly but may occur at any age, especially as sequelae to joint trauma, chronic inflammatory arthritis, or congenital malformation. OA of the spine may lead to spinal stenosis (neurogenic claudication), with aching or pain in the legs or buttocks on standing or walking.

TREATMENT

- **Acetaminophen** in a dosage of up to 1000 mg qid is the initial pharmacologic treatment.
- **Low-dose NSAIDs or selective COX-2 inhibitors** are the next step, followed by full-dose treatment (see Treatment under the Basic Approach to Rheumatic Diseases section). Because this patient population is often elderly and may have concomitant renal or cardiopulmonary disease, NSAIDs should be used with caution.
- The data for **glucosamine sulfate and chondroitin sulfate** are contradictory. Some studies suggest it may reduce symptoms as well as the rate of cartilage deterioration, whereas others have shown that these agents have little benefit in patients with OA. Glucosamine should not be administered to patients who are allergic to **shellfish**. Synthetic and naturally occurring hyaluronic acid derivatives can be administered intra-articularly and may reduce pain and improve mobility in select patients. Commercially, hyaluronan preparations currently available in the United States include sodium hyaluronate (**Hyalgan, Supartz, and Euflexxa**) and hylan G-F 20 (**Synvisc**).
- **Intra-articular glucocorticoid injections** often are beneficial but probably should not be given more than every 3–6 months (see General Principles under Basic Approach to the Rheumatic Diseases section). Systemic steroids should be avoided.
- **Tramadol**, a μ-opioid agonist, may be useful as an alternative analgesic agent. Narcotics may be useful for short-term pain relief and in patients in whom other therapeutic modalities are contraindicated, but in general, they should be avoided for long-term use.
- **Topical NSAIDs, lidocaine, or capsaicin** may provide symptomatic relief with minimal toxicity.
- **Gabapentin** has also been used to help with neural pain modification in patients with severe symptoms of arthritis who are unresponsive to the previously mentioned modalities.
- **Duloxetine** has been approved by the US Food and Drug Administration (FDA) for treatment of OA and chronic lower back pain.

Nonpharmacologic Therapies

- Activities that involve excessive use of the joint should be identified and avoided. Poor body mechanics should be corrected, and misalignments such as pronated feet may be aided by orthotics. An exercise program to prevent or correct muscle atrophy can also provide pain relief. When weight-bearing joints are affected, support in the form of a cane, crutches, or a walker can be helpful. Weight reduction may be of benefit, even for non–weight-bearing joints. Thumb splints may be useful for OA of the first carpometacarpal joint. Consultation with occupational and physical therapists may be helpful.

- **OA of the spine** may cause radicular symptoms from pressure on nerve roots and often produces pain and spasm in the paraspinal soft tissues. Physical supports (cervical collar, lumbar corset), local heat, and exercises to strengthen cervical, paravertebral, and abdominal muscles may provide relief in some patients.
- **Epidural steroid injections** may reduce radicular symptoms.

Surgical Management

- **Surgery** can be considered when patients suffer from disabling pain or deformity. Joint replacement surgery usually relieves pain and increases function in selected patients.
- **Laminectomy and spinal fusion** should be reserved for patients who have severe disease with intractable pain or neurologic complications.

Spondyloarthropathies

The **spondyloarthropathies** are an interrelated group of disorders characterized by one or more of the following features: spondylitis, sacroiliitis, enthesopathy (inflammation at sites of tendon insertion), and asymmetric oligoarthritis. Extra-articular features of this group of disorders may include inflammatory eye disease, urethritis, and mucocutaneous lesions. The spondyloarthropathies aggregate in families, where they are associated with HLA-B27 antigen.

Ankylosing Spondylitis

DIAGNOSIS

- **Ankylosing spondylitis** clinically presents as inflammation and ossification of the joints and ligaments of the spine and sacroiliac joints.
- Patients are usually young men who classically describe low back pain and prolonged morning stiffness, which improve with exercise.
- Hips and shoulders are the peripheral joints that are most commonly involved. Progressive fusion of the apophyseal joints of the spine occurs in many patients and cannot be predicted or prevented.

TREATMENT

Behavioral

- Physical therapy emphasizing extension exercises and posture is recommended to minimize possible late postural defects and respiratory compromise.
- Patients should be instructed to sleep supine on a firm bed without a pillow and to practice postural and deep-breathing exercises regularly.
- Cigarette smoking should be strongly discouraged.

Medications

- **Nonsalicylate NSAIDs**, such as indomethacin, are used to provide symptomatic relief, and **selective COX-2 inhibitors** are also effective (see General Principles under Basic Approach to the Rheumatic Diseases section).
- **Methotrexate and sulfasalazine** provide benefit for peripheral disease in some patients (see Treatment under Rheumatoid Arthritis section).
- **TNF blockade** has been shown to be of benefit even in some patients with apparent fixed deformities.
- **Pamidronate**, a bisphosphonate, may provide modest clinical benefits. Systemic glucocorticoids are not commonly used and can worsen osteopenia.

Surgical Management

Many patients develop osteoporosis in the fused spondylitic spine and are at risk of spinal fracture. Surgical procedures to correct some spine and hip deformities may result in significant rehabilitation in carefully selected patients.

Arthritis of Inflammatory Bowel Disease

GENERAL PRINCIPLES

Arthritis of inflammatory bowel disease occurs in up to 46% of patients with either Crohn disease or ulcerative colitis (*Autoimmun Rev 2014;13(1):20*). It may also occur in some patients with intestinal bypass and diverticular disease.

DIAGNOSIS

Clinical features include **spondylitis**, **sacroiliitis**, and **peripheral arthritis**, particularly in the knee and ankle. Peripheral joint and spinal disease may not always correlate with the activity of the colitis.

TREATMENT

- **NSAIDs** relieve joint pain and inflammation in patients with arthritis due to inflammatory bowel disease (IBD). However, GI intolerance due to NSAIDs may be increased among this group of patients, and NSAIDs may exacerbate underlying IBD.
- **Sulfasalazine, methotrexate, azathioprine, and systemic glucocorticoids** may also be effective (see Treatment under Rheumatoid Arthritis section).
- **TNF antagonists** may benefit both the colitis and arthritis.
- Local **injection of glucocorticoids and physical therapy** are useful adjunctive measures.

Reactive Arthritis

GENERAL PRINCIPLES

- **Reactive arthritis** refers to the inflammatory arthritis that occasionally follows certain GI or genitourinary infections. The triad of arthritis, conjunctivitis, and urethritis was formerly referred to as **Reiter syndrome**.
- *Chlamydia trachomatis* is the most commonly implicated genitourinary infection. *Shigella flexneri, Salmonella* spp., *Yersinia enterocolitica*, or *Campylobacter jejuni* are the most commonly implicated GI infections. *Clostridium difficile* can also trigger the arthritis.
- Of patients, 50–80% are HLA-B27 positive. Males and females are equally affected after GI infections, although males more commonly develop the above classic triad after a *Chlamydia* infection.

DIAGNOSIS

Clinical Presentation

The clinical syndrome may include **asymmetric oligoarthritis**, **urethritis**, **conjunctivitis**, and characteristic **skin and mucous membrane lesions**. The syndrome is usually transient, lasting from 1 to several months, but chronic arthritis may develop in 4–19% of patients.

Diagnostic Testing

The triggering infection may have been asymptomatic. Testing for stool pathogens is low yield if the diarrheal illness has resolved, but urine testing for *Chlamydia* may be helpful if the clinical syndrome is consistent with reactive arthritis.

TREATMENT

- Conservative therapy is indicated for control of pain and inflammation in these diseases.
- Spontaneous remissions are common, making evaluation of therapy difficult.
- **NSAIDs** (especially indomethacin) are often useful, and **selective COX-2 inhibitors** also provide relief (see General Principles under Basic Approach to the Rheumatic Diseases section).
- **Sulfasalazine** or **methotrexate** may be of benefit for arthritis that does not resolve after several months (see Treatment under Rheumatoid Arthritis section).
- Trial of an **anti–TNF-α** agent might be considered in patients who do not respond to sulfasalazine or methotrexate.
- In unusually severe cases, **glucocorticoid therapy** may be required to prevent rapid joint destruction (see General Principles under Basic Approach to the Rheumatic Diseases section).
- Treatment for chlamydia infection, if detected, is appropriate. Prolonged empiric antibiotic therapy has not been shown to be beneficial.
- **Conjunctivitis** is usually transient and benign, but ophthalmologic referral and treatment with topical or systemic glucocorticoids are indicated for **iritis**.

Psoriatic Arthritis

GENERAL PRINCIPLES

Classification

Five major patterns of joint disease occur: (a) asymmetric oligoarticular arthritis, (b) distal interphalangeal joint involvement in association with nail disease, (c) symmetric rheumatoid-like polyarthritis, (d) spondylitis and sacroiliitis, and (e) arthritis mutilans.

Epidemiology

Prevalence varies; however, it has been reported that as many as 30% of patients with psoriasis have some form of inflammatory arthritis (*Rheumatology (Oxford) 2015; 54(1):20*).

TREATMENT

- **NSAIDs,** particularly indomethacin, are used to treat the arthritic manifestations of psoriasis, in conjunction with appropriate measures for the skin disease.
- **Intra-articular glucocorticoids** may be useful in the oligoarticular form of the disease, but injection through a psoriatic plaque should be avoided. Severe skin and joint diseases generally respond well to **methotrexate** (see Treatment under Rheumatoid Arthritis section).
- **Sulfasalazine and leflunomide** may also have disease-modifying effects in polyarthritis.
- **TNF-α blockers** may produce dramatic improvement in both skin and joint disease.
- **Ustekinumab** is a human monoclonal antibody to the shared p40 subunit of IL-12 and IL-23 that interferes with receptor binding to immune cells. It is administered subcutaneously. In patients who weigh less than 100 kg, the dose is 45 mg SC at week 0 and 4.

It is then given every 12 weeks. For patients who weigh more than 100 kg, the dose is 90 mg SC given at the same intervals as the lower dose. It may be administered alone or in combination with methotrexate. Patients should be screened for TB prior to initiating this medication and periodically while on it. Monitor for infections and injection site reactions. Monitor all patients for the development of nonmelanoma skin cancer because this has been reported.

- **Apremilast** is an orally administered phosphodiesterase-4 inhibitor. It suppresses multiple proinflammatory cytokines involved in the innate and adaptive immunity. Initial starting dose is 10 mg daily, which is slowly uptitrated to a maximum dose of 30 mg twice daily. GI upset and headaches have commonly been reported.

COMPLICATIONS

Colonization of psoriatic skin with *S. aureus* increases the risk of wound infection after reconstructive joint surgery.

Systemic Lupus Erythematosus

GENERAL PRINCIPLES

Definition

SLE is a multisystem disease of unknown etiology that primarily affects women of child-bearing age. The female-to-male ratio is 9:1. It is most common in the second and third decades of life and in African Americans.

Pathophysiology

Pathophysiology is multifactorial and incompletely understood, with interplay of genetic predisposition and environmental factors.

DIAGNOSIS

- Disease manifestations are protean, ranging in severity from fatigue, malaise, weight loss, and fever, to potentially life-threatening cytopenias, nephritis, cerebritis, vasculitis, pneumonitis, myositis, and myocarditis.
- Current American College of Rheumatology classification criteria are used primarily for research purposes but are helpful to review when suspicion arises. Based on the classification criteria, the presence of 4 or more of the 11 findings are required.
  - Malar rash
  - Discoid rash
  - Photosensitivity
  - Oral or nasopharyngeal ulcers
  - Arthritis
  - Serositis
  - Proteinuria and cellular casts
  - Seizures, psychosis, or other neurologic manifestations
  - Autoimmune hemolytic anemia, leukopenia or lymphopenia, and thrombocytopenia
  - Antinuclear antibodies (ANA)
  - Anti–double-stranded DNA antibodies, anti-Smith (SM) antibodies, or antiphospholipid antibodies
- Commonly associated serology includes anti-SSA (Ro) and anti-SSB (La) antibodies in approximately 30% of patients and anti-RNP in 40% of patients.

- Some classification criteria also include alopecia, low complement, and a positive direct Coombs test (*Arthritis Rheum 2012;64:2677*).

TREATMENT

Medications

- **NSAIDs** usually control SLE-associated arthritis, arthralgias, fever, and mild serositis but not fatigue, malaise, or major organ system involvement. The response to **selective COX-2 inhibitors** is similar. Hepatic and renal toxicities of NSAIDs appear to be increased in SLE.
- **Hydroxychloroquine** 200 mg bid may be effective in the treatment of rash, photosensitivity, arthralgias, arthritis, alopecia, and malaise associated with SLE and in the treatment of **discoid and subacute cutaneous lupus erythematosus**. The drug is not effective for treating fever or major organ manifestations, but long-term usage may decrease incidence of flares and risk of thrombosis, as well as renal and CNS involvement. For the potential ophthalmologic complications, patients need regular eye examination.
- **Glucocorticoid therapy**
  - **Indications** for systemic glucocorticoids include life-threatening manifestations of SLE, such as glomerulonephritis, CNS involvement, thrombocytopenia, hemolytic anemia, and debilitating manifestations of SLE that are unresponsive to conservative therapy.
  - **Dosage:** Patients with severe or potentially life-threatening complications of SLE should be treated with prednisone, 1–2 mg/kg PO daily, which can be given in divided doses. After disease is controlled, prednisone should be tapered slowly, with the dosage being reduced by no more than 10% every 7–10 days. More rapid reduction may result in relapse. **IV pulse therapy** in the form of methylprednisolone, 500–1000 mg IV daily for 3–5 days, has been used in SLE in such life-threatening situations as rapidly progressive renal failure, active CNS disease, and severe thrombocytopenia. Patients who do not show improvement with this regimen probably are unresponsive to steroids, and other therapeutic alternatives must be considered. A course of oral prednisone should follow completion of pulse therapy.
- **Immunosuppressive therapy**
  - Indications for immunosuppressive therapy in SLE include life-threatening manifestations of SLE such as glomerulonephritis, CNS involvement, thrombocytopenia, hemolytic anemia, and the inability to reduce corticosteroid dosage or severe corticosteroid side effects.
  - Choice of an immunosuppressive therapy is individualized to the clinical situation. Often, **cyclophosphamide** is used for life-threatening manifestations of SLE. High-dose monthly IV pulse cyclophosphamide ($0.5–1.0$ g/m^2) may be less toxic but is also less immunosuppressive than low-dose daily oral cyclophosphamide (1.0–1.5 mg/kg/d). **Azathioprine** (1–3 mg/kg/d) and **mycophenolate mofetil** (500–1500 mg bid) are also used as steroid-sparing agents for serious lupus manifestations. There is increasing evidence that mycophenolate mofetil may be as effective as cyclophosphamide in certain classes of lupus nephritis with fewer side effects, and it is particularly preferred in the younger population where fertility maintenance is a concern. **Methotrexate** (7.5–20.0 mg weekly) is often used for musculoskeletal and skin manifestations. **Rituximab** has been shown in uncontrolled observational studies to be effective in cases of severe SLE not responding to conventional treatment; however, placebo-controlled studies have been disappointing. **Belimumab** inhibits B-lymphocytic stimulator (BLyS) signaling, thereby decreasing B cell survival, and differentiation into immunoglobulin-producing plasma cells. It was approved by the FDA in 2012 for the treatment of adult autoantibody-positive lupus patients who are receiving standard therapy after it was

shown in trials to reduce SLE disease activity and flares. The efficacy of belimumab has not been evaluated in patients with severe lupus nephritis or CNS lupus, and it has not been studied in combination with other biologics or cyclophosphamide.

Nonpharmacologic Therapies

- **Conservative therapy** alone is warranted if the patient's manifestations are mild.
- **General supportive measures** include adequate sleep and fatigue avoidance.
- All patients, not just those with photosensitive rashes, are advised on use of sunscreens with sun protection factor (SPF) of 30 or greater, protective clothing, and sun avoidance. Isolated skin lesions may respond to **topical steroids**.
- Consider prophylaxis against *Pneumocystis* pneumonia in patients treated with cyclophosphamide. Also consider adding prophylaxis for the prevention of bladder and gonadal toxicity from this agent. Appropriate immunizations should be considered prior to initiation of immunosuppressive therapy, especially against influenza and pneumococcus. Immunization with live vaccines is contraindicated in immunosuppressed patients, but varicella-zoster vaccine may be recommended prior to initiation of therapy.

SPECIAL CONSIDERATIONS

- Patients with lupus have accelerated **coronary and peripheral vascular disease**, especially with high disease activity and chronic steroid use, and cardiovascular risk factors should be managed aggressively.
- **Transplantation and chronic hemodialysis** have been used successfully in SLE patients with renal failure. Clinical and serologic evidence of disease activity often remits when renal failure ensues.
- **Pregnancy in SLE:** An increased incidence of second-trimester spontaneous miscarriages and stillbirths has been reported in women with antibodies to cardiolipin or lupus anticoagulant. SLE patients may experience flares during pregnancy if the lupus is active at the time of conception. Differentiation between active SLE and preeclampsia is often difficult. Women in whom SLE is well controlled are less likely to have a flare of disease during pregnancy.
- **Neonatal lupus** may occur in offspring of anti-SSA– or anti-SSB–positive mothers, with skin rash and heart block as the most common manifestations.
- **Drug-induced lupus** typically has a sudden onset and is associated with serositis and musculoskeletal manifestations. Renal and CNS manifestations are rare. Serology includes positive ANA and **antihistone antibodies**, negative anti-SM and anti–double-stranded DNA antibodies, along with normal complement levels. The disease usually resolves with drug discontinuation. Offending drugs include procainamide, hydralazine, minocycline, diltiazem, isoniazid, chlorpromazine, quinidine, methyldopa, and anti-TNF biologics.

Systemic Sclerosis

GENERAL PRINCIPLES

Definition

Systemic sclerosis (scleroderma) is a systemic illness characterized by progressive fibrosis of the skin and visceral organs. The etiology is unknown, but many manifestations of scleroderma are secondary to vasculopathy.

Classification

- Scleroderma can be subdivided based on anatomic skin distribution into **localized scleroderma** (morphea and linear scleroderma) and **systemic sclerosis** (diffuse cutaneous, limited cutaneous, and systemic sclerosis sine scleroderma). The limited cutaneous form involves the extremities distal to the knees and elbows as well as the face. Diffuse cutaneous scleroderma involves the skin of the proximal extremities and the trunk. Systemic sclerosis sine scleroderma affects the internal organs without skin involvement. The **CREST syndrome** is **c**alcinosis, **R**aynaud phenomenon, **e**sophageal dysmotility, **s**clerodactyly, and **t**elangiectasias.

- **Nephrogenic systemic fibrosis** is a potential complication of MRI with gadolinium contrast in patients with renal failure. It is associated with skin thickening and internal organ fibrosis resembling scleroderma, without Raynaud phenomenon or ANA positivity.

DIAGNOSIS

Clinical Presentation

- Nearly all patients with systemic sclerosis have **Raynaud phenomenon**. It is typically the presenting feature. Nail fold capillary changes are also common.
- **Diffuse scleroderma** is associated with scleroderma "renal crisis," and multiple internal organs are affected. Long-term survival is poor.
  - **GI involvement:** Decreased gut motility can occur, leading to bacterial overgrowth, malabsorption, diarrhea, and weight loss. Occasionally, severe constipation and intestinal pseudo-obstruction occur. Classic endoscopic findings include colonic wide mouth diverticula, patulous esophagus, esophageal strictures, and gastric antral vascular ectasia, also known as watermelon stomach.
  - **Renal involvement:** The appearance of sudden hypertension and renal insufficiency indicates potential scleroderma renal crisis. It is associated with a microangiopathic hemolytic anemia and carries a poor prognosis.
  - **Cardiopulmonary involvement:** Patchy myocardial fibrosis can result in heart failure or arrhythmias. Pulmonary involvement includes pleural effusions and inflammatory alveolitis leading to interstitial fibrosis and pulmonary hypertension.
  - **Other organ systems: Skin** involvement appears initially with edematous and erythematous "salt and pepper" pigmentation changes before progressing to skin tightening and thickening. **Musculoskeletal** manifestations range from arthralgias to arthritis with joint contractures due to the regional skin involvement.
- **Limited scleroderma** is more often associated with primary pulmonary hypertension in the absence of ILD or biliary cirrhosis

Diagnostic Testing

More than 95% of scleroderma patients are ANA positive, and 20–40% are anti–Scl-70 positive (associated with diffuse disease). Up to 40% of patients with limited scleroderma have anticentromere antibody. RNA polymerase III antibody has been found to increase the risk of scleroderma renal crisis.

TREATMENT

Therapeutic options for scleroderma are limited. Treatment focuses on organ involvement and symptoms.

- **Skin:** No therapeutic agent is effective for these cutaneous manifestations. **Physical therapy** is important to retard and reduce joint contractures.
- **GI involvement**
  - Reflux esophagitis generally responds to standard therapy (e.g., **H²-receptor antagonists**, **proton pump inhibitors**, and **promotility agents**).

○ Treatment with broad-spectrum antimicrobials in a rotating sequence including **metronidazole** often improves malabsorption. Metoclopramide may reduce bloating and distention.

○ Occasionally, esophageal strictures require mechanical **esophageal dilation**.

• **Renal involvement:** Aggressive blood pressure control with **ACE inhibitors** may delay, prevent, or even reverse renal failure in patients with suspected scleroderma renal crisis. ARBs do not appear to be as effective.

• **Cardiopulmonary involvement:** Coronary artery vasospasm can cause angina pectoris and may respond to calcium channel antagonists. Pulmonary involvement, such as pulmonary hypertension, is treated with standard therapies for these conditions (see Chapter 10, Pulmonary Diseases). Patients with pulmonary parenchymal disease may benefit from glucocorticoids and cyclophosphamide.

Raynaud Phenomenon

GENERAL PRINCIPLES

Raynaud phenomenon is a vasospasm of the digital arteries and can result in ischemia of the digits. It manifests as repeated episodes of color changes of the digits after cold exposure or emotional stress. Primary Raynaud disease has no predisposing factors and is milder. Secondary Raynaud disease occurs in individuals with a predisposing factor, usually a collagen vascular disease.

TREATMENT

Medications

• **Calcium channel antagonists** (of the dihydropyridine group) are the preferred initial agents, although they may exacerbate gastroesophageal reflux and constipation.

• Alternative vasodilators such as prazosin are occasionally helpful but can have limiting side effects, including orthostatic hypotension.

• Other agents that might improve vasospasm include **topical nitroglycerin** applied to the dorsum of the hands, phosphodiesterase inhibitor (e.g., **sildenafil**), and endothelin receptor antagonist (e.g., **bosentan**).

• Daily low-dose aspirin therapy is often prescribed for its antiplatelet effects.

• Patients with severe ischemic digits should be hospitalized, and conditions such as macrovascular disease, vasculitis, or a hypercoagulable state should be ruled out. An IV infusion of a prostaglandin or prostaglandin analog may be considered.

• Patients should be instructed to avoid exposure to cold, protect the hands and feet from trauma, limit caffeine intake, and discontinue cigarette smoking.

Surgical Management

• **Sympathetic ganglion blockade** with a long-acting anesthetic agent may be useful when a patient has progressive digital ulceration that fails to improve with medical therapy.

• Surgical digital sympathectomy may be beneficial.

Necrotizing Vasculitis

GENERAL PRINCIPLES

• **Necrotizing vasculitis** is characterized by inflammation of blood vessels, leading to tissue damage and necrosis. This diagnosis includes a broad spectrum of disorders with various causes that involve vessels of different types, sizes, and locations. The immunopathologic process may involve immune complexes.

- Although in most cases the inciting agent has not been identified, some are associated with chronic hepatitis B and C.
- Vasculitis "mimics" should be considered, including bacterial endocarditis, HIV infection, atrial myxoma, paraneoplastic syndromes, cholesterol emboli, and cocaine and amphetamine use.

DIAGNOSIS

Systemic manifestations including fever and weight loss are common. Table 25-1 summarizes the clinical features and diagnostic and treatment approaches of the most common forms of vasculitis.

TREATMENT

The response to therapy and long-term prognosis of these disorders are highly variable.

- **Glucocorticoids** are the initial therapy. Although vasculitis that is limited to the skin may respond to lower doses of corticosteroids, the initial dosage for visceral involvement should be high (prednisone, 1–2 mg/kg/d). If life-threatening manifestations are present, a brief course of high-dose pulse therapy with methylprednisolone, 500 mg IV q12h for 3–5 days, should be considered.
- Strong immunosuppressives are used in the induction treatment of necrotizing vasculitis when major organ system involvement is present. **Cyclophosphamide** has historically been the initial choice. **Rituximab** is now an approved alternative for remission induction.
- **Methotrexate**, **azathioprine**, and **mycophenolate mofetil** can be used for maintenance therapy and as initial therapy in less severe presentations.

Polymyalgia Rheumatica

DIAGNOSIS

Clinical Presentation

Polymyalgia rheumatica (PMR) presents in elderly patients as proximal limb girdle pain, morning stiffness lasting at least 30 minutes, and constitutional symptoms. It is associated with **temporal arteritis (TA)** in up to 40% of patients (see Table 25-1).

Diagnostic Testing

- There is no established diagnostic criterion. The diagnosis remains clinical.
- The erythrocyte sedimentation rate (ESR) is >50 mm/h.

TREATMENT

- If PMR is present without evidence of TA, **prednisone**, 10–15 mg PO daily, usually produces dramatic clinical improvement within a few days.
- Patients who are suspected of having TA should be treated promptly with high-dose steroids to prevent blindness, and rheumatology should be consulted immediately.
- The ESR should return to normal during initial treatment. Subsequent therapeutic decisions should be based on ESR and clinical status.
- Glucocorticoid therapy can be tapered gradually to a maintenance dosage of 5–10 mg PO daily but should be continued for at least 1 year to minimize the risk of relapse.

TABLE 25-1   Clinical Features and Diagnostic and Treatment Approaches to Vasculitis

Vasculitic Syndrome	Clinical Features	Diagnostic Approach	Treatment
Large-vessel involvement			
Temporal arteritis	Headache, located temporally in >50% Jaw claudication Commonly associated with PMR	ESR >50 mm/h Temporal artery biopsy	Prednisone, 60–80 mg/d
Takayasu arteritis (affects the aorta and primary branches)	Women more commonly affected Greatest prevalence in Asians Commonly presents between ages 20–30 Constitutional symptoms Finger ischemia Arm claudication	Aortic arch arteriogram	Prednisone, 60–80 mg/d
Medium-vessel involvement			
Polyarteritis nodosa	Skin ulcers Nephritis Mononeuritis Mesenteric ischemia	Skin biopsy Renal biopsy Sural nerve biopsy Mesenteric angiogram Hepatitis B, C testing ANCA negative	Prednisone 60–100 mg/d Cyclophosphamide 1–2 mg/kg/d can be added
Kawasaki disease	Seen in children Fever Conjunctivitis Lymphadenopathy Mucocutaneous erythema Coronary aneurysms	Clinical Coronary angiogram	IV immunoglobulin Aspirin Anticoagulation

Small-vessel involvement

Condition	Clinical features	Diagnostic tests	Treatment
Granulomatosis with polyangiitis (c-ANCA vasculitis)	Sinusitis Pulmonary infiltrates Nephritis	c-ANCA, sinus biopsy Lung biopsy Renal biopsy	Prednisone 60–100 mg/d *and* cyclophosphamide 1–2 mg/kg/d Rituximab Plasmapheresis
Microscopic polyangiitis	Pulmonary infiltrates Nephritis	p-ANCA Renal biopsy	Prednisone 60–100 mg/d Cyclophosphamide 1–2 mg/kg/d can be added
Churg-Strauss syndrome	Asthma, allergic rhinitis Fleeting pulmonary infiltrates Mononeuritis multiplex	p-ANCA Peripheral eosinophilia Elevated IgE levels Biopsy (sural nerve/skin) with eosinophilic granulomas	Prednisone 60–100 mg/d Cyclophosphamide if renal, GI, CNS, or cardiac involvement
Vasculitis in SLE or RA	Skin ulcers Polyneuropathy	Skin or sural nerve biopsy	Prednisone 60–80 mg/d Cyclophosphamide 1–2 mg/kg/d can be added
Cutaneous leukocytoclastic vasculitis	Palpable purpura	Skin biopsy	NSAIDs, antihistamine, colchicines, dapsone Low-dose prednisone Discontinue inciting drug
Henoch-Schönlein purpura	Palpable purpura Nephritis Mesenteric ischemia	Skin biopsy Renal biopsy IgA immune complex deposition	Supportive treatment Prednisone 20–60 mg/d may be needed

ANCA, antineutrophil cytoplasmic antibodies; c-ANCA, cytoplasmic antineutrophil cytoplasmic antibodies; CNS, central nervous system; ESR, erythrocyte sedimentation rate; GI, gastrointestinal; p-ANCA, perinuclear antineutrophil cytoplasmic antibodies; PMR, polymyalgia rheumatica; RA, rheumatoid arthritis; SLE, systemic lupus erythematosus.

Cryoglobulin Syndromes

GENERAL PRINCIPLES

Cryoglobulins are serum immunoglobulins that reversibly precipitate in the cold. Cryoglobulins are categorized as type 1 (monoclonal, no RF activity) or as those with RF activity, the "mixed" types 2 (monoclonal) and 3 (polyclonal).

Etiology

- Patients with **type 1** usually have an underlying hematologic disorder such as myeloma, lymphoma, or Waldenström macroglobulinemia.
- **Types 2 and 3** are associated with small-vessel vasculitis and can be present in patients with chronic inflammatory diseases such as hepatitis B and C virus infection, endocarditis, SLE, and RA. The majority of patients with mixed cryoglobulinemia have hepatitis C, although only 5% of patients with hepatitis C and cryoglobulins develop vasculitis.
- **"Essential"** cryoglobulinemia (cryoglobulinemia without an etiology) has become exceedingly rare since the discovery of hepatitis C.

DIAGNOSIS

- Symptoms in monoclonal cryoglobulinemia are related to hyperviscosity (blurring of vision, digital ischemia, headache, lethargy).
- Clinical manifestations of mixed cryoglobulinemia are mediated by immune complex deposition (arthralgias, palpable purpura, glomerulonephritis, and neuropathy).

TREATMENT

- Secondary cryoglobulinemia responds to **treatment of the underlying disorder**. It may recur when treatment is stopped.
- Patients with progressive renal failure, distal necrosis, advanced neuropathy, or other severe manifestations should be treated aggressively with **prednisone** and immunosuppression.
- **Plasmapheresis** can be used in addition to immunosuppression in severe disease.

Polymyositis and Dermatomyositis

GENERAL PRINCIPLES

- **Polymyositis (PM)** is an inflammatory myopathy that presents as weakness and occasionally tenderness of the proximal musculature.
- **Dermatomyositis (DM)** is an inflammatory myopathy associated with proximal muscle weakness and a characteristic skin rash. Gottron papules and a heliotrope rash are hallmark features of DM, but other skin manifestations may be seen.
- PM and DM can occur alone or in association with a variety of neoplasms. Patients with rheumatic diseases such as SLE or RA can also have myositis.

DIAGNOSIS

- Elevated muscle enzyme levels (creatine kinase, aldolase, transaminases, lactate dehydrogenase [LDH]).
- Myositis-specific or -associated antibodies such as Jo-1. Anti–Jo-1 antibodies are strongly associated with ILD, Raynaud phenomenon, and arthritis. These antibodies have therapeutic and prognostic implications and should be assessed in all patients.

- Characteristic findings can be seen on electromyogram (EMG), but these changes are not specific and can be seen in infectious or metabolic myopathies.
- A muscle biopsy can establish the diagnosis but may not be required if myositis-related antibodies are present in the right clinical setting. MRI is useful for the detection of inflammation and necrosis and can aid in identifying a biopsy location.
- Screening for common neoplasms, such as colon, lung, breast, and prostate cancer, should be considered in these patients as well as individual risk-based assessment. Risk factors for malignancy in the setting of myositis include the presence of DM, cutaneous vasculitis, male sex, and advanced age.

TREATMENT

- When PM or DM occurs without associated disease, it usually responds well to **prednisone**, 1–2 mg/kg PO daily. Systemic complaints, such as fever and malaise, respond first, followed by muscle enzymes, and finally, muscle strength. Once serum enzyme levels normalize, the prednisone dosage should be reduced slowly to maintenance levels of 10–20 mg PO daily. Appearance of steroid-induced myopathy and hypokalemia may complicate therapeutic assessment.
- Patients who do not respond to glucocorticoids or who need steroid-sparing treatment may respond to **methotrexate, mycophenolate mofetil,** or **azathioprine.**
- IV infusion of **immunoglobulin** may hasten improvement of severe dysphagia.
- Severe cases are typically treated with **rituximab.**
- PM or DM associated with neoplasia tends to be less responsive to glucocorticoid therapy but may improve after removal of the malignant tumor.
- **Physical therapy** is essential in the management of myositis.

26

Medical Emergencies

Rebecca Bavolek, Evan S. Schwarz, and Jason Wagner

AIRWAY EMERGENCIES

Emergent Airway Management

GENERAL PRINCIPLES

Recognition of the need to manage a patient's airway must be made in a timely and rapid fashion. Respiratory failure can range from immediate to insidious. Increasing evidence shows that inexperienced intubators frequently do more harm than good.

Etiology

The need to emergently manage an airway typically arises for one of three reasons.
- Loss of airway protective reflexes
- Respiratory failure
- Cardiopulmonary arrest

TREATMENT

- If you are not prepared to manage a definitive airway, there are several things that can be done to either temporarily support the airway or help maximize success.
- Inexperienced intubators should maintain the airway with the best device immediately available. Evidence suggests the following order from most effective to least.
  - High-flow nasal cannula oxygen at 15 L/min (apneic oxygenation increases desaturation time)
  - Non-rebreather oxygen mask (NRB) at 15 L/min
  - Bag-valve mask (BVM)
  - Supraglottic airway devices (laryngeal mask airway, Combitube, King Tube)
- While awaiting definitive airway expertise, there are steps that can be taken to improve success during intubation.
  - Place the patient upright to decrease dependent lung volume before intubation.
  - Place the patient on NRB for 3 minutes if possible.
  - If you cannot delay for 3 minutes, then deliver eight vital capacity breaths via BVM.
  - Place a positive end-expiratory pressure valve set to 5–20 cm H_2O on an NRB adding positive pressure to both bagging and passive oxygenation.

Performing the above steps will maximize your chances of success in nearly all airway situations, whether you are the one managing the airway or someone else.

Emergent Airway Adjuncts

- **Gum elastic bougie** is a flexible rubbery stick with a hockey stick tip. The bougie can be used blindly but is better suited for direct laryngoscopy where the intubator cannot visualize the cords. The goal is to obtain the best view possible and for the coude tip of the bougie to be distal and anterior. When the bougie is in the trachea, you can often feel the tracheal rings as you slide the bougie back and forth. Alternatively, you can push the bougie down the oropharynx as deep as possible without losing control of it. If in the esophagus, the bougie will slide all the way down past the stomach with minimal resistance. If in the trachea, the bougie will quickly hit a bronchus and meet resistance. Once you are in the trachea, you can simply slide an endotracheal tube (ETT) over the bougie and verify placement as you normally would.

- **Laryngeal mask airway (LMA)** is an easy-to-use rescue device for nearly all airway events. It is an ETT with a balloon at the end that is inflated to cup the trachea while occluding the esophagus. Note that it should not be used in patients with upper airway obstruction that cannot be cleared or patients with excessive airway pressures such as with chronic obstructive pulmonary disease (COPD), asthma, or pregnancy. There are models of LMAs (which are preferred) that allow an ETT to be passed through them when a definitive airway is desired. Be cautious with excessive bagging because this can lead to emesis.
- **Supraglottic airway devices** are placed blindly in the oropharynx and inflated with air. An upper balloon obstructs the oropharynx while a lower balloon obstructs the esophagus, allowing ventilation in a similar fashion to an LMA with the same limitations. Note that you cannot intubate through a supraglottic device as you can with intubating LMAs.
- **Fiberoptic/digital airway devices** are considered by many the new standard of care. These devices allow the intubator to get a view of the vocal cords via a camera or fiberoptic scope without having to view it through the mouth, making intubation much easier. Excessive secretions or blood can obstruct the camera, so the person using these devices needs to be capable of direct laryngoscopy as well as indirect fiberoptic laryngoscopy.

Pneumothorax

GENERAL PRINCIPLES

- Pneumothorax may occur spontaneously or as a result of trauma.
- **Primary spontaneous pneumothorax** occurs without obvious underlying lung disease.
- **Secondary spontaneous pneumothorax** results from underlying parenchymal lung disease including COPD and emphysema, interstitial lung disease, necrotizing lung infections, *Pneumocystis jirovecii* pneumonia, TB, and cystic fibrosis.
- **Traumatic pneumothoraces** occur as a result of penetrating or blunt chest wounds.
- **Iatrogenic pneumothorax** occurs after thoracentesis, central line placement, transbronchial biopsy, transthoracic needle biopsy, and barotrauma from mechanical ventilation and resuscitation.
- **Tension pneumothorax** results from continued accumulation of air in the chest that is sufficient to shift mediastinal structures and impede venous return to the heart. This results in hypotension, abnormal gas exchange, and ultimately, cardiovascular collapse.
  - Causes include barotrauma due to mechanical ventilation, a chest wound that allows ingress but not egress of air, or a defect in the visceral pleura that behaves in the same way ("ball-valve" effect).
  - Suspect tension pneumothorax when a patient experiences hypotension and respiratory distress on mechanical ventilation or after any procedure in which the thorax is pierced by a needle.

DIAGNOSIS

Clinical Presentation
History
- Patients commonly complain of ipsilateral chest or shoulder pain, usually of acute onset. A history of recent chest trauma or medical procedure can suggest the diagnosis.
- Dyspnea is usually present.

Physical Examination

- Although examination of the patient with a small pneumothorax may be normal, classic findings include decreased breath sounds and a more resonant percussion note on the ipsilateral side.
- With a larger pneumothorax or with underlying lung disease, there may be tachypnea and respiratory distress. The affected hemithorax may be noticeably larger (due to decreased elastic recoil of the collapsed lung) and relatively immobile during respiration.
- If the pneumothorax is very large, and particularly if it is under tension, the patient may exhibit severe distress, diaphoresis, cyanosis, and hypotension. In addition, the patient's trachea may be shifted to the contralateral side.
- If the pneumothorax is the result of penetrating trauma or pneumomediastinum, subcutaneous emphysema may be felt.
- Clinical features alone do not predict the relative size of a pneumothorax, and in a stable patient, further diagnostic studies must be used in order to guide treatment strategy. However, tension pneumothorax remains a clinical diagnosis, and if suspected in the appropriate clinical scenario, immediate intervention should be undertaken prior to further testing.

Diagnostic Testing

Electrocardiography

An **ECG** may reveal diminished anterior QRS amplitude and an anterior axis shift. In extreme cases, tension pneumothorax may cause electromechanical dissociation.

Imaging

- A **CXR** will reveal a separation of the pleural shadow from the chest wall. If the posteroanterior radiograph is normal and pneumothorax is suspected, a lateral or decubitus film may aid in diagnosis (*Thorax 2003;58(suppl II):ii39*). Air travels to the highest point in a body cavity; thus, a pneumothorax in a supine patient may be detected as an unusually deep costophrenic sulcus and excessive lucency over the upper abdomen caused by the anterior thoracic air. This observation is particularly important in the critical care unit, where radiographs of the mechanically ventilated patient are often obtained with the patient in supine position.
- Although tension pneumothorax is a clinical diagnosis, radiographic correlates include mediastinal and tracheal shift toward contralateral side and depression of the ipsilateral diaphragm.
- **Ultrasonography** is a useful tool for bedside diagnosis of pneumothorax, especially on patients who must remain supine or who are too unstable to undergo CT scanning. Placement of the probe in the intercostal spaces provides information regarding the pleura and underlying lung parenchyma. During normal inspiration, the visceral and parietal pleura move along one another and produce a "sliding sign" phenomenon. In addition, the air-filled lung parenchyma below the pleura produces a ray-like opacity known as "comet tails." Presence of the sliding sign and comet tails on ultrasound during inspiration rule out a pneumothorax with high reliability at the point of probe placement. Conversely, absence of these signs is a highly reliable predictor for the presence of pneumothorax. Several places on the chest should be evaluated, including places that air is most likely to accumulate such as the anterior and lateral chest (*Chest 2012;141:1099*). Studies have shown that in the hands of an experienced clinician with ultrasound training, chest ultrasound is more sensitive than CXR (*Emerg Radiol 2013;20:131*).
- Chest CT is the gold standard for diagnosis and determining the size of pneumothorax. Although not always necessary, it may be particularly useful for differentiating pneumothorax from bullous disease in patients with underlying lung conditions (*Thorax 2003;58(suppl II):ii42*).

TREATMENT

Treatment depends on cause, size, and degree of physiologic derangement.

- **Primary pneumothorax**
  - A small, primary, spontaneous pneumothorax without a continued pleural air leak may resolve spontaneously. Air is resorbed from the pleural space at roughly 1.5% daily, and therefore, a small (approximately 15%) pneumothorax is expected to resolve without intervention in approximately 10 days.
  - Confirm that the pneumothorax is **not increasing in size** (repeat the CXR in 6 hours if there is no change in symptoms) and send the patient home if he or she is asymptomatic (apart from mild pleurisy). Obtain follow-up radiographs to confirm resolution of the pneumothorax in 7–10 days. Air travel is discouraged during the follow-up period, because a decrease in ambient barometric pressure results in a larger pneumothorax.
  - If the pneumothorax is **small but the patient is mildly symptomatic,** far from home, or unlikely to cooperate with follow-up, admit the patient and administer high-flow oxygen; the resulting nitrogen gradient will speed resorption.
  - If the patient is **more than mildly symptomatic or has a larger pneumothorax,** simple aspiration is a reasonable initial management strategy. However, aspiration may not be successful for very large pneumothoraces. In patients in whom aspiration fails, proceed with thoracostomy tube insertion (*Thorax 2003;58(suppl II):ii39*).
  - **Pleural sclerosis** to prevent recurrence is recommended by some experts but, in most cases, is not used after a first episode unless a persistent air leak is present.
- **Secondary pneumothorax**
  - Individuals with a secondary spontaneous pneumothorax are usually symptomatic and require lung reexpansion.
  - Often, a bronchopleural fistula persists and a larger thoracostomy tube and suction are required.
  - **Consult a pulmonologist** about pleural sclerosis for persistent air leak and to prevent recurrence.
  - **Surgery** may be required for persistent air leak and should be considered for high-risk patients for prevention of recurrence.
- **Iatrogenic pneumothorax**
  - Iatrogenic pneumothorax is generally caused either by introducing air into the pleural space through the parietal pleura (e.g., thoracentesis, central line placement) or by allowing intrapulmonary air to escape through breach of the visceral pleura (e.g., transbronchial biopsy). Often, no further air leak occurs after the initial event.
  - If the pneumothorax is small and the patient is minimally symptomatic, he or she can be managed conservatively. If the procedure that caused the pneumothorax required sedation, admit the patient, administer oxygen, and repeat the CXR in 6 hours to ensure the patient's stability. If the patient is completely alert and the CXR shows no change, the patient can be discharged.
  - If the patient is symptomatic or if the pneumothorax is too large for expectant care, a pneumothorax catheter with aspiration or a one-way valve is usually adequate and can often be removed the following day.
  - Iatrogenic pneumothorax due to barotrauma from mechanical ventilation almost always has a persistent air leak and should be managed with a chest tube and suction.
  - **Tension pneumothorax**
    - When the clinical situation and physical examination strongly suggest this diagnosis, decompress the affected hemithorax immediately with a 14-gauge needle. Place the needle in the second intercostal space, midclavicular line, just superior to the rib. Release of air with clinical improvement confirms the diagnosis.
    - Recognize that an obese patient or a patient with a large amount of breast tissue may not have resolution of tension with a standard angiocatheter due to inability to reach

the chest wall or weight of the tissue kinking off the air escape path. These patients may require a longer needle than a standard angiocatheter in order to reach the intrathoracic space for decompression or require insertion of a larger gauge reinforced catheter to stent open the pathway for air release.

- If long-needle decompression or reinforced catheter insertion is unsuccessful, and the diagnosis is highly probable in an unstable patient, surgical decompression can be performed by incision of the pleura in the fourth to fifth anterior axillary line above the rib in the same space in which thoracostomy tubes are inserted. This technique has been shown to be effective; however, safety and complication rates are not able to be determined due to lack of studies (*Resuscitation 2007;72(1):11*). The full technique for this procedure is beyond the scope of this book.
- Seal any chest wound with an occlusive dressing and arrange for placement of a thoracostomy tube.

HEAT-INDUCED INJURY

Heat Exhaustion

GENERAL PRINCIPLES

Heat exhaustion occurs through water or sodium depletion but is often a combination of both. Water depletion heat exhaustion often occurs in the elderly or persons working in hot environments with limited water replacement. Salt depletion occurs in unacclimatized individuals who replace fluid losses with large amounts of hypotonic solution.

DIAGNOSIS

- The patient presents with headache, nausea, vomiting, dizziness, weakness, irritability, and/or cramps.
- The patient may have postural hypotension, diaphoresis, and normal or minimally increased core temperature.

TREATMENT

- Treatment consists of resting the patient in a cool environment, accelerating heat loss by fan evaporation, and repleting fluids with salt-containing solutions.
- If the patient is not vomiting and has stable blood pressure, an oral, commercial, balanced salt solution is adequate.
- If the patient is vomiting or hemodynamically unstable, check electrolytes and give 1–2 L of 0.9% saline IV.
- The patient should avoid exercise in a hot environment for 2–3 additional days.

Heat Syncope

GENERAL PRINCIPLES

- Heat syncope is a variant of postural hypotension.
- Exercise in a hot environment results in peripheral vasodilation and pooling of blood, with subsequent loss of consciousness. The affected individual has normal body temperature and regains consciousness promptly when supine. These factors separate this syndrome from heat stroke.

TREATMENT

Treatment consists of resting in a cool environment and fluid repletion.

Heat Stroke

GENERAL PRINCIPLES

- Heat stroke occurs in two varieties, classic and exertional. Both varieties present with high core temperatures that result in direct thermal tissue injury. Secondary effects include acute renal failure from rhabdomyolysis. Even with rapid therapy, mortality rates can be very high for body temperatures above 41.1°C (106°F). The distinction between classic and exertional heat stroke is not important because the therapeutics goals are similar in both and a delay in cooling increases mortality rate.
- The cardinal features of heat stroke are **hyperthermia (>40°C [104°F]) and altered mental status.** Although patients presenting with classic heat stroke may have anhidrosis, this is not considered a diagnostic criterion, because 50% of patients are still diaphoretic at presentation.
- The central nervous system (CNS) is very vulnerable to heat stroke with the cerebellum being highly sensitive. Ataxia may be an early sign. Seizures are common. Neurologic injury is a function of maximum temperature and duration of exposure (*N Engl J Med 2002;346:1978*).

DIAGNOSIS

Diagnosis is based on the history of exposure or exercise, a core temperature usually of 40.6°C (105°F) or higher, and changes in mental status ranging from confusion to delirium and coma.

Differential Diagnosis

- Drug associated
  - Toxicity
    - Anticholinergic
    - Stimulant toxicity
    - Salicylate toxicity
  - Neuroleptic malignant syndrome (NMS) associated with antipsychotic drugs. It is worth noting that NMS and malignant hyperthermia are both accompanied by severe muscle rigidity.
  - Serotonin syndrome
  - Malignant hyperthermia
  - Drug withdrawal syndrome (ethanol withdrawal)
  - Drug fever
- Infections
  - Generalized infections (sepsis, malaria, etc.)
  - CNS infections (meningitis, encephalitis, brain abscess)
- Endocrine
  - Thyroid storm
  - Pheochromocytoma
- Hypothalamic dysfunction due to stroke or hemorrhage
  - Status epilepticus
  - Cerebral hemorrhage (*Emerg Med Clin North Am 2013;31(4):1097*)

Diagnostic Testing

Laboratories
- Laboratory studies should include complete blood count (CBC); partial thromboplastin time; prothrombin time; fibrin degradation products; electrolytes; blood urea nitrogen (BUN); creatinine, glucose, calcium, and creatine kinase levels; liver function tests (LFTs); arterial blood gases (ABGs); urinalysis; and ECG.
- If an infectious etiology is suspected, obtain appropriate cultures.

Imaging
If a CNS etiology is considered likely, CT imaging followed by spinal fluid examination is appropriate.

TREATMENT

- **Immediate cooling** is necessary.
  - The best method of cooling is controversial. A systematic review showed that ice water immersion decreases body temperature twice as quickly as passive cooling and is the procedure of choice when exertional heat stroke is anticipated (long-distance races, military training). If that cannot be achieved, continuous water spray accompanied by fanning has been shown to be adequate for most patients with exertional heat stroke (*Int J Sports Med 1998;19(suppl 2):S150; Ann Intern Med 2000;132:678; J Athl Train 2009;44(1):84*).
  - If response is insufficiently rapid, submerge the patient in ice water, recognizing that this may interfere with resuscitative efforts (*Am J Emerg Med 1996;14:355*).
  - Most emergency facilities that do not care for large numbers of heat illness cases are not equipped for this treatment. In this case, mist the patient continuously with tepid water (20–25°C [68–77°F]). Cool the patient with a large electric fan with maximum body surface exposure.
  - Ice packs should be placed at points of major heat transfer, such as the groin, axillae, and chest, to further speed cooling.
  - Antipyretics have no indication.
- **Dantrolene sodium** does not appear to be effective for the treatment of heat stroke (*Crit Care Med 1991;19:176*).
- Monitor core temperatures continuously by rectal probe because oral and tympanic membrane temperature may be inaccurate.
- Discontinue cooling measures when the core temperature reaches 39°C (102.2°F), which should ideally be achieved within 30 minutes. A temperature rebound may occur in 3–6 hours and should be retreated.
- **For hypotension, administer crystalloids:** If refractory, treat with vasopressors and monitor hemodynamics. Avoid pure α-adrenergic agents, because they cause vasoconstriction and impair cooling. Administer crystalloids cautiously to normotensive patients.

COMPLICATIONS

- **Rhabdomyolysis** may occur. Treat as described in Chapter 13, Renal Diseases.
- **Hypoxemia and acute respiratory distress syndrome** may occur. Treat as described in Chapter 8, Critical Care.
- Treat seizures with benzodiazepines and phenytoin.

MONITORING/FOLLOW-UP

Patients should be placed on telemetry.

COLD-INDUCED ILLNESS

Exposure to the cold may result in several different forms of injury. A risk factor is accelerated heat loss, which is promoted by exposure to high wind or by immersion. Extended cold exposure may result from alcohol or drug abuse, injury or immobilization, and mental impairment.

Chilblains

GENERAL PRINCIPLES

- Chilblains are among the mildest form of cold injury and result from exposure of bare skin to a cold, windy environment (0.6–15.6°C [33–60°F]).
- The ears, fingers, and tip of the nose typically are injured, with itchy, painful erythema on rewarming.

TREATMENT

Treatment involves rapid rewarming (see Frostnip section), moisturizing lotions, analgesics, and instructing the patient to avoid reexposure.

Immersion Injury (Trench Foot)

GENERAL PRINCIPLES

Immersion injury is caused by prolonged immersion (longer than 10–12 hours) at a temperature <10°C (<50°F).

TREATMENT

Treat by rewarming followed by dry dressings. Treat secondary infections with antibiotics.

Frostnip (Superficial Frostbite)

GENERAL PRINCIPLES

Superficial frostbite involves the skin and SC tissues.

DIAGNOSIS

Areas with first-degree involvement are white, waxy, and anesthetic; have poor capillary refill; and are painful on thawing. Second-degree involvement is manifested by clear or milky bullae.

TREATMENT

The **treatment of choice** is rapid rewarming. Immerse the affected body part for 15–30 minutes; hexachlorophene or povidone-iodine can be added to the water bath. Narcotic analgesics may be necessary for rewarming pain. Typically, no deep injury ensues and healing occurs in 3–4 weeks.

Deep Frostbite

GENERAL PRINCIPLES

- Deep frostbite involves death of skin, SC tissue, and muscle (third degree) or deep tendons and bones (fourth degree).
- Diabetes mellitus, peripheral vascular disease, an outdoor lifestyle, and high altitude are additional **risk factors**.

DIAGNOSIS

- The tissue appears frozen and hard.
- On rewarming, there is no capillary filling.
- Hemorrhagic blisters form, followed by eschars. Healing is very slow, and demarcation of tissue with autoamputation may occur.
- The majority of deep frostbite occurs at temperatures <6.7°C (44°F) with exposures longer than 7–10 hours.

TREATMENT

- The treatment is rapid rewarming as described earlier. **Rewarming should not be started until there is no chance of refreezing.**
- Administer analgesics (IV opioids) as needed.
- Early surgical intervention is not indicated.
- **Elevate** the affected extremity, prevent weight bearing, separate the affected digits with cotton wool, prevent tissue maceration by using a blanket cradle, and prohibit smoking.
- Update tetanus immunization.
- Intra-arterial vasodilators, heparin, dextran, prostaglandin inhibitors, thrombolytics, and sympathectomy are not routinely justified.
- Role of antibiotics is unclear (*Tintinalli's Emergency Medicine Manual. 7th ed. New York: McGraw-Hill, 2010: Chapter 202: Frostbite and Other Localized Cold Injuries*).
- Amputation is undertaken only after full demarcation has occurred.

Hypothermia

GENERAL PRINCIPLES

Definition
Hypothermia is defined as a core temperature of <35°C (95°F).

Classification
Classification of severity by temperature is not universal. One scheme defines hypothermia as mild at 34–35°C (93.2–95°F), moderate at 30–34°C (86–93.2°F), and severe at <30°C (86°F).

Etiology
- The most common cause of hypothermia in the United States is cold exposure due to alcohol intoxication.
- Another common cause is cold water immersion.

DIAGNOSIS

Clinical Presentation

Presentation varies with the temperature of the patient on arrival. All organ systems can be involved.

- **CNS effects**
  - At temperatures **below 32°C (89.6°F)**, mental processes are slowed and the affect is flattened.
  - At **32.2°C (90°F)**, the ability to shiver is lost, and deep tendon reflexes are diminished.
  - At **28°C (82.4°F)**, coma often supervenes.
  - **Below 18°C (64.4°F)**, the electroencephalogram (EEG) is flat. On rewarming from severe hypothermia, central pontine myelinolysis may develop.
- **Cardiovascular effects**
  - After an initial increased release of catecholamines, there is a decrease in cardiac output and heart rate with relatively preserved mean arterial pressure. ECG changes manifest initially as sinus bradycardia with T-wave inversion and QT interval prolongation and may manifest as atrial fibrillation at temperatures of <32°C (<89.6°F).
  - Osborne waves (J-point elevation) may be visible, particularly in leads II and V_6.
  - An increased susceptibility to ventricular arrhythmias occurs at temperatures **below 32°C (89.6°F)**.
  - At temperatures of **30°C (86°F)**, the susceptibility to ventricular fibrillation is increased significantly, and unnecessary manipulation or jostling of the patient should be avoided.
  - A decrease in mean arterial pressure may also occur, and at temperatures of **28°C (82.4°F)**, progressive bradycardia supervenes.
- **Respiratory effects**
  - After an initial increase in minute ventilation, respiratory rate and tidal volume decrease progressively with decreasing temperature.
  - ABGs measured with the machine set at 37°C (98.6°F) should serve as the basis for therapy without correction of pH and carbon dioxide tension (PCO_2) (*Ann Emerg Med 1989;18:72; Arch Intern Med 1998;148:1643*).
- **Renal manifestations:** Cold-induced diuresis and tubular concentrating defects may be seen.

Differential Diagnosis

- Cerebrovascular accident
- Drug overdose
- Diabetic ketoacidosis
- Hypoglycemia
- Uremia
- Adrenal insufficiency
- Myxedema

Diagnostic Testing

Laboratories

- Basic laboratory studies should include CBC, coagulation studies, LFTs, BUN, electrolytes, creatinine, glucose, creatine kinase, calcium, magnesium, amylase levels, urinalysis, ABGs, and ECG.
- Obtain toxicology screen if mental status alteration is more profound than expected for temperature decrease.
- Serum potassium is often increased.
- Elevated serum amylase may reflect underlying pancreatitis.

- Hyperglycemia may be noted but should not be treated because rebound hypoglycemia may occur with rewarming.
- Disseminated intravascular coagulation may also occur.

Imaging
Obtain chest, abdominal, and cervical spine radiographs to evaluate all patients with a history of trauma or immersion injury.

TREATMENT

Medications
- Administer supplemental oxygen.
- Give **thiamine** to most patients with cold exposure, because exposure due to alcohol intoxication is common.
- Administration of **antibiotics** is a controversial issue; many authorities recommend antibiotic administration for 72 hours, pending cultures. In general, the patients with hypothermia due to exposure and alcohol intoxication are less likely to have a serious underlying infection than those who are elderly or who have an underlying medical illness.

Other Nonpharmacologic Therapies
- **Rewarming:** The patient should be rewarmed with the goal of increasing the temperature by 0.5–2.0°C/h (32.9–35.6°F/h), although the rate of rewarming has not been shown to be related to the outcome.
- **Passive external rewarming**
  - ○ This method depends on the patient's ability to shiver.
  - ○ It is effective only at core temperatures of **32°C (89.6°F) or higher**.
  - ○ Remove wet clothing, cover patient with blankets in a warm environment, and monitor.
- **Active external rewarming**
  - ○ Application of heating blankets (40–45°C [104–113°F]) or warm bath immersion may cause paradoxical core acidosis, hyperkalemia, and decreased core temperature, as cold stagnant blood returns to the central vasculature (*J R Nav Med Serv 1991;77:139*), although Danish naval research supports arm and leg rewarming as effective and safe (*Aviat Space Environ Med 1999;70:1081*).
  - ○ Pending further investigation, active rewarming is best reserved for young, previously healthy patients with acute hypothermia and minimal pathophysiologic derangement.
- **Active core rewarming is preferred for treatment of severe hypothermia**, although few data are available on outcomes (*Resuscitation 1998;36:101*).
  - ○ **Heated oxygen** is the initial therapy of choice for the patient whose cardiovascular status is stable. This therapeutic maneuver can be expected to raise core temperatures by 0.5–1.2°C/h (32.9–34.2°F/h) (*Ann Emerg Med 1980;9:456*). Administration through an ETT results in more rapid rewarming than delivery via face mask. Administer heated oxygen through a cascade humidifier at a temperature of 45°C (113°F) or lower.
  - ○ **IV fluids** can be heated in a microwave oven or delivered through a blood warmer; give fluids only through peripheral IV lines.
  - ○ **Intravascular heat exchange via catheter** is a recent addition to the options on this list. Less invasive and more familiar to most physicians than the more extreme options, this option can increase body temperature up to 3°C/h. This is simply a central venous catheter placed by the familiar modified Seldinger technique. After placement, warm fluids are run through the catheter (not into the venous system) allowing for cool blood to rewarm as it passes.
  - ○ **Heated nasogastric or bladder lavage** is of limited efficacy because of low-exposed surface area and is reserved for the patient with cardiovascular instability.
  - ○ **Heated peritoneal lavage** with fluid warmed to 40–45°C (104–113°F) is more effective than heated aerosol inhalation, but it should be reserved for patients with cardiovascular

instability. Only those who are experienced in its use should perform heated peritoneal lavage, in combination with other modes of rewarming.

○ **Closed thoracic lavage** with heated fluid by thoracostomy tube has been recommended but is unproved (*Ann Emerg Med 1990;19:204*).

○ **Hemodialysis** can be used for the severely hypothermic, particularly when due to an overdose that is amenable to treatment in this way.

○ **Extracorporeal circulation** (cardiac bypass) is used only in hypothermic individuals who are in cardiac arrest; in these cases, it may be dramatically effective (*N Engl J Med 1997;337:1500*). Extracorporeal circulation may raise the temperature as rapidly as 10–25°C/h (50–77°F/h) but must be performed in an intensive care unit (ICU) or operating room.

Resuscitation

• Maintain airway and administer oxygen.
• If intubation is required, the most experienced operator should perform it (see Airway Management and Tracheal Intubation section in Chapter 8, Critical Care).
• Conduct **cardiopulmonary resuscitation (CPR)** in standard fashion. Perform simultaneous vigorous core rewarming; as long as the core temperature is severely decreased, it should not be assumed that the patient cannot be resuscitated. Reliable defibrillation requires a core temperature of 32°C (89.6°F) or higher; prolonged efforts (to a core temperature of 35°C [95°F]) may be justified because of the neuroprotective effects of hypothermia. **Do not begin CPR if an organized ECG rhythm is present**, because inability to detect peripheral pulses may be due to vasoconstriction, and CPR may precipitate ventricular fibrillation.
• Do not perform Swan-Ganz catheterization, because it may precipitate ventricular fibrillation.
• If ventricular fibrillation occurs, begin CPR as per the advanced cardiac life support (ACLS) protocol (Appendix C). Amiodarone may be administered as per the protocol, although there is no evidence to support its use or guide dosage; some experts suggest reducing the maximum cumulative dose by half. Avoid procainamide because it may precipitate ventricular fibrillation and increase the temperature that is necessary to defibrillate the patient. Rewarming is key.
• Monitor ECG rhythm, urine output, and, possibly, central venous pressure in all patients with an intact circulation.

Disposition

• Admit patients with an underlying disease, physiologic derangement, or core temperature <32°C (<89.6°F), preferably to an ICU.
• Discharge individuals with mild hypothermia (32–35°C [89.6–95°F]) and no predisposing medical conditions or complications when they are normothermic and an adequate home environment can be ensured.

MONITORING/FOLLOW-UP

• Monitor core temperature.
• A standard oral thermometer registers only to a lower limit of 35°C (95°F). Monitor the patient continuously with a rectal probe with a full range of 20–40°C (68–104°F).

OVERDOSES

Overdose, General

Below is a brief review of three of the most common toxicologic emergencies physicians encounter in the United States. For more information about these exposures and other toxicologic conditions, please refer to Chapter 28, Toxicology, an online chapter.

Acetaminophen

GENERAL PRINCIPLES

N-Acetyl-para-aminophenol (APAP) is available worldwide as an over-the-counter analgesic and antipyretic. It is the most common cause of toxicologic fatalities and liver failure in the United States (*Clin Toxicol (Phila) 2014;52(10):1032; Hepatology 2005;42(6):1364*).

DIAGNOSIS

Clinical Presentation

- Patients can initially present with nausea, vomiting, and abdominal pain. However, patients can be asymptomatic, even after potentially toxic ingestions.
- As toxicity progresses, patients develop transaminase elevation, metabolic acidosis, renal failure, and a coagulopathy.
- Patients may eventually develop fulminant hepatic failure, cerebral edema, and sepsis.
- Acetaminophen combination products (such as opioids, antihistamines) can cause additional symptoms such as opioid toxicity and anticholinergic delirium.

History

To predict the risk of hepatotoxicity after acute overdose and use the Rumack-Matthew nomogram, a reliable time of ingestion must be obtained from the patient or family/friends.

Physical Examination

Assess airway, breathing, and circulation (ABCs) and mental status. Especially in patients who are nauseated or vomiting, the assessment of mental status is crucial to prevent aspiration pneumonitis.

Diagnostic Criteria

- Obtain an APAP serum concentration at 4 hours or later after an acute ingestion.
- Plot the APAP concentration on the Rumack-Matthew nomogram (APAP serum concentration vs. time after ingestion) to assess the possibility of hepatic toxicity. Note: The nomogram can only be used for acute ingestions.
- In general, an APAP dose of 150 mg/kg is the potentially toxic limit that requires therapeutic intervention. This limit includes an added 25% safety margin that was added by the US Food and Drug Administration (*BMJ 1998;316(7146):1724*).
- If the time of ingestion is unknown or the ingestion occurred over multiple days or hours, the Rumack-Matthew nomogram cannot be used. The clinician must use the history and laboratory results to determine if the patient is at risk for hepatic injury.

Diagnostic Testing

- **APAP serum level at 4 hours** after ingestion or later (see above).
- **LFT, international normalized ratio, coagulation tests**—aspartate aminotransferase (AST) is a relatively sensitive nonprognostic marker for hepatic injury.

TREATMENT

- *N*-**Acetylcysteine (NAC):** NAC is the antidote to prevent APAP-related hepatotoxicity (*Toxicol Sci 2004;80(2):343*). It should be administered early (i.e., within 8 hours after ingestion) to prevent liver injury but still offers some protection if its administration is delayed (*N Engl J Med 1988;319(24):1557*).
- NAC can be administered either orally or IV.

- **Oral dosing:** Loading dose of 140 mg/kg PO, then 70 mg/kg PO every 4 hours for a total of 17 doses.
- **IV dosing:** Per the package insert, NAC is administered using a three-bag approach: bag 1: 150 mg/kg over 1 hour; bag 2: 50 mg/kg administered over 4 hours; bag 3: 100 mg/kg over 16 hours. The infusion is then continued if there are signs of toxicity. To simplify the approach, hospitals have developed their own protocols. At Barnes-Jewish Hospital, the protocol is to administer the loading dose over 1 hour followed by a continuous infusion at 14 mg/kg/h for the next 20 hours.
- **NAC indications:** NAC treatment should be started in the following:
  - Any patient after acute poisoning with a toxic APAP level according to the nomogram.
  - Patients who present beyond 8 hours after acute ingestion. Start NAC therapy while awaiting the initial APAP serum concentration and LFTs. Continue treatment if the serum concentration is in the toxic range per nomogram or the LFTs are elevated.
  - Patients who present more than 24 hours after acute ingestion and still have a detectable serum APAP level or elevated AST.
  - Patients with chronic APAP exposure (i.e., >4 g/d in adults, >120 mg/kg/d in children) who present with elevated acetaminophen concentrations and transaminases or a concerning history.
  - Patients with signs of fulminant hepatic failure. NAC treatment should be started immediately and transfer to a transplant center arranged without fail. NAC is shown to improve survival of patients in fulminant hepatic failure (*Lancet 1990;335(8705):1572; N Engl J Med 1991;324(26):1852; BMJ 1991;303(6809):1026*).

Opioids

DIAGNOSIS

Clinical Presentation
Symptoms of opioid overdose are respiratory depression, a depressed level of consciousness, and **miosis**. However, the pupils may be dilated with acidosis or hypoxia or following an overdose with meperidine, propoxyphene, or dextromethorphan.

Diagnostic Testing
Laboratories
Drug concentrations and other standard laboratory tests are of little use. Urine drug screens are associated with multiple false positives and negatives. Opioid intoxication is a clinical diagnosis.

Imaging
A CXR should be obtained if pulmonary symptoms are present or there is concern for aspiration.

TREATMENT

- Treatment includes airway maintenance, ventilatory support, and naloxone, an opioid antagonist.
- Limit use of whole-bowel irrigation to body packers. Body packers rarely require surgery, except in cases of intestinal obstruction. This should only be done in consultation with a poison center or medical toxicologist.

Medications
- **Naloxone hydrochloride** is indicated for opioid-induced respiratory depression. It should not be used to reverse decreased mental status.

- The lowest effective dose should be used. The goal of treatment is adequate spontaneous respiration and not necessarily alertness. The initial dose is 0.04–2 mg IV, although the lowest effective dose should be used.
- Larger doses (up to 10 mg IV) may be required to reverse the effects of methadone.
- If multiple doses of naloxone are required, an IV infusion should be initiated. The infusion should be started at two-thirds of the dose required to reverse respiratory depression.
- In the absence of an IV line, naloxone can be administered sublingually (*Ann Emerg Med 1987;16:572*), intranasally (*Emerg Med J 2006;23:221*), or IM. Isolated opioid overdose is unlikely if there is no response to a total of 10 mg of naloxone.
- **Disposition**
  ○ Patients should be observed for at least an hour following naloxone administration.
  ○ Patients requiring a naloxone infusion should be admitted to an ICU.
  ○ Body packers should be admitted to an ICU for close monitoring of the respiratory rate and level of consciousness and remain in the ICU until all packets have passed, as documented by CT.

Salicylates

GENERAL PRINCIPLES

Definition

- Salicylate toxicity may result from **acute or chronic** ingestion of acetylsalicylic acid (aspirin is a generic name in the United States, but a brand name in the rest of the world).
- Toxicity from chronic ingestion typically occurs in elderly patients with chronic underlying medical conditions. They can present similarly to patients with sepsis.

DIAGNOSIS

Clinical Presentation

- Nausea, vomiting, tinnitus or hearing changes, tachypnea, tachycardia, diaphoresis, hyperpnea, and malaise are common in acute toxicity.
- Severe intoxications may include lethargy, noncardiogenic pulmonary edema, seizures, and coma, which may result from cerebral edema and energy depletion in the CNS.

Diagnostic Testing

- Obtain electrolytes, BUN, creatinine, and glucose.
- Obtain either ABGs or venous blood gases.
- Obtain a serum salicylate concentration. Patients generally require treatment for concentrations >30 mg/dL. **Note: Units may be different at other institutions. For the purposes of this chapter, salicylate concentrations are in mg/dL.**
- Salicylate concentrations >100 mg/dL are very serious and often fatal.
- Salicylate concentrations of 10–30 mg/dL often do not require treatment. However, patients should receive serial evaluations to make sure that the concentration is appropriately decreasing.
- Chronic ingestion can cause toxicity at lower salicylate concentrations than acute ingestions.

TREATMENT

Medications

- **Multidose charcoal** may be useful in severe overdose (*Pediatrics 1990,85:594*) or in cases in which salicylate concentrations fail to decline as absorption tends to be delayed due to bezoar formation and pylorospasm.

- Patients are often volume depleted and require 1–2 L of normal saline.
- **Urine alkalinization** is indicated for patients with salicylate concentrations >30 mg/dL.
- Administer 150 mEq (three ampules) sodium bicarbonate in 1000 mL 5% dextrose in water (D5W) at 1.5–2 times maintenance.
- Maintain alkalinization and titrate to a goal urine pH of 7.5–8. Patients with hypokalemia cannot effectively have their urine alkalinized.
- **Use caution in patients who cannot handle large volumes of fluid such as the elderly, patients with renal failure, patients with heart failure, or patients with cerebral or pulmonary edema.**
- Alkalinization can be stopped once the serum concentration is <30 mg/dL. The patient should have a repeat salicylate concentration drawn 4–6 hours after all treatment is stopped. If it is declining appropriately (approximately half of previous concentration), the patient does not require further treatment.
- **Hyperventilate any patient requiring endotracheal intubation.** Intubation should be avoided if at all possible in these patients, because they require complex ventilatory settings. The ventilator should be set at their maximal respiratory rate. Any worsening of their acidosis due to improper ventilator settings can result in rapid deterioration and death.
- **Treat altered mental status with IV dextrose** even with a normal blood glucose.
- Treat **seizures** with a **benzodiazepine**. Standard antiepileptics will not be effective.

Hemodialysis

Indications include:
- Salicylate concentrations >100 mg/dL in acute toxicity
- Salicylate concentrations >80 mg/dL or rising despite treatment
- Salicylate concentrations >60 mg/dL in chronic toxicity
- Patients with pulmonary edema, cerebral edema, or seizures
- Patients requiring intubation
- Patients who cannot receive large amounts of fluid and have potentially toxic ingestions

Appendix A

Immunizations and Postexposure Therapies

Abigail L. Carlson and Carlos A. Q. Santos

- **Active immunization** promotes the development of a durable primary immune response (B-cell proliferation, antibody response, T-cell sensitization) such that subsequent exposure to the pathogen results in a secondary response that protects against the development of disease (Table A-1).
- **Passive immunization** involves the administration of immune globulin that results in transient protection against infection. It is usually used in a host with limited capacity to mount a primary immune response, when exposure to a pathogen occurs in a previously unvaccinated host, or to protect against toxin-mediated disease.
- **Postexposure prophylaxis** is therapy given following exposure to a pathogen to prevent the development of disease. This can include active immunization, passive immunization, and/or antimicrobial therapy (Tables A-2 and A-3).
- **Adverse events potentially related to vaccination** should be reported through the Vaccine Adverse Event Reporting System (VAERS) at *http://vaers.hhs.gov/* or 1-800-822-7967.
- **More information,** including the adult vaccine schedule, recommendations regarding travel, and guideline updates, can be found at the Centers for Disease Control and Prevention (CDC) website, *http://www.cdc.gov/*. Additional guidance for specific clinical questions can be obtained by contacting the CDC at 1-800-232-4636 or NIPINFO@cdc.gov.

TABLE A-1 Selected Adult Immunization Recommendations in the United States

Vaccine, Dose	Indications	Contraindications	Precautions
Haemophilus influenzae type b (Hib) 0.5 mL IM	**1 dose:** adults not previously vaccinated with anatomic or functional asplenia, with sickle cell disease, or undergoing elective splenectomy **3 doses:** hematopoietic stem cell transplant recipients 6–12 mo after successful transplant (separate doses by ≥4 wk)	Severe allergic reaction to any vaccine component or after a previous dose	Moderate or severe acute illness with or without fever
Hepatitis A Single-antigen vaccine (Havrix, Vaqta): 1 mL IM Hepatitis A/hepatitis B combined vaccine (Twinrix): 1 mL IM	**Any adult seeking protection from hepatitis A virus (HAV)** **Specific indications:** men who have sex with men (MSM); illicit drug use; laboratory workers exposed to HAV; chronic liver disease; receipt of clotting factor concentrates; travelers to countries with high or intermediate endemicity of HAV; persons who anticipate close personal contact with an adoptee from a country with high or intermediate endemicity during the first 60 d after arrival. **Dosing:** Havrix: 2 doses at 0 and 6–12 mo Vaqta: 2 doses at 0 and 6–18 mo Twinrix: 3 doses at 0, 1, and 6 mo	Severe allergic reaction to any vaccine component or after a previous dose	Moderate or severe acute illness with or without fever

Hepatitis B

Recombivax HB Single-Antigen Vaccine, Standard (10 µg/mL)
Formulation: 1 mL IM
Recombivax HB Single-Antigen Vaccine, High Dose (40 µg/mL)
Formulation: 1 mL IM
Engerix-B Single-Antigen Vaccine (20 µg/mL): 1 mL IM
Twinrix: See Hepatitis A

Any adult seeking protection from hepatitis B virus (HBV)

Specific indications: sexually active persons not in long-term, mutually monogamous relationship; persons seeking evaluation or treatment for a sexually transmitted disease (STD); injection drug users; MSM; **health care personnel;** public safety workers potentially exposed to blood or body fluids; persons age <60 with diabetes (and those age ≥60 at discretion of treating clinician); end-stage renal disease (ESRD); HIV infection; chronic liver disease; household contacts and sex partners of persons with chronic HBV infection; travelers to countries with high or intermediate prevalence of HBV; clients and staff of institutions for persons with developmental disability

Vaccinate all adults in the following settings: facilities providing STD treatment, HIV testing and treatment, or drug abuse treatment and prevention services; health care settings targeting services to injection drug users or MSM; correctional facilities; ESRD programs and facilities for chronic hemodialysis (HD) patients; institutions and nonresidential day care facilities for persons with developmental disabilities

Standard dosing: 3 doses Recombivax HB or Engerix-B at 0, 1, and 4 mo

HD patients or other immunocompromised: 3 doses high-dose Recombivax HB at 0, 1, and 6 mo or 8 doses of Engerix-B given as four 2-dose (2 mL) injections at 0, 1, 2, and 6 mo

Twinrix: See hepatitis A

Severe allergic reaction to any vaccine component or after a previous dose

Moderate or severe acute illness with or without fever

(continued)

A-3

TABLE A-1 Selected Adult Immunization Recommendations in the United States (*Continued*)

Vaccine, Dose	Indications	Contraindications	Precautions
Human papillomavirus (HPV) Quadrivalent (HPV4) or bivalent (HPV2): 0.5 mL IM	**Females (HPV4 or HPV2):** adults (including **immune compromised**) through age 26 yr if not previously vaccinated **Males (HPV4 Only):** adults through age 21 yr if not previously vaccinated; through age 26 yr if MSM or **immune compromised** Administer 3-dose series, with 2nd dose at 4–8 wk, 3rd dose at 24 wk (16 wk after 2nd dose)	Severe allergic reaction to any vaccine component or after a previous dose	Moderate or severe acute illness with or without fever; **pregnancy**
Influenza Intramuscular inactivated or recombinant influenza vaccine (IIV or RIV): 0.5 mL IM Intradermal IIV: 0.1 mL ID Live attenuated influenza vaccine (LAIV): 0.2 mL intranasal	**Everyone** 1 dose annually prior to influenza season; consider high-dose regimen in elderly Standard dose quadrivalent and trivalent IIV: all persons Intradermal trivalent IIV: 18–64 yr High-dose IIV: age ≥65 yr Cell culture-based IIV: age ≥18 yr RIV: age ≥18 yr, **safe for persons with egg allergy** LAIV: age 2–49 yr without contraindications **Health care personnel** who receive LAIV should avoid providing care for severely immune suppressed persons (i.e., requiring protective environment) for 7 d after vaccination	Severe allergic reaction to any vaccine component or after a previous dose All except RIV: severe allergic reaction to egg protein LAIV only: **pregnancy, immune suppression,** persons who have taken influenza antiviral medications within previous 48 hr	Moderate to severe illness with or without fever; history of Guillain-Barré syndrome (GBS) within 6 wk of previous influenza vaccination LAIV only: asthma; chronic medical conditions that may predispose to higher risk of influenza-related complications (e.g., lung disease, cardiovascular disease, diabetes, renal or hepatic disease)

Measles, mumps, rubella (MMR)
0.5 mL SC

Adults born after 1957: 1 dose if no documentation of prior vaccination (e.g., in childhood) or laboratory confirmation of immunity to all 3 viral components; for measles/mumps nonimmune, 2nd dose of MMR, administered at ≥28 d after 1st dose, recommended for students in postsecondary educational institutions, **health care personnel**, and international travelers

Persons who received inactivated (killed) measles vaccine or measles vaccine of unknown type from 1963–1967, or persons vaccinated before 1979 with either killed mumps vaccine or mumps vaccine of unknown type who are at high risk for mumps infection (e.g., **health care personnel**) should be considered for revaccination with two doses of MMR vaccine

Women of childbearing age: Rubella immunity should be determined. If no immunity and nonpregnant, give 1 dose of MMR; **pregnant women with no rubella immunity:** 1 dose on completion or termination of pregnancy and before discharge from the health care facility

Health care personnel born before 1957: If no documentation of vaccination or laboratory confirmation of immunity or disease, consider vaccination (2 doses if measles or mumps nonimmune, 1 dose if rubella nonimmune)

Severe allergic reaction to any vaccine component or after a previous dose; known **severe immunodeficiency** (e.g., hematologic and solid tumors, receipt of chemotherapy, congenital immunodeficiency, long-term immunosuppressive therapy, HIV infection with CD4$^+$ <200 cells/μL); **pregnancy**

Moderate or severe acute illness with or without fever; Recent (≤11 mo) receipt of antibody-containing blood product; history of thrombocytopenia or thrombocytopenic purpura; need for tuberculin skin testing within 4 wk of vaccination (measles component may temporarily suppress reactivity)

(continued)

TABLE A-1 Selected Adult Immunization Recommendations in the United States (*Continued*)

Vaccine, Dose	Indications	Contraindications	Precautions
Meningococcal (*Neisseria meningitidis*) Quadrivalent meningococcal conjugate vaccine (MenACWY) or meningococcal polysaccharide vaccine (MPSV4): 0.5 mL SC	**Adults with high risk for infection** **1 dose MenACWY:** microbiologists routinely exposed to isolates of *N. meningitidis*; military recruits, persons who travel to or live in countries where meningococcal disease is hyperendemic or epidemic, first-year college students age ≤21 living in residence halls if no vaccination since 16th birthday **2 doses MenACWY:** anatomic or functional asplenia, persistent complement component deficiency, HIV-infected with another indication for vaccination **Revaccination every 5 yr:** if high-risk condition persists (e.g., asplenia, microbiologist) **MPSV4:** use only if age ≥56 yr, have never received MenACWY, and only 1 dose needed	Severe allergic reaction to any vaccine component or after a previous dose	Moderate or severe acute illness with or without fever

Pneumococcal (*Strepto-coccus pneumoniae*)
13-Valent pneumococcal conjugate vaccine (PCV13): 0.5 mL IM
23-Valent pneumococcal polysaccharide vaccine (PPV23): 0.5 mL IM or SC

Adults ≥65 yr of age: 1 dose PCV13, followed by 1 dose PPSV23 at 6–12 mo

- If prior PPV23 given at age ≥65 yr: give 1 dose PCV13 at least 1 yr after last PPV23
- If prior PPV23 given at age <65 yr: give 1 dose PCV13 at least 1 yr after last PPV23, followed by 1 dose PPV23 at 6–12 mo
- If prior PCV13 at age <65: 1 dose PPV23 at least 6–12 mo after last PCV13
- If prior PCV13 and PPV23 at age <65: 1 dose PPV23 at least 6–12 mo after last PCV13 and 5 yr after last PPV23

Adults 19–64 yr of age AND:

- Immune compromise, anatomic or functional asplenia: 1 dose PCV13, followed by 1 dose PPV23 at ≥8 wk and 2nd dose at ≥5 yr after 1st PPV23
  - If prior dose PPV23 given: give 1 dose PCV13 ≥1 yr after PPV23, give 2nd dose PPV23 once ≥8 wk after PCV13 and ≥5 yr after PPV23
  - If 2 prior doses PPV23 given: 1 dose PCV13 ≥1 yr after last PPV23 dose
  - If prior PCV13 given: 1 dose PPV23 at ≥8 wk after PCV13 and 2nd dose at ≥5 yr after 1st PPV23
  - If prior PCV13 and 1 dose PPV23 given: 1 dose PPV23 at ≥5 yr after 1st PPV23 dose
- Cerebrospinal fluid leak or cochlear implant: 1 dose PCV13, followed by 1 dose PPV23 at ≥8 wk
- Chronic heart, lung, or liver disease, alcoholism, diabetes mellitus, smoke cigarettes, or reside in nursing home/long-term care facility: 1 dose PPV23

Severe allergic reaction after a previous dose or to a vaccine component PCV13 only: severe allergic reaction to any vaccine containing diphtheria toxoid

Moderate or severe acute illness with or without fever

(continued)

TABLE A-1 Selected Adult Immunization Recommendations in the United States (*Continued*)

Vaccine, Dose	Indications	Contraindications	Precautions
Tetanus, diphtheria (Td)/ tetanus, diphtheria, pertussis (Tdap) 0.5 mL IM (Other formulations [e.g., diphtheria and tetanus toxoids and acellular pertussis (DTaP)] not recom- mended for adult use)	**Everyone** Td: Every 10 years Tdap: One dose after age 18 yr as substitute for one Td booster; **pregnant women**: one dose every pregnancy (preferably at 27–36 wk gestation) Adults with unknown or incomplete (<3-dose) history of primary vaccination series with Td-containing vaccines: begin or complete primary vaccination series including at least 1 dose of Tdap Postexposure prophylaxis: see Table A-2	Severe allergic reaction to any vaccine component or after a previous dose Tdap only: encepha- lopathy (e.g., coma, prolonged seizures) not attributable to other cause within 7 d of ad- ministration of previous dose of Tdap, DTaP, or diphtheria and tetanus toxoids and pertussis (DTP) vaccine	Moderate or severe acute illness with or without fever; GBS within 6 wk after previous dose of tet- anus toxoid–containing vaccine; history of Arthus-type (type III) hypersensitivity reac- tions after previous dose of diphtheria toxoid– containing vaccine Tdap only: progressive or unstable neurologic disorder, uncontrolled seizures, or progressive encephalopathy until treatment regimen established and condition stabilized

Vaccine	Recommendation	Contraindications	Precautions
Varicella (chickenpox) 0.5 mL SC For shingles (herpes zoster) vaccine: see Zoster	**Everyone without evidence of immunity** 2 doses, 4–8 wk apart; if 1 dose given previously, give 2nd dose only Evidence of immunity: • Documented vaccination (2 doses >4 wk apart) • U.S. born before 1980 **except** if pregnant or health care personnel • Varicella or zoster infection documented by health care provider • Laboratory confirmation of immunity or disease	Severe allergic reaction to any vaccine component or after a previous dose; known **severe immunodeficiency** (e.g., hematologic and solid tumors, receipt of chemotherapy, congenital immunodeficiency, long-term immunosuppressive therapy, HIV infection with $CD4^+$ <200 cells/μL); **pregnancy**	Recent (≤11 mo) receipt of antibody-containing blood product; moderate or severe acute illness with or without fever; receipt of specific antivirals (i.e., acyclovir, famciclovir, valacyclovir) 24 h before vaccination, avoid use for 14 d after vaccination
Zoster 0.65 mg SC For varicella (chickenpox) vaccine: see Varicella	**Adults ≥60 yr of age** 1 dose regardless of prior episodes of herpes zoster	Severe allergic reaction to a vaccine component; known **severe immunodeficiency** (e.g., hematologic and solid tumors, receipt of chemotherapy, congenital immunodeficiency, long-term immunosuppressive therapy, HIV infection with $CD4^+$ <200 cells/μL); **pregnancy**	Moderate or severe acute illness with or without fever; receipt of specific antivirals (i.e., acyclovir, famciclovir, valacyclovir) 24 h before vaccination, avoid use for 14 d after vaccination

Adapted from Centers for Disease Control and Prevention. Advisory Committee on Immunization Practices Recommended Immunization Schedule for Adults Aged 19 Years or Older—United States, 2015. *MMWR Morb Mortal Wkly Rep* 2015;64(4):91–92; *http://www.cdc.gov/vaccines/schedules/downloads/adult/adult-combined-schedule.pdf*.

TABLE A-2	Selected Adult Postexposure Prophylaxis Recommendations
Disease	**Indications and Therapy**
Anthrax	Indicated for all contacts. Either ciprofloxacin 500 mg PO bid (preferred for **pregnant women**), or doxycycline 100 mg PO bid for 60 d and anthrax vaccine absorbed (AVA) SC series (obtained from the CDC): First dose administered as soon as possible, second and third doses administered at 2 and 4 wk after the first dose. (Alternative antibiotic regimens available; see CDC website.)
Botulinum toxin	Close observation of exposed person; treat with heptavalent botulinum antitoxin (equine immunoglobulin) at first sign of illness (obtained via consultation with state health department).
Diphtheria	Indicated for close (e.g., household) contacts: Benzathine penicillin G 1.2 million units IM once or erythromycin (base) 500 mg PO bid for 7–10 d and tetanus and diphtheria (Td) booster vaccine (see Table A-1). Diphtheria antitoxin (DAT) 10,000 units IM/IV (after appropriate sensitivity testing) used for prophylaxis only in exceptional circumstances, obtained in consultation with the CDC (770-488-7100).
Hepatitis A	For healthy persons **<40 years**: Single-antigen hepatitis A vaccine (see Table A-1). For **persons ≥40 years, immune compromised,** or with chronic liver disease: Immune globulin (IG), 0.02 mL/kg IM once. Administer **within 14 d** of exposure. Indicated for unvaccinated household and sexual contacts of infected individual; coworkers of infected food handlers; all staff and children at day care centers caring for diapered children where ≥1 case has occurred or when cases occur in ≥2 households of center attendees; only classroom contacts in centers not caring for diapered children.
Hepatitis B	**Nonoccupational:** If exposure source is known surface antigen positive, unvaccinated or incompletely vaccinated persons should receive vaccine (see Table A-1) and hepatitis B immune globulin (HBIG) 0.06 mL/kg IM once. Vaccinated persons without serologic confirmation of immunity should receive 1 vaccine dose. If exposure source antigen status is unknown, unvaccinated persons should receive the vaccine series, and incompletely vaccinated persons should receive the remaining doses. Vaccinated persons require no further treatment. **Occupational:** See Table A-3.

(continued)

TABLE A-2	Selected Adult Postexposure Prophylaxis Recommendations (*Continued*)
Disease	**Indications and Therapy**
HIV	**Nonoccupational:** Indicated within 72 h of exposure to HIV-infected blood, urogenital secretions, or other body fluids (e.g., condomless sexual intercourse, needle sharing). Administer tenofovir-emtricitabine 300 mg/200 mg (1 tablet) PO daily and raltegravir 400 mg PO bid for 28 d. Test for HIV at presentation and ensure follow-up for repeat HIV testing at 6 weeks. If alternative regimens desired, recommend consultation with an HIV specialist. **Occupational:** See Table A-3.
Measles	**Nonoccupational:** If nonimmune (see Table A-1), give measles, mumps, rubella (MMR) vaccine within 72 h of initial exposure. For **pregnant women** (if nonimmune) or severely **immunocompromised** (regardless of prior immunity), give immunoglobulin 400 mg/kg IV (IVIG) once within 6 d of exposure. Monitor for signs/symptoms for at least 1 incubation period. **Occupational:** See Table A-3.
Meningococcus (*Neisseria meningitidis*)	Indicated for close contacts of patients with invasive meningococcal disease, including household contacts, child care center contacts, and persons directly exposed to the patient's oral secretions. Administer ciprofloxacin 500 mg PO once, rifampin 600 mg PO bid for 2 d, or ceftriaxone 250 mg IM once (preferred in **pregnancy**).
Pertussis (*Bordetella pertussis*, whooping cough)	Indicated for all household contacts, persons with high risk of severe illness (e.g., **immunocompromised**, third trimester of **pregnancy**, asthma), or those who will have contact with high-risk persons (including infants age <12 mo). Administer a macrolide antibiotic (azithromycin 500 mg PO day 1, 250 mg PO daily days 2–5; erythromycin 500 mg PO q6h for 14 d; clarithromycin 500 mg PO bid for 7 d) within 21 d of symptom onset in exposure source.
Plague	Indicated for close contacts of pneumonic plague patients or persons with direct contact with infected body fluids or tissues (for **pregnant women**, weigh prophylactic benefits with antibiotic risks): doxycycline 100 mg PO bid or ciprofloxacin 500 mg PO bid for 10 days.
Rabies	See Rabies Postexposure Prophylaxis section of this appendix.

(continued)

TABLE A-2	Selected Adult Postexposure Prophylaxis Recommendations (*Continued*)
Disease	**Indications and Therapy**
Tetanus	**For clean, minor wounds:** If vaccination history unknown or <3 doses tetanus toxoid-containing vaccine, give Tdap and complete catch-up vaccination (see Table A-1). If ≥3 doses and >10 yr since last dose, give Tdap (if not yet received) or Td. **For all other wounds:** If vaccination history unknown or <3 doses tetanus toxoid-containing vaccine, give tetanus immune globulin 250 units IM once, as well as Tdap (at separate site) and complete catch-up vaccination. If ≥3 doses and >5 years since last dose, give Tdap (if not yet received) or Td.
Tularemia	Routine prophylaxis not recommended. If exposure in bioterrorism or mass casualty setting, give doxycycline 100 mg PO bid or ciprofloxacin 500 mg PO bid (preferred in **pregnant women**) for 14 d.
Smallpox	Indicated in setting of intentional release of smallpox (variola virus) for exposed persons and persons with contact with infectious materials from smallpox patients, weighing risks and benefits for those with relative contraindications. Vaccinate with vaccinia vaccine (available from the CDC Drug Service at 404-639-3670) ideally within 3 d of exposure; vaccination 4–7 d after exposure may offer some protection.
Varicella	Indicated for exposed persons without evidence of immunity. Vaccinate (see Table A-1) within 3 d of exposure (possibly effective up to 5 d of postexposure). If contraindication to vaccination and at high risk of severe infection (e.g., **pregnant women, immunocompromised**), give varicella-zoster immune globulin (VariZIG) 12.5 international units (IU)/kg IM once (minimum, 125 IU; maximum, 625 IU) within 10 d of exposure, which can be obtained from FFF Enterprises (800-843-7477, *http://www.fffenterprises.com*).

CDC, Centers for Disease Control and Prevention; Tdap, tetanus, diphtheria, pertussis.

TABLE A-3	Selected Postexposure Guidelines for Health Care Personnel[a]

Pathogen	Treatment
HIV	Indicated for exposure to HIV-infected blood, tissue, or body fluids (e.g., semen, vaginal secretions, amniotic fluid)[b] via percutaneous injury, contact with mucous membranes, or contact with nonintact skin. Administer as soon as possible within 72 h after exposure (can consider up to 1 wk in very-high-risk cases). Preferred regimen is tenofovir-emtricitabine 300 mg/200 mg (1 tablet) PO daily and raltegravir 400 mg PO bid for 28 d or until exposure source tests negative for HIV (unless acute seroconversion is suspected).[c] Test exposed workers at baseline, 6 wk, 12 wk, and 6 mo for HIV (baseline, 6 wk, and 4 mo if using 4th-generation test). Assistance with choosing a regimen may be obtained by calling the National Clinicians' Post-Exposure Prophylaxis Hotline (PEPline) at 1-888-448-4911 or an HIV expert.
Hepatitis B	For percutaneous injury with blood or blood-contaminated fluids from known surface antigen–positive source: Unvaccinated health care worker: Administer hepatitis B immunoglobulin (HBIG), 0.06 mL/kg IM, within 96 h of exposure AND start hepatitis B vaccine series (see Table A-1). Vaccinated health care worker: Known responder: no treatment Nonresponder after initial vaccination: HBIG × 1 and revaccinate Nonresponder after revaccination: HBIG × 2 doses 1 mo apart Antibody response unknown: check anti-HBs titer; if ≥10 IU/mL: no therapy; if <10 IU/mL: HBIG × 1 and vaccine booster.
Hepatitis C	Immunoglobulin and postexposure prophylaxis not effective. Ensure occupational health follow-up for baseline and subsequent follow-up testing.
Measles	If no documented evidence of immunity, give MMR vaccine within 72 h of initial exposure. For **pregnant women** (if nonimmune) or severely **immunocompromised** (regardless of prior immunity), give immunoglobulin 400 mg/kg IV (IVIG) once within 6 d of exposure. Monitor for signs/symptoms for at least 1 incubation period. Health care personnel without evidence of immunity should be off duty from day 5 after first exposure to day 21 after last exposure, regardless of whether prophylaxis was given.

[a]All blood and body fluid exposures should be reported to the occupational health department. Source patients should be tested for HIV (with consent), hepatitis B surface antigen (HbsAg), and hepatitis C antibody (anti-HCV).
[b]Body fluids not considered infectious include feces, urine, vomitus, saliva, and tears, unless these are visibly contaminated with blood.
[c]Multiple alternative antiretroviral regimens are available if exposed worker has contraindications to or is otherwise unable to use the preferred regimen, or if the exposure source is known to have resistant virus. See *Infect Control Hosp Epidemiol 2013;34:875.* Consultation with an HIV specialist is recommended in such cases.

Rabies Postexposure Prophylaxis

- For all suspected rabies exposures, consultation with local or state health officials is recommended. Contact information can be found at *http://www.cdc.gov/rabies/resources/contacts.html*.
- Postexposure prophylaxis is generally indicated only for bite wounds from mammals. (*MMWR Recomm Rep 2008;57:1*)
  - Bites from bats, skunks, raccoons, foxes, and most other carnivores warrant immediate prophylaxis unless the animal is confirmed to be rabies negative by laboratory testing. Animals should not be held for observation but euthanized as soon as possible.
  - Bites from dogs, cats, and ferrets that are rabid or suspected to be rabid also warrant immediate prophylaxis. If the animal is healthy and can be observed for 10 days, do not begin prophylaxis but observe. If signs or symptoms of rabies develop in the animal, prophylaxis should begin immediately. For bites where the status of the animal is unknown, consult with public health officials
  - Bites from all other sources (e.g., rodents, hares, livestock) should be considered on an individual basis and prophylaxis initiated only in consultation with public health officials.
- Postexposure prophylaxis consists of wound care, a vaccination series, and in certain situations, administration of human rabies immune globulin (HRIG) (Table A-4) (*MMWR Recomm Rep 2010;59(RR02):1–9*).
  - All wounds should be cleaned thoroughly with soap and water and irrigated with a virucidal solution such as povidone-iodine.
  - Human diploid cell vaccine (HDCV) or purified chick embryo cell vaccine (PCECV) 1 mL IM should be administered in the deltoid, which is the only acceptable site for vaccination in adults.
  - If HRIG is indicated, give 20 IU/kg IM once. Do not administer in same syringe as vaccine. When possible, infiltrate as much of the product as able around and into the wound(s). The remaining volume can be administered intramuscularly at any site anatomically distant from the site of vaccination. However, vaccine doses on subsequent days can be given at the same site as previous HRIG.

TABLE A-4	Rabies Postexposure Prophylaxis Recommendations	
	Therapy	
Vaccination Status	**Vaccine**	**HRIG**
Not previously vaccinated	Yes, on days 0, 3, 7, and 14	Yes, once on day 0
Previously vaccinated	Yes, on days 0 and 3	No

HRIG, human rabies immune globulin.

Appendix B

Infection Control and Isolation Recommendations
Abigail L. Carlson and Carlos A. Q. Santos

- **Standard precautions** should be practiced on all patients at all times to minimize the risk of nosocomial infection.
  - **Perform hand hygiene** with an alcohol-based hand sanitizer before and after patient contact (including after gloves are removed), after contact with the patient's environment, and in between caring for different patients. Soap and water should be used for visibly contaminated hands and after contact with patients with confirmed or suspected *Clostridium difficile* infection if the alcohol-based preparation used is not active against *C. difficile* spores.
  - **Wear gloves** when direct contact with body secretions or blood is anticipated.
  - **Wear a gown** when clothing may be in contact with body fluids.
  - **Wear a mask** when prolonged procedures, including puncture of the spinal canal, are performed (e.g., myelography, epidural anesthesia, intrathecal chemotherapy).
  - **Wear a mask and protective eyewear** when splashes of body fluid are possible.
  - **Use proper respiratory hygiene and cough etiquette** (applies to health care workers as well as all patients and visiting family or friends). Mouth and nose must be covered when coughing, and tissues must be disposed of properly. Hand hygiene must be performed after contact with respiratory secretions.
  - **Safely dispose** of sharp instruments, needles, wound dressings, and disposable gowns.
- **Specific isolation procedures** must be performed in addition to standard precautions depending on the major mode of microorganism transmission in health care settings.
  - **Contact precautions** are used when microorganisms can be transmitted via direct contact between patients and health care workers or by contact between patients and contaminated objects. In addition to standard precautions, the following must be done:
    - Assign the patient to a **private room** if possible. Cohorting is allowed if necessary.
    - **Wear gown and gloves** to enter the room; remove them before leaving the room.
    - Use a **dedicated stethoscope and thermometer**.
    - Minimize environmental contamination during patient transport (e.g., patient can be placed in a gown).
  - **Droplet precautions** are used when microorganisms can be transmitted by respiratory secretion particles larger than 5 μm. Droplets remain suspended in the air for limited periods, and exposure of ≤3 feet (1 meter) is usually required for human-to-human transmission. In addition to standard precautions, the following must be done:
    - Assign the patient to a **private room**. The door must be kept closed as much as possible. Rooms with special air handling systems are **not** required.
    - Wear a **surgical mask** within 6 feet of patients.
    - Limit patient transport and activity outside their room. If transporting the patient outside the room is necessary, the patient must wear a surgical mask.
  - **Airborne precautions** must be used when microorganisms can be transmitted by respiratory secretion particles <5 μm. These airborne particles remain suspended in the air for extended periods. In addition to standard precautions, the following must be done:
    - Assign the patient to a **negative-pressure room**. Doors must remain closed.
    - Wear a **tightly fitting respirator** that covers the nose and mouth with a filtering capacity of 95% (e.g., N95 mask) to enter the room. Susceptible individuals should not enter the room of patients with confirmed or suspected measles or chickenpox.
    - Limit patient transport and activity outside their room. If transporting the patient outside the room is necessary, the patient must wear a surgical mask. Higher level respirator masks (e.g., N95) are **not** required for the patient.

TABLE B-1	Health Care Isolation Recommendations for Specific Infections	
Infection/Condition	**Type**	**Duration, Comments**
Adenovirus, pneumonia	Droplet, contact	Duration of illness In immunocompromised hosts, extend duration of precautions due to prolonged viral shedding
Anthrax	Standard	Duration of illness Contact precautions indicated if wound with uncontained copious drainage. Alcohol hand rubs ineffective against spores; use soap and water or 2% chlorhexidine gluconate solution for hand hygiene. If aerosolizable spore-containing substance (e.g., powder) is present, wear respirator, protective clothing until decontamination complete.
Botulism	Standard	Duration of illness
Burkholderia cepacia, pneumonia or colonization	Contact	Unknown Recommendations will vary by institution. Avoid exposure to persons with cystic fibrosis. Private room preferred.
Clostridium difficile	Contact	Duration of hospitalization and future hospitalizations Recommendations for initiation and discontinuation of precautions will vary by institution.
Conjunctivitis, acute viral	Contact	Duration of illness
Diphtheria		
Cutaneous	Contact	Until off antimicrobial treatment and two cultures taken 24 h apart are negative
Pharyngeal	Droplet	Same as for cutaneous diphtheria
Ebola virus disease		See Viral hemorrhagic fevers
Hepatitis, viral	Standard	Duration of illness For hepatitis A and E, contact precautions are indicated for diapered or incontinent individuals.

(continued)

TABLE B-1	Health Care Isolation Recommendations for Specific Infections (*Continued*)

Infection/Condition	Type	Duration, Comments
Herpes simplex virus		
Encephalitis	Standard	Duration of illness
Mucocutaneous, recurrent (skin, oral, genital)	Standard	Duration of illness
Mucocutaneous, severe (disseminated or primary)	Contact	Until lesions dry and crusted
Herpes zoster		See Varicella
Human metapneumovirus	Contact	Duration of illness
Influenza	Droplet	Immunocompetent: 7 d after illness onset or until 24 h after resolution of symptoms, whichever is longer Immunocompromised: Duration of illness Respiratory protection equivalent to an N95 respirator is recommended during aerosol-generating procedures.
Lice		
Head (pediculosis)	Contact	Until 24 h after start of therapy
Body	Standard	Duration of illness Can be transmitted via infested clothing. Wear gown and gloves when handling clothing.
Pubic	Standard	Duration of illness
Measles (rubeola)	Airborne	Immunocompetent: 4 d after onset of rash Immunocompromised: Duration of illness[a]
Middle eastern respiratory syndrome coronavirus (MERS-CoV)	Airborne, contact	Determine on a case-by-case basis in consultation with local, state, and federal public health authorities

(*continued*)

TABLE B-1	Health Care Isolation Recommendations for Specific Infections (*Continued*)	
Infection/Condition	**Type**	**Duration, Comments**
Meningitis, *Haemophilus influenzae* type B or *Neisseria meningitidis*	Droplet	Until 24 h after start of therapy For other etiologies of meningitis, standard precautions can be used.
Meningococcal disease (*N. meningitidis*)	Droplet	Until 24 h after start of therapy If colonization without active disease, standard precautions can be used.
Monkeypox	Airborne, contact	Airborne: Until monkeypox confirmed and smallpox excluded Contact: Until lesions crusted
Multidrug-resistant organisms, infection or colonization (e.g., MRSA, VRE, ESBLs)	Contact	Duration of hospitalization and future hospitalizations Recommendations for initiation and discontinuation of precautions will vary by institution and organism.
Mumps (infectious parotitis)	Droplet	Until 5 d after onset of symptoms[a]
Mycoplasma, pneumonia	Droplet	Duration of illness
Parvovirus B19 (erythema infectiosum)	Droplet	Immunocompromised patient: Duration of hospitalization Transient aplastic crisis or red cell crisis: 7 d
Pertussis (*Bordetella pertussis*, whooping cough)	Droplet	Until 5 d after start of therapy
Plague (*Yersinia pestis*)		
Bubonic	Standard	Duration of illness
Pneumonic	Droplet	Until 48 h after start of therapy
Poliomyelitis	Contact	Duration of illness
Respiratory syncytial virus	Contact	Duration of illness In immunocompromised hosts, extend duration of precautions due to prolonged viral shedding.
Rhinovirus	Droplet	Duration of illness Add contact precautions if copious moist secretions.

(*continued*)

TABLE B-1	Health Care Isolation Recommendations for Specific Infections (*Continued*)

Infection/Condition	Type	Duration, Comments
Rubella (German measles)	Droplet	Until 7 d after onset of rash[a] Pregnant women who are not immune should not care for these patients.
Scabies	Contact	Until 24 h after start of therapy For Norwegian scabies: 8 d or 24 h after the second treatment with scabicide
Severe acute respiratory syndrome coronavirus (SARS)	Airborne, droplet, contact	Duration of illness plus 10 d after resolution of fever if respiratory symptoms are absent or improving Eye protection (goggles, face shield) also recommended.
Smallpox (variola)	Airborne, contact	Duration of illness; until all scabs have crusted and separated (3–4 wk)[a] For vaccine complications, see Vaccinia.
Streptococcus group A	Droplet	Until 24 h after start of therapy For endometritis or limited skin, wound, or burn infection, standard precautions can be used.
Tuberculosis (*Mycobacterium tuberculosis*)		Recommendations regarding initiation and discontinuation of precautions will vary by institution.
Extrapulmonary, draining lesion	Airborne, contact	Until patient is improving clinically and drainage has ceased or there are 3 consecutive negative cultures of drainage Rule out active pulmonary disease.
Extrapulmonary, without draining lesion	Standard	Duration of illness Rule out active pulmonary disease.

(*continued*)

TABLE B-1	Health Care Isolation Recommendations for Specific Infections (*Continued*)	
Infection/Condition	**Type**	**Duration, Comments**
Pulmonary or laryngeal disease, confirmed	Airborne	Until patient is on effective therapy, is improving clinically, and has 3 consecutive sputum smears negative for acid-fast bacilli collected on separate days
Pulmonary or laryngeal disease, suspected	Airborne	Until likelihood of infectious tuberculosis is deemed negligible and either there is another diagnosis that explains the clinical syndrome or the results of 3 sputum smears for AFB are negative Each of the sputum specimens should be collected 8–24 h apart, and at least one should be an early-morning specimen
Tularemia	Standard	Duration of illness
Vaccinia	Standard	Duration of illness[a] Contact precautions recommended for eczema vaccinatum, fetal vaccinia, generalized vaccinia, progressive vaccinia, and blepharitis or conjunctivitis with significant drainage. If unvaccinated, only health care workers without contraindications to vaccine should provide care.
Varicella		
Varicella disease (chickenpox)	Airborne, contact	Until lesions dry and crusted[a] In immunocompromised host, prolong duration of precautions for duration of illness.
Herpes zoster, localized (shingles)	Standard	Duration of illness[a] In immunocompromised host, use airborne and contact precautions until disseminated disease ruled out.
Herpes zoster, disseminated	Airborne, contact	Duration of illness[a]

(*continued*)

TABLE B-1	Health Care Isolation Recommendations for Specific Infections (Continued)

Infection/Condition	Type	Duration, Comments
Viral hemorrhagic fevers		
Ebola virus disease	Droplet, contact	Discontinue only in consultation with local, state, and federal public health officials In addition to droplet and contact precautions, a powered air-purifying respirator (PAPR) or N95 respirator, examination gloves with extended cuffs, and fluid-resistant or impermeable gowns, aprons, and boot covers are recommended. Detailed information and updated recommendations can be found at *http://www.cdc.gov/vhf/ ebola/healthcare-us/hospitals/ infection-control.html*
Lassa, Marburg, and Crimean-Congo fever viruses	Droplet, contact	Duration of illness Single-patient room preferred. Emphasize use of sharps safety devices and safe work practices, hand hygiene, barrier protection against blood and body fluids, including goggles or face shields and appropriate waste handling. Use N95 or higher respirators when performing aerosol-generating procedures.

AFB, acid-fast bacilli; ESBL, extended-spectrum β-lactamase; MRSA, methicillin-resistant *Staphylococcus aureus*; VRE, vancomycin-resistant enterococcus.
[a]Susceptible health care workers should not enter room if immune caregivers are available.
Adapted from Siegel JD, Rhinehart E, Jackson M, et al. 2007 Guideline for isolation precautions: Preventing transmission of infectious agents in healthcare settings. *Am J Infect Control* 2007;35:S65–S164.

Appendix C

Advanced Cardiac Life Support Algorithms
Mark Gdowski

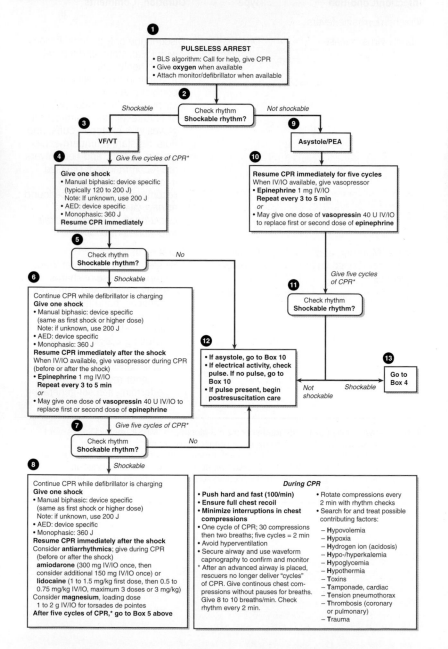

1
PULSELESS ARREST
• BLS algorithm: Call for help, give CPR
• Give **oxygen** when available
• Attach monitor/defibrillator when available

2
Shockable — Check rhythm **Shockable rhythm?** — _Not shockable_

3
VF/VT

9
Asystole/PEA

4 _Give five cycles of CPR*_
Give one shock
• Manual biphasic: device specific (typically 120 to 200 J)
  Note: If unknown, use 200 J
• AED: device specific
• Monophasic: 360 J
Resume CPR immediately

10
Resume CPR immediately for five cycles
When IV/IO available, give vasopressor
• **Epinephrine** 1 mg IV/IO
  Repeat every 3 to 5 min
  _or_
• May give one dose of **vasopressin** 40 U IV/IO to replace first or second dose of **epinephrine**

5
Check rhythm **Shockable rhythm?** — _No_
Shockable

6
Continue CPR while defibrillator is charging
Give one shock
• Manual biphasic: device specific (same as first shock or higher dose)
  Note: if unknown, use 200 J
• AED: device specific
• Monophasic: 360 J
Resume CPR immediately after the shock
When IV/IO available, give vasopressor during CPR (before or after the shock)
• **Epinephrine** 1 mg IV/IO
  Repeat every 3 to 5 min
  _or_
• May give one dose of **vasopressin** 40 U IV/IO to replace first or second dose of **epinephrine**

Give five cycles of CPR*

11
Check rhythm **Shockable rhythm?**

Give five cycles of CPR*

12
• If asystole, go to Box 10
• If electrical activity, check pulse. If no pulse, go to Box 10
• If pulse present, begin postresuscitation care

Not shockable — _Shockable_

13
Go to Box 4

7 _Give five cycles of CPR*_
Check rhythm **Shockable rhythm?** — _No_
Shockable

8
Continue CPR while defibrillator is charging
Give one shock
• Manual biphasic: device specific (same as first shock or higher dose)
  Note: if unknown, use 200 J
• AED: device specific
• Monophasic: 360 J
Resume CPR immediately after the shock
Consider **antiarrhythmics**; give during CPR (before or after the shock)
  amiodarone (300 mg IV/IO once, then consider additional 150 mg IV/IO once) or
  lidocaine (1 to 1.5 mg/kg first dose, then 0.5 to 0.75 mg/kg IV/IO, maximum 3 doses or 3 mg/kg)
Consider **magnesium**, loading dose 1 to 2 g IV/IO for torsades de pointes
After five cycles of CPR,* go to Box 5 above

During CPR
• **Push hard and fast (100/min)**
• **Ensure full chest recoil**
• **Minimize interruptions in chest compressions**
• One cycle of CPR: 30 compressions then two breaths; five cycles = 2 min
• Avoid hyperventilation
• Secure airway and use waveform capnography to confirm and monitor
* After an advanced airway is placed, rescuers no longer deliver "cycles" of CPR. Give continous chest compressions without pauses for breaths. Give 8 to 10 breaths/min. Check rhythm every 2 min.

• Rotate compressions every 2 min with rhythm checks
• Search for and treat possible contributing factors:
  – Hypovolemia
  – Hypoxia
  – Hydrogen ion (acidosis)
  – Hypo-/hyperkalemia
  – Hypoglycemia
  – Hypothermia
  – Toxins
  – Tamponade, cardiac
  – Tension pneumothorax
  – Thrombosis (coronary or pulmonary)
  – Trauma

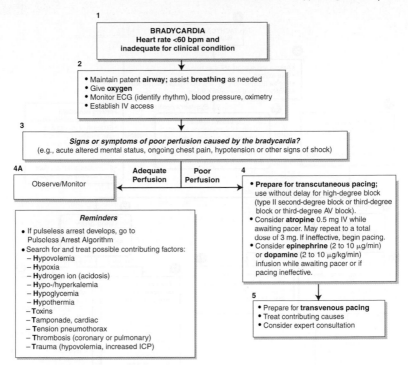

Figure C-2. Bradycardia algorithm. AV, atrioventricular; bpm, beats per minute; ICP, intracranial pressure. (From American Heart Association in collaboration with the International Liaison Committee on Resuscitation. Guidelines 2010 for cardiopulmonary resuscitation and emergency cardiovascular care. *Circulation* 2010;122:S729–S767.)

Figure C-1. Advanced cardiac life support pulseless arrest algorithm. AED, automated external defibrillator; BLS, basic life support; CPR, cardiopulmonary resuscitation; IO, intraosseous; PEA, pulseless electrical activity; U, unit; VF, ventricular fibrillation; VT, ventricular tachycardia. (From American Heart Association in collaboration with the International Liaison Committee on Resuscitation. Guidelines 2010 for cardiopulmonary resuscitation and emergency cardiovascular care. *Circulation* 2010;122:S729–S767.)

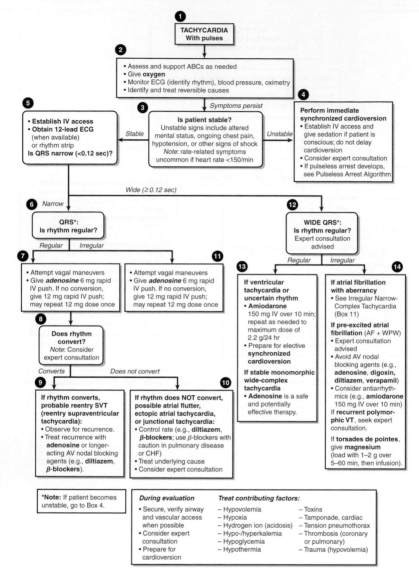

Figure C-3. Advanced cardiac life support tachycardia algorithm. AF, atrial fibrillation; AV, atrioventricular; CHF, congestive heart failure; SVT, supraventricular tachycardia; VT, ventricular tachycardia; WPW, Wolff-Parkinson-White syndrome. (From American Heart Association in collaboration with the International Liaison Committee on Resuscitation. Guidelines 2010 for cardiopulmonary resuscitation and emergency cardiovascular care. *Circulation* 2010;122:S729–S767.)

Index

Page numbers in italic denote online chapters and page numbers followed by an *f* or *t* denote figures and tables, respectively.